FOR REFERENCE

Do Not Take From This Room

ENCYCLOPEDIA OF
BIOETHICS

ENCYCLOPEDIA OF
BIOETHICS

REVISED EDITION

Warren Thomas Reich

EDITOR IN CHIEF

Georgetown University

Volume 1

MACMILLAN LIBRARY REFERENCE USA
SIMON & SCHUSTER MACMILLAN
NEW YORK

SIMON & SCHUSTER AND PRENTICE HALL INTERNATIONAL
LONDON   MEXICO CITY   NEW DELHI   SINGAPORE   SYDNEY   TORONTO

Simon & Schuster Macmillan
866 Third Avenue, New York, NY 10022

PRINTED IN THE UNITED STATES OF AMERICA

printing number
   2   3   4   5   6   7   8   9   10

LIBRARY OF CONGRESS CATALOG-IN-PUBLICATION DATA
Encyclopedia of bioethics / Warren T. Reich, editor in chief. — Rev.
   ed.
      p. cm.
      Includes bibliographical references and index.
      ISBN 0-02-897355-0 (set)
      1. Bioethics—Encyclopedias.   2. Medical ethics—Encyclopedias.
   I. Reich, Warren T.
   QH332.E52   1995
   174′.2′03—dc20
                                            94-38743
                                            CIP

Lines from the poem "The Scarred Girl" by James Dickey, quoted in the entry on "Interpretation," originally appeared in *Poems, 1957–1967,* © 1978 by James Dickey, Wesleyan University Press, and have been reprinted here by permission of the University Press of New England.

The paper used in this publication meets the minimum requirements of American National Standard for Information Sciences—Permanence of Paper for Printed Library Materials, ANSI Z39.48-1984.

Contents

Editorial and Production Staff

Georgetown University

Coordinating Editor
Mary B. Evans

Assistant Editors
Courtney S. Campbell
Sandra M. Hass
Nancy S. Jecker
Drew Leder

Administrative Editor
Jessica B. Marshall

Administrative Officer
Seth R. Kaufman

Editorial and Research Assistants
Frank Chessa
Lauren Deichman
James J. Doyle
Stephen Hanson
Kevin T. Keith
Tysha Lupe
Patricia Mazzarella
Kathryn McGinness
Estela B. Mendoza
Maria H. Murray
Kristin Nelson-Jones
Leanne R. Pearce
Mary Kay Scott
Carol Mason Spicer
Susan Stark
Rachael Yocum

Appendix Editor
Carol Mason Spicer

Appendix Advisory Group
Glenn C. Graber, Chair

Patricio Figueroa
Doris Goldstein
Rihito Kimura

Editorial Advisory Board

Preface

In the preface to the first edition of this Encyclopedia (1978) I called attention to the unique problems associated with creating the first encyclopedia for a field of learning and what it takes to accomplish such a task. In the mid-1980s, when I began contemplating preparation of a revised edition, I was inclined to think that the task would indeed be challenging but easier than producing the first edition. After all, the hard questions about setting the parameters of the field of bioethics, organizing this body of knowledge, preparing a comprehensive set of entries on basic topics and practical issues, establishing scholarly and editorial criteria, and selecting appropriate terminology for the field had been faced by a superb group of associate editors and authors. The task would be that of improving an already existing and well-received reference work; and the experience acquired in preparing the first edition would greatly facilitate preparation of a revision. Some parts of the highly regarded first edition—such as articles dealing with history and some basic concepts—it was felt, might require only minor revisions. All these factors, I thought, would make the task of revision easier than preparation of the first edition.

I was to discover that my assumptions were quite mistaken. Preparation of the revised edition has been at least twice as difficult as assembling the first edition, partly because we felt constrained to match if not exceed the demanding standards that we set for the first edition. Other factors that rendered preparation of the revised edition exceptionally difficult were the surprisingly extensive changes that had occurred in the field; the enormous expansion of literature on many topics; the appearance of many new issues; the competitiveness and divisiveness that have emerged among various schools of thought; the importance of including all voices, new and old, in as evenhanded a way as possible; and the high standards we set for the new edition in response to all these elements. In a word, preparation of this edition has been demanding because the pressures were great to produce a work that would speak usefully and accurately to a second generation of the field of bioethics that looks and acts quite differently from the first. The editors hope this goal has been achieved.

Planning for a revised edition

Having conceived the idea of developing the first edition of this work and having orchestrated its preparation between 1971 and 1978, I had a strong interest in seeing it kept alive, as did the publisher. Consequently, I carried out an intensive planning stage for a revised edition between 1985 and 1987, with the assistance of a creative, devoted, and highly intelligent administrative editor, Jessica B. Marshall. We sought answers to two questions: What has been the significance and usefulness of the first edition? Precisely what sort of revision, if any, is needed for this Encyclopedia?

Evaluations of the first edition solicited from a wide range of leading bioethics scholars not connected with the work in any direct way nor with the university that first sponsored its development convinced us of the need to keep this work alive. We launched a lengthy inquiry to identify the extent of the need for revision and the format and methods for best implementing it. Our method of proceeding included a survey of all eight associate editors and virtually all 285 contributors to the first edition; two specially assembled conferences of leading U.S. scholars in bioethics, held at Georgetown University; a consultation on the international aspects of the Encyclopedia, involving bioethics scholars who had been invited to participate in a conference at the Sorbonne in Paris; an informal survey of people active in bioethics; and discussions with the publisher.

The planning phase led to the conclusion that preparation of an updated version of the *Encyclopedia of Bioethics* was not simply a desirable project but one that was crucial to the future of the field. The research of the preliminary planning phase provided us with a detailed and extensive analysis of the revision that was needed, as well as the best format and methods to accomplish the revision.

Even by 1985, at least 50 percent of all articles in the first edition were in need of significant revision. By the time we actually began the project in January 1990, it was clear that scarcely a single topic in the original edition had been unaffected by profound changes not only in science, technology, and ethics but even in the way in which moral problems are perceived. Consequently, what we have prepared in this revised edition is a fresh, new work.

The task of producing this new work required strong and committed support; an outstanding Board of Editors who could collaborate as a team; meticulous planning; extensive consultation with Advisory Board members and other advisers; selection of the best possible authors; an atmosphere of freedom of inquiry for authors and editors; a first-rate editorial staff; extensive and meticulous reviews; and high editorial standards.

The editors and the editorial plan

An outstanding Board of Editors designed a detailed plan and evaluated the manuscripts. Because the field of bioethics had become so specialized within its first generation, the fourteen area editors comprising the Board of Editors were selected partly on the basis of their knowledge of special areas of bioethics. They were also chosen on the basis of their knowledge of the field of bioethics in general and the diversity of their intellectual, professional, and methodological backgrounds. They contributed to this project a level of expertise, dedication, and patience that could scarcely have been matched by any other group. Their names are listed on the page opposite the title page.

The area editors and I, working collaboratively, exercised full autonomy in giving shape to this collection of often controversial topics. We established editorial policies, determined the basic list of topics, selected contributors, and reviewed both the initial and the revised manuscripts.

The first task of the Board of Editors was to establish a plan comprised of entry and article titles, article scope notes, and a list of possible authors and reviewers for each of the topics. With a manifest sense of service to the whole field of bioethics, the editors developed their basic plan in two meetings held at the Cosmos Club in Washington, D.C., on April 27–29 and September 14–16, 1990.

We then engaged a large number of scholars to offer horizontal, or cross-sectional, evaluations of this "vertical" listing of topics to assure comprehensive and accurate coverage from the perspectives of many disciplines and interests. The evaluations and recommendations of these reviewers pertained to such perspectives as minority concerns, women's interests, gay and lesbian issues, mental-health issues, care of animals, public health, environmental health, law, philosophy, history, feminist thought, behavioral sciences, world religions, literature, and so forth.

Together with the staff at Georgetown University, I had the task of refining, coordinating, and completing the editorial plan, as well as setting standards and establishing project procedures. The plan was constantly adapted to accommodate new ideas and meet emerging needs; in a sense, the "final plan" for the Encyclopedia was completed four and one-half years after commencement of the project, with the submission of the last article in mid-1994.

The Editorial Advisory Board, whose names are listed on pp. ix–xi, is a richly interdisciplinary and international group of distinguished scholars and professionals who supported the project in a variety of ways. For example, they provided valuable service on author selection, the geography of bioethics in various parts of the world, and how to solve some troublesome editorial problems. They also offered important comments from the perspective of the major disciplines that historically are the "parent disciplines" of bioethics.

The day-to-day work of preparing this edition entailed collaboration between two teams: the academic team based at Georgetown University and the publisher's team in New York. The Georgetown-based staff was responsible for the contents, methods, and quality standards of the Encyclopedia as an organic whole, the reviewing process, the cross-referencing, and so on. The publisher's editorial team operationalized the intellectual plan. They commissioned all the articles, maintained contact with all authors, did substantive and copy-editing of all manuscripts, coordinated the outside reviews, checked revised manuscripts and bibliographies, and prepared all materials for production.

Our review process was unusually thorough and meticulous. Each manuscript was reviewed by four editors and one or more outside reviewers for appropriateness of scope, accuracy of content, and clarity of style. The editor in chief or a scholarly editor working with him prepared a master review with revision instructions for the author. The role of the outside reviewers, which was a key element in our review process, assured a high degree of accuracy. Every article was reviewed by a scholar who was an expert on the specific topic dealt with in the article. An article on rape had to be read by an expert on rape; an article on medical ethics in the Renaissance had to be read by a Renaissance scholar; et cetera. In addition, an interdisciplinary bioethics article that contained a section, say, on economics, was reviewed by an economist. These special reviewers, whose names are listed on p. lxiii, made an important contribution to the accuracy of the Encyclopedia.

Acknowledgments

Georgetown University provided a supportive academic environment, excellent research resources, and the administrative services required for carrying out this project. We are particularly indebted to two presidents of the University, Timothy S. Healy, S.J., and Leo J. O'Donovan, S.J., for their faith in this project; to Robert M. Veatch, director of The Joseph and Rose Kennedy Institute of Ethics for his support; to Edmund D. Pellegrino, director of the Center for Clinical Bioethics and former director of the Center for the Advanced Study of Ethics; and to Irene McDonald, executive assistant to the director of the Kennedy Institute. An extraordinarily helpful research, documentary, and bibliographic service was rendered to this project by Doris M. Goldstein, director; Tamar Joy Kahn, senior bibliographer; and the entire staff of the Library and Information Services of the Kennedy Institute of Ethics. Finally, I express my appreciation to Seymour Perry, former chair; Jay Siwek, acting chair; and Jane Beer, administrator of the Department of Family Medicine, for their constant support; and to George Schreiner and Murray Feshbach for their assistance.

We are most grateful for the support received from the following donors, whose grants supported the work of a small, part-time editorial staff at Georgetown University. (The Macmillan Publishing Company covered all other expenses related to the project.)

For the preliminary planning phase:

National Endowment for the Humanities
Joseph P. Kennedy, Jr., Foundation

For the revision project:

National Endowment for the Humanities
National Science Foundation
Hillsdale Fund
Frank J. Lewis Foundation
The Davis Fund
The Sherwick Fund
General Service Foundation
The Greenwall Foundation
The Commonwealth Fund
Masamichi Sakanoue, M.D.
Shigeo Morioka, Yamanouchi Pharmaceutical Co., Ltd.

We are especially grateful that the National Endowment for the Humanities (NEH), which had supplied key funding for the first edition, provided the groundwork for funding of the revision project by awarding both an outright grant and matching gifts to encourage contributions from the private sector. In particular, I express my appreciation for the assistance of Helena C. Agüera and Martha B. Chomiak of the Reference Materials Section, Division of Research Programs, of the NEH; Stephen Veneziani and David J. Wallace of the NEH grants office; and Rachelle D. Hollander, director of Ethics and Values Studies, National Science Foundation.

For valuable advice and assistance in achieving support for this project, I want to thank Shattuck W. Hartwell, of the Cleveland Clinic Foundation; Eunice Kennedy Shriver and Robert Montague of the Joseph P. Kennedy, Jr., Foundation; Michael Hoffman of the Cleveland Foundation; Associate Editor Stephen G. Post; the project's area editors, Professor Rihito Kimura of the Kennedy Institute of Ethics at Georgetown University; and Mary Anne Hohman, director of Foundation Relations of the Georgetown University Office of Alumni and University Relations.

We are extremely grateful to the following persons who submitted detailed reviews of our first-draft plan: Annette C. Baier, Troyen A. Brennan, Peter G. Brown, Robert W. Daly, Dena S. Davis, Rebecca Dresser, Paul T. Durbin, Rem B. Edwards, Ruth Faden, Renée C. Fox, Sara T. Fry, Jorge Garcia, Willard Gaylin, Eugene C. Hargrove, Richard P. Haynes, Kathryn Montgomery Hunter, Charles B. Keely, Mary B. Mahowald, Robert Michels, Jonathan D. Moreno, Seyyed Hossein Nasr, F. Barbara Orlans, Carroll Pursell, Charles H. Reynolds, William J. Richardson, Daniel N. Robinson, Marian Secundy, Earl Shelp, Susan Sherwin, Robert C. Solomon, Lawrence E. Sullivan, Stephen Viederman, and Robert Weir.

We are also grateful to the members of the Cleveland Area Task Force on Bioethics, who critiqued our plans and manuscripts on the occasion of several meetings. Members of the Task Force included faculty and staff members from Case Western Reserve University, The Cleveland Clinic, John Carroll University, Cleveland State University, Northeastern Ohio Universities College of Medicine, The Cleveland Foundation, Hiram College, the Allen Memorial Library, Ursuline College, St. Mary Seminary, and the University of Akron.

We were fortunate that Mary Solberg was the publisher's project editor. A true intellectual and a highly experienced editor, she skillfully edited every manuscript and maintained an excellent working relationship with all authors and editors. We were also fortunate in being able to create a symbiosis of the academic and publisher's teams. Elly Dickason, editor in chief of Macmillan Reference, supervised the project and moved it deftly to production; and Philip Friedman, president and publisher of Macmillan Reference, manifested exceptional professional skills in shepherding this project from a mere idea to publication.

Significant portions of this project were carried out at the Center for Biomedical Ethics at the Case Western Reserve University (CWRU) in Cleveland, Ohio, where I collaborated with Stephen G. Post, the associate editor of the Encyclopedia. Professor Post, who shared many of my responsibilities, brought to the project a rich and broad knowledge of the humanities, good judgment in bioethics, and direct experience with the biomedical sciences. I am indebted to him for having been a delightful and supportive partner. Thomas H. Murray, director of the CWRU Center and member of the Editorial Advisory Board, gave valuable advice and support to the project and was instrumental in helping to organize the Cleveland Area Task Force for Bioethics, which served as a sounding board for this project.

The assistant editors—knowledgeable in bioethics, skilled as scholarly writers, and judicious in their judgment—rendered an indispensable service by reviewing manuscripts and preparing detailed guides for individual authors in the task of revising manuscripts. They are: Courtney Campbell of Oregon State University, Sandra Hass of the American Psychiatric Association, Nancy Jecker of the University of Washington, and Drew Leder of Loyola College in Baltimore.

Key to the success of the Georgetown team were the outstanding organizational, editorial, and interpretational skills of Coordinating Editor Mary B. Evans and the extraordinary administrative and support skills of Seth Kaufman. I am grateful to them for their daily cooperation and forbearance.

Credit for the quality of the articles must go principally to the contributors. They accommodated themselves generously to the plan, the purpose, the scholarly standards, the sought-for writing style, and the demanding schedule of the Encyclopedia. The following standards guided us in the selection of contributors: that they should have highly respected qualifications to write on the topic as well as the ability to write well, and that as a group they should include diverse intellectual backgrounds and appropriate geographical and institutional representation. The names of the contributors are listed on p. xliii. We are especially grateful to those contributors who prepared excellent articles on extremely short notice as we approached the end of the project.

Finally, I want to express my appreciation to Laurence B. McCullough and George A. Kanoti for sharing their sanity and broad vision with me; and to Ronald Goldfarb for his practical advice in charting the course.

Dedicatory acknowledgments

While it is not customary for an encyclopedia to contain a dedication, four special, dedicatory acknowledgments are in order.

First, we honor by the labors invested in this revised edition the memory of the late André E. Hellegers, who died a few months after publication of the first edition. To repeat what I wrote in the Preface of the first edition, "This encyclopedia could not have been developed had it not been for the intellectual vision and continuing labors of André E. Hellegers, first director of The Joseph and Rose Kennedy Institute of Ethics at Georgetown University. His constant supportive efforts made possible the launching and sustaining of this project." I hope his sharp instinct for identifying the kernel of complex interdisciplinary problems and his ability to bring together the right kind of people who are equipped to examine them from a multidisciplinary perspective will be found reflected in this revised edition.

Second, I want to acknowledge and praise the two colleagues who have worked closest with me on the first two editions of this Encyclopedia and without whom they would not have appeared: Mary B. Evans, the coordinating editor of this edition, and Sandra M. Hass, the managing editor of the first edition. They placed the highest priority on the completion of the Encyclopedia; insisted daily on the implementation of the finest standards; and created a respectful and effective spirit of teamwork. Their intelligence, good judgment, and remarkable loyalty—not to mention their rare ability to prod their closest colleagues inspiringly—are deeply appreciated.

Finally, on behalf of all the editors, who functioned in a rather familial fashion, I want to acknowledge with sorrow the passing in August 1994 of Georgia Childress, wife of Area Editor James Childress. May Georgia and Jim be in peace.

Warren Thomas Reich
Editor in Chief

Introduction

When the *Encyclopedia of Bioethics* was first published in 1978, it was the first encyclopedia in its field. Some seventeen years later, it is now widely acknowledged that it has been a major force in the establishment of the field, giving to its topics definition, background, and prospect for a more integrated role in human learning. This new edition collects the advances of the last twenty years and, its editors hope, will influence the scholarship of the coming decades.

Since the appearance of the first edition, bioethics has become much more firmly established as a field of learning. One can now more clearly identify standards of professional competence in the field. A number of peer-review journals exist; graduate programs in bioethics have multiplied; subspecialties have developed; at least four professional societies for bioethics exist in the United States alone; most colleges and universities regularly include bioethics offerings in their curricula; faculty members are hired specifically for their competence in this field; it is required in all U.S. medical schools and in the graduate training of a number of medical specialties; most schools of nursing require bioethics, as do some programs in health-care administration. It is widely taught in the professional schools for other health professions and graduate and professional schools in the life sciences. Over two hundred bioethics research institutes exist throughout the world; and governmental agencies and professional organizations regularly include bioethicists in the commissions charged with developing policies related to the life sciences and health. The fact that scientists, health-care professionals, economists, theologians, philosophers, lawyers, sociologists, and others contribute to the field of bioethics in increasing numbers—often in their own disciplinary journals—attests to the multidisciplinarity and vitality of the field.

Although bioethics began in the United States, it has found fertile soil in many nations. The first edition of this Encyclopedia provided the seeds for international bioethics; but scholars in other nations have made unique contributions. Not only have they drawn upon their own cultural understanding of ethics, of health, and of science but their social situations have posed problems quite different from those in the United States. For example, Third World countries criticize the excessive emphasis in U.S. bioethics on technology's grip on questions of life and death, insisting that issues such as the ethics of poverty, the depletion of resources for future generations, and the development of effective public-health measures are more important to them. The international and intercultural dimensions of bioethics are fast becoming a salient feature of the field.

Whether bioethics has become a fully established discipline remains debatable. It can, of course, be called a discipline in the minimal dictionary sense of "a field of learning." Some would call it a discipline in the full sense of the word, that is, as having its own distinctive and agreed-upon subject matter, methods, body of literature, standards for professional admissibility, and so forth. The previous two paragraphs indicate that many of the characteristics of an academic discipline are beginning to appear.

However, I would say it is still a nascent discipline, not a discipline in the full sense of the word. In its course of development it has drawn on many established academic disciplines: theology, philosophy, sociology, anthropology, law, literature, medicine, the life sciences, and others. Its scholars have come from various disciplines, and its scholarly writings simultaneously fall under the title of several disciplines. It is characterized by a variety of methodologies. Thus, bioethics has been evolving as a multidisciplinary field of learning. Indeed, much of the challenge and interest in bioethics is traceable to the fact that one finds in it the approaches and mentalities of a number of disciplines.

In recent years interest has arisen in whether there is a distinctive method in bioethics. The methods of analytic, principle-based moral philosophy have contributed enormously to the establishment of bioethics in its first generation in the United States. The fact that numerous alternative approaches are now being pursued contributes immeasurably to the richness of the field. Whether bioethics will come to be regarded as a distinctive and major discipline probably depends on how it develops its interdisciplinary methods.

Whether bioethics is called a field or a discipline, there is no doubt that it enjoys broad public influence, provides intense intellectual interest in many settings, and has turned the basic normative disciplines—philosophical, theological, religious, and legal—in newer, more vital directions.

The origins of bioethics have become more apparent in the past two decades. Although moral teachings and ethical inquiries regarding health and what are now called the life sciences have existed in religious and secular settings for centuries, and medical ethics has long existed in various religious and professional forms, a distinctive ethical interest in health and the life sciences arose in the 1950s and 1960s.

During this period of the immediate "prehistory" of bioethics, deliberate control of human fertility was perceived as having profound implications for physical and mental health and economic well-being; people became aware of the threat posed to human health and well-being by the massive pollution of the environment; and the "new genetics" raised the possibility of manipulating physical and behavioral human characteristics. Unprecedented advances in biomedicine, such as the first heart transplants, the first clinical use of kidney dialysis and of respiratory support, with their increased technological capacity to prolong life, raised ethical problems that the old medical ethics never encountered. These developments stimulated a renaissance of traditional medical ethics and, simultaneously, fostered unprecedented, new interdisciplinary conversations. Theology, philosophy, law, and sociology had previously engaged issues arising from medicine, health care, and the life sciences, but rarely in dialogue. By 1970 the disciplines now contributing to bioethics were finding one another.

The revelation of three or four notorious instances of research abuses in the United States (unconsented research involving risk to life) coupled with spreading public discussions of therapeutic abuses (e.g., unconsented surgery) created a sense of moral outrage around the same time. These abuses were felt to be violations of the sense of human rights that had emerged since the Nuremberg trials following World War II in which Nazi atrocities were condemned; and they also offended against the idea of civil rights that had emerged strongly in the United States in the 1950s and 1960s.

As the 1970s began, something distinctive occurred: The word "bioethics" was begotten (by the oncologist Van Rensselaer Potter); ethics came to be regarded—in the public forum of the United States—as a legitimate part of the humanities distinct from religion (though still embracing religious elements); and the various, aforementioned historical strands came together in the emergence of the field of bioethics. Stimulated in part by the heuristic power of the new word "bioethics," the field of bioethics came into being when some creative thinkers (Potter, André Hellegers, Daniel Callahan, Paul Ramsey, and others) suggested that the language, logic, and wisdom of ethics be combined with the language, logic, data, and values of the life sciences and health care. The preparation of the *Encyclopedia of Bioethics* began within the first year after the coining of "bioethics"; it was designed to embrace within bioethics the full range of what constitutes ethics and the most inclusive interpretation of what constitutes the life sciences.

The revised edition has a purpose quite similar to the first: to present, in integrated fashion, what is known about the scientific and clinical state of the art; to synthesize, analyze, and compare a full range of ethical positions taken on the problems of bioethics, as well as the social, legal, and policy options in matters dealing with the life sciences and health care; to establish and explore the scope and methods of the field; to identify new and emerging issues and voices; to supply the reader with additional resources, especially bibliographies and important documents included in the Appendix; and to indicate where our knowledge of the ethics of the life sciences and health care is deficient and requires deeper exploration.

Yet there are some significant differences between this edition and the original. The 1978 edition offered 315 articles by 285 contributors in four volumes, this edition is expanded to 464 articles by 437 contributors in five volumes. All articles are original, signed contributions never before published. Very few articles are carried over from the first edition; among these are Pedro Laín Entralgo's Professional–Patient Relationship: Historical Aspects, the late Talcott Parsons's Death in the Western World, and Jay Katz's Legal and Ethical Issues of Consent in Health Care. We have appended to the latter two articles postscripts by leading authors who bring the original articles up to date.

There are remarkable differences in the substantive contents of the two editions. A discussion of the contents of this work and the ways in which it differs from the first edition can best be explained against the background of discussions about the definition of the field of bioethics.

Bioethics: Its meaning and scope

Bioethics is a composite term derived from the Greek words *bios* (life) and ēthikē (ethics). It can be defined as *the systematic study of the moral dimensions—including moral vision, decisions, conduct, and policies—of the life sciences and health care, employing a variety of ethical methodologies in an interdisciplinary setting.* The moral dimensions that are examined in bioethics are constantly evolving, but they tend to focus on several major questions: What is or what might be one's (or a society's) moral vision? What sort of person should one be, or what sort of society should we be? What ought to be done in specific situations? And how are we to live harmoniously?

I will comment, first, on the part of the definition dealing with the scope of bioethics (moral dimensions of the life sciences and health care). Later I will comment on the part of the definition that deals with methods.

Many scholars and much of the public tend to identify the scope of bioethics in a somewhat narrow medical sense; in this approach bioethics would be a slightly expanded medical ethics, including the ethics of biomedical research. But the editors of both the first and the revised editions opted for a broader scope that would embrace the social, environmental, and global issues of health and the life sciences. Thus, we see the field of bioethics as going beyond biomedical ethics to embrace health-related and science-related moral issues in the areas of public health, environmental health, population ethics, and animal care. To emphasize these broader areas more thoroughly, we were fortunate to have among our area editors leading specialists in the bioethical issues in these topical areas.

Those who first coined and made public use of the word "bioethics" understood the word in this broader sense; and in more recent years there has been a growing interest in these broader, social dimensions of bioethics.

There are several good reasons for joining the medical with the social/global areas of the life sciences and health. An excessively narrow medical orientation tends to medicalize and technologize the field of bioethics, thus making its agenda and even its methods more easily shaped by the current forms of clinical technologies and by powerful medical institutions. Yet the plight of human illness is far more pervasively affected by international food and migration policies and public-health practices than by the worries and diseases that bring people to highly technologized hospitals. This same medicalization of bioethics has tended to minimize the ethics of nursing and other health professionals, and especially the nonprofessional ethics of families and other communities. The linking of environmental with clinical concerns in bioethics makes sense for two additional reasons. The choice to introduce pollutants into the environment is the choice to cause deadly diseases. Thus, to attend only to the moral problems associated with treating the disease (e.g., forgoing ventilatory support for persons with terminal lung disease) and to neglect the moral problems raised by the social, environmental, and economic causes of the disease (e.g., tobacco and other environmental pollutants) distorts the moral enterprise regarding health. Furthermore, human, animal, and plant life are not only interdependent, they also compete for the resources required for good health. Hence, if we are to understand our responsibility to take care of the health of humans, we must critically examine it in this interdependent and competitive context.

Scholars may never agree on the precise scope of the field. Since the dramatic biomedical issues are the ones most readily identified with bioethics, many books on bioethics will be devoted almost exclusively to biomedical problems. No harm is done by that. But there are now signs of an increasing interest in dialogue between medical and clinical bioethics, on the one hand, and environmental bioethics, on the other. In the meantime, this Encyclopedia attempts to offer both diversity and unity for the field.

These comments on the scope of the field of bioethics prompt a description of the scope of this revised edition—in terms of the specific problem-areas covered—and how it differs substantially from that of the first edition. The following topical survey of the revised edition notes some of the more salient new materials, section by section, while calling attention to familiar topics that have been recast and updated.

One broad category of entries deals with concrete, normative questions regarding what decisions, actions, policies, or attitudes ought or ought not be adopted in the following fifteen topical areas.

Professional–Patient Relationship: Remarkable changes have occurred in this category. The first edition, surprisingly, contained no entry on autonomy, although autonomy was discussed in the entry on paternalism. No published review criticized us for that omission, undoubtedly because the ethical principle of autonomy had not achieved the prominence that it did in the bioethics of the 1980s. Yet within a few short years the entire field of medical bioethics seemed to be dominated by the one principle of patient autonomy. Debates then ensued on whether physician beneficence has at least as much moral importance as patient autonomy; a backlash occurred when physicians and other scholars began setting moral limits to what the patient could request in terms of treatment that professionals found morally objectionable because of their futility; and this was followed by attempts to mediate—both theoretically and through practical dialogue—between the two sometimes conflicting elements.

On a much larger scale, the years since 1978 have witnessed the flourishing of a broader interest in professional ethics on the part of all health-related professions. Physicians, nurses, and ethicists began to discuss—among themselves and with patients, families, and other parties—the ethical decisions raised by particular cases, giving rise to the subspecialty of clinical ethics. Clinical ethics committees proliferated exponentially, expanding institutional involvement in bioethics and stimulating distinctive methodologies for case analysis. Ethics consultations were formalized, suggesting questions about the professional competence of clinical ethicists.

One finds in this edition a number of new issues discussed in the category of professional–patient relationship, for example, patients' responsibilities, conflict of interest, impaired professionals, privileged communications, sports, and sexual standards for the professional relationship. The art of medicine is a new topic that subsumes medical decision making. Topics familiar from the first edition receive a fresh perspective, such as confidentiality, information disclosure (in place of the term "truth-telling"), informed consent, medical malpractice, medical codes and oaths, patients' rights, and unorthodoxy in medicine.

Finally, we have assembled an expanded group of articles dealing with some dominant health-care professions and occupations, including medicine, nursing, mental-health professions, dentistry, surgery, pharmacy, social work, public-health workers, allied health professions, pastoral care providers, biomedical engineers, scientific publishers, death educators, genetic counselors, genetic engineers, health officials, and occupational-health-care providers.

Public health: Fascination with the ethical issues in the clinical setting, such as discontinuing medical treatment so as to allow the patient to die, has, unfortunately, overshadowed the moral choices to be made in the community setting, where many more lives and the quality of life and health are at stake. This edition considerably expands coverage of public-health ethics, with the assistance of an area editor who specializes in the ethics of public health.

A small group of core entries examines the determinants of public health, its history, its philosophy, and its methods; the international dimensions of public health; and the law, legal philosophy, and legal moralism that have tended to shape public understandings and behaviors in public-health issues as varied as the prohibition of alcoholic beverages, immunization, and sexually transmitted diseases. Another cluster of articles examines global questions such as health promotion, health education, health screening and testing, occupational safety and health, injury and injury control, and epidemics. A few entries examine even more specific topics, such as the public-health ethics issues surrounding AIDS, the disposal of toxic wastes, and the responsibilities of health officials. Several articles examine warfare in terms of the moral responsibility to take care of the public's health in consideration of the vast global morbidity and mortality rates that it causes, comparable to illness and death caused in times past by epidemics.

Other sociopolitical issues in bioethics: The revised edition revisits, from the perspective of the 1990s, first-edition topics such as racism and torture. But new topics also tackle long-neglected social issues in human health, such as sexism, prostitution, female circumcision (or, more correctly, genital mutilation), interpersonal abuse (child abuse, abuse between domestic partners, elder abuse), rights of children, child custody, adoption, disabilities (medical, sociological, philosophical, theological, and legal aspects), and the death penalty.

Health care: This edition contains a thorough treatment of the issues involved in health-care delivery systems. It includes discussion of the larger social and ethical issues: health-care allocation, health-care financing and economics, commercialism, the quality of health care, health policy, and the international dimensions of health care. It also includes a comprehensive discussion of the principles of justice and beneficence and the right to health care that would govern the reform of health-care systems. This revised edition also contains new material on the health-care–related issues pertaining to AIDS, alternative therapies, chronic care, and the institutional setting of health care: health-care institutions, the hospital, academic health centers, laboratories, medical information systems, the pharmaceutical industry, and nursing homes.

The reader will also find updated discussions of topics that appeared in the first edition regarding the health care of special populations: fetuses, infants, children, adolescents, women, the aged, the disabled (only the "mentally handicapped" were discussed in the first edition), prisoners, and prostitutes. A single first-edition article on medical ethics education has been replaced by a series of articles on bioethics education at every level and for a variety of professions.

Fertility and human reproduction: The first edition contained articles about the ethics of in vitro fertilization (IVF), in spite of the fact that, at the time of their writing, the procedure had not yet been performed. At that time, the scientific situation strongly influenced the ethical response. For example, the appropriate article reported on the ethical argument regarding IVF: Because it was regarded as entailing unknown hazards to the one being procreated, the procedure would be an objectionable form of human experimentation, for it would be done without the consent of the subject. In July 1978, just before publication of the first edition, Louise Brown, the first "test-tube baby," was born; tens of thousands of humans have been conceived in this way in the intervening years. While the basic question of the morality of IVF procedures is still debated, there has been a shift of emphasis from safety and consent to such questions as the just distribution of this service, honesty about its outcomes, and the various forms of obtaining, storing, and using human gametes and embryos.

In addition, a host of more recently developed reproductive technologies—including the use of surrogate wombs and the cyropreservation of sperm, ova, and human embryos—have brought about increasingly complex fertility-related human relationships that raise ethical questions far more complex than did IVF. Fetal research is being intensely debated; the meaning of the maternal–fetal relationship has come under reassessment, partly under the influence of feminist thought; and the collection of articles on abortion manifest continued and constantly shifting ethical, religious, and legal debates. Even medical perspectives on abortion are constantly shifting. All these issues and more are given careful, contemporary analysis in this revised edition from the perspectives of secular and religious ethics, medicine, science, law, and public policy.

Biomedical and behavioral research: The first edition, in tune with its times, used the term "human experimentation," and made a strong distinction between biomedical and behavioral research, which were discussed in separate entries. In this edition, the term human research is used in place of human experimentation; and the editors merged biomedical and behavioral research into one set of articles dealing simply with research. From an ethical perspective, the distinction seemed no longer warranted. New topics on the ethics of research include research issues in AIDS, biotechnology, commercialism in scientific research, minorities as research subjects, multinational research, research bias, research ethics committees, research with vulnerable groups, and xenografts. Basic methodological issues are covered in entries on research methodology and research policy. The interrelated topics of fraud, theft, and plagiarism are given a new currency in this edition; and some of the well-established topics—such as informed consent in research, and research in special populations such as children, fetuses, women, and the aged—are extensively revised.

Mental health and behavioral issues: The revised edition had to fight against the continuing assumption that health care means physical medicine—an assumption that has the effect of marginalizing ethical and social issues in mental health and mental-health care. Thus, to correct the impression that health-care distribution means the distribution of physical health care, this edition has separate articles on mental-health services: their settings, their programs, and the ethics of their provision. Whereas psychosurgery was one of the most hotly contested issues in bioethics at the time of the first edition, in this edition the topic is discussed mostly from a historic perspective; the entry notes shifts in medical practices and attitudes, as well as in ethical positions being taken. This edition also presents a new generation of thought on such topics as mental patients' rights, commitment to mental institutions, institutionalization and deinstitutionalization, the mentally disabled, and substance abuse.

Sexuality and gender: Current insights into sexual development, sexual identity, and gender identity—which have pervasive bioethical implications—are characteristic of this small cluster of articles. A master article on sexual ethics provides an overall guide to ethical reflection on a wide range of ethical issues associated with human sexuality.

Death and dying: In the early to mid-1970s, the guidelines and policies that offered standards for discontinuing medical treatment, allowing patients to die, and performing active euthanasia could be contained in a single, slim file folder. In the intervening years the professional and public policies, policy recommendations, and other scholarly writings on these issues have become so voluminous that one of our tasks for the revised edition was simply to summarize the vast literature on the topic. This can be found in the large and important entry on "Death and Dying: Euthanasia and Sustaining Life," where the reader can also find an explanation of the ethical and legal aspects of advance directives (a term that did not exist at the time of the first edition).

Neurological, philosophical, ethical, and legal aspects of the definition and determination of death have undergone considerable developments; this edition explains them and offers the key arguments. Suicide, which has taken on new significance with the interest in assisted suicide, is discussed in a new entry on that topic. New topics, in addition to advance directives, include hospice, end-of-life care, and death education.

The dramatic ethical questions surrounding technology and termination of life are certainly not the only important questions pertaining to death and dying. Because the moral dimensions of death and dying are likely to be as broad as the realities of death and dying themselves, the cultures surrounding them, and the moment-by-moment internal and external choices to be made by the dying and all of us who anticipate dying and caring for the dying, we have included core articles on background topics that could have the effect of expanding our moral vision of what it means to die. Those basic articles deal with death in Eastern and Western philosophical and religious thought, anthropological perspectives on death and dying, and the "art of dying." A historical article on *Ars moriendi* is paired with one on the art of dying in our contemporary culture. Undoubtedly, future editions will examine more of the history and contemporary analysis of this important topic.

Genetics: The scientific and ethical aspects of genetics are dramatically different today as compared with the times almost twenty years ago when the first edition was being prepared. Gene therapy, genome mapping and sequencing, genetic engineering, genetic testing and screening, and the patenting of organisms—some of the most rapidly developing areas of genetic ethics—are included in this edition. The coverage is thorough. For example, an entry on scientific, ethical, and legal dimensions of genetic testing and screening includes articles on preimplantation and prenatal diagnosis, newborn screening, carrier screening, and predictive and workplace testing; another entry considers the ethics of genetic engineering in plants, animals, and humans. Additional new topics and newly revisited first-edition topics include such areas as eugenics (from the perspectives of history, ethics, and religious law), the practice of medical genetics, genetic counseling, and the relationship of genetics to human behavior generally and specifically to racial minorities. The core articles that explain and analyze the scientific, philosophical, and attitudinal background information on the entire area of human genetics are those dealing with evolution, genetics and environment, genetics and human self-understanding, and genetics and the law.

Population ethics: Ethical issues arising in the context of the relationship of population dynamics to human health have not been constantly in the forefront of public awareness or ethical scholarship during the period that has elapsed since the appearance of the first edition. Yet there have been important new developments in this area, many of which are gaining more attention due to the 1994 United Nations meeting on population issues in Cairo, Egypt.

With this edition's entries on population ethics it was not our purpose to cover every ethical question that arises in reference to population dynamics and population studies; our focus is the ethical implications of population issues that relate to human health. Fertility control, which is a major element in population studies, presents extensive scientific and ethical issues relating to human health. The revised edition examines this topic from the perspectives of major world religions, secular norms, and the law; and special fertility-related problems are discussed: the use of compulsion, strong persuasion, incentives, and disincentives in fertility control strategies; the corporate responsibilities of donor agencies; and the health effects of various fertility control methods. However, this edition goes beyond fertility control to consider another major component of population studies: migration. Articles in this edition examine health-related ethical issues of migration at a time when approximately 100 million international migrants—a sizable proportion of whom are refugees—are the suffering, visible face of what may well be the major human crisis of our age.

Organ and tissue transplantation and artificial organs. In the 1970s, the ethical questions dealt with justification of the procedures, risks versus benefits, and the need to preserve individuality as technology grafted foreign living and nonliving substances onto the human body. In this new edition, after transplants and implants have become much more common, the articles on these topics tend to emphasize the just distribution of organs and the development of regional, national, and international systems of organ allocation. The ethical and legal aspects of organ procurement have been thoroughly examined from such perspectives as whether specific consent is required from the person from whom organs are harvested before or after death, and the procurement of organs from living donors and cadavers. An interdisciplinary entry was required to examine transplantation of organs from medical, psychological, social, cultural, ethical, and legal perspectives. In addition, the reader finds an examination of commercialism in the sale and/or surgical transplantation of human body parts.

Welfare and treatment of animals: The first edition had a single entry on animals; it dealt with animal experimentation in the context of its possible benefit to humans. In the meantime, the importance of broader issues in the care of animals has emerged as a topic of major concern in bioethics, prompting us to include an entirely new concentration of articles on the whole area of the health and welfare of nonhuman animals and human responsibilities for them.

The core article in this section is the lead article in the entry on animal welfare and rights: ethical perspectives on the treatment and status of animals. Other articles discuss the welfare and treatment of animals in every setting: in the wild, in hunting, as endangered species, as pets and companion animals, in zoos, in agriculture and factory farming, and in research. Finally, we include a new entry on veterinary ethics.

Environment: The breadth of this edition—and of the discipline of bioethics that it represents—is typified by two contrasting articles. One is an article on autonomy, a highly individualistic theme discussed above in the section on the patient–professional relationship; and the other, in the section on environment, is the article on sustainable development, a decidedly global issue. Typical of the entries on environment, the article on sustainable development deals with the economic, developmental, environmental, demographic, and justice-related goals that will benefit the health and well-being of future generations. This Encyclopedia tries to sustain a healthy balance between individual and global issues in bioethics.

Environmental issues in bioethics deal with global problems related to health and the life sciences; and these problems may be viewed as global on the part of the entire human species, all nonhuman nature, or the biosphere as a whole. In our entries we have tried to avoid opting for one to the exclusion of the others; but we probably have given most emphasis to ethical issues related to human environmental health. Our articles deal with specific global-ethical issues such as what to do with hazardous wastes and toxic substances; endangered species and biodiversity; and climatic change. But the main focus of this collection of articles is found in topics that explain the setting, the values, the principles, and the law involved. For example, the central article on environmental ethics gives an overview of this area of bioethics; it then discusses the theories of deep ecology, land ethic, and ecofeminism. Other core topics covered in this edition are on the relationship between genetics and environment in health care; environment and religion; and environmental policy and law.

Codes, oaths, and other directives: An important and completely revised element is the Appendix, which offers documentation with brief commentaries on "Codes, Oaths, and Directives Related to Bioethics." Three articles offer analytic and historical background for the consideration of these sources of bioethics: two articles on medical codes and oaths in the body of the Encyclopedia; and, introducing the Appendix, an article on the nature and role of codes and other ethics directives.

It may not be surprising to discover that, since appearance of the first edition, directives on the rights of patients and on the rights of people to health care have multiplied; more unusual is the appearance of documents on the responsibilities of patients and the professional freedom of physicians. Key documents in this category are found in the first section of the Appendix.

The second section of the Appendix contains ethical directives for the practice of medicine dating from the fourth century B.C.E. to 1994. Many countries are represented in this section; all foreign-language documents have been translated into English. Ethical directives for other health-care professions—nursing, dentistry, chiropractic, psychology, social work, dietetics, pastoral care, pharmacy, and so forth—are found in the third section. The fourth section contains ethical directives for human research, beginning with the pre–Nazi-era German Guidelines on Human Experimentation, and including documents from the United States and many other countries. The final two sections are on topics not included in the first-edition Appendix: They contain important ethical directives pertaining to the welfare and use of animals, including veterinary medicine and research involving animals; and ethical codes and declarations pertaining to the environment, environmental health, and environmental professionals.

Bioethics: Its basic tools and methods

The Introduction to the first edition offered this definition of bioethics: "the systematic study of human conduct in the area of the life sciences and health care, insofar as this conduct is examined in the light of moral values and principles." This definition was widely quoted in many parts of the world as the foundational definition of bioethics.

A sign of the vitality of this new field is that in the intervening years controversy has surrounded this definition. Some authors have claimed that inclusion of the word "principles" in the first edition's definition helped to move the field of bioethics in its initial stages toward an "applied" ethics model. In this model, principles, understood as normative rules devised and perfected by moral philosophers, are simply applied to moral problems, whatever those problems may be. This model has had the effect of implying that normative moral knowledge focuses almost exclusively on ethical principles, thus ruling out relationships, emotions, narratives, images, the attitudes and convictions of people involved in medical cases, and so on, as serious sources of moral knowledge and norms.

This criticism of the first-edition definition of bioethics manifests a confusion about the meaning of the word "principles." The definition in the first edition used a meaning of "principle" that is etymological: It signified "source" or "origin." By saying that in bioethics, certain kinds of conduct (that associated with the life sciences and health care) are examined in the light of the *principles* of morality, it meant examined in the light of the sources of morality or ethics, that is, the sources of moral knowledge and judgment, whatever those sources might be.

This meaning of "principle" was common in ethics for centuries, and is found in the titles of textbooks such as *The Principles of Ethics, Principles of Moral Philosophy,* and *Principles of Moral Theology.* Indeed, the term is used with the same meaning in virtually every field of learning and has long been used in the titles of hundreds upon hundreds of textbooks and brief reference works, including those for the basic sciences and medicine, such as *Principles of Anatomy, Principles of Pathology,* and *Principles of Neurology.*

At the time the first edition of the Encyclopedia appeared, this meaning of "principles" was still current. I used the term "principles" in the meaning of source quite deliberately in the Encyclopedia's original definition of bioethics, because I wanted a definition that would leave the field of bioethics open to any past or future methodology. In particular, I wanted a definition that would encourage the use of sources of meta-ethical and normative moral knowledge that were not current in the 1970s, when the narrowly conceived deontological/teleological framework of rule-based ethics was so popular. The word "values" was included in the first definition to accentuate this openness to all sources of moral knowledge: Whereas the primary "principles" (sources) of a field of learning were generally understood to be those that could be summarized systematically in a textbook, I added the word "values" to suggest that among the sources of ethical knowledge some are actually experienced as values and exercise a normative function before they are fully analyzed in textbooks.

Soon after the appearance of the first edition, however, the more constrained meaning of principle became the dominant one, namely, a concise statement of a rule or norm of behavior, an "action guide." This more recent meaning has caused a direct reversal of the intent of openness to the widest possible range of sources of moral knowledge that was signified by the "principles" of the first definition. Consequently, the definition employed in this edition (articulated above) drops the word "principles" and speaks simply of "a variety of ethical methodologies in an interdisciplinary setting."

This commentary on sources of knowledge for bioethics invites some comments on what we call the "basic topics" in the revised edition. Like the first edition, the revised edition places major emphasis on the basic knowledge needed for bioethics; it is no mere anthology of articles on areas of ethical controversy. Furthermore, there are significant changes in these underlying topics, indicative of the profound changes that have occurred in ethics itself—its methodologies and assumptions—over the past decade and a half.

Basic concepts and approaches. There are two articles in the revised edition on bioethics. One is called simply bioethics. The other is contained in the long entry on Medical Ethics, History of, in the section on The Americas; the article "United States in the Twentieth Century" describes the rise and salient features of bioethics. These two articles should be the starting point for anyone seeking an explanation of the discipline of bioethics, its methods, and its scope. Both articles are sensitive to the many changes that have occurred in the field.

The core entry on ethics has been reduced from twelve articles in the first edition to five articles here: on the task of ethics, moral epistemology, normative ethical theories, social and political theories, and religion and morality. We believe this arrangement for describing what ethics is all about will provide an excellent groundwork for the reader.

Various basic features of ethics and special approaches to ethical reasoning (with special reference to their bearing on bioethics) are pursued under such familiar topics as natural law, double effect, utility, rights, law and morality, law and bioethics, and public policy and bioethics. New topics in this category include virtue (long a traditional part of moral philosophy and theology, it had been neglected by thinkers of the nineteenth and twentieth centuries and has only recently experienced a renaissance), value and valuation, interpretation, and narrative (which deals with the moral experiences and stories that shape the lives of people and cultures, and how they are interpreted as ethically significant), responsibility (which makes important connections between moral rules and the moral agent), feminism (which challenges bioethical assumptions across the board), and casuistry (a late medieval and Renaissance approach to ethics that is currently transforming discussions about case-based reasoning).

Certain concepts and ideas are ingredient in or presupposed to critical bioethical reflection. Many of these topics are new to this edition; all are given a fresh, new approach. They include authority, body, care, conscience, emotions, freedom and coercion, harm, healing, health and disease, life, love, nature, obligation and supererogation, pain and suffering, race and racism, and tragedy.

Finally, a cluster of entries on principles and virtues offer contemporary considerations of such topics as beneficence, autonomy, compassion, fidelity and loyalty, informed consent, justice, paternalism, trust, and the like. Even a traditional topic like justice reveals new dimensions, such as the debate about the communitarian ideal of the common good versus a welfare liberal conception of justice, and the call of feminist justice for assigning rights and duties according to a gender-free standard.

Religious traditions. Bioethical beliefs, norms, teachings, and practices of the dominant world religions are thoroughly covered in this edition. Separate entries introduce the reader to the worlds of African Religion, Buddhism, Confucianism, Eastern Orthodox Christianity, Hinduism, Islam, Jainism, Judaism,

Native American religions, Protestantism, Roman Catholicism, Sikhism, and Taoism. Certain entries, such as those on abortion and eugenics, contain special articles on the perspectives especially of the world religions that are most dominant in the United States.

Historical perspectives.   The editors were convinced that a historical perspective is often essential for a proper interpretation of bioethical issues. Consequently, in this edition we offer new topics: The history of childhood, the history of the care of infants, and historical perspectives on women are examples. Other entries offer the history of the idea of death, care, health and disease, and the professional–patient relationship.

A monumental historical entry can be found in the book-length set of articles on the history of medical ethics. Its thirty-four articles, designed to be read either separately or in sequence, are divided into six sections: Near and Middle East; Africa; South and East Asia; Europe; the Americas; and Australia and New Zealand. Each section contains articles in chronological sequence, with such titles as: Ancient Near East; Prerepublican China; Sub-Saharan Africa; Greece and Rome; Renaissance and Enlightenment; and a survey of the contemporary history of medical ethics and bioethics in a variety of countries and groups of countries in various parts of the world.

Disciplines bearing on bioethics: The assumption underlying this work is that all the contributing disciplines are concerned with an evaluative endeavor and that each discipline brings a different competence and methodology to such questions as: What should be done? Who should decide? What virtues and values should guide society in these areas? In assembling this revised edition, we have been guided by the special competence of each discipline. In an attempt both to explain and contribute to the interdisciplinarity of bioethics, we offer entries that survey an entire discipline while revealing some important connections to bioethics. In this category the reader will find entries on the philosophy of biology, the philosophy of science, economics, law, literature, anthropology of medicine, philosophy of medicine, and sociology of medicine.

Special features of the Encyclopedia

The international and interdisciplinary character of the Encyclopedia is evident from the fact that the 437 contributors are from every continent and represent many fields of learning including ethics, biology, medicine and many other health professions, psychology, philosophy, religion, theology, sociology, regional studies, feminist scholarship, language, literature, anthropology, law, policy science, demography, and history.

We are aware that we have not achieved the level of interdisciplinarity to which we had aspired. We attempted to achieve an interdisciplinary approach through several means. First, we urged authors to take a decidedly interdisciplinary approach, taking account of the nature of the topic. Second, we used the device of juxtaposing articles from the perspectives of various disciplines throughout this work. Yet interdisciplinarity is not achieved by mere juxtaposition. Authors were asked to shape their articles to address the contents of companion articles within the same entry; and in virtually every case, authors either read the companion articles or were instructed regarding their contents.

Contributors were asked to make all topical presentations at least somewhat international. Cultural, ethical, and legal differences make a completely international article virtually impossible. Nonetheless, this edition offers a strong international component through its inclusion of separate international topics, articles on bioethics in various parts of the world, and an international subdivision within a number of topical articles. Whenever possible, articles on historical and current issues in bioethics in various parts of the world, as well as the articles on world religions, were written by indigenous authors, many of them the pioneers of bioethics in their own countries.

All encyclopedias must face the problem of bias, which affects even the most distinguished scholars in all fields of learning. In an encyclopedia dealing exclusively with ethics and values related to sensitive issues of life, health, and death, the presumption is that biases and ideologies might insinuate themselves even more easily. The editors insisted that the contributors give fair representation to a variety of ethical views on a given topic. Frequently the perspective of the individual author cannot be entirely concealed, nor should it be. When an element of bias does appear in some articles, we believe this is counterbalanced by the breadth of perspectives offered in related entries.

Every effort has been made to offer a clear and direct exposition of the material for the uninitiated reader and to avoid the use of undefined technical terms. However, in a few instances prior knowledge of the subject will prove helpful.

Organization of the Encyclopedia

Entries are arranged alphabetically. To achieve a systematic and multidisciplinary coherence among related topics, some *entries* are composed of several *articles*. For example,

ORGAN AND TISSUE TRANSPLANTS

    I. MEDICAL OVERVIEW
   II. SOCIOCULTURAL ASPECTS
 III. ETHICAL AND LEGAL ISSUES

The reader seeking information on ethical aspects of organ transplantation would do well to read all three articles, for they represent an interlocking bioethical analysis of all the salient features of this question.

The bibliographies following each article are an important resource. They were prepared by the contributors and were verified and edited by the publisher's bibliographic editor. Generally, we have attempted to keep the bibliographies fairly brief and representative; but the purposes of bibliographies can vary from article to article, and we intended bibliographies as resources for further research. On a topic for which few if any secondary sources exist, it has been advisable to list the primary sources in the bibliography. Other articles require listing of extensive documentation, because for that topic they are the key resources. The bibliographic items refer the reader to sources used by the contributor, some of which have been cited in the text in parentheses, for example: (Smith, 1972, p. 50).

Use of the Encyclopedia is facilitated by a carefully worked-out system of cross-references that lead the reader to other entries or to parts of the Appendix that offer further information relevant to the article at hand. The principal cross-referencing device is found in a paragraph following each article. Here the reader is referred to other articles, which are listed in categories of descending importance as regards their relevance to the present article. We have used a uniform style in the cross-references, to help the reader differentiate between the titles of entries and of articles. Entry titles use large capitals for the first letter of each main word; article titles use all small capitals:

For further discussion of topics mentioned in this article, see the entry HEALTH AND DISEASE, *article on* HISTORY OF THE CONCEPTS.

An additional device to assist the reader in locating materials is the "blind entry" or "see entry." Significant topics that readers may be likely to seek out but that do not have their own entry are listed alphabetically, with a reference to the entry or entries where that information can be found. For example,

IN VITRO FERTILIZATION   *See* REPRODUCTIVE TECHNOLOGIES, *articles on* IN VITRO FERTILIZATION AND EMBRYO TRANSFER, ETHICAL ISSUES, *and* LEGAL AND REGULATORY ISSUES.

The alphabetical arrangement of the entries, the cross-referencing, and the blind entries make the entire body of the Encyclopedia self-indexing. Nonetheless, an indispensable tool is its thorough index: Many specific topics and names can be found only by making use of the index. Furthermore, the index creatively organizes and subdivides interesting clusters of topically related information.

This second and much expanded edition of the *Encyclopedia of Bioethics* manifests the extraordinary vitality of the field of bioethics; the coming-of-age of a whole new generation of highly diversified scholars; the evolution of major, new perspectives in the sciences and health care; the constant addition of new topics and ethical viewpoints; and the challenging evolution of moral ideas and the conversations and arguments that deal with them.

Warren Thomas Reich
Editor in Chief

Alphabetical List of Article Titles

List of Contributors

Adams, Paul L.
  University of Tennessee
  Sexual Development

Aird, John S.
  U.S. Bureau of the Census (retired)
  Population Policies, *section on* Strategies of Fertility
    Control, *article on* Compulsion

Allen, Anita L.
  Georgetown Law Center
  Abortion, *section on* Contemporary Ethical and Legal
    Aspects, *article on* Legal and Regulatory Issues;
    Privacy in Health Care

Amundsen, Darrel W.
  Western Washington University
  Medical Ethics, History of, *section on* Near and Middle
    East, *article on* Ancient Near East; *section on* Europe,
    Ancient and Medieval, *articles on* Greece and Rome,
    Early Christianity, *and* Medieval Christian Europe

Anderson, W. French
  National Institutes of Health, Bethesda, Maryland
  Gene Therapy, *article on* Strategies for Gene Therapy

Anderson, Gerard F.
  Johns Hopkins University
  Health Policy, *article on* Health Policy in International
    Perspective

Andolsen, Barbara Gilkert
  Monmouth College
  Marriage and Other Domestic Partnerships

Angell, Marcia
  New England Journal of Medicine
  Fraud, Theft, and Plagiarism

Annas, George J.
  Boston University
  Patients' Rights, *article on* Origin and Nature of Patients'
    Rights

Arnold, Robert M.
  University of Pittsburgh
  Bioethics Education, *article on* Medicine; Informed
    Consent, *article on* Clinical Aspects of Consent in
    Health Care

Aroskar, Mila A.
  University of Minnesota
  Bioethics Education, *article on* Nursing

Asch, Adrienne
  Wellesley College
  Disability, *article on* Attitudes and Sociological
    Perspectives

Bakar, Osman
  Malaya University, Kuala Lumpur
  Abortion, *section on* Religious Traditions, *article on*
    Islamic Perspectives

Baker, George T., III
  Shock Aging Research Foundation, Silver Spring, Maryland
  Aging and Aged, *article on* Theories of Aging and Life
    Extension

Baker, Robert
  Union College
  Mental Illness, *article on* Conceptions of Mental Illness

Banja, John D.
  Emory University
  Rehabilitation Medicine; Disability, *article on* Health
    Care and Physical Disability

Banks, Joanne Trautmann
Pennsylvania State University
Literature

Baran, Annette
Psychotherapist, Los Angeles
Adoption

Basch, Paul F.
Stanford University
International Health

Bassett, William
University of San Francisco
Eugenics and Religious Law, *article on* Christianity

Battin, Margaret Pabst
University of Utah
Suicide

Bayer, Ronald
Columbia University
AIDS, *article on* Public-Health Issues

Bayley, Corrine
St. Joseph Health System, Orange, California
Hospital, *article on* Contemporary Ethical Problems

Beary, John F., III
Pharmaceutical Research and Manufacturers of America
Pharmaceutics, *article on* Pharmaceutical Industry

Beauchamp, Dan E.
State University of New York, Albany
Health Promotion and Health Education; Lifestyles and Public Health; Public Health, *article on* Philosophy of Public Health; Public Health and the Law, *article on* Legal Moralism and Public Health

Beauchamp, Tom L.
Georgetown University
Informed Consent, *articles on* History of Informed Consent, *and* Meaning and Elements of Informed Consent; Paternalism

Bedau, Hugo Adam
Tufts University
Civil Disobedience and Health Care

Benatar, Solomon R.
University of Cape Town, South Africa
Medical Ethics, History of, *section on* Africa, *article on* South Africa

Benjamin, Martin
Michigan State University
Conscience

Berg, Kåre
Institute of Medical Genetics, Oslo, Norway
Medical Genetics, *article on* Practice of Medical Genetics

Bickel, Janet
Association of American Medical Colleges, Washington, D.C.
Women, *article on* Women as Health Professionals: Contemporary Issues

Biesecker, Barbara Bowles
University of Michigan
Genetic Counseling, *article on* Practice of Genetic Counseling

Bishop, Anne H.
Lynchburg College
Nursing, Theories and Philosophy of; Nursing as a Profession

Bishop, Laura Jane
Georgetown University
Medical Ethics, History of, *section on* Europe, *article on* Contemporary Period: German-Speaking Countries and Switzerland

Blasszauer, Bela
Medical University of Pecs, Hungary
Medical Ethics, History of, *section on* Europe, *article on* Contemporary Period: Central and Eastern Europe

Bloch, Sidney
University of Melbourne, Australia
Psychiatry, Abuses of

Bloom, Peter B.
University of Pennsylvania
Hypnosis

Bloom, Samuel W.
Mount Sinai School of Medicine, New York
Professional–Patient Relationship, *article on* Sociological Perspectives

Bondolfi, Alberto
University of Zurich, Switzerland
Medical Ethics, History of, *section on* Europe, *article on* Contemporary Period: German-Speaking Countries and Switzerland

Bonnicksen, Andrea L.
Northern Illinois University
Reproductive Technologies, *article on* In Vitro Fertilization and Embryo Transfer

Bosk, Charles L.
University of Pennsylvania
Health and Disease, *article on* Sociological Perspectives

Botkin, Jeffrey R.
University of Utah

Circumcision, *article on* Male Circumcision; Genetic Testing and Screening, *article on* Ethical Issues

Bouchard, Larry D.
University of Virginia

Tragedy

Bouillon-Jensen, Cindy
Washington State Department of Social and Health Services

Infants, *article on* History of Infanticide

Bowman, James E.
University of Chicago

Genetics and Racial Minorities

Boxer, Marilyn J.
San Francisco State University

Women, *article on* Historical and Cross-Cultural Perspectives

Branson, Roy
Washington Institute, Washington, D.C.

Prisoners, *article on* Research Issues

Brennan, Troyen A.
Harvard University

Informed Consent, *article on* Issues of Consent in Mental-Health Care; Medical Malpractice

Breslow, Lester
University of California, Los Angeles

Public Health, *article on* Determinants of Public Health

Bresnahan, James F.
Northwestern University

Death: Art of Dying, *article on* Contemporary Art of Dying

Brieger, Gert H.
Johns Hopkins University

Medicine as a Profession

Brock, Dan W.
Brown University

Death and Dying: Euthanasia and Sustaining Life, *article on* Ethical Issues; Public Policy and Bioethics

Brody, Baruch A.
Baylor College of Medicine

Law and Morality

Brody, Howard
Michigan State University

Clinical Ethics, *article on* Elements and Methodologies; Patients' Responsibilities, *article on* Duties of Patients; Placebo

Browder, J. Pat
Kaiser Permanente, Raleigh, North Carolina

Healing

Brown, Alan P.
University of Massachusetts

Informed Consent, *article on* Issues of Consent in Mental-Health Care

Brown, Douglas
Louisiana State University

Mental Health, *article on* Mental Health and Religion

Brown, Kate H.
Creighton University

Information Disclosure, *article on* Attitudes Toward Truth-Telling

Bulger, Roger J.
Association of Academic Health Centers, Washington, D.C.

Academic Health Centers; Health-Care Delivery, *article on* Health-Care Institutions

Bunker, John P.
Stanford University

Artificial Organs and Life-Support Systems

Burns, Chester R.
University of Texas, Galveston

Medical Ethics, History of, *section on* The Americas, *article on* Colonial North America and Nineteenth-Century United States

Cahill, Lisa Sowle
Boston College

Abortion, *section on* Religious Traditions, *article on* Roman Catholic Perspectives

Caldwell, John C.
National Centre for Epidemiology and Population Health, Canberra, Australia

Population Policies, *section on* Strategies of Fertility Control, *article on* Changes in Attitude and Culture

Callahan, Daniel
Hastings Center, Briarcliff Manor, New York

Bioethics

Callicott, J. Baird
University of Wisconsin, Madison

Environmental Ethics, *articles on* Overview, *and* Land Ethic

Campbell, Courtney S.
Oregon State University

Utility

Cantor, Norman L.
Rutgers University

Life, Quality of, *article on* Quality of Life in Legal
Perspective

Cao, Antonio
University "degli Studi" of Cagliari, Italy

Genetic Testing and Screening, *article on* Carrier
Screening

Caplan, Arthur L.
University of Pennsylvania

Artificial Hearts and Cardiac Assist Devices; Organ and
Tissue Transplants, *article on* Ethical and Legal Issues

Capron, Alexander Morgan
University of Southern California

Death, Definition and Determination of, *article on* Legal
Issues in Pronouncing Death; Death and Dying:
Euthanasia and Sustaining Life, *article on* Professional
and Public Policies; Law and Bioethics

Caranasos, George J.
University of Florida, Gainesville

Pharmaceutics, *article on* Issues in Prescribing

Carson, Hampton L.
University of Hawaii

Evolution

Carson, Ronald A.
University of Texas, Galveston

Interpretation

Carter, Albert Howard, III
Eckerd College

Self-Help

Carter, Michele A.
University of Texas, Galveston

Mental-Health Services, *article on* Ethical Issues

Cassel, Christine K.
University of Chicago

Health-Care Delivery, *article on* Health-Care
Institutions; Health-Care Financing: Introduction

Cassell, Eric J.
Cornell University

Medicine, Art of; Pain and Suffering

Chapple, Christopher Key
Loyola Marymount University

Jainism

Charo, R. Alta
University of Wisconsin, Madison

Reproductive Technologies, *article on* Legal and
Regulatory Issues

Childress, James F.
University of Virginia

Metaphor and Analogy; Organ and Tissue Procurement,
article on Ethical and Legal Issues Regarding Cadavers

Chill, Julia C.
Carnegie Corporation of New York

Prisoners, *article on* Torture and the Health Professional

Christakis, Nicholas A.
University of Pennsylvania

Multinational Research

Christiansen, Drew
United States Catholic Conference, Washington, D.C.

Food Policy

Christoffel, Tom
University of Illinois, Chicago

Homicide

Churchill, Larry R.
University of North Carolina, Chapel Hill

Beneficence

Ciccone, J. Richard
University of Rochester

Expert Testimony

Cohen, Cynthia B.
*National Advisory Board on Ethics in Reproduction,
Washington, D.C.*

Reproductive Technologies, *article on* Ethical Issues

Cole, Thomas R.
University of Texas, Galveston

Aging and the Aged, *article on* Old Age

Coleman, Eli
University of Minnesota

Homosexuality, *article on* Clinical and Behavioral
Aspects

Cook, Harold J.
University of Wisconsin, Madison

Medical Ethics, History, *section on* Europe, *article on*
Renaissance and Enlightenment

Cook-Deegan, Robert Mullan
National Academy of Sciences, Washington, D.C.

Genome Mapping and Sequencing

Copenhaver, Brian
University of California, Los Angeles

Death: Art of Dying, *article on* Ars Moriendi

Cranford, Ronald E.
University of Minnesota
Death, Definition and Determination of, *article on* Criteria for Death

Crigger, Bette-Jane
Hastings Center, Briarcliff Manor, New York
Communication, Biomedical, *article on* Media and Bioethics

Csordas, Thomas J.
Case Western Reserve University
Body, *article on* Cultural and Religious Perspectives

Culver, Charles M.
Coral Gables, Florida
Commitment to Mental Institutions; Electroconvulsive Therapy

Curran, Charles E.
Southern Methodist University
Fertility Control, *article on* Ethical Issues; Roman Catholicism

Dagi, Teodoro Forcht
Uniformed Services University of the Health Sciences
Autoexperimentation

Dalton, Clare
American University
Sexuality in Society, *article on* Legal Approaches to Sexuality

Davis, Anne J.
University of California, San Francisco
Bioethics Education, *article on* Nursing

DeJong, Gerben
National Rehabilitation Hospital, Bethesda, Maryland
Disability, *article on* Health Care and Physical Disability

Dell, Ralph
Institute of Laboratory Animal Resources, Washington, D.C.
Animal Research, *article on* Law and Policy

Dellinger, Anne M.
Hogan and Hartson, Washington, D.C.
Infants, *article on* Public Policy and Legal Issues

Desai, Prakash N.
V.A. Medical Center, Chicago
Medical Ethics, History of, *section on* South and East Asia, *article on* India

De Ville, Kenneth Allen
East Carolina University
Commercialism in Scientific Research

Dooley, Dolores
University College, Cork, Ireland
Medical Ethics, History of, *section on* Europe, *article on* Contemporary Period: Republic of Ireland

Dougherty, Charles J.
Creighton University
Clinical Ethics, *article on* Institutional Ethics Committees; Whistleblowing in Health Care

Drane, James F.
Edinboro University of Pennsylvania
Alternative Therapies, *article on* Ethical and Legal Issues

Dubler, Nancy Neveloff
Albert Einstein College of Medicine
Fertility Control, *article on* Legal and Regulatory Issues; Prisoners, *article on* Health-Care Issues

Duffy, John
University of Maryland
Public Health, *article on* History of Public Health

Dunlap, Julie
Freelance writer, Columbia, Maryland
Animal Welfare and Rights, *article on* Zoos and Zoological Parks

Dyer, Allen R.
East Tennessee State University
Advertising

Edwards, Rem B.
University of Tennessee
Behaviorism, *article on* Philosophical Issues; Freedom and Coercion

Eisenberg, Rebecca S.
University of Michigan
Patenting Organisms

Elliott, Carl
McGill University, Montreal, Canada
Mentally Disabled and Mentally Ill Persons, *article on* Research Issues

Elliott, Deni
University of Montana
Communication, Biomedical, *article on* Media and Medicine

Elshtain, Jean Bethke
Vanderbilt University
Ethics, *article on* Social and Political Theories

Engel, J. Ronald
Meadville/Lombard Theological School
Environment and Religion; Sustainable Development

Engelhardt, Dietrich von
Institute for Medicine and the History of Science, Lübeck, Germany

Health and Disease, *article on* History of the Concepts; Medical Ethics, History of, *section on* Europe, *article on* Contemporary Period: Introduction

Engelhardt, H. Tristram, Jr.
Baylor College of Medicine

Health and Disease, *article on* Philosophical Perspectives; Medicine, Philosophy of

Erde, Edmund L.
University of Medicine and Dentistry of New Jersey

Freedom and Coercion

Esposito, John L.
Georgetown University

Population Ethics, *section on* Religious Traditions, *article on* Islamic Perspectives

Evans, Mark I.
Wayne State University

Genetic Testing and Screening, *article on* Prenatal Diagnosis

Evans, Richard J.
University of London, England

Epidemics

Faden, Ruth R.
Johns Hopkins University

Informed Consent, *articles on* History of Informed Consent, *and* Meaning and Elements of Informed Consent

Farley, Margaret A.
Yale University

Sexual Ethics

Feldman, David M.
Jewish Center of Teaneck, New Jersey

Abortion, *section on* Religious Traditions, *article on* Jewish Perspectives; Eugenics and Religious Law, *article on* Judaism; Population Ethics, *section on* Religious Traditions, *article on* Jewish Perspectives

Ferngren, Gary B.
Oregon State University

Medical Ethics, History of, *section on* Near and Middle East, *article on* Ancient Near East

Flanagin, Annette
American Medical Association, Chicago

Communication, Biomedical, *article on* Scientific Publishing

Fletcher, John C.
University of Virginia

Clinical Ethics, *article on* Elements and Methodologies; Evolution

Flew, Antony
University of Reading, England

Genetics and Human Self-Understanding

Forrow, Lachlan
Harvard University

Bioethics Education, *article on* Medicine; Warfare, *article on* Nuclear Warfare

Fox, Renée C.
University of Pennsylvania

Organ and Tissue Transplants, *article on* Sociocultural Aspects

Franklin, Sarah
University of California, Santa Cruz

Life

Franks, Cyril M.
Rutgers University

Behavior Modification Therapies

Freedman, Benjamin
Jewish General Hospital of Montreal, Canada

Research, Unethical

Friedmann, Theodore
University of California, San Diego

Gene Therapy, *article on* Strategies for Gene Therapy

Fry, Sara T.
Boston College

Nursing Ethics

Fuller, Robert C.
Bradley University

Alternative Therapies, *article on* Social History

Gaines, Atwood D.
Case Western Reserve University

Mental Illness, *article on* Cross-Cultural Perspectives; Race and Racism

Garbarino, James
Cornell University

Children, *article on* Mental-Health Issues

Garcia, Jorge L. A.
Rutgers University

Double Effect

Garland, Michael J.
Oregon Health Sciences University
Health-Care Financing, article on Health-Care Insurance

Gervais, Karen Grandstrand
Minnesota Center for Health Care Ethics
Death, Definition and Determination of, article on Philosophical and Theological Perspectives

Gevitz, Norman
University of Illinois, Chicago
Unorthodoxy in Medicine

Gillon, Raanan
University of London, England
Medical Ethics, History of, section on Europe, article on Contemporary Period: United Kingdom

Gin, Nancy E.
North Orange County Community Clinic, Anaheim, California
Health Policy, article on Politics and Health Care

Glass, Richard M.
American Medical Association, Chicago
Communication, Biomedical, article on Scientific Publishing

Glick, Shimon M.
Ben Gurion University of the Negev, Beersheva, Israel
Medical Ethics, History of, section on Near and Middle East, article on Israel

Glover, Jacqueline J.
George Washington University
Health-Care Delivery, article on Health-Care Systems

Gold, Mark S.
University of Florida
Substance Abuse, article on Addiction and Dependence

Gomez, Carlos F.
University of Virginia
Disability for Public Office

Gorman, Robert F.
Southwest Texas State University
Population Policies, section on Donor Agencies, article on Migration and Refugees

Gostin, Lawrence O.
Georgetown University/Johns Hopkins University Program on Law and Public Health
Disability, article on Legal Issues

Gracia, Diego
Complutense University of Madrid, Spain
Medical Ethics, History of, section on Europe, article on Contemporary Period: Southern Europe

Gracia, Teresa
Complutense University of Madrid, Spain
Medical Ethics, History of, section on Europe, article on Contemporary Period: Southern Europe

Grad, Frank P.
Columbia University
Public Health and the Law, article on Philosophy of the Law of Public Health

Green, Ronald M.
Dartmouth College
Population Ethics, section on Religious Traditions: Introduction

Greenlick, Merwyn R.
Oregon Health Sciences University
Health-Care Financing, article on Health-Care Insurance

Greenwold, Mary
National Institute for Healthcare Research, Rockville, Maryland
Mental Health, article on Mental Health and Religion

Grim, John A.
Bucknell University
Native American Religions

Grobstein, Clifford
University of California, San Diego
Fetus, article on Human Development from Fertilization to Birth

Guy, R. Kent
University of Washington
Medical Ethics, History of, section on South and East Asia: General Survey

Haddad, Amy Marie
Creighton University
Pharmacy

Hallak, Mordecai
Lady David Carmel Hospital, Haifa, Israel
Genetic Testing and Screening, article on Prenatal Diagnosis

Handyside, Alan H.
University of London, England
Genetic Testing and Screening, article on Pre-Implantation Embryo Diagnosis

Harakas, Stanley S.
Holy Cross Greek Orthodox School of Theology
Eastern Orthodox Christianity; Population Ethics, *section on* Religious Traditions, *article on* Eastern Orthodox Christian Perspectives

Harrison, Beverly Wildung
Union Theological Seminary
Abortion, *section on* Religious Traditions, *article on* Protestant Perspectives

Harrison, James
Clinical psychologist, New York
Homosexuality, *article on* Ethical Issues

Hartung, William D.
New School for Social Research
Warfare, *article on* International Weapons Trade

Hathout, Hassan
Islamic Center of Southern California, Pasadena
Medical Ethics, History of, *section on* Near and Middle East, *article on* Contemporary Arab World

Hauerwas, Stanley
Duke University
Virtue and Character

Hawes, Joseph M.
University of Memphis
Children, *article on* History of Childhood

Haynes, Richard P.
University of Florida, Gainesville
Agriculture

Hehir, J. Bryan
Harvard University
Population Ethics, *section on* Religious Traditions, *article on* Roman Catholic Perspectives

Heyd, David
Hebrew University of Jerusalem, Israel
Obligation and Supererogation

Hiner, N. Ray
University of Kansas, Lawrence
Children, *article on* History of Childhood

Hittinger, Russell
Catholic University of America
Natural Law

Hoffman, Catherine
Institute for Health and Aging, San Francisco
Health-Care Financing, *article on* Medicaid

Holder, Angela Roddey
Yale University
Adolescents; Informed Consent, *article on* Legal and Ethical Issues of Consent in Health Care: A Postscript

Holstein, Martha
University of Texas, Galveston
Aging and the Aged, *article on* Old Age

Horwitz, Allan V.
Rutgers University
Mental-Health Services, *article on* Settings and Programs

Humphreys, Paul W.
University of Virginia
Science, Philosophy of

Hunter, Kathryn M.
Northwestern University
Narrative

Hunter, Rodney J.
Emory University
Pastoral Care

Iden, Sara
Columbia University
Abortion, *article on* Medical Perspectives

Jacobsberg, Lawrence B.
Cornell University
Mental Illness, *article on* Issues in Diagnosis

Jaggar, Alison M.
University of Colorado
Human Nature

Jameton, Andrew
University of Nebraska
Information Disclosure, *article on* Ethical Issues; Medical Ethics, History of, *section on* The Americas, *article on* The United States in the Twentieth Century

Jamieson, Dale
University of Colorado
Climatic Change

Jecker, Nancy S.
University of Washington
Aging and the Aged, *article on* Societal Aging; Care, *article on* Contemporary Ethics of Care

Joffe, Carole
University of California, Davis
Fertility Control, *article on* Social Issues

Johnson, Dawn E.
U.S. Department of Justice
Maternal–Fetal Relationship, *article on* Legal and Regulatory Issues

Johnson, Mark P.
Wayne State University
Genetic Testing and Screening, *article on* Prenatal Diagnosis

Jonsen, Albert R.
University of Washington
Casuistry; Medical Ethics, History of, *section on* South and East Asia, *article on* China: Contemporary China; *section on* The Americas, *article on* The United States in the Twentieth Century

Juengst, Eric
Case Western Reserve University
Gene Therapy, *article on* Ethical and Social Issues

Kahn, Jeffrey
Medical College of Wisconsin
Animal Research, *article on* Law and Policy

Kane, Rosalie A.
University of Minnesota
Long-Term Care, *article on* Concept and Policies

Kanoti, George A.
Cleveland Clinic Foundation, Cleveland, Ohio
Clinical Ethics, *article on* Clinical Ethics Consultation

Kellert, Stephen R.
Yale University
Animal Welfare and Rights, *article on* Zoos and Zoological Parks

Kelly, Kevin V.
Cornell University and Columbia University
Psychoanalysis and Dynamic Therapies

Kennedy, Louanne
California State University, Northridge
Blood Transfusion

Kesel, M. Lynne
Colorado State University, Fort Collins
Veterinary Ethics

Kevles, Daniel J.
California Institute of Technology
Eugenics, *article on* Historical Aspects

Kilner, John F.
Center for Bioethics and Human Dignity, Bannockburn, Illinois
Health-Care Resources, Allocation of, *articles on* Macroallocation, *and* Microallocation

Kimura, Rihito
Georgetown University, and Waseda University, Tokyo, Japan
Medical Ethics, History of, *section on* South and East Asia, *article on* Japan: Contemporary Japan

King, Nancy M. P.
University of North Carolina, Chapel Hill
Privacy and Confidentiality in Research

Kirkland, Russell
University of Georgia
Taoism

Kitagawa, Joseph Mitsuo (deceased)
University of Chicago
Medical Ethics, History of, *section on* South and East Asia, *article on* Japan: Through the Nineteenth Century

Klein, Ellen R.
University of North Florida
Animal Welfare and Rights, *article on* Hunting

Kleinman, Arthur
Harvard University
Medicine, Anthropology of

Kliever, Lonnie D.
Southern Methodist University
Death, *article on* Western Religious Thought

Knight, James Allen
Texas A&M University
Divided Loyalties in Mental-Health Care

Kopelman, Loretta M.
East Carolina University
Children, *article on* Health-Care and Research Issues; Research Methodology, *article on* Controlled Clinical Trials; Research Policy, *article on* Risk and Vulnerable Groups

Kopolow, Louis E.
George Washington University
Patients' Rights, *article on* Mental Patients' Rights

Koshuta, Monica
Hospice of Washington, Washington, D.C.
Hospice and End-of-Life Care

Koso-Thomas, Olayinka A.
University of Nairobi, Kenya
Circumcision, *article on* Female Circumcision

Kost, Kathryn
Alan Guttmacher Institute, New York
Population Policies, *article on* Health Effects of Fertility
Control

Kuszler, Patricia C.
Hogan and Hartson, Washington, D.C.
Infants, *article on* Public Policy and Legal Issues

Laín Entralgo, Pedro
Complutense, University of, Madrid, Spain
Professional–Patient Relationship, *article on* Historical
Perspectives

Lamb, H. Richard
University of Southern California
Institutionalization and Deinstitutionalization

Lang, Joan A.
University of Texas, Galveston
Sexual Development

Lantos, John D.
University of Chicago
Abuse, Interpersonal, *article on* Child Abuse; Infants,
article on Medical Aspects and Issues in the Care of
Infants

Lappé, Marc
University of Illinois, Chicago
Eugenics, *article on* Ethical Issues

Larson, David B.
*National Institute for Healthcare Research, Rockville,
Maryland*
Mental Health, *article on* Mental Health and Religion

Last, John M.
University of Ottawa, Ontario, Canada
Health Officials and Their Responsibilities

Lavin, Michael
University of Arizona
Substance Abuse, *article on* Smoking

Lebacqz, Karen
McGill University, Montreal, Canada
Feminism; Patients' Responsibilities, *article on* Virtues of
Patients; Sexual Ethics and Professional Standards

Leder, Drew
Loyola College
Bioethics Education, *article on* Secondary and
Postsecondary Education; Health and Disease, *article
on* The Experience of Health and Illness

Lederer, Susan E.
Pennsylvania State University
Military Personnel as Research Subjects

Lennox, James G.
University of Pittsburgh
Nature

Levenstein, Charles
University of Massachusetts, Lowell
Occupational Safety and Health, *article on* Ethical Issues

Levine, Carol
Orphan Project, City of New York
Research Policy, *article on* Subject Selection

Levine, Robert J.
Yale University
Informed Consent, *article on* Consent Issues in Human
Research; Multinational Research; Research Ethics
Committees

Lezotte, Dennis
University of Colorado
Medical Information Systems

Lichtenberg, Judith
University of Maryland, College Park
Population Policies, *article on* Migration and Refugees

Lidz, Charles W.
Western Psychiatric Institute, Pittsburgh, Pennsylvania
Informed Consent, *article on* Clinical Aspects of
Consent in Health Care

Lidz, Victor
Medical College of Pennsylvania and Hahnemann University
Death, *articles on* Anthropological Perspectives, *and*
Death in the Western World: A Postscript

Lifton, Betty Jean
Psychologist, New York
Adoption

Lindahl, B. I. B.
University of Stockholm, Sweden
Medical Ethics, History of, *section on* Europe, *article on*
Contemporary Period: Nordic Countries

Linzey, Andrew
University of Oxford, England
Animal Welfare and Rights, *articles on* Vegetarianism, *and* Pet and Companion Animals

Lo, Bernard
University of California, San Francisco
AIDS, *article on* Health Care and Research Issues

Loftin, Robert W. (deceased)
University of North Florida
Animal Welfare and Rights, *article on* Hunting

Lohr, Kathleen N.
Institute of Medicine, Washington, D.C.
Health Care, Quality of

Looney, Barbara L.
Georgetown University and Johns Hopkins University
Disability, *article on* Legal Issues

Lovin, Robin W.
Southern Methodist University
Ethics, *article on* Religion and Morality

Lowenthal, David T.
University of Florida, Gainesville
Pharmaceutics, *article on* Issues in Prescribing

Lustig, B. Andrew
Texas Medical Center
Compassion

Lynn, Joanne
Dartmouth-Hitchcock Medical Center
Death and Dying: Euthanasia and Sustaining Life, *article on* Advance Directives; Hospice and End-of-Life Care

Lysaught, M. Therese
Park Ridge Center, Chicago
Body, *article on* Social Theories

Macklin, Ruth
Albert Einstein College of Medicine
Abortion, *section on* Contemporary Ethical and Legal Aspects, *article on* Contemporary Ethical Perspectives; Rights, *article on* Rights in Bioethics

Maehle, Andreas-Holger
University of Durham, England
Medical Ethics, History of, *section on* Europe, *article on* Nineteenth Century: Europe

Mahowald, Mary B.
University of Chicago
Fetus, *article on* Philosophical and Ethical Issues; Organ and Tissue Procurement, *article on* Ethical and Legal Issues Regarding Living Donors; Person

Mainetti, José Alberto
National University of La Plata, Argentina
Medical Ethics, History of, *section on* Americas, *article on* Latin America

Marmor, Theodore R.
Yale University
Health-Care Financing, *article on* Medicare

Marsh, Frank H.
University of Tennessee
Medical Information Systems

Martin, George R.
National Institutes of Health, Bethesda, Maryland
Aging and the Aged, *article on* Theories of Aging and Life Extension

Mastroianni, Luigi
University of Pennsylvania
Reproductive Technologies: Introduction

Maxwell, Stephanie L.
Johns Hopkins University
Health Policy, *article on* Health Policy in International Perspective

Mbiti, John S.
University of Bern, Switzerland
African Religion

McCarthy, Charles R.
National Institutes of Health, Bethesda, Maryland
Research Policy, *article on* General Guidelines

McCullough, Laurence B.
Baylor College of Medicine
Long-Term Care, *article on* Nursing Homes

McEwen, Jean E.
Shriver Center for Mental Retardation, Waltham, Massachusetts
Genetic Testing and Screening, *article on* Legal Issues

McGough, Lucy S.
Louisiana State University
Children, *article on* Child Custody

McLaughlin, Martin M.
United States Catholic Conference, Washington, D.C.
Food Policy

McLeod, W. H.
University of Otago, Dunedin, New Zealand
Sikhism

McNicoll, Geoffrey
Population Council, New York
Population Policies, *section on* Strategies of Fertility Control, *article on* Strong Persuasion

Mechanic, David
Rutgers University
Medicine, Sociology of

Menzel, Paul T.
Pacific Lutheran University
Economic Concepts in Health Care

Merskey, Harold
University of Western Ontario, London, Canada
Psychosurgery, *article on* Ethical Issues

Michler, Robert E.
Columbia University
Xenografts

Miller, Barbara D.
George Washington University
Population Ethics, *section on* Religious Traditions, *article on* Hindu Perspectives

Miller, Bruce L.
Michigan State University
Autonomy; Students as Research Subjects

Miller, Timothy S.
Salisbury State University
Hospital, *article on* Medieval and Renaissance History

Milliken, Nancy
University of California, San Francisco
Maternal–Fetal Relationship, *article on* Medical Aspects

Mitcham, Carl
Pennsylvania State University
Technology, *article on* Philosophy of Technology

Momeyer, Richard W.
Miami University
Death, *article on* Western Philosophical Thought

Moore, Allison W.
New York Theological Seminary
Abuse, Interpersonal, *article on* Abuse Between Domestic Partners

Morgan, John D.
University of Western Ontario, London, Canada
Death, Attitudes Toward; Death Education

Morreim, E. Haavi
University of Tennessee
Conflict of Interest; Life, Quality of, *article on* Quality of Life in Health-Care Allocation

Moseley, Kathryn L.
Henry Ford Hospital, Detroit, Michigan
Infants, *article on* Medical Aspects and Issues in the Care of Infants

Moskop, John C.
East Carolina University
Laboratory Testing

Moss, Alvin H.
West Virginia University
Kidney Dialysis

Motulsky, Arno G.
University of Washington
Genetics and Environment in Human Health

Murphy, Timothy F.
University of Illinois, Chicago
Gender Identity and Gender Identity Disorders

Murray, Robert F., Jr.
Howard University
Genetic Counseling, *article on* Ethical Issues

Murray, Thomas H.
Case Western Reserve University
Authority; Genetic Testing and Screening, *article on* Ethical Issues; Occupational Safety and Health, *article on* Testing of Employees; Sports

Musto, David F.
Yale University
Substance Abuse, *article on* Legal Control of Harmful Substances

Nadelson, Carol C.
Harvard University and Tufts University
Women, *articles on* Health-Care Issues, *and* Women as Health Professionals: History

Naess, Arne
University of Oslo, Norway
Environmental Ethics, *article on* Deep Ecology

Nakasone, Ronald Y.
Graduate Theological Union
Buddhism

Ndinya-Achola, Jeckoniah O.
University of Nairobi, Kenya
Medical Ethics, History of, *section on* Africa, *article on* Sub-Saharan Countries

Nelkin, Dorothy
New York University
Health Screening and Testing in the Public Health Context

Nelson, Hilde Lindemann
Hastings Center, Briarcliff Manor, New York
Family

Nelson, James Lindemann
Hastings Center, Briarcliff Manor, New York
Family

Newell, Nanette
Oregon Biotechnology Association, Portland
Biotechnology

Newton, Lisa H.
Fairfield University
Licensing, Discipline, and Regulation in the Health Professions

Nicholson, Linda J.
State University of New York, Albany
Sexual Identity

Nightingale, Elena
Carnegie Corporation of New York
Prisoners, *article on* Torture and the Health Professional

Norton, Bryan G.
Georgia Institute of Technology
Future Generations, Obligations to

Notman, Malkah T.
Harvard University
Women, *articles on* Health-Care Issues, *and* Women as Health Professionals: History

Novak, David
University of Virginia
Judaism

Oakley, John C.
Northwest Neuroscience Institute, Seattle, Washington
Electrical Stimulation of the Brain; Psychosurgery, *article on* Medical and Historical Aspects

Oakley, Justin
Centre for Human Bioethics, Melbourne, Australia
Medical Ethics, History of, *article on* Australia and New Zealand

Ogletree, Thomas W.
Yale Divinity School
Responsibility; Value and Valuation

Olshansky, S. Jay
University of Chicago
Aging and the Aged, *article on* Life Expectancy and Life Span

Omenn, Gilbert S.
University of Washington
Genetic Testing and Screening, *article on* Predictive and Workplace Testing; Genetics and Environment in Human Health

Osborne, Richard W.
Saratoga Therapy and Training, Saratoga Springs, New York
Substance Abuse, *article on* Alcoholism

Ozar, David T.
Loyola University of Chicago
Dentistry; Profession and Professional Ethics

Panuska, J. A.
Scranton University
Cryonics

Parkinson, Michael D.
Bureau of Health Professions, Rockville, Maryland
Health Officials and Their Responsibilities

Parsons, Talcott (deceased)
Harvard University
Death, *article on* Death in the Western World

Pawlson, L. Gregory
George Washington University
Health-Care Delivery, *article on* Health-Care Systems

Pellegrino, Edmund D.
Georgetown University
Medical Education

Petersen, William
Ohio State University
Population Ethics, *section on* Elements of Population Ethics, *article on* History of Population Theories

Peterson, Lynn M.
Harvard University
Surgery

Petrie, William M.
Psychiatric Consultants, Nashville, Tennessee
Psychopharmacology

Pinches, Charles R.
University of Scranton
Action

Pisaneschi, Janet I.
Western Michigan University
Allied Health Professions

Policar, Michael
Solano Partnership Healthplan, Suisun, California
Fertility Control, *article on* Medical Aspects

Porter, Roy
Wellcome Institute for the History of Medicine, London, England
Medical Ethics, History of, *section on* Europe, *article on* Nineteenth Century: Great Britain

Post, Stephen G.
Case Western Reserve University
Bioethics Education: Introduction; Love

Povar, Gail J.
George Washington University
Women, *article on* Women as Health Professionals: Contemporary Issues

Proctor, Robert N.
Pennsylvania State University
National Socialism

Prottas, Jeffrey M.
Brandeis University
Organ and Tissue Procurement, *article on* Medical and Organizational Aspects

Purtilo, Ruth B.
Creighton University
Bioethics Education, *article on* Other Health Professions; Professional-Patient Relationship, *article on* Ethical Issues; Teams, Health-Care

Qiu, Ren-Zong
Chinese Academy of Social Sciences, Beijing, China
Medical Ethics, History of, *section on* South and East Asia, *article on* China: Contemporary China

Quirk, Michael J.
New School for Social Research
Ethics, *article on* Moral Epistemology

Ratanakul, Pinit
Mahidol University, Bangkok, Thailand
Medical Ethics, History, *section on* South and East Asia, *article on* Southeast Asian Countries; Population Ethics, *section on* Religious Traditions, *article on* Buddhist Perspectives

Ratner, Adam J.
Columbia University
Xenografts

Reamer, Frederic G.
Rhode Island College
Social Work in Health Care

Redmond, Geoffrey P.
Foundation for Developmental Endocrinology, Cleveland, Ohio
Eugenics and Religious Law, *article on* Hinduism and Buddhism

Regan, Tom
North Carolina State University
Animal Welfare and Rights, *article on* Ethical Perspectives on the Treatment and Status of Animals

Reich, Warren Thomas
Georgetown University
Care, *articles on* History of the Notion of Care, Historical Dimensions of an Ethics of Care in Health Care, *and* Contemporary Ethics of Care

Reilly, Philip R.
Shriver Center for Mental Retardation, Waltham, Massachusetts
Genetics and the Law; Genetic Testing and Screening, *article on* Legal Issues

Reiser, Stanley Joel
University of Texas, Houston
Technology, *article on* History of Medical Technology

Reitemeier, Paul
University of Nebraska
Strikes by Health Professionals

Relman, Arnold S.
Brigham and Women's Hospital, Boston
Health-Care Financing, *article on* Profit and Commercialism

Rhymes, Jill A.
Baylor College of Medicine
Long-Term Care, *article on* Nursing Homes

Risse, Günter B.
University of California, San Francisco
Hospital, *article on* Modern History

Robertson, John A.
University of Texas, Austin
Reproductive Technologies, *article on* Cryopreservation of Sperm, Ova, and Embryos

Robinson, Daniel N.
Georgetown University
Behaviorism, *article on* History of Behavioral Psychology

Rollin, Bernard E.
Colorado State University, Fort Collins
Animal Welfare and Rights, *article on* Animals in Agriculture and Factory Farming; Genetic Engineering, *article on* Animals and Plants

Rolston, Holmes, III
Colorado State University, Fort Collins

Animal Welfare and Rights, *article on* Wildlife Conservation and Management; Endangered Species and Biodiversity

Room, Robin
Addiction Research Foundation of Ontario, Toronto, Canada

Substance Abuse, *article on* Alcohol and Other Drugs in a Public-Health Context

Rose, Eric A.
Columbia University

Xenografts

Rosenfield, Allan
Columbia University

Abortion, *article on* Medical Perspectives

Rosser, Sue V.
University of South Carolina

Research Bias

Rotgers, Frederick
Rutgers University

Behavior Modification Therapies

Rothman, David
Columbia University

Research, Human: Historical Aspects

Rowland, Diane
Johns Hopkins University

Health-Care Financing, *article on* Medicaid

Roy, David J.
Clinical Research Institute of Montreal, Canada

Medical Ethics, History, *section on* The Americas, *article on* Canada

Ruse, Michael
University of Guelph, Ontario, Canada

Biology, Philosophy of

Sachedina, Abdulaziz
University of Virginia

Eugenics and Religious Law, *article on* Islam; Islam; Medical Ethics, History of, *section on* Near and Middle East, *article on* Iran

Sachs, Greg A.
University of Chicago

Aging and the Aged, *article on* Health-Care and Research Issues

Sagoff, Mark
University of Maryland

Environmental Policy and Law

Sari, Nil
Cerrahpasa Medical Faculty, Istanbul, Turkey

Medical Ethics, History of, *section on* Near and Middle East, *article on* Turkey

Sass, Hans-Martin
Ruhr University, Bochum, Germany

Medical Ethics, History of, *section on* Europe, *article on* Contemporary Period: German-Speaking Countries and Switzerland

Savitt, Todd L.
East Carolina University

Minorities as Research Subjects

Schaffner, Kenneth F.
George Washington University

Research Methodology, *article on* Conceptual Issues

Schmitz, Phyllis
Hospice of Washington, Washington, D.C.

Hospice and End-of-Life Care

Schöne-Seifert, Bettina
Georg-August University, Göttingen, Germany

Harm; Medical Ethics, History of, *section on* Europe, *article on* Contemporary Period: German-Speaking Countries and Switzerland; Risk

Schopp, Robert F.
University of Nebraska, Lincoln

Behavior Control

Schrag, Francis
University of Wisconsin, Madison

Children, *article on* Rights of Children

Scofield, Giles R.
Pace University, White Plains, New York

Impaired Professionals

Scudder, John R., Jr.
Lynchburg College

Nursing, Theories and Philosophy of

Seashore, Margaretta R.
Yale University

Genetic Testing and Screening, *article on* Newborn Screening

Sherman, Nancy
Georgetown University

Emotions

Tong, Rosemarie
    Davidson College
    Reproductive Technologies, *article on* Surrogacy

Toole, Michael J.
    Centers for Disease Control and Prevention, Atlanta, Georgia
    Warfare, *article on* Public Health and War

Tronto, Joan C.
    Hunter College
    Sexism

Turnbull, Sharon K.
    East Tennessee State University
    Sex Therapy and Sex Research, *articles on* Scientific and Clinical Perspectives, *and* Ethical Issues

Ubel, Peter A.
    University of Pittsburgh
    Organ and Tissue Procurement, *article on* Ethical and Legal Issues Regarding Living Donors

Unschuld, Paul U.
    Munich University, Germany
    Confucianism; Medical Ethics, History of, *section on* South and East Asia, *article on* China: Prerepublican China

Vance, Richard
    Bowman Gray School of Medicine
    Healing

Vanderpool, Harold Y.
    University of Texas, Galveston
    Death and Dying: Euthanasia and Sustaining Life, *article on* Historical Aspects

Vaux, Kenneth L.
    University of Illinois, Chicago
    Cryonics

Veatch, Robert M.
    Georgetown University
    Medical Codes and Oaths, *articles on* History, *and* Ethical Analysis; Population Policies, *section on* Strategies of Fertility Control, *article on* Incentives and Disincentives

Verbrugge, Lois M.
    University of Michigan
    Chronic Care

Verhey, Allen
    Hope College
    Protestantism

Wachbroit, Robert S.
    University of Maryland
    Genetic Engineering, *article on* Human Genetic Engineering

Wachter, Maurice A. M. de
    Institute for Bioethics, Maastricht, Netherlands
    Medical Ethics, History of, *section on* Europe, *article on* Contemporary Period: The Benelux Countries

Wadell, Paul J.
    Catholic Theological Union
    Friendship

Wadlington, Walter
    University of Virginia
    Reproductive Technologies, *article on* Artificial Insemination

Waitzkin, Howard
    North Orange County Community Clinic, Anaheim, California
    Health Policy, *article on* Politics and Health Care

Walker, Bailus, Jr.
    Howard University
    Occupational Safety and Health, *article on* Occupational Health-Care Providers

Wallace, Edwin R., IV
    Medical College of Georgia
    Mental Health, *article on* Meaning of Mental Health

Wallwork, Ernest
    Syracuse University
    Sexuality in Society, *article on* Social Control of Sexual Behavior

Walter, James J.
    Loyola University of Chicago
    Life, Quality of, *article on* Quality of Life in Clinical Decisions

Walters, LeRoy
    Georgetown University
    Fetus, *article on* Fetal Research; Gene Therapy, *article on* Ethical and Social Issues

Warren, Karen J.
    Macalester College
    Environmental Ethics, *article on* Ecofeminism

Warwick, Donald P.
    Harvard University
    Population Ethics, *section on* Elements of Population Ethics, *articles on* Definition of Population Ethics, *and* Is There a Population Problem?; *and article on* Normative Approaches; Population Policies, *section on* Donor Agencies, *article on* Fertility Control

Wasserman, David
University of Maryland
DNA Typing

Webb-Mitchell, Brett P.
Duke University
Disability, *article on* Philosophical and Theological Perspectives

Weir, Robert F.
University of Iowa
Infants, *article on* Ethical Issues

Weiss, Mitchell G.
University of Toronto, Canada
Hinduism

Wellman, Carl
Washington University
Rights, *article on* Systematic Analysis

Wenz, Peter S.
Sangamon State University
Environmental Health

Wertz, Dorothy C.
Shriver Center for Mental Retardation, Waltham, Massachusetts
Medical Genetics, *article on* Ethical and Social Issues; Reproductive Technologies, *article on* Sex Selection

Wetle, Terrie
University of Connecticut
Long-Term Care, *article on* Home Care

Wettstein, Robert M.
University of Pittsburgh
Competency

Whitbeck, Caroline
Massachusetts Institute of Technology
Biomedical Engineering; Trust

White, Amanda
Montefiore Medical Center, Bronx, New York
Fertility Control, *article on* Legal and Regulatory Issues

Whitney, Glayde
Florida State University
Genetics and Human Behavior, *article on* Scientific and Research Issues

Whorton, James C.
University of Washington
Animal Research, *article on* Historical Aspects

Wikler, Daniel
University of Wisconsin, Madison
Health Promotion and Health Education; Lifestyles and Public Health

Wildes, Kevin Wm.
Georgetown University
Health and Disease, *article on* Philosophical Perspectives; Medicine, Philosophy of

Williams, John R.
Canadian Medical Association, Ottawa, Ontario, Canada
Medical Ethics, History of, *section on* The Americas, *article on* Canada

Wilson, Ann L.
University of South Dakota
Women, *article on* Research Issues

Winslade, William J.
University of Texas, Galveston, and University of Houston
Confidentiality; Privileged Communications

Winslow, Gerald R.
Pacific Union College
Triage

Wogaman, J. Philip
Wesley Theological Seminary
Population Ethics, *section on* Religious Traditions, *article on* Protestant Perspectives

Wolf, Rosalie S.
Medical Center of Central Massachusetts, Worcester
Abuse, Interpersonal, *article on* Elder Abuse

Wolf, Susan M.
University of Minnesota
Iatrogenic Illness and Injury

Wood, Glenn
National Institute for Healthcare Research, Rockville, Maryland
Mental Health, *article on* Mental Health and Religion

Young, Allan
McGill University, Montreal, Canada
Health and Disease, *article on* Anthropological Perspectives

Special Reviewers

To assure accuracy of content, articles in this encyclopedia were subject to review not only by the editors but also by specialists in the numerous fields of learning discussed in the articles. More than 350 special reviewers were called upon to examine manuscripts for accuracy and comprehensiveness, and, on occasion, to recommend alternate authors and reviewers. These reviewers represent fields as diversified as surgery, Islamic studies, philosophy, environmental sciences, theology, psychiatry, law, public health, anthropology of medicine, geriatrics, policy studies, genetics, history, psychology, demography, health-care administration, agriculture, medical economics, medicine, nursing, and dentistry. We are indebted to the following scholars, from a number of different countries, who drew on their specialized knowledge to offer detailed assessments of this work:

George Agich
Darrel W. Amundsen
Ronald Anderson
Lori Andrews
Marcia Angell
George J. Annas
Paul S. Appelbaum
Mila A. Aroskar
John Arras
Ali Asani
Adrienne Asch
Nicholas Ashford
Samuel P. Asper
Robert Bach
Annette Baier
Osman Bakar
Robert Baker
Joanne Trautmann Banks
William J. Barber
David Barnard
Ronald Bayer
Corrine Bayley
Tom L. Beauchamp
Mark Beers

Martin Benjamin
Barbara Berkman
A. Purusholtama Bilimoria
Robert H. Binstock
J. David Bleich
Michael Bliss
Lawrence Blum
Jeffrey Blustein
Edouard Boné
Andrea L. Bonnicksen
Richard Bonnie
Larry D. Bouchard
Donna Lee Bowen
Andrew Brennan
Troyen A. Brennan
Dan W. Brock
Howard Brody
Peter G. Brown
Don S. Browning
Allen Buchanan
Rodolfo Bulatao
Chester R. Burns
Lisa Sowle Cahill
Sir Roy Calne

Alastair V. Campbell
Courtney S. Campbell
Arthur L. Caplan
Fred Carney
Kim Carney
Christine K. Cassel
Robert C. Cefalo
Gary Chiodo
Paul Chodoff
Larry R. Churchill
A. W. Clare
June Clark
Ellen Wright Clayton
K. Danner Clouser
John B. Cobb
C. Edward Coffey
Cynthia B. Cohen
Thomas Cole
Gary Comstock
Martin Cook
Rebecca Cook
Robert Mullan Cook-Deegan
Barbara B. Crane
Carl F. Cranor

Kenneth Crispell
Charles E. Curran
Robert Daly
Nancy Davis
Leonardo D. de Castro
David DeGrazia
Joe DeMarco
Prakash Desai
William Doty
Charles J. Dougherty
James F. Drane
Rebecca Dresser
Nancy Neveloff Dubler
John Duffy
Gerald Dworkin
Allen R. Dyer
David Ehrenfeld
Sherman Elias
Ezekiel Emanuel
J. Ronald Engel
Horacio Fabrega, Jr.
Ruth R. Faden
Margaret A. Farley
J. E. Ferguson, II
Gary B. Ferngren
Frederick Ferré
John Field
Caleb E. Finch
Harvey Fineberg
Joseph Fink
Norman J. Finkel
George P. Fletcher
Marsha Fowler
Daniel M. Fox
Renée C. Fox
Joel Frader
Benjamin Freedman
Sara T. Fry
Sally Gadow
Atwood D. Gaines
Fred Gifford
Norman Girardot
Mitchell Golbus
Samuel Goldstein
Gabriel Gomes
Irving Gottesman
Glenn Graber
Bradford H. Gray
Ronald M. Green
Paul J. Griffiths
Richard M. Gula
Vigen Guroian
Amy Marie Haddad
Jack Hadley
F. Terry Hambrecht

Alan Harwood
Stanley Hauerwas
Leonard Hayflick
Peter Heath
J. Bryan Hehir
Hilde Hein
Donald Hernandez
Neville Hicks
Kurt Hirschhorn
Kimberly Hoagwood
James Holstein
Kazumasa Hoshino
Edmund Howe
David Hufford
David Hull
Edward Hundert
Kathryn M. Hunter
Stephen L. Isaacs
Wes Jackson
Dale Jamieson
Bruce Jennings
Howard W. Jones, Jr.
Albert R. Jonsen
Yoshio Kawakita
Stephen R. Kellert
Seymour Kessler
Daniel J. Kevles
Edward W. Keyserlingk
Chin-Tai Kim
Jeffrey C. King
Nancy M. P. King
Michael Klare
Michael A. Kligman
Robert Kolodny
Rosalind Ladd
Thomas L. Lalley
Marc Lappé
John La Puma
Jennifer Leaning
Karen Lebacqz
Drew Leder
Susan E. Lederer
Gregory K. Lehne
Charles M. Leslie
Robert J. Levine
Harvey L. Levy
Norman B. Levy
Janet Lewis
Alan Lockwood
Erich Loewy
Robert W. Loftin
Fernando Lolas
Edward LeRoy Long, Jr.
Kenneth M. Ludmerer
George Lundberg

Joanne Lynn
Houston Macintosh
Ruth Macklin
Mary B. Mahowald
Jean-Francois Malherbe
Richard Marrs
Frank H. Marsh
Leo Marx
Luigi Mastroianni, Jr.
William E. May
William F. May
Charles R. McCarthy
Richard A. McCormick
Laurence B. McCullough
Enda McDonough
Lucy S. McGough
Ernan McMullin
Gilbert Meilaender
Curt Meine
James Melius
Paul T. Menzel
Roger Meyer
Robert Michels
Myriam Miedzian
Bruce L. Miller
Peter Miller
Richard Miller
Timothy S. Miller
Harry R. Moody
Michael S. Moore
E. Haavi Morreim
John C. Moskop
Arno G. Motulsky
Nancy Murphy
James J. Murray
Thomas H. Murray
David F. Musto
James Muyskens
Carol C. Nadelson
Ronald Y. Nakasone
Stephen Nathanson
Robert A. Neimeyer
Dorothy Nelkin
Lawrence Nelson
Linda J. Nicholson
Elena O. Nightingale
Robert Nirschl
Bryan G. Norton
David Novak
Lloyd Novick
Ron Numbers
John C. Oakley
Robert Olick
Gilbert S. Omenn
John O'Neil

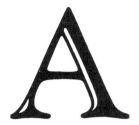

ABORTION

I. MEDICAL PERSPECTIVES

Medical information and perspectives on abortion are not just data untinged by values. Throughout history medical facts and moral values regarding abortion have been inextricably intertwined, and the current era is no exception.

People interested in the ethics of abortion turn to medicine and medical practitioners for the following sort of information and perspectives, which will be considered in this article: (1) whether medical knowledge clarifies the moral status of the fetus as a human being; (2) whether medical information on abortion confirms it to be safe for the woman; (3) what the medical perspectives are on performing early versus late abortions (and the attendant question of the fetus that survives an abortion); and (4) what the public health and international perspectives are on abortion.

Medical knowledge regarding status of the fetus

However much information biomedical investigation may provide regarding pregnancy, fetal development, and abortion, it cannot provide a determination as to when human life begins. The answer to that question—which deals with the moral status of the fetus—is arrived at by a process that entwines medical facts with experiences, values, religious and philosophical beliefs and attitudes, perceptions of meaning, and moral argument. Such a process extends beyond the special competency of medicine. For example, medicine has never had the ability to establish when ensoulment—an ancient criterion involving the "infusion" of the soul into the body of the fetus, thus conferring moral status on the fetus—occurs. Similarly, today there is disagreement among some physicians over the moral status of the fetus and the permissibility of abortion.

There is some confusion about the definition of abortion. Spontaneous abortion, or what is commonly termed a miscarriage, refers to a spontaneous loss of a pregnancy before viability (at about 25 or 26 weeks of gestation). Losses after that point in a pregnancy are termed "preterm deliveries," or, in the case of the delivery of a fetus who has already died, "stillbirths." The terminology commonly used in relation to induced abortion is different. Here, viability is not the key point. Rather, any termination of a pregnancy by medical or surgical means is termed an abortion, regardless of the stage of the pregnancy.

Safety and harm for the woman

Possible physical harm. There is a close tie between medical information on the safety of abortion practices and ethical positions on abortion. For example, at a time when abortions were frequently harmful to women—such as when legal restrictions increased recourse to untrained practitioners—opponents of abortion appealed to information on the likelihood of medical harm to the woman and risks of future pregnancies as arguments against abortion (Kunins and Rosenfield, 1991).

At the present time, induced abortions performed within the first twelve weeks of pregnancy are among the safest and simplest forms of surgery and, based on maternal mortality ratios (number of deaths per 100,000 live births), both first- and second-trimester abortion, when performed by properly trained personnel, in general are safer than carrying a pregnancy to term (Cates and Grimes, 1981). As a result, ethical arguments against abortion now tend to be restricted to areas other than maternal safety. Nonetheless, some aspects of medical safety and harm—including possible complications and psychological sequelae—continue to be important for ethical discourse, especially since a basic tenet of medical ethics is to avoid harm.

The major immediate complications of induced abortion, listed in order of frequency, are infection, hemorrhage, uterine perforation, and anesthesia-related complications. Overall complication rates for legal first-trimester abortions are less than 0.5 deaths per 100,000 abortions performed (as compared to more than four per 100,000 in the early 1970s, before the U.S. Supreme Court decision *Roe v. Wade* (1973) permitted medically supervised abortions).

Medical complications associated with induced abortion are directly related to gestational age and the type of procedure used to terminate the pregnancy. Most abortions (over 90 percent) done in the United States are performed within the first twelve weeks of pregnancy, when abortion is safest. More serious complications may occur in procedures done later in pregnancy.

Abortion procedures. Information on abortion procedures often sheds light on questions of safety as well as on other aspects of abortion that are relevant to ethics. The most common early-trimester abortion procedure (done between seven and twelve weeks gestation) is suction curettage, in which a thin plastic tube (canula) is inserted through the cervix and, by negative pressure vacuum, the contents of the uterus are aspirated. Usually, following the aspiration procedure, a curettage (using a sharp, spoon-shaped surgical instrument, a curette) is performed to ensure that all fetal tissue has been removed.

Complications of suction curettage procedures are rare, and even when they occur, are usually not serious. General anesthesia is considered by many to be an unnecessary additional risk, since local anesthesia, injected into the cervix, often is quite effective (Grimes et al., 1979). A short course of prophylactic antibiotics is sometimes prescribed, although postabortion infection is uncommon with suction curettage. Because of its safety, suction curettage is performed most often in free-standing clinics or outpatient centers in hospitals.

At twelve to twenty weeks' gestation, the most common method used for abortion is dilation and evacuation (D&E), which uses specially designed forceps in conjunction with vacuum aspiration to facilitate the removal of the uterine contents. Prior to initiating the procedure, the cervix is dilated gradually over a number of hours using spongelike materials that expand as they absorb local cervical fluids. Though still considered a minor surgical procedure, D&E is clearly more involved and invasive than suction curettage, and a trained and skilled clinician is essential. Although it is possible to use only local anesthesia for D&E, the procedure is considerably more uncomfortable than suction curettage, and general anesthesia is often used, making the procedure more risky. The D&E procedure can be performed in free-standing clinics, but often ambulatory surgical services in a hospital setting are chosen for the procedures performed later in pregnancy (after the fourteenth week) because emergency care can be quickly provided in case of a complication. Informed-consent procedures require that the various methods of abortion be discussed as well as the possible anesthesia alternatives.

The other abortion procedure used fairly commonly in the second trimester is instillation abortion, in which a solution instilled into the amniotic cavity through the abdomen via amniocentesis results in the death of the fetus and termination of the pregnancy. Uterine contractions signaling labor begin twelve to twenty-four hours later and culminate with the expulsion of the fetus. Anesthesia is not commonly used for instillation procedures. Discomfort varies widely among patients, usually in relation to the length of labor and the time before complete expulsion of the fetus and placenta. More serious complications can occur during instillation procedures, including inadvertent introduction of the solution into the mother's bloodstream, excessive bleeding at the time of expulsion of the fetus, or retention of placenta, and for this reason hospital admission is usually advised. Instillation procedures are now used mainly for procedures beyond the twentieth week of gestation. All late-pregnancy abortion procedures carry significant risk if carried out by physicians not specially trained in the technique.

A promising alternative to surgical abortion for early first-trimester terminations of pregnancy is chemical abortion. For example, the antiprogestin drug RU-486 works by blocking progesterone production by the ovaries, an essential hormone in the early stages of pregnancy and in the implantation of the embryo. The drug is given within the first forty-nine days of a confirmed pregnancy and is used in conjunction with a prostaglandin, which produces uterine contractions and subsequent expulsion of the uterine contents. A follow-up visit is necessary eight to twelve days later to ensure that complete termination of the pregnancy has occurred. Thus, in the United States—assuming that the drug will be approved by the USFDA as expected—three visits will be necessary for this medical means of pregnancy termination: the first to make the diagnosis and to give the RU-486, the second, two days later, for the prostaglandin, and the third for the final follow-up. In France, a fourth visit is required by law since a one-week delay between the diagnosis of pregnancy and the initiation of an abortion procedure is mandated.

As a result of the requirement for three visits (or four in France) and because there may be a few days before the abortion occurs and as many as ten or more days of vaginal bleeding thereafter, many women in France still prefer suction curettage as their method of choice, and this may well prove to be the case in the United States when the drug becomes available. However, there is anticipation that many women will still prefer a medical means of abortion, not wishing to undergo surgery (albeit a minor procedure) or to be subjected to the harassment that may occur outside some clinic facilities.

Successful termination has been shown to occur in 96 percent of patients, with the remaining patients requiring suction curettage for complete removal of the products of conception. For surgical procedures, less than 1 percent require a second curettage because the procedure was incomplete. In France, RU-486 is provided only through clinic facilities. One of the questions that needs to be answered in the new clinical investigation trials being undertaken in the United States is whether or not it is safe and efficient to provide RU-486 plus prostaglandin in a private doctor's office. Most women develop strong cramping after taking the prostaglandin (because the drug induces uterine contractions) and usually have the abortion within a few hours after receiving prostaglandin. In a clinic setting, this often occurs during the same four hours women remain

in the clinic after taking the prostaglandin. However, some French physicians believe that a clinic setting is not essential.

Although RU-486 has been used primarily to interrupt a pregnancy after the missed period, there are also studies assessing its effectiveness as a "morning after" pill, for use after unexpected midcycle intercourse.

Availability of abortion providers. The majority of abortion procedures in the United States are provided by obstetrician-gynecologists, with a small percentage performed by other providers such as family practice physicians, midwives, or nurse practitioners. There are serious concerns about the provision of abortion procedures in the future for several reasons. Although most obstetrician-gynecologists believe that women should have the right to choose to terminate a pregnancy, at the same time, most do not wish to perform them. As a result, approximately 80 percent of counties in the United States do not have an abortion facility. A majority of ob/gyn residency training programs do not offer abortion training routinely; rather, most provide it on an optional basis, making abortion the only gynecological surgical procedure that is considered an elective part of training. As a result, a majority of graduating residents have little or no training in this area.

Finally, even where training has taken place, the increasing incidence of harassment and even violence (including the 1993 and 1994 murders of abortion providers in Florida) has resulted in more reluctance on the part of physicians to be involved in the provision of this service. This raises serious ethical questions as to the social responsibility of professionals in this field to make certain that this procedure is available to all patients.

Possibly harmful effects on subsequent pregnancies. Questions have been raised about possible long-term harmful effects of induced abortion, especially for women who have had multiple abortions. Much of the concern centers on subsequent pregnancies, following one or more induced abortions. Medical evidence has consistently shown that a woman who has one properly performed induced abortion in the first trimester of pregnancy has the same chance of a normal outcome of a subsequent pregnancy as a woman who has never had an abortion. The evidence is less definitive for women who have had more than one induced abortion or an abortion with complications, although there is no reason to believe that additional abortion procedures, carried out by well-trained professionals, will have a long-term adverse effect. Overall, in terms of medical risk, abortion procedures, particularly those carried out in the first trimester of pregnancy, are among the safest of all surgical procedures.

Psychological effects. A much grayer area is that of the psychological consequences of induced abortion. It is difficult to generalize about the emotional responses of patients to pregnancy termination but, like physical complications, psychological complications may be related to the type of procedure and the gestational age at the time of termination, with earlier suction curettage theoretically leading to fewer psychological complications than later procedures.

However, most studies in this area suffer from methodological problems, including a lack of consensus about symptoms, inadequate study design, and lack of adequate follow-up. Furthermore, the so-called postabortion syndrome does not meet the American Psychiatric Association's definition of trauma (Gold, 1990).

Despite the many problems with most investigations, "the studies are consistent in their findings of relatively rare instance of negative responses after abortion and of decreases in psychological distress after abortion compared to before abortion" (Adler et al., 1990). Former U.S. Surgeon General C. Everett Koop, at the request of the White House, undertook a major assessment of the literature on this topic and concluded in a 1989 congressional hearing that "the data were insufficient . . . to support the premise that abortion does or does not produce a postabortion syndrome and that emotional problems resulting from abortion are minuscule from a public health perspective" (Koop, 1989a). Given Koop's personal opposition to abortion, the conclusions of his assessment are of particular importance.

Approximately 10 percent of induced abortions in the United States take place between twelve and twenty weeks of gestation, and less than 1 percent take place between twenty and twenty-four weeks. This means that more than 150,000 second-trimester procedures occur each year, a much larger number than in other developed nations where abortion is legal. Most would agree that decreases in the total numbers of abortions would be highly desirable, particularly decreases in second-trimester procedures.

The most common reasons for these later procedures, particularly among younger teens, are indecision about termination and failure to recognize (or denial of) pregnancy. A much smaller percentage of these later abortions occur because of medical or genetic reasons, which theoretically may correlate with greater psychological distress.

Choosing to terminate a pregnancy is a serious decision that is rarely made lightly. In addition to complete information about abortion procedure options, counseling should be made available to women faced with a decision about an unplanned pregnancy.

Early versus late abortions: Controversies in medicine

Medical practitioners often have more difficulty with late abortions as compared to earlier ones, both because the procedures are more difficult to perform in late abortions and because of the more advanced state of fetal development. A particularly difficult issue relates to the survival of a fetus in which instillation procedure has been the method of termination. Although this is rare, when it does occur, most physicians would take all steps to treat the surviving premature newborn. With the D&E procedure, no fetus survives, due to the destructive nature of the technique.

Medical attitudes toward abortion have constantly been shaped by the medical profession's knowledge of and attitude toward the stage of development of the fetus, interacting with local cultural, religious, and legal ideas and beliefs. Together, these factors have had a significant impact on medical practice.

Prior to the latter half of the nineteenth century, abortion was available in the United States under the doctrines of British common law that permitted termination of a pregnancy until the time of "quickening" (detection of fetal movement). However, medical knowledge available at that time made it difficult to confirm a pregnancy with certainty prior to "quickening," for it was only this detection of fetal movement that confirmed the existence of a living human fetus. There is little in the historical literature that describes how physicians in that era actually felt about abortions, although based on the information discussed below, one can assume that there were concerns about abortion.

By the second half of the nineteenth century, as scientific knowledge grew, so did the realization that fetal development occurs on a continuum, suggesting that the fetus is a living entity before fetal movement is felt. Prompted by this new medical knowledge, physicians, particularly those who were members of the newly formed American Medical Association (AMA), began openly to oppose abortion and urged its criminalization as an immoral practice. As a basis for this change, the Hippocratic Oath was used to oppose abortion at any time during pregnancy.

The concept of the fetus as a human entity separate from the mother has long been the subject of ethical concern within the medical profession. The AMA's *Principles of Medical Ethics* permit physicians to perform abortions, provided they are done in accordance both with the law and with "good medical practice" (Council on Ethical and Judicial Affairs, 1994, Opinion 2.01). In general, for the last 100 years or more, and especially since the 1973 U.S. Supreme Court decision in *Roe* v. *Wade* greatly liberalized the legal permissibility of abortion, medical practitioners have tended to place the value of the life of the mother above that of the fetus and there has been general agreement that abortion is permissible in those cases where the health of the mother is seriously compromised by a pregnancy.

However, just as *Roe* v. *Wade* allowed for some restrictions on abortions in the second trimester, so the medical profession has shown a reluctance to perform abortions later in pregnancy. In addition to new ethical dilemmas over fetal and maternal rights, many medical professionals remain ambivalent about the morality of abortion, a conflict that is heightened by increased technological sophistication in the field of perinatology and genetics.

Depending on the technology available to a physician and the condition of the individual fetus (gestational age and any developmental deformity), it is now routinely possible to save the lives of premature babies born at thirty weeks gestation. Babies born at twenty-six to twenty-seven weeks and earlier have survived with intensive neonatal intervention and support, though often with some degree of functional impairment. With abortions occasionally performed up to twenty-five or twenty-six weeks gestation, one can see the conflict within medicine: Fetuses that might be aborted by one group of physicians are aggressively supported as patients by another group.

Physicians who provide abortion services prefer to do early abortions, that is, up to twelve weeks, for several reasons. First, it is generally agreed that, though a fetus may exhibit primitive reflexes before twenty weeks gestation, there is no evidence that the brain and neurological system are developed enough even at twenty-four weeks for the fetus to experience pain. Second, as discussed earlier, second-trimester techniques that might appear to be more humane or to show more respect for the fetus, generally entail more danger for the woman. Third, the physicians who are committed to offering abortion procedures are intent on offering the safest procedures for the woman and regard the benefit to the woman as superseding the goal of minimalization of harm to the fetus.

Most abortion practitioners do not perform abortions past twenty-four weeks, and even then, usually only when the fetus has a condition incompatible with life outside the uterus. Extremely few U.S. practitioners will perform elective late abortions (beyond twenty-four weeks). Antiabortion activists often single out these atypical practitioners for their demonstrations.

With early abortion methods, such as dilation and curettage (D&C) or suction curettage, the fetus is destroyed. In instillation abortion procedures, where the viability of the fetus may be an issue, the fetus occasionally survives an abortion; and the further question sometimes arises in bioethics of whether the abortion technique chosen should be that which maximizes the possibility of fetal survival. Again, techniques that could possibly terminate a pregnancy without causing fetal death are more risky for the woman; in fact, in very late abortions the appropriate procedure for the woman may require inducing fetal death prior to delivery. Because of the medical commitment to benefit the mother, and since most physicians who have a high level of respect for the life and survival of the fetus do not engage in the practice of abortion, very few fetuses are aborted alive. It is assumed that abortion will always entail the death of the fetus: The goal of that medical practice is deliberately to accomplish the death of the fetus while terminating the pregnancy. However, most institutions require that fetuses surviving the procedure be provided with immediate neonatal care.

Public-health and international perspectives

Abortion is widely available with varying restrictions throughout the industrialized world. In recent years, there also has been a trend toward liberalization of abortion laws in many developing countries, such as in India, where abortion has been legalized; and in Bangladesh, where an early first-trimester procedure called menstrual regulation (which is really an early suction curettage) has been officially sanctioned by the government even though abortion per se has not been legalized. Abortion laws are most restrictive in Latin America, sub-Saharan Africa, and Central Asia.

Many of these countries have high rates of maternal mortality, and complications of illegal abortions are one of its leading causes. According to the World Health Organization, as many as 100,000 or more maternal deaths occur each year as a result of complications of an unsafe, usually illegal abortion attempt. Even in the United States, some illegal abortions continue to be performed in cases where women are without the resources to obtain a legal abortion. Although reliable incidence data are lacking as to the number of illegal abortions performed worldwide, there clearly is a strong demand for abortion, a demand that will probably always exist. As evidenced by the estimated number of women who undergo illegal abortion attempts, most women who are so determined to terminate a pregnancy will attempt to do so either by themselves or with assistance.

Consequently, the public-health concerns about the complications of unsafe abortion attempts, coupled with the complex issues relating to the reproductive and autonomy rights of women versus the rights of the fetus, suggest the continuing importance that must be given by the field of bioethics to abortion, particularly to the question of whether abortion should be made available equally to all persons requesting it regardless of national citizenship, ethnic or racial identity, or economic status.

ALLAN ROSENFIELD
SARA IDEN

Directly related to this article are the other articles in this entry: CONTEMPORARY ETHICAL PERSPECTIVES, LEGAL AND REGULATORY ISSUES, JEWISH PERSPECTIVES, ROMAN CATHOLIC PERSPECTIVES, PROTESTANT PERSPECTIVES, *and* ISLAMIC PERSPECTIVES. *For a further discussion of top-*

ics mentioned in this article, see the entries ADOLESCENTS; AUTONOMY; FETUS, *especially the article on* PHILOSOPHICAL AND ETHICAL ISSUES, HARM; INFORMED CONSENT; LAW AND BIOETHICS; MATERNAL–FETAL RELATIONSHIP; MEDICAL ETHICS, HISTORY OF, *section on* SOUTH AND EAST ASIA, *article on* INDIA; PUBLIC HEALTH; PUBLIC POLICY AND BIOETHICS; RIGHTS; VALUE AND VALUATION; *and* WOMEN, *article on* HEALTH-CARE ISSUES. *For a discussion of related ideas, see the entries* CONFLICT OF INTEREST; DOUBLE EFFECT; HEALTH-CARE RESOURCES, ALLOCATION OF; HEALTH POLICY; *and* ROMAN CATHOLICISM.

Bibliography

ADLER, NANCY E.; DAVID, HENRY P.; MAJOR, BRENDA N.; ROTH, SUSAN H.; RUSSO, NANCY F.; and WYATT, GAIL E. 1990. "Psychological Responses After Abortion." *Science* 248:41–44.

BERGER, GARY S.; BRENNAR, WILLIAM E.; and KEITH, LOUIS G., eds. 1981. *Second Trimester Abortion.* Littleton, Mass.: PSG.

CATES, WILLARD, JR., and GRIMES, DAVID A. 1981. "Morbidity and Mortality of Abortion in the United States." In *Abortion and Sterilization: Medical and Social Aspects,* pp. 155–180. Edited by Jane E. Hodgson. London: Academic Press.

CORSON, STEPHEN L.; SEDLACEK, THOMAS V.; and HOFFMAN, JEROME J. 1986. "Suction Dilation and Evacuation." In their *Greenhill's Surgical Gynecology.* 5th ed., pp. 350–353. Edited by Richard H. Lampert. Chicago: Year Book Medical.

COUNCIL ON ETHICAL AND JUDICIAL AFFAIRS. AMERICAN MEDICAL ASSOCIATION. 1994. *Code of Medical Ethics: Current Opinions with Annotations: Including the Principles of the Medical Ethics, Fundamental Elements of the Patient-Physician Relationship, and Rules of the Council on Ethical and Judicial Affairs.* Chicago: Author.

GOLD, RACHEL BENSON. 1990. *Abortion and Women's Health: A Turning Point for America?* New York: Alan Guttmacher Institute.

GRIMES, DAVID A. 1992. "Surgical Management of Abortion." In *Te Linde's Operative Gynecology,* 8th ed., pp. 317–339. Edited by John D. Thompson and John A. Rock. Philadelphia: J. B. Lippincott.

GRIMES, DAVID A.; SCHULTZ, KENNETH F.; CATES, WILLARD, JR.; and TYLER, CARL W., JR. 1979. "Local Versus General Anesthesia: Which Is Safer for Performing Suction Curettage Abortions?" *American Journal of Obstetrics and Gynecology* 135, no. 8:1030–1035.

HENSHAW, STANLEY K. 1990. "Induced Abortion: A World Review, 1990." *Family Planning Perspectives* 22, no. 2: 76–89.

KOOP, C. EVERETT. 1989a. *Hearings before the Human Resources and Intergovernmental Relations Subcommittee of the Committee on Governmental Operations, House of Representatives.* 101st Congress, 1st session.

——. 1989b. *Medical and Psychological Effects of Abortion on Women.* Washington, D.C.: U.S. Department of Health and Human Services.

KUNINS, HILLARY, and ROSENFIELD, ALLAN. 1991. "Abortion: A Legal and Public Health Perspective." *Annual Review of Public Health* 12:361–382.

Roe v. Wade. 1973. 410 U.S. 113.

II. CONTEMPORARY ETHICAL AND LEGAL ASPECTS

A. CONTEMPORARY ETHICAL PERSPECTIVES

There is probably no issue in bioethics more controversial and more difficult to resolve than that of abortion. There are several reasons for this, reasons that are more political than they are matters of ethical principle. The first is that unlike many ethical issues in biology and medicine, the abortion debate is not limited to scholars and practitioners but has engulfed the entire society in the United States. Candidates for public office feel compelled to take a stand on abortion. In the legal and regulatory sphere, there is constant activity in state and federal courts, in bills introduced into legislatures, and in regulations promulgated by the Department of Health and Human Services and other government agencies.

A second reason for the intractability of the abortion issue is that at the extremes, both proponents and opponents of the right to abortion hold views more akin to ideologies than to rationally held positions. Opponents at one extreme defend an absolute prohibition of abortion, while proponents at the opposite extreme support the absolute right of women to procure an abortion on demand. The rhetoric used by both sides reveals the ideological character of the debate. Spokespersons for opponents of abortion adopted for their side the label "pro-life," thereby implying that anyone willing to allow abortion is "anti-life." Supporters of the right of women to have an abortion, for their part, selected a label that reflects the cherished American value of freedom to choose, calling themselves "pro-choice." The ideological battle lines of the controversy are thus drawn, with one side charging the other with being against life in slogans that proclaim "Abortion is murder," and the other side contending that foes of abortion are against free choice and the right of women to control their own bodies. When ethical positions assume the characteristics of an ideology, rational argument is no longer possible. The fundamental stakes in this debate are revealed by the use of rights language by the opposing factions: "right to life" and "right to choose."

A third reason for the impossibility of reaching agreement about the ethics of abortion stems from roots of the pro-life position in religious beliefs. Although opponents of abortion do not always identify the religious underpinnings of their views, a demographic analysis links the antiabortion movement with particular religions and denominations, chiefly Roman Catholicism and fundamentalist Protestantism. It is also true, however, that many people on the pro-choice side are deeply religious, believing in the sacredness of life and humanity created in the image of God, for example. If it is impossible to argue about the rightness or wrongness of fundamental religious convictions, so too will it be impossible to mount a rational argument about an ethical position that is deeply rooted in a religious worldview. Dogmatic adherence to an ideology, whether religious or secular, tends to make people unwilling to argue rationally in defense of their positions.

Between these extremes, however, is a range of moderate positions on the morality of abortion. These positions acknowledge that abortion is ethically problematic yet can be justified. Scientific advances in prenatal diagnosis now make it possible to detect numerous abnormalities in utero. All but the extreme pro-life faction agree that abortion is ethically justifiable in cases of serious, uncorrectable disorders detected by amniocentesis, chorionic villus sampling, sonography, and other diagnostic techniques. Less agreement exists regarding minor abnormalities or cases in which the genetic disease is eventually lethal but the affected individual could live for many years. However, profound disagreement surrounds the practice of prenatal diagnosis followed by abortion for the purpose of selecting the sex of the child. Advances in knowledge of human genetics continue to increase the number and kinds of different genetic abnormalities that can be detected in utero, giving rise to worries that the sheer number of abortions will multiply as more and more information becomes available.

The contemporary controversy surrounding abortion focuses on three central ethical issues: the moral standing of embryonic and fetal life, the conflict of "rights" between the pregnant woman and her fetus, and whether the harmful consequences for women likely to result from restricting their right to an abortion outweigh the negative consequences of terminating fetal life.

Somewhat less prominent in the overall debate, but related to those major issues, is a question of social justice. Ample evidence exists to show that restrictive policies on abortion adversely affect more minority-group and poor women than white middle-class or wealthy women. The most prominent disagreements in the abortion controversy focus on the rights of the individual woman and the permissible role of government in restricting those rights. Nevertheless, questions of social justice are also ethical concerns, whether they involve women's access to information about abortion services,

access to the services themselves, or government funding for abortions for poor women.

Personhood and the abortion debate

The question of the "personhood" of the fetus is one of the central questions in the abortion controversy (Garfield and Hennessy, 1984). However, one feminist line of thought contends that too much emphasis has been placed on that question, to the detriment of concerns about women, including their physical and mental health and their prospects for social equality and independence (Sherwin, 1992). The latter approach affirms the capacity of women for moral agency and thus places little emphasis on the search for objective criteria for defining when personhood begins.

At the most fundamental level, the personhood question is whether an entity resulting from fertilization of a human egg by human sperm can properly be said to have rights—in particular, a right to life—at any point during the nine-month gestational period. This question gives rise to the related yet different question: "What is a person?" or "When does personhood begin?" The two questions are joined because of the underlying premise that persons are legitimate bearers of rights. Therefore, it is argued, if an embryo or fetus can be termed a person, it can be said to have rights. However, the problem of arriving at a consensus on criteria for personhood has proved as difficult as resolving the abortion issue itself.

That difficulty was acknowledged by the U.S. Supreme Court in its landmark decision in 1973 in the case of *Roe v. Wade*. The Court decided that a fetus is not a person for the purposes of the Fourteenth Amendment to the Constitution, but declined to embark on the task of defining "personhood": "We need not resolve the difficult question of when life begins. When those trained in the respective disciplines of medicine, philosophy, and theology are unable to arrive at any consensus, the judiciary, at this point in the development of man's knowledge, is not in a position to speculate as to the answer." The fundamental disagreement on which the abortion controversy rests concerns the point at which human life acquires moral standing, a point typically characterized as the beginning of personhood.

The answers offered at opposite poles of this debate are that personhood begins at conception, and so a very early embryo has rights, and that personhood begins at the moment of birth or later, thus disqualifying all prenatal life from the category of personhood. Philosophers, theologians, and others who contribute to the literature on this topic hold as many different views about when personhood begins as they do on the topics of fetal rights and the right of women to have an abortion. Even if everyone agrees that rights can properly be ascribed only to persons, that agreement would not settle the abortion debate because of sharp disagreements over the proper criteria for personhood.

The difficulty of reaching agreement on a set of defining criteria for personhood stems from the value-laden quality of the concept of personhood, no matter which definition is adopted. For example, one position holds that at no stage of development does the fetus meet criteria of personhood. The philosopher Mary Anne Warren proposes a set of criteria for personhood so rigorous that even a newborn infant might not fulfill them. For ease of reference, we may call this a "strict" standard of personhood. The following traits, Warren argues, are those "most central to the concept of personhood, or humanity in the moral sense" (Warren, 1978, p. 224):

1. Consciousness (of objects and events external or internal to the being) and in particular the capacity to feel pain.
2. Reasoning (the developed capacity to solve new and relatively complex problems).
3. Self-motivated activity (activity that is relatively independent of either genetic or direct external control).
4. The capacity to communicate, by whatever means, messages of an indefinite variety of types—that is, not just with an indefinite number of possible contents but on many indefinite, possible topics.
5. The presence of self-concepts and self-awareness, individual or racial or both.

At the opposite end of the spectrum are criteria for personhood that are easy to fulfill. Again, for ease of reference, let us term this a "lenient" standard of personhood. This position is also value-laden, resting on a traditional set of religious values. John T. Noonan, arguing that personhood begins at conception, identifies this as "the Christian position as it originated" (Noonan, 1983, p. 304). Noonan contends that this position does not depend on a narrow theological or philosophical concept, although many Christian theologians and historians disagree with his contention. Noonan's criterion for personhood is "simple and all-embracing: if you are conceived by human parents, you are human" (Noonan, 1983, p. 304). Although Noonan refers to "humanity" rather than to "personhood," it is clear that he takes these two concepts to be equivalent, since the moral question related to when a being is human is "When is it lawful to kill?" Noonan and others, such as the Protestant theologian Paul Ramsey (1975), have thus adopted a very lenient standard of personhood, which they further buttress with modern scientific findings. Conception is the "decisive moment of humanization" because that is when the new being receives the genetic code; "a being with a human genetic code is man" (Noonan, 1983, p. 307).

Between these two extremes lies a range of other criteria for personhood, some of which are matters of traditional belief while others have been introduced more recently as a result of scientific developments. An example of the former is "quickening," the time at which a pregnant woman first feels fetal movement. Another example is "animation"; Thomas Aquinas and early Christian authors talked about "ensoulment," the time at which the embryo or fetus becomes infused with a soul.

An example of a criterion that relies on modern scientific knowledge is the presence of electroencephalographic (brainwave) activity. This criterion, defended by the philosopher Baruch Brody (1978), has the feature of symmetry, as it can be used to determine the beginning as well as the end of "human life." One interpretation of this criterion holds that the onset of encephalographic activity is the time when the fetus becomes a person (about six weeks' gestational age), just as the cessation of brainwave activity serves as a determination of death, even if other vital functions are sustained by artificial life supports. However, this interpretation has been contested in another account of the significance of brainwave activity. Nancy Felipe Russo asks, "Why can't we agree on access to abortion before the developing human becomes 'brain alive'?" Yet she contends that "being able to produce a squiggle is not [the same as] having a human brain wave. Cortical functioning that is comparable to human brain waves doesn't happen until much later. There is debate on when—connections to the cortex are established certainly before thirty weeks, but also certainly after twenty weeks" (Russo, 1992, p. 21).

Viability—the capability of surviving outside the womb with or without artificial support—is one other point between conception and birth that many people hold to be the time at which the fetus acquires moral standing. Although the U.S. Supreme Court declined to define "personhood," the importance accorded to "viability" in *Roe v. Wade* (1973) appears to have underwritten the position that the fetus becomes a person at the point of viability. Yet it is important to recall that the Supreme Court's decision did not prohibit abortion, the termination of fetal life, after viability. Instead, the Court used viability as a place to draw a line beyond which the state may interfere with a woman's "right to privacy":

With respect to the State's important and legitimate interest in potential life, the "compelling" point is at viability. This is so because the fetus then presumably has the capability of meaningful life outside the mother's womb. . . . If the State is interested in protecting fetal life after viability, it may go so far as to proscribe abortion during that period, except when it is necessary to preserve the life or health of the mother.

The tendency to confuse ethics and law is found in the abortion controversy, as in other bioethical debates. The ethics of abortion, including attempts to specify when a fetus acquires personhood, must be kept distinct from Supreme Court rulings and other legal developments. After a period of increasing liberalization of abortion laws in the United States, the 1980s and early 1990s saw a tightening of restrictions. Nevertheless, despite wide variations in state laws regulating abortion, fetal viability remains the point where many people draw a moral line. Beyond that point, the fetus is thought to be a person or—what amounts to the same thing in these ethical arguments—acquires rights. Even outside the abortion context, arguments that pit maternal rights against fetal rights invoke viability: for example, the issue of whether a pregnant woman has the right to refuse a medical procedure. Medical professionals frequently argue that before viability, they are obligated to accept a pregnant woman's refusal of treatment but that once the fetus becomes viable, their obligation shifts to the second "patient" and requires them to act to preserve fetal life or health. Thus the concept of fetal viability, used in a 1973 Supreme Court decision to mark the point at which the state acquires an interest in potential life, has been elevated to a criterion for according moral standing to the fetus.

One approach to the personhood of prenatal life has been termed the "developmental" view. This approach denies that there is a single point or a sharp line that distinguishes personhood from an intrauterine existence that lacks moral standing. Lisa Sowle Cahill contends that "an individual member of the species does not self-evidently have exactly the same status morally and therefore in terms of 'rights' that other members at other stages may have." Cahill finds a developmental view of fetal status most convincing and states that "even at conception the fetus has very considerable value, simply because of its human identity and immense potentiality." The difficulty for Cahill is "how to assign an amount or degree of value, whether at the beginning or at a later point" (Cahill, 1992, p. 24). Although the developmental view is likely to be appealing to many people, its shortcoming lies in the difficulty, if not impossibility, of translating it into public policy.

A final strategy for defining "personhood" makes use of the potentiality principle. It is simply the *potential for* developing into an adult human being that confers on a fertilized ovum the moral status of a full-fledged adult. This strategy thus takes the moment of conception as marking the beginning of personhood. John T. Noonan (1983) embraces this argument explicitly, while Michael

Tooley, Baruch Brody, and Mary Anne Warren argue directly against it. Judith Jarvis Thomson does not offer an argument against using the potentiality principle but observes that similar things might be said about the development of an acorn into an oak tree: ". . . it does not follow that acorns are oak trees, or that we had better say they are. . . . A newly fertilized ovum, a newly implanted clump of cells, is no more a person than an acorn is an oak tree" (Thomson, 1978, p. 199).

The wide range of criteria proposed for defining "personhood" should serve to demonstrate the impossibility of using this strategy to resolve the abortion controversy. Proponents of choice advocate freedom and equality for women and propose a strict definition of "personhood," thereby giving women a wide moral latitude for terminating pregnancy. Opponents of abortion tend to favor sex-appropriate social roles and an idealized, traditional family, and adopt a lenient definition that identifies a woman as a "mother" immediately after fertilization. The futility of trying to resolve the abortion controversy by appealing to the concept of a person can best be shown by noting that proponents of both extreme standards believe that agreement about personhood is crucial for settling the abortion issue. Warren and Tooley propose criteria for personhood that a newborn infant cannot meet, while Noonan adopts a criterion that a newly fertilized ovum can meet. The questionable utility of defining "personhood" is further demonstrated by Thomson's argument that abortion may be morally justified even if it is acknowledged that the fetus is a person from the moment of conception. The reason the task of trying to arrive at objective criteria for personhood is bound to fail is that the values people already hold about abortion are imported into the debate over when personhood begins.

Nor is any progress made toward a resolution when analogies are used to buttress a right-to-life argument. Arguments from analogy are often flawed, and the following example is a case in point. Some foes of abortion argue that refusal to recognize the rights of embryos or fetuses has historical analogues in refusal to recognize the rights of blacks who were enslaved or Jews who were killed in the Holocaust. One Roman Catholic theologian, Richard John Neuhaus, uses this analogy when he asks: "*If* one believes that 20 million abortions are equivalent to 20 million instances of the taking of innocent human life, does not the analogy with the Holocaust become more appropriate? Perhaps even inevitable?" (Neuhaus, 1992, p. 222).

Neuhaus does believe that abortion is the taking of innocent human life, so for him the analogy is apt. As he notes, however, supporters of the right to abortion are "understandably outraged" when those abortions are compared with the Holocaust. No one who does not already subscribe to the view that embryos and fetuses have rights will be convinced by an argument from analogy citing the doctrine of the Third Reich that Jews, gypsies, homosexuals, Slavs, and others were not human beings in the full meaning of the term. By using this analogy, Neuhaus attempts to show that like those people then, fetuses today are not included in the community of legal rights, protections, and entitlements.

In spite of all the difficulties with these arguments and analogies, appeals to the personhood of the fetus are unlikely to disappear from the abortion debate. This is because the contention that the fetus is a person is the basis for ascribing rights, including the right to life.

Rights and the abortion controversy

Ascribing rights to the fetus poses two profound problems: first, whether the fetus is a type of entity to which rights can properly be assigned and, second, how to resolve conflicts of rights assigned to the fetus with those ascribed to the pregnant woman.

The initially promising path of trying to ascertain whether a fetus is a person and therefore possesses rights is evidently of little use. It is no less controversial to bypass the intermediate step of defining "personhood" and go directly to ascribing rights to an embryo or fetus. The position that human life acquires moral standing from the moment of conception is an article of religious faith for some people and an absurd proposition for others. The latter group finds it impossible to construct a rational defense of the assertion that a cluster of cells attached to the lining of the womb should be granted the rights normally accorded living children and adult human beings. Yet despite the lack of any similarity between the properties of a conceptus and those of a woman, man, or child, opponents of abortion contend that human life deserves protection from the moment of conception.

In the abortion debate, the rights of the fetus are typically pitted against the rights of the pregnant woman. In the political debate carried on first in the United States and later in other countries, feminists adopted the phrase "a woman's right to control her own body," identifying a right that could presumably override the right to life of the fetus. "The right to control one's own body" is a way of specifying the right to self-determination.

In the international sphere, the basic right to control reproduction has been ascribed both to couples and to individuals. In 1974 in Bucharest, a fundamental right was agreed upon as part of the World Population Plan of Action. Representatives of 136 governments stated that "all couples and individuals have the basic right to decide freely and responsibly the number and spacing of their children and to have the information,

education, and means to do so" (United Nations, 1975). In order for this potential right to become an actual right, individuals, groups, and governments would have to refrain from interfering with the freedom of women or couples to make and carry out family-planning decisions, including the decision to have an abortion. Despite the efforts of some religious and political groups in various countries to curtail this basic right, it has been reaffirmed by statements such as the Convention on the Elimination of All Forms of Discrimination Against Women (U.N. General Assembly, 1980).

The underlying basis for this reproductive right is the right to liberty. The principle of liberty dictates that individuals have a right to freedom of decision and action, to the extent that their actions do not interfere with the rights of others. Opponents in the abortion controversy do not disagree on the soundness of that fundamental ethical principle itself, yet they disagree profoundly over its application: Foes of abortion claim that the act of terminating a pregnancy does interfere with the rights of another (the fetus), while advocates of a woman's right to procure an abortion deny that killing a fetus is a violation of rights.

As is true of any conflict of rights, this one might be resolved in favor of either party—the woman or the fetus. If a right to life is ascribed to fetuses and a right to terminate a pregnancy is assigned to women, a higher priority could be given to the rights of the woman. However, as important as the value of liberty is in Western philosophical and political thought, only rarely is it held to outweigh the value of human life when the two values conflict. Therefore, the most reasonable way to resolve this apparent conflict of rights in favor of the woman is to deny that the fetus can properly be considered an entity having rights.

Still, an argument in support of assigning the right to choice a higher priority than the right to life has been put forward. Thomson constructs an argument using a fanciful analogy that has become well known among readers of the abortion literature. She posits that you awake one morning to find yourself hooked up to the body of a famous violinist, who needs the help of your kidneys to sustain his own life for a period of nine months. After that, the violinist will have recovered. The violinist is a person, and so he has a right to life. Your life is not endangered, but your freedom to move about for nine months is drastically inhibited. The analogy invites us to consider the violinist as an analogue to a fetus, and you and your kidneys as analogous to a pregnant woman and her life supports for the fetus. If your right to liberty—that is, to disconnect yourself from the violinist—overrides his right to life, the argument goes, should it not follow that a woman's right to terminate her pregnancy overrides the fetus's right to life? That conclusion rests on an appeal to the intuition that no one should have to remain involuntarily hooked up to another person, even to sustain that person's life (Thomson, 1978).

Thomson's philosophical imagination notwithstanding, the soundness of her analogy has been rejected by both opponents and proponents of the right to abortion. Arguing in general against the use of artificial cases in the abortion debate, Noonan decries this one in particular, claiming that "the similitude to pregnancy is grotesque" (Noonan, 1978, p. 210). Taking the opposite side from Noonan in the abortion debate, Warren criticizes Thomson's analogy on the grounds that it is too weak to do the work required for defending women's right to abortion: "The Thomson analogy can provide a clear and persuasive defense of an abortion only with respect to those cases in which the woman is in no way responsible for her pregnancy, e.g., where it is due to rape" (Warren, 1978, p. 221). The trouble with philosophical arguments that rely on the use of analogies is that they stand or fall with the strength of the analogy.

Liberal feminists like Warren rest their defense of a right to abortion on the premise that the fetus is not a person and therefore lacks a right to life. In contrast, a more radical line of feminist thought defends the moral rightness of abortion itself. Catharine MacKinnon contends that "the abortion choice should be available and must be *women's*, but not because the fetus is not a form of life. In the usual argument, the abortion decision is made contingent on whether the fetus is a form of life. I cannot follow that. Why should not women make life or death decisions?" (MacKinnon, 1984, p. 46). The matter of women's moral agency is the central issue in this defense of women's right to choose.

This line of feminist analysis emphasizes the interests and experiences of women. Susan Sherwin identifies as the central moral feature of pregnancy the fact that it takes place in women's bodies and has profound effects on women's lives: "Unlike nonfeminist accounts, feminist ethics demands that the effects of abortion policies on the oppression of women be of principal consideration in our ethical evaluation" (Sherwin, 1992, pp. 104–105). This feminist approach seeks to avoid an exclusive focus on rights and other "masculinist conceptions of freedom (such as privacy, individual choice, and individuals' property rights with respect to their own bodies)" (Sherwin, 1992, p. 100).

There is another, quite different problem underlying the abortion debate framed as a conflict of rights between the pregnant woman and the fetus. This is a moral inconsistency, which only a few pro-life advocates acknowledge to be a problem. Many opponents of abortion, holding that a right to life outweighs a right to choose, are nonetheless prepared to grant exceptions in the case of pregnancies resulting from rape and incest. Why should such exceptions be permitted? If the fetus has a genuine right to life in virtue of the type of entity it is, why should the circumstances that led to its existence alter that right? A thoroughly consistent opposition to abortion that rests on the right to life of the fetus would not grant the priority of the right of the woman to choose simply because the pregnancy occurred as the result of rape or incest.

This conclusion becomes evident when we reflect on what is ethically permissible in the case of individuals whose right to life is unquestioned and undisputed. If it were discovered that the mother of a five-year-old child, or even a one-year-old infant, had borne the child as the result of rape or incest, that would not grant the woman (or anyone else) moral license to kill the child. The fact that in such cases the child is no longer in the womb should make no moral difference if a fetal right to life is the basic premise of the antiabortion position. Right-to-life advocates Jack and Barbara Willke state their disagreement with those who "would return the violence of killing an innocent baby for the violence of rape" (Willke and Willke, 1988, p. 151) and ask, regarding the case of incest: "Isn't it a Twisted Logic that would Kill an Innocent Unborn Baby for the Crime of his Father?" (Willke and Willke, 155).

Opponents of abortion who are prepared to grant exceptions to the priority of the right to life of fetuses in the case of rape and incest must account for an apparent moral inconsistency. Either they must explain why a fetus that results from rape or incest has a lower moral status or less of a right to life than other fetuses or they must adopt the more restrictive but consistent position that all fetuses have a right to life, regardless of the way they came into being. Those who ascribe an absolute value to fetal life cannot consistently allow exceptions in the case of rape or incest. More moderate opponents of abortion are not inconsistent in allowing such exceptions, but they must then provide a cogent account of their basis for holding that abortion is morally wrong.

Consequentialist arguments

Both in the bioethics literature and in the political arena, the abortion debate in the United States has been carried out almost exclusively in the language of rights. Yet consequentialist ethical arguments, those that appeal to the good and bad results of actions or social practices, provide an alternative mode of ethical analysis. The long history of women's deaths and diseases from self-induced abortions, along with data about the persistence of morbidity and mortality resulting from clandestine abortions, documents the harmful consequences of antiabortion policies. These consequences affect not only women but also the children they bear and the entire society in countries where population growth strains monetary and natural resources. Thus the negative consequences of restricting access to safe abortions are a compelling factor to consider in an ethical assessment.

Since safe, legal abortions have been available to most women in the United States at least since 1973, and in some states even before *Roe v. Wade* (1973), the consequences of a prohibitionist or highly restrictive policy on abortion as a contemporary issue can best be evaluated by looking at less developed countries. An estimated 200,000 or more Third World women die every year as a result of botched abortions (Germain, 1989). In Bangladesh alone, reports indicate that at least 7,800 women die each year due to abortion complications (Kabir, 1989). In most African countries, where safe abortion either is not available or is legally restricted, illegal abortion is the only solution for women with unwanted pregnancies. Complications of these abortions include hemorrhage, infection, abdominal perforations, and secondary infertility (Mashalaba, 1989). Infertility itself produces catastrophic consequences in Africa, and is almost always blamed on the woman, especially in rural areas (Mashalaba, 1989). Similar reports from Latin American countries document that most abortions are performed in sordid and clandestine conditions and that physicians use medicines such as hormone shots to induce menses, or unsafe curettage that can be harmful to women's health (Toro, 1989).

The negative consequences of enforcing restrictive policies on abortion are not limited to risks to the lives and health of women but extend also to the children they bear. Close spacing of children produces more high-risk pregnancies, premature births, and low-birth-weight infants. The very large number of "street children" (millions in Brazil alone) is a clear testimony to another dramatic consequence of unwanted pregnancies (Pinotti and Faúndes, 1989). Reports from developed as well as less developed countries and assessments by experts in the field of reproductive health throughout the world leave no room for doubt that women will continue to seek to end unwanted pregnancies regardless of legal or religious prohibitions.

It is instructive to compare the consequences for women's lives and health in countries that have changed their abortion laws in the past few decades. Legalization of abortion has tended to reduce maternal mortality, while making laws more restrictive has had the opposite effect. For example, in Czechoslovakia abortion laws were made less restrictive during the 1950s, and abortion-related mortality fell by 56 percent and 38 percent in the periods 1953–1957 and 1958–1962, respectively. In contrast, in Romania a restrictive abortion law was enacted in 1966, resulting in a sevenfold increase in deaths from abortion. The abortion mortality per million women aged 15 to 44 rose from 14.3 in 1965 to 97.5 in 1978 (Hagenfeldt, 1989).

Compared with the rights-based framework in which the debate is typically cast in the United States, the discussion in many nations is carried on in terms of the consequences of permitting or prohibiting abortion. This point was emphasized by Fred T. Sai, an African scholar who is one of the leading world authorities on reproductive health, and Karen Newman, working at International Planned Parenthood Federation in London:

> The ethical arguments about abortion are complex, although often presented simplistically. Often debated is a woman's "right" to control over her body and to refuse to carry to term a pregnancy she does not want. However, not often considered is the ethics of withholding the benefits of a technology which is less hazardous than carrying a pregnancy to term. Nineteenth-century anti-abortion laws were generally designed to save women from the dangerous, and often experimental, surgical procedures of the time. However, this reason is no longer valid, and today the effect of applying anti-abortion laws is to increase rather than reduce risk to women's lives and health. (Sai and Newman, 1989, p. 162)

Even in places where abortion is a legally available option, antiabortion feelings and behavior can violate the rights and harm the interests of women. Both within and outside the United States, some women who seek abortions are denied information about their options, while others who succeed in procuring abortions are treated punitively by physicians or other health-care workers. Whether the punitive behavior consists of failure to give adequate pain medication, delaying treatment, or simply being rude, women still suffer indignities despite the availability of safe, legal abortions.

Consequences of the medical method of abortion. Until the late 1980s, the only available methods for performing abortions were surgical, requiring instruments to remove the products of conception from the uterus. The development of a medical abortifacient, antiprogestin drugs (for example, the French "abortion pill," RU-486), accompanied by the hormone prostaglandin, has stimulated some new features in the debate. Although a careful analysis reveals that, for the most part, the ethical issues are not new or different, the politics of abortion has led to suggestions that antiprogestins bear ethical hazards of a novel sort.

A central ethical issue regarding the introduction of any new technology is the assessment of its risks and benefits. It is important not to overstate the comparative benefits of this medical method over the traditional surgical alternatives. On the one hand, unlike vacuum aspiration or curettage, RU-486 does not involve insertion of instruments into the uterus and thus poses no risk of accidental perforation and infection from unclean instruments. It does not require the same degree of technical skill as the surgical techniques used to terminate pregnancy, so in this respect a medical method of abortion poses less risk to women than existing alternatives. On the other hand, RU-486 requires a follow-up visit to the clinic forty-eight hours later for administration of prostaglandin. Failure to follow the antiprogestin with prostaglandin could lead to greater risks than surgical methods; women may suffer the complications of incomplete abortion and lack proper medical supervision.

In making comparative risk–benefit assessments, it is important to use appropriate data for the locale in which the technology is to be used, since data about risks and benefits gathered about women in developed countries may not be strictly applicable to women in less developed countries. Other local or regional differences can also affect the risk–benefit ratios. Consider two examples.

First, in a society that has an adequate number of properly trained health-care workers, the risks of septic abortion and other complications of termination of pregnancy are much lower than they are in countries with too few or inadequately trained workers. Second, in regions where adequate follow-up is difficult to attain, a method like RU-486, which requires a second visit to the clinic at a prescribed interval, may well have lower safety and efficacy than elsewhere.

Risk–benefit assessments have a built-in relativity. Depending on the characteristics of the providers, the nature of the service delivery systems, and the demographic and cultural features of a country or region, the benefit–risk ratio of a particular method of abortion may vary. The risks include not only the medical and psychological risks of the method itself but also the risk of not having safe, effective, or otherwise acceptable methods available, including backup services to offer surgical abortion in case the medical method fails.

One feature of antiprogestins does raise a novel ethical issue. Antiprogestins work by preventing implantation of the fertilized ovum. Étienne-Émile Baulieu, the French scientist responsible for the research leading to development of RU-486, has proposed the term "contragestion" (a contraction of "contra-gestation") to emphasize that it falls somewhere between contraception and abortion (Baulieu, 1989). Construed as a "contragestive," RU-486 might thus be acceptable to some opponents of abortion who object to termination of pregnancy.

Women who have religious reasons for avoiding or restricting termination of pregnancy can use RU-486 after fertilization has occurred but before implantation of the embryo. At that point, the woman is arguably not yet pregnant. Once the embryo is implanted in a woman's uterus, she is pregnant and removal of the embryo terminates that pregnancy. However, there is debate over whether a woman whose egg has been fertilized should be considered pregnant in the brief time before implantation. Based on current medical knowledge, it is widely held that conception is a process that properly includes both fertilization and implantation (Baulieu, 1989).

The plausibility of this view is heightened by experience following the introduction of in vitro fertilization (IVF). A woman's egg can be fertilized in a dish, but she is not pregnant until the "preembryo" (before implantation) becomes attached to her uterus. Evidence that it is pregnancy, not fertilization, that matters to some from a moral point of view comes from Mexico and other Latin American countries, where physicians are opposed to abortion but not to disposing of ova fertilized by means of IVF.

Consequences of nonsurgical abortion methods. The prospect that this method could become widely available has influenced the political debate surrounding abortion. Opponents of abortion have expressed two worries: that a medical method will make abortion too easy to procure (Cook, 1991; Grimes, 1991) and psychologically easier for women to choose to have them (Callahan, 1991). Both worries stem from the concern that introduction of antiprogestins will lead to the performance of more abortions. Like any argument that rests on probable consequences, this one must be subjected to empirical scrutiny.

One question is whether nonsurgical abortions are "easier" for women to undergo than surgical ones; a second, quite different question is whether less discomfort from the procedure is likely to induce more women to procure abortions. With regard to the empirical likelihood that introduction of medical methods will lead to an increase in the number of abortions, there seems to be no factual basis. As one international authority on abortion observes:

> There is no evidence that access to non-surgical abortion encourages abortions that would not otherwise occur, or leads to an increase in abortions. . . . Indeed, the Netherlands, with publicly funded abortion services widely available, has the lowest abortion rate in the industrialized world. That's because the Dutch also have access to sex education and information as well as contraceptive and voluntary sterilization services. (Cook, 1991, p. B7)

Evidence from one set of clinical trials indicates that women who used RU-486 found it "far less violent" than surgical methods they had previously undergone (Grimes, 1991). Although this psychological evidence clearly counts as a benefit of RU-486 over other methods, opponents of abortion have argued that pain and suffering are just deserts for women who choose to have abortions. Underlying this view is the moral judgment that women are guilty because it is their sexual behavior that results in unwanted pregnancies. Those who argue that it is a good thing when a method of abortion has punishing consequences object to RU-486, among other reasons, on grounds that the consequences are less punitive for women than those of other methods.

This argument against RU-486 distorts the well-established means of calculating the risks and benefits of medical procedures. That there are fewer side effects, normally judged to be advantageous in the usual assessment of risks versus benefits, is taken here to be a *disadvantage*. There is no reasonable reply to an argument that construes increased pain and suffering resulting from a medical intervention as a benefit to the patient rather than a harm. In making risk–benefit calculations, taking pain and suffering to be a benefit rather than a harm is a perverse weighing of consequences.

In addition to "more readily procurable," "easier" can also mean "psychologically more acceptable." One opponent of abortion refers to the "moral ambiguity" of RU-486, arguing that this medical method makes it psychologically easier for women to choose abortion. "This ambiguity is present if the woman taking a 'morning-after pill' or a pill like RU-486 that produces an 'overdue period' is not sure whether she is aborting a fertilized embryo" (Callahan, 1991, p. B7). The possibility that this "ambiguity" may make it emotionally easier for some women to choose abortion does not count as a moral advantage of RU-486 for foes of abortion, despite the evident benefits to women of decreased psychological stress. This is because they believe that "taking a human life that has already begun" is morally unacceptable (Callahan, 1991, p. B7). Inability to agree on that fundamental premise—the moral status of a fertilized ovum—is what prevents any compromise in the intractable abortion debate, regardless of the method of pregnancy termination. It also leads to a perverse transformation of what are normally counted as risks into benefits, and to the reverse.

A similar twist has occurred with respect to the value of privacy, a key ingredient in the abortion debate. As a drug that can be prescribed by physicians and taken by women in the doctor's office or even in their own homes, RU-486 clearly offers the opportunity for greater privacy and more control by women than methods that require a visit to a clinic. It has been surmised that if abortions with RU-486 become widely available in physicians' offices, "opponents of abortion might lose their targets for picketing, harassment, and violence. For example, since 1977, 110 abortion clinics have been burned or bombed in this country" (Grimes, 1991, p. B5). If the resulting decreased incidence of disruption and violence is viewed as a *disadvantage* of a medical method of abortion, that is another irrational weighing

of harms and benefits. In any rational calculation of harms and benefits, lowering the potential loss of lives, dignity, or property can only reasonably be viewed as a benefit.

Abortion and the issue of justice

A principle of social justice holds that all persons within a given society deserve equal access to goods and services that fulfill basic human needs. A country might have liberal laws pertaining to abortion services, such as those in developed countries that permit women to procure an abortion up to the time of fetal viability. But if a government does not provide financial assistance to poor women who seek abortions, those women are denied equal access to a procedure that is available to financially better-off women. In that situation, a legally guaranteed right to abortion services will be a right in name only. Many rights presuppose the existence of corresponding obligations on the part of persons, agencies, or governments to act in ways that enable those rights to be realized. In the delivery of health care generally, the principle of justice is violated when health services are available only to those with the ability to pay. Feminists emphasize the broader issues of the accessibility and delivery of abortion services in their ethical analysis of abortion (Sherwin, 1992).

Equally problematic from the standpoint of justice are proposals that would deny government-sponsored assistance to family-planning clinics providing information to clients about abortion. If some women are denied access to information about the availability of abortions and the means to procure them, they will lack access to services that are available to women who are better educated or financially better off. The same conclusion holds for population assistance programs that cross national boundaries. For wealthier donor nations to restrict or deny funds to recipient countries that provide abortion services as a component of their family-planning programs is to violate this principle of justice.

The principle of justice mandates that all individuals who need them should have equitable access to health services, including the means to procure an abortion. "Equitable access" means that use of these services should not be based on an ability to pay for them. And a precondition for access is information about the existence and nature of the services. To fulfill the requirements of justice, it is necessary to have the widest possible distribution of reproductive health services, ensuring equitable access for everyone.

These conclusions apply both to developed and to less developed countries. Poor women disproportionately bear the burden of restrictive abortion laws and inadequate or nonexistent public services. Describing the situation in Africa, Sai and Newman identify a form of injustice that exists worldwide: "Wealthy women, who can afford private doctors or travel to countries where abortion is legal and safe, can get abortions almost free of risk; but poor women often pay for abortions with their health, their future fertility and possibly their lives" (Sai and Newman, 1989, p. 162).

Whether motivated by political or religious concerns, opponents of abortion erect obstacles that are difficult for providers of abortion services, as well as for women seeking those services, to surmount. An example is the problem women may face in obtaining abortions even in countries with liberal abortion laws. In the United States, a strong, vocal minority not only maintains an opposition to abortion for members of its own religious communities but also seeks to change existing laws to prohibit abortions altogether. These groups disrupt political speeches and heckle candidates for elected office. In the extreme, some antiabortion groups resort to violence, bombing abortion clinics and using physical force to prevent women from entering physicians' offices.

In developed as well as in less developed countries, the tactics used by extreme opponents of abortion have a disproportionate impact on poor women, compounding the existing injustice of the gap between rich and poor. In some countries with liberal abortion laws, lack of medical personnel and facilities or the behavior of physicians and hospital administrators have the effect of curtailing access to abortion services, especially for economically or socially deprived women. Examples include parts of Austria, France, India, Italy, and the United States (Tietze and Henshaw, 1986). This serves as a reminder that the mere existence of laws on the books is not sufficient to ensure ethically just practices.

Is abortion an insoluble moral problem?

It is reasonable to wonder whether abortion poses an insoluble moral problem. As a political issue in a pluralistic society, abortion does appear to be unresolvable. Political compromise, the usual mode of settling disagreements in a pluralistic society, is not a satisfactory method for resolving deep moral controversy. Those who believe that a fetus is truly a person, with a right to life equivalent to that of a child or an adult, cannot permit some abortions, under some circumstances, without compromising their moral integrity. Similarly, those who argue that a woman has moral standing at least equal to that of a fetus, and who affirm that women's full moral agency grants them the right to terminate an unwanted pregnancy, see no reason to compromise that principle.

As a matter of individual moral choice, however, the question of whether to have an abortion is taken seriously and has been decided by millions of women.

Some women choose to abort only fetuses discovered by prenatal diagnosis to be abnormal. Other women decide to seek an abortion following failed contraception, after determining that they cannot, for financial or emotional reasons, have more children. Within marriage, that choice is typically made by the couple, not by the woman alone. Couples who choose abortion for the purpose of selecting the sex of their child are reflective about their decision but are nonetheless criticized by those who find their reason frivolous or otherwise morally unacceptable.

Few people have argued that abortion poses no moral issues whatsoever. However, even if it is acknowledged that a morally preferable alternative would be to prevent a large number of abortions from taking place, there will always be unwanted pregnancies, and women in those circumstances will risk their lives and their health, if necessary, to have an abortion. It is evident that neither the U.S. Supreme Court's 1973 abortion ruling that granted women constitutional protection nor subsequent laws and judicial decisions that have increasingly eroded that protection have silenced the ethical and political debate surrounding abortion. According to one contemporary line of thought, as long as the moral status of the embryo and fetus cannot be resolved, the abortion debate will not be laid to rest. And according to a feminist critique, as long as oppression of women is ignored or tolerated, abortion will remain one among many social problems whose resolution can be achieved only by increasing the power of women and freeing them from domination based on their sex.

RUTH MACKLIN

Directly related to this article is the companion article, CONTEMPORARY ETHICAL AND LEGAL ASPECTS: B. LEGAL AND REGULATORY ISSUES, *and the other sections in this entry:* MEDICAL PERSPECTIVES, *and* RELIGIOUS TRADITIONS, *articles on* JEWISH PERSPECTIVES, ROMAN CATHOLIC PERSPECTIVES, PROTESTANT PERSPECTIVES, *and* ISLAMIC PERSPECTIVES. *Also directly related is the entry* FERTILITY CONTROL. *For a further discussion of topics mentioned in this article, see the entries* ETHICS, *especially the articles on* TASK OF ETHICS, *and* RELIGION AND MORALITY; FEMINISM; FETUS; JUSTICE; LIFE; MATERNAL–FETAL RELATIONSHIP; PERSON; RIGHTS; SEXISM; UTILITY; *and* WOMEN, *article on* HEALTH-CARE ISSUES. *For a discussion of related ideas, see the entries* AUTONOMY; METAPHOR AND ANALOGY; RISK; *and* VALUE AND VALUATION. *Other relevant material may be found under the entries* ADOPTION; CONFLICT OF INTEREST; ECONOMIC CONCEPTS IN HEALTH CARE; FAMILY; PROFESSIONAL–PATIENT RELATIONSHIP; REPRODUCTIVE TECHNOLOGIES; *and* WOMEN, *article on* HISTORICAL AND CROSS-CULTURAL PERSPECTIVES.

Bibliography

BAULIEU, ÉTIENNE-ÉMILE. 1989. "RU-486 as an Antiprogesterone Steroid: From Receptor to Contragestation and Beyond." *Journal of the American Medical Association* 262, no. 13:1808–1814.

BRODY, BARUCH A. 1978. "On the Humanity of the Foetus." In *Contemporary Issues in Bioethics*, pp. 229–240. Edited by Tom L. Beauchamp and LeRoy Walters. Encino, Calif.: Dickenson.

CAHILL, LISA SOWLE. 1992. "Defining Personhood: A Dialogue." *Conscience* 13 (Spring):19–28.

CALLAHAN, SIDNEY. 1991. "The First Stage of Life *Is* Life." *Los Angeles Times*, June 19, p. B7.

COOK, REBECCA. 1991. "Is a Flat Ban Ethical?" *Los Angeles Times*, June 18, p. B7.

GARFIELD, JAY L., and HENNESSEY, PATRICIA, eds. 1984. *Abortion: Moral and Legal Perspectives*. Amherst: University of Massachusetts Press.

GERMAIN, ADRIENNE. 1989. "The Christopher Tietze International Symposium: An Overview." *International Journal of Gynecology and Obstetrics* 30 (suppl. 3):1–8.

GRIMES, DAVID. 1991. "RU-486: Politics and Science Collide." *Los Angeles Times*, June 17, p. B5.

HAGENFELDT, KERSTIN. 1989. "Ethics and Human Values in Family Planning: European and North American Perspectives." In *Ethics and Human Values in Family Planning: Conference Highlights, Papers, and Discussion: XXII CIOMS Conference, Bangkok, Thailand, 19–24 June 1988*, pp. 184–207. Edited by Z. Bankowski, José Barzelatto, and Alexander M. Capron. Geneva: Council for International Organizations of Medical Sciences.

KABIR, SANDRA M. 1989. "Causes and Consequences of Unwanted Pregnancy from Asian Women's Perspectives." *International Journal of Gynecology and Obstetrics* 130 (suppl. 3):9–14.

MACKINNON, CATHARINE. 1984. "*Roe v. Wade*: A Study in Male Ideology." In *Abortion: Moral and Legal Perspectives*, pp. 45–54. Edited by Jay L. Garfield and Patricia Hennessey. Amherst: University of Massachusetts Press.

MACKLIN, RUTH. 1983. "Personhood in the Bioethics Literature." *Milbank Memorial Fund Quarterly/Health and Society* 61, no. 1:35–57.

MASHALABA, NOLWANDLE NOZIPO. 1989. "Commentary on the Causes and Consequences of Unwanted Pregnancy from an African Perspective." *International Journal of Gynecology and Obstetrics* 30 (suppl. 3):15–19.

NEUHAUS, RICHARD JOHN. 1992. "The Way They Were, the Way We Are." In *When Medicine Went Mad: Bioethics and the Holocaust*, pp. 211–230. Edited by Arthur L. Caplan. Totowa, N.J.: Humana.

NOONAN, JOHN T., JR. 1978. "How to Argue About Abortion." In *Contemporary Issues in Bioethics*, pp. 210–217. Edited by Tom L. Beauchamp and LeRoy Walters. Encino, Calif.: Dickenson.

———. 1983. "An Almost Absolute Value in History." In *Moral Problems in Medicine*. 2d ed., pp. 303–308. Edited by Samuel Gorovitz, Ruth Macklin, Andrew L. Jameton, John M. O'Connor, and Susan Sherwin. Englewood Cliffs, N.J.: Prentice-Hall.

PALCA, JOSEPH. 1989. "The Pill of Choice?" *Science* 245, no. 4924:1319–1323.

PINOTTI, JOSÉ ARISTODEMO, and FAÚNDES, ANIBAL. 1989. "Unwanted Pregnancy: Challenges for Health Policy." *International Journal of Gynecology and Obstetrics* 30 (suppl. 3):97–102.

RAMSEY, PAUL. 1975. "The Morality of Abortion." In *Moral Problems: A Collection of Philosophical Essays*. 2d ed., pp. 37–58. Edited by James Rachels. New York: Harper & Row.

Roe v. Wade. 1973. 410 U.S. 113, 159.

RUSSO, NANCY FELIPE. 1992. "Defining Personhood: A Dialogue." *Conscience* 13 (Spring): 19–28.

SAI, FRED T., and NEWMAN, KAREN. 1989. "Ethics and Human Values in Family Planning: Africa Regional Perspective." In *Ethics and Human Values in Family Planning: Conference Highlights, Papers, and Discussion: XXII CIOMS Conference, Bangkok, Thailand, 19–24 June 1988*, pp. 143–166. Edited by Z. Bankowski, José Barzelatto, and Alexander M. Capron. Geneva: Council for International Organizations of Medical Sciences.

SHERWIN, SUSAN. 1992. *No Longer Patient: Feminist Ethics and Health Care*. Philadelphia: Temple University Press.

THOMSON, JUDITH JARVIS. 1978. "A Defense of Abortion." In *Contemporary Issues in Bioethics*, pp. 199–209. Edited by Tom L. Beauchamp and LeRoy Walters. Encino, Calif.: Dickenson.

TIETZE, CHRISTOPHER, and HENSHAW, STANLEY K. 1986. "Abortion Laws and Policies." In their *Induced Abortion: A World Review*, 6th ed., pp. 11–28. New York: Alan Guttmacher Institute.

TOOLEY, MICHAEL. 1983. "Abortion and Infanticide." In *Moral Problems in Medicine*, 2d ed., pp. 308–323. Edited by Samuel Gorovitz, Ruth Macklin, Andrew L. Jameton, John M. O'Connor, and Susan Sherwin. Englewood Cliffs, N.J.: Prentice-Hall.

TORO, OLGA LUCIA. 1989. "Commentary on Women-Centered Reproductive Health Services." *International Journal of Gynecology and Obstetrics* 30 (suppl. 3):119–123.

UNITED NATIONS. 1975. "World Population Plan of Action." In vol. 1 of *The Population Debate: Dimensions and Perspectives: Papers of the World Population Conference, Bucharest, 1974*, pp. 155–167. New York: Author.

———. GENERAL ASSEMBLY. 1980. *Resolution Adopted by the General Assembly on the Report of the Third Committee (A/34/830 and A/34/L.61): Convention on the Elimination of All Forms of Discrimination Against Women*. A/RES/34/18D.

WARREN, MARY ANNE. 1978. "On the Moral and Legal Status of Abortion." In *Contemporary Issues in Bioethics*, pp. 217–228. Edited by Tom L. Beauchamp and LeRoy Walters. Encino, Calif.: Dickenson.

WILLKE, JACK C. and WILLKE, BARBARA. 1988. *Abortion: Questions & Answers*. Rev. ed. Cincinnati, Ohio: Hayes.

B. LEGAL AND REGULATORY ISSUES

Most contemporary legal systems regulate the practice of abortion (Petersen, 1993; Sachdev, 1988; Glendon,

1987). Governments around the world legislate whether, when, why, and how the estimated 40 million abortions that occur each year may or must occur. In some countries, such as Belgium and Denmark, abortion is governed primarily by national laws; in others, such as Australia, abortion is governed mainly by state or regional laws. The belief that abortion is unsafe, irreligious, immoral, unjust, or genocidal has tended to push regulation in the direction of laws that expressly prohibit some or all abortions. The conviction that abortion can alleviate overpopulation, avert economic hardship, protect women's health, promote sex equality, or eliminate undesirable progeny has tended to produce laws that permit, guarantee, or even compel abortion.

An international survey of existing law reveals four basic patterns or "models" of express abortion regulation: (1) a model of prohibition; (2) a model of permission; (3) a model of prescription; and (4) a model of privacy. Under the model of prohibition, the laws of a jurisdiction punish most abortions as criminal offenses, as in Ireland. Under the model of permission, laws permit abortions that meet more or less stringent criteria established by government and designated third-party decision makers, as in Germany. Under the model of prescription, laws specifically require or encourage the termination of pregnancies falling into certain specific categories, as in China. Finally, under the model of privacy, laws restrain government from enactments that criminalize or severely restrict medically safe abortions, as in the United States under *Roe* v. *Wade* (1973). The model of privacy treats abortion decisions as substantially a matter of private choices rather than public law.

As with law developed in response to other practices, abortion law is subject to change from one era to the next. Countries under the sway of the model of prohibition in one generation have moved toward the model of privacy in subsequent generations. For example, when the Supreme Court of the United States declared in *Roe* v. *Wade* that the nation's constitution bars statutes categorically criminalizing all abortions, it announced a national standard for state and federal law that ushered out the model of prohibition and ushered in the model of privacy.

Yet, beginning in 1989, a number of Supreme Court rulings critical of *Roe* v. *Wade* moved the United States away from the model of privacy toward a model of permission. Public-opinion surveys conducted between 1987 and 1991 show that a "majority of Americans . . . approved limited legal access to abortion" (Cook et al., 1992). Some polls indicate an overwhelming approval rate for abortion privacy among highly educated and affluent women (Sachdev, 1988), and among African-American, Asian-American, and Native American women (National Council of Negro Women, 1991). A national poll conducted in 1994 by Barna Research

Groups showed that 78 percent of the adults surveyed approved the legalization of some (49%) or all (29%) abortions. An even higher approval rate was obtained in a 1994 survey conducted by Yankelovich Partners, Inc. In this survey 85 percent said a woman should be able to obtain an abortion no matter what the reason (46%) or in certain circumstances (39%). A CBS News/New York Times poll conducted in 1994 found that 77 percent of those surveyed favored "generally available" abortion (40%) or abortion with "stricter limits" (37%); only 21 percent said abortion "should not be permitted." Despite widespread public support for keeping some abortions legal, organized opponents of abortion rights continue to pressure lawmakers to reinstate blanket prohibitions.

The model of prohibition

The model of prohibition governs official abortion policy in many African, Latin American, and Islamic countries, including Bangladesh, Indonesia, and Nigeria (Sachdev, 1988). Chile, in South America, and Sri Lanka, in southern Asia, permit abortion only to save the life of the woman. Most jurisdictions in Europe and North America reject the model of prohibition; they permit abortion, if only where pregnancy results from rape or incest or where the continuation of pregnancy threatens the health of the woman (Petersen, 1993; Glendon, 1987).

Ireland, a largely Roman Catholic nation, is one of the few Western countries—Belgium and Malta are two others—whose laws continued beyond the 1970s to criminalize abortions either absolutely or subject to a strictly limited number of exceptions (Solomons, 1992). Under a 1983 amendment to the Irish constitution, Irish law permits abortion only to save the life of the woman. Overturning a ruling that a teenage rape victim who credibly threatened suicide could not travel to England for an abortion, the Irish Supreme Court found in 1992 that abortion would be permissible "if it is established as a matter of probability that there is a real and substantial risk to the life as distinct from the health of the mother, which can only be avoided by the termination of her pregnancy."

Jurisdictions whose laws reflect the model of prohibition often assert a strong religious or humanitarian policy interest in protecting what are thought to be the rights and interests of unborn children. However, other objectives have also prompted strict abortion prohibition. For example, during the nineteenth and twentieth centuries, abortion opponents in the United States have cited the need to protect pregnant women from medical and psychological risks of abortion. There can be no doubt that unskilled, unsanitary abortion procedures are a health risk, and that some women who obtain abortion experience medical complications and emotional anguish. However, some lawyers and judges doubt that medical abortion performed during the first three months of pregnancy is less safe than pregnancy and childbirth (Tribe, 1990; Rhode, 1989). They similarly doubt that elective medical abortion poses a serious risk of psychological harm. Although one writer has concluded that "psychological problems occur in the lives of almost all aborted women" (Reardon, 1987), a report of the American Psychological Association concludes that "severe emotional reactions" rarely follow abortion, even in the case of minors (Melton and Pliner, 1986).

Countries whose populations have been ravaged by war and genocide have sometimes proscribed abortion in an effort to increase the birth rate. Strict abortion prohibition has had the additional, if only implicit, goal of reinforcing social roles. The cultural assumption that motherhood is the appropriate social role for women buttressed Joseph Stalin's 1936 abortion prohibitions enacted to furnish the former Soviet Union with "a new group of heros" (Sachdev, 1988). The belief that bearing children is women's natural destiny may lead some to assume that birth control and abortion are both immoral and unhealthful. After 1933, Adolf Hitler prohibited contraception and declared abortion a capital offense on the belief that birth control was unhealthful. On the other hand, abortion prohibitions adopted in Germany in 1943 aimed at the "vitality of the German people" and excluded from criminality abortions performed on "racially" undesirable women (Sachdev, 1988).

The reach of laws prohibiting abortion can be broad. Obtaining an abortion has been subject to criminal penalty in some instances, and so too has distributing abortion information. Provisions of the famous Comstock Law enacted by the Congress of the United States in 1873 and later rescinded, outlawed abortion-related implements and information as "obscene" and "immoral" (Garrow, 1994; Rhode, 1989). Offenders of the Comstock Law faced imprisonment with hard labor and monetary fines. Jurisdictions prohibiting abortion generally aim at the conduct of third-party abortion providers. However, some abortion statutes also criminalize pregnant women's own conduct, making it a punishable offense to obtain or seek abortions from third parties. Legal systems rarely punish medical abortion as the full equivalent of felonious unjustified murder.

Criminalizing self-induced abortion poses special problems of detection and law enforcement. Self-induced abortion has often involved risky procedures, such as inserting knitting needles, wire coat hangers, or other foreign objects through the cervix. Many self-induced abortions are detected because they end tragically in medical and police emergencies. In 1989, a health-care group in California promulgated a videotape demonstrating "menstrual extraction," a nonmedical abortion

technique trainers say women can learn to perform safely at home with the help of a friend. To the extent that they are workable, abortion procedures that can be performed without medical assistance fall beyond the practical reach of law.

Prohibitive abortion law requires lawmakers to define what counts as abortion, and therefore what is subject to criminal penalties. The surgical and medical procedures generally in use by physicians in licensed hospitals and clinics in Europe and the United States plainly qualify as abortion. However, certain forms of birth control not viewed as abortion could conceivably fall under the scope of strict abortion prohibitions. Popularly viewed as a form of contraception, the intrauterine device (IUD) may function as a kind of abortifacient, blocking implantation of a fertilized egg, rather than preventing ovulation or fertilization. Étienne-Émile Baulieu's drug, RU-486, named for its French manufacturer, Roussel Uclaf, poses a related difficulty of definition. Described by French Minister of Health Claude Levin as "the moral property of women, not just the property of the drug company," RU-486 arrived on the European scene in the 1980s. Unlike pharmaceutical contraceptives that prevent fertilization or ovulation, RU-486 acts to block the successful implantation of a fertilized egg. Rejecting the popular "abortion pill" label, Baulieu has suggested that RU-486 is neither contraception nor abortion but something new—"contragestation." Still, it seems unlikely that a jurisdiction that strictly prohibits abortion would view "contragestation" as anything other than early abortion.

In South Africa, Latin America, the Caribbean, and Korea, abortion flourishes under regimes of prohibitive abortion law because the laws are not aggressively enforced (Sachdev, 1988). The criminal code of Bangladesh strictly prohibits most abortions; but physicians commonly induce abortion by performing a uterine evacuation procedure known as "menstrual regulation" on women who are many weeks pregnant. Prohibitive abortion laws commonly fall short of their stated goals and public expectations because governments are unwilling or unable to enforce the letter of the law. The prohibitive laws that governed abortion in the United States prior to *Roe* v. *Wade* were enacted to preserve unborn life and women's physical and mental health (Garrow, 1994). It has been argued that the aim of fetal preservation was at least partly undermined by the large number of clandestine abortions performed notwithstanding prohibitive laws (Tribe, 1990). Although most abortions were illegal in much of the United States prior to 1973, American women obtained an estimated 200,000 to 1,200,000 abortions each year in the 1960s and early 1970s (Tietze et al., 1988), compared to about 1,500,000 each year throughout the 1980s and early 1990s. David Reardon (1987) puts the number of abortions pre-*Roe* at merely 100,000 to 200,000 per year. The aim of preserving women's health may have been frustrated under the regime of prohibition because clandestine abortions were commonplace but were not always performed by skilled practitioners in hygienic settings. This was especially true of the illegal abortions obtained by African-American women, who accounted for a disproportionate number of the victims of illegal procedures. (Twenty percent of the deaths related to pregnancy and childbirth in the United States in 1965 were attributed to illegal abortions.) Legalization of abortion probably resulted in a small-to-moderate increase in the number of abortions, but it appears to have greatly decreased the incidence of abortion-related infertility and death.

Model of permission

The model of permission became the pervasive one around the world in the final quarter of the twentieth century. Under the model of permission, abortion is legally available, but only with the approval of government officials or officially designated decision makers, such as administrative boards, committees, physicians, or judges. In some permission-model jurisdictions, officials grant permission pro forma in nearly every case. In Norway, prior to 1975 reforms that liberalized abortion, as many as 94 percent of the requests for abortions made to Abortion Boards were routinely granted (Olsnes, 1993). Official decision makers in permissive jurisdictions rely upon a handful of factors to determine which abortions to permit and which abortions to prohibit (Petersen, 1993; Sachdev, 1988; Glendon, 1987).

The stage of pregnancy is very frequently a factor. Officials called upon to implement legal norms or exercise discretion often permit "early" abortions and prohibit "late" ones. This no doubt helps to explain the statistic that 90 percent of reported abortions take place within the first three months of pregnancy. Another factor decision makers commonly consider is the woman's medical or social status. Restrictive laws require that officials deny permission to abort for reasons other than medical hardship. Liberal laws often require that officials allow abortions because pregnancy or childbirth would involve social or economic hardship for the woman. In many jurisdictions grounds for social hardship include rape, incest, or the age and marital status of the woman. The health or condition of the fetus can be a third factor in permitting or prohibiting abortion. The law may premise access to abortion on evidence that a child would be born with serious physical or mental abnormalities. With advances in prenatal testing that enable detection of the sex of a fetus, it is now possible for a pregnant woman to abort selectively unwanted male or female offspring. In some instances, abortion for sex se-

lection may be tied to a desire to avoid giving birth to a child with a gender-related genetic disease. However, abortion for sex selection per se is presumably, if not explicitly, illegal in all models of permission jurisdictions. In principle, model of privacy jurisdictions permit early abortion for any reason, including sex selection. The U.S. Supreme Court has not specifically determined whether states must permit abortion for purposes of sex selection.

For some portion of the twentieth century, a number of countries have governed abortion under highly bureaucratic versions of the model of permission (Sachdev, 1988). For a time in the eastern European countries of Hungary, Romania, Poland, and Bulgaria, abortion was lawful only if approved by a state board or committee. These countries reportedly permitted abortion in almost every case through the fourth month of pregnancy. Romania reverted to a prohibitive policy in 1966 in response to concerns about underpopulation and the health effects of multiple abortions. It prohibited most contraception and abortion for women who did not have at least four, and eventually five, children. Abortion prohibition was accompanied by a significant incidence of mortality related to illegal abortion. In the mid-1980s, 86 percent of the women in Romania who died as a consequence of pregnancy or childbirth died as a result of illegal abortions, compared with, for example, 29 percent in the former Soviet Union and 13 percent in Sri Lanka.

Other historical instances of the bureaucratic model of permission are the laws and administrative regulations in force in Denmark from 1939 to 1973, and in Sweden from 1939 to 1974. In Denmark, local and national committees consisting of teams of social workers, physicians, and psychiatrists evaluated the applications of women seeking legal abortions. Scandinavian officials on boards or committees charged with decision making typically assessed the impact of childbirth and child care on the mental or physical health of the woman, and the woman's living conditions. Israeli Ministry of Health regulations enacted in 1978 permitted hospitals and clinics to form committees consisting of two physicians and a social worker for deciding whether to grant women's abortion requests. Although living conditions, such as other children and economic hardship, were initially an authorized basis for granting abortion requests, Israel amended the law in 1980 under pressure from religious groups and in response to concerns about a declining population rate.

Today, a number of countries in Asia, South America, Europe, and North America make a woman's obtaining an abortion dependent upon the approval of one or more physicians, a judge, or one or both parents. Great Britain and countries whose abortion law was modeled on Great Britain's—Hong Kong, Zambia, and

Australia—are examples of countries whose laws place decision making in the hands of physicians. The law of Great Britain was transformed over a great many centuries from a law of prohibition, to a law of permission, and even privacy. Early English common law embodied the model of prohibition, at least for abortions taking place after the first few months of pregnancy. The common law proscribed abortion after "quickening," about the fourth month of pregnancy, when fetal "animation" or "ensoulment" was deemed to have taken place. In 1861 the statutory abortion law of Great Britain defined as a felony any act intended to cause abortion, whether induced by the woman herself, if she were pregnant, or by others, whether or not she was in fact pregnant. The Abortion Act of 1967 abolished the nineteenth-century felony. The act's liberal provisions permit an abortion where any two medical practitioners certify in good faith that pregnancy "would involve risk to the life of the pregnant woman, or of injury to the physical or mental health of the pregnant woman or any existing children of her family, greater than if the pregnancy were terminated." Under this rule, qualifying for abortion poses no practical difficulty for women with the money to pay private physicians. As English law illustrates, the model of permission can have the distinct effect of empowering the medical and psychiatric professions to govern reproduction in accordance with their profession's internal standards of judgment.

In the Australian states (Petersen, 1993), abortions are permitted under common law or criminal codes if one or two physicians believe in good faith that it is necessary to save the life of the woman or to protect her mental or physical health. In New South Wales, social and economic conditions are deemed relevant to the assessment of impact on a woman's health. In South Australia and the Northern Territory, abortion is also lawful where there is a risk of a seriously disabled child. In India, the Medical Termination Pregnancy law enacted in 1971 permits abortions that one or, if the woman is more than twelve weeks pregnant, two physicians certify. Grounds for certification are liberal. Abortion may be obtained to preclude a risk to the pregnant woman's mental or physical health, or a risk of the birth of a child with serious mental or physical abnormalities. No abortions after twenty weeks are legal under the law. A woman's mental health is considered at risk in cases of economic hardship and where pregnancy resulted from failed contraception. The 1975 Abortion and Sterilization Act made many abortions lawful in the Republic of South Africa, on the certification of two physicians that statutory requirements are met. The law requires that where abortion is sought on grounds of risk to mental health, one of two certifying physicians be a psychiatrist willing to attest to danger of permanent mental harm.

In contrast to South African, Indian, Australian, English, and most western European law, French law permits women to make their own judgments (early in pregnancy) about whether they are entitled to abortion on grounds of hardship. In this respect, French law resembles the federal law of the United States under *Roe v. Wade*. French regulations enacted in 1975 are representative of international responses to the judicial transformation of United States law with *Roe v. Wade* in 1973. Reflecting the aspirations of both the model of permission and the model of privacy, the French enactment begins with a declaration that the law guarantees respect for every human being from the beginning of life, and that this principle is to be sacrificed only in case of necessity and according to specific conditions. But the law authorizes any woman who is ten weeks pregnant or less to request a physician for an abortion if she believes pregnancy or childbirth will create hardship. Moreover, at any stage of pregnancy, right up to the moment of birth, abortion is lawful if two physicians, one of them from an official list, certify that continuation of pregnancy would put the woman's health gravely in peril, or that there is a strong possibility that the child would suffer from an incurable condition.

The French abortion law imposes numerous conditions on all abortions. Attending physicians must inform women of the medical risks of abortion and give them an official guide to the forms of assistance available to families, mothers, and children, and to relevant social service organizations. Women must then consult one of the listed social services. Women wishing to proceed with abortion must confirm their request in writing, after a one-week waiting period. Abortions must be performed by physicians in a public or recognized private hospital and must be reported to the regional health authorities. Hospitals must provide women who have obtained abortions with birth control information.

The model of privacy may best describe the overall aspiration of *Roe v. Wade*. However, the model of permission is arguably more descriptive of United States abortion law pertaining to unemancipated minors. The Supreme Court has taken the position that minors have a constitutional right to privacy and may terminate their pregnancies without parental consent, but that minors may not object on constitutional grounds to parental notification requirements and waiting periods. Individual justices on the Court have argued that requiring pregnant minors to notify family members of pregnancy and abortion, in effect, gives veto powers to third parties in a way that is inconsistent with the spirit of *Roe v. Wade*. Yet, a majority held in *Hodgson v. Minnesota* (1990) that states providing a "judicial by-pass procedure" may attempt to involve one or both parents in minors' abortion decision making by requiring minors or their physicians to contact parents in advance of abortion. In judicial bypass procedures, minors must be permitted to ask a judge to waive parental notification requirements. The judge is expected to waive the requirement if he or she determines that the minor is mature or that notification is not in the minor's best interests. Justices in the minority have objected that bypass procedures are unwarranted, since most minors notify parents or other responsible adults of pregnancy and abortion, and most minors seeking judicial waiver obtain it. In addition, the practical effect of mandatory notification is that some teens will delay abortion, increasing costs and medical risks. Some justices have argued that laws requiring parental involvement place minors with abusive parents or broken homes at a disadvantage and even at mortal risk.

Model of prescription

Under the models of permission and privacy, government permits some or all of the abortions women want. Under the model of prescription, government compels or virtually compels women to obtain abortions the government wants. Far-reaching compulsory abortion laws have been rare in the modern world. In the West, policymakers frown upon official and unofficial policies of mandatory abortion for poor and mentally incompetent women. Although health-care providers reportedly recommend abortion in some instances—for example, when a pregnant woman is addicted to cocaine or infected with the AIDS virus—the United States government does not officially recommend or mandate abortion for any class of pregnancy. Under a penal code adopted in 1979, Cuban law proscribes abortion performed without the permission of the woman.

In an effort to control overpopulation and protect its economy, China began adopting "planned birth" family-planning measures in 1953. These measures aggressively encourage abortion through a system of penalties and rewards. Under the Chinese constitution, both the government and individuals are responsible for the planned-birth policy. In 1974, couples were limited to two children. Since 1979 couples wishing to bear children have been authorized to have only one child, and then only after securing a government permit. To encourage compliance, abortion is offered at no cost and may entitle the woman to a two-week paid leave of absence; women who have an IUD inserted or a tubal ligation along with abortion may receive additional paid leave. The effect of the planned-birth policy on the abortion rate in China is not known in the West. However, female infanticide and abortion for sex selection are reported. Chinese families have reportedly resorted to infanticide and selective abortion to ensure that their one-child quota is filled by a child of the culturally preferred male sex.

Model of privacy

Under the model of privacy, the law rarely compels abortion and permits all or virtually all abortions, as long as they are performed by medically qualified persons in clinics, hospitals, or other qualified facilities. Safety is a frequent goal of legal systems characterized by the model of privacy, although safety is not necessarily suggested by "privacy" nomenclature. The former Soviet Union adopted the model of privacy on safety and privacy grounds in 1920, more than a half century before the model came to dominate understandings of U.S. law. The goal of the Soviet decree legalizing any abortion performed by a physician in a state hospital was both to keep women safe from unskilled abortionists and to secure women's freedom and equality in work, education, and marriage. In 1936, the decree was rescinded in favor of a law prohibiting abortion other than to spare the life or health of the woman or prevent transmission of an inheritable disease. The shift back to the models of prohibition and permission seems to have been motivated by concern about declining birthrates, health effects of medical abortions, and diminished regard for marriage and childbearing. But in 1955, the Soviet law moved back toward the model of privacy, again to protect women from unskilled abortionists and to give women themselves an opportunity to decide whether to become mothers (Sachdev, 1988).

In Japan, abortion has been legal since the government passed Eugenic Protection Laws in 1948 to protect women's health and deter the birth of what were considered undesirable offspring. The lack of trust by government and the medical profession in oral contraceptives has led to abortion becoming a major form of birth control in Japan. In practice, abortion is available to women upon request. The law does limit abortion, but the limitations are extremely liberal. Abortion is permitted when performed by designated physicians to avert mental and physical disease or abnormalities; when pregnancy results from violence; or when the woman's health would be impaired for physical or economic reasons. Functionally, one can view Japan as a model of privacy jurisdiction; yet women's autonomy and equality are not the express policy objectives of its liberal abortion law. Japan follows the model of permissions insofar as laws restrict abortion and have not been designed specifically to promote autonomous, private decision making.

In the United States, abortion policy since the early 1970s has been directed to women's rights. During the early 1970s, the United States and a number of other countries adopted laws approximating the model of privacy. The theory that during the first trimester abortion ought to be available without any restrictions gained popularity. In effect, it was adopted in the former East Germany in 1972, Denmark in 1973, Sweden in 1974, France in 1975, and Norway in 1978 (Sachdev, 1988; Olsnes, 1993). "Fetal viability," the point at which, in some of these countries, the interests of the woman cease to be accorded overriding weight, is variously fixed between twenty weeks and twenty-eight weeks. In Norway, under 1978 amendments to a 1975 law, a woman "shall herself make the final decision concerning termination of pregnancy provided that it is possible to perform the operation before the twelfth week of pregnancy has elapsed." After the twelfth week, abortion sought for a number of medical or social indications is available upon successful application to an "Abortion Board" (Olsnes, 1993).

In *Morgentaler et al.* v. *The Queen* (1988), the Supreme Court of Canada found by a margin of five to two that provisions of the Criminal Code infringed Section 7 of the Canadian Charter of Rights and Freedoms promising "life, liberty and security of the person." The Canadian justices argued that personal security, and with it bodily integrity, human dignity, and self-respect, were threatened by interference with reproductive choices (Morton, 1993). The Canadian legislature remains free to regulate abortion consistent with the *Morgentaler* decision. However, in 1990 a bill to restrict abortion access to women whose physicians certified a health-related need for the procedure failed. The government thereafter announced that it would not seek new abortion legislation (Morton, 1993).

In Canada, the United States, and other model-of-privacy jurisdictions, liberal abortion law permits autonomous choices about matters that profoundly affect women's bodies, lifestyles, and equality. However, it is now generally recognized that laws that decriminalize and deregulate abortion do not guarantee that every woman who desires an abortion will get one. Abortion is costly, and may or may not be covered by the health insurance of women who have insurance. The U.S. Supreme Court has repeatedly held that state and federal governments may encourage childbirth over abortion by refusing to include abortion among Medicaid and other entitlements awarded the poor. As a consequence, public funding for abortion is not available as a matter of right; publicly funded civilian and military hospitals are not required to perform abortion services; and states may prohibit physicians employed by public hospitals from performing abortions.

Focus: The United States

The Constitution of the United States does not mention "abortion" by name. However, the Supreme Court has consistently held since *Roe* v. *Wade* (1973) and *Doe* v. *Bolton* (1973) that the due process clause of the Fourteenth Amendment guarantees American women a fundamental right to obtain medically safe abortions. States may not categorically ban abortion or unduly burden women's fundamental constitutional right to terminate pregnancy.

The state of Connecticut passed the first American legislation against abortion in 1821 (Garrow, 1994). At first, American law did not penalize early (pre-quickening) abortion. However, between 1827 and 1860, twenty states or territories passed statutes against abortion at all stages of pregnancy. By 1868, thirty-six states or territories had antiabortion statutes in place, enforcement of which was often lax. In 1965, all fifty states treated abortion and attempted abortion at all stages of pregnancy as felonies, subject to certain exceptions. In forty-six states and the District of Columbia, the relevant statutes explicitly permitted abortion to save the mother's life, while in two of the other four states a similar exception was recognized by the courts.

Between 1967 and early 1973, a dozen jurisdictions in the United States adopted somewhat permissive abortion laws patterned on the model legislation suggested in 1962 by the influential American Law Institute. These laws permitted abortion when performed by a licensed physician who determined that there was a substantial risk that pregnancy would seriously injure the physical or mental health of the mother; that the child would be born with grave physical or mental defect; or that the pregnancy resulted from rape or incest. Almost all of the other reforming jurisdictions nevertheless sought to strengthen the institutionalization of abortion practice by stipulating that an abortion would be lawful only if performed in an accredited hospital after approval by a committee established in the hospital for that purpose.

The decriminalization of abortion on the national level lagged behind the decriminalization of contraception. In 1965 the Supreme Court decided *Griswold* v. *Connecticut,* holding that states may not outlaw a married woman's use of birth control. The Court based its ruling on an unenumerated constitutional "right to privacy" implicit in the Bill of Rights and the Fourteenth Amendment. This same right to privacy was invoked in 1973 in *Roe* v. *Wade* to limit government interference with abortion. The right to privacy was, and is, controversial among lawyers and judges reluctant to recognize novel unenumerated rights. However, both the American Medical Association and the American College of Obstetricians and Gynecologists favored legalization of abortion. The immediate effect of *Roe* v. *Wade* and *Doe* v. *Bolton*, its simultaneously decided, lesser-known companion case, was to invalidate the laws regulating abortion in every state, except perhaps the already very permissive laws adopted in 1969 and 1970 in New York, Alaska, Hawaii, and Washington.

Roe and *Doe* established that (1) no law can restrict the right of a woman to have a physician abort her pregnancy during the first three months, or first trimester, of her pregnancy; (2) during the second trimester the abortion procedure may be regulated by law only to the extent that the regulation reasonably relates to the preservation and protection of maternal health; (3) at the point at which the fetus becomes "viable," a law may prohibit abortion, but only subject to an exception permitting abortion whenever necessary to protect the woman's life or health (including any aspects of her physical or mental health); and (4) no law may require that all abortions be performed in a hospital, or that abortions be approved by a hospital committee or by a second medical opinion, or that abortions be performed only on women resident in the state concerned.

The Court in *Roe* and *Doe* concluded that the Constitution does not accord legal personhood status to the fetus. Critics of this conclusion point out that the unborn are implicitly treated as legal persons in several other areas of the law. The unborn are taken into account in the allocation of property rights and the attribution of criminal and civil responsibility. For example, the unborn can inherit property. Negligently killing or injuring a fetus can give rise to civil liability for wrongful death, wrongful birth, battery, and other torts.

Roe made clear that women were not to be ascribed a right to exclusive control over their bodies during pregnancy. Yet the case signaled that the Constitution limits the role government may play in abortion decisions. In the first decade and a half after *Roe*, the Court struck down numerous state abortion restrictions. States attempted to control abortion through advertising restrictions; zoning restrictions; record-keeping and reporting requirements; elaborate "informed consent" and physician-counseling requirements; mandatory waiting periods; bans on abortions for sex selection; the requirement of the presence of a second physician during the abortion procedure; the requirement that physicians employ methods of abortion calculated to save the lives of viable fetuses; the oversight requirement that physicians send all tissue removed during an abortion to a laboratory for analysis by a certified pathologist; the requirement that insurance companies offer at a lower cost insurance that does not cover most elective abortion; legislating a statewide information campaign to communicate an official state policy against abortion; legislating criminal sanctions for physicians who knowingly abort viable fetuses; and requirements that some or all abortions after the first trimester be performed in a hospital. However, the Supreme Court has repeatedly validated state and federal government policies that prefer childbirth to abortion by declining to pay for the abortions of poor women entitled to welfare benefits for prenatal care and childbirth.

A major reaffirmation of *Roe*, *Thornburgh v. American College of Obstetricians and Gynecologists* (1986), held that states were not permitted to indirectly prohibit abortion by encumbering the decision to seek abortion with unnecessary regulations. A series of highly publicized Court decisions handed down since 1989 appear to permit more extensive regulation of first- and second-

trimester abortions than *Roe* and *Doe* seemed to contemplate. *Webster v. Reproductive Services* (1989) permitted legislation requiring viability testing and limits on publicly funded physician care. The Court declined in *Webster* to decide the constitutionality of the declaration in the preamble of a Missouri statute that "[the] life of each human being begins at conception," and that "unborn children have protectable interests in life, health and well being" because the state had not yet sought to limit abortion by appeal to it. Encouraged by the *Webster* decision, several states and the territory of Guam sought between 1989 and 1992 to ban or discourage abortion through aggressive new regulation and enforcement. Anticipating that the Supreme Court would welcome an opportunity to overrule *Roe* in the 1990s, Guam enacted legislation prohibiting most abortion and its advocacy. A federal judge quickly declared Guam's law unenforceable under *Roe*.

In two 1990 cases critical of *Roe*, *Hodgson v. Minnesota* and *Ohio v. Akron Center for Reproductive Health*, the Court upheld parental notification requirements for minors. *Rust v. Sullivan* (1991) upheld a federal "gag rule" statute, subsequently eliminated by Congress, prohibiting abortion counseling by physicians in federally supported facilities. *Planned Parenthood v. Casey* (1992) affirmed *Roe v. Wade* as the law of the land and invalidated spousal notification. However, the case upheld a twenty-four-hour waiting period as part of a state's "informed consent" procedures. *Casey* shed the trimester framework of *Roe*, opening the door to regulation at any stage of pregnancy. *Casey* also announced a weaker standard of review in abortion cases that promised to permit more state regulation. Under *Roe*, abortion statutes were to be struck down if they did not further a "compelling" state interest. Under *Casey*, statutes "rationally related" to a "legitimate" state interest are to be upheld, assuming they do not "unduly burden" the abortion right.

This weakening of the standard of review in abortion cases underscores that constitutional abortion law in the United States hovers uneasily between the models of permission and privacy. For this reason, it seems likely that the Supreme Court will be asked again and again to clarify the extent to which the state and federal government may restrict abortion rights.

As long as it stands, *Roe v. Wade* will serve to provide a national abortion law standard for the United States. Since *Roe* in 1973, several attempts have been made in both houses of the national Congress to undercut the judicial decision through legislation. One attempt, premised on the idea of "states' rights," involved legislation which, if adopted, would have established that no right to an abortion is secured by the Constitution and, therefore, that the fifty states are free to adopt restrictions on abortions. A second attempt, premised on "fetal personhood," would have expanded the definition of "person" under the due process and equal protection clauses of the Fifth and Fourteenth Amendments. The fetal personhood legislation would have declared that the right to personhood attaches from the moment of conception.

Supporters of *Roe* in Congress have attempted to legislate the holding of *Roe* through a federal statute. The Freedom of Choice Act was introduced into Congress several times after *Webster,* beginning in November 1989. Its passage by Congress would prohibit states from enacting restrictions on the right to abortion before fetal viability. A 1994 survey conducted by the Hickman-Brown Research Company found that 56 percent of those polled "strongly" or "somewhat" favored passage of a Freedom of Choice Act, while 38 percent somewhat or strongly opposed such a law. Initiatives to amend the federal constitution to include pro-life or pro-choice strictures have not advanced far beyond the drafting table.

State statutes and state constitutions are an increasingly significant source of protection for abortion rights. With *in re T.W.,* the Florida Supreme Court invalidated that state's parental consent requirement, relying upon the state constitution (*T.W.,* 1989). As a result of this decision, Florida recognized a fundamental abortion right independent of *Roe* v. *Wade.* A Maryland referendum endorsed by voters in 1992 similarly established state abortion rights not tied to the fate of *Roe* v. *Wade* in the Supreme Court.

The implications of abortion law

The liberalization of abortion law establishes rights for women who wish to terminate their pregnancies. The full implications of those rights for (1) the disposal of fetal remains and eggs fertilized in vitro; (2) the enforceability of surrogate contract; (3) the criminalization of pregnant women's conduct; and (4) organized protest at abortion cites are unclear. An important set of issues spawned by liberal regulation surrounds the disposition of fetal remains. Do women who elect to abort have a familial, proprietary, or other interest in fetal tissue remains? State statutes typically require that abortion providers dispose of fetal remains in the way physicians dispose of other excised tissues. Yet some effort has been made to treat abortion tissues and fetuses differently, either because of their possible commercial value for research into the treatment of diabetes, leukemia, Alzheimer's disease, and Parkinson's disease; or because of their possible value as lost "children." In 1984, a federal judge in Louisiana held that a statute requiring abortion providers to present patients with the option of burial or cremation was an unconstitutional burden on freedom of choice. Over 90 percent of all abortions performed in the United States, and other countries, are performed during the first trimester. The court implied that women might be discouraged from first-trimester abortions on the mistaken belief that extracted tissue would resemble a baby. American courts and legislators are unlikely to permit outright sales of abortion tissues for research purposes. Indeed, federal agency policies adopted in the 1980s declared a moratorium on the use of abortion tissues derived from elective abortions partly out of concern that women might be encouraged to abort for gain. Signaling a change in policy, in 1993, very early in his administration, Democratic President Bill Clinton issued an executive order lifting the moratorium on fetal tissue research.

Technology has spawned perplexing questions about the need to regulate the disposal of unwanted fertilized eggs and "frozen" embryos. Should abortion strictures apply? The liberal tenor of *Roe* may imply that neither pregnant women nor laboratory technicians do wrong to destroy potential life in its early stages of development. In jurisdictions where early abortion is strictly prohibited or restricted, some decision must be made about whether to regard fertilized eggs and frozen embryos as human beings or as merely potential human beings comparable to gametes. For some, extending abortion prohibitions to, for example, a frozen embryo suggests an exaggerated respect for human life. For others, failure to dignify laboratory-based potential human life with ethical and legal concern suggests an egregious want of humanity.

Hundreds of men and women have been parties to commercial surrogate motherhood contracts in recent decades. Commercial surrogacy agreements commonly obtain provisions in which the would-be surrogate undertakes that she will not obtain an abortion should she become pregnant as a result of the surrogacy transactions. In the celebrated *Baby* M case, MaryBeth Whitehead agreed in writing that she would "not abort the child once conceived" unless a physician determined it necessary to protect her health or "the child has been determined . . . to be physiologically abnormal." Although the Supreme Court of 'New Jersey refused to enforce the surrogacy contract in *Baby* M, other jurisdictions have not done so and face questions about the commercial alienability of constitutional abortion rights.

Another set of issues relates to the extent to which abortion rights may prevent government from intervening to enjoin or punish risky behavior by pregnant women who, for example, smoke cigarettes, consume alcohol, abuse drugs, and fail to heed medical advice. In a number of isolated cases in the United States, judges have jailed pregnant women they feared would abuse or neglect their fetuses. A somewhat different concern is the legal implications of government intervention in the event that a pregnant woman refuses a blood transfusion needed to save her life, or a cesarean delivery physicians believe to be in the best medical interest of the unborn. Some view *Roe v. Wade* as holding by implication that women have a broad right to control—and even abuse—their own bodies without regard to fetal well-being. Yet a plausible counterview is that *Roe* does nothing more than immunize women from prosecution for early abortions, if they choose to have them.

Abortion is controversial in many countries, and the controversy is highly politicized. Violence aimed at abortion providers has occurred both in Canada and the United States. In May 1992, a bomb blast blamed on antiabortion radicals destroyed the Morgentaler abortion clinic in Toronto. Rare in Canada, dozens of abortion clinic bombings and fires have occurred in the United States. Pro-life antiabortion activists throughout the United States have demonstrated at abortion sites to focus attention on their concerns. Generally peaceful, these demonstrations have sometimes become blockades that interfere with the ability of patients and staff to utilize facilities where abortions are believed to take place. Demonstrators have sometimes resorted to harassment, noise nuisance, property damage and violence. The shooting deaths of two Florida physicians outside abortion facilities in 1993 and again in 1994 dramatized the conflict between protesters and clinics. The United States Congress passed the Freedom of Access to Clinic Entrances Act of 1994 in an effort to assure freedom of access to reproduction services. The act makes acts of obstruction and interference at places providing reproductive services a federal offense punishable by fines and imprisonment.

Abortion rights and free-speech rights clash in the context of conflicts over abortion clinic protests. Women have a legal right to seek abortion and to protection from physical assault and harassment. But antiabortion protesters have a First Amendment right to freedom of speech and expression. In 1990, a Maryland court applying the First Amendment upheld a state law proscribing a religious protestor's "loud and unseemly" antiabortion litany. In light of First Amendment values, some federal courts have been reluctant to enjoin abortion protestors accused of actual or threatened violence on the basis of state or federal statutes, such as the Ku Klux Klan Act, not clearly enacted for that purpose. In *National Organization for Women v. Scheidler*, however, the Supreme Court determined that the federal Racketeer Influences and Corrupt Organizations (RICO) statute could apply to a coalition of antiabortion groups alleged to be members of a nationwide conspiracy to close abortion clinics. The alleged conspirators unsuccessfully argued that RICO applies only to conspiracies in which the alleged racketeers act for the sake of economic gain rather than out of religious, moral, or political conviction. The Court found that acts that did not generate income for alleged racketeers but that adversely affected businesses such as abortion clinics were potentially conspiratorial under the RICO statute. In sum, the practice of abortion raises numerous legal issues in the jurisdictions that permit it. Because so many oppose abortion on religious and moral grounds, abortion-related questions of legal policy will remain especially complex in the United States and other pluralistic societies. In addition, should reproductive technologies for creating, preserving, and terminating gametes and fetuses continue to proliferate, the number of legal concerns about reproductive rights and responsiblilties is as likely to expand as to contract.

ANITA L. ALLEN

Directly related to this article is the companion article, CONTEMPORARY ETHICAL AND LEGAL ASPECTS: A. CONTEMPORARY ETHICAL PERSPECTIVES, *and the other sections in this entry:* MEDICAL PERSPECTIVES, *and* RELIGIOUS TRADITIONS, *articles on* JEWISH PERSPECTIVES, ROMAN CATHOLIC PERSPECTIVES, PROTESTANT PERSPECTIVES, *and* ISLAMIC PERSPECTIVES. *For a further discussion of topics mentioned in this article, see the entries* CHILDREN, *article on* RIGHTS OF CHILDREN; EUGENICS; EUGENICS AND RELIGIOUS LAW; FERTILITY CONTROL; FETUS; HEALTH-CARE RESOURCES, ALLOCATION OF; POPULATION ETHICS, *section on* ELEMENTS OF POPULATION ETHICS, *articles on* DEFINITION OF POPULATION ETHICS, *and* HISTORY OF POPULATION THEORIES; POPULATION POLICIES, *sections on* STRATEGIES OF FERTILITY CONTROL, *and* HEALTH EFFECTS OF FERTILITY CONTROL; PRIVACY IN HEALTH CARE; RACE AND RACISM; REPRODUCTIVE TECHNOLOGIES, *articles on* SEX SELECTION, SURROGACY, *and* CRYOPRESERVATION OF SPERM, OVA, AND EMBRYOS; *and* WOMEN, *articles on* HISTORICAL AND CROSS-CULTURAL PERSPECTIVES, *and* HEALTH-CARE ISSUES. *Other relevant material may be found under the entries* AUTONOMY; FREEDOM AND COERCION; JUSTICE; NATIONAL SOCIALISM; PATERNALISM; RESPONSIBLITY; RIGHTS; *and* SEXISM.

Bibliography

Baby M, in re. 1988. 109 N. J. 396, 537 A.2d 1227.

COHEN, SHERRILL, and TAUB, NADINE, eds. 1989. *Reproductive Laws for the 1990s.* Clifton, N.J.: Humana Press.

COOK, ELIZABETH A.; JELEN, TED G.; and WILCOX, CLYDE. 1992. *Between Two Absolutes: Public Opinion and the Politics of Abortion.* Boulder, Colo.: Westview Press.

Doe v. Bolton. 1973. 93 S. Ct. 739.

GARFIELD, JAY L., and HENNESSEY, PATRICIA. 1984. *Abortion: Moral and Legal Perspectives.* Amherst: University of Massachusetts Press.

GARROW, DAVID J. 1994. *Liberty and Sexuality: The Right to Privacy and the Making of Roe v. Wade.* New York: Macmillan.

GLENDON, MARY ANN. 1987. *Abortion and Divorce in Western Law.* Cambridge, Mass.: Harvard University Press.

Griswold v. Connecticut. 1965. 381 U.S. 479, 483.

Hodgson v. Minnesota. 1990. 110 S. Ct. 2926.

JOHNSEN, DAWN E. 1986. "The Creation of Fetal Rights: Conflicts with Women's Constitutional Rights to Liberty, Privacy, and Equal Protection." *Yale Law Journal* 95, no. 3:599–625.

KING, PATRICIA A. 1979. "The Juridical Status of the Fetus: A Proposal for the Legal Protection of the Unborn." *Michigan Law Review* 77 (August):1647.

LUKER, KRISTIN. 1984. *Abortion and the Politics of Motherhood.* Berkeley: University of California Press.

MALOY, KATE, and PATTERSON, MARGARET JONES. 1992. *Birth or Abortion? Private Struggles in a Political World.* New York: Plenum Press.

MANIER, EDWARD; LIU, WILLIAM; and SOLOMON, DAVID, eds. 1977. *Abortion: New Directions for Policy Studies.* Notre Dame, Ind.: University of Notre Dame Press.

MELTON, GARY B., and PLINER, ANITA J. 1986. "Adolescent Abortion: A Psycholegal Analysis." In *Adolescent Abortion: Psychological and Legal Issues,* pp. 1–39. Edited by Gary B. Melton. Lincoln: University of Nebraska Press.

MICHEL, AARON E. 1981–82. "Abortion and International Law: The Status and Possible Extension of Women's Right to Privacy." *Journal of Family Law* 20, no. 2:241–261.

MORTON, FREDERICK LEE. 1993. *Pro-Choice vs. Pro Life: Abortion and the Courts in Canada.* Norman: University of Oklahoma Press.

NATIONAL COUNCIL OF NEGRO WOMEN AND COMMUNICATIONS CONSORTIUM MEDIA CENTER. 1991. *Women of Color Reproductive Health Poll.* New York: Author.

Ohio v. Akron Center for Reproductive Health. 1990. 110 S. Ct. 2972.

OLSNES, RAGNHILD. 1993. "The Right to Self Determined Abortion." In *Birth Law,* pp. 65–91. Edited by Anne Hellum. Oslo: Scandinavian University Press.

PETCHESKY, ROSALIND P. 1990. *Abortion and Women's Choice: The State, Sexuality and Reproductive Freedom.* Rev. ed. Boston: Northeastern University Press.

PETERSEN, KERRY A. 1993. *Abortion Regimes.* Brookville, Vt.: Dartmouth.

Planned Parenthood v. Casey. 1992. 112 S. Ct. 2791.

REARDON, DAVID C. 1987. *Aborted Women: Silent No More.* Chicago: Loyola University Press.

RHODE, DEBORAH L. 1989. *Justice and Gender: Sex Discrimination and the Law.* Cambridge, Mass.: Harvard University Press.

RICHARDS, DAVID A. J. 1986. *Toleration and the Constitution.* New York: Oxford University Press.

ROBERTSON, JOHN A. 1983. "Procreative Liberty and the Control of Contraception, Pregnancy, and Childbirth." *Virginia Law Review* 69, no. 3:405–464.

Roe v. Wade. 1973. 410 U.S. 113.

Rust v. Sullivan. 1991. 111 S. Ct. 1759.

SACHDEV, PAUL, ed. 1988. *International Handbook on Abortion.* New York: Greenwood.

SIEGEL, REVA. 1992. "Reasoning from the Body: A Historical Perspective on Abortion Regulation and Questions of Equal Protection." *Stanford Law Review* 44 (January):261–381.

SOLOMONS, MICHAEL. 1992. *Pro Life? The Irish Question.* Dublin: Lilliput.

Thornburgh v. American College of Obstetricians and Gynecologists. 1986. 106 S. Ct. 2169.

TIETZE, CHRISTOPHER; FORREST, JACQUELINE DARROCH; and HENSHAW, STANLEY K. 1988. "United States of America." In *International Handbook on Abortion,* pp. 473–494. Edited by Paul Sachdev. New York: Greenwood Press.

TRIBE, LAURENCE H. 1990. *Abortion, the Clash of Absolutes.* New York: W. W. Norton.

T. W., in re. 1989. 551 S. 2d. 1186 (Fla.).

Webster v. Reproductive Services. 1989. 109 S. Ct. 3040.

WEDDINGTON, SARAH R. 1992. *A Question of Choice.* New York: Putnam.

III. RELIGIOUS TRADITIONS

A. JEWISH PERSPECTIVES

The following article is a revision of "Abortion: Jewish Perspectives" by David M. Feldman that appeared in the first edition of the Encyclopedia of Bioethics *(1978). Portions of the original appear in the revised article.*

The abortion question in Talmudic law begins, but does not remain, with an examination of the legal status of the fetus. For this the Talmud has a phrase, *ubar yerekh immo;* the fetus, that is, is "part of the mother," rather than an independent entity. This designation says nothing about the right of abortion; the term is found only in theoretical contexts. It defines, for example, ownership in the case of an embryo found in a purchased animal; as intrinsic to its mother's body, the embryo belongs to the buyer. On the human level, in religious conversion of a pregnant woman to Judaism, her unborn child is automatically included and requires no added ceremony.

Nor does the fetus have power of acquisition; gifts or transactions made on its behalf, except by its parents, are not binding, and it inherits from its father naturally, without transaction or legal transfer. Germane as such technical information might seem to the question of abortion, it tells us only that the fetus, in Jewish as in Roman law, has no "juridical personality" of its own.

Palestinian and Alexandrian thought

In Judaism, the morality of abortion is a function of the legal attitude to feticide, as distinguished from homicide or infanticide. The law of homicide in the Torah, in one of its several formulations (Exod. 21:12), reads: "*Makkeh ish* . . ." (One who slays a man . . .). Does "man" here include any human, say, a day-old child? Yes, says the Talmud, pairing it with another text (Lev. 24:17): *ki yakkeh kol nefesh adam* (If one slays any *nefesh adam,* any human person). The "any" is understood to include the day-old child, but the *nefesh adam* is taken to exclude the fetus in the womb, for the fetus in the womb is *lav nefesh hu*, not a person, until born. In the words of Rashi, the classic commentator (with authority of legal pronouncement) on Bible and Talmud, only when the fetus "comes into the world" is it a "person" (Sanhedrin 72b).

The basis, then, for denying capital-crime status to feticide in Jewish law is scriptural. Alongside the *nefesh adam* source-text is another basic one, in Exod. 21:22, 23: "If men strive together, and wound a pregnant woman, expelling her progeny, with no harm befalling [her], then [the offender] shall surely be punished [by fine]. But if harm befall [her], then shalt thou give life for life." The Talmud makes explicit the teaching of this passage: Only monetary compensation is exacted of him who causes a woman to miscarry. And though the abortion spoken of here is accidental, the passage is still a source for the teaching that feticide is not a capital crime. Neither murder nor accidental homicide can be expiated by monetary fine.

This fundamental passage has an alternative rendering in the Septuagint, the Greek translation of the Bible produced in the third century B.C.E. One word change there yields an entirely different statute on miscarriage. Viktor Aptowitzer's essays analyze the difference; the school of thought represented by the Septuagint he calls the Alexandrian view, as opposed to the Palestinian—that is, the Talmudic—view set forth above. The word in question is *ason*, rendered above as "harm"; hence, "if no harm [i.e., death] befall [her, the mother], then shall [he] be fined. . . ." The Greek sees the word *ason* as "form," yielding instead something like: "If no form [to the fetus], then punishment by fine; if form, then life for a life." The "life for life" clause is thus applied to the fetus, not just the mother, and a distinction is made—as Augustine later formulated it—between *embryo informatus* and *embryo formatus*. For the latter, though not yet born, the text so rendered prescribes the death penalty (Aptowitzer, 1924).

Among the Christian church fathers, the consequent doctrine of feticide as murder was preached by Tertullian, who accepted the Septuagint, and by Jerome, whose classic Bible translation nonetheless renders this passage according to the Hebrew text official within the Church. Closer to the main body of the Jewish community, we find the Samaritans and Karaites reflecting the Alexandrian view, and more important, so does Philo, the popular first-century philosopher of Alexandria. On the other hand, Philo's younger contemporary, Josephus, bears witness to the Palestinian (*halakhic*) tradition. Aside from its textual warrant, the Palestinian is the more authentic reading, Aptowitzer declares, while the other is a later tendency, "which, in addition, is not genuinely Jewish but must have origi-

nated in Alexandria under Egyptian-Greek influence" (Aptowitzer, 1924, p. 88).

Noahide restrictions

In the rabbinic tradition, then, abortion remains a noncapital crime at worst. But a curious factor further complicates the question of the criminality of the act. One more biblical text, this one in Genesis and hence "before Sinai" and part of the Commandments of the "Descendants of Noah," served as the source for the teaching that feticide is indeed a capital crime—for non-Jews. Gen. 9:6 reads, "One who sheds the blood of man, through man [i.e., through the human court of law] shall his blood be shed." The Hebrew (*shofekh dam ha-adam ba-adam . . .*) allows for a translation of "man, in man" as well as "man, through man" (or "person, in person"). The Talmud records the exposition of Rabbi Ishmael: "What is this 'man, in man'? It must refer to a fetus in its mother's womb" (Sanhedrin 57b). The locus of this text in Genesis, standing as it does without the qualifying balance of the Exodus (Sinaitic) passage, made feticide a capital crime for the rest of the world (i.e., those not heir to the Sinaitic covenant) in Jewish law. Some modern scholars hold this exposition to be more sociological than textually inherent, representing a reaction to abuse. In view of rampant abortion and infanticide, they claim, Rabbi Ishmael expounded the above exegesis of the Genesis text in order to render judgment against the Romans.

Regardless of its rationale, this teaching associated with Rabbi Ishmael remains part of codified Jewish law, as Moses Maimonides (1135–1204), for example, formulates it: "A 'Descendant of Noah' who killed a person, even a fetus in its mother's womb, is capitally liable." His Legal Code goes on to describe the court, whose members are to be Israelites or the resident aliens themselves. The stricture, however, does not extend to life-saving ("therapeutic") abortion nor, according to some, to abortion during the first forty days of pregnancy. Implications of this anomaly—a different law for the "Descendants of Noah"—were dealt with in a Responsum (a unit in a series of Responsa, formal answers to questions of Jewish law submitted to rabbinic authority) of the eighteenth century. "It is not to be supposed," writes Rabbi Isaac Schorr, "that the Torah would consider the embryo as a person [*nefesh*] for them [Noahides] but not a person for us. The fetus is not a person for them either; the Torah was just more severe in its practical ruling in their regard. Hence, therapeutic abortion would be permissible to them, too" (Responsa *Koach Shor*, No. 20).

In the rabbinic system, then, abortion is not murder. Nor is it more than murder, as would be the case if "ensoulment" were at issue. Talmudic discussions raise the possibility of the moment—conception, birth, post-birth—at which the soul joins the body. However, this is seen to be irrelevant to the abortion question, because the soul is immortal no matter when it enters or leaves the body. And, more important than being immortal, it is a pure soul, free of the taint of "original sin." In the words of the Talmud, cited verbatim in the Daily Prayer Book, "My God, the soul with which Thou has endowed me is pure."

Broader legal discussion

Murder (killing of the innocent) is always forbidden in Jewish law, even to save life. The three cardinal sins that call for martyrdom instead of transgression are idolatry, adultery-incest, and murder. "For all sins in the Torah, ya-avor v'al ye-hareg (let one transgress rather than endanger one's life). But, for idolatry, adultery, and murder—ye-hareg v'al ya-avor (let him surrender his life rather than transgress)." Abortion, then, would require martyrdom if it were deemed murder, and, having been removed from that category, it becomes permissible and, where indicated, even mandated. The Mishnah sets forth the basic Talmudic law in this regard:

> If a woman has [life-threatening] difficulty in child-bearing, the embryo within her should [even] be dismembered limb by limb. For, her life takes precedence over its life. Once its head (or its greater part) has emerged, it may not be touched.
>
> For, we may not set aside one life [nefesh] for another life. (Mishnah, Oholot, 7:6)

In its analysis of such provisions, the Talmud had suggested that the reason for ever permitting abortion is that the fetus may be in the category of an "aggressor," that is, its life would be forfeited under the law that permits killing a "pursuer" in order to save the intended victim. An attacker, not being innocent, forfeits protection under "Thou shalt not murder." The Talmud proceeds to dismiss this reasoning, since the fetus is quite innocent, with no malice aforethought. Also, since we cannot know "who is pursuing whom," the predicament must be deemed an "act of God"—she is "being pursued from Heaven"—and the pursuer provision cannot apply. Yet, in his great Law Code, Maimonides reintroduced the possibility, which became, incidentally, the source for Aquinas of the "aggressor" idea in the Christian tradition. Maimonides formulates the Mishnaic rule as follows:

> This, too, is a (Negative) Commandment—not to "take pity" on the life of a pursuer. Therefore, the Sages ruled that when a woman has [life-threatening] difficulty in childbearing, the fetus in her womb is to be removed—either with drugs or by surgery—because it is like a pursuer seeking to kill her.
>
> Once its head has emerged, it may not be touched, for we do not set aside one life for another; this is the natural course of the world. (Mishneh Torah, Laws of Murder and Preservation of Life, 1:9)

Commentators to Maimonides' Code suggest, in view of the obvious difference between his conclusion and that of the Talmud, that his point is the gravity of abortion. Though technically not murder, the deed is so grave that it is comparable; hence, he writes, "the fetus is *like* a pursuer."

Maternal welfare

The subsequent rabbinic tradition seems to align itself either to the right, in the direction of Maimonides, or to the left, toward Rashi, above. The first approach can be identified especially with the late Chief Rabbi of Israel, Issar Unterman, who sees any abortion as "akin to homicide" and therefore allowable only in cases of corresponding gravity, such as saving the life of the mother. This approach then builds *down* from that strict position to embrace a broader interpretation of lifesaving situations, which include a threat to her health, for example, as well as a threat to her life.

The second approach, associated with another former Chief Rabbi of Israel, Ben Zion Uziel, and others, assumes that no explicit prohibition against abortion exists—other than an antiprocreational one—and builds *up* from that permissive position to safeguard against indiscriminate abortion. This includes the example of Rabbi Yair Bacharach in the late seventeenth century, whose classic Responsum saw no legal bar to abortion in the case before him, but disallowed it on other grounds. The case was one of a pregnancy conceived in adultery; the woman, "in deep remorse," wanted to destroy the fruit of her sin. The author refuses to allow it, not on legal but social grounds, as a safeguard or deterrent against immorality. Other authorities in the "lenient" line disagreed on this point, reaffirming the legal sanction of abortion for the woman's welfare, whether life or health or mental health, or even avoidance of "great pain." Rabbi Jacob Emden (d. 1776) suggested the latter justification would even include the case of unmarried pregnancy, since there is no greater pain than shame.

The criterion in both approaches remains maternal rather than fetal welfare. A principle in these matters is *tza'ara d'gufah kadim,* that is, avoidance or prevention of "her pain should be the first consideration." The mother's welfare is primary, and hence maternal indications rather than fetal ones—or, remarkably, rather than the husband's wishes—are determinative. Rabbinic rulings on abortion are thus amenable to the following generalization: If a possibility or probability exists that a child may be born with abnormalities, and the mother seeks abortion on grounds of pity for the life of such a child, the consulted rabbi would decline permission. If, however, an abortion for that same potentially deformed child were sought on grounds of severe anguish suffered now by the mother, permission would be granted. The fate of the fetus is unknown, future, potential, part of "the secrets of God"; the mother's condition is known, she is present and asking for compassion.

In the matter of genetic diseases such as Tay-Sachs disease, rabbinic authorities recommend screening before rather than during pregnancy. (A computerized registry, called *Dor Yesharim*, allows for determination before marriage of carrier status.) This is to avoid amniocentesis after the first trimester, with possible abortion on the basis of its findings. Such abortion, for fetal rather than maternal reasons, would not ordinarily be sanctioned by Jewish law. Yet the one can blend into the other: Fetal risk can mean mental anguish for the mother; the fetal indication becomes a maternal one. The woman's welfare is thus the key to warrant for abortion. A recent rabbinic opinion on terminating a pregnancy caused by rape or incest reflects this position. Unlike "Mother Earth," which receives and fructifies seed planted by the farmer, writes Rabbi Yehudah Perilman of nineteenth-century Minsk, the woman's humanity dictates that she "not be asked to nurture seed implanted within her against her will" (Responsa *Or Gadol*, No. 31).

Implicit in the Mishnah cited above is the teaching that the rights of the fetus are secondary to the rights of the mother until the moment of birth. This principle is obscured by the contemporary phrase "right to life." In the abortion context, the issue is not right to life but right to be born. The right to be born is relative—to the welfare of the mother, for example—while the right to life, of existing persons, is absolute. "Life" may begin before birth, but prehuman life, like animal life or plant life, has a status different from human life. Rabbinic law has determined that human life begins with birth; or, to put it more aptly, life begins to be called human only at birth. This is neither a medical nor a legal judgment, but a metaphysical one, and it serves only to give the mother, who is actual, priority over the fetus, which is potential, in any mortal clash.

According to the same Mishnah, this disparity ends at the moment of birth. "Once the fetus has emerged . . . we may not set aside one life for another." Now the "sanctity of life" principle means that the infant is inviolable, regardless of supposed "quality of life" differences. A mortal clash of rights is no longer resolved in her favor; mother and newborn baby are equal from the moment of birth, and the right to continued life even of a defective child is absolute.

Pronatalism

Procreation ("Be fruitful") is an affirmative commandment in the Jewish legal system, and even the neglect to father or conceive is termed "bloodshed," very much in the figurative sense. The pronatalist attitude of Judaism helps account for its abhorrence of casual abortion, not to mention the self-brutalizing effect. There may be legal sanction for recourse to abortion where necessary, but the position remains one of hesitation before the sanctity of even potential life and a pronatalist reverence for the gift of life.

Accordingly, abortion for "population control" is repugnant to the Jewish mind, as is abortion for reasons other than deeply serious ones, parallel to the gravity of the deed. Orthodox, Conservative, and Reform Jews, though different in the degree of their respective adherence to ritual law, share this attitude to the moral question. Termination of pregnancy for economic reasons is not admissible, either. Whereas taking precaution by birth control or abortion against physical threat remains a *mitzvah*, this is not the case when the fear is financial hardship. In the state of Israel, abortion is illegal according to its secular statutes, unless approved by a hospital committee for any of the following circumstances: age of mother, her single status, rape/incest, danger to her health, or fetal deformity, which exclude financial or other considerations. But "Just One Life"—from the Talmudic teaching that "If one saves just one life, it is as if he saved an entire world"—is an agency in the voluntary sector that provides an alternative: economic assistance and counseling for childbirth and child care.

In the Jewish community today, with a conscious or unconscious impulse to replenish ranks decimated by the European Holocaust, contemporary rabbis invoke not the more lenient but the more stringent Responsa of the earlier and later authorities. Even the permissive decisions, they point out, presupposed a natural hesitation to resort to abortion. Against a contemporary background of rights claimed for their own sake, consulted rabbis tend to move away from Rashi's position and its followers, closer to that of Maimonides and those who uphold it, allowing abortion only for the gravest of reasons.

DAVID M. FELDMAN

Directly related to this article are the companion articles in this section, ROMAN CATHOLIC PERSPECTIVES, PROTESTANT PERSPECTIVES, *and* ISLAMIC PERSPECTIVES, *and the articles in the other sections in this entry:* MEDICAL PERSPECTIVES, *and* CONTEMPORARY ETHICAL AND LEGAL ASPECTS, *articles on* CONTEMPORARY ETHICAL PERSPECTIVES, *and* LEGAL AND REGULATORY ISSUES. *Also directly related to this article are the entries* EUGENICS AND RELIGIOUS LAW, *article on* JUDAISM; FETUS, *article on* PHILOSOPHICAL AND ETHICAL ISSUES; INFANTS, *article on* HISTORY OF INFANTICIDE; JUDAISM; LIFE; MEDICAL ETHICS, HISTORY OF, *section on* NEAR AND MIDDLE EAST, *article on* ISRAEL; *and* PERSON. *Other relevant material may be found under the entries* ETHICS, *article on* RELIGION AND MORALITY; LIFE; MATERNAL–FETAL RELATIONSHIP; *and* WOMEN, *article on* HISTORICAL AND CROSS-CULTURAL PERSPECTIVES.

Bibliography

APTOWITZER, VICTOR. 1924. "Observations on the Criminal Law of the Jews." *Jewish Quarterly Review* 15:55–118.

BLEICH, J. DAVID. "Abortion in Halakhic Literature." In *Jewish Bioethics*, pp. 134–177. Edited by Fred Rosner and J. David Bleich. New York: Hebrew Publishing.

FELDMAN, DAVID M. 1968. *Birth Control in Jewish Law: Marital Relations, Contraception, and Abortion as Set Forth in the Classic Texts of Jewish Law.* New York: New York University Press.

———. 1986. *Health and Medicine in the Jewish Tradition: L'hayyim—To Life.* New York: Crossroad.

HERRING, BASIL F. 1984. "Abortion." In his *Jewish Ethics and Halakhah for Our Time: Sources and Commentary*, pp. 25–45. New York: Ktav.

JAKOBOVITZ, IMMANUEL. 1967. *Jewish Medical Ethics: A Comparative and Historical Study of the Jewish Religious Attitude to Medicine and Its Practice.* New York: Bloch.

KLEIN, ISAAC. 1975. "Abortion." In his *Responsa and Halakhic Studies.* New York: Ktav.

ROSNER, FRED. 1986. *Modern Medicine and Jewish Ethics.* New York: Ktav.

B. ROMAN CATHOLIC PERSPECTIVES

The following is a revision and update of the first edition article "Abortion: Roman Catholic Perspectives" by John R. Connery.

The Roman Catholic tradition has always treated abortion as a serious sin. Yet Catholic teaching on abortion has not always centered on the "right to life" of the individual fetus, nor has it always viewed all abortion as homicide. For several centuries, early abortion in particular was characterized more as a sexual sin than as killing, and was condemned as an interference in the natural outcome of the reproductive process, often assuming as its context an illicit sexual liaison.

The fact that Catholic views of the precise status of the fetus as human life have changed over time, and that the church's position has a philosophical rather than a religious basis, are key to late-twentieth-century church teaching on abortion. That teaching is that the fetus must be given the benefit of the doubt, and be treated as if it were a person from conception onward. This teaching is not stated as a sectarian religious proposition, but as a humanistic and philosophical truth to be recognized in civil laws guaranteeing appropriate protection to fetal life. Although exhortations to protect life

in the womb have often been supported with religious allusions (for instance, to the will of the Creator or to the image of God in humanity), the duties to continue pregnancy and to sustain infants have been grounded primarily in the "natural law," understood as a shared human morality innate to all persons and knowable by reason.

In examining the foundations and development of the Catholic position, it is important to place modern teaching in the context of changing views of women's roles in family and society. Other factors influencing debates about Roman Catholicism and abortion are the relation of scientific knowledge about the beginnings of human life to the moral status of life; the relation among civil law, morality, and the church as an institutional actor; and contraception and population, especially in international perspective.

Historical development

Although Catholic claims about abortion are not narrowly religious, certain biblical and early Christian characterizations of life in the womb no doubt have contributed to an ethos in which abortion is viewed negatively. The Hebrew Scriptures (Old Testament) did not treat the killing of a fetus as the killing of an infant (Exod. 21:22), although the Greek Septuagint translation of the Hebrew (early third century B.C.E.) adds a distinction between the formed and the unformed fetus, and presents abortion of the former as homicide. This distinction reflects the ancient Greek view (Aristotle) that the matter and form of any being must be mutually appropriate (the "hylomorphic theory"), and that the embryo or fetus could not have a human soul ("form") until the body ("matter") was sufficiently developed. Often quoting the Septuagint, patristic and medieval theologians maintained this distinction, which remained a key component of Roman Catholic discussion of abortion until at least the eighteenth century.

The Gospels do not address abortion explicitly, though the infancy narratives manifest interest in the importance of the individual before birth, at least in respect of God's will for him or her in the future (Matt. 1:18–25; Luke 1:5–45). In Paul's Letter to the Galatians (5:20) and in Revelation (9:21), condemnations of magical drugs (*pharmakeia*) associated with various forms of immorality, including promiscuity and lechery, may very likely extend to abortifacients. The connection is made clear in two early Christian texts, the *Didache* and the *Epistle to Barnabas.* "'You shall not kill. You shall not commit adultery. You shall not corrupt boys. You shall not fornicate. You shall not steal. You shall not make magic. You shall not practice medicine (*pharmakeia*). You shall not slay the child by abortions (*phthora*). You shall not kill what is generated. You shall not desire your neighbor's wife' (*Didache* 2.2)" (Noonan, 1970, p. 9).

Contraceptive and abortifacient drugs, as well as infanticide, were certainly used widely in the ancient world, not only to conceal sexual crimes but also to limit family size and conserve property. Early Christian authors such as Tertullian, Jerome, and Augustine in the Western church, and Clement of Alexandria, John Chrysostom, and Basil in the Eastern church, repudiated these practices. They did not, however, challenge their patriarchal social context, with its requirement that female sexuality serve the good of the family and its assumption that women seeking to avoid pregnancy were usually guilty of sexual infidelity. Local councils tended to support this stand. In 303 c.e., on the Iberian Peninsula, the Council of Elvira excluded from the church for the rest of her life any woman who had obtained an abortion after adultery. In 314, the Eastern church, at the Council of Ancyra (Ankara), reduced the period of penance to ten years, although it retained the lifetime ban for voluntary homicide. Such church laws made no distinction between the formed and the unformed fetus, but Tertullian, Jerome, and Augustine considered that the sin of abortion might not be homicide until after ensoulment. (The fetus was considered by many ancient writers to receive a soul only after the body had "formed," or reached an appropriate level of development, at about three months.)

Formation of the fetus became a consideration in assigning penance in private confession during the seventh century, but it was not universally recognized in church law until the decree *Sicut ex* of Innocent III in 1211. The decree dealt with irregularity, which could be incurred for homicide. An irregularity is a canonical impediment that bars a man from receiving or exercising holy orders. Irregularities are based on defects (such as mental or physical illness) or crimes (including attempted suicide, murder, and abortion). According to the decree, irregularity would not be incurred for abortion unless the fetus was animated. Since the time of animation was identified with formation, the decree implied that only abortion of the formed fetus was considered homicide. Following Aristotle, forty and ninety days were accepted as the time of animation for the male and the female fetus, respectively. Confusion arose, however, from a parallel tradition that extended the notion of homicide not only to the abortion of the unformed fetus but also to sterilization. Both traditions claimed a factual base, the one in the premise that the "man" is contained in miniature in the male seed, and the other in Aristotle's reported observation of aborted fetuses. During the Middle Ages, the distinction between formed and unformed was generally accepted, notably by Thomas Aquinas, and only the abortion of the

formed fetus was classified as homicide, even in reference to sacramental penances. Earlier abortions were not murder, but they were still forbidden as serious sins because they interfered with the procreative outcome of sexual acts.

In the early fourteenth century, the Dominican John of Naples introduced an exception, subsequently accepted by several others: It would be permissible to abort the unformed fetus in order to save the life of the mother. Later theologians, particularly Thomas Sánchez (sixteenth century), used the argument of self-defense against an unjust aggressor (so characterizing the fetus) or the principle of totality (looking on the fetus as part of the mother). In 1588, Sixtus V reaffirmed a more rigid position, classifying even sterilization as homicide, and (in the decree *Effraenatam*) making excommunication a penalty of the universal church for the sin of abortion. A modification in 1591 again limited the provision to the case of the animated fetus, at either forty or ninety days. This legislation remained in effect until 1869, when Pius IX extended it to all direct abortion. Twenty years later, the Holy Office of the Vatican declared that neither craniotomy nor any other action to destroy the fetus directly would be permitted, even if without it both mother and child would die. Until that point, the exception to save maternal life had been debated by the theologians without receiving official condemnation. While theologians sought a balance of the value of the fetus with other values, especially the life of the mother, papal legislation moved toward a reinforcement of the abortion prohibition.

A moderating influence that continues today was exerted via the "principle of double effect." This principle, pertaining to acts that have both good and evil effects, permits a moral distinction between direct and indirect abortion. Only direct abortions are absolutely prohibited in official Roman Catholic teaching. Indirect (permitted) abortions are those operations that have as their primary effect the saving of the mother's life, with the death of the fetus a foreseen but not directly intended secondary effect. The classic example is the removal of the cancerous uterus of a woman who is pregnant. In this case, the death of the fetus is neither in itself the desired outcome of the intervention, nor even willed and caused as the means by which the woman's life is saved. The removal of the cancer, not the fetus, heals. Double effect may also be applied to the removal of a fallopian tube in the case of an ectopic pregnancy. The premise behind the justification of indirect abortion is that while the direct killing of an innocent human being is immoral, the woman's life is at least equal in value to that of her unborn offspring, so that she has no duty to assume serious risk to her own life in order to sustain the child.

Contemporary teaching

In his 1930 encyclical on marriage, *Casti connubii*, Pius XI affirmed the equal sacredness of mother and fetus, but condemned the destruction of the "innocent child" in the womb, who can in no way be considered an "unjust assailant." (The sticking point here, of continuing interest to moralists, is whether it is necessary to have an unjust intention to qualify as an unjust aggressor, or whether unintentionally posing an unjust danger to another is sufficient. Soldiers in war, for instance, may have noble personal intentions, yet validly be viewed by their opponents as unjust attackers.) The Second Vatican Council (*Gaudium et spes*, no. 51) referred to abortion and infanticide as "unspeakable crimes." The complex agenda of and challenges to current church teaching are well focused by the 1974 Vatican "Declaration on Abortion."

This document is a response to changed Western abortion laws, as well as to population measures in developing nations. Even as it resists these pressures, it adapts its message on abortion to cultural and legal contexts characterized by the emancipation of women and the need to control births. The document responds to the Western political value of free choice by asserting that "freedom of opinion" does not extend further than the rights of others, especially the right to life. It observes that while ensoulment has been debated historically, abortion has always been condemned. Most important, the document insists that human reason can and should recognize respect for human life as the most fundamental of all goods, and the condition of their realization. It sees modern science as confirming that human life begins with fertilization, though allowing that science can never definitively settle what is properly a philosophical question. Still, "it is objectively a grave sin to dare to risk murder" if there is doubt as to whether the fetus is fully a human person.

The "Declaration on Abortion" recognizes that pregnancy can pose serious burdens for the health and welfare of women, families, and children themselves. It advocates that individuals and nations exercise "responsible parenthood" by natural means of avoiding conception. It also exhorts "all those who are able to do so to lighten the burdens still crushing so many men and women, families and children, who are placed in situations to which in human terms there is no solution" (no. 23). It excludes abortion as an answer but also concludes that what is necessary "above all" is to "combat its causes" through "political action" (no. 26). The "Declaration" anticipates later efforts, notably by the U.S. episcopacy, to advocate moral consistency on killing, in that it contrasts growing protests against war and the death penalty with the social vindication of abortion.

From the standpoint of both the Vatican and the U.S. bishops, the unborn should be included within a greater respect for life in general, and be protected by more stringent social limits on killing of all kinds.

Critical debates

Among the debated questions regarding the Roman Catholic tradition on abortion are certainly the following. First, is it reasonable and scientifically sound to urge that the fetus be treated as a "person" from conception onward, especially if to do so will have dire consequences for the woman who bears it? While most Roman Catholic theologians assume a conservative attitude toward the value of prenatal life, not all accept that full value is present at the outset; rather, it increases in some developmental fashion, at least through the earlier stages. Several authors (Carol Tauer, 1984; Richard McCormick, 1984; Thomas Shannon and Allan Wolter, 1990) have pointed to the time of implantation, at about fourteen days, as a "line" after which individuality appears more settled (the possibility of "twinning" being past) and the chance of survival greatly magnified (for a discussion, see Cahill, 1993).

Second, is the equality of women, and the substantive legal, social, and material support for women and families enjoined by the "Declaration," really as high on the practical pro-life agenda of Roman Catholicism as is the enactment of punitive sanctions for abortion? A deep skepticism about whether this is so gives the "abortion rights" cry of many feminists its immense symbolic value in the struggle for gender and sexual equality. While some Catholic feminists believe that sexual self-determination and effective birth control is a better way to ensure women's liberation than recourse to a form of killing, other Catholic feminists insist that the choice to terminate pregnancy must be available to women as long as a patriarchal church and society identify women's roles as reproductive and domestic in order to constrain women's moral agency and to exclude women from the range of social participation available to men.

Third, even granted that the fetus has significant value, can and should restrictive abortion laws be kept in place—or reenacted in nations that have moved toward liberalization? John Courtney Murray (1960, ch. 7) distinguishes between law and morality. Morality in principle governs all human conduct, while law pertains to the "public order," the minimum moral requirements of healthy social functioning. Modern nations vary in the degree of restraint on abortion choice they see public order as requiring (see Glendon, 1987). Abortion policy debates, especially in more lenient systems like that of the United States, challenge Roman Catholicism to reshape the social consensus about the value of the unborn. Any legislation not backed by a consensus favoring enforcement will lead both to disrespect for the law and to the proliferation of unregulated extralegal alternatives. A precondition for a less permissive abortion consensus is the creation both of avenues other than "abortion rights" for the exercise of women's social and personal freedoms, and of social supports encouraging women and families to raise children.

A major point of debate within Roman Catholicism is the level of legal compromise acceptable to those who would accord the fetus more value than does the current consensus. Following the principle that law and morality are not coterminous, some argue that a policy that encourages early abortion and restricts it to "hard cases" (e.g., threat to life or health, rape, incest, serious birth defects) could command enough broad support to justify it as a practical advance in the limitation of abortion. Advocates of a more stringent position insist that the full weight of the church's moral authority be marshaled behind a policy that would outlaw abortion altogether.

Finally, can the church credibly defend its anti-abortion position while disallowing the most effective forms of birth control? It is relevant to this question that many nations' aspirations to economic and cultural prosperity are plagued by limited freedom for women in marriage and family, and by increasing overpopulation. In the industrialized countries, the abortion controversy tends to focus on individual rights, either of the fetus or of the mother, with Roman Catholic proponents framing the issue in terms of a legally protectable right to life. In such nations, the church tends to address itself to the absolutization of private choice over what it sees as human life, and the trivialization of the abortion decision as it becomes a substitute for sexual responsibility and contraception.

However, the Roman Catholic church is an international organization, with a substantial or growing membership in, for example, Latin America, the Philippines, and Africa. In many nations, the question of women's freedom to combine family with public vocation as the context for the abortion debate is overshadowed by dire poverty; the inaccessibility of education, adequate employment, and health care; the ambiguous economic implications of a large family in rural, agricultural settings; and the radically disadvantaged position of girls and women within the family in some traditional cultures. Especially in the absence of ready access to contraception, abortion may appear to such women, to families, and even to government agencies to be a desperate but necessary means of controlling fertility. As the 1974 "Declaration on Abortion" indicates, the global Roman Catholic position on abortion must go beyond the condemnation of abortion as murder to address personal and social situations in which abortion

appears as the only viable answer to deprivation or oppression.

LISA SOWLE CAHILL

Directly related to this article are the companion articles in this section, JEWISH PERSPECTIVES, PROTESTANT PERSPECTIVES, *and* ISLAMIC PERSPECTIVES, *and the articles in the other sections in this entry:* MEDICAL PERSPECTIVES, *and* CONTEMPORARY ETHICAL AND LEGAL ASPECTS, *articles on* CONTEMPORARY ETHICAL PERSPECTIVES, *and* LEGAL AND REGULATORY ISSUES. *Also directly related are the entries* ROMAN CATHOLICISM; POPULATION ETHICS, *section on* RELIGIOUS TRADITIONS, *article on* ROMAN CATHOLIC PERSPECTIVES; NATURAL LAW; *and* DOUBLE EFFECT. *For a further discussion of topics mentioned in this article, see the entries* FERTILITY CONTROL, *articles on* SOCIAL ISSUES, ETHICAL ISSUES, *and* LEGAL AND REGULATORY ISSUES; LAW AND MORALITY; LIFE; POPULATION POLICIES, *section on* STRATEGIES OF FERTILITY CONTROL, *article on* CHANGES IN ATTITUDE AND CULTURE; *and* WOMEN, *article on* HISTORICAL AND CROSS-CULTURAL PERSPECTIVES. *Other relevant material may be found under the entries* FETUS, *articles on* HUMAN DEVELOPMENT FROM FERTILIZATION TO BIRTH, *and* PHILOSOPHICAL AND ETHICAL ISSUES; MATERNAL–FETAL RELATIONSHIP, *article on* ETHICAL ISSUES; *and* PERSON. *See also the* APPENDIX (CODES, OATHS, AND DIRECTIVES RELATED TO BIOETHICS), *section* II: ETHICAL DIRECTIVES FOR THE PRACTICE OF MEDICINE, ETHICAL AND RELIGIOUS DIRECTIVES FOR CATHOLIC HEALTH FACILITIES *of the* UNITED STATES CATHOLIC CONFERENCE, *and selections from the* HEALTH CARE ETHICS GUIDE *of the* CATHOLIC HEALTH ASSOCIATION OF CANADA.

Bibliography

ABBOTT, WALTER M., ed. 1966. *The Documents of Vatican II: All Sixteen Texts Promulgated by the Ecumenical Council, 1962–1965.* New York: America Press.

ASHLEY, BENEDICT, and O'ROURKE, KEVIN D. 1978. *Health Care Ethics: A Theological Analysis.* St. Louis: Catholic Hospital Association.

CAHILL, LISA SOWLE. 1993. "The Embryo and the Fetus: New Moral Contexts." *Theological Studies* 54, no. 1:124–142.

CONNERY, JOHN R. 1977. *Abortion: The Development of the Roman Catholic Perspective.* Chicago: Loyola University Press.

GLENDON, MARY ANN. 1987. *Abortion and Divorce in Western Law: American Failures, European Challenges.* Cambridge, Mass.: Harvard University Press.

GRISEZ, GERMAIN G. 1970. *Abortion: The Myths, the Realities, and the Arguments.* New York: Corpus.

JUNG, PATRICIA BEATTIE, and SHANNON, THOMAS A., eds. 1988. *Abortion and Catholicism: The American Debate.* New York: Crossroad.

McCORMICK, RICHARD A. 1984. *Health and Medicine in the Catholic Tradition: Tradition in Transition*. New York: Crossroad.

MURRAY, JOHN COURTNEY. 1960. *We Hold These Truths: Catholic Reflections on the American Proposition*. New York: Sheed & Ward.

NOONAN, JOHN T., JR., ed. 1970. *The Morality of Abortion: Legal and Historical Perspectives*. Cambridge, Mass.: Harvard University Press.

PIUS XI, POPE. 1930. *Casti Connubii*. In *Matrimony*, pp. 219–291. Translated by Michael J. Byrnes. Papal Teachings Series. Selected and arranged by the Benedictine monks of Abbaye Saint-Pierre de Solesmes. Boston: St. Paul Editions, 1963.

SHANNON, THOMAS A., and WOLTER, ALLAN B. 1990. "Reflections on the Moral Status of the Pre-Embryo." *Theological Studies* 51, no. 4:603–626.

TAUER, CAROL A. 1984. "The Tradition of Probabilism and the Moral Status of the Early Embryo." *Theological Studies* 45, no. 1:3–33.

VATICAN CONGREGATION FOR THE DOCTRINE OF THE FAITH. 1974. "Declaration on Abortion." *Origins* 4:386–392.

C. PROTESTANT PERSPECTIVES

Reviews of the history of Protestant teaching on abortion focus most often upon specific comments regarding abortion in the writings of leaders of the various church reform movements in European Christianity beginning in the sixteenth century. Several of the most effectual Reformation leaders, including Martin Luther (1483–1546) and John Calvin (1509–1564), were powerful both in reconceiving church practice and in articulating reformulations of Christian theological and ethical teaching. Consequently, for many of their followers and spiritual heirs, their teaching has remained uniquely authoritative in discerning Protestant truth claims. The formal criteria for discerning Christian truth proposed by these reformers, however, is best characterized as privileging the role of Christian scripture (usually referred to by Protestants as the Old and New Testaments) in adjudicating doctrinal and moral disputes. This primacy of scripture as theological and moral norm also characterized the teaching of most other sixteenth-century reformers, including the theological leaders of the many Anabaptist movements.

Since the sixteenth century, all dissent from authoritative Roman Catholic teaching and practice, including newly emergent Christian movements, receives the label "Protestant." The rapidly growing Pentecostal movements in Latin America, indigenous Christian movements in Asia, and the African indigenous churches that are now numerically preponderant among Christians on that continent all fall under this rubric. As a result, extreme caution needs to be exercised in characterizing "Protestant" moral teaching in any contem-

porary moral dilemma. Even when interpreters are familiar with very diverse Protestant cultural traditions, those who identify themselves as Protestants interpret the meaning of conformity to scriptural norms in a wide variety of ways, and reveal wide differences in biblical "hermeneutics," or principles of interpretation, of sacred texts. The diversity of hermeneutical options available accounts in part for the complexity of Protestant voices on abortion today.

Before identifying contemporary Protestant hermeneutical diversity and therefore the range of existing contemporary Protestant viewpoints on abortion, it is important to clarify the cultural roots of Protestantism that shape them.

Early Protestant views of abortion

Martin Luther's and John Calvin's theological and moral reforms were shaped by their reconceptions of both the meaning of Christian life and Christian ritual practice. Neither could be said to have proposed shifts in the foundational notions of human nature embedded in late medieval Christianity. Traditional notions of human nature, including gender and human species reproduction, were not in dispute and did not shift at the time of the Reformation. What is notable among Protestant reformers is the paucity of comment on any questions about human sexuality and reproduction, including abortion. Martin Luther, a prolific preacher and writer, did not mention abortion at all. Had he done so, he likely would have presumed its moral wrongness because he was educated as an Augustinian monk and was learned in the available theological texts of the period, including especially *Sentences* by the twelfth-century theologian Peter Lombard, which contained collations of opinions on abortion by earlier theologians. The lists included the judgments of many who associated abortion with sexual immorality, especially with adultery, and condemned the practice.

John Calvin also knew this authoritative tradition that explicitly condemned abortion, as his commentaries on Gen. 38:10 make clear. His remarks on Exod. 21:22 further attest that he believed abortion to be wrong morally. Modern critical biblical exegetes agree that Exod. 22:21 is the only text in Christian scripture that explicitly refers to abortion, albeit to abortion that occurs because of injury to a pregnant woman. The issue in this passage was not elective abortion. Even so, Calvin used the occasion of comment on this text to make known his view that the fetus is already a person, a matter the text does not address.

On gender, sexuality, and reproduction, these reformers maintained continuity with earlier traditions. Both Luther and Calvin also followed what they took to be early Christian theological consensus, that divine ensoulment (i.e., the point of spiritual animation of human beings by God) of human life occurs at conception, though not all the Protestant theologians who followed them agreed. Modern conservative historical interpreters construe Calvin and Luther's views on this point as confirming their own current belief that Protestant teaching agrees with modern papal teaching, namely, that full human life occurs at conception. Caution needs to be exercised here, however. Although the majority of Protestant theologians followed the view that ensoulment occurred when the "seed" was planted in utero, their perspectives were not developed in relation to questions about human gestation. To argue that these views speak to the value of fetal life is misleading, since their opinions were developed as aspects of the theological debate about sin and salvation, and not in relation to modern embryological understanding. In any case, Protestant ritual practice suggests that commonsense norms were in fact applied to actual fetuses. Protestants, like Roman Catholics, did not practice baptism in relation to miscarriages or aborted fetuses.

Modern Protestant views on abortion

Specific comment on abortion is rare in most Reformation traditions until the twentieth century. Perhaps in deference to the lack of biblical discussion, most reformers considered matters regarding the morality of abortion, like matters governing all sexual and reproductive behavior, to be ordered by human rational discernment. They were issues of "natural morality" rather than of revealed truth. Despite emphasis on recovering the meaning of Christian biblical tradition, Lutherans, Calvinists, and Anglicans (post-Roman Church of England adherents) maintained the view, long-standing in western Christianity, that much moral knowledge, including the order of human sexuality and reproduction, falls within the purview of "natural" human knowledge, that is, they are matters for rational deliberation and discernment. Contrary to the trend of modern Protestant fundamentalist biblicism in discussions of abortion, most Protestant traditions tended to embrace a type of reasoning that accepted human rational (and therefore "scientific") data as relevant to these moral judgments on these issues. The Anabaptists were often exceptions methodologically, however. They sought guidance on moral issues exclusively from scripture without reference to other sources. However, Anabaptists also stressed freedom of conscience in deliberating moral dilemmas, and often resisted fixed ecclesiastical standards on questions such as abortion. Not surprisingly, contemporary Anabaptist heirs often oppose with great adamance state-prescribed policies making abortion illegal.

It is not too much to say that Protestantism possessed neither an explicitly developed tradition of moral reasoning about abortion nor any elaborated body of teaching on the ethics of so-called medical practice until well into the nineteenth century. Reproduction in Protestant communities, as in all premodern communities, was shaped by female cultural practice and midwifery until at least the very late nineteenth century. Contemporary cultural historians agree that nearly all female subcultures encouraged some means of fertility control, and that most took recourse to abortifacients (substances that induce abortions) in extreme cases. Such methods were primitive and dangerous, however, and documentation regarding the range and scope of their use is all but nonexistent. The fact that women, and not men, both comprised and knew the culture of reproduction probably limited public awareness in prevailing practices. Knowledge about available interventions in pregnancies may not have been widely shared, and such knowledge may have been quite rare among male theologians until the "medicalizing" of pregnancy and reproduction in the twentieth century. In the nineteenth century, male medical practitioners increasingly attempted to discredit midwifery, frequently on the grounds that midwives practiced abortion, but Protestant clergy in the United States showed great reluctance to support such efforts.

The major impact of the Reformation in shaping Protestant attitudes on abortion is rarely mentioned in traditional historiography. The most important influence of Protestantism in the abortion debate arose from the changes in spiritual practice initiated by Reformation Christianity; these changes in turn led to a powerful shift in how socialization into Christian faith took place. Initiation into Christianity moved from a locus in the church-based penitential system to the Christian family, which gradually became the basic social unit of Christian piety. Protestant spirituality was pervasively formed by this embrace of the family as the proper site for transmission of both faith and morals. The change engendered by the Reformation overturned celibacy not only as the proper norm for clerical life but also as the norm of optimal Christian piety. The Reformation movements made the sexually monogamous, procreation-centered family both the center of their basic community and their strongest metaphor for divine blessing. For Calvinists, explicitly from the outset, and for Lutherans, Anglicans, and Anabaptists more slowly, adherence to this form of social practice came to be taught as a Christian duty. Parents were to oversee their children's successful entrance into procreative-centered marriage literally as a mandate of faith.

This shift in the structure of Christian sociology, more than any change in explicit moral teaching, shaped subsequent moral sensibilities toward abortion among Protestants. This new emphasis on the sacerdotal character of the family reinforced the appeal of Protestant Christianity in traditionalist non-European cultures as well. Both ancient Hebraic and Jewish and pre-Protestant Christian sources had at times equated procreation and biological fertility or fruitfulness as signs of divine blessing, and such pronatalist sentiments had had some influence in earlier Christian attitudes toward abortion. However, the rise of Protestantism made such sensibilities powerful in European cultures and central to modern Christian moral sensibility about reproduction. This portended a deep suspicion regarding elective abortion when the practice became widespread and safe.

Many modern Protestants arrive at their judgments about the morality of abortion from a deep-seated sense that any pregnancy is intrinsically a sign of divine blessing and that to deny this is impious. So deep does the equation of fertility and divine blessing run in Protestant cultures that western Christianity itself has strongly reinforced traditional patriarchal norms that female "nature" is centered in and fulfilled only through maternity. Today, traditional Protestant cultures (those untouched by religious pluralism) tend to experience any weighing of questions about the status of fetal life as expressing a "secular" or "antireligious" mindset.

Despite the strong pronatalist disposition of traditional Protestant spirituality, however, critical historians have also noted a certain tension between Protestant teaching on abortion and Protestant pastoral practice. Even in traditionalist Protestant cultures, where moral and theological discourse is unequivocal in condemning abortion, pastoral practice is frequently far less censorious. Scattered evidence exists that Protestant priests, pastors, and elders often treated those who had abortions or administered them with a surprising degree of compassion or even leniency. There is no evidence that the practice of abortion was deemed "an unforgivable sin," as some ancient church canons insisted, or that abortion was equated with "murder" or "unjustified killing." Even among contemporary Protestant fundamentalists, historians have observed this tension between formal moral condemnation and more permissive ecclesiastical practice. Theological and moral condemnation notwithstanding, noncelibate clergy may be in touch with many of the concrete conditions and dilemmas of pregnancy and reproduction that shape women's lives. In any case, the general stance of Protestant traditionalism and of the newer, postmodernist biblical hermeneutics is toward a degree of pastoral compassion, even if abortion is starkly condemned at the formal level.

All current available data suggest that the rate of recourse to abortion among women who are part of Christian communities that formally condemn abortion—Protestant traditionalist, Protestant fundamentalist, or Roman Catholic—is at least as great as it is among women who come from liberal Protestant and Jewish communities or who are nonpracticing with regard to religion.

The most typical contemporary Protestant attitude toward abortion remains a traditionalist, pronatalist negativity toward the practice, with a reluctant recognition that abortions do occur frequently, even within the Protestant communities of faith. Such cautious negativity is maintained without strong, elaborated moral justification, chiefly because the strong cultural ethos of the existing family-centered sociology of the Protestant churches gives this view such plausibility. Traditionalist consensus tends to break down, however, whenever Protestant communities are confronted with debates shaped by conflicts within the wider culture or from newly articulate dissent within these Protestant communities themselves. Such debate is now ongoing in all churches rooted in the continental Reformation. For the most part the debate reflects the divisions in biblical hermeneutics already mentioned.

Three newer hermeneutical positions appear in the abortion debate. First, there is a quite unprecedented biblical fundamentalist hermeneutic asserting itself in many Protestant cultural contexts. This new fundamentalism is developed particularly to resist change in issues involving gender, sexuality, family, and reproduction. On all of these issues, restoration of a premodern interpretation of sex/gender and the reproductive system is the primary goal. Human gender and sexual identity, this approach insists, are rooted in "nature" and in "divine decree" central to the presumed "biblical" message. Using both the language of natural law and tradition of the mandate of divine revelation as synonymous and as equally legitimated by scripture, the new fundamentalists contend that the essence of the biblical witness is the biological-religious "givenness" of male/female nature and the revealing of the proper "telos," or end, of human sexuality. Abortion is unthinkable, a violation of all of the norms of faith and morals. This hermeneutic aims to make even the discussion of abortion taboo in Protestant theological and moral discourses, to make it literally unthinkable. This approach tends to drive from the field several generations of historical-critical study by Protestant theological liberals. Previously, liberal biblical scholarship had successfully persuaded interpreters of the Bible within mainline Protestantism that interpretation of scriptural texts had to be guided by awareness of different historical times and variations among cultures. Liberals recognized that biblical worldviews do not presuppose modern ideas about the origin and nature of the universe and its inhabitants. Such considerations undergirding previous Protestant biblical interpretation, once widely accepted, are often forgotten in the wake of the force of the new fundamentalist hermeneutic.

Second, although the new fundamentalism gains force in Protestant communities, most "oldline" Protestant denominations (rooted in Europe) remain informed by historical-critical methods of scriptural interpretation and continue to speak in a voice consistent with conclusions of the earlier liberal biblical hermeneutic. Broadly speaking, these churches acknowledge that biogenetic and other scientific knowledge must be given its due in deliberating the morality of abortion. Most concede that decisions to have abortions are justified in some cases and can be consistent with biblical faithfulness. This casts several major Protestant denominations on the side of the public policy debate that supports limited legality of abortions. Although several of the "old line" denominations have been strongly pressed by fundamentalists and traditionalists in their ranks to shift to antiabortion public-policy positions, Lutherans, Anglicans, Methodists, Presbyterians, and United Church of Christ denominations, among others, have maintained their public positions. Discussion of what may constitute "justifiable reasons" for choosing abortion is decidedly underdeveloped in such Protestant communions. A strong consensus prevails that supports abortions in cases of pregnancies due to sexual violence (rape and incest); in cases where the life or physical health of the mother is at stake; and, perhaps, in cases where prospective parents lack the spiritual and physical resources to rear an additional child. There are also important historical reasons why old-line liberal Protestant communities place a strong emphasis on "responsible parenthood," but that story is outside the scope of this article. This too is an important and largely unexamined chapter in understanding Protestant views on both family planning and abortion.

Finally, in nearly all contemporary Protestant communities/cultures, another hermeneutic for interpreting the Christian abortion tradition is emerging. It may be called a "liberationist" or even a "profeminist liberationist" principle of interpretation. Although it is still a decided minority position within formalized Protestant theological-moral discourse, this hermeneutic is influencing many, especially women. It calls upon Protestant theology and ethics to reformulate moral and religious judgments with special attention to concerns for women's well-being and in recognition that Christian teaching on gender, sexuality, and reproduction is embedded in a wider system of social control of women's lives. Acknowledging internal contradictions within scripture, a liberation hermeneutic refuses authority to culturally repressive male-supremacist readings of biblical texts and postscriptural theological interpretations. Like liberals, proponents of the emerging liberation hermeneutic represent a spectrum of convictions about what reasons might justify specific acts of abortion, but strongly con-

cur that the Protestant Christian moral voice must actively advocate broad-based social change to enable women to shape their reproductive capacity. They contend that the moral evaluation of abortion must not be predicated on discourse that obscures women's full standing as moral agents or that fails to include realism about the historical pressures surrounding biological reproduction in women's lives. Among Protestants, only Unitarian/Universalists have adopted such a hermeneutic officially.

The contesting voices characterized here are most visible and most intense within Protestant Christian communities in the United States. However, analogous dynamics are at work in Protestant communities in other areas of the globe, as they are within Roman Catholic, Orthodox, and other religious communities. The struggle over which hermeneutical voice shall prevail in Protestant teaching on abortion remains unresolved.

BEVERLY WILDUNG HARRISON

Directly related to this article are the companion articles in this section, JEWISH PERSPECTIVES, ROMAN CATHOLIC PERSPECTIVES, *and* ISLAMIC PERSPECTIVES, *and the articles in the other sections in this entry:* MEDICAL PERSPECTIVES, *and* CONTEMPORARY ETHICAL AND LEGAL ASPECTS, *articles on* CONTEMPORARY ETHICAL PERSPECTIVES, *and* LEGAL AND REGULATORY ISSUES. *Also directly related are the entries* PROTESTANTISM; NATURAL LAW; *and* ETHICS, *article on* RELIGION AND MORALITY. *For further discussion of topics mentioned in this article, see the entries* BODY; FAMILY; FETUS; LIFE; *and* WOMEN. *Other relevant material may be found under the entries* AUTONOMY; FEMINISM; JUSTICE; RESPONSIBILITY; *and* SEXUAL IDENTITY.

Bibliography

BROWN, PETER R. L. 1988. *The Body and Society: Men, Women, and Sexual Renunciation in Early Christianity.* New York: Columbia University Press.

COHEN, SHERRILL, and TAUB, NADINE, eds. 1989. *Reproductive Laws for the 1990s.* Clifton, N.J.: Humana.

CONNERY, JOHN R. 1977. *Abortion: The Development of the Roman Catholic Perspective.* Chicago: Loyola University.

GORDON, LINDA. 1976. *Woman's Body, Woman's Right: A Social History of Birth Control in America.* New York: Grossman.

GROBSTEIN, CLIFFORD. 1988. *Science and the Unborn: Choosing Human Futures.* New York: Basic Books.

HARRISON, BEVERLY WILDUNG. 1983. *Our Right to Choose: Toward a New Ethic of Abortion.* Boston: Beacon Press.

JONES, JACQUELINE. 1986. *Labor of Love, Labor of Sorrow: Black Women, Work, and the Family. From Slavery to the Present.* New York: Vintage.

KENNEDY, DAVID M. 1970. *Birth Control in America: The Career of Margaret Sanger.* New Haven, Conn.: Yale University Press.

McLAREN, ANGUS. 1990. *A History of Contraception from Antiquity to the Present Day.* Oxford: Basil Blackwell.

MOHR, JAMES. 1979. *Abortion in America: The Origins and Evolution of Public Policy: 1800–1900.* Cambridge, Mass.: Harvard University Press.

NOONAN, JOHN T., JR., ed. 1970. *The Morality of Abortion: Legal and Historical Perspectives.* Cambridge, Mass.: Harvard University Press.

OLASKY, MARVIN. 1992. *Abortion Rites: A Social History of Abortion in America.* Wheaton, Ill.: Crossways.

RAPP, RAYNA, and SCHNEIDER, JANE, eds. 1995. *Articulating Hidden Histories: Exploring the Influence of Eric R. Wolf.* Berkeley: University of California Press.

RICH, ADRIENNE C. 1976. *Of Woman Born: Motherhood as Experience and Institution.* New York: W. W. Norton.

ROUSSELLE, ALINE. 1988. *Porneia: On Desire and the Body in Antiquity.* New York: Basil Blackwell.

D. ISLAMIC PERSPECTIVES

Since ancient times every human society has dealt with the issue of abortion. The way each treats the issue has depended on the way each views fundamental questions of individual and societal life, such as the meaning and sanctity of human life, sexuality and gender relations, the role of marriage and family, the meaning of human freedom, and the related issues of rights and responsibilities of the individual.

The roles of medicine and law in the Islamic debate on abortion

Islam's response to abortion during the fourteen centuries of its existence has been documented mostly in the jurisprudential works of its doctors of law and the medical writings of its physicians. Islamic perspectives on abortion have been shaped directly by both its theology and its revealed law (Shari'a). Because of the centrality of the latter as a practical guide in the religious and spiritual life of Muslims, however, they depend heavily on the deliberations and ethico-legal decrees (*fatwās*) of experts whenever practical problems arise in society. The main practical role of theology is to provide the necessary spiritual and intellectual framework within which ethico-legal debates are pursued.

Since the Divine Law of Islam refuses to make a separation between law and ethics, the traditional Muslim jurist (*faqih*) is at once an ethicist and a legal expert. The physician's duty in matters concerning abortion is to provide medical advice and recommendations befitting each individual case, as Islamic law generally permits abortion on medical and health grounds up to a certain stage of pregnancy. Close collaboration between medicine and law in Islam has generated a well-developed branch of Islamic jurisprudence that deals with many biomedical issues, including contraception and abortion.

In all cases of abortion, the physician is an important witness. The idea of the testimony of a trustworthy physician is well known in Islam, since Islamic law puts great emphasis on the idea of a trustworthy witness, whom it always defines in terms of believing in God and having a good moral character. The close rapport between medicine and law in Islam is further strengthened by the fact that this religion has produced a sizeable number of jurists who either practiced medicine or at least possessed a sound general knowledge of the subject. Ibn Rushd (known by the Latin name Averröes, d. 1198), Ibn al-Nafīs (d. 1288), the discoverer of the minor circulation of the blood, Ibn Ḥazm (d. 1064), Fakhr al-Dīn Rāzī (d. 1209), and in more recent times, Ḥasan al-'Aṭṭar al-Khalwatī (d. 1835), a rector of the prestigious al-Azhar University in Cairo, were some of the most famous jurists–medical practitioners. Al-Shāfi'ī (d. 820), the founder of one of the four Sunni schools of law, is credited in traditional sources with knowledge of medicine.

Conversely, there have been many Muslim physicians who were well versed with the philosophy of the Shari'a and the ethical teachings of the Qur'an and hadiths (i.e., recorded sayings, behavior, and actions attributed to the Prophet, and in the case of the Shi'ite branch of Islam, also to the Imams, their foremost spiritual leaders), but who were never recognized as jurists in the technical sense of the term. The most famous of these was Ibn Sīnā (d. 1037). These physicians were generally knowledgeable in embryology. As scholars of natural philosophy, of which psychology is a part, many of these physicians also developed a comprehensive theory of the soul that includes a treatment of the problem of identifying the stage of pregnancy when the ensoulment of the body takes place in the womb. The connection between embryology and psychology is therefore of great practical interest to Islamic law.

At ensoulment a fetus attains the legal status of a human being, with all the rights accorded by the Shari'a. Although Muslim jurists rely substantially on the Qur'an and prophetic medicine for their knowledge of embryology, they also demonstrate a positive attitude toward the scientific embryology of the philosopher-physicians, since they do not see any basic contradiction between the two sources.

The theological context

The abortion debate in Islam takes place in a particular religious environment created by the divinely revealed teachings of the religion. These teachings are accepted by Muslims as sacred and immutable and have remained unquestioned in the debate over the centuries. The most important of these teachings concerns the meaning and purpose of human life.

Islam teaches that human life is sacred because its origin is none other than God, who is the Sacred and the ultimate source of all that is sacred. Human beings are God's noblest creatures by virtue of the fact that he has breathed his spirit into every human body, male and female, at a certain stage of its embryological development. This breathing of the divine spirit into the human fetus is called its ensoulment; it confers on the human species the status of theomorphic beings. Islam shares with Judaism and Christianity the teaching that God has created humans in his own image.

Islam teaches that a human is not just a mind–body or soul–body entity that has come into existence through an entirely physical, historical, or evolutionary process. He or she is also a spirit whose reality transcends the physical space–time complex and even the realm of the mind. This spiritual substance present in each human individual, to which Muslim philosophers and scientists refer as the most excellent part of the rational soul and which has cognitive powers to the extent of being able to know itself, God, and the spiritual realm in general, is what distinguishes humans from the rest of earthly creatures.

The Qur'an refers more than once to the ensoulment of the human body, almost always in the context both of describing God's creation of Adam, the first ancestor of the human race, and of affirming the superiority of humans over the rest of creation, including the angels (for example, at 15:28–30). There is also a more specific reference to the ensoulment of the human fetus that is made as part of its description of the process of pregnancy and birth. The Qur'anic passage quoted perhaps most often in the abortion debate is, "We [i.e., God and his cosmic agents] have created man out of an extraction of clay [the origin of semen]; then we turn it into semen and settle it in a firm receptacle. We then turn semen into a clot [literally, something which clings] which we then fashion into a lump of chewed flesh. Then we fashion the chewed flesh into bones and we clothe the bones with intact flesh. Then we develop out of it another creature. So blessed be God, the best of creators" (23:12–14).

Both ancient and modern commentators on the Qur'an generally agree that the last stage in the formation of the human fetus as indicated by the phrase "develop out of it another creature" mentioned in this Qur'anic passage refers to the ensoulment of the fetus, resulting in its transformation from animal into human life. As to exactly when the ensoulment of the fetus takes place, the Qur'an does not provide any information. The prophetic hadiths contain a detailed periodi-

zation of each of the different stages of fetal growth mentioned in the Qur'an. In theology as in law, matters on which the Qur'an is either silent or held to be less explicit than the hadith, the latter takes a decisive role. Thus it is the testimony of the hadith concerning the ensoulment of the fetus that has proved decisive in the formulation of Islamic theological doctrine concerning abortion.

According to one hadith, organ differentiation in the fetus does not begin to take place until six weeks after the time of fertilization. According to another, an angel who is a divine agent of ensoulment of the fetus is sent to breathe a distinctively human soul into it after 120 days of conception have passed. In his commentary on the Qur'anic verse on human reproduction cited above, basing his views on hadiths as well as on the findings of physicians, Jalāl al-Dīn al-Suyutī (d. 1505), an encyclopedist and author of a popular work on prophetic medicine, declared, "All wise men are agreed that no soul is breathed in until after the fourth month" (Elgood, 1962, p. 240).

If God has given a theomorphic nature to human persons and has created them in the best of molds (Qur'an, 95:4), having unique faculties not enjoyed by creatures of other species, it is not without a noble purpose. According to the Qur'an, human beings have been created to know God and to be God's servants and representatives on Earth in accordance with his own wishes as revealed to all branches of the human family through his prophets and messengers. One of the six fundamental articles of the Islamic creed is belief in a future life—not in this world of sensual experience and mental images, but in another world whose space–time complex is entirely different from the one we presently experience.

In the Qur'anic view, human life does not end with death. In reality, death is only a passage between two parts of a continuous life, namely the present and the posthumous. How we fare in that future life depends on how we conduct ourselves in this present life. By leading a spiritually, ethically, and morally healthy life in this world, we will attain salvation and prosperity in the after-death life. The previously cited verse on human conception and birth is immediately preceded by a reference to life in paradise and immediately followed by a statement on the certainty of death and resurrection. Muslims understand from this and other verses that there is a grand divine scheme for humans that they have no right to disturb. On the contrary, they are to participate fully in this cosmic scheme as helpers of God in both their capacities as his servants and representatives.

Human reproduction, birth, and death are part of this grand divine scheme. Indeed, the Qur'anic view is that there is even a preconception phase of human existence. The Qur'an refers to a covenant between God and all the human souls in the spiritual world before the creation of this world. God addressed the souls collectively, asking them "Am I not your Lord?" Without hesitation they all bore witness to his Lordship, thus implying that God-consciousness is in the very nature of the human soul.

The general implication of the Islamic teachings on the meaning and purpose of life for reproduction and abortion is clear. Although reproduction is not explicitly commanded in the Qur'an, it does appear to be encouraged. A few hadiths are explicit in their encouragement of procreation. The most popular is the hadith that says that, on the Day of Resurrection, the Prophet would be proud of the numbers of his community compared with other communities and that he admonishes his followers to reproduce and increase in number.

One can say with certainty that the general religious climate that prevailed in Muslim societies throughout the ages even until modern times is one in which procreation is encouraged and abortion very much discouraged. Cyril Elgood observes that "in Islamic countries moral approval of the practice of abortion was not readily given" (Elgood, 1970) although procurement of abortion, of which there were many cases, was not necessarily considered a criminal act. When he further says that "it is almost universally recognized by civilized nations that abortion is to be practiced only on the rarest of occasions" (Elgood, 1970, p. 240), the majority of Muslims would make the spontaneous response that this is precisely the Islamic view of abortion.

If Islam encourages the propagation of the human species, then it also insists that every human life be given due protection. (Abortion, however, is not considered the ending of a human life unless ensoulment of the fetus has occurred.) One of the fundamental goals of Islamic law is the protection of human life. Islam takes a serious view of the taking of human lives (except in cases that have been legitimized by the Divine Law itself) and of all acts injurious to life. One of the five basic human rights enshrined in the Shari'a is the protection by the state of every human life. The Qur'an asserts that "whosoever kills a [single] human for other than murder or other than the corruption of the earth [i.e. war], it is as though he has killed all humankind and whosoever has saved one human, it is as though he has saved all humankind" (5:35). The phrase "other than murder" in this verse refers to justifiable homicide, like self-defense and capital punishment as prescribed under the Islamic law of equality (qisas).

The Islamic view of marriage and sexuality also casts a long shadow on the abortion debate. Human reproduction should take place within the framework of the sacred institution of marriage. Islam describes marriage as "half of religion" and strongly condemns sexual relations outside of marriage. The main purpose of the institution of marriage is the preservation of the human species, although Islam also recognizes the spiritual, psychological, and socioeconomic functions of marriage. That there is indeed much more to marriage than just procreation or sexual fulfillment has been amply clarified by many classical Muslim thinkers.

One of the best treatises on the wisdom of marriage in all its dimensions was composed by the prominent jurist, theologian, and Sufi, al-Ghazzālī (d. 1111). This highly influential religious scholar and critic of Aristotelian philosophy defends the permissibility of married couples' practicing contraception on the ground of their need to secure a happy marriage. He goes so far as to hold that a man who fears that his wife's bearing children might affect her health or good looks and that he might therefore begin to dislike her, should refrain from having children (Rahman, 1987). Al-Ghazzālī's view clearly suggests that procreation is not the sole purpose of marriage.

Islamic discussion of abortion is always related to the question of the rights and responsibilities of both the husband and the wife. One of the major issues in contemporary debate on abortion in the West concerns the rights of women to procure abortion. Islam answers the question not only by appealing to its theological doctrines on the meaning and scope of human rights and responsibilities, but also to its religious theory of conception based on revealed data and hadith teachings. The Qur'an stresses the idea that everything in the heavens and on earth belongs to God. Metaphysically speaking, humans do not own anything, not even their own bodies. It is God who has apportioned rights and responsibilities to males and females, husbands and wives, fathers and mothers. Men and women in Islam obtain their mutual rights through the arbitration of the Divine Law.

In general, Muslim jurists pay great attention to women's rights in the practice of contraception and the procurement of abortion. In the words of Basim F. Musallam, "One can speak of a classical Islamic opinion on contraception generally and consistently adopted in Islamic jurisprudence, regardless of school. This classical opinion was the sanction of coitus interruptus with a free woman provided she gave her permission" (Musallam, 1983). A "free woman" is a nonslave and married. Islamic jurisprudence treats coitus interruptus under three categories, namely (1) with a wife who is a free woman; (2) with a wife who is a slave of another party; and (3) with a man's own slave or concubine. All schools of Islamic law consider coitus interruptus permissible. The majority of them insist on the woman's consent only if she belongs to the first category, since Islamic law recognizes her basic rights to children and sexual fulfillment. No permission is needed from a slave woman. In the case of abortion, the Hanafis granted the pregnant woman the right to abort even without her husband's permission provided she has a valid reason in the eyes of the Shari'a. (The Hanafis are followers of the Islamic school of law founded by the prominent jurist Abu Hanifah and are mainly found in Turkey and the Indian subcontinent.) The Qur'anic teaching that children are not created of the man's semen alone, but of both parents together, has a bearing also on Muslim discussion of the mutual rights of husband and wife in the permissibility of abortion.

Islamic law and abortion

The Islamic view of fetal development based on the Qur'an and hadith is central to the Muslim arguments on abortion. All Muslim jurists believe that the fetus becomes a human being after the fourth month of pregnancy. Consequently, abortion is prohibited after that stage (Musallam, 1983). However, the jurists differ in their views concerning the permissibility of abortion during the first four months of pregnancy, that is, the period prior to the ensoulment of the fetus.

Jurists of the Hanafi school of law allowed abortion to be performed at any time during the four-month period. A special document compiled by 500 Hanafi 'ulamā' (religious scholars), decrees that "the woman has the right to adopt some method of obtaining abortion if quickening of the fetus has not occurred, which happens after 120 days of conception" (Abedin, 1977, p. 121).

Most Maliki jurists, by contrast, prohibit abortion absolutely. Their main argument is that although the fetus does not become a human until after its ensoulment, one should not tamper with the natural process of conception once the semen has settled in the womb, since the semen is destined for ensoulment. A minority of Maliki jurists, however, allow abortion of a fetus up to forty days old. Other schools of Islamic jurisprudence, among both Sunnis and Shi'ites, agree with the Hanafis in their tolerance of abortion, although again they differ on the specifics.

It is important to emphasize the fact that there is a specific theological and ethico-legal context in which abortion has been permitted in Islam. Muslim jurists classify all human acts into five categories, namely (1) the obligatory (wājib), (2) the recommended (mandūb), (3) the allowable or the indifferent (mubāh), (4) the blameworthy or the discouraged (makrūh), and (5) the forbidden (harām). Abortion, at the most liberal level, has been placed by jurists in the third category, that of the allowable. Jurists have deliberated on the special conditions under which abortion is permitted, apart from the biological factor of ensoulment. They have also discussed cases of criminal abortion and types of penalties to be imposed on convicted wrongdoers.

Muslim jurists permit abortion mostly on medical and health grounds. One of the valid reasons often mentioned is the presence of a nursing infant. It is feared that a new pregnancy would put an upper limit on lactation. The jurists believe that if the mother could not be replaced by a wet nurse, the infant would suffer, if not die.

Contemporary Muslim society is faced with the reality that the practice of abortion is on the rise. In a number of Muslim countries, many unwanted pregnancies result from illicit sexual relations as well as from rapes. There are also related issues of birth control or family planning as a national policy, easy access to modern contraceptives, and the challenge to traditional Islamic doctrines on abortion and contraception arising from advances in genetics and biomedical technology. A well-defined Islamic response to these contemporary challenges has not yet emerged, but interest in these subjects is gaining momentum. As contemporary Muslim intellectuals and religious scholars debate these problems, traditional sources on contraception and abortion will be of immense value.

OSMAN BAKAR

Directly related to this article are the companion articles in this section: JEWISH PERSPECTIVES, ROMAN CATHOLIC PERSPECTIVES, *and* PROTESTANT PERSPECTIVES, *and the articles in the other sections of this entry:* MEDICAL PERSPECTIVES, *and* CONTEMPORARY ETHICAL AND LEGAL ASPECTS, *articles on* CONTEMPORARY ETHICAL PERSPECTIVES, *and* LEGAL AND REGULATORY ISSUES. *For a further discussion of Islamic religious tradition, see the entries* EUGENICS AND RELIGIOUS LAW, *article on* ISLAM; ISLAM; MEDICAL ETHICS, HISTORY OF, *section on* NEAR AND MIDDLE EAST, *articles on* IRAN, TURKEY, *and* CONTEMPORARY ARAB WORLD; *and* POPULATION ETHICS, *section on* RELIGIOUS TRADITIONS, *article on* ISLAMIC PERSPECTIVES. *Other relevant material may be found under the entries* ETHICS, *article on* RELIGION AND MORALITY; INFANTS, *article on* HISTORY OF INFANTICIDE; MATERNAL–FETAL RELATIONSHIP; *and* WOMEN, *article on* HISTORICAL AND CROSS-CULTURAL PERSPECTIVES.

Bibliography

ABEDIN, SALEHA MAHMOOD. 1977. "Islam and Muslim Fertility: Sociological Dimensions of a Demographic Dilemma." Ph.D. thesis, University of Pennsylvania.

ANEES, MUNAWAR AHMAD. 1989. *Islam and Biological Futures: Ethics, Gender and Technology.* London: Mansell.

BAKAR, OSMAN. 1991. *Tawhid and Science: Essays on the History and Philosophy of Islamic Science.* Penang–Kuala Lumpur: Secretariat for Islamic Philosophy and Science.

BOUHDIBA, ABDELWAHAB. 1985. *Sexuality in Islam.* Translated by Alan Sheridan. London: Routledge & Kegan Paul.

EBRAHIM, ABUL FADL MOHSIN. 1988. *Biomedical Issues: Islamic Perspective.* Mobeni: Islamic Medical Association of South Africa.

ELGOOD, CYRIL. 1962. "Tibb-ul-Nabbi or Medicine of the Prophet: Being a Translation of Two Works of the Same Name." *Osiris* 14:33–192.

———. 1970. *Safavid Medical Practice; or, The Practice of Medicine, Surgery and Gynaecology in Persia Between 1500 A.D. and 1750 A.D.* London: Luzac.

MAUDOODI, ABUL A'LA. 1968. *Birth Control: Its Social, Political, Economic, Moral, and Religious Aspects.* 3d ed. Lahore, Pakistan: Islamic Publications.

MUSALLAM, BASIM. 1983. *Sex and Society in Islam: Birth Control Before the Nineteenth Century.* Cambridge: At the University Press.

RAHMAN, FAZLUR. 1987. *Health and Medicine in the Islamic Tradition: Change and Identity.* New York: Crossroad.

SAYYID-MARSOT, AFAF LUTFI, ed. 1979. *Society and the Sexes in Medieval Islam.* Malibu, Calif.: Undena.

ABUSE, INTERPERSONAL

I. Child Abuse
    John D. Lantos
II. Abuse Between Domestic Partners
    Allison Moore
III. Elder Abuse
    Rosalie S. Wolf

I. CHILD ABUSE

Current pediatrics and social-work textbooks generally include chapters on child abuse that describe the epidemiology, clinical manifestations, differential diagnosis, and treatment of abused children. They usually discuss the legal requirement to notify state child-protection agencies of suspected abuse, and may describe the investigations such reports trigger. It is accepted by most pediatricians, social workers, and laymen that investigations may result in legal actions against parents and other responsible adults. Children may be removed from their homes. Parents may have their custodial rights terminated, and may face criminal charges. The entire process of diagnosis and intervention for child abuse is presented as both necessary and morally compelling.

Changing attitudes on child abuse

However, within this seeming consensus of moral sentiment lies a mystery. Until the twentieth century, much of what we now consider to be child abuse was regarded as morally acceptable and legally permissible. In fact, people generally argued not only that it was permissible to oppress and punish children to the point of physical abuse, but also that such abuse was necessary for the children's moral edification (Radbill, 1974). Thus, "Spare the rod and spoil the child." Parents and teachers had absolute authority over children's lives. They could, and did, physically and sexually abuse children with an impunity so complete that such acts were seldom recognized or acknowledged.

Our current approaches to child abuse reflect a radical change in our moral view of the family. Until the twentieth century, families were usually seen as small, autocratic moral universes. Parents (in most cases, fathers) could use children (and wives) as they saw fit. Children had no independent moral rights. The movement to recognize and prevent child abuse, and to punish abusers, reflects a partial empowerment of the child. Such a sea change in moral sentiment raises important questions about the timelessness of moral principles affecting the care of children. Either child abuse was always wrong but not recognized as wrong, suggesting that our moral sensitivities are improving over time, or child abuse became wrong only recently, suggesting that moral values are not timeless and immutable but transient and constantly evolving.

Whether moral principles, such as those designed to guide the care of children, have changed over time or whether people have gradually become more or less virtuous in the treatment of children will be debated elsewhere in this work. Currently, attempts to formulate standards for appropriate ethical and legal responses to child abuse can be seen as efforts to craft social and legal policies that reflect our views of how children should be cared for and reared. But parents and other caregivers receive conflicting messages from current social policies; whereas our society currently restricts child abuse, its institutions and laws condone other activities—such as sexual activity during early teenage years and exposure to violence in television, films, and daily life—that would have been regarded as morally problematic in societies of previous eras and are so regarded in non-U.S. societies today. From one perspective, these conflicting efforts can be seen as experiments in social policy; from another perspective, selective legal interventions in the area of child abuse are viewed as justified by the legal doctrine of *parens patriae.* In this doctrine the state claims an interest in protecting the lives and well-being of children, even if this means limiting parental autonomy and infringing on family privacy.

Nevertheless, physical and sexual abuse of children is still common; in most instances, abuse is never reported or discovered.

Defining child abuse

Definitions of abuse are notoriously variable, circular, or designed to leave room for interpretation on a case-by-case basis. In the United States, the Child Abuse Prevention and Treatment Act of 1974 (PL93-247) defines abuse and neglect as

> the physical and mental injury, sexual abuse, negligent treatment or maltreatment of a child under the age of 18 by a person who is responsible for the child's welfare under circumstances which indicate that the child's health and welfare is harmed or threatened thereby. . . .

State definitions based on this law vary. Arguments about whether a particular act constitutes abuse under such a definition may focus on the nature of the act itself, whether the act caused harm, whether there was or should have been prior recognition that the act would cause harm, and whether the caretaker might have prevented the harm.

In both physical and sexual abuse, different individuals or communities distinguish acceptable from unacceptable behaviors using different criteria. In physical abuse, a distinction must be made between acceptable forms of discipline or punishment and abuse. As Kim Oates (1982) points out, definitions must specify whether abuse should be defined in terms of particular actions or particular effects. He describes two children who are pushed roughly to the ground by their fathers. One falls against a carpeted floor, the other hits a protruding cupboard door. The second sustains a skull fracture, the first is uninjured. If an act must cause harm to be abuse, then the second child was clearly abused, while the first may not have been. Acts that leave no physical marks are harder to classify as abuse, and it is generally harder to sustain criminal convictions or obtain civil sanctions in such cases, even though an unmarked child may sustain as much or more psychological harm as from actions that cause physical signs of abuse.

In sexual abuse, definitional problems also arise. Child sexual abuse is generally intrafamilial, and falls under the rubric of incest. While prohibitions against incest are universal, different cultures define incest to include, or exclude, different activities. "Parent-child nudity, communal sleeping arrangements, and tolerance for masturbation and peer sex play in children coexist with stringent incest taboos. . . . (M)others in many cultures use genital manipulation to soothe and pleasure infants. Some cultures prescribe the deflowering of pubertal girls by an adult male or by the father" (Goodwin, 1988, p. 33). Exotic cultural differences may be mirrored by different beliefs in our own culture. Some parents may sleep with their children, bathe with them, or take pictures of the children naked on the beach. In some jurisdictions, these activities may be defined as illegal or morally inappropriate.

Cultural or religious differences may also play a role in evaluating what constitutes medical neglect. Christian Scientists, for example, may claim that it is appropriate not to take their sick children to a doctor, while courts may determine that such behavior constitutes neglect. Some Native Americans believe that organ transplantation is prohibited, and so may refuse life-sustaining treatment for their children in liver failure. Similarly, Jehovah's Witnesses may, on the basis of their belief, seek to refuse consent for blood transfusions for their children, even if transfusions would preserve life. In situations like these, judgments must be made about the relative importance of respecting religious and cultural diversity, on the one hand, and protecting the interests of vulnerable children, on the other.

In addition to cultural differences in defining what behaviors are or are not permissible, serious moral problems arise when we attempt to determine whether, in any particular case, a behavior that is clearly not permissible in fact occurred. Court cases may turn on the rules governing the collecting and presentation of evidence. Even in adult rape cases, victims have difficulty convincing juries that they have been raped. Such difficulties are compounded in child-abuse cases, where young children often cannot testify convincingly on their own behalf.

In summary, both physical abuse and sexual abuse of children exist along a spectrum, from obvious cruelty and exploitation to grayer areas of corporal punishment or sexual game playing. The strong moral arguments against egregious abuse of children often lose strength as the definition of abuse expands along a spectrum including activities that may be considered morally praiseworthy, morally acceptable, morally forgivable, or immoral but noncriminal.

Reporting child abuse

Most laws are vague in defining the reporting requirements for child abuse. Generally, they require reporting if someone "has reasons to believe that a child has been subjected to abuse." Such laws do not attempt to quantify the degree of suspicion, the quality of the evidence, or the likelihood of abuse that must be present to compel a report. In the crafting of such laws, it seems that the goal was to protect people who report abuse by allowing broad latitude to individuals in defining what they mean by a "suspicion" of abuse. A utilitarian calculus seems to be at work—that it would be better to have reports made that prove to be groundless than to allow subtle cases of abuse to go unreported. Even with such vague and permissive requirements, evidence suggests that abuse is underreported rather than overreported.

There are a number of reasons why people might not report child abuse even though they believe it to be wrong. Child abuse may be ignored because people have difficulty defining and recognizing it (Besharov, 1981; Zellman, 1992). It may go undiscovered because adults who are aware that a child is being abused are reticent to get involved and do not report it (Dhooper et al., 1991). Or professionals may feel reticent to threaten what they perceive as a therapeutic relationship with the adult or adults involved. When abuse is reported, health professionals and legal agencies need to weigh the relative risks and benefits of preserving the family against those of removing the child from it (Zellman, 1990).

Reticence to report suspected child abuse may be based on the sociology of health-care delivery, on respect for confidentiality in the doctor–parent relationship, on unwillingness to stigmatize parents when there is doubt about the actual occurrence of abuse, or on a desire to preserve a therapeutic relationship or avoid the perception that professionals are enemies.

Pediatricians in private practice are paid by the parents or other adults responsible for the children to whom they provide care, and often develop long-term relationships with these adults and the children. In such situations, relationships must be based on mutual trust. Pediatricians may give adults the benefit of the doubt regarding injuries that may be associated with abuse. They may also be fearful that child-abuse reports will be bad for business. These factors may partially explain why reports of abuse are more likely to come from hospital emergency rooms than from private doctors' offices (Badger, 1989).

In addition to economic considerations, moral aspects of the doctor–parent (or other adult) relationship may impede reporting. Generally, doctors promise confidentiality, and the moral reasons for confidentiality are compelling. Adults must confide in doctors, and may need to tell them information that would be embarrassing or damaging were it known by others. However, this promise of confidentiality may conflict with a pediatrician's concern about the child's best interest. Although the law requires doctors to report suspected child abuse, reporting is quite sporadic and inconsistent (Dhooper et al., 1991; Zellman, 1990; Oates, 1982). Studies of pediatricians reveal that older doctors are less likely to report child abuse than are younger doctors, and males are less likely to report it than females (Keen and Dukes, 1991). None of the studies that document inconsistent reporting disentangle the economic, moral, and legal considerations that lead doctors and other child-welfare professionals to report or not to report abuse.

Reticence to report may also result from a lack of faith in the efficacy of interventions. Many child-protection agencies are underfunded and understaffed. In times of tight budgets, they may not receive the highest legislative priority. As a result, they may be unable to provide counseling and supervision services to every child or family reported to them. In some states, child-protection agencies operate under court supervision because they have been found to neglect the children in their custody. While such agencies clearly provide excellent services to most children, highly publicized cases in which they have failed to provide adequate protection may lead to skepticism about the efficacy of reporting.

Risks and benefits of intervention

Because society only recently recognized the problem of child abuse, there has been little time to evaluate the effects of different responses to abuse. Three types of responses have been attempted: (1) those designed to prevent abuse; (2) those designed to deal with the psychological consequences of abuse; and (3) those designed to punish offenders.

Preventive programs are difficult to evaluate because of almost insurmountable ethical and methodological problems (Conte, 1987). Abuse is a hidden problem. Assessing whether heightened awareness of the problem leads to increased reporting or decreased occurrence would require intrusive evaluation and follow-up for enormous numbers of people (Reppucci and Haugaard, 1989; Fink and McCloskey, 1990). Generally, studies focus on surrogate outcome measures, such as "ability to discriminate safe from unsafe situations," rather than on actual decreases in the incidence of sexual abuse (Hazzard et al., 1991, p. 134).

Intervention for children who have suffered abuse requires a delicate balance between trying to protect the child, trying to help the parents, and trying to preserve the family. Parents who abuse children often have been abused themselves, and may have a higher incidence of psychiatric problems (Steele and Pollack, 1974). Many parents regret their actions, desire psychiatric help, and comply with treatment programs. However, 5 to 30 percent of abused children who stay in their family are subject to further episodes of abuse (Jellinek et al., 1992). At present, there are no reliable indicators of which parents will continue to abuse their children and which are likely to respond to therapy. Furthermore, any data that might address this issue will necessarily be probabilistic. Thus, decisions about the value of such data in an individual case will incorporate normative values about the degree of risk appropriate for a particular child facing a particular custody decision.

Programs designed to punish child abusers are driven less by considerations of the risks and benefits of interventions and more by the dictates of the legal system. Evidence against alleged abusers seldom establishes guilt beyond a reasonable doubt. As a result, criminal prosecution is rare, and conviction even rarer (Peters, 1989). Furthermore, it is unclear whether stricter laws or harsher punishments decrease the incidence of child abuse. As in other areas of criminal law, the justification for criminal prosecution seems to derive more from a notion of punitive justice than from a calculation of the degree to which punishment of offenders deters potential future offenders. Debate about this issue must take place in the context of more general debates about the morality of incarceration or the potential for rehabilitation in any criminal situation.

Conclusion

An apparent consensus about child abuse masks profound disagreements about the proper boundaries of family privacy, the obligations of parents and health professionals, and governmental responsibility to oversee the care and nurturing of children. These disagreements are reflected in difficulties in defining child abuse, difficulties in enforcing compliance with mandatory reporting requirements, and difficulties in evaluating the effects of interventions. Thus, while the law requires that child abuse be reported if it is suspected, health professionals can create their own index of suspicion. Some providers may report ambiguous cases, while others rarely report suspected abuse at all.

Individuals who work with children must balance their legal and ethical obligations to children, to their parents or caretakers, and to society. Professionals who have a higher regard for familial privacy and parental authority may develop a stricter standard or a higher threshold for suspecting abuse, and thus may be less likely to report it. Professionals who believe more strongly in the independent rights of children may develop a lower threshold for suspecting abuse, and may thus be more likely to report it. Current legal and moral approaches, while theoretically compelling, are quite recent, and have not been thoroughly evaluated. The principle that children deserve protection and nurturance is generally accepted, but the means by which the principle is to be brought to fruition remain uncertain.

JOHN D. LANTOS

Directly related to this article are the other articles in this entry: ABUSE BETWEEN DOMESTIC PARTNERS, *and* ELDER ABUSE. *Also directly related is the entry* CHILDREN, *especially the articles on* RIGHTS OF CHILDREN, *and* HEALTH-CARE AND RESEARCH ISSUES. *For a further discussion of topics mentioned in this article, see the entries* CONFIDENTIALITY; FAMILY; PROFESSIONAL–PATIENT RELATIONSHIP; SEXUAL ETHICS; *and* SOCIAL WORK IN HEALTH CARE. *For a discussion of related ideas, see the entries*

HARM; INFORMATION DISCLOSURE; *and* PRIVACY IN HEALTH CARE. *Other relevant material may be found under the entries* ADOLESCENTS; BEHAVIOR CONTROL; *and* SEXUAL DEVELOPMENT.

Bibliography

BADGER, LEE W. 1989. "Reporting of Child Abuse: Influence of Characteristics of Physician, Practice, and Community." *Southern Medical Journal* 82, no. 3:281–286.

BESHAROV, DOUGLAS J. 1981. "Toward Better Research on Child Abuse and Neglect: Making Definitional Issues an Explicit Methodological Concern." *Child Abuse and Neglect* 5, no. 4:383–390.

CONTE, JON R. 1987. "Ethical Issues in Evaluation of Prevention Programs." *Child Abuse and Neglect* 11, no. 2:171–172.

DHOOPER, SURJIT S.; ROYSE, DAVID D.; and WOLFE, L. C. 1991. "A Statewide Study of the Public Attitudes Toward Child Abuse." *Child Abuse and Neglect* 15, nos. 1–2: 37–44.

FINK, ARLENE, and McCLOSKEY, LOIS. 1990. "Moving Child Abuse and Neglect Prevention Programs Forward: Improving Program Evaluations." *Child Abuse and Neglect* 14, no. 2:187–206.

GOODWIN, JEAN M. 1988. "Obstacles to Policymaking About Incest: Some Cautionary Folktales." In *Lasting Effects of Child Sexual Abuse*, pp. 21–37. Edited by Gail Elizabeth Wyatt and Gloria Johnson Powell. Newbury Park, Calif.: Sage.

HAZZARD, ANN; WEBB, CAROL; KLEEMEIER, CAROL; ANGERT, LISA; and POHL, JUDY. 1991. "Child Sexual Abuse Prevention: Evaluation and One-Year Follow-up." *Child Abuse and Neglect* 15, nos. 1–2:123–138.

JELLINEK, MICHAEL S.; MURPHY, J. MICHAEL; POITRAST, FRANCIS; QUINN, DOROTHY; BISHOP, SANDRA J.; and GOSHKO, MARILYN. 1992. "Serious Child Mistreatment in Massachusetts: The Course of 206 Children Through the Courts." *Child Abuse and Neglect* 16, no. 2:179–185.

KEAN, ROBERT B., and DUKES, RICHARD L. 1991. "Effects of Witness Characteristics on the Perception and Reportage of Child Abuse." *Child Abuse and Neglect* 15, no. 4: 423–435.

OATES, KIM. 1982. "Child Abuse: A Community Concern." In *Child Abuse—A Community Concern*, pp. 1–12. Edited by Kim Oates. London: Butterworths.

PETERS, JAMES M. 1989. "Criminal Prosecution of Child Abuse: Recent Trends." *Pediatric Annals* 18, no. 8:505–506, 508–509.

RADBILL, SAMUEL X. 1974. "A History of Child Abuse and Infanticide." In *The Battered Child*, 2d ed., pp. 3–21. Edited by Ray E. Helfer and C. Henry Kempe. Chicago: University of Chicago Press.

REPPUCCI, N. DICKON, and HAUGAARD, JEFFREY J. 1989. "Prevention of Child Sexual Abuse: Myth or Reality." *American Psychologist* 44, no. 10:1266–1275.

STEELE, BRANDT F., and POLLACK, CARL. 1974. "A Psychiatric Study of Parents Who Abuse Infants and Small Children." In *The Battered Child*, 2d ed., pp. 89–133. Edited by Ray E. Helfer and C. Henry Kempe. Chicago: University of Chicago Press.

ZELLMAN, GAIL L. 1990. "Report on Decision-Making Patterns Among Mandated Child Abuse Reporters." *Child Abuse and Neglect* 14, no. 3:325–336.

———. 1992. "The Impact of Case Characteristics on Child Abuse Reporting Decisions." *Child Abuse and Neglect* 16, no. 1:57–74.

II. ABUSE BETWEEN DOMESTIC PARTNERS

Common sense suggests that abuse between domestic partners is "just plain wrong." Nonetheless, domestic violence only began to be recognized as an ethical issue because of the advocacy work of grass-roots battered-women's movements and of feminist and liberationist movements in theology, ethics, and the social sciences. This article defines domestic violence, explores some of the reasons it is difficult for women to escape abuse, and outlines some of the underlying social and ethical issues.

Definition of domestic violence and its broader social context

The term "domestic partners" implies some serious bond, such as marriage, a child in common, cohabitation, or financial ties. It also usually implies emotional and sexual connections between people who have chosen to be with each other. Emotional, legal, and material connections make it difficult to end the relationship once abuse occurs. Police, lawmakers, medical professionals, and the general public have found it difficult to acknowledge the prevalence of domestic violence or act to prevent it because of the voluntary, emotional nature of a relationship based in the private rather than the public sphere and because of patriarchal assumptions about women and marriage.

In any intimate relationship people may hurt each other, but abuse occurs when one person systematically hurts, threatens, rapes, manipulates, tries to kill or kills the other, and when fear replaces trust and respect as the basis of the relationship. Physical violence, with the intent of one spouse to cause harm to the other, is the accepted definition of spouse abuse in all countries where spouse abuse has been studied (Gelles and Cornell, 1983). Consistent insults, criticism, disregard for one partner's needs, isolation, damage to property and pets, and withholding money, food, or other necessities are other ways abusers try to dominate and control the relationship. The overwhelming majority of spousal abuse throughout the world is by men against women (Gelles and Cornell, 1983; Levinson, 1989).

It is hard to document the extent of domestic abuse for several reasons. First, until recently, very few countries have kept records of it—violence has to be reported to some authority in order to be recorded (Gelles and Cornell, 1983). Second, the information kept (e.g., percentage of police calls related to family disputes, homicide statistics, number of women served by shelters, percentage of people reporting violence in surveys) varies widely. In most countries awareness and research about domestic abuse against women tend to lag behind awareness and research about child abuse. Most research studies have analyzed family violence in a single country, using approaches that provide no basis for cross-cultural comparison (Gelles and Cornell, 1983).

A sampling of international statistics hints at the magnitude of the problem of domestic abuse. Analysis of ninety small-scale and peasant societies found that wife beating was the most common type of family violence and that adult women were at the greatest risk of severe injury and death (Levinson, 1989). Seventy percent of the murders in Portugal occur in the home (Gelles and Cornell, 1983). In many U.S. states and in most regions of the world, it is not illegal for husbands to rape their wives. In Japan, wife beating is the second most frequent cause of divorce initiated by women. In Peru, 70 percent of all crimes reported to the police are of women beaten by their husbands. Federal Bureau of Investigation records in the United States estimate that a woman is beaten every eighteen seconds (Wetzel, 1992). In the United States, domestic violence is the single largest cause of injury to women ("Special Report," 1990), and over half of all female homicide victims are murdered by male partners compared with 12 percent of male victims killed by female partners (Council on Ethical and Judicial Affairs, 1992).

Yet awareness of domestic abuse is increasing. The U.S. Department of State highlighted the problem of rampant discrimination against women for the first time in 1993 in its annual report on human-rights abuses. Examples cited included physical abuse against women in all countries; "honor killings" for alleged adultery by wives, especially in South America; denial in many countries of political, civil, or legal rights in voting, marriage, travel, testifying in court, inheriting and owning property, and obtaining custody of children; forced prostitution and the refusal to recognize marital rape as a crime on several continents; genital mutilation in many African countries; sexual and economic exploitation of domestic servants in Southeast Asia; and dowry deaths (murder of a bride when her family cannot give her husband's family the expected dowry) in Bangladesh and India. In 1993 the U.N. General Assembly adopted the Declaration on the Elimination of Violence Against Women and established a Special Rapporteur on Violence Against Women (U.S. Department of State, 1994).

The psychological and social context of domestic abuse

The changes that occur in a battered woman's sense of self-esteem and competence are often more lasting and more damaging to women than the actual physical abuse. Battered women learn to pay attention to their partner's needs instead of their own in hopes of reducing the violence. They begin to distrust their own judgment and their own abilities to provide for themselves and their children (if they have children). They may eventually come to believe that they deserve the abuse they receive. When family, friends, religious leaders, and helping professionals disbelieve, blame, or trivialize battered women's experiences and do not respond to their appeals for help, women feel even more trapped and convinced that abuse is inevitable. Chances to escape abusive relationships or find a loving relationship begin to seem impossible (Moore, 1990).

Another psychological dynamic first described by Lenore Walker also explains why it is so difficult for battered women to decide to leave an abusive relationship (Walker, 1979). Walker documents a three-part cycle of (a) a violent episode; (b) regret by the abuser, love, attention, reparation, and promises never to be abusive again (the "honeymoon period"); and (c) cessation of loving attention and a period of escalating tension between partners leading to another violent episode. Battered women yearn for the honeymoon period of love and attention that reinforces their initial hopes for the relationship. Unfortunately, over time, the honeymoons become shorter and the severity and frequency of abuse increase, sometimes resulting in death. Walker also describes the "learned helplessness syndrome," where women lose faith in their ability to act effectively because batterers respond so unpredictably and illogically to so many of their actions (Walker, 1979).

The emotional, psychological, and physical consequences of abuse must be understood in their larger context of sexism, patriarchy, and paternalistic dominance (Lerner, 1986). Gerda Lerner defines sexism as "the ideology of male supremacy, of male superiority, and of beliefs that support and sustain it" (Lerner, 1986, p. 240). Sexism undergirds patriarchy, "the institutionalization of male dominance over women and children in the family and the extension of male dominance over women in society in general (Lerner, 1986, p. 239). A sociological study of domestic abuse in Scotland documents the connection between domestic violence and patriarchal marriage. The researchers argue that the law, the church, economic opportunities, appeals to science or to "the natural order," and social customs all promote women's subordinate status in marriage. Women find their struggle to resist domination, including violence, within marriage labeled "wrong, immoral, and a violation of the respect and loyalty a wife is supposed to give her husband" (Dobash and Dobash, 1979, p. ix). A study of ninety small-scale societies found that economic inequality, inequality of domestic decision-making authority, and restrictions on women's freedom to divorce were the strongest predictors of wife beating (Levinson, 1989). The major religious faiths have traditionally taught male superiority, the duty of women to obey men, and the sin of divorce even in the case of extreme abuse, which only exacerbates religious women's difficulties in escaping abuse.

Women's subordination is ostensibly mitigated by the unwritten contract for exchange of services in marriage, which Lerner calls "paternalistic dominance": Men are expected to provide economic support and protection from harm in exchange for obedience, sexual service, and unpaid domestic service, including care of dependent family members (Lerner, 1986). These expectations are built into marriage and divorce laws (Weitzman, 1981) and help define women's roles, opportunities, and sense of self (Degler, 1980). The perception and public rhetoric that women's subordination is "normal," "necessary," and even desirable for women may contradict women's lived experiences. Yet without language and communities in which women may define their own experience, subordination often goes unchallenged.

Karen Lebacqz offers a powerful analysis of the role-conditioning of men and women that contributes to domestic abuse in marital or nonmarital relationships. She argues that "'normal' patterns of male–female sexual relating in U.S. culture are defined by patterns of male dominance over women," so that women come to expect male domination and the possibility of violence in heterosexual relations (Lebacqz, 1990, p. 3). Many recent studies (Fortune, 1983; McGillis, 1989 [cited in Lebacqz, 1990]) find that women have often experienced undesired forced sexual relations with male acquaintances which neither women nor men considered to be rape. Male power over women is eroticized in mainstream media and pornography and comes to be perceived as sexually desirable, even when women know their experiences of abuse are not desirable (Lebacqz, 1990).

Expectations of male dominance in private heterosexual relations are reinforced by men's greater access to economic, political, religious, and cultural power in public life. Christine Firer Hinze analyzes how the creation and maintenance of distinct public and private realms tends to keep women dependent on male earning power and status. "A 'feminized' private realm confers indirect status and informal power in childbearing, homemaking, and other personalized nurturing, caretaking and consumption tasks . . . a separate, 'masculinized' public arena disperses public status and formal power in cultural, political, and economic matters" (Hinze, 1992, p. 283). Even within the public realm, women are most frequently employed in domestic service and in technical service and sales occupations with lower status and salaries than male employment. In the United States, women of color are disproportionately represented in the lowest-paid positions in domestic service compared with white women (U.S. Department of Labor, 1986). The differences between male and female access to power become especially apparent when women who decide to leave abusive partners try to find adequate jobs, housing, medical care, child care, and education for their children.

Emerging awareness of domestic violence as a social and clinical problem

The understanding of the *paterfamilias* with life and death control over wife (wives), children, slaves, and property is found in most every culture throughout the world: in ancient Greek and Roman society, in the Middle Eastern cultures represented in Christian, Jewish, and Muslim scriptures, and in Confucian understandings of the family, to name a few examples. Religious values have played an ambiguous role, sometimes perpetuating, sometimes condemning domestic abuse. For instance, trends in Christian history that attribute to women responsibility for the presence of evil in creation also sanctioned public torture and murder of women accused of being witches or heretics (Brown and Bohn, 1989; Fortune, 1983). Yet ideals in all religions, such as the intrinsic worth of all people in Christianity or of special obligations of husbands toward wives and vice versa in Christianity and Judaism, have also condemned domestic abuse. The emergence of religious and secular movements to prevent child abuse and violence against women could not occur until women and children began to be seen as individuals in their own right.

The gradual shift in attention from silent acceptance of abuse to its recognition as a problem can be illustrated by examining the history of changing laws in the United States. Until the late nineteenth century, the assumptions underlying laws and social policy in the United States came from English common law, where the husband was considered the head of the house with absolute control over his wife and children. The term "rule of thumb" comes from a modification of English common law that gives husbands the right to beat wives "provided that he used a switch no bigger than his thumb" (Martin, 1983, p. 32). From 1874 until the 1970s, the prevailing U.S. court precedents held that although husbands do not have the legal right to chastise their wives, the courts should not interfere in do-

mestic affairs except when permanent injury, malice, cruelty, or dangerous violence can be proven (Martin, 1983). In the 1970s, growing recognition of the severity of abuse against women, due largely to the "women's liberation movement," led most states to offer women legal protection against abuse by their husbands or by the fathers of their children. In many states, however, access to information about legal options, advocates to clarify procedures and support women, and affordable remedies are still hard to find.

The first battered women's shelters were established in the 1970s in England and the United States when women who had suffered abuse came to newly formed women's support groups asking for a place to stay (Schecter, 1982). Judith Herman describes the interaction of consciousness-raising groups, increased public awareness, and changes in social policy and the treatment of female victims of rape and domestic violence by medical and psychological professionals in the U.S., beginning in the 1970s (Herman, 1992). Public discussion of domestic violence gave its victims the language, the courage, and the end to isolation that enabled them to decide that abuse against them was wrong even when prevailing social norms had led them to accept abuse as normal and justifiable (Herman, 1992; Schecter, 1982; Russell, 1984).

"Why don't women just leave?" is a frequent query. Unlike children or the elderly, adult women are expected to be able to protect themselves, so women who "choose" to remain with an abuser are often blamed for their situation. Men and women are—in theory—peers in a relationship of mutual equality and need, although the reality of male privilege undermines genuine equality. The long-term effects of abuse by a chosen lover, the economic, social, and legal barriers faced by women living independently or with children, the fear of even greater violence or death for the woman or for other family members if she leaves, and the pressure on women to sustain intimate relationships with men reduce the options available to women who want abuse to end. These same factors also reduce battered women's ability to recognize and act on existing options.

Legislative issues

Legislation affecting battered women varies widely within the United States, and even more widely among nations. The 1979 Convention on the Elimination of All Forms of Discrimination Against Women bars discrimination against women by private persons or organizations. Compliance with this convention is monitored by the U.N. Committee on the Elimination of Discrimination Against Women (U.N. General Assembly, 1979). In 1992 specific recommendations were added that prohibit battering, rape, mental suffering, and other violence perpetuated against women. The recommendations urge governments to develop criminal penalties and civil remedies for domestic abuse, to abolish the honor defense (exoneration of husbands who, to protect their honor, kill wives suspected of adultery), and to provide services to ensure women's safety (U.N. Document HRI/GEN/1, 1992). Concerns of particular states and nations include: the definition of rape (e.g., can women be raped within marriage?); legal restraints that exist on abusers' activity; accessibility of legal protection; whether spouse abuse is considered a misdemeanor or a felony; how orders of protection or restraining orders, which limit an abuser's contact with the woman he has hurt, are enforced; and sentencing patterns in family court, civil court, and criminal court cases. All of these legal practices can reflect patriarchal attitudes and ignorance on the part of judges and the police of the relevant social and psychological issues.

Some current ethical and legal issues under discussion in many different U.S. states include custody arrangements when one parent has abused the other and may continue to do so: What criteria are used to determine whether fathers who abuse their children's mother are "fit parents"? Lawyers and social workers question the use of the "battered woman's defense" in criminal cases where women hurt or kill their abuser in self-defense, or who do not intervene to protect their abused children because they fear for their own lives. At what point does abuse render women incapable of caring for themselves or their children? Men who kill female partners often receive much shorter jail sentences than women who kill male partners because men are likely to murder without forethought while, often, women calculate when their abusers will be most vulnerable (Browne, 1987). Local battered women's shelters and legal assistance programs have the most current information on these issues.

Medical care

Questions about the possibility of domestic violence should be part of all regular medical histories for all women in all settings where women come for medical care. Domestic violence affects women of all economic groups, educational levels, ethnic groups, religions, and ages. Routinely asking about violence and childhood sexual abuse may help abused women recognize that they are not alone and that help is available. Questions should be posed so that they do not impute blame to women. Women who are abused may well deny their abuse out of fear, shame, or distrust. This is far more likely when their partners accompany them to doctors' offices or emergency rooms: Women need to be asked about abuse when they are alone, or at least when their partners are not able to hear their responses. Informa-

tion about resources for battered women should be prominently displayed and easily available for women to take without their asking.

Battered women who have left their abusers are also likely to return more than once before they are ready to leave permanently. This can be frustrating to medical professionals who treat a particular woman's injuries repeatedly, and can lead them to blame the woman, who needs to take her own time to decide how she can live in safety. Accurate medical records, including clinical reasons for suspecting abuse, are essential evidence for women who may eventually press criminal or civil charges against their abusers. No laws require reporting suspected abuse against women (there are such laws for suspected child abuse), because women are not "dependent." Nonetheless, if medical professionals incorporate questions and information about domestic violence into their routine treatment of women, they will address some of the social barriers that keep battered women from finding safety.

Ignorance about domestic violence and childhood sexual abuse also plagues psychotherapists, psychiatrists, and clergy who do not understand the emotional or material barriers that make leaving difficult. Often, they either blame women for remaining in dangerous relationships or they consistently ignore signs of abuse and refuse to pay serious attention to women who talk about abuse. Couples therapy often tries to assign responsibility for problems equally to each partner in the relationship, which ignores the reality of violence and the fear of the abuser that makes abusive relationships inherently unequal. Attributing responsibility for the violence to the offender, and specific treatment for the batterer in individual therapy or groups, is essential if abuse is to end. Fear of retaliation by the abuser can also prevent counseling professionals from intervening in situations of domestic abuse.

Treatment resources for male abusers are scarce. Most abusers deny they have a problem. Most batterers only participate in treatment groups for batterers when they are ordered to do so by a legal or judicial authority. Months of consistent participation may pass before they acknowledge their responsibility (Gondolf, 1985). Inconsistent prosecution, enforcement, and sentencing often reinforce abusers' beliefs that their abuse is not a serious problem. Local battered women's shelters and family courts often know about resources for abusers.

Conclusion

Ethical issues raised by abuse between domestic partners fall into categories of treatment and prevention. Treatment includes breaking the silence that surrounds domestic violence; holding abusers legally accountable for their actions and requiring them to cease their violence;

listening to victims; helping victims recognize their strengths and believe they are worthy to live in safety; and working with them to navigate through social, economic, legal, and religious barriers to safety (NiCarthy, 1982). The balance between active intervention in order to keep women from being hurt or killed, and respecting their need to decide how and when to end an abusive relationship, is difficult to find.

Prevention includes challenging the prevailing social norms of sexism and patriarchy, of private spheres for women's work and public roles for men, of violence against women, and of violence as a way of resolving conflict between people or groups of people. No woman will be safe until social, political, and economic institutions ensure her access to the material resources she needs to support herself and her children.

ALLISON MOORE

Directly related to this article are the other articles in this entry: CHILD ABUSE, *and* ELDER ABUSE. *For a further discussion of topics mentioned in this article, see the entries* MARRIAGE AND OTHER DOMESTIC PARTNERSHIPS; SEXISM; *and* WOMEN, *articles on* HISTORICAL AND CROSSCULTURAL PERSPECTIVES, *and* HEALTH-CARE ISSUES. *For a discussion of related ideas, see the entries* CONFIDENTIALITY; *and* PATERNALISM. *Other relevant material may be found under the entries* FAMILY; FEMINISM; HOMICIDE; *and* INFORMATION DISCLOSURE, *article on* ETHICAL ISSUES.

Bibliography

BROWN, JOANNE CARLSON, and BOHN, CAROLE R., eds. 1989. *Christianity, Patriarchy and Abuse: A Feminist Critique.* New York: Pilgrim.

BROWNE, ANGELA. 1987. *When Battered Women Kill.* New York: Free Press.

COUNCIL ON ETHICAL AND JUDICIAL AFFAIRS. AMERICAN MEDICAL ASSOCIATION. 1992. "Physicians and Domestic Violence: Ethical Considerations." *Journal of the American Medical Association* 267, no. 23:3190–3193.

DEGLER, CARL N. 1980. *At Odds: Women and the Family in America from the Revolution to the Present.* New York: Oxford University Press.

DOBASH, R. EMERSON, and DOBASH, RUSSELL. 1979. *Violence Against Wives: A Case Against the Patriarchy.* New York: Free Press.

FORTUNE, MARIE M. 1983. *Sexual Violence: The Unmentionable Sin.* New York: Pilgrim.

GELLES, RICHARD J., and CORNELL, CLAIRE PEDRICK, eds. 1983. *International Perspectives on Family Violence.* Lexington, Mass.: D. C. Heath.

GONDOLF, EDWARD W. 1985. *Men Who Batter: An Integrated Approach for Stopping Wife Abuse.* Holmes Beach, Fla.: Learning.

HERMAN, JUDITH LEWIS. 1992. *Trauma and Recovery.* New York: Basic Books.

HINZE, CHRISTINE FIRER. 1992. "Power in Christian Ethics: Resources and Frontiers for Scholarly Exploration." *Annual of the Society of Christian Ethics, 1992:277–290.*

KUMARI, RANJANA. 1989. *Brides Are Not for Burning.* New Delhi: Radiant.

LEBACQZ, KAREN. 1990. "Love Your Enemy: Sex, Power, and Christian Ethics." *Annual of the Society of Christian Ethics, 1990:3–26.*

LERNER, GERDA. 1986. *The Creation of Patriarchy.* New York: Oxford University Press.

LEVINSON, DAVID. 1989. *Family Violence in Cross-Cultural Perspective.* Newbury Park, Calif.: Sage.

MARTIN, DEL. 1983. *Battered Wives.* Rev. ed. New York: Pocket Books.

McGILLIS, KELLY. 1989. *Against Her Will: Rape on Campus.* Northbrook, Ill.: Learning Corporation of America. Videotape reporting the results of a study of 6,000 college students by the National Institutes of Health and *Ms.* magazine; quoted in Lebacqz, 1990.

MOORE, ALLISON. 1990. "Moral Agency of Women in a Battered Women's Shelter." *Annual of the Society of Christian Ethics, 1990:131–148.*

NiCARTHY, GINNY. 1982. *Getting Free: A Handbook for Women in Abusive Relationships.* Seattle, Wash.: Seal. Seal Press offers many self-help handbooks for battered women, including books about African-American and Latina women's issues.

PIZZEY, ERIN. 1974. *Scream Quietly or the Neighbors Will Hear.* London: If Books.

ROY, MARIA. 1988. *Children in the Crossfire.* Deerfield, Fla.: Health Communications.

RUSSELL, DIANA E. H. 1984. *Sexual Exploitation: Rape, Child Sexual Abuse, and Workplace Harassment.* Beverly Hills, Calif.: Sage.

SCHECHTER, SUSAN. 1982. *Women and Male Violence: The Visions and Struggles of the Battered Women's Movement.* Boston: South End.

"Special Report: Everyday Violence Against Women." 1990. *Ms.,* September–October, pp. 33–56.

U.N. GENERAL ASSEMBLY. 1979. *Convention on the Elimination of All Forms of Discrimination Against Women.* New York: Author.

———. 1993. Declaration on the Elimination of Violence Against Women. General Assembly Resolution 48/104 of 20 Dec. 1993; United Nations Document A/C.3/48/L.5.

U.S. DEPARTMENT OF LABOR. OFFICE OF THE SECRETARY, WOMEN'S BUREAU. 1986. "Twenty Facts About Women Workers." Fact Sheet 86–2.

U.S. DEPARTMENT OF STATE. 1994. *Country Reports on Human Rights Practices for 1993: Report Submitted to the Committee on Foreign Affairs.* Washington, D.C.: Author.

WALKER, LENORE E. 1979. *The Battered Woman.* New York: Harper & Row.

WEITZMAN, LENORE J. 1981. *The Marriage Contract: Spouses, Lovers, and the Law.* New York: Free Press.

WETZEL, JANICE WOOD. 1992. *The World of Women: In Pursuit of Human Rights.* New York: New York University Press.

III. ELDER ABUSE

The phenomenon known as elder abuse first appeared in the British scientific literature in 1975 (Burston) to describe the physical abuse of an elderly dependent person by a caregiving family member. In the years that followed, the definition broadened to include acts of commission (physical, psychological, and financial abuse) and omission (neglect) that result in harm to a person sixty-five years (in some states, sixty years) or older by a relative or a person with whom the elder has a trusting relationship.

Policy development

In the United States interest in elder abuse was sparked by testimony on battering of parents before a U.S. House of Representatives subcommittee investigating family violence in 1978. The growing numbers of elderly persons in society, the rising political power of the older population, and the existing state bureaucracies for delivering protective services lent legitimacy to making elder abuse a public issue. Despite the efforts of a few representatives to pass national legislation throughout the 1980s, no action was taken by the Congress. Nevertheless, federal agencies did incorporate elder abuse into their agendas, but not at the funding level of the U.S. Children's Bureau program for child abuse.

Without a national focus, a knowledge base, or model statutes, the states developed their own laws, definitions, and reporting procedures. Some used existing adult protective legislation; others, domestic violence acts. Still others passed specific elder abuse laws. By the late 1980s, each of the fifty states had a system in place for receiving reports and investigating, assessing, and monitoring cases. Forty-three of the fifty states adopted the child-abuse approach, making it mandatory for health and social-service professionals and others who work with older persons (the list varies in each of the forty-three states) to report suspected cases of abuse and neglect, subject to a fine or imprisonment or both. In the other states, reporting is voluntary.

However, not all gerontologists agree that elder abuse is an issue. Some believe that society would be better served if, instead of creating a separate response system for a very narrow segment of the older population (whose problems, they say, could be addressed under the rubric of domestic violence or family caregiving), attention were focused on expanding income protection, medical care, and social services for all frail, elderly persons (Crystal, 1986; Callahan, 1986).

Theoretical considerations

Early attempts to understand the nature of elder abuse were influenced by the child-abuse model. Victims were viewed as very dependent older women mistreated by well-meaning but overburdened adult daughters. Later findings suggested that spouse abuse might be a more useful framework for study, since the individuals involved were legally independent adults. To some health researchers, however, using the family violence paradigm, with its emphasis on harm, intentionality, and responsibility, was counterproductive, particularly in cases that involved elders with unmet needs (Phillips, 1986; Fulmer and O'Malley, 1987). They recommended that elder abuse be considered from the perspective of family caregiving. None of these interpretations are sufficient in and of themselves. Neither the child abuse nor the spouse abuse model takes into consideration the impact of the aging process, while the family caregiving theory cannot explain abusive situations in which the victim has no unmet physical needs. It has been suggested that the concept of elder mistreatment may be too complex to be encompassed in one unifying theoretical model (Stein, 1991).

Risk factors and characteristics

Although early studies were useful in documenting the existence of the problem and promoting state elder abuse policies, they were generally based on data collected from agency files; used small, unrepresentative samples; and lumped together the various types of abuse. Karl Pillemer (1986) sought to overcome some of these methodological weaknesses by interviewing victims directly, adding a nonabused comparison group, and limiting the investigation to physical abuse. He selected five risk factors from the family violence and gerontological literature as the most plausible for his investigation: psychopathology of the perpetrator, dependency and exchange relationships between victim and perpetrator, external stress, social isolation, and the intergenerational transmission of violence. His results showed that the abusers were much more likely than the comparison group of caregivers to have mental, emotional, and/or alcohol problems and to be dependent on the victims. Conversely, the abused elders were not more functionally dependent than the control group in carrying out their activities of daily living; in fact, they were less impaired in a number of ways. The families in which abuse occurred tended to have fewer outside contacts and were less satisfied with them than were their non-abuse counterparts. Neither of the other two risk factors (external stress and intergenerational transmission of violence) was supported by the findings. Similar results have been reported by other researchers (Phillips, 1986; Bristowe and Collins, 1989; Anetzberger, 1987).

A comparison of 328 cases by abuse type (physical, psychological, financial, neglect) revealed three distinct profiles (Wolf et al., 1986). Perpetrators of physical/psychological abuse were more likely than those of neglect to have a history of mental illness and alcohol abuse, and to be dependent on the victim for financial resources. The victims were apt to be in poor emotional health but relatively independent in the activities of daily living. Since these types of abuse involved family members who were most intimately related and emotionally connected, it was likely that this form of maltreatment had its underpinnings in long-standing, pathological family dynamics and interpersonal processes that became more highly charged when the dependent relationship was altered by illness or financial needs.

In contrast with the cases of physical/psychological and financial abuse, those involving neglect appeared to be very much related to the dependency needs of the victim. Neither psychological problems nor financial dependency was a significant factor in the lives of these perpetrators; instead, the victims were a source of stress. Financial abuse represented still another profile. The victims were generally widowed and had few social supports. The perpetrators had financial problems and histories of substance abuse. Rather than interpersonal pathology or victim dependency, the salient factor in explaining these cases was the desire for money.

Prevalence

Although knowledge about the extent of elder abuse is sorely needed to guide policy and planning activities, by 1992 only three prevalence studies were reported. Using a methodology that had been validated in two national family violence surveys, Karl Pillemer and David Finkelhor (1988) surveyed 2,020 noninstitutionalized elders living in the metropolitan Boston area and found that 3.2 percent had experienced physical abuse, verbal aggression, and/or neglect in the period since they reached sixty-five years. Spouse abuse was more prevalent (58 percent) than abuse by adult children (24 percent), the proportion of victims was roughly equally divided between males and females, and economic status and age were not related to the risk of abuse. A national prevalence survey of elder abuse in Canada repeated the Boston methodology but added financial abuse (Podnieks, 1992). Four percent of Canadian elders able to respond on the telephone were found to have recently experienced one or more forms of mistreatment. Again, the rates of victimization for men and women were about equal. However, an epidemiological study of abuse experienced by persons sixty-five years or older in a small semi-industrialized town in west-central Finland produced a prevalence rate of 2.5 percent for men, 7.0 percent for women, and 5.4 percent for both sexes (Kivelä et al., 1992).

Treatment and ethical issues

A number of potential conflicts face practitioners who are handling elder abuse cases. While tangible proof may be obtainable in situations involving physical and financial abuse, psychological abuse and neglect are far more difficult to verify. Symptoms of sexual abuse may elude the investigator who is not aware that not only old but also very old people can be so victimized. Cultural biases and lack of full knowledge about the circumstances involved in a case may lead a worker to conclude, falsely, that abuse has occurred. The instability of the mental and physical status of the victim and/or the perpetrator and the dynamics of their relationship may add to case uncertainty. The individual who at first appears to be the victim may actually be the perpetrator. The issue of competency can be particularly troublesome. There may be resistance on the part of the victim to undergo medical assessment, or of the perpetrator to allow it, or even of the medical profession to make a decision.

An individual who under the law is mandated to report a case of suspected abuse may hesitate because the details of the situation have not been fully documented. Whether the problem is civil or criminal may be unclear. Certainly, the unwillingness of the victim to press charges has been a major hindrance to intervention efforts. Even though the law may require an investigation, the older person may not wish to cooperate or to accept the services that are offered. This negative response brings the worker face to face with a dilemma: the interest of the state, professionals, and society in protecting vulnerable persons versus the individual's right to self-determination; in terms of ethical principles, the tension between autonomy and beneficence. To the degree that family caregiving issues are involved, elder mistreatment violates the virtues of care, compassion, benevolence, and respect for parents. It is a reminder, at a time when the care of older persons is viewed as primarily a family function, that the community cannot abrogate its responsibility.

Conclusion

Advances in understanding the nature of elder abuse will necessitate examining the problem from many perspectives. Not only must distinctions be made among the various types of abuse and neglect, but more attention must be paid to differences based on gender, race, culture, relationships, and circumstances. The awakening interest in the problem among social scientists and medical personnel all over the world is a welcome sign. The results of their efforts should be very constructive in building the theoretical and empirical base for successful treatment and prevention programs.

ROSALIE S. WOLF

Directly related to this article are the other articles in this entry: CHILD ABUSE, *and* ABUSE BETWEEN DOMESTIC PARTNERS. *Also directly related is the entry* AGING AND THE AGED. *For a further discussion of topics mentioned in this article, see the entry* FAMILY. *This article will find application in the entries* LONG-TERM CARE, *articles on* NURSING HOMES, *and* HOME CARE. *For a discussion of related ideas, see the entries* COMPASSION; HARM; RESPONSIBILITY; *and* TRUST.

Bibliography

ANETZBERGER, GEORGIA. 1987. *The Etiology of Elder Abuse by Adult Offspring.* Springfield, Ill.: Charles C. Thomas.

BRISTOWE, ELIZABETH, and COLLINS, JOHN B. 1989. "Family Mediated Abuse of Non-Institutionalized Frail Elderly Men and Women Living in British Columbia." *Journal of Elder Abuse & Neglect* 1, no. 1:45–64.

BURSTON, G. R. 1975. "Granny-battering." *British Medical Journal* 3, no. 5983:592.

CALLAHAN, JAMES J., JR. 1986. "Guest Editor's Perspective." *Pride Institute Journal of Long Term Home Health Care* 5, no. 4:2–3.

CRYSTAL, STEPHEN. 1986. "Social Policy and Elder Abuse." In *Elder Abuse: Conflict in the Family,* pp. 331–339. Edited by Karl A. Pillemer and Rosalie S. Wolf. Dover, Mass.: Auburn House.

FULMER, TERRY, and O'MALLEY, TERRENCE. 1987. *Inadequate Care of the Elderly: A Health Care Perspective on Abuse and Neglect.* New York: Springer.

JOHNSON, TANYA. 1986. "Critical Issues in the Definition of Elder Mistreatment." In *Elder Abuse: Conflict in the Family,* pp. 167–196. Edited by Karl A. Pillemer and Rosalie S. Wolf. Dover, Mass.: Auburn House.

KIVELÄ, SIRKKA-LIISA; KÖNGÄS-SAVIARO, PÄIVI; KESTI, ERKKI; PAHKAL, KIMMO; and IJÄS, MAIJA-LIISA. 1992. "Abuse in Old Age—Epidemiological Data from Finland." *Journal of Elder Abuse & Neglect* 4, no. 3:1–12.

PHILLIPS, LINDA R. 1986. "Theoretical Explanations of Elder Abuse: Competing Hypotheses and Unresolved Issues." In *Elder Abuse: Conflict in the Family,* pp. 197–217. Edited by Karl A. Pillemer and Rosalie S. Wolf. Dover, Mass.: Auburn House.

———. 1988. "The Fit of Elder Abuse with the Family Violence Paradigm and the Implications of a Paradigm Shift for Clinical Practice." *Public Health Nursing* 5, no. 4: 222–229.

PILLEMER, KARL A. 1986. "Risk Factors in Elder Abuse: Results from a Case-Control Study." In *Elder Abuse: Conflict in the Family,* pp. 239–264. Edited by Karl A. Pillemer and Rosalie S. Wolf. Dover, Mass.: Auburn House.

PILLEMER, KARL A., and FINKELHOR, DAVID. 1988. "The Prevalence of Elder Abuse: A Random Sample Survey." *Gerontologist* 28:51–57.

PODNIEKS, ELIZABETH. 1992. "A National Survey on the Abuse of the Elderly in Canada." *Journal of Elder Abuse & Neglect* 4, no. 1/2:1–25.

STEIN, KAREN. 1991. "A National Agenda for Elder Abuse and Neglect Research: Issues and Recommendations." *Journal of Elder Abuse & Neglect* 3, no. 3:91–108.

WOLF, ROSALIE S.; GODKIN, MICHAEL A.; and PILLEMER, KARL A. 1986. "Maltreatment of the Elderly: A Comparative Analysis." *Pride Institute Journal of Long Term Home Health Care* 5, no. 4:10–17.

ACADEMIC HEALTH CENTERS

The definition of the modern American academic health center adopted by the Association of Health Academic Centers is "an institution having either an allopathic or osteopathic medical school, at least one other health-professional educational program or school, and at least one associated teaching hospital" (Association of Academic Health Centers, 1992). Most academic health centers comprise three or more professional schools, the most common being nursing, dentistry, allied health, pharmacy, and public health, in addition to medicine. Of the 126 allopathic and 15 osteopathic medical schools in the United States, 121 institutions meet the requirements of this definition. Academic health centers may be university-based or freestanding universities of the health sciences. Two-thirds are public institutions and one-third are private. Taken together, academic health centers are responsible for the majority of government-funded biomedical research and the great majority of postbaccalaureate health professional education, and they provide half of the nation's uncompensated hospital care (Association of Academic Health Centers, 1994).

Since the end of World War II, U.S. health and biomedical science policy has been characterized by expansion. Federal policies have focused on basic and applied biomedical research, including personnel training to increase the number of well-qualified scientists and capital expansion of laboratory capacity. Almost all of this increased public support has been funneled into universities, with the largest concentration directed to academic health centers. As a consequence, there has been a substantial increase in the number of university-based and university-related teaching hospitals, and many existing institutions have been refurbished. Together, these institutions have become the most advanced network of high-technology medicine in the world.

Societal policies and preferences for a diversified and largely private health-financing system have provided strong financial incentives to enhance specialization and further technologic invention. And federal and state policies from the late 1940s until the early 1990s generally encouraged sharp increases in the number of health professionals educated in academic health centers. In 1970, for example, the federal government offered annual capitation payments (a fixed amount for each enrolled student) to medical schools that significantly increased the sizes of their entering classes. This, plus the development of a large number of new medical schools, led to a virtual doubling of the number of medical school graduates between the mid-1960s and the mid-1980s (Association of American Medical Colleges, 1993).

Despite their enormous growth and success, academic health centers find themselves in the eye of a storm that has been triggered most recently by trends in health-care reform in the 1990s. It may seem paradoxical that a political movement toward reorganization and refinancing of national health services should highlight a conflict in values within the academic health center and its university. The explanation of this apparent paradox may open the way for an appropriate debate on the future role of academic health centers. Simply put, the explanation for the paradox is that health-care reform will serve to separate more precisely the teaching, research, and education functions and will highlight conflicts of commitment and interest at both institutional and individual faculty levels. The remainder of this entry will elaborate on this explanation.

Until very recently, there was no doubt in the public mind that the academic health centers were meeting the public's expectations by doubling the output of very well-trained specialist physicians, biomedical scientists, and other advanced-degree health professionals. The expansion of specialty medicine was closely linked to the advances in basic and applied research; this linkage made university hospitals the centerpieces of the U.S. health-care system. During the 1980s and early 1990s, medical-school clinical faculty expanded in number and prospered under the prevailing technologically oriented, procedure-oriented, fee-for-service payment system. Many of these dollars were used for the operation and advancement of the institutions as well as for the payment of the earners' salaries.

Moreover, there has been a major cross-subsidization of education and research by clinical earnings. Clinical revenue now provides the single largest source of support for medical schools, averaging about 31 percent of their budgets nationwide (Association of American Medical Colleges, 1993). Similarly, research and education funds have enhanced the clinical enterprise of the health-science center. For example, federal payments for graduate medical education that support medical residents and their educational costs are of economic benefit to the teaching hospitals because of the huge service load borne by the residents.

Through five decades of overall prosperity and growth, academic health centers were able to use the three biggest sources of funding (education, research, and service dollars) in highly effective and synergistic ways. If, from time to time, one funding stream was temporarily reduced, the other two could more than make up the difference. With health-care reform in the mid-1990s, the trend to managed care and capitated health plans became dominant. This trend toward capitation (health plans receiving fixed payment amounts to provide services to meet an individual's needs) is driving providers into networks of care in which the high-cost teaching hospital becomes a financial drain instead of a fiscal bonanza. This dramatic alteration in the fiscal landscape of the academic health center is taking place very rapidly and comes at a time when the other two financial streams are being reduced or stringently limited (U.S. Physician Payment Review Commission, 1993). As a result, there is growing concern, especially in the academic community, about the vulnerability and fragility of these institutions. Given the extent to which academic health centers are leveraged financially and depend upon multiple sources of external funds over which they have little or no control, faculty and administrators may appear to be worrying more about the economic viability of their institutions than about the quality of the education or care they provide (Lombardi, 1991).

The threat of continuing cutbacks, job losses, and role redefinitions serves to stimulate widespread faculty anxiety. In medical schools especially, where expansion has been most dramatic, the financial threat is enhanced by the growing external criticism of what they have been doing and failing to do.

While faculties have been progressing with successful research on the frontiers of molecular disease and therapy, powerful forces in society have been roused to question the high cost of "high-tech" medical care and the propriety of the degree of specialty domination of American health care. Although teaching hospitals already provide 50 percent of the nation's uncompensated care, many critics believe that academic health centers have seriously failed to do what they could and should have done to raise the health status of the underserved and disadvantaged populations in their local communities. They are criticized for their relative lack of emphasis on such issues as prevention and chronic, long-term care. In return for government support, academic health centers are being asked to reorient their activities and expand their horizons into community-based public health, which for many is alien to their basic sciences focus (Schroeder et al., 1989; Inui, 1992). The argument for social responsibility of academic health centers is that they have received large amounts of taxpayer support for building their research empires, yet little of their success is returned to certain constituencies in the form of preventive care or community-based public-health services. This argument applies to public as well as private institutions that also receive some public support.

In addition to being held accountable for the public's health, medical schools are being asked by many states and in several federal health-reform proposals to ensure that half their graduates enter primary care. This, too, is intended to meet a social goal—improved access to care and reduced costs. Funding for medical schools in some states has already been made contingent on this outcome; student loans may also be tied to primary care. While this is a worthy goal in some ways, it is also problematic in several respects. First, it will dramatically alter the work force available in the teaching hospitals, many of which are national or regional resources for specialty care. Second, such public policies could be seen to infringe on the rights of individuals. U.S. society does not dictate career decisions to lawyers, professors, or others. Is medicine intrinsically different? Third, if student loans are tied to career commitments in primary care, will economically disadvantaged students be disproportionately affected by being steered into the lower-paid, lower-status ranges of the profession? Fourth, the "50 percent primary-care physician" dictum fails to take account of all the other health professionals, many of whom can play significant roles in primary care. The threat of such a policy may already be having some interesting, and perhaps unintended, consequences as more physician assistants and nurse-practitioners pursue specialty careers (Fowkes, 1993). And fifth, when all citizens have access to health care, we may find severe shortages of at least some kinds of specialists, especially in the traditionally underserved areas.

Thus, the expectations for academic health centers are expanding even as the resources shrink. Clearly, this is a time of challenge and stress for academic health centers. Some may go out of business. While some may be able to continue to emphasize biomedical research and specialty medicine, most will have to reexamine their basic premises and the nature of their relationship to the society and constituencies that nurture them (Bulger, 1990). Most will have to do some painful reconfiguring that will involve an appropriate involvement with at least some of the broader concerns of the society. These institutions, born and bred within universities with academic values, have now become important players in a social movement to reform health care. As the academic health centers reconsider and reinvent themselves, the tension between the basic university values and those of a service-oriented business that increasingly characterize the teaching hospitals and related patient-care activities will need to reach a new balance (Bulger, 1992). The stress of that tension may be so great that some institutions will sell their hospitals and clinics to a private health-service provider system and refocus their attention on teaching and research.

In other instances it may be possible to strike a new balance between the values of academe and the values of the society. For example, since health care for the underserved has been a traditional concern of university programs, academic health centers might successfully stimulate, participate in, and help evaluate new programs of health-care delivery to the chronically underserved. Several initiatives along these lines are taking shape, building upon outreach through primary-care outpatient sites, telecommunications, and new organizational forms to facilitate coordination of services among existing providers in a region (Association of Academic Health Centers Task Force, 1992). These and other creative health-service ideas will emerge and be implemented in many academic institutions, even as they seek to enhance their educational and research efforts.

ROGER J. BULGER

For a further discussion of topics mentioned in this entry, see the entries ALLIED HEALTH PROFESSIONS; HEALTH CARE, QUALITY OF; HEALTH-CARE DELIVERY, *especially the article on* HEALTH-CARE INSTITUTIONS; HEALTH-CARE FINANCING; HEALTH POLICY, *article on* POLITICS AND HEALTH CARE; *and* MEDICAL EDUCATION. *For a discussion of related ideas, see the entries* AUTONOMY; *and* VALUE AND VALUATION. *Other relevant material may be found under the entries* COMMERCIALISM IN SCIENTIFIC RESEARCH; HOSPITAL; RESEARCH METHODOLOGY; *and* RESEARCH POLICY.

Bibliography

ASSOCIATION OF ACADEMIC HEALTH CENTERS. 1992. *Charter and By-Laws of the Association of Academic Health Centers.* Rev. ed. Washington, D.C.: Author.

———. 1994. *Critical Data About Academic Health Centers: Survey Report.* Washington, D.C.: Author.

ASSOCIATION OF ACADEMIC HEALTH CENTERS TASK FORCE ON HUMAN RESOURCES FOR HEALTH. 1992. *Avoiding the Next Crisis in Health Care.* Washington, D.C.: Author.

ASSOCIATION OF AMERICAN MEDICAL COLLEGES. 1993. *Association of American Medical Colleges Data Book: Statistical Information Related to Medical Education.* Washington, D.C.: Author.

BULGER, ROGER J. 1990. "Covenant, Leadership and Value Formation in Academic Health Centers." In *Integrity in Health Care Institutions: Humane Environments for Teaching, Inquiry and Healing,* pp. 3–17. Edited by Ruth Ellen Bulger and Stanley Joel Reiser. Iowa City: University of Iowa Press.

———. 1992. "The Role of America's Academic Health Centers in a Reformed Health System." *Journal of American Health Policy* 2, no. 6:35–38.

FOWKES, VIRGINIA. 1993. "Meeting the Needs of the Underserved: The Roles of Physician Assistants and Nurse Practitioners." In *The Roles of Physician Assistants and Nurse Practitioners in Primary Care*, pp. 69–84. Edited by D. Kay Clawson and Marian Osterweis. Washington, D.C.: Association of Academic Health Centers.

INUI, THOMAS S. 1992. "The Social Contract and the Medical School's Responsibilities." In *The Medical School's Mission and the Population's Health: Medical Education in Canada, the United Kingdom, the United States, and Australia*, pp. 23–59. Edited by Kerr L. White and Julia E. Connelly. New York: Springer-Verlag.

LOMBARDI, JOHN V. 1991. "Science, Doctors, and the University: New Alliances for a Competitive Age." In *Preparing for Science in the 21st Century*, pp. 51–61. Edited by Donald C. Harrison, Marian Osterweis, and Elaine R. Rubin. Washington, D.C.: Association of Academic Health Centers.

SCHROEDER, STEVEN A.; ZONES, JANE S.; and SHOWSTACK, JONATHAN A. 1989. "Academic Medicine as a Public Trust." *Journal of the American Medical Association* 262, no. 6:803–812.

U.S. PHYSICIAN PAYMENT REVIEW COMMISSION. 1993. *Annual Report to Congress*. Washington, D.C.: Author.

ACCESS TO HEALTH CARE

See HEALTH-CARE RESOURCES, ALLOCATION OF. See also HEALTH-CARE DELIVERY; and HEALTH-CARE FINANCING.

ACTING AND REFRAINING

See ACTION. For discussion of the concepts in withdrawing and withholding treatment, see DEATH AND DYING: EUTHANASIA AND SUSTAINING LIFE.

ACTION

Discussion in bioethics typically concentrates on whether a particular action is morally right or wrong. It is easy to presume, therefore, that actions are constants and that it is the business of ethics to assign to them variable modifiers such as "right" or "wrong," "good" or "bad." Closer inspection reveals this is not the case. Moral disagreements often hinge as much on what a specific action is as on whether it is right or wrong. Virtually without exception the major problems in bioethics involve questions regarding how actions are appropriately described.

While questions related to action and action description may seem abstruse, it is important to see that they arise quite quickly and naturally in routine discussions of issues in medical ethics. The simple demand that someone "define his terms" in a discussion of eu-

thanasia, for instance, asks for greater clarity about what the action "euthanasia" designates. What makes an act of euthanasia an act of euthanasia?

Initially we might note that "euthanasia" is brought into a discussion with regard only to patients who are terminally ill, in a persistent vegetative state, or in intractable pain. Beyond that, it designates an action involving the death of these patients—involvement of a specific sort. In this regard, consider if someone, call her S, kills patient P—who is in the final stages of bone cancer and enduring excruciating pain—not because S pities him but because she stands to gain from his death. Her action might masquerade as euthanasia but almost certainly is not. Clearly, then, motive and/or intent in acting partly determine what is or is not euthanasia. Intention, especially, can be quite subtle; we may need further distinctions to proceed, such as one separating indirect from direct intention, or possible outcome foreseen from outcome intended. For example, suppose in another case S acts to relieve P's pain but, in so doing, knowingly risks his death . . . and P dies. Is this euthanasia?

In another vein, suppose S does not act at all but stands by while P dies from something S's intervention might have prevented, perhaps from cardiac arrest. S purposefully did not act to preserve P's life. Is this euthanasia? There are reasons to think so, for S refrained from acting partly because she thought P would be better off dead. Perhaps euthanasia need include no bodily movements at all but only a purely mental act. If movement is required, what of another case? Suppose S's movement was to disconnect a respirator, and P subsequently died. Did S euthanize P in this case?

Returning to our imagined discussion, clearly the move to "define one's terms" involves complexities about action and action description that cannot be settled with hasty stipulations. Yet in the rush to proceed to judgments about right or wrong we are tempted to pass quickly over this vast territory of inquiry. If we do, it is likely that our discussions will end in confusion rather than genuine agreement or disagreement, for we will be unable to tell what actions the judgment "euthanasia is wrong (or right)" specifies. In what follows below, we pause within this vast territory, briefly attempting to outline its largely uncharted regions.

The philosophical discussion

Discussion of questions regarding action and action description has been ongoing in analytic philosophy as "action theory," with increased activity since the 1960s. Philosophers have typically begun their analysis with *events*, suggesting that actions are a species of events, one in which human actors are involved in some special way (see Zimmerman, 1984). A common intuition, perhaps morally based, encourages this pattern of analysis: From among the myriad events constantly occurring in our world, we seek to identify those in which human involvement is decisive. Involving choice and agency, these events easily become the chief object of our moral judgment. Events as actions admit of moral evaluation; events that are not actions do not, or at least not so clearly.

A discussion of events may also serve to moor actions ontologically. Events, along with individual things and properties, have been thought by some philosophers to exist irreducibly. We think of this as a temporal existence—events have a life, they begin and end in time—but at least one philosopher, Roderick Chisholm (1976), has suggested they are perhaps better classed as proposition-like entities. As such they can recur. So the single event "the sun's rising" (expressed in this proposition-like form) happened yesterday and today, and will happen tomorrow. For dealing with actions as we are wont to—generalizing and grouping them, assessing them morally, attributing the same action to different agents—some move such as Chisholm's seems necessary. For example, if Jack stabbed John to death and Jill poisoned Judy to death, we want to say of both that they killed. If each deed is understood only as a unique particular, this would be difficult.

Some analytic philosophers have worked around this problem by distinguishing act types from act tokens. An act token is a particular act performed by a particular person at a particular time. An act type is more like an event as described above on Chisholm's accounting, a recurring entity that can be done by different persons in different circumstances. In action theory, more discussion has been devoted to act tokens than to act types. Specifically at issue has been the matter of how a particular act (act token) is individuated. The difficulties are occasioned by at least two complexities to be found in any particular act: that it is composed of smaller parts, each which might be considered an act; and that as a piece of human behavior it can be described variously, for example, in terms of the intentions of the person who did it, its results, short and long term, or its physical movements. So we might find that "S's taking target practice at time t" yields the following list of descriptions:

1. S's willingness to move her finger at t
2. S's moving her finger at t
3. S's pulling the trigger at t
4. S's firing a gun at t
5. S's shooting at the bull's-eye at t
6. S's violating an ordinance prohibiting firearm use at t.

Philosophers have come to call these elaborations of particular actions "action trees." Controversy has arisen over the relation between the various discrete acts within them. Are we to say, for example, that "S's moving her finger at t" is the same act as "S's shooting at the bull's-eye"? The unity approach, championed by Donald Davidson (1980) and G. E. M. Anscombe, claims that they are the same action, under different descriptions (Anscombe, 1981). Against the unity approach some, notably Alvin Goldman (1970), have argued that dissimilarities between each description prohibit them from being so understood. (For example, we can say that 2 caused 4, but evidently 6 did not.) To these objectors, it seems better to adopt a pluralist approach that construes each of the above designations as applying to a distinct act. Since this leaves unexplained the obvious close relation between them, various alternatives that reconnect the discrete acts have been offered by "pluralists," among them Judith Thomson's (1977) attempt to re-collect the various actions as parts of one larger whole or Goldman's (1970) notion that they are related in a special *by* relation (for instance, S shot at the bull's-eye *by* pulling the trigger).

Whether or not the descriptions in the action tree are one or many actions, it is plain that the character of the descriptions differs in tone or focus. In 2, S moves her finger, for what reason we do not know until we attend to 5, which relates the finger moving to the intentional human world. Further disagreement among philosophers arises at this point regarding how this human world—that in which people have purposes, intentions, and motives, and give reasons for action—relates to the impersonal world of events governed, as it is supposed, by strict causal laws. Controversy here reflects a larger and older controversy concerning freedom and determinism, although the disagreement cannot be so easily characterized. No one argues that action descriptions do not presume basic conceptions of agency, intentionality, justification, and the like; on all accounts the presence of these things is necessary for events rightly to be labeled "actions." Rather, differences arise about *precisely* which of these broadly intentional features makes an action an action and about how the action, once identified, is to be fit into the ongoing stream of events surrounding it. Even among analytical philosophers, discussion of this matter has often turned mysterious. So Carl Ginet (1990) defines actions in terms of something he calls an "actish phenomenal character," something we all experience in acting but cannot describe clearly. Even Davidson, who argues that to act is to cause something, suggests that we cannot generally identify the causal laws under which "mental events" (such as rememberings and decisions, as well as actions) are to be subsumed.

As Davidson's influential causal theory illustrates, when considering the identity of an action, it is common to look *before* the action for some act of willing, some mental event. The presumption, both strong and ancient, seems to be that if human action is anything, it is voluntary. No doubt, voluntariness is an important consideration in understanding actions; but it is not entirely clear that all acts must be preceded or accompanied by some distinct act of the will.

Inadvertent acts are acts that include no such willing; they involve a movement of the body that involuntarily brings about some noteworthy result. ("While reaching for the salt, I inadvertently spilled the wine.") It may be, of course, that inadvertent acts are not full-fledged acts. Nonetheless, we do regret inadvertent acts, in a way that we do not regret movements of our bodies that are entirely forced (see Austin, 1957).

It is true that we rarely persist in blaming someone for an inadvertent act. ("I'm sorry I spilled the wine." "Oh, that's all right. You didn't mean to.") Nonetheless, as Aristotle pointed out, some actions are not strictly voluntary, that is, that are accompanied by no clear act of the will, for which we do ascribe blame. These belong to the class of acts he called "not voluntary." Certain human actions done in ignorance are not completely voluntary, since the ignorance bars the agent from knowing fully what he or she did, yet they are also not completely involuntary, since the agent was ignorant because of some prior (voluntary) disposition not to know what in fact should have been known. So if a physician prescribes a drug that she did not know (but could and should have known) was dangerous to certain patients, and the drug kills the patient, while we might not accuse her of voluntarily killing the patient, we would blame her nonetheless for the patient's death.

This analysis suggests that the retrospective judgments of an agent or of members of his or her community do as much to determine what description is assigned to an action as do prior or accompanying acts of will. As Anscombe implies, reasons for action are often discovered by the agent or members of his or her community *after* an action—but are nonetheless appropriately included in a description of it. It suggests as well that it is not only for actions that agents are held morally accountable. For while the ignorant physician was wrong to prescribe the drug, we blame her not so much for her action as for her prior *inaction* that led to the ignorance.

Acting and refraining

The discussion so far may invite the impression that actions primarily involve the voluntary movement of the body. Yet as discussion of inadvertent acts and culpable ignorance has just indicated, moral assessment is often offered in cases of inaction. This truth is not much emphasized in American criminal law, where it is usually required that prosecution follow only upon someone's

doing something (acting) when he or she should not have, passing over other cases in which someone *did not do* something that evidently should have been done (Glendon, 1991). With regard to medicine and the law, however, negligence is a main ground for medical malpractice. Negligence implies a lack, and fits as easily with *refraining from acting* as with acting, for example, refraining from providing certain life-preserving treatments to a terminally ill patient.

A refraining may be thought of as a kind of action in itself, insofar as it involves some specific act of the will, or mental event. That is, one (actively) decided not to x, so we say that person refrains from x. Yet Saint Thomas Aquinas, who wrote extensively on these matters, was concerned as well with refrainings of another sort. He held that one could have duties of which one was unaware and so might be oblivious to occasions when one should have acted upon them. The ignorant physician discussed above serves as an illustration. She at no point decided not to prescribe a safer available drug—there was no specific act of the will. Nevertheless, we single out her failure to do so, for it is something she should have done and did not. Aquinas, the Christian theologian, would call this failure of duty a "sin of omission." It is importantly termed *sin* rather than *act* of omission—a more contemporary usage (D'Arcy, 1963)—since it is precisely the failure of duty by which it is identified.

To the question of whether sins of omission are by themselves less serious than those of commission, since they involve no active bodily movements, Aquinas answers negatively: "Omission and commission are found in the same species of sin" (I-II, Q. 72, Art. 6). Which is to say that there is nothing about acting as one should not that makes it morally different from not acting as one should. James Rachels, a contemporary proponent of euthanasia, concurs. He says that no moral significance can be assigned to the "bare fact" that in one case one acted and in the other case one did not (1981, p. 465). He illustrates his point with the example of Smith, who kills his young cousin by drowning him in the bath, and Jones, who watches his cousin drown (1975). Jones, it turns out, was planning to do just what Smith did, but was aided by the lucky coincidence that his cousin slipped and hit his head. So Jones needed only to stand by, refraining from rescuing him.

Narrowly understood, the point is that there is nothing about the bodily motion itself—the motion that goes along with killing someone—that makes the act of killing in itself worse than the nonaction or lack of bodily motion that accompanies letting someone die. It does not necessarily follow, however, that "killing" taken as a general action is not prima facie morally worse than letting die, as has been maintained by Rachel's opponent Phillipa Foot (1977) and others. For Aquinas's point is merely that the bodily motion involved in the sinful action is not determinative of the type of sin under which it is finally classified. Killing taken as an action of the killer implies that he did something: He moved his body in some way that resulted in a death. But this is not to say that killing is the same thing as the movement. As has been said, actions are more than events, more than human bodily movements, for they have their rightful place in the human world of intentions, purposes, moral praise and blame, and so on. To say, therefore, that no moral significance should be attributed to the bare difference between moving one's body and not moving it is quite another thing than to say that there is no moral significance in the difference between killing and letting die.

Aquinas's view is best appreciated when we note that (for him at least) an action is not determined by the specific bodily movement it involves. Bodily movements connected with killing can be as diverse as those involving injecting with a syringe, strangling with a rope, writing a signature (to a death warrant), and so on. An action is instead determined by what its actor aims at in his bodily movement, by his primary intention. With the action "killing" this is someone's death. So killing could be defined simply as successfully moving one's body in order to bring about someone's death. (Sometimes we refer loosely to killing "done" by falling trees or by a driver involved in an auto accident. It is less clear, however, that these are instances of the *action* killing, with which we are concerned here.)

What of letting die? Should we define it as *not* moving one's body in order to bring about someone's death? Rachels has helpfully illustrated that *some* lettings die are this—and there is no reason to think these are any less morally blameworthy than killings. Yet it is possible to hold that while all killings necessarily involve the intention that someone die, the refraining from action we have come to call letting die does not, for when we let die, we often do not aim at someone's death but at something else, such as a patient's comfort while dying. If one held, as do many Christian moralists (see Sullivan, 1977), that it is always wrong directly to intend the death of a human being, and insofar as all killings involve this intention necessarily, while not all cases of letting die do, it could make sense to say that killing (the general description, not a specific killing) is morally worse than letting die.

Killing, letting die, and the role of the doctor

A "refraining" cannot logically be defined simply as not acting. The consequences would be quite absurd, for everyone would be refraining from an infinite set of actions when at rest—or even when acting. (For example, while reading an encyclopedia article one is refraining from driving a car, mailing a letter, treating a patient, composing a sonnet, and so on, infinitely.) Better to circumscribe "refraining" in another way; perhaps by identifying some case in which some "refraining" was involved and working backward. Many wish to say, for instance, that someone refrained from offering lifesaving treatment to Infant Doe, the newborn with Down syndrome who died in 1982 in an Indiana hospital due to an obstruction in the esophagus that surgeons could easily have corrected. Yet clearly it was not everyone who did not act to save his life, for again this would be a huge class of individuals. Who, then, let Infant Doe die? His parents? his doctors? his nurses? anyone who viewed him in the hospital? the governor of Indiana?

The problem here is that, unlike cases of an action such as killing, it is less apparent to whom the description "he or she refrained" rightly applies. For in cases of killing, one or more persons move their bodies to bring about the death; they designate themselves as the killers. There is no such self-designation in cases of letting die. That the designation is clearer in cases of action than of nonaction is largely due to the causal relation that obtains between an action and its result. So to determine if "P killed Q" is true, we first look to see if some movement P made led causally to Q's death. (For instance, knife in hand, P thrust his arm forward; the knife penetrated Q's body; Q began bleeding; Q died from loss of blood.) In cases of the refraining "letting die," this causal chain cannot be traced in the same way to point specifically to some human agent, and that is the problem.

Using the notion of cause more broadly than most contemporary analysts, Aquinas supposes that in a certain way refrainings *do* cause things to occur.

> Now one thing proceeds from another in two ways. First, directly, in which something proceeds from another inasmuch as the other acts; for instance heating from heat. Second, indirectly; in which sense something proceeds from another through this other not acting; thus the sinking of a ship is set down to the helmsman from his having ceased to steer.—But we must take note that the cause of what follows from want of action is not always the agent as not acting; but only . . . when the agent can and ought to act. For if the helmsman were unable to steer the ship or if the ship's helm be not entrusted to him, the sinking of the ship would not be set down to him. . . . (I-II, Q. 6, Art. 3)

Many people did not steer the ship that sank; but only one, the helmsman, "caused" the ship to sink by not steering it. The reason is plain: He was in a unique role with respect to the ship's course. As helmsman he was responsible for steering the ship. This is the beginning point of Aquinas's analysis, beyond which he proceeds to make two further points: First, he not only must be the helmsman but it must have been his responsibility in the specific incident of the ship's sinking to steer it, and, second, it must have been within his power so to do.

Applied to cases of refraining from acting collected under the description "letting die," for someone to be thought to "let die," it must be in his or her power to act so as to prevent the death. This eliminates some candidates in the Infant Doe case and also explains why we do not look for people who "let die" if the death could not have been humanly prevented. More important, however, the person must be in the right role with respect to the dying patient, not only generally but in the specific incident of the death. In current social-political arrangements in the West, this is more often than not the patient's physician and immediate family. So we say Infant Doe's parents and his doctor(s) let him die.

One need not argue that it is always wrong for someone (anyone) in his or her action to aim at (directly intend) the death of a human person in order to claim it is always wrong for a physician to do so with respect to a patient. As John Casey (1971) has pointed out, this might be done specifically with reference to the role of the doctor, the role in this sense circumscribing the range of actions physicians could countenance. It would follow that a physician should never kill as a physician, even if it would leave open the question whether someone else might rightly kill, someone who stands in a different role with respect to the patient, such as family members.

To cover cases of letting die, more about the role might be said. If, like the helmsman with the ship, it is decided that the physician's role is to do everything in her power to extend life, then when she does not and could have, she has failed in her role. It would follow that all cases of letting die would be culpable. On the other hand, if one defined the role of physician in a different way, one that included the notion that she should comfort a dying patient but not extend his life at all costs, then cases where the patient dies and the physician does nothing to prevent it are not culpable cases of letting die. Indeed, one might even refuse to name them lettings die by saying, like Aquinas's helmsman, that it is wrong to "set down to" the doctor the death in such a case since it is not part of her role to prevent it. Such a logic would restrict the description "letting die" to culpable cases only, perhaps those like Infant Doe— or of some other sort, depending upon the specific nature of the role designation.

While the modern language of "letting die" could have taken this course, it has not. Analysis of sins of omission, therefore, is not enough to cover it. Since for Aquinas omissions were necessarily culpable failures to act, the specific "not doing" was identified and individuated by the culpability. In modern medicine there seems to be a need for a broader application of the term "letting die," since technological advances have provided the means to extend almost any given life almost indefinitely. This forces a conscious decision not to extend a life. "Letting die" in present usage generally covers all such conscious decisions, some morally culpable, some not. The moral burden shifts from determining whether a physician is guilty of a "sin of omission" (that is, "refrains from preserving a life" in the more restricted and necessarily negligent sense of "refrain") to when letting die is culpable.

The two senses of letting die—culpable and non-culpable—can be helpfully organized by employing another distinction from Aquinas. He suggests that voluntariness applies to an agent when he does not act in two circumstances: (1) when he wills not to act and (2) when he does not will to act. Cases of (1) involve deliberation; they imply that it is in the agent's power to act, that he knows this, and that he consciously decides not to act. Cases of (2) involve no such thought; the agent does not decide not to act, he merely does not act, although he could have acted. For (2) to avoid the danger of applying to too broad a class of agents, it must be circumscribed by a role that includes rules for right action for those who stand within it. So described, cases of (2) would necessarily involve culpability—they are like sins of omission. With (1), however, it is not so much the role that identifies the refraining but the agent's performance of an "interior act" of willing not to act. Applied to a physician who "let die" in this first sense, an inward act occurs, known first to the physician, but later also to those with whom he converses regarding his deliberation or, most plainly to the modern setting, to those he gives a Do Not Resuscitate (DNR) order. His performance of this willing—so long as it is clear that he has the power to act to extend the life, which is a necessary condition for either sense of voluntary refraining to apply—is enough to make the description "letting die" appropriately apply. Whether or not he is right to let die in a particular case remains an open question, one that cannot be answered without a further delineation of the nature of the physician's role with respect to patients who are dying or irreversibly comatose or in a persistent vegetative state or (some would include) in intractable pain.

Intention, action description, and double effect

Perhaps the most widely debated moral principle in medical ethics, the principle of double effect (PDE), relies essentially upon a distinction between a given action and some, if not all, of its effects. The principle stipulates that it is morally permissible to engage in some action that will cause an evil effect so long as four conditions are satisfied: (1) The act itself, prescinded from the evil caused, is good or at least neutral; (2) the good effect of the act is what the agent intends directly, only permitting the evil effect; (3) the good effect must not be caused by means of an evil effect; (4) there must be some proportionately grave reason for permitting the evil effect to occur.

From condition (1), the locution "the act itself"; from (2), "intends directly"; from (3), "an effect caused"; and from (4), "reason for permitting"—none of these can be understood without some prior discussion of what an action is and how it is related to its various effects and what it "causes" (which need not be the same), and the intention of the actor within the action and his or her reasons for doing it (which also need not be the same). PDE has been much maligned by thinkers sympathetic with utilitarianism (such as Fletcher, 1973), which is not surprising, since this theory maintains that the sum of the consequences of an action entirely determines its rightness or wrongness. In response to these directions, moralists of other persuasions have accused utilitarians (or situationists, as in Fletcher's case) of grossly distorting the nature of human action (see Ramsey, 1967, 1968).

While many who grant the importance of PDE have emphasized its proportionality requirement rather than its stipulation that no evil effect be directly intended (see McCormick, 1979), PDE in any form presumes an essential distinction between direct and indirect intention, or, as it is perhaps more profitably put, intention and foresight. This demands, of course, some discussion of what intention is.

In her book *Intention*, G. E. M. Anscombe (1963) describes an intentional action as that which falls in the range of actions to which the question "why?" (directed to the actor) can be fit. (As she understands it, the exchange "Why did you kick me?—Sorry, my leg jerked" involves a rejection of the question "why?" and thus a rejection of the action as intentional.) One might think that this sort of explanation of intention connects to an interior act of the will over which the agent presides and that he or she alone can decipher. On this notion of intention, double effect could not but become superfluous, at least for the purposes of judging the rightness or wrongness of an action. So we might say, for example, that only President Harry S. Truman knew if, when he ordered the bombing of Hiroshima, he intended to kill eighty thousand people. If we continue to count intention as central to moral assessment, it would follow that only Truman could assess his act. Otherwise we could do nothing other than propose a new ground for such assessment, as utilitarians do with their exclusive emphasis upon consequences (Smart, 1973).

Yet Anscombe rejects this strongly inner notion of intention. In the first place, the answer to "why?" is often appropriately given retrospectively. Less a revelation of an internal state of mind, it is an interpretation of the action, as narrated by the actor looking back. It is a mistaken bifurcation of internal thought and external action, as Stuart Hampshire has argued (1983), that has led to the link between intention and the inner and private.

Further, Anscombe notes that the action itself is made intelligible within a description that provides the relevant intention. That is, we do not treat actions as putty, assigning new intentions to them. Private thought cannot transform a bombing, for example, into an action in which the destruction of property and human lives is not intended, for that intention is embedded in the action of bombing. Insofar as actions are more than mere movements and include intentions, specifically named actions include specific intentions.

In some cases one might *redescribe* the particular action, either by giving it a new name or by eliding it into a broader action description that replaces the description under which the action is morally evaluated (see Ramsey, 1968; Pinches 1991). Frequently done, this cannot but render PDE superfluous. If the "bombing of Hiroshima" is elided into Truman's professed larger objective, "ending the war," the arguments one might level (using PDE) against the bombing are rendered ineffectual, for they were formed to apply to "an act of bombing an entire city" now replaced with "an act of ending the war."

These considerations bring up the question of whether there is something like the ultimate description of an action, one that takes precedence over all other possible descriptions. It is related as well to the problem of the individuation of action discussed earlier. Instead of pressing for one primary description, proponents of PDE can limit the proliferation of descriptions by emphasizing that any action must be understood within a community of shared webs of beliefs and practices that impart meaning to it. So Alasdair MacIntyre holds that the concept of an intelligible action is more fundamental than that of an action as such (1981). Intelligible actions are made possible largely by our shared language of description, which in turn rests upon the shared beliefs and practices of our communities.

If someone walks to a public phone, inserts a coin, and presses the numbered buttons, I assume he or she is "making a telephone call." I can describe, and the person can engage in, this action because we both know and make use of telephones, coins, conversations, and so on. If I discover the person is not making a call but is playing a tune with the buttons, that person's action is no longer intelligible—not because I do not understand the action "playing a tune" but because I have lost a sense of what the agent who performed it in this case is up to. (This is illustrated by the fact that I will ask further questions: Do you do that often? What made you do it just now?)

Returning to the questions of individuation, this example illustrates that we can identify an action as discrete and meaningful only because we have a form of life and a language that reflects it which identify slices of human bodily movement in relation to the shared purposes or concerns of the people who live it. Because the end of a human life (death) is of the greatest concern to us, we have actions and words such as "killing," "abortion," "letting die," "murder," "suicide," "fratricide," and so on to describe various sorts of human involvement with it. In applying PDE, its advocates in effect attempt to limit any redescription of human behavior that relegates descriptions like these and the concerns that underlie them (such as directly killing) to a secondary level of importance. So Truman cannot call "ordering the bombing of Hiroshima" an "act of ending the war," for what lies between is the killing of eighty thousand (innocent) humans, something that is—or should be—of the greatest importance to Truman the human actor and to us humans who describe his action.

Julius Kovesi (1967) extends this point by noting that morality is contained in action descriptions (and so in actions themselves); it is not something we add to actions after they are described. A murder is not first identified and then assessed morally; in describing it as murder we judge it morally. While we may try to neutralize the description by drawing it out ("he purposefully thrust the knife into his body"), this misdirects us, for our concern is with a human's death, and with the intent of the agent who caused it.

Similar attempts at neutralization are not uncommon in medicine—an abortion might be redescribed as "surgically removing foreign tissue from the uterus"—but since the activities of medicine have intelligibility and meaning in relation to concerns of the people of the communities in which they are performed, the force of these communities' descriptions cannot be escaped by such technicalization. If, on the other hand, certain descriptions change in these communities—as "abortion" may be changing in certain contexts to "termination of pregnancy"—medicine is sometimes forced into a dilemma. Under which descriptions should medicine understand its activities? Indeed, the biomedical moral issues of our time often ride on the status of a particular action (for instance, abortion, euthanasia, lying, suicide, contraception): how it is to be described and interpreted, in conjunction with how it is to be morally evaluated.

CHARLES R. PINCHES

For a further discussion of topics mentioned in this entry, see the entries DEATH AND DYING: EUTHANASIA AND SUSTAINING LIFE; DOUBLE EFFECT; ETHICS, article on NORMATIVE ETHICAL THEORIES; FREEDOM AND COERCION; RESPONSIBILITY; and UTILITY. For a discussion of related ideas, see the entries ABORTION; and BEHAVIOR CONTROL.

Bibliography

ANSCOMBE, G. E. M. 1963. *Intention.* 2d ed. Ithaca, N.Y.: Cornell University Press.

———. 1981. "'Under a Description.'" In her *Metaphysics and the Philosophy of Mind*, pp. 208–223. Minneapolis: University of Minnesota Press.

AQUINAS, ST. THOMAS. *Summa Theologica*, I-II Q. 1–21, 71–73.

ARISTOTLE. *Nicomachean Ethics.* Book 3.

AUSTIN, J. L. 1957. "A Plea for Excuses." In vol. 56 of *Proceedings of the Aristotelian Society 1956*, pp. 1–30. London: Harrison and Sons.

CASEY, JOHN. 1971. "Actions and Consequences." In *Morality and Moral Reasoning: Five Essays in Ethics*, pp. 155–205. Edited by John Casey. London: Methuen.

CHISHOLM, RODERICK M. 1976. *Person and Object: A Metaphysical Study.* La Salle, Ill: Open Court.

D'ARCY, ERIC. 1963. *Human Acts: An Essay in Their Moral Evaluation.* Oxford: At the Clarendon Press.

DAVIDSON, DONALD. 1980. *Essays on Actions and Events.* Oxford: At the Clarendon Press.

FOOT, PHILLIPA. 1977. "Euthanasia." *Philosophy and Public Affairs* 6, no. 2: 85–112.

FLETCHER, JOSEPH. 1973. "Ethics and Euthanasia." In *To Live and to Die: When, Why and How*, pp. 113–122. Edited by Robert H. Williams. New York: Springer-Verlag.

GINET, CARL. 1990. *On Action.* New York: Cambridge University Press.

GLENDON, MARY ANN. 1991. *Rights Talk: The Impoverishment of Political Discourse.* New York: Free Press.

GOLDMAN, ALVIN. 1970. *A Theory of Human Action.* Englewood Cliffs, N.J.: Prentice-Hall.

HAMPSHIRE, STUART. 1983. *Thought and Action.* New ed. Notre Dame, Ind.: University of Notre Dame Press.

KOVESI, JULIUS. 1967. *Moral Notions.* London: Routledge & Kegan Paul.

MacINTYRE, ALASDAIR. 1981. *After Virtue.* Notre Dame, Ind.: University of Notre Dame Press.

McCORMICK, RICHARD A. 1979. "Ambiguity in Moral Choice." In *Doing Evil to Achieve Good*, pp. 7–53. Edited by Richard A. McCormick and Paul Ramsey. Chicago: Loyola University Press.

PINCHES, CHARLES. 1991. "Principle Monism and Action Descriptions: Situationism and Its Critics Revisited." *Modern Theology* 7:249–268.

RACHELS, JAMES. 1975. "Active and Passive Euthanasia." *New England Journal of Medicine* 292, no. 2:78–80.

———. 1981. "Reasoning About Killing and Letting Die." *Southern Journal of Philosophy* 19:465–473.

RAMSEY, PAUL. 1967. *Deeds and Rules in Christian Ethics*, pp. 145–240. New York: Scribner.

———. 1968. "The Case of the Curious Exception." In *Norm and Context in Christian Ethics*, pp. 67–135. By Gene Outka, Paul Ramsey, and Frederick S. Carney. New York: Scribner.

SMART, J. J. C. 1973. *Utilitarianism: For and Against*, pp. 30–42. New York: Cambridge University Press.

SULLIVAN, THOMAS D. 1977. "Active and Passive Euthanasia: An Impertinent Distinction?" *Human Life Review* 3, no. 3:40–46.

THOMSON, JUDITH JARVIS. 1977. *Acts and Other Events*. Ithaca, N.Y.: Cornell University Press.

ZIMMERMAN, MICHAEL J. 1984. *An Essay on Human Action*. New York: Peter Lang.

ACTIVE EUTHANASIA

See DEATH AND DYING: EUTHANASIA AND SUSTAINING LIFE; *and* INFANTS, *articles on* HISTORY OF INFANTICIDE, *and* ETHICAL ISSUES. *See also* SUICIDE.

ADDICTION AND DEPENDENCE

See SUBSTANCE ABUSE, *article on* ADDICTION AND DEPENDENCE. *For a discussion of addiction programs, see* MENTAL-HEALTH SERVICES.

ADOLESCENTS

Adolescents in the United States, defined as persons between thirteen and eighteen, today have much greater rights to make health-care decisions than they did a generation ago.

General consent to medical procedures

Under British common law—the system by which cases decided by judges and then used as precedents were far more important than statutes enacted by Parliament, a system that the United States retained when it declared its independence—a minor was effectively a chattel of his or her parents. A "minor" meant someone under twenty-one until the Twenty-sixth Amendment in 1971 gave voting rights to eighteen-year-olds, to whom the states then granted majority.) Child abuse was not against the law anywhere in the United States until 1903 because it interfered with parental rights of discipline. A physician who treated a minor without parental consent except in a life-threatening emergency could be liable, even in cases of a satisfactory medical outcome, to the child's father for interference with his control of his child. (Married women, until about the time of World War I, could not bring lawsuits, for themselves or for their children.)

Beginning in the early 1960s, however, physicians urged state legislators to recognize that adolescents were contributing to an epidemic of venereal disease in this country. Because adolescents knew that physicians were reluctant to treat them without parental consent, these young people were not seeking medical care. They were afraid, with cause, that parents would be notified of the diagnosis even if no treatment was provided, so they refused to enter the health-care system. By the end of the 1960s, all states had enacted statutes permitting treatment of minors for venereal disease without parental notification. In the early 1970s, legislatures provided the same protection for physicians who dealt with adolescents' problems involving drug and alcohol abuse. Also beginning in the 1960s, many states enacted statutes providing that minors of a given age (from fourteen to sixteen) might consent generally to medical or surgical care.

Regardless of statutory authority, however, it has been at least forty years since any court in the United States has allowed parents of a child of fifteen or older to recover damages from a physician for treating their adolescent without their consent, when consent was given by the child. Courts in these cases now uphold treatment given when the patient is mature enough to understand the medical information and to give the same sort of informed consent that would be accepted from an adult patient. This has become known as the "mature minor" rule. The decision to treat an adolescent without parental involvement, of course, depends as much on the nature of the illness and the risks of the treatment as it does on the age of the patient. Although most physicians would treat an adolescent on his or her own for a sore throat or earache, it is not likely that an oncologist would accept as a patient an adolescent with leukemia who refused to involve his or her parents.

In any case, these decisions rarely involve critical illness because hospitals, for financial reasons, refuse to admit minors without parental consent except in emergencies. Since adolescents, if they are insured, are insured as dependents on their parents' health insurance policies, the consent of the policyholders is required for nonemergency admission. Thus issues about treatment of adolescents without parental involvement almost always are confined to outpatient care given in clinics and physicians' offices where the health-care provider will accept whatever payment the young person can make on his or her own.

Even at common law, children of any age (including infants) can be treated without parental consent in an emergency—"emergency" being broadly defined to include anything requiring immediate care, even if not life-threatening. Thus a two-year-old with a fracture or laceration who is brought to the emergency room by a twelve-year-old baby-sitter would be treated even if parents could not be located.

The other exception at common law—and today an exception to requirements for parental consent to treatment—is the "emancipated minor," a concept since the early days of English law. Its modern definition covers minors who are married, who are in military service, or who are not living at home and are not financially dependent on their parents. In some states minors living at home but self-supporting are considered emancipated. In almost all states unmarried minor mothers, as young as eleven or twelve, are emancipated even if they are living with their parents; and in some states pregnant minors of any age are emancipated.

Adolescents who meet the definition of emancipation in the states where they are living may consent to or refuse any medical care, buy and sell real estate, and sue or be sued without appointment of a guardian. The parent is not financially responsible for supporting the emancipated minor and is not obliged to provide any further parental care to him or her.

Refusal of treatment.   Another issue arises when minors wish to refuse treatment that their parents wish to be provided. In the context of "necessary" medical care, when an adolescent's life is not at stake, most courts will permit the young person to decide.

Only one case has reached the appellate level in which an adolescent, a Jehovah's Witness, wished to refuse life-saving treatment. She had leukemia and needed blood transfusions, which are forbidden by her religious beliefs. The trial judge decided that the patient understood her situation, understood that she would die without treatment, and that her refusal was based on her religious convictions and not on parental coercion or fear of abuse if she consented. He therefore allowed her to refuse on the same basis that an adult would be allowed to refuse. The decision was upheld on appeal (*In the Interests of E.G.*, 1987/1989).

The limits of an adolescent's right to refuse life-saving treatment are ill-defined in law. At least one court has held that a young adolescent and her parents had no right on religious grounds to refuse treatment for her bone cancer, and ordered it provided (*Hamilton*, 1983). This situation is so rarely presented to courts—although it obviously must occur at least occasionally within the health-care system—that no one knows whether oncologists and other physicians caring for adolescents with life-threatening conditions are adept at dealing with the psychosocial issues, such as appearance, that arise with these patients, and at resolving the issue with the adolescent. How much weight should be given to a fourteen-year-old's conviction that he would rather die than lose his leg as part of the treatment of his bone cancer?

Perhaps the oncologists who deal with these young people are able to resolve the issues through decisions that respect the patients' autonomy while preserving their lives. Are these adolescents treated over their objections but with parental consent, no outsider such as a judge ever knowing about it? Or are these adolescents being allowed to refuse treatment? Since no studies exist of such cases, there is no information on which to base conclusions.

Confidentiality.   If an adolescent is accepted for treatment without the knowledge of his or her parents, the next question is what information, if any, the parents are entitled to have. Once the young person is accepted for treatment, presumably because the physician feels confident that the patient can give informed consent, it appears that a promise of confidentiality has been given. If the physician is not comfortable dealing with the adolescent alone, then he or she should not agree to provide the treatment without parental involvement.

The statutes of most states providing for treatment of minors for venereal diseases, drug abuse, or alcohol problems without parental consent forbid disclosure to parents, without the patient's consent, that the treatment has been provided or the condition exists. Some of these statutes forbid sending a bill to the parents for the care, lest they question the adolescent about the reason for the visit to the physician or clinic.

The urgent question today about confidentiality of adolescent patients in terms of disclosures to parents concerns HIV infection. On one hand, not only is the HIV-infected young person confronted with a life-threatening problem for which he or she should receive loving support, but the cost of medications (such as AZT) to delay the onset of full-blown AIDS is usually far beyond the reach of a teenager without parental assistance and insurance coverage from the parent. On the other hand, AIDS clinics serving adolescent patients have ample evidence that, as was true about venereal disease in the 1960s, adolescents will not come for testing or for care unless they trust clinic personnel not to involve their parents. Long-term follow-up studies from New York City indicate that teenagers whose parents do not know they are HIV-positive fare as well as those whose parents are involved (Kipke and Hein, 1990). In order to get adolescents into testing and treatment, if discussions over time do not result in the adolescent's agreement to let his or her family be involved, some hospital clinics are providing these young people with free medications.

It is likely that in any serious medical situation, from a positive pregnancy test to a diagnosis of HIV-positivity, physicians and nurses urge adolescents to tell their parents and agree to help them do it. It is also likely that, confronted with a crisis, most adolescents eventually agree to involve a family member. Physicians and nurses who care for adolescents, however, know that for the remainder, "My father will kill me" may not be hyperbole. Moreover, adolescents in problematic, unsupportive families will not seek care unless they know that their confidences will be protected.

Contraception.   In 1965 the U.S. Supreme Court held that state statutes forbidding the prescription of contraceptives to a married woman violated her and her husband's constitutional right of privacy. In 1972 the Court applied the same rule to unmarried adults. In 1977 the Supreme Court held that minors have the same constitutional right of privacy and that state statutes making it a criminal offense to provide contraceptives to minors were unconstitutional.

Title X of the U.S. Public Health Service Act of 1970 requires that family-planning services be available at federally funded clinics without regard to age, as well as religion, race, or other attribute. In 1978 Title X was amended specifically to include adolescents, but in 1981 it was again amended to read, "To the extent practical, entities which receive grants or contracts under Title X shall encourage family participation in projects assisted under this subsection." Federal regulations were then enacted that required any entity receiving federal funds for family-planning services to notify parents within ten days that their minor daughter had received contraceptive services, but these regulations were immediately declared unconstitutional on the grounds that they violated congressional intent as expressed in the act. Thus a minor has the right to obtain contraceptive services from an entity receiving federal funds. This statute does not apply to a physician in private practice, who thus—when asked to provide contraceptives to an adolescent—is legally able to refuse on the basis of ethical objections.

Abortion.   Although recent decisions give state legislatures more power to regulate abortions than they had after *Roe v. Wade*, the Supreme Court has preserved the basic principles of its initial decision. The rationale of the Supreme Court in the 1973 decision was that a woman's right to privacy and her right to control her own body give her the right to decide whether to bear a child. All the women bringing the 1973 cases were adults, and the rights of minors to have abortions have been the subject of many appellate decisions since then.

Beginning in 1979 (*Bellotti v. Baird*) and continuing in a line of cases that has not yet resolved the issue, the Supreme Court has held that if a state wishes to enact legislation requiring parental consent to a minor's abortion, it must provide an alternative forum to permit the young woman to bypass the requirement by seeking approval of her choice from a judge. The judge's view of

abortion is to be irrelevant—his or her role is to determine whether the young woman is sufficiently mature to make an informed decision. If she is sufficiently mature, she has a right to a court order permitting an abortion.

To put this issue in its social and ethical context, the Children's Defense Fund notes that in the United States every day twenty-seven thirteen- and fourteen-year-olds have their first baby, and thirteen sixteen-year-olds have their second child.

In discussion of a minor's right to decide about contraception or abortion, it should be remembered that an adolescent mother, no matter how immature, has always been considered emancipated for the purpose of releasing her baby for adoption, even over the objections of her parents, and parents have never been able to force a daughter to surrender the baby for adoption. In the context of discussions about minors' rights to choose to have abortions, it should also be noted that no matter how young the adolescent mother, she assumes the same responsibilities and decision-making authority for her child as a woman of twenty-five. Her parents have no obligation whatever to support or care for her baby, except in Wisconsin, where a statute imposes this obligation until the minor mother is eighteen. In many states, since she becomes emancipated by virtue of having a baby, her parents have no further obligations to support or care for her. And if they have prevented her abortion, they are legally free to expel an eleven-year-old and her infant from the family home. The compelling ethical issue in this area, which is almost never mentioned in the literature, is this dichotomy between decision making and responsibility for the long-term effects of that decision.

The rationale for state legislatures' enaction of statutes requiring parental consent or judicial bypass for abortion is the belief that young women are "too immature" to make this decision for themselves. If a girl requires parental consent to choose abortion, does she have the right to refuse an abortion her parents wish her to have? If she is "too immature" to decide for herself, and her parent or parents must agree with her decision to have an abortion in order "to protect her interests," is she also too immature to decide to have her baby and to refuse abortion if the parental assessment is that she is too young to be a mother and should abort? In the few cases where parents have tried to obtain court orders to force an adolescent daughter to have an abortion, courts have held that the girl had the right to make the decision. None of these decisions, however, have come from states with parental consent statutes.

Sexual abuse.   Most child-abuse statutes requiring mandatory reporting by health-care providers of abuse or well-founded suspicion of abuse apply to all minors. Sexual activity may, of course, constitute child abuse. If a young child "consents" to sexual activity of any sort, it is legally reportable abuse; but in the teen years, whether sexual activity—heterosexual or homosexual—constitutes abuse may be much more problematic.

In 1984 the California attorney general issued an opinion that all sexual activity by children under fourteen had to be reported as child abuse, regardless of whether the minor was the victim of abuse or was engaged in voluntary sexual contact. Anyone under fourteen who was "treated for venereal disease, birth control, for pregnancy or for abortion" was to be reported as "abused." Planned Parenthood and several physicians brought suit to challenge that ruling, on the grounds that it invaded the minors' privacy rights. The Court of Appeals of California declared the ruling unconstitutional and held that child-abuse reporting laws do not require professionals who have no knowledge or suspicion that actual abuse has occurred to report such activities solely because the minor is under fourteen, if he or she indicates that the activity was voluntary, consensual, and with another minor of "similar age" (*Planned Parenthood Affiliates of California* v. *Van de Kamp*, 1986).

It should be remembered that if an adolescent is reported as abused, child-welfare agencies begin investigations with home visits. There is then no possibility that pregnancy or venereal disease (in spite of specific statutory provisions of confidentiality) will not be revealed to parents. This being the case, young teens in need of treatment for sexually related problems will usually not present themselves for medical care.

Mental-health issues

Consent to treatment. The issue of the young person's right to seek mental-health treatment is unlikely to involve private psychotherapy, since the parent can refuse to pay the bill and in most cases a young person cannot afford it. A more practical question involves an adolescent's right of access to a community mental-health facility, a drug treatment center, or a counseling center for troubled adolescents. Community mental-health centers are probably covered by the normal rules of minor consent that apply to other medical treatment, since those institutions, most of which receive federal funds, must be careful to comply with requirements of proper licenses and credentials for all staff.

In some cases, however, treatment may be offered by caregivers without formal medical credentials. In drug rehabilitation centers, for example, many of the personnel may be former drug addicts without formal mental-health training. Although this may be a viable method of treating addiction, it complicates the issue of the legal right of the adolescent to seek care. All statutes granting adolescents specific authority to consent to medical treatment, and all cases in which these issues have been decided, have dealt with the rights of young people to receive treatment from physicians, nurses, and other heath-care providers who fall within the boundaries of "mainstream medicine." Minor treatment statutes quite specifically refer to treatment given by physicians. Although there are no cases on the point, it is unlikely that courts would extend these rights of consent to encompass an unemancipated minor's right to seek treatment from a chiropractor; it is even more unlikely that a court would hold that an adolescent's right to consent to care would apply to situations where the minor would choose to consult an alternative healer such as a naturopath. Parents in many cases have been found guilty of child neglect if they refused treatment from physicians and took their children to alternative healers, so it is most improbable that the young person has the right to go to the same practitioners on his or her own. Drug-rehabilitation clinics not directed by physicians and nurses and places where therapy is provided by persons outside the credentialed health-care system, undoubtedly would be held to fall into the same category.

Refusal of psychiatric treatment. Many forms of behavior that may seem perfectly rational to an adolescent can be interpreted by a parent as sufficiently abnormal to warrant psychiatric intervention, at least on an outpatient basis. By definition, this discussion involves those minors who would generally be considered "normal neurotics" in adult psychiatry. Such adolescents are functional and are not engaging in criminal or dangerous antisocial behavior. They have not engaged in definitive delinquent behavior and are not dangerous to themselves or others.

As discussed above, if minors have the right to consent to treatment, a court would probably hold that they have the right to refuse it. More to the point, however, as a fact of psychiatric practice, although it might be possible to subdue a teenager physically in order to remove his or her appendix, it is absolutely impossible to carry out any form of effective psychotherapy on an unwilling patient. The patient will simply refuse to discuss anything. At least one court has held that a school system violates the minor's right of privacy if it sets up a system of routine psychological evaluations in the absence of any behavior that indicates serious emotional disturbance that may require treatment.

Confidentiality and psychiatric treatment. What is the psychiatrist's obligation of confidentiality to a minor patient? There are only a few state court decisions on confidentiality in regard to any right a minor may have to keep statements to physicians protected from invasion by parental curiosity.

Since young children are almost never treated outside a family-centered therapeutic situation, this conflict probably arises infrequently with them, but it does arise often with adolescent patients. In a parent–adolescent conflict, the parent and child may be genuinely adversarial parties because of the nature of their relationship, and the psychiatrist must frequently assume that anything told to the parent will be used against the child.

Some authorities seem to take the position that a psychiatrist is perfectly free to, and probably should, discuss anything she or he chooses with the parents of minor patients—from young children through adolescents—and, moreover, to discuss the situation with patients' teachers. This is a violation of any child's right of privacy and may also be questionable therapeutically. Particularly where an outside person such as a teacher is involved, merely telling the teacher that the student is in psychiatric treatment may elicit a negative attitude toward the student and may cause the fact of treatment to be entered on the permanent school record for anyone to see. Except in cases where the psychiatrist is or should be convinced that the college student, adolescent, or younger child will do harm to himself or herself or to others, the minor should have the same right of confidentiality that exists in any psychotherapeutic relationship. Thus, as would be true of any adult patient, information should be given to parents or others only with permission of the patient.

What constitutes an emergency for justified revelation to a parent or other person is, in the last analysis, a matter of professional judgment; but in the past few years courts have begun to hold psychiatrists to a duty to warn potential victims if a patient communicates plans to harm them. The problem, of course, is to establish whether the patient really intends harm to others. If it is decided that a psychiatrist had reasonable cause to have thought that danger actually existed but neither committed the patient nor warned the victims and harm then occured, the psychiatrist may be found liable in an action brought by the victims or their survivors.

A parent's right to know is less restricted than any right to know of anyone else. And the level of suspicion that something is wrong necessary for disclosure to the parent of a child should probably be far lower than in the case of a psychiatrist trying to assess a duty to warn or to divulge information involving an adult patient. If the young person is threatening suicide or injury to another person, the psychiatrist's decision to report the information to the parents should be based on a far less stringent prediction of probability than would be necessary to divulge the information to the police, the threatened victim, or anyone other than a parent.

In-patient treatment. There are two distinct standards for commitment of adult patients to mental institutions. Involuntary commitment of adults is reserved for those persons who are "dangerous to themselves or others" or are considered "gravely mentally disabled," the legal definition of which is that as the result of mental illness, the patient cannot provide the necessities of life—food, clothing, shelter, and medical care—for himself or herself. Voluntary commitment occurs when the patient and his or her physician agree that treatment would be beneficial.

Minors of any age fall into an altogether different category. By statute many states allow "voluntary" commitment of children by their parents. Minors who are committed as "voluntary" patients at their parents' behest are less protected legally than are adult patients. Adult voluntary patients in a mental hospital can leave at will unless, after arrival at the hospital, they are deemed to fall within the category of "dangerousness" or "disability" applied to involuntary patients, at which point a judge must hold a hearing and the patient must be civilly committed or allowed to leave. Involuntary patients, on the other hand, have a right to a judicial hearing at the time of admission to the hospital and the right to release when no longer dangerous to themselves or others. Most states, however, provide that minors may not leave a mental hospital without the approval of their parents. If parents choose not to have their child released, the patient cannot legally leave the hospital. Thus, on a standard of reasonable due process of law, hospitalized minors are in a far more restricted legal position than adults.

The case law indicates that there are many situations in which abusive parents have sought to incarcerate their children in mental hospitals for reasons having nothing to do with the children's condition. In the 1960s, for example, some male adolescents were confined to hospitals for months or years because they refused to cut their hair (see, e.g., *Sealy*, 1969 and cases cited in Ellis, 1974). In many cases, it has become clear that adolescents have been committed to mental hospitals without any serious attempt by admitting psychiatrists to discover whether the young people are really mentally ill (see cases cited in Lessem, 1974).

If a child or adolescent has conflicts with a parent, society apparently concludes that the young person, not the parent, is the one with the problem. This is not necessarily true. In particular, as many judicial decisions have indicated, a parent cannot be assumed to have the best interests of a child at heart when commitment proceedings are undertaken.

In the early 1970s, several cases held that children do have certain minimal rights of due process before being committed to a mental institution, and a right to be released from a mental hospital or an institution for the retarded on constitutional grounds if they have been denied a fair hearing and representation by counsel (*Roger S.*, 1977; *Melville v. Sabbatino*, 1973; *Sippy*, 1953; *Long*, 1975; and cases cited in Weithorn, 1988).

As a result of these decisions, many states enacted statutes providing that younger children (under thirteen or fourteen) could be admitted "voluntarily" to mental hospitals by their parents, but minors over the statutory age had a right to a hearing, counsel, and due process, either at the minor's request or automatically. Where those statutes exist, the rights conferred by them are enforceable in the state courts under state constitutional rights of due process.

In 1979, however, the U.S. Supreme Court held that if a state legislature did not choose to enact such a statute, a minor's federal constitutional rights were not violated by "voluntary" admission to a mental hospital by a parent, even if the minor was not free to leave the institution thereafter. The court held that to protect minors from abuses of parental authority, the decision to admit had to be reviewed by a "neutral fact finder," but the fact finder could be a staff physician, "so long as he or she is free to evaluate independently the child's mental and emotional condition and need for treatment" (*Parham v. J.R.*, 1979). After that decision, virtually no more states enacted due process statutes for minor mental patients. In those states that have not enacted statutes providing for judicial intervention in a minor's commitment, the young person has no right to be evaluated by an independent psychiatrist or to consult a lawyer and may be denied the right even to contact a grandparent or other relative for help.

As press reports in 1991 indicated, some profit-making mental hospitals admitted any adolescent patient whose parents sought admission. Some paid high school guidance counselors bounties to convince parents that their children needed hospitalization and then, after the unsuspecting parents admitted them, refused to release the patients for weeks or months (Cowley, 1991; Darnton, 1989). If any malpractice suits have been filed against these institutions, they have not yet been resolved and reported. The possibility of abuse of this population is a very serious one—because, once hospitalized, the patients can be totally isolated from outside contact. State legislators and judges have been unwilling to deal with the problems of bad-faith actions by either parents or physicians.

An increasingly important problem today involves the rights of young people whose parents have admitted them to an alcohol or drug treatment facility. The courts in at least two states have held that since these institutions do not claim to be "mental hospitals," any rights to judicial intervention the minor may have under state law if admitted to a mental hospital do not apply, and

the courts will not question the parent's right to admit the adolescent, even in the absence of an institutional definition of "addiction" to which the adolescent presumably conforms (*R.J.D. v. The Vaughn Clinic*, 1990; *Department of Health and Rehabilitative Services v. Straight*, 1986). Thus a minor unjustly confined in a mental hospital or addiction facility may have no recourse to, or even a right to contact, outside help of any sort. By contrast, if the parent wishes to turn for help to the juvenile court system and have the child declared "unmanageable" for precisely the same behavior, the child has a presumption of innocence, the right to counsel, and the right to a full hearing.

Participation in research

In 1974 Congress passed the National Research Act, establishing the National Commission for the Protection of Human Subjects of Biomedical and Behavioral Research. Congress mandated that the commission study the problems of biomedical research and report to the secretary of health, education, and welfare (now health and human services) on what ethical principles should be applied in research funded by or performed under the direction of the federal government. The commission was also specifically mandated to consider the ethical and regulatory issues involved in research on a variety of "special populations" deemed particularly vulnerable, including children. The commission issued significant studies and regulatory recommendations on each of the groups. Most of the recommendations are now federal regulations.

In general, research on minors is permissible if it involves no greater than minimal risk (defined as "the probability and magnitude of physical or psychological harm that is normally encountered in the daily lives, or in the routine medical or psychological examination, of healthy children"); or, when greater risk is involved, if there is likely to be a direct benefit to the young person. Parental permission is required for research on most preadolescent children. The commission's recommendations and the final regulations permit adolescents to participate in some research projects without parental consent. If the local institutional review board (IRB) determines that a research protocol is designed for a subject population for which parental or guardian permission is not a reasonable requirement, the researcher may include adolescents as subjects without parental involvement. Any waiver of parental permission must be accompanied by the IRB's acceptance of a substitute mechanism for the protection of adolescent subjects or a finding that they are not placed at any risk. The discretion afforded to the IRB by the regulations for protecting the rights and welfare of the human subjects of all ages in its institution make it extremely unlikely that research that could endanger an adolescent would ever be approved. It is most improbable that any IRB would waive parental permission for adolescent participation in any project that included a serious risk of even minimal harm.

The three following types of research normally involve adolescents who participate without parental consent:

1. Research in which adolescence is relevant. For example, a researcher might wish to question pregnant teenagers coming to a prenatal clinic about their knowledge of contraception at the time they became pregnant.
2. Research in which adolescence is irrelevant. For example, a researcher might wish to draw small amounts of blood from volunteers, and a sixteen-year-old, seeing the poster, volunteers.
3. Research that involves an attempt to recruit subjects from all age groups. For example, an epidemiologist might wish to do a community survey about knowledge of HIV infection, and some of the people she approaches in the local shopping mall are adolescents.

It is likely that an IRB would approve these studies as suitable for adolescent consent without parental involvement. However, there is a fourth type that normally requires parental involvement:

4. Research that is not related to the patient's age but involves investigational therapy. If an adolescent patient has a disease for which his or her physician-researcher wishes to administer such therapy, parental permission would almost certainly be sought. Investigational therapies that involve risk (and most do, at least to the same degree that comparable standard treatment does) are reserved for the treatment of serious illness. It is most unlikely that a physician would be caring for an adolescent ill with the sort of serious condition on which this type of research is done without involvement of parents. It is most unlikely that an IRB would approve this even if the investigator wished to deal with the adolescent patient alone.

Research in schools involving "normal educational practices" is exempt from requirements of either IRB review or of parental permission. The secretary of health and human services held that this type of research carries no risk of harm. While most research on instructional methods may be innocuous, some psychological research may have harmful consequences. For example, research using unproven testing methods that classify children as "bright," "slow learners," "hyperkinetic," "depressed," or "uncoordinated" may be entered into school records and follow students for years. Some of this research may have much more harmful consequences than much of the minimal-risk biomedical research (such as a finger prick for a blood sample) for which consent from the parent, the subject, or both is required.

Federal regulations require that in any research funded by or submitted to the federal government, prospective subjects must be advised that they may refuse to participate without penalty or loss of benefits.

Although the National Commission recommended that even young children should have the right to refuse to participate in any intervention that is not for their benefit, the regulations governing research on children omitted the provision. If an adolescent is considered sufficiently mature to agree to participate, however, his or her refusal should be accepted as would a refusal from an adult who is a prospective research subject. It is also quite likely that a court would grant adolescents a greater right to refuse participation in the trial of an investigational drug or therapy than the same adolescents would have to refuse a standard treatment—even if their parents or physician thought the investigational treatment would be more likely to alleviate the illness.

Transplantation

In the early days of organ transplantation, minors were occasionally kidney donors for siblings. Given the terrible dilemmas that faced a family who had to put one child at risk in surgery to save another, medical institutions required court approval of parental consent to the removal of a donor child's kidney. Courts usually approved the procedures, on the grounds that the healthy child derived benefit from the continued existence of the sick sibling (*Hart v. Brown,* 1972; *Little v. Little,* 1979; *Richardson,* 1973; see also discussions of the first, and unpublished, decisions involving twin kidney donors in Curran, 1959). However, the immediate risk of surgery to the donor child was not the only concern; additional concerns involved the quality of the donor child's life with one kidney and the possibility that some injury to that kidney would occur later in life. As transplantation techniques and drugs to fight organ rejection have improved, the use of kidneys from cadavers instead of from live donors has become virtually universal.

Today minors are involved primarily in bone marrow donations to siblings. Since the risk to the donor is minimal and since his or her bone marrow will regenerate so that the donor has no permanent impairment, different issues are presented. Most transplant centers do not feel it necessary to involve the courts in these transplants.

Certainly no prospective donors should be coerced into donating against their will, but within the family unit, it is difficult to see how to prevent reality from having a coercive effect. If no adult is a compatible donor, it is a fact that without a donation of bone marrow from the sibling, the ill child will probably die. Given that situation, prospective donors, adolescent or adult, cannot help feeling "responsible" if they wish to refuse.

Conclusion

The U.S. political system ignores the rights of those who cannot vote. Instead of adequate drug treatment facilities, teenagers are told, "Just say no" (even if they have already said yes and are in desperate need of help). While politicians make speeches about adolescent girls' inability to decide for themselves about abortion, many girls are on their own with their babies as two generations of throwaway children. Many political figures apparently would prefer to see adolescents die of AIDS than to have them educated about safe sex and condom use. Even with ample evidence that some mental hospitals have paid employees of high schools to bring them patients, legislators have made no change in the commitment laws for minors. While most parents attempt to love and be responsible for their children at any age, some do not. Health-care providers who treat adolescents try to respect their dignity, their autonomy, and their privacy, but the care they receive is administered within the boundaries of a society that seems to be growing increasingly hostile to their interests.

ANGELA RODDEY HOLDER

Directly related to this entry is the entry CHILDREN, *articles on* HISTORY OF CHILDHOOD, RIGHTS OF CHILDREN, HEALTH-CARE AND RESEARCH ISSUES, MENTAL-HEALTH ISSUES, *and* CHILD CUSTODY. *For a further discussion of topics mentioned in this entry, see the entries* ABORTION, *section on* CONTEMPORARY ETHICAL AND LEGAL ASPECTS, *article on* CONTEMPORARY ETHICAL PERSPECTIVES; ABUSE, INTERPERSONAL, *article on* CHILD ABUSE; COMMITMENT TO MENTAL INSTITUTIONS; FERTILITY CONTROL, *article on* SOCIAL ISSUES, *and* ETHICAL ISSUES; INFORMED CONSENT, *article on* LEGAL AND ETHICAL ISSUES OF CONSENT IN HEALTH CARE (*with its* POSTSCRIPT); MENTAL-HEALTH SERVICES; MENTALLY DISABLED AND MENTALLY ILL PERSONS; ORGAN AND TISSUE TRANSPLANTS, *article on* ETHICAL AND LEGAL ISSUES; PATIENTS' RIGHTS; RESEARCH METHODOLOGY; *and* RESEARCH POLICY. *For a discussion of related ideas, see the entries* AUTOMONY; COMPETENCY; CONFIDENTIALITY; FAMILY; INFORMATION DISCLOSURE; INFORMED CONSENT; PATERNALISM; *and* PRIVACY IN HEALTH CARE.

Bibliography

Bellotti v. Baird. 1976. 424 U.S. 952; 443 U.S. 622 (1979).

CHILDREN'S DEFENSE FUND. 1988. *A Call for Action to Make Our Nation Safe for Children: A Briefing Book on the Status of American Children in 1988.* Washington, D.C.: Author.

CONGRESS OF THE UNITED STATES. OFFICE OF TECHNOLOGY ASSESSMENT. 1991. *Adolescent Health*, vol. 1, *Summary and Policy Options*, No. OTA-H-468. Washington, D.C.: U.S. Government Printing Office. Vol. 2, *Background and the Effectiveness of Selected Prevention and Treatment Services*. No. OTA-H-466. Washington, D.C.: U.S. Government Printing Office. Vol. 3, *Crosscutting Issues in the Delivery of Health and Related Services*. No. OTA-H-467. Washington, D.C.: U.S. Government Printing Office.

COWLEY, GEOFFREY. 1991. "Money Madness." *Newsweek*, November 4, pp. 50–52.

CURRAN, WILLIAM J. 1959. "A Problem of Consent: Kidney Transplantation in Minors. *NYU Law Review* 34:891–898.

DARNTON, NINA. 1989. "Committed Youth." *Newsweek*, July 31, pp. 66–72.

Department of Health and Rehabilitative Services v. Straight. 1986. 497 So. 2d 692 (Fla.).

ELLIS, JAMES W. 1974. "Volunteering Children: Parental Commitment of Minors to Mental Institutions." *California Law Review* 62:840–916.

GAYLIN, WILLARD, and MACKLIN, RUTH, eds. 1982. *Who Speaks for the Child? The Problem of Proxy Consent.* New York: Plenum.

Hamilton, In re. 1983. 657 S. W. 2d 425 (Tenn.).

Hart v. Brown. 1972. 289 A. 2d 386 (Conn.).

HEIN, KAREN, and DiGERONIMO, THERESA FOY. 1989. *AIDS: Trading Fears for Facts: A Guide for Teens.* Mount Vernon, N.Y.: Consumers Union.

HOLDER, ANGELA R. 1985. *Legal Issues in Pediatrics and Adolescent Medicine.* 2d ed. New Haven, Conn.: Yale University Press.

———. 1988. "Constraints on Experimentation: Protecting Children to Death." *Yale Law and Policy Review* 6:137–156.

In the Interests of E. G. 1987. 161 Ill. App. 3d 765, 113 Ill. Dec. 477, 515 N.E. 2d 286; 549 N.E. 2d 322 (1989).

KIPKE, MICHELE, and HEIN, KAREN. 1990. "Acquired Immunodeficiency Syndrome (AIDS) in Adolescents." *Adolescent Medicine: State of the Art Reviews* 1, no. 3:429–449.

KOPELMAN, LORETTA M., and MOSKOP, JOHN C., eds. 1989. *Children and Health Care: Moral and Social Issues.* Boston: Kluwer Academic Publishers.

LESSEM, LOUIS. 1974. "On the Voluntary Admission of Minors." *University of Michigan Journal of Law Reform* 8:189–216.

LEVINE, ROBERT J. 1988. *Ethics and Regulation of Clinical Research.* 2d ed. New Haven, Conn.: Yale University Press.

Little v. Little. 1979. 576 S. W. 2d 493 (Tex.).

Long, In re. 1975. 214 S. E. 2d 626 (N.C.).

MELTON, GARY B.; KOOCHER, GERALD P.; and SAKS, MICHAEL J. 1983. *Children's Competence to Consent.* New York: Plenum.

Melville v. Sabbatino. 1973. 313 A. 2d 886 (Conn.).

Morrissey, James M.; Hofmann, Adele D.; and Thrope, Jeffrey C. 1986. *Consent and Confidentiality in the Health Care of Children and Adolescents: A Legal Guide.* New York: Free Press.

National Research Council. 1987. *Risking the Future: Adolescent Sexuality, Pregnancy and Childbearing.* Washington, D.C.: National Academy Press.

Parham v. J. R. 1979. 442 U.S. 584, 99 S. Ct. 2493, 61 L. Ed. 2d 101.

Planned Parenthood Affiliates of California v. Van de Kamp. 1986. 226 Cal. Rptr. 361 (Cal.).

Richardson, In re. 1973. 284 So. 2d 185 (La.).

R. J. D. v. The Vaughn Clinic. 1990. 572 So. 2d 1225 (Ala.).

Roe v. Wade. 1973. 410 U.S. 113.

Roger, S., In re. 1977. 569 P. 2d 1286, 141 Cal. Rptr. 298.

Sealy, In re. 1969. 218 So. 2d 765 (Fla.).

Sippy, In re. 1953. 97 A. 2d 455 (D. C. Mun. Ct.).

Weithorn, Lois A. 1988. "Mental Hospitalization of Troublesome Youth: An Analysis of Skyrocketing Admission Rates." *Stanford Law Review* 40:773–838.

ADOPTION

Historical background

Adoption is an institution as old as civilization. It may be defined as a social transaction through which a person belonging by birth to one family or kinship group acquires, through legal means, a new family or new kinship ties.

In its broadest sense, the term "adoption" may be used to describe the taking in, nurturing, and rearing of biologically unrelated children in need of protection and care. The terms "adoption" and "fostering" are used interchangeably in some countries, but in the United States adoption, in contrast to temporary foster arrangements, is a legal and permanent transaction.

Shaped by the laws and cultures of each society, adoption was seldom concerned primarily with rescuing abandoned children but rather with the transfer of a child or adult from one set of parents to another in order to ensure property rights or family continuity. Yet the perception of adoption has always wavered between the legal fiction that a child is reborn into the adoptive family and the folk belief that blood is thicker than water. The Egyptians and the Hebrews practiced adoption; the Old Testament chronicles the story of Moses, who was adopted by the daughter of the Pharaoh but later returned to his people and led them out of bondage.

Roman law, the foundation of institutionalized legal adoption, was concerned primarily with property and inheritance rights but permitted birth parents to reclaim their abandoned children if they paid expenses incurred by the adoptive parents (Boswell, 1988). The Code of Napoleon, enacted in 1804, which was the beginning of modern adoption legislation and is still a major influence in French and Latin American law, allowed adoptees to have knowledge of family background and the option to retain their original name. The modern French government social security system provides for both "simple" (open) adoption and "complete" (closed) adoption.

English common law, the basis for U.S. law, stressed blood lineage and did not legalize stranger adoption, the total legal transfer of the child to nonrelatives, until 1926. Until then, a form of apprenticeship existed in which children lived with and worked under the master training them. Orphans were sent as indentured servants to the American colonies to help with the labor shortage. Economic considerations superseded any concern for the welfare of the individual child.

From the mid-nineteenth century until the beginning of the twentieth century, New York City street urchins were routinely rounded up and loaded into boxcars on "orphan trains" that carried them to "God-fearing" farm families in the West. There were no legal contracts or protections for the children who, once severed from their families, were regarded as orphans and forced into a life of domestic or manual labor thousands of miles away.

The transition from apprenticeship and indenture to present-day adoption was gradual in the United States, but by 1929 every state had some form of statutory adoption. Licensed adoption agencies established in the 1920s investigated prospective adoptive families to try to ensure the well-being of adopted children. Adoption records were open, but in the late 1930s a few states began to close them.

After World War II, U.S. adoption shifted its focus from the needs of homeless children to the desires of infertile couples to adopt healthy white newborns. Adoption became the means for the childless to create a family. As state after state closed their records, the adopted child's birth certificate was sealed and replaced with an amended document that named the adoptive parents as the birth parents. The original intent was to spare the child the stigma of illegitimacy, not to cut him or her off from the birth heritage. Over the years the rationale of protecting the confidentiality of the birth mother was added, but an even greater concern was the protection of the adoptive parents, who feared the birth parents might reappear to reclaim their biological, though no longer legal, child. By 1994 all but two states, Alaska and Kansas, had sealed records.

Contemporary adoption practice in the United States

The social upheavals of the 1960s and 1970s had a major impact on adoption practice. The legalization of abortion, along with the widespread use of contraceptives and the increased tendency of unmarried mothers to keep their children, led to a shortage of white, adoptable newborns. At the same time, there was a rise in infertility among couples who delayed having children.

The states regulate adoption practice; most states permit both independent and agency adoption. As the shortage of white, adoptable babies grew more acute, adoption became a commercial enterprise. Lawyers and "baby brokers" took over most infant adoptions from the agencies, frequently using newspaper advertisements to entice pregnant women and couples to give up their children with offers of money and other benefits.

Without regulation by the child-welfare field, there is little protection for the baby and both sets of parents. Prospective adopters may spend a great deal of money for medical, living, and legal costs only to have the pregnant woman change her mind and keep the baby or choose another family. Conversely, a birth mother who has been promised open communication with the adoptive parents and the child may find herself cut off once the adoption is finalized. Or the birth mother may break her promise to stay in touch with the family if she finds visits too difficult to continue. Safeguards for the baby are lacking when the investigation of the family by an agency occurs after the infant is already in the home and petition has been filed for legal adoption.

Special needs and biracial adoption

In the 1990s adoption agencies, both private and public, focus primarily on finding families for "hard to place" children, a category that includes older children, sibling groups, disabled children, and biracial or minority racial children. The American Public Welfare Association estimated in 1992 that 429,000 children lived in foster care in the United States, a 53 percent increase from 1987. About 85,000 children were reported to be legally free for adoption. Many child-welfare specialists believe that if sufficient effort were expended, homes could be found for them. Some states offer subsidies to families who are willing to adopt and raise disabled children. Single persons and gay and lesbian couples, not generally approved for newborn babies, are often considered acceptable for placement of children who otherwise might not find permanent homes. This remains a controversial issue in some parts of the United States, as a number of individuals and groups question the ability of these nontraditional adoptive parents to raise healthy, normal children.

In 1972 the National Association of Black Social Workers (NABSW) launched a campaign against allowing white families to adopt black or biracial children. The NABSW called this practice genocide. They maintained that, with enough effort and focus, black families could be found for these children. Proponents of inter-

racial adoption argue that the benefits children gain from having permanent and loving homes outweigh the social and psychological difficulties they may face because of society's prejudice toward mixed-race families. Mental-health professionals generally agree that permanency, whether with legal adoption or long-term placement, is a paramount need for all children; they believe that growing up without roots and a stable home is a primary cause of lifelong problems. Many child advocates prefer that a child be placed with his or her extended family or within his or her community of race or religion, but accept the fact that biracial placement is preferable to no permanency as long as the families are sensitive to biracial issues and seek integrated communities in which to raise their children.

Adoption of Native American children is a related and equally controversial issue. Many Native Americans believe that adoption by Caucasians robs them of their children and robs the children of their native heritage. When Congress enacted the Indian Child Welfare Act of 1978, giving tribal courts exclusive jurisdiction over adoption proceedings involving Native American children, each tribe developed its own guidelines concerning the Native American lineage a child needed to qualify as a member. Children identified as members of a particular tribe must be placed for adoption with a family of that tribe.

Intercountry adoption

The shortage of desirable adoptable babies in the United States has led many who wish to adopt to seek children in other countries. The first "international adoptions" generally involved Amerasian children, that is, those fathered by GIs in Japan during and after World War II, in Korea during and after the Korean War, and in Vietnam during the U.S. involvement there. These adoptions were first sponsored by church groups and then by licensed adoption agencies (Lifton, 1994).

Since the middle of the 1980s, international adoption has shifted from the rescue of war orphans to the legal or (in some cases) illegal trafficking in children. Most of the children are drawn from Korea, Latin America, and Eastern Europe because these countries have made the emigration of children more accessible. Human-rights organizations report that many children are taken away from their families without formal relinquishments (Mantaphon, 1993). Studies of intercountry adoptions suggest that children cut off from their own culture and transplanted into a totally foreign environment may be more vulnerable to emotional problems (Verhulst et al., 1990a, 1990b). Many have difficulty in attaching to their new family or feeling part of the community, where they may not find full acceptance because of racial differences.

The 1989 U.N. Convention on the Rights of the Child addressed the rights of the adopted child along with the rights of all children. According to the convention, each child has a right to receive a name, to acquire a nationality, and, as far as possible, to know and be cared for by his or her parents. A child placed outside of his or her family of origin has the right to maintain contact with his or her birth parents.

The sealed-record controversy

For over half a century, closed adoption (i.e., with sealed records) was viewed by U.S. society as beneficial to everyone: The homeless child born out of wedlock was given a second chance in a new family, the infertile couple was able to become "real" parents, and the birth mother was free to go on with her life as if she had never had a child. Yet research conducted since the mid-1970s has consistently indicated that the secrecy in the closed-adoption system can often create lifelong psychological problems for everyone involved (Sorosky et al., 1978).

Although adopted children comprise less than 5 percent of the population, the percentage of adopted children in mental-health facilities and residential treatment centers has been reported to be as high as 30 percent. Some researchers have found that adopted children score lower in academic achievement and social skills than the nonadopted, have a high incidence of learning disabilities, and display behavior characterized as impulsive, aggressive, and antisocial (Schecter et al., 1964; Brodzinsky and Schecter, 1992; Brinich, 1989). Psychotherapists have postulated that an adopted child's perception of rejection and abandonment by the birth mother can cause low self-esteem. Ignorance of origins ("genealogical bewilderment") can lead a child to rebellion against the adoptive parents and society, and eventually to delinquency (Wellisch, 1952; Sants, 1964; Kirschner and Nagel, 1988).

Women who relinquish their infants often suffer a profound loss and experience lifelong difficulties. Like the child, they are encouraged by society to deny and repress the feelings that accompanied giving up their children for adoption. Some studies indicate that these women never forgive themselves. Some may feel they have no right to a happy marriage and other children, while others may try without success to have other children as replacements for the one that they relinquished (Deykin et al., 1984; Millen and Roll, 1985).

The closed-adoption system also encourages adoptive parents to deny their grief at not being able to produce a child that will carry on their lineage. They are expected to conceal their unresolved conflicts over infertility as they pretend that adopting a child is the same as giving birth (Blum, 1983). Adoptive parents who are able to acknowledge the differences between an adoptive and birth family, instead of denying them, have been shown to have better communication and closer relationships with their children (Kirk, 1964).

The closed-adoption system tends to pit the right of the adopted child to know the identity of his or her birth parents against the right of the birth mother to confidentiality, and against the right of the adoptive parents to maintain exclusive parental roles. The National Council for Adoption (NCFA), a lobbying organization representing traditional adoption agencies, contends that sealed records protect the privacy of the birth mother, who was promised confidentiality (Caplan, 1990). A national birth-parent group, Concerned United Birth Parents (CUB), argues that the majority of birth mothers did not ask for confidentiality and in fact want to have knowledge of or some contact with the children they gave birth to. Until 1976, birth fathers had no rights, only responsibilities. At that time, the U.S. Supreme Court gave birth fathers equal right of consent with birth mothers in adoption arrangements.

Search and reunion

One of the effects of the civil-rights movement of the 1960s was the emergence of an adoption-reform movement led by adult adoptees. Its rallying cry was that the civil rights of the adopted had been violated when their original birth records were sealed, denying them access to information available to nonadopted people. Adoption support groups have been established across the United States to provide emotional support, lobby for open records, and facilitate the search for birth parents.

Some states, rather than open their previously sealed adoption records, have established "reunion registries" that will connect adoptees with their birth parents if both register and indicate their mutual desire. In other jurisdictions, there is an intermediary system, in which the court, or an adoption agency is empowered to search for the birth mother if an adoptee requests a reunion. The birth mother retains the right of refusal of contact. Adopted activists believe that both registries and intermediaries violate their right to information and the ability to make direct contact with birth relatives.

More adopted women search for their birth parents than adopted men. The quest to find the birth mother is usually stronger than the need to locate the birth father. Adoptees tend to begin their search when they become aware of formerly repressed feelings that often surface at times of life transitions, such as impending marriage, parenthood, or death of adoptive parents (Sorosky et al., 1978; Lifton, 1988).

The secrets inherent in the closed-adoption system make reunion difficult for both birth mother and adoptee. To return to each other is to return to their earlier traumas. The adoptee experiences grief, anger, and divided loyalties; the birth mother relives the unresolved sadness, guilt, and humiliation she felt at the time of pregnancy, birth, and relinquishment (Lifton, 1994).

No matter whom adoptees find—a loving, a withholding, or even a deceased parent—the opportunity to heal arises when they can integrate the past with the present. Adoptees' relationship to their adoptive parents is usually strengthened once they have resolved their identity issues. Reality replaces their fantasies, and they are able to recognize the important role of their adoptive parents (Gonyo and Watson, 1988; Sorosky et al., 1978; Lifton, 1994). Birth parents also enter a healing process after reunion because they have the opportunity to explain to their child why they relinquished him or her and to forgive themselves and be forgiven (Gediman and Brown, 1989).

Some adoptees and birth parents develop close, ongoing kinship ties. Others maintain a more distant relationship that may involve little more than exchanging holiday cards. A few, after one or two meetings, close off contact. Whatever follows the reunion, however, the individuals involved have been able to take control of this important aspect of their lives.

Open versus closed adoption

Since the early 1980s there has been a trend toward openness in adoption. In the placement of older children, good adoption practice dictates providing each child with a "life book" that has information and photographs about their history. Often these children are encouraged to maintain contact with the previous foster mother and with relatives, such as grandparents, in the extended birth family.

In infant adoption, a birth mother may choose the parents for her baby, but completely open arrangements—where there is an ongoing relationship between birth and adoptive families—are still rare. Semi-open adoption is more usual. It may vary from little more than a single meeting between the birth mother and adoptive parents, with no disclosure of names or discussion of future contact, to annual exchanges of photographs and information and the promise of more contact when the child grows up (McRoy et al., 1988). Professionals describe open-adoption arrangements as a process in which all parties move at their own pace over the years (Silber and Dorner, 1989).

Opponents of open adoption argue that it makes it difficult for the birth mother to accept that she has given up a child, that it hinders adoptive parents in forming secure ties with an infant, and that it deprives the child of a sense of permanence with the adoptive family (Caplan, 1990). Proponents of open adoption believe that birth mothers who take an active part in the placement process can resolve their guilt and grief about giving up their baby; that it obviates adoptive parents' fantasies about the child's background because they have facts; that it permits adopted children to know that their birth parents are real persons, not ghosts; and that they were not given up because there was something wrong with them (Silber and Dorner, 1990).

Court battles between birth parents and adoptive parents

Since the mid-1980s the number of contested adoption cases has multiplied. Many have been brought by birth mothers (and increasingly by birth fathers) who feel that they did not receive proper counseling or enough time, or were coerced into signing relinquishment papers. When the birth mother seeks the return of the child, lawyers for the adoptive parents may delay action in order to prolong the child's presence in the adoptive home. The longer that period, the stronger the argument that it is in the best interests of the child to stay in the only home he or she has ever known. Adoptive-parent lobbies now seek to limit the time that birth parents may have to revoke their consent or relinquishment. There is also a strong movement to develop uniform state laws that would limit the problems of interstate placements and decrease the legal conflicts of different jurisdictions.

Conclusion

The adoption field is betwixt and between stasis and change. The records remain sealed in most states, but the traditional closed system is gradually giving way to a more open one that allows birth parents and adoptive parents to meet and even maintain contact over the years for the sake of the child.

Adoption practice is no longer exclusively concerned with healthy white newborns. Adoptees now include transracial and biracial children and older handicapped children with special needs. Standards for adoptive parents, once modeled on white, middle-class, heterosexual couples, have changed to include single parents, homosexual couples, and minority and biracial couples of any age.

Uniform state laws are necessary to regulate adoption practice, but there is much disagreement about the relative importance of birth-parent versus adoptive-parent rights. The term "best interests of the child" has come to mean whatever people want it to mean. Prospective adoptive parents and birth parents find themselves in adversarial roles where their own best interests may conflict with the best interests of the child.

Adoption-reform activists believe it is in the best interests of the child to have adoption practice limited to nonprofit agencies and child-welfare specialists. They stress the need for adequate legal and psychological counseling for both birth parents and adoptive parents before and after the birth of the baby and especially before finalizing relinquishment plans.

Reformers would like to see adoption records unsealed so that adopted children can integrate their dual heritage and avoid many of the psychological problems that are caused by secrecy. They advocate a nationwide program that would promote sex education, pregnancy prevention, family preservation, and legally enforced open-adoption arrangements when relinquishment and placement are necessary.

ANNETTE BARAN
BETTY JEAN LIFTON

For a further discussion of topics mentioned in this entry, see the entries ABORTION; CHILDREN, *articles on* RIGHTS OF CHILDREN, *and* HEALTH-CARE AND RESEARCH ISSUES; CONFIDENTIALITY; FAMILY; FERTILITY CONTROL; INFANTS, *articles on* ETHICAL ISSUES, *and* PUBLIC-POLICY AND LEGAL ISSUES; PRIVACY IN HEALTH CARE; *and* RACE AND RACISM. *For a discussion of related ideas, see the entry* INFORMATION DISCLOSURE. *Other relevant material may be found under the entries* ADOLESCENTS; *and* MATERNAL–FETAL RELATIONSHIP.

Bibliography

BARAN, ANNETTE, and PANNOR, REUBEN. 1990. "Open Adoption." In *The Psychology of Adoption*, pp. 316–331. Edited by David M. Brodzinsky and Marshall D. Schechter. New York: Oxford University Press.

BLUM, HAROLD P. 1983. "Adoptive Parents: Generative Conflict and Generational Continuity." *Psychoanalytic Study of the Child* 38:141–163.

BOSWELL, JOHN. 1988. *The Kindness of Strangers: The Abandonment of Children in Western Europe from Late Antiquity to the Renaissance.* New York: Pantheon.

BOWLBY, JOHN. 1982. *Attachment and Loss.* 2d ed. New York: Basic Books.

BRINICH, PAUL. 1989. "Psychoanalytic Psychotherapy with Adoptees." Paper presented at the 36th Annual Meeting of the American Academy of Child and Adolescent Psychiatry, New York, October 13.

BRODZINSKY, DAVID M., and SCHECHTER, MARSHALL D. 1992. *Being Adopted, The Lifelong Search for Self.* New York: Doubleday.

CAPLAN, LINCOLN. 1990. *An Open Adoption.* New York: Farrar Straus Giroux.

DEYKIN, EVA Y; CAMPBELL, LEE; and PATTI, PATRICIA. 1984. "The Postadoption Experience of Surrendering Parents." *American Journal of Orthopsychiatry* 54, no. 2:271–280.

ERIKSON, ERIK H. 1980. *Identity and the Life Cycle: Selected Papers.* New York: W. W. Norton.

GAYLORD, C. LESTER. 1976. "The Adoptive Child's Right to Know." *Case and Comment* 81, no. 2:38–44.

GEDIMAN, JUDITH S., and BROWN, LINDA P. 1989. *Birthbond: Reunions Between Birthparents and Adoptees—What Happens After.* Far Hills, N.J.: New Horizon.

GONYO, BARBARA, and WATSON, KENNETH W. 1988. "Searching in Adoption." *Public Welfare* 46, no. 1:14–22.

KINGSOLVER, BARBARA. 1993. *Pigs in Heaven: A Novel.* New York: HarperCollins.

KIRK, H. DAVID. 1964. *Shared Fate: A Theory of Adoption and Mental Health.* New York: Free Press.

KIRSCHNER, DAVID, and NAGEL, LINDA S. 1988. "Antisocial Behavior in Adoptees: Patterns and Dynamics." *Child and Adolescent Social Work* 5, no. 4:300–314.

LIFTON, BETTY JEAN. 1988. *Lost and Found: The Adoption Experience.* New York: Perennial Library.

———. 1994. *Journey of the Adopted Self: A Quest for Wholeness.* New York: Basic Books.

MANTAPHON, WITHIT. 1993. *Sale of Children: Report.* Geneva: U.N. Economic and Social Council.

MCKENZIE, JUDITH K. 1993. "Adoption of Children with Special Needs." *Future of Children* 3, no. 1:62–76.

MCROY, RUTH G.; GROTEVANT, HAROLD D.; and WHITE, KERRY L. 1988. *Openness in Adoption: New Practices, New Issues.* New York: Praeger.

MILLEN, LEVERETT, and ROLL, SAMUEL. 1985. "Solomon's Mothers: A Special Case of Pathological Bereavement." *American Journal of Orthopsychiatry* 55, no. 3:411–418.

RYNEARSON, EDWARD K. 1982. "Relinquishment and Its Maternal Complications: A Preliminary Study." *American Journal of Psychiatry* 139, no. 3:338–340.

SANTS, H. J. 1964. "Genealogical Bewilderment in Children with Substitute Parents." *British Journal of Medical Psychology* 37, pp. 131–141.

SCHECTER, MARSHALL D.; CARLSON, PAUL V.; SIMMONS, JAMES Q., III; and WORK, HENRY H. 1964. "Emotional Problems in the Adoptee." *Archives of General Psychiatry* 10, no. 2:109–118.

SILBER, KATHLEEN, and DORNER, PATRICIA. 1990. *Children of Open Adoption and Their Families.* San Antonio, Tex.: Corona.

SOROSKY, ARTHUR D.; BARAN, ANNETTE; and PANNOR, REUBEN. 1978. *The Adoption Triangle: The Effects of the Sealed Record on Adoptees, Birth Parents and Adoptive Parents.* New York: Anchor.

VERHULST, FRANK C.; ALTHAUS, MONIKA; and VERSLUIS-DEN BIEMAN, HERMA J. 1990a. "Problem Behavior in International Adoptees: I. An Epidemiological Study." *Journal of the American Academy of Child and Adolescent Psychiatry* 29, no. 1: 94–103.

———. 1990b. "Problem Behavior in International Adoptees: II. Age of Placement." *Journal of the American Academy of Child and Adolescent Psychiatry* 29, no. 1: 104–111.

WELLISCH, ERICH. 1952. "Children Without Genealogy: A Problem of Adoption." *Mental Health* 13:41–42.

WINNICOTT, DONALD W. 1955. "Adopted Children in Adolescence." In Report of the Residential Conference Held at Roehampton, July 8–11, 1953, pp. 33–41. Roehampton, U.K.: A. Rampton.

ADVANCE DIRECTIVES

See Death and Dying: Euthanasia and Sustaining Life, *articles on* advance directives, ethical issues, *and* professional and public policies.

ADVERTISING

As the cost of health care becomes an increasing focus of attention, advertising becomes an increasing object of concern. At its best, advertising can provide information to help consumers make informed choices. Conversely, it can inflate expectations, create demand, manipulate desire, transform wants into perceived needs, and increase utilization and cost of health-care services. In the not-too-distant past, health care was understood as medical care. The activities of physicians were regulated by standards of ethics that eschewed commercialism. Although there has always been an economic aspect (usually a fee) associated with the physician–patient encounter, the revolution in the financing of health-care delivery is transforming the personal doctor–patient relationship into a socially complex interaction in which physicians are cast among a multitude of providers, and patients are transformed into consumers. The obligations and interests of these providers may be motivated by their desire to serve the public or to make a profit for an institution's shareholders. The focus on the economics of health care underscores the commercial aspects of health-care delivery by both physicians and other providers. Although physicians and not-for-profit institutions should be responsive to a service ethic, they compete in the same economic arena as for-profit organizations and often behave similarly. Furthermore, patients may not be the consumers at all. Services may be purchased by employers, alliances, the state (especially mental-health services), or other contracting entities, whose interests may not entirely coincide with those of the patient.

The effect of appeals for business through advertising may be judged by the standards of business ethics: truthfulness, nondeceitfulness, nonexploitativeness, and profitability. But health care is not strictly a commodity to be sold effectively for profit to the public. The care of health is also a fundamental human endeavor binding the caregiver and the careseeker in reciprocal ways. Otto Guttentag, noting the essential human quality of health care, defines medicine as "the care of health of human beings by human beings" (Guttentag, 1963). Lawrence Nelson and colleagues argue that several key features distinguish caring for the sick from other commercial products: (1) patients are in a distinctive position of vulnerability and dependency on those providing the products or services; (2) their well-being—perhaps even life—is at stake in the encounter with the provider; and (3) their relationship with the provider may become an important aspect of the healing encounter. All of these elements suggest that health-care providers have special obligations that go beyond the usual obligations of the seller to the buyer (Nelson et al., 1989).

Traditional prohibitions against medical advertising attempted to minimize the commercialization of the encounter (Relman, 1978). According to the traditional view, physicians and other professionals should obtain business by developing a reputation for quality service, or getting referrals from satisfied patients/clients or from others who know their work, not from any kind of self-promotion.

The major ethical issue in advertising in a market economy is truthfulness. If given adequate information, the consumer should make appropriate choices: what kind of health care, where, when, provided by whom, at what cost. A larger question concerns the justice of a market system of choice based on individual self-interest. Proponents view advertising in health care as a way to promote competition and thus reduce cost in the highly regulated health-care industry. Opponents criticize advertising for inflating expectations and thus increasing cost. Others suggest that the quality of care has been lowered by making cost rather than quality the focus of allocation decisions (Rodning and Dacso, 1987).

The high cost of health care in the United States has prompted a search for ways of reducing both the cost of medical services and the percentage of Gross National Product devoted to health care without appreciably lowering quality of care. Advertising is located at the crossroads between cost and quality, between regulated markets with an emphasis on quality and free markets with an emphasis on cost and choice. Regulations that provide standards for training, licensure, specialty certification, and hospital accreditation have resulted in high-quality, but expensive, health care. Market solutions, such as encouraging advertising to promote competition, have been seen as a way of reducing cost.

Historical background

The origins of professionalism.   Modern professional organizations, defined by their codes of ethics and regulating themselves by ethical principles, take their origin from the Aesculapian societies of the fourth century b.c.e. and in particular from the Oath of Hippocrates, which bound its members to ethical standards that did not apply to society as a whole. The Hippocratic Oath emphasized the principle of patient benefit, placing the patient at the center of the physician's concern.

By the nineteenth century, when the British Medical Association (BMA) and the American Medical Association (AMA) were founded, the concept of a profession organized around explicit standards of ethics was well established. Prohibitions against advertising were among the first professional standards because treatments based on scientific knowledge distinguished physicians from their main competitors, itinerant salesmen promoting often dubious products with even more dubious claims. Advertising was expressly prohibited as unprofessional and undignified in virtually all countries where physicians had established their professional identity and organized like the Aesculapian physicians of old around a code of ethics (Havighurst, 1978; Dyer, 1985). In the United States the actual license to practice is granted and regulated by each state, but the task of enforcing the ethics codes falls to professional associations such as the AMA or specialty societies.

The antitrust challenge to the professions. The health-care professions in the United States have always maintained a delicate balance between altruism and economic self-interest (Jonsen, 1990). As the medical profession became more scientifically effective and better organized, it developed regulations (licensure, specialty certification, and accreditation) that guaranteed a virtual monopoly on health-care delivery. Health care became synonymous with medical care. Although the Sherman Antitrust Act banned monopolies in 1891, the learned professions were considered exempt from the Sherman Act, which applied only to businesses. However, the business aspects of medicine have received increasing attention, and the learned professions exemption under the Sherman Act ended in 1975 with the U.S. Supreme Court's *Goldfarb* decision, in which Virginia lawyers were found guilty of charges of price fixing of the fees charged for title searches (*Goldfarb* v. *Virginia State Bar,* 1975).

The *Goldfarb* decision heralded a flurry of antitrust activity in the professional arena, most notably the 1975 suit by the Federal Trade Commission (FTC) against the AMA, holding that the AMA was in restraint of trade because its code of ethics prohibited advertising. The 1957 AMA Principles of Medical Ethics then in effect said, simply, "[A physician] shall not solicit patients," meaning that a physician should not attempt to obtain patients by deception or false advertising. The 1980 revision eliminated all reference to advertising. Nonetheless, in 1982 the U.S. Supreme Court decided the case in favor of the FTC, barring the AMA from making any reference to advertising and the solicitation of patients, and further prohibiting the AMA from "formulating, adopting and disseminating" any ethical guidelines without first obtaining "permission from and approval of the guidelines by the Federal Trade Commission" (*American Medical Association* v. *Federal Trade Commission,* 1980).

The FTC suit hinged on questions of cost, advertising, and the mercantile aspects of medical practice. The position of the FTC was that costs were high because doctors had a monopoly on health-care delivery and could thus maintain artificially high costs for their own profit. If doctors were not prohibited from advertising, it was argued, prices would come down because patients could shop for the best prices. In other words, medicine could be better controlled if it were regulated as a business rather than as a profession (Pertshuk, 1978).

In the mid-1980s the British Monopolies and Mergers Commission (MMC) addressed a similar issue with the BMA, whose General Medical Council opposed the efforts of a general practitioner to advertise his holistic medical practice in local newspapers. Presumably the interest of the MMC in allowing the general practitioner to advertise was to promote consumer choice rather than to lower costs, since under the National Health Service costs are controlled by fixed budgets and by using the general practitioner as "gatekeeper" to specialty services (Gillon, 1989; Colman, 1989).

The ethics and goals of advertising

Advertising serves two very distinct and divergent objectives: (1) dissemination of information, and (2) product differentiation, which economists define as public perception of differences between two products, even though such differences may not in fact exist.

Dissemination of information provides the facts on which rational consumers can make informed choices. In health care, information about the services provided, location, hours of service, fees charged, and languages spoken are examples of services that might be advertised. Arguments in favor of advertising in health care are based on an understanding of advertising as dissemination of information.

Advertising also serves to differentiate products, and the methods for doing so can be ethically more problematic. How can the claim be made and justified that one product is better than another? The FTC requires that any claims of product differentiation be empirically measurable. In order to claim that a particular mouthwash "kills germs on contact by millions," it is necessary to be able to count killed germs. Usually advertisers attempt to differentiate products not on the basis of objective criteria about the product, but by manipulating unconscious wishes and fantasies (youth, power, beauty, sex, affluence), associating the product with images of attractive people in beautiful surroundings. The consumer is left to feel tremendous anxiety about the possible consequences of making the wrong choice of dentifrice, antiperspirant, or health plan.

Though many physicians have been reluctant (or averse) to advertise, health-care institutions have readily accepted the imperative to advertise in an attempt to create markets, capture market share, and find niches in the marketplace. Notable in this regard is advertising directed at target populations, for example, women, cancer patients, and those needing psychiatric and substance-abuse services.

Truth in advertising was the concern when the field of advertising itself attempted to follow the course of professionalism in the early part of the twentieth century. At issue were the values that distinguished professional advertisers from retail-space merchants. The American Marketing Association established university training programs and codes of ethics that promoted the scientific ideal of detachment and statistical analysis. The scientific vision of community and definition of people as consumers replaced the older, empathic, and value-laden world in which a merchant understood what customers (not consumers) wanted and needed because everyone lived in the same community (Christians et al., 1978; Schultze, 1981).

Professional advertising is an illustrative example because medicine's traditions of professionalism are derived from an era in which the physician participated in the life of the community in which he or she practiced. Knowledge of the patient as a person, as well as the patient's life history and social situation, has traditionally been deemed essential to quality care. At issue today for medicine is whether it will be possible to preserve the values of individualized care that characterized the ideals of an earlier era.

Gender and advertising in health care

The use of gender in advertising illustrates some of the broader issues in health-care advertising. Statistical analysis of advertisement content reveals that men and women are imaged differently (Rudman and Hagiwara, 1992; Hawkins and Aber, 1988; Wallace, 1985; see also Stage, 1979; Kiefer, 1980). Women are placed in positions submissive to men; ads focus on the sexuality of the user rather than on the product. Women are more likely than men to be portrayed as depressives requiring medical treatment (Courtney and Whipple, 1983). Female patients are more likely than men to be pictured naked.

Content analysis raises some fundamental ethical questions about health-care advertising. Are these gender discrepancies a legitimate attempt to market to women, who do make more visits to physicians, have more surgery, and receive more psychotropic drugs (Fidell, 1980)? Alternatively, do negative images of women portrayed in advertising actually contribute to women's views of themselves? If so, are these advertisements contributing to the very problems their products purport to cure?

Cosmetic surgery advertising for procedures (face lifts, breast and penile implants, liposuction, and tummy tucks) to enhance some ideal physical image appeals to both men and women. These ideals are also created by advertisements for clothes, perfumes, and travel (Wolf, 1991). The informed consumer should be alert to the subtle or subliminal influences of advertising that attempts to create and manipulate wants and needs and transform marginal wants into perceived needs (Galbraith, 1967, 1988). Such advertising is most effective when its effect is not conscious and not subject to volitional control. As such it is antithetical to the traditional medical ethic of beneficence. It is also antithetical to the bioethical principle of autonomy in that the subliminal messages of advertising work to diminish the consumer's ability to make free and consciously reflected choices. Advertising of this sort is ethically in direct variance with ideals and goals of health care that seek to promote autonomy by helping the patient gain more control over his or her life.

Conclusion

One ethical issue regarding advertising focuses on truthful dissemination of information and objectively measurable standards for judging the truth of advertising claims. A more problematic issue is the way in which advertising plays upon people's unconscious wishes and fantasies: sex, greed, and the quest for power, status, and perfection. The scientific basis for advertising rests on the ability to identify and manipulate such longings and fears. When we speak of "the market" or "market forces" or "demand," we are generally talking about human wants and wishes manipulated in this way.

Key concerns facing the ethics of advertising in health care include: standards or regulations that should govern the placement of advertisements; whether the free expression of any appeal is legitimate so long as it does not mislead, make false claims, or actually harm; whether the promotion of unhealthful products such as tobacco or alcohol could be so morally offensive that government might be persuaded to extend the scope of regulation in advertising, such as by limiting advertising to the dissemination of information; and whether the effectiveness of a psychology of persuasion is sufficient to justify advertisements, or whether some higher principle should be brought to bear. Advertising itself should be subjected to the first principle of Hippocratic ethics, *primum non nocere:* First do no harm.

ALLEN R. DYER

Directly related to this entry are the entries COMMUNICATION, BIOMEDICAL, *article on* MEDIA AND MEDICINE; ECONOMIC CONCEPTS IN HEALTH CARE; CONFLICT OF INTEREST; *and* HEALTH-CARE FINANCING, *article on* PROFIT AND COMMERCIALISM. *For a further discussion of topics mentioned in this entry, see the entries* BENEFICENCE; HEALTH PROMOTION AND HEALTH EDUCATION; HOS-

PITAL, *article on* CONTEMPORARY ETHICAL PROBLEMS; PROFESSION AND PROFESSIONAL ETHICS; *and* SEXISM. *Other relevant material may be found under the entries* COMMERCIALISM IN SCIENTIFIC RESEARCH; FREEDOM AND COERCION; HEALTH-CARE RESOURCES, ALLOCATION OF; HEALTH POLICY, *article on* POLITICS AND HEALTH CARE; *and* PHARMACEUTICS.

Bibliography

American Medical Association v. *Federal Trade Commission.* 1980. 639 F. 2d 433 (2d Cir.); 102 S. Ct. 1744 (1982).

CHRISTIANS, C. G.; SCHULTZE, Q. J.; and SIMMS, N. H. 1978. "Community, Epistemology, and Mass Media Ethics." *Journalism History* 5:38–41, 65–67.

COLMAN, RICHARD D. 1989. "The Ethics of General Practice and Advertising." *Journal of Medical Ethics* 15, no. 2:86–89, 93.

COURTNEY, ALICE E., and WHIPPLE, THOMAS W. 1983. *Sex Stereotyping in Advertising.* Lexington, Mass.: Lexington Books.

DYER, ALLEN R. 1985. "Ethics, Advertising and the Definition of a Profession." *Journal of Medical Ethics* 11, no. 2: 72–78.

———. 1988. *Ethics and Psychiatry: Toward Professional Definition.* Washington: American Psychiatric Press.

FIDELL, LINDA S. 1980. "Sex Role Stereotypes and the American Physician." *Psychology of Women Quarterly* 4, no. 3:313–327.

GALBRAITH, JOHN KENNETH. 1967. *The New Industrial State*, pp. 270–273. Boston: Houghton Mifflin.

———. 1988. "Economics and Advertising: Exercise in Denial." *Advertising Age*, November 9, pp. 80–84.

GILLON, RAANAN. 1989. "Advertising and Medical Ethics." *Journal of Medical Ethics* 15, no. 2:59–60, 85.

Goldfarb v. *Virginia State Bar.* 1975. 421 U.S. 773.

GUTTENTAG, OTTO E. 1963. "On Defining Medicine." *Christian Scholar* 46, no. 3:200–211.

HAVIGHURST, CLARK. 1978. "Advertising by Medical Professionals." In vol. 1 of *Encyclopedia of Bioethics*, pp. 44–48. Edited by Warren T. Reich. New York: Macmillan.

HAWKINS, JOELLEN W., and ABER, CYNTHIA S. 1988. "The Content of Advertisements in Medical Journals: Distorting the Image of Women." *Women's Health* 14, no. 2: 43–59.

JONSEN, ALBERT R. 1990. *The New Medicine and the Old Ethics.* Cambridge, Mass.: Harvard University Press.

KIEFER, TONA. 1980. "The 'Neurotic Woman' Syndrome: How Drug Companies Feed the Fantasies of the Male Medical Establishment." *The Progressive* 44, no. 12:26–29.

MORREIM, E. HAAVI. 1988. "A Moral Examination of Medical Advertising." *Business and Society Review* no. 64:4–6.

NELSON, LAWRENCE J.; CLARK, H. WESTLEY; GOLDMAN, ROBERT L.; and SCHORE, JEAN E. 1989. "Taking the Train to a World of Strangers: Health Care Marketing and Ethics." *Hastings Center Report* 19, no. 5:36–43.

PERTSHUK, MICHAEL. 1978. "Remarks." In *Competition in the Health Care Sector: Past, Present, and Future*, pp. 11–13.

Edited by Warren Greenberg. Washington, D.C.: U.S. Government Printing Office.

RELMAN, ARNOLD S. 1978. "Professional Directories—But Not Commercial Advertising—As a Public Service." *New England Journal of Medicine* 299, no. 9:476–478.

RODNING, CHARLES B., and DACSO, CLIFFORD C. 1987. "A Physician/Advertiser Ethos." *American Journal of Medicine* 82, no. 6:1209–1212.

RUDMAN, WILLIAM J., and HAGIWARA, AKIKO F. 1992. "Sexual Exploitation in Advertising Health and Wellness Products." *Women and Health* 18, no. 4:77–89.

SCHULTZE, QUENTIN J. 1981. "Professionalism in Advertising: The Origin of Ethical Codes." *Journal of Communication* 31, no. 2:64–71.

STAGE, SARAH. 1979. *Female Complaints: Lydia Pinkham and the Business of Women's Medicine.* New York: W. W. Norton.

WALLACE, CYNTHIA. 1985. "Women's Healthcare Spending New Target of Hospitals' Ads." *Modern Healthcare* 15, no. 6:52, 56.

WOLF, NAOMI. 1991. *The Beauty Myth: How Images of Beauty Are Used Against Women.* New York: Morrow.

AFRICA

See MEDICAL ETHICS, HISTORY OF, *section on* AFRICA.

AFRICAN RELIGION

This article presents a brief, general picture of Africa's traditional religious heritage, focusing on the major beliefs because these underlie the general attitudes of individuals and society and shape their worldview. Various terms are used to refer to the indigenous religious heritage, including African Religion, African Traditional Religions, African Indigenous Religions, and African Religious Traditions. This article makes use of the most current term, "African Religion." It is clear that in such a vast continent, there are diversities of religious life and concepts, but there are also similarities that make it possible to give a general picture.

After a brief word on the origin of African Religion, this entry considers it in terms of belief in God and other spiritual beings, mystical power, and the continuation of human life after death. It describes how human beings are seen to be at the center of the world, and traces the journey of individual life from birth to death and beyond. Moral and ethical values are shown to regulate people's relationships with one another, nature, and God. African peoples give health and related problems much attention, for both their physical and their spiritual welfare. Religions originating outside of Africa, together with the influences of "modern" life, also have an impact upon the traditional religious heritage.

Origin and sources of African religion

African Religion evolved gradually as people experienced different life situations, raising questions and reflecting on such mysteries of life as birth and death, joy and suffering, the forces of nature, and the purpose of life. Its history is bound up with the history of each people or tribe, and goes back to prehistoric times. Some elements distinguish it from Christianity and Islam, the other major religions of Africa, while other elements resemble them. African Religion is practiced today mostly in the southern two-thirds of Africa, including Madagascar, where Christianity is statistically dominant. In the northern one-third, dominated by Islam, African Religion exists beneath the surface, among indigenous peoples, despite their having been subjugated and dominated by Arab immigrants for many centuries.

African Religion is found primarily in oral sources, including stories, myths, proverbs, prayers, ritual incantations, songs, names of people and places, and the specialized and carefully guarded knowledge of religious personages. Other sources are art and language; ceremonies and rituals; religious objects and places like shrines, altars, and ceremonial symbols; and magical objects and practices. It also emerges among Christians and Muslims in times of crisis like severe illness or death, disputes, political and sports competitions, examinations, and the search for employment. Since the nineteenth century these sources have increasingly been recorded in writing, and since the second half of the twentieth century, on film and on audiotapes and videotapes.

African Religion spread to the western hemisphere through African peoples who were forcibly transplanted to the West Indies and the Americas by the slave trade. It settled there and survived in a mixture with Christianity, despite the influence of other cultures and environments. For example, the spirit possessions that abound among people of African descent in Brazil and the West Indies have their origins in Africa. Voodoo in the Caribbean and *macumba* in Brazil are remnants of African Religion that have been modified to suit local practice. Some names of people in Jamaica, like Cudjoe, Acheampong, Kwaku, and Obi are originally African, but these are said to be disappearing. After careful study of the American scene, Gayraud Wilmore concludes that "an essential ingredient of Afro-American Christianity prior to the Civil War was the creative residuum of the African Religions," characterized by a spirituality of response to the reality of the spirit world and its reaction with objective reality (1983, p. 26).

Major beliefs in African religion

As an all-embracing worldview, African Religion has a number of beliefs held in common by the community. Individuals cannot reject a particular belief, since beliefs are part and parcel of the wider community. The term "community" is used here to refer to a grouping of persons in a particular area who lead a fairly similar cultural life, within a given people or in a town.

Belief in God.   Belief in God is found among all African peoples. The Creator and Preserver of all things, God is invisible, but the ongoing work of creation points to God's existence and involvement in the world. There are no atheists in African traditional society; belief in God is part of the common knowledge of everyone, including children. There are no pictorial or other representations of God by African peoples. Oral appellations of God include Father, Mother, Parent, Friend, Savior, Protector, Giver of Children, Giver of Rain, the Shining One, the Kind One, and the Everlasting One. God is good, compassionate, just, and loving to all people. The overall picture of God is of one who is above gender classification, neither male nor female, since God is Spirit. To grasp some aspects of God, people find anthropomorphic concepts useful and, according to the situation, may speak of God in male or female terms for that purpose. Furthermore, many African languages do not distinguish gender grammatically.

People express their belief in and awareness of God through prayers, invocations, sacrifices and offerings, praise songs, and dedication of children to God. In some areas priests and priestesses officiate at religious ceremonies, pray on behalf of their communities, and pass on the theological, philosophical, and practical knowledge of their religion. They are, or should be, morally upright. In Nigeria and Uganda, priestesses regard themselves as "married" (i.e., wholly dedicated) to God for a given period of time in their life, but later marry human husbands.

Belief in other spiritual beings.   There is widespread belief in the existence of other spiritual beings created by and subject to God. The spirits can be considered in two categories: those associated with nature and those that are remnants of human beings after death. Nature spirits are personifications of heavenly or earthly objects and phenomena: the stars, the sun, thunder, rain and storms, mountains, earthquakes, lakes, waterfalls, and caves.

Some communities, especially in West Africa, have "divinities," spirit functionaries prominent in the life of the community. This particularly reflects the political structure, with the queen or king at the top and various chieftains or ministers below. Some "divinities" are said to have assisted God in the ordering of the world; others, to be in charge of aspects of nature like the weather, earthquakes, and epidemics. But many African peoples do not have divinities in their cosmology.

Most of the human spirits are those of people who died more than five generations ago; the others are of persons who are remembered by name and known collectively as the "living dead," since they are regarded as part of the family. When they "appear" to the living, either directly or through a medium, they are recognized by name, and what they communicate, in the form of requests, instructions, or warnings, is taken very seriously by their families. However, the spirits of the departed generally have little or no place in the beliefs of nomadic peoples, probably because they do not remain for years on the land where they bury their dead.

Spirits of the unknown dead are sometimes called upon or otherwise used in divination and medical practice, but otherwise they have no personal family ties to the living. They are said to possess people or animals, and are often featured in folk stories in which they perform great feats, although sometimes they are depicted as stupid or as fearful of the living. Many stories are told about spirits, resulting in an integration of their world into the world of living human beings.

Humanity at the center of the world. African Religion places humans at the center of the world. It is believed throughout Africa that God created human beings, and thousands of stories and myths visualize how this happened. According to some, humans were created at the end of the primal creation, formed from clay as husband and wife (or as two pairs), or created in heaven (sky) and lowered to the earth. Others say that husband and wife were created in a vessel, in water, or in the fruit of a tree.

Creation stories relate that the original state of humanity was one of bliss, in which people were endowed with immortality, rejuvenation (if they became old), or resurrection (if they died). The earth was directly linked to heaven (the sky); God and humans lived close to each other, as a family. For various reasons these gifts were lost; death, disease, and suffering appeared, as well as the separation between heaven and earth, between God and humans. However, God did not abandon humans, but he endowed them with various abilities and knowledge, so that they could survive. Through sacrifices and prayers humans still have access to God at any time. Through prayers people praise and thank God, and solicit God's help in the fight against disease, suffering, danger, and death.

A strong feature of African cosmology is the recognition of the world as comprising two interlinked realities: the visible and the invisible, the physical and the spiritual. Both are bound together in a primordial unity. They interact, and Africans do not make a strong dis-

tinction between the two. This helps to explain African awareness of and insights into the spiritual realm, an awareness at both shallow and deep levels ranging from visions, dreams involving spiritual objects or beings or messages, contact with the living dead and spirits, and divination to concepts about and experiences of God.

The life journey of the individual is marked with rites, particularly at birth, initiation, marriage, and death. Birth and name-giving ceremonies express joy in the family and gratitude to God for the child. Children are the symbol and actualization of immortality; they counteract death with new life and old age with rejuvenation. At adolescence, initiation ceremonies are performed, often followed by a period of seclusion for the initiated, during which they learn matters pertaining to adult life. Initiation ceremonies serve, among other things, to give the individual an identity as a member of the community to which he or she is thereby mystically bound. The most dramatic involve circumcision for boys and clitoridectomy for girls. The personal shedding of blood forges mystical links to the ground, to the land.

Marriage is a religious duty that, under normal circumstances, everyone is obliged or expected to fulfill. The bearing of children is the central part of marriage, and no efforts are spared to ensure that there are children in each marriage; otherwise, the couple fails to become a family. In effect the family never dies; only its members do. If, for example, the husband is impotent, his "brother" (in the wider sense of kinship ties) will (must) sleep with his wife so that she will bear him children. If the wife is barren, her husband will marry another wife, who will be expected to bear children for both wives. Polygamy is an accepted and respected form of marriage in about 15 percent of African families. Children knit the community into a vast network of relationships: brothers, sisters, cousins, parents, grandparents, uncles, aunts, and many distant relatives. The basic philosophy says "I am because we are, and since we are therefore I am."

Burial and funeral rites serve, among other things, to send the departed in peace to the spirit world, and to express condolences to the bereaved. Various symbols and acts speak of death and the continuation of life: normal activities are stopped for a day following a death or funeral; hair on the head is shaved; the house of the departed is closed or even abandoned; clothes of colors that symbolize bereavement (white, black, or red) are worn; the bodies of surviving members of the family are smeared with mud or white chalk; cattle are driven away from the homestead of the departed; people fast; and fires in the home are extinguished. Some societies bury a few personal belongings with the dead, such as spears, cooking pots, ornaments, money, and clothes. Among other groups the property of the deceased is distributed—by force if need be—among relatives or clan members.

Life after death.   Belief in the continuation of life after death is held all over Africa. The next world is pictured as being like the present one, inhabited by spirits and located in thick forests, desert places, underground, or on mountains. There is neither reward for a good life on earth nor punishment for an evil life. The departed retain their human characteristics and the living dead are still part of their earthly families, to whom they appear in dreams, in waking, or through divination, particularly if there is a major family event.

The living show remembrance of the departed through such acts of affection as naming new children after them, taking care of their graves, and pouring libations of beer, wine, milk, or tea and placing bits of food on the floor, on the graves, or in a family altar. People who die without children are considered most unfortunate, since they have no descendants to "remember" them, something that the extended family only rarely does. In some societies people invoke departed members of the family, especially parents and grandparents, and ask them to relay their requests further, until they reach God. There is thus a unity and a line of communication between the living, the departed, and God. Harmony is necessary to maintain this unity in a healthy spiritual condition.

Belief in mystical power.   There is a deeply rooted belief in a mystical power or force in the universe that derives from God. This power is used in medical practice, divination, protecting people and property, predicting where to find lost articles, and foretelling the outcome of an undertaking. It is also employed in the practice of magic, sorcery, and witchcraft. Diviners, traditional doctors, and witches know better than others how to employ it. The belief in and practice of magic causes much fear in African life, which leads to accusations, quarrels, fights, and countermeasures in families and communities. The positive use of this mystical power is cherished and plays a major role in regulating ethical relations in the community and in supplying answers to questions about the causes of good luck and misfortune.

Sacred places and objects.   Sacred places and objects—including mountains, caves, waterfalls, rocks, trees, rainmaking stones, and certain animals, as well as altars, sacrificial pots, masks, drums, and colors—are set aside for religious activities. Some places are kept as sanctuaries in which no human beings or animals may be killed, and where no trees may be felled. Some homesteads have family altars or graves that serve as sacred spots where prayers, offerings, and small sacrifices are made. Nature is often personalized in order that humans may communicate and live in harmony with it. If humans hurt nature, nature hurts them. Humans are the

priests of nature, indeed of the universe; this is a sacred trust given to them by God, who endowed them with more abilities than other creatures on earth.

Ethics and morals.   The ethics and morals of African Religion are embedded in values, customs, traditional laws, and taboos. God is ultimately the giver of morality. Moral offenses include disrespect toward elderly people, sexual transgressions (incest, rape, intercourse with children, adultery, and homosexual intercourse), murder, stealing, robbery, telling lies, deliberately causing bodily harm, and the use of sorcery and witchcraft. Such acts are punished by making the offender and his or her family feel shame or ostracism, or pay a fine; sometimes the offender is beaten or stoned to death.

On the other hand, kindness, friendliness, truthfulness, politeness, generosity, hospitality, hard work, caring for elderly parents, respect for elderly people and the weak and retarded, and protection of children and women are virtues that earn praise and admiration in the community. Women are regarded and treated as full moral agents; they are also protected against maltreatment by men, since they are considered to be less able or equipped to defend themselves physically, especially when they are pregnant or aged. Society rewards the good and punishes the evil. The spirits of the living dead maintain interest in the morals of their descendants, and may punish offenders by causing failure in undertakings, sickness, and bad dreams as warnings or deterrents. God is ultimately watching over the moral life of the community, society, and humankind. From time to time, if moral order is severely broken, God may punish the wider society or give warnings through calamities, epidemics, drought, war, and famine.

The home and the community convey moral teaching, generally from the older to the younger members, through word and example. Initiation ceremonies (some of which may last several years) are the formal communal occasions for instilling moral values in young people. Stories, proverbs, and taboos are employed in the teaching of morals. Where the basic philosophy of life is "I am because we are," it is extremely important that the two dimensions of "I am" and "We are" be carefully observed and maintained for the survival of all, through moral values. The individual is very much exposed to the community, and anonymity is virtually out of the question.

African Religion affirms and celebrates life. Laughter is heard even in the most difficult situations. Communal festivals filled with rejoicing—laughter, eating, dancing, singing, and drumming—renew and strengthen community ties. Even sad occasions like funerals are communal events that bring many people together to share in mourning, and thus lighten the burden of bereavement.

Health and medicine

Life in African communities is often a struggle against forces of destruction: illness, disease, accidents, childlessness, suffering, misfortune, spirit possession, quarrels, war, and death. Natural threats such as drought, earthquakes, epidemics, famines, and locust invasions affect the whole community. When these forces of destruction strike the individual or the family, people ask "who" has caused it to happen. Even if there are physical explanations of how an accident has occurred, or how a disease like malaria or AIDS is caused, human agents are believed to be behind it. These agents are said to use mystical power—magic, witchcraft, sorcery, the spell, the curse, or broken taboos—following quarrels, acting out of jealousy, hatred, greed, or evil intentions. Health is seen as a fundamentally ethical question pointing to relationships in the family, in the community, and between people and nature.

Medicine women and men (traditional doctors) are found in every village. Their work is highly appreciated and in constant demand. They undergo long training and apprenticeship to acquire knowledge of herbs, roots, fruits, shells, insects, and juices, especially of their medicinal properties. They learn to diagnose illnesses and complaints that affect not only human beings but also animals and fields. They use divination to communicate with the invisible world at the psychic level of consciousness. They perform healing rituals and invocations. Their "medicine" is directed not only against the disease or misfortune in question but also to the removal and prevention of its mystical cause, such as witchcraft. The human or spirit agent "behind" the problem is usually named, and part of the healing process involves coming to terms with the "diagnosed offender." The process of diagnosis, cure, and preventive measures is often carried out in the presence of the family or community, which thus participates in the healing.

African society generally shows great care toward handicapped and retarded people. Part of this special treatment comes from the fear that if you mistreat or fail to help the handicapped, you or members of your family will become similarly handicapped. Likewise, the issue of abortion is partly undergirded by the fear that a major misfortune, such as the failure to bear more children, will befall the family of a woman who has an abortion. Furthermore, the high rate of infant mortality has probably contributed to the great value that people attach to children and their consequent abhorrence of abortion. There are extremely few written references to abortion, and in some societies a woman who has had one is killed by the community or a curse is placed on her. There are, however, areas where twins were traditionally considered to bring misfortune, and consequently one or both children would be killed for the protection of the community. On the other hand, in certain areas twins were (and still are) considered to be special people, bearers of blessings or extraordinary abilities, and even called "children of God." Written information on so-called mercy killing is scanty, but suicide and homicide occur in many areas. From time to time the community is provoked beyond endurance and a mob kills by stoning, beating, or burning an offender, such as someone accused of stealing and robbery (nearly always men), practicing witchcraft (nearly always women), or committing sexual offenses like incest, intercourse with children, or rape (only men). In such cases the community undergoes a healing process, physically and ethically. The life and dignity of the community are thereby placed above the lives of individual members who do not maintain its values and order.

"Medicine" is also used to bring good fortune (health, success, loving relations, protection against danger). In their practice, traditional doctors hold that it is God who heals or brings about good results, and some of them regularly invoke God for healing and the welfare of the individuals and community. These doctors are upright, trustworthy, and respected members of their community, the symbols of its welfare and health. Through them, folk medical knowledge and practice have been passed on through many generations. Since modern or Western medicine and its wonders are too expensive for most Africans, the traditional doctors continue to respond to the health needs of many people, and complement or even replace the services of modern medicine. As in other spheres of religious life, women are very active in health matters and are believed to show deeper sensitivities than men, especially since they carry human life in their own bodies and are more attuned to the spiritual dimension of health. In many communities female traditional doctors outnumber their male counterparts, and nearly all mediums are women.

Conclusion

African Religion has encountered other religions, notably Christianity and Islam, and other cultures, especially Western. Many of its adherents convert to Christianity or Islam. But conversion does not mean abandoning the world of traditional religiosity. On the contrary, many Christians derive rich spirituality from African Religion. Translations of the Bible into some seven hundred African languages (as of 1992) use religious terms and concepts of African Religion. But while it seems to find ways of surviving and of accommodating to contemporary life, there are changes in social, political, educational, technological, and scientific life for which it has not prepared itself.

In the nineteenth century African Religion was studied almost exclusively by foreigners: missionaries, anthropologists, colonial rulers, and self-styled African experts. On the whole it was presented negatively, often interpreted falsely, and ridiculed by those with racist attitudes. However, since about the middle of the twentieth century, a more objective approach has gained ground not only in Africa but also in the New World, where peoples of African descent find in it a meaningful part of their heritage. The African religious heritage in North America provided the cultural, social, and spiritual setting for modeling Christianity among African-Americans—for example, the place of the church as a focal point of community life, the dynamic worship tradition, and the assimilation of African cultural traits. In Latin America, especially in Brazil, African Religion has blended firmly with Roman Catholicism, so much so that many people do not know where to draw the line (if need be). Some of the healing practices called "folk medicine" are traceable to those of traditional doctors in Africa. Gayraud Wilmore (1983), Roger Bastide (1978), and Leonard Barrett (1976), among others, have documented the survival and strong impact of African Religion in the New World.

We are in a much better position to understand African Religion academically today than at the beginning of the twentieth century. Just as it has survived since prehistoric times and has done so in new social and cultural environments across the oceans, we may presume that it will survive in new forms in the coming generations.

JOHN S. MBITI

Directly related to this entry is the entry MEDICAL ETHICS, HISTORY OF, *section on* AFRICA. *For a further discussion of topics mentioned in this entry, see the entries* ABORTION; CIRCUMCISION; DEATH, *article on* ANTHROPOLOGICAL PERSPECTIVES; ISLAM; MARRIAGE AND OTHER DOMESTIC PARTNERSHIPS; NARRATIVE; NATURE; PROTESTANTISM; ROMAN CATHOLICISM; *and* WOMEN, *article on* HISTORICAL AND CROSS-CULTURAL PERSPECTIVES. *This entry will find application in the entry* ENVIRONMENT AND RELIGION. *For a discussion of related ideas, see the entries on* BODY, *article on* CULTURAL AND RELIGIOUS PERSPECTIVES; LIFE; *and* VALUES AND VALUATION.

Bibliography

AWOLALU, J. OMOSADE, and DOPAMU, P. ADELUMO. 1979. *West African Traditional Religion.* Ibadan, Nigeria: Onibonoje Press.

BARRETT, LEONARD E. 1976. *The Sun and the Drum: African Roots in Jamaican Folk Tradition.* Kingston, Jamaica: Sanster's.

BASTIDE, ROGER. 1978. *The African Religions of Brazil: Toward a Sociology of the Interpenetration of Civilizations.* Translated by Helen Sebba. Baltimore: Johns Hopkins University Press.

HARJULA, RAIMO. 1980. *Mirau and His Practice: A Study of the Ethnomedical Repertoire of a Tanzanian Herbalist.* London: Tri-Medi.

IDOWU, E. BOLAJI. 1973. *African Traditional Religion. A Definition.* London: SCM Press.

MBITI, JOHN S. 1990. *African Religions and Philosophy.* 2d ed. Oxford: Heinemann.

———. 1991. *Introduction to African Religion.* 2d ed. Oxford: Heinemann.

MULAGO, GWA CIKATA. 1980. *La religion traditionelle des Bantu et leur vision du monde.* 2d ed. Kinshasa, Zaire: University of Kinshasa.

OBBO, CHRISTINE. 1980. *African Women: Their Struggle for Economic Independence.* London: Zed Press.

OLUPONA, JACOB K., ed. 1991. *African Traditional Religions in Contemporary Society.* New York: International Religious Foundation.

OPOKU, KOFI A. 1978. *West African Traditional Religion.* Accra, Ghana: Far Eastern Publishers.

PARRINDER, E. GEOFFREY. 1962. *African Traditional Religion.* 2d ed. London: SPCK.

RANGER, TERENCE O., and KIMAMBO, ISAIAH, eds. 1972. *The Historical Study of African Religion: With Special Reference to East and Central Africa.* London: Heinemann.

SEMPEBWA, JOSHUA W. 1983. *African Traditional Moral Norms and Their Implications for Christianity: A Case Study of Ganda Ethics.* St. Augustin, Germany: Steyler.

SETILOANE, GABRIEL M. 1976. *The Image of God Among the Sotho-Tswana.* Rotterdam: A. A. Balkema.

WILMORE, GAYRAUD S. 1983. *Black Religion and Black Radicalism: An Interpretation of the Religious History of Afro-American People.* 2d ed. Maryknoll, N.Y.: Orbis.

AGEISM OR AGE DISCRIMINATION

See AGING AND THE AGED, *article on* SOCIETAL AGING.

AGING AND THE AGED

I. THEORIES OF AGING AND LIFE EXTENSION

"Aging" can be defined as the accumulation of chronological events that render an organism more susceptible to the stresses of life and thereby increase the probability of death. However, there are also changes in such areas as integrative skills, which improve with age. The "senescent period" is that period of the adult life span, usually the last third, during which the processes of aging become manifest. "Maximum life span" refers to the longest lived individual of a given species. "Mean life span" is the average that members of a species can expect to live. Based on actuarial data, "life expectancy" indicates the amount of time an average individual can expect to live and is usually calculated from birth. "Gerontology" is a field of scientific study that examines the biological, medical, and psychosociological processes of aging. The field of gerontology is also concerned with the well-being, care, and treatment of the elderly and extends to geriatric health care (Baker and Shock, 1991).

Rates of aging

Aging occurs as the result of events that damage molecules, cells, and tissues, thereby exhausting reparative processes and ultimately resulting in decreased physiological performance. Rates of aging are governed by two major factors: (1) the specific genetic background of the species and (2) its interaction with the environment. The mean life span of a species is related to the processes of aging in that the accumulation of deleterious events reduces the ability of the organism to survive environmental insults, including lessening of individual defense systems and increasing the susceptibility to many diseases. In humans, some age-associated problems, such as alterations in visual capacity, may begin early in life (five to eight years of age) and progressively worsen thereafter (Baker and Shock, 1991). Other systems, such as the immune response and the ovarian-pituitary changes at the time of menopause, may show a more sudden decline in midlife. Such changes, however, may not become clinically significant until much later in life.

Life expectancy in technologically advanced societies has virtually doubled in the last hundred years due, in large measure, to enhanced sanitation, the advent of antibiotics and vaccines, and improved clinical interventions. Maximum life span of humans, however, appears not to have changed dramatically at least over the period of recorded time (Olshansky et al., 1990). Current estimates suggest that even the elimination of heart disease and cancer would have only a modest effect on mean life span and no effect on the maximum life span of the species unless the causes and rates of aging are affected.

It is not clear how aging and life span evolved. Most remarkably, the life span of certain species of the same group (phylogenetic class), such as humans and shrews, exhibit a 100-year difference in maximum longevities, although these animals have only recently diverged in evolutionary time, and their cells are virtually identical in organization and function (Finch, 1990). A number of concepts have been developed to explain the variations in life span based on variations in host defenses to environmental damage. Chronic diseases in humans, such as diabetes, shorten life span, but at least some aspects of these changes, as in adult-onset diabetes, result from inactivity and weight gain and can be prevented or even reversed (Reaven, 1988). Disease can accelerate the rates of aging. Aging is not a disease to be cured but rather a complex series of biological alterations to be understood. Only through understanding of the processes of aging can effective interventions be developed.

Causes of aging

Many factors, both internal to the organism and environmental, cause molecular and cellular damage and contribute to aging of the organism. These factors that accelerate the rates of aging processes include radiation, toxins, oxygen radicals, stress hormones, modified lipids and proteins, cytokines, and even glucose that progressively modifies proteins and causes multiple degenerative changes (Stadtman, 1992).

Cellular senescence. Tumor cells have an unlimited capacity to divide both in cell culture outside the body and in the body. Normal cells, however, exhibit only a limited number of cell divisions in culture and then enter a senescent, nondividing state (Hayflick, 1992). For example, normal human skin cells, called fibroblasts, taken from very young individuals will undergo some fifty to sixty population doublings in cell culture, enter a senescent phase, and then die. The older the individual from whom these cells are taken, the fewer the cell divisions. The loss of this ability of cells to divide outside the body with time is believed to be relevant to aging and has been much studied (Cristofalo and Pignolo, 1993). Senescent cells do not express cell-cycle regulating genes (i.e., those factors called protoncogenes that regulate cell division and initiate DNA synthesis), as do younger cells, thereby causing a blockage in cell division (McCormick and Campisi, 1991).

Recent studies indicate that the repeating end regions of chromosomes, called telomeres, shorten measurably each time cells divide in culture (Harley et al., 1992). It has been postulated that the loss of the telomeric ends combined with the absence of a specific enzyme to replace them eventually destabilizes chromosomal structure and may induce cellular senescence.

These observations provide an attractive molecular genetic mechanism to explain limited cell division with biological age as well as uncontrolled proliferation of cells (cancer) in the presence of the enzyme that replaces lost telomeres. Although this phenomenon has not been universally observed, a similar shortening of telomeres has been reported in aging animal tissues and may be fundamental to the diminished repair capacity for certain tissues with age.

Mitochondrial damage.   The major site of energy production in the cell takes place in mitochondria. These are independently replicating cell organelles that increase their number in response to exercise and other stimuli. Energy, in the form of adenosine triphosphate (ATP), produced by mitochondria requires molecular oxygen. In the process, some of the oxygen can form oxygen radicals, highly reactive forms of oxygen molecules with unpaired electrons, that are potentially very damaging to proteins, DNA, and other cellular molecules. Mitochondria contain circular DNA molecules that code for some of its essential components. Recent studies show that with age an increasing number of mitochondria in some cells have significant portions of their DNA deleted (Wallace, 1992). These deletions are believed to result from damage from oxygen radicals (Linnane et al., 1989). Such deletions are postulated to cause a progressive reduction in metabolism and to be an important age-related deficit particularly in tissues like muscle and brain.

Natural defenses against aging

The ability of cells to resist, adapt to, and repair damaged molecules is a key factor in their survival and, thereby, the longevity of the organism. Numerous biochemicals, for example, Vitamin C, tocopherols (Vitamin E), beta-carotene, glutathione, and uric acid, among others, are scavengers of free radicals and serve a critical, protective role (Ames, 1991). In addition to these chemical defenses, cells can respond to damage by increasing the production of antioxidant enzymes, antistress proteins, and various repair enzymes that protect the cell. Some of these genetic responses become attenuated with age and lead to an increased sensitivity and accelerated aging (Udelsman et al., 1993).

Theories of aging

Many theories have been proposed to account for aging. A number are called "stochastic" theories because they propose random damage from myriad environmental insults. These include the Somatic Mutation Theory (Szilard, 1959), Error Catastrophe Theory (Orgel, 1963), Free-Radical Theory (Harman, 1956), Crosslinkage

Theory (Bjorksten, 1968), Redundant Message Theory (Medvedev, 1990), and Glycation Theory (Cerami, 1985), among others, which propose that limitations in the repair of molecular damage is an important cause of aging.

"Programmed" theories suggest that life span is under active, genetic control, for example, by processes that limit cell division as discussed above. Most of these theories have not been substantiated by experimental evidence as the ultimate cause of aging. It would appear that numerous factors are involved in the processes of aging, including molecular damage from external or internal factors (oxygen radicals, glucose, radiation, infections, etc.), declines in energy production due to mitochondrial dysfunction, declining hormone production, and so forth (Adelman and Roth, 1982). Thus, aging is both stochastic and programmed, involving both environmental and genetic factors.

Potential interventions into aging processes

Genetic background, lifestyle, and nutritional factors can either accelerate or retard the rates of aging. In humans, long-lived parents may confer a three- to four-year average increase in life span to their offspring (Finch, 1990), whereas lifestyle factors can reduce life expectancy. Selection experiments in genetic alteration among lower animals, fruit flies, and nematodes have resulted in almost doubling life span by genetic alterations (Arking et al., 1993). Such studies, as well as evidence that demonstrates a decline in mortality at older ages in fruit flies (Curtsinger et al., 1992) and medflies (Carey et al., 1992), suggest that the limits on life span are not immutable. While it is unrealistic to expect dramatic increases in human life span in the near future, we can expect advances in interventions that will retard or ameliorate age-related declines and the incidence and severity of age-associated diseases. Such strategies can be classified into four general types: (1) lifestyle alterations; (2) pharmacological interventions; (3) biological enhancement; and (4) molecular-genetic interventions.

Lifestyle interventions.   Lifestyle interventions relate primarily to factors that affect the risk of acquiring diseases, such as smoking, lack of exercise, and poor nutrition. Exercise and weight reduction can prevent or even correct various metabolic disturbances. A proper diet provides not only adequate nutrition but also a variety of chemicals that protect the body against noxious environmental agents known to cause cancer and to contribute to certain degenerative diseases. In the future, the optimal levels of dietary supplements will be assessed by measuring their ability to retard molecular damage. Diet restriction has been demonstrated to extend life span by 30 to 50 percent and to enhance physiological performance in a number of laboratory animals (Weindruch and Walford, 1988). The increase in life span is related primarily to reduced caloric intake rather than any particular food component. Animals maintained on a calorically restricted diet show less decline in neuroendocrine and immune function with age, lower rates of cancer and other degenerative diseases, as well as less damage from oxygen radicals and glucose than animals allowed to eat all they want.

Pharmacological interventions.   Pharmacological interventions include those that reduce the progression of diseases, such as L-DOPA in Parkinson's disease. Recent developments hold promise that many such agents can be used to enhance functional impairments with age, particularly in the central nervous system. Experimentation on the use of synthetic chemical agents to prevent damage from oxygen radicals and other potentially harmful products of cellular metabolism are also yielding promising results.

Biological interventions.   Biological interventions include hormone replacement, such as estrogen therapy in postmenopausal women. The use of growth hormones to reverse age-related declines in muscle mass in humans was one of the first and encouraging uses of biological materials specific to age-related changes (Rudman et al., 1990). Such therapy could include the use of various hormones involved in the growth and maintenance of cells, for example, those that could slow nerve-cell loss in Alzheimer's disease patients.

Molecular-genetic interventions.   Molecular-genetic interventions may find their greatest use in preventing age-related declines in biochemical or physiological systems. Molecular-genetic techniques have been used to increase the levels of antioxidant-enzyme systems in lower organisms with promising success (Orr and Sohal, 1994). Gene therapies for various human diseases, such as cystic fibrosis, are currently being tested. There is great potential as new factors are identified and techniques refined to intervene and improve genetic systems that are ultimately responsible for age-related physiological declines in humans. Although the extrapolations of findings from one organism to another are often scientifically unjustified, they do point to exciting avenues for scientific exploration to enhance the quality and span of human life.

GEORGE R. MARTIN
GEORGE T. BAKER III

Directly related to this article are the other articles in this entry: LIFE EXPECTANCY AND LIFE SPAN, SOCIETAL AGING, HEALTH-CARE AND RESEARCH ISSUES, *and* OLD AGE. *Other relevant material may be found under the entries* DEATH, ATTITUDES TOWARDS; FUTURE GENERATIONS,

OBLIGATIONS TO; LIFESTYLES AND PUBLIC HEALTH; *and* POPULATION ETHICS, *section on* ELEMENTS OF POPULATION ETHICS.

Bibliography

ADELMAN, RICHARD C., and ROTH, GEORGE S., eds. 1982. *Testing of Theories of Aging.* Boca Raton, Fla.: CRC Press.

AMES, BRUCE N. 1991. "Endogenous DNA Damage as Related to Nutrition and Aging." In *The Potential for Nutritional Modulation of Aging Processes: Proceedings of an International Conference,* pp. 251–261. Edited by Donald K. Ingram, George T. Baker III, and Nathan W. Shock. Trumbull, Conn.: Food and Nutrition Press.

ARKING, ROBERT; DUKAS, STEVEN, P.; and BAKER, GEORGE T., III. 1993. "Genetic and Environmental Factors Regulating the Expression of an Extended Longevity Phenotype in a Long Lived Strain of *Drosophila.*" *Genetica* 91, nos. 1–3:127–142.

BAKER, GEORGE T., III, and SHOCK, NATHAN W. 1991. "Theoretical Concepts Governing Gerontological Research." In *The Potential for Nutritional Modulation of Aging Processes: Proceedings of an International Conference,* pp. 3–15. Edited by Donald K. Ingram, George T. Baker III, and Nathan W. Shock. Trumbull, Conn.: Food and Nutrition Press.

BJORKSTEN, JOHAN. 1968. "The Crosslinkage Theory of Aging." *Journal of the American Geriatrics Society* 16, no. 4:408–427.

CAREY, JAMES R.; LEIDO, PABLO; OROZCO, DINA; and VAUPEL, JAMES W. 1992. "Slowing of Mortality Rates at Older Ages in Large Medfly Cohorts." *Science* 258, no. 5081:457–461.

CERAMI, ANTHONY. 1985. "Hypothesis: Glucose as a Mediator of Aging." *Journal of the American Geriatrics Society* 33, no. 9:626–634.

CRISTOFALO, VINCENT J., and PIGNOLO, ROBERT J. 1993. "Replicative Senescence of Human Fibroblast-like Cells in Culture." *Physiological Reviews* 73, no. 3:617–638.

CURTSINGER, JAMES W.; FUKUI, HIDENORI H.; TOWNSEN, DAVID R.; and VAUPEL, JAMES W. 1992. "Demography of Genotypes: Failure of the Limited Life-Span Paradigm in *Drosophila Melanogaster.*" *Science* 258, no. 5081:461–463.

FINCH, CALEB E. 1990. *Longevity, Senescence, and the Genome.* Chicago: University of Chicago Press.

HARLEY, CALVIN B.; VAZIRI, HOMAYOUIN; COUNTER, CHRISTOPHER M.; and ALLSOPP, RICHARD C. 1992. "The Telomere Hypothesis of Cellular Aging." *Experimental Gerontology* 27, no. 4:375–382.

HARMAN, DENHAM. 1956. "Aging: A Theory Based on Free-Radical and Radiation Chemistry." *Journal of Gerontology* 11, no. 3:298–300.

HAYFLICK, LEONARD. 1992. "Aging, Longevity, and Immortality in Vitro." *Experimental Gerontology* 27, no. 4: 363–368.

McCORMICK, ANN, and CAMPISI, JUDITH. 1991. "Cellular Aging and Senescence." *Current Opinion in Cell Biology* 3, no. 2:230–234.

MEDVEDEV, ZHORDES A. 1990. "An Attempt at a Rational Classification of Theories of Aging." *Biological Reviews* 65, no. 3:375–398.

OLSHANSKY, S. JAY; CARNES, BRUCE A.; and CASSEL, CHRISTINE. 1990. "In Search of Methuselah: Estimating the Upper Limits to Human Longevity." *Science* 250, no. 4981:634–640.

ORGEL, LESLIE E. 1963. "The Maintenance of the Accuracy of Protein Synthesis and Its Relevance to Ageing." *Proceedings of the National Academy of Science* 49, no. 4:517–521.

ORR, WILLIAM C., and SOHAL, RAJINDAR S. 1994. "Extension of Life-Span by Overexpression of Superoxide Dismutase and Catalase in *Drosophila Melanogaster.*" *Science* 263, no. 5150:1128–1130.

REAVEN, GERALD M. 1988. "Role of Insulin Resistance in Human Disease." *Diabetes* 37, no. 12:1595–1607.

RUDMAN, DANIEL; FELLER, AXEL G.; NAGRAJ, HOSKOTE S.; GERGANS, GREGORY A.; LALITHA, PARDEE Y.; GOLDBERG, ALLEN F.; SCHLENKER, ROBERT A.; COHN, LESTER; RUDMAN, INGE W.; and MATTSON, DALE E. 1990. "The Effects of Human Growth Hormone in Men over 60 Years Old." *New England Journal of Medicine* 323:1–6.

STADTMAN, EARL R. 1992. "Protein Oxidation and Aging." *Science* 257, no. 5074:1220–1224.

SZILARD, LEO. 1959. "On the Nature of the Aging Process." *Proceedings of the National Academy of Science* 45, no. 1: 30–45.

UDELSMAN, ROBERT; BLAKE, MICHAEL J.; STAGG, CAROLE A.; LI, DING-GANG; PUTNEY, D. JAMES; and HOLBROOK, NIKKI J. 1993. "Vascular Heat Shock Protein Expression in Response to Stress: Endocrine and Autonomic Regulation of This Age-Dependent Response." *Journal of Clinical Investigation* 91, no. 2:465–473.

WALLACE, DOUGLAS C. 1992. "Mitochondrial Genetics: A Paradigm for Aging and Degenerative Diseases?" *Science* 256, no. 5057:628–632.

WEINDRUCH, RICHARD, and WALFORD, ROY L. 1988. *The Retardation of Aging and Disease by Dietary Restriction.* Springfield, Ill.: Charles C. Thomas.

II. LIFE EXPECTANCY AND LIFE SPAN

In the United States in 1900, the average life expectancy (also referred to as longevity) of a newborn baby was 47.7 years—46.4 for males and 49.0 for females. By 1990 the average life expectancy increased to 75.4 years—78.8 for females and 72.0 for males. Why did life expectancy increase so rapidly in the twentieth century, and what are the prospects for increasing it further? Perhaps more important, has the overall health of the population improved or worsened during this transition, and what are the health consequences of further increases in life expectancy?

The measure of life expectancy at birth is a statistic that represents the expected duration of life for babies born during a given time period, usually one calendar year. Calculated from death rates observed at every age, it is based on the critical assumption that the age-specific risks of death observed during a given year will prevail for all babies born in that year, for the remainder of their lives. In contrast, life span is the theoretical upper limit to life that would be observed if everyone in the population adopted ideal lifestyles from birth to death and if external threats to life were eliminated. Some researchers believe that there is no biologically determined life span per se (Carey et al., 1992), but rather a series of time-dependent physiological declines that may eventually be subject to modification.

Life expectancy in today's developed nations increased rapidly during the twentieth century because of rapid declines in death rates (usually expressed as the number of deaths per 100,000 population over one year) at younger and middle ages. This transformation in death rates, which has occurred to some extent in every nation, is referred to as the epidemiologic transition (Omran, 1971). During this transition, death rates from infectious and parasitic diseases, which tend to kill at younger ages, decline rapidly and the saved population lives to older ages, at which they are exposed to aging-related disorders such as vascular diseases and cancer. Although a small fraction of the population has always survived to older ages, the epidemiologic transition allows over 90 percent of all babies born to survive past the age of sixty-five. The redistribution of death from younger and middle ages to older ages is a general characteristic of the epidemiologic transition, although varying degrees of decline in death rates are experienced by different nations and subgroups of populations within nations.

Mortality transition patterns

There are two interesting patterns in the epidemiologic transition of the United States. In 1900 the average life expectancy for women was 2.6 years greater than that of men. By 1990 this difference had increased to 6.8 years. Although the increasing gender gap in longevity is attributable to more rapid declines in death rates for women at every age and for most causes of death, it is unclear why the mortality transition of women has proceeded at a faster pace than that of men. The prevailing explanation for the widening gender gap in life expectancy in the twentieth century is a combination of lifestyle characteristics among men that make them more prone to vascular diseases and cancer, and, with extended longevity, the increased expression of genetic differences.

Another interesting pattern in the U.S. mortality transition is the difference observed in historical trends in longevity between blacks and whites. In the early part of the twentieth century, the expectation of life at birth was lower for blacks than for whites by about ten years because blacks had higher death rates than whites. The difference in death rates between blacks and whites is thought to be due to a combination of biological, social, and environmental factors, but scientific studies to date have not adequately determined the relative importance of these factors. In the later twentieth century the racial gap in longevity has been reduced to seven years. This indicates that the mortality transition for blacks was faster than that of whites—particularly for black females. However, it is important to remember that because blacks had considerably higher mortality at most ages than whites early in the century, larger reductions in death rates were required for blacks to close the racial gap in longevity.

An interesting aspect of racial trends in longevity is that at older ages (i.e., at ages seventy and older), the death rates for blacks are currently lower than those of whites. This is caused either by poor data quality, resulting in an underestimation of old-age mortality for blacks, or by selective survival, in which only the most robust segment of the black population survives to older ages. Also interesting is the trend since 1984 toward declining life expectancy for blacks, while life expectancy for the rest of the population continues to increase. This unexpected trend is a direct result of increasing death rates for blacks between the ages of fifteen and forty-four—a product of higher mortality from accidents, homicides, and AIDS.

Extending life expectancy

The prospect for increasing life expectancy further is a subject of intense scientific debate. Projections of life expectancy can have a significant influence on anticipated changes in social programs, such as Social Security and Medicare, that are influenced by the future size and health status of the older population. Some scientists have argued that life expectancy at birth for humans cannot practically exceed about eighty-five years (Olshansky et al., 1990). This conclusion is based on the facts that (1) survival up to and beyond the age of 110 is as rare today as it has always been; (2) the rapid increase in death rates from aging-related diseases that begins in the second decade of life has not changed in recorded history—instead, death rates have shifted down at comparable rates for most age groups; (3) the reduction in death rates required at every age to increase average life expectancy at birth to eighty-five years is extremely large—in fact, larger than what would occur with the elimination of cancer and heart disease; and (4) life expectancy has been shown to be a demographic statistic that becomes less sensitive to declining death

rates as it approaches higher levels. Taken together, these facts point clearly to the difficulty in achieving the reduction in death rates required to increase life expectancy past eighty-five years.

Other researchers have argued that theoretically, average life expectancy at birth could reach 100 years (Manton et al., 1991; Ahlburg and Vaupel, 1990). Several conditions are required for this to occur. Under one scenario, everyone in the population would have to adopt an "optimal" risk-factor profile, maintain their physical functioning throughout life, retain the risk-factor status of a thirty-year-old for the duration of life, and respond in the same beneficial way to a fixed regime of risk-factor modifications (Manton et al., 1991). This means that everyone would have to eliminate behaviors such as smoking, drinking, and overeating, and somehow avoid the health problems, such as arthritis and sensory impairments, that now tend to compromise physical functioning in older ages.

In a second scenario, a life expectancy of 100 could be achieved if death rates declined by 2 percent at every age for every year for the next century (Ahlburg and Vaupel, 1990). Recent evidence indicates that mortality declines of this magnitude have been rare in the historical record of the United States (Olshansky and Carnes, 1994), and that such models lead to death rates that are inconsistent with evolutionary theories about the onset and progression of death rates from aging-related causes (Carnes and Olshansky, 1993). It is doubtful that either of these scenarios is practicably achievable, although they do represent laudable goals for health-care planners.

Effects of extended life expectancy on general population

Observing historical trends in mortality, and anticipating future improvements, raises the question of how the overall health of the population is influenced by these trends. From a historical perspective, there is little doubt that the thirty-year increase in life expectancy in the twentieth century was a result of trading one set of diseases and causes of death for another. The epidemiologic transition allowed much larger proportions of each birth cohort to survive to older ages, something that had never before been experienced by the human population. There is little doubt this was a worthwhile trade. Now that the focus of modern medicine is to attack the causes of death that were traded for earlier in the century, we are faced with the same sort of question: What do we get in return for reducing the risk of death from vascular diseases and cancer? This is a particularly interesting question, since successful efforts to reduce the death rate from today's fatal diseases will produce much smaller gains in life expectancy than those achieved earlier in the century, when primarily the younger population was saved from early death.

This question of how future declines in old-age mortality will influence the health status of the population is also an area of intense scientific debate. The debate is framed around what is generally referred to as the expansion versus compression of morbidity hypotheses. Those who follow the *compression-of-morbidity* hypothesis believe that improved lifestyles and advances in medical technology will postpone the onset of disease to older ages, thus compressing the period of disease and disability into a shorter time before death (Fries, 1980). With this hypothesis the critical assumption is that both fatal diseases, and nonfatal but highly disabling age-dependent diseases, will simultaneously be postponed and compressed against a biologically fixed and immutable upper limit to life.

The *expansion-of-morbidity* hypothesis, however, points out that factors that are known to reduce the risk of death from fatal diseases do not alter the age at onset or progression of the most debilitating diseases of old age, such as Alzheimer's disease and hearing and vision loss. Further reductions in old-age mortality from present levels are therefore hypothesized to allow much larger segments of the population to survive to the oldest ages (over eighty-five), where the risk of age-related disabling diseases is particularly high and currently immutable (Verbrugge, 1984; Olshansky et al., 1991). The empirical data used to test these competing hypotheses indicate that morbidity and disability may in fact be declining for those under the age of eighty-five, but after that age the risk of disability and its duration appear to be increasing. However, it is not yet possible to draw definitive conclusions about these hypotheses because of deficiencies in the available data.

Is it possible to extend the human life span beyond current practical limits and achieve an increase in the duration of healthy life among the older population? Answers to these questions may be found in work now under way in molecular biology. Based on a current understanding of the process of senescence, extending the human life span would require slowing down the aging rate itself. There is no definitive evidence at this time to indicate that the life span of humans can be modified by any means. However, there is suggestive evidence to indicate that dietary restriction could postpone many of the physiological decrements associated with aging—including those associated with both fatal and nonfatal diseases of aging (Weindruch and Walford, 1988). Although it is not practical to expect that human experiments will be conducted on the longevity benefits associated with dietary restriction, or that enough people will actually restrict their diets to influence national statistics, research in this area may eventually reveal the underlying physiological mechanisms that link dietary restriction to increased longevity. In this way it may eventually become possible to imitate the effects of dietary restriction without actually altering diet.

Scientists debate these issues on scientific grounds, but there are important moral issues close to the surface in the discussions. For example, we know that a lower life expectancy observed among subgroups of the population is linked to poverty and minority status. If we are interested in preventing premature death, then social conditions may be a more direct target than efforts to manipulate the basic rate of aging. Also, the definition of "premature death" is no longer obvious, and raises questions about the value of length of life compared with quality of life when extreme longevity is also associated with the expression of frailty and disability.

Since societies do not have homogeneous views on these competing values, whose values should prevail? Further, societies almost always provide public support for infirm elderly people. How shall we value policies in the context of increasing life expectancy when many other social goods and needs are unfulfilled? This question is stated most clearly in the intergenerational equity debate. That is, should we be donating so much of our resources to the old when so many children live in poverty, when public schools are so needy? Some would argue that increasing longevity is a triumph of modern society, and if we work hard enough on prevention, we can eliminate old-age disability. But even for those who believe this is theoretically possible, it does not seem likely in the foreseeable future. Finally, the push toward increasing life expectancy raises fundamental resource-allocation questions for those concerned about the problems posed by global population growth. For example, it is inescapable that in the long run (i.e., beyond the middle of the twenty-first century), gains in longevity beyond those already expected will accelerate growth rates that, even at current rates of increase, will inevitably lead to a doubling of the size of the human population by the year 2050.

The impact of science on life expectancy

Population aging also has implications in the context of human evolution. Scientists in the field of evolution biology have hypothesized, in nonhuman species, a link between reproduction and the rate of senescence (Finch, 1990). Although it is unlikely that the physiological mechanisms regulating human reproduction will be altered intentionally to postpone senescence, it may eventually become possible to manipulate the genome to achieve the same effect. In fact, the mapping of the human genome may eventually reveal these and other aging-related genes that could be manipulated by methods being developed in molecular biology. There is reason to believe that breakthroughs in this area are forthcoming and that by controlling genes that influence diseases of aging, it may become possible to allow more people to survive longer and healthier than is currently the case. Just how much longer and healthier people can survive through manipulating the genome is the subject of intense debate. It may also become possible to achieve increases in longevity by introducing pharmaceuticals that alter the environment in which the genome operates. One example is the current effort to introduce into the human diet natural and artificial antioxidants (i.e., substances that reduce the amount of damage caused by the presence of free radicals, products of normal metabolism implicated in the aging process). The result may be a general deceleration of the entire aging process.

If methods of increasing human longevity are realized by manipulating the genome or introducing pharmaceuticals, then a new set of questions will arise: How would such developments influence the age structure of the human population and the social and economic institutions that have been developed under the assumption that human longevity is limited? These may prove to be a much more difficult set of problems than those we face today.

S. JAY OLSHANSKY

Directly related to this article are the other articles in this entry: THEORIES OF AGING AND LIFE EXTENSION, SOCIETAL AGING, HEALTH-CARE AND RESEARCH ISSUES, *and* OLD AGE. *Also directly related is the entry* PUBLIC HEALTH, *especially the article on* PUBLIC-HEALTH METHODS: EPIDEMIOLOGY AND BIOSTATISTICS. *For a further discussion of topics mentioned in this article, see the entries* GENETICS AND ENVIRONMENT IN HUMAN HEALTH; HEALTH-CARE RESOURCES, ALLOCATION OF, *article on* MICROALLOCATION; LIFE, QUALITY OF, *article on* QUALITY OF LIFE IN HEALTH-CARE ALLOCATION; *and* LIFESTYLES AND PUBLIC HEALTH. *This article will find application in the entries* GENETIC ENGINEERING, *article on* HUMAN GENETIC ENGINEERING; POPULATION ETHICS, *especially the section on* ELEMENTS OF POPULATION ETHICS; *and* POPULATION POLICIES. *For a discussion of related ideas, see the entries* DEATH, ATTITUDES TOWARD; FUTURE GENERATIONS, OBLIGATIONS TO; HEALTH PROMOTION AND HEALTH EDUCATION; *and* VALUE AND VALUATION.

Bibliography

AHLBURG, DENNIS A., and VAUPEL, JAMES W. 1990. "Alternative Projections of the U.S. Population." *Demography* 27, no. 4:639–652.

CAREY, JAMES R.; LIEDO, PABLO; OROZCO, DINA; and VAUPEL, JAMES W. 1992. "Slowing of Mortality Rates at Older Ages in Large Medfly Cohorts." *Science* 258, no. 5081:457–461.

CARNES, BRUCE A., and OLSHANSKY, S. JAY. 1993. "Evolutionary Perspectives on Human Senescence." *Population and Development Review* 19, no. 4:793–806.

FINCH, CALEB E. 1990. *Longevity, Senescence, and the Genome.* Chicago: University of Chicago Press.

FRIES, JAMES F. 1980. "Aging, Natural Death, and the Compression of Morbidity." *New England Journal of Medicine* 303. no. 3:130–135.

MANTON, KENNETH G.; STALLARD, ERIC; and TOLLEY, H. DENNIS. 1991. "Limits to Human Life Expectancy: Evidence, Prospects and Implications." *Population and Development Review* 17, no. 4:603–637.

OLSHANSKY, S. JAY, and CARNES, BRUCE A. 1994. "Demographic Perspectives on Human Senescence." *Population and Development Review* 20, no. 1:57–80.

OLSHANSKY, S. JAY; CARNES, BRUCE A.; and CASSEL, CHRISTINE K. 1990. "In Search of Methuselah: Estimating the Upper Limits to Human Longevity." *Science* 250, no. 4981:634–640.

OLSHANSKY, S. JAY; RUDBERG, MARK A.; CARNES, BRUCE A.; CASSEL, CHRISTINE K.; and BRODY, JACOB A. 1991. "Trading Off Longer Life for Worsening Health: The Expansion of Morbidity Hypothesis." *Journal of Aging and Health* 3, no. 2:194–216.

OMRAN, ABDEL R. 1971. "The Epidemiologic Transition: A Theory of the Epidemiology of Population Change." *Milbank Memorial Fund Quarterly* 49, no. 4:509–538.

VERBRUGGE, LOIS M. 1984. "Longer Life but Worsening Health? Trends in Health and Mortality of Middle-Aged and Older Persons." *Milbank Memorial Fund Quarterly/Health and Society* 62, no. 3:475–519.

WEINDRUCH, RICHARD, and WALFORD, ROY L. 1988. *The Retardation of Aging and Disease by Dietary Restriction.* Springfield, Ill.: Charles C. Thomas.

III. SOCIETAL AGING

A society is said to age when its number of older members increases relative to its number of younger members. The societies of the United States and of many other industrialized nations have been aging since at least 1800. In 1800, the demographic makeup of developed countries was similar to that of many Third World countries in the early 1990s, with roughly half the population under the age of sixteen and very few people living beyond age sixty. Since that time, increases in life expectancy, combined with declines in fertility rates, have dramatically increased the proportion of older persons in developed nations. By contrast, the age profile in many Third World countries is still heavily weighted toward younger age groups, even though the increase in actual numbers of old people is even greater in many developing countries than it is in the developed world. What future societies will regard as distinct about population aging in the twentieth and twenty-first centuries is the rapid pace at which it is occurring. Those over the age of eighty-five are the fastest-growing age group in the United States. Since 1900, this group has become twenty-one times as numerous, and there has been an eightfold increase in the number of people over the age of sixty-five.

During the last century or more that population records have been kept, women's life expectancy has always exceeded men's (Cassel and Neugarten, 1988). Although at younger ages there are more men than women, by old age women far outnumber men (Cassel and Neugarten, 1988). In the group aged sixty-five and older, there are 68 men per 100 women. For ages eighty-five and over, there are 45 men per 100 women. Although demographic predictions have sometimes been proven wrong by subsequent facts, demographers today predict this sex differential will increase until the year 2050, at which time it will level off; but before it does, there will be only 38.8 men per 100 women aged eighty-five and over.

Ethical implications

The rapid increase in the number of older persons relative to younger ones carries important implications for society. In the area of health care, societal aging will increase costs and exert greater pressure to ration services. It will therefore bring to the fore questions regarding a just distribution of health care between young and old. The population's aging will also alter the nature of health services by increasing the number of patients who have chronic and disabling conditions that are not life-threatening. This, in turn, will change the face of bioethical debate, from a focus on acute life-and-death medical decisions made at a particular instant in time, to an emphasis on ongoing and often relatively mundane problems spanning many years. Finally, societal aging portends changes for family life. Already, the imbalance between young and old is placing strains on offspring who undertake caregiving responsibilities and is prompting questions about the scope and limits of filial duties. To the extent that family members play an increasing role in elder care, their role in health-care decision making is a significant and vigorously debated question.

Health-care rationing.   The aging of society will increase health-care expenditures simply because persons over the age of sixty-five consume far more health care than other age groups do. In the United States, persons sixty-five and over account for roughly 12 percent of the population but utilize one-third of the country's total personal health-care expenditures (exclusive of research costs). In an era of fiscal constraints, this makes the elderly an obvious target for health-care rationing. The financial savings that would accrue if the

elderly were disfranchised from various forms of health care is disproportionately high, because the elderly are more frequent utilizers of health care. According to one estimate, if those over the age of fifty-five were excluded from treatment for renal disease in the United States, 45 percent of the costs of the renal-disease program would be saved. In many other areas a large financial saving could be achieved through excluding elderly persons.

Arguments supporting age-based rationing and the shifting of scarce resources from old to young groups have been advanced by Daniel Callahan (1987), Norman Daniels (1988), Richard Lamm (1987), and Samuel Preston (1984), among others. Callahan, for example, proposes rationing publicly funded life-extending care based on old age. Such a proposal might be implemented once society comes to accept the idea that "government has a duty, based on our collective social obligation, to help people live out a natural life span, but not actively to help extend life beyond that point" (Callahan, 1987, p. 137). Both Lamm and Preston favor directing fewer resources to older age groups and more to younger persons as a necessary condition of meeting duties to younger and future generations. They maintain that unless we limit health-care expenditures for the old, we will eventually impoverish health services and other social goods for the young. Finally, Daniels urges us to think about justice between the young and old from a first-person point of view. According to him, when we succeed in viewing our lives as a whole, rather than from a particular point in time, it will sometimes be prudent for us to prefer a health-care plan that distributes fewer services to our old age in exchange for more services earlier in life.

Critics of age-based rationing object, for example, to the implications of age-based rationing for women (Jecker, 1991a); to the violation that age-based rationing implies of the moral thrust of both Judaism and Christianity (Post, 1991); and to the message that age-based rationing conveys about the meaning and worth of the lives of aged persons (Murray, 1991).

Long-term care.   In addition to increasing health-care expenditures, societal aging will increase the number of disabled persons and the need for long-term care, including adult day care, in-home services, and care in resident facilities, convalescent homes, and intermediate and skilled nursing facilities. Several factors will contribute to a greater need for long-term care. First, the ratio of older women to older men is expected to increase, and older women experience a greater incidence of morbidity and disability than older men. Second, the population over age eighty-five constitutes the fastest-growing portion of the population, and the oldest old are the heaviest users of long-term care, with more than 70 percent of those eighty-five and over requiring some kind of assistance with one or more activities of daily living. Finally, fewer offspring will be available to serve as informal caregivers for future generations of elderly persons. This is because individuals are having fewer children than previous generations did, and greater numbers of women are joining the paid labor force.

The growing need for long-term care raises social and policy questions concerning the just allocation of funds between acute hospital care and "low technology" supportive services for chronic disabling conditions. In addition, it alters the nature of clinical ethical cases by changing the sorts of decisions faced and the age, gender, and health profile of the affected population. According to one commentator (Moody, 1992), bioethical analysis has tended to emphasize a principle of individual autonomy and respect for persons' self-determination. Yet this principle begins to break down as the patient population becomes increasingly geriatric, increasingly dependent, and increasingly disabled. In this environment, it is argued, the ideals of human dignity and self-respect, ideals that are intimately linked to human relationship and community, will assume greater significance. Yet others suggest, to the contrary, that the values of autonomy and privacy must retain their central importance because such values are inextricably linked to assuring a good quality of life in old age.

Family relationships.   The rapid aging of society will reshape relationships within the family as parent–child relationships extend over many more years and pose new challenges in later life. Although most agree that parents undertake special duties toward offspring, there are different opinions as to whether grown children have corresponding duties toward aging parents. On the other hand, Jane English denies that adult offspring owe their parents anything by virtue of being their offspring. Instead, she defends the idea that "the duties of grown children are those of friends, and result from love between them and their parent, rather than being things owed in repayment for the parents' earlier sacrifices" (English, 1991, p. 147). Others object to special duties of any form, whether founded on friendship, filial status, citizenship, or other bases. The favoritism implied by special duties is sometimes considered logically or psychologically at odds with the ethical requirements of impartiality and equal respect for persons (Meyers et al., 1993).

On the other side of this debate are those who defend special duties. Various underpinnings for adult children's responsibilities toward aging parents have been offered, including gratitude, reciprocity, and duties to the vulnerable (Meyers et al., 1993).

Historical and cultural perspectives

An aging society, defined as a society in which the population of older individuals is increasing relative to the population of younger individuals, presupposes that individuals can be separated into meaningful categories of old and young. Although contemporary Western society tends to conceive of youth, adolescence, middle age, and old age as unique life stages with distinct sets of problems, this perspective is hardly universal. Indeed, present conceptions of the life course are a relatively recent phenomenon. Thomas Cole traces the metaphor of life's stages to the cities of northern Europe in the sixteenth and seventeenth centuries, where the current life-stage metaphor first emerged. Picturing life as a series of ordered stages represents the life course as in conformity with the order of the universe and makes it possible for every individual to "step outside of his own life experiences and view it as a whole" (Cole, 1992, p. 25).

Just as our recognition of aging reflects our historical and cultural traditions, so our beliefs about the meaning and value of old age bespeak our historical and cultural heritage. The social rank of elderly persons varies during different historical and culture periods, depending upon the perceived cost of supporting older age groups and the contribution they are thought to make (Amoss and Harrell, 1981). For example, the Akamba people of Africa believe that "the older a person becomes, the more intricately interwoven that person becomes in the lives of others, and the greater the damage done if that person is removed. At the same time, the older person has wisdom—a perspective on life that comes only with age—which is considered to be a particularly important social resource" (Kilner, 1984, p. 19). By contrast, U.S. society has traditionally valued "pragmatism, action, power, and the vigor of youth over contemplation, reflection, experience and the wisdom of age"; hence, ageism (age discrimination) is especially evident in U.S. society (Butler, 1969, p. 243).

Despite different cultural conceptions of aged persons and their role in society, anthropologists identify common biological and cultural features of aging. Thus, every known society has "a named category of people who are old—chronologically, physiologically, or generationally. In every case these people have different rights, duties, privileges, and burdens from those enjoyed or suffered by their juniors" (Amoss and Harrell, 1981, p. 3). This suggests that people in culturally distinct societies may face similar ethical questions concerning relationships among people of different ages.

NANCY S. JECKER

Directly related to this article are the other articles in this entry: THEORIES OF AGING AND LIFE EXTENSION, LIFE EXPECTANCY AND LIFE SPAN, HEALTH-CARE AND RESEARCH ISSUES, *and* OLD AGE. *For a further discussion of topics mentioned in this article, see the entries* CHRONIC CARE;

FAMILY; HEALTH-CARE RESOURCES, ALLOCATION OF, *article on* MICROALLOCATION; LIFE, QUALITY OF, *article on* QUALITY OF LIFE IN HEALTH-CARE ALLOCATION; LONG-TERM CARE; *and* POPULATION ETHICS, *section on* ELEMENTS OF POPULATION ETHICS. *For a discussion of related ideas, see the entries* FUTURE GENERATIONS, OBLIGATIONS TO; *and* JUSTICE.

Bibliography

AMOSS, PAMELA T., and HARRELL, STEVAN, eds. 1981. *Other Ways of Growing Old: Anthropological Perspectives.* Stanford, Calif.: Stanford University Press.

BUTLER, ROBERT N. 1969. "Age-Ism: Another Form of Bigotry." *Gerontologist* 9, no. 3:243–246.

CALLAHAN, DANIEL. 1987. *Setting Limits.* New York: Simon and Schuster.

CASSEL, CHRISTINE K., and NEUGARTEN, BERNICE L. 1988. "A Forecast of Women's Health and Longevity: Implications for an Aging America." *Western Journal of Medicine* 149, no. 6:712–717.

COLE, THOMAS R. 1992. *The Journey of Life: A Cultural History of Aging in America.* New York: Cambridge University Press.

DANIELS, NORMAN. 1988. *Am I My Parents' Keeper? An Essay on Justice Between the Young and the Old.* New York: Oxford University Press.

ENGLISH, JANE. 1991. "What Do Grown Children Owe Their Parents?" In *Aging and Ethics: Philosophical Problems in Gerontology,* pp. 147–154. Edited by Nancy S. Jecker. Clifton, N.J.: Humana.

FONER, NANCY. 1984. *Ages in Conflict: A Cross-Cultural Perspective on Inequality Between Old and Young.* New York: Columbia University Press.

JECKER, NANCY S. 1991a. "Age-Based Rationing and Women." *Journal of the American Medical Association* 266, no. 25:3012–3015.

———, ed. 1991b. *Aging and Ethics.* Clifton, N.J.: Humana.

KANE, ROSALIE A., and CAPLAN, ARTHUR L., eds. 1990. *Everyday Ethics: Resolving Dilemmas in Nursing Home Life.* New York: Springer.

KILNER, JOHN F. 1984. "Who Shall Be Saved? An African Answer." *Hastings Center Report* 14, no. 3:18–22.

LAMM, RICHARD D. 1987. "Ethical Care for the Elderly: Are We Cheating Our Children?" In *Should Medical Care Be Rationed by Age?* pp. xi–xv. Edited by Timothy M. Smeeding, Margaret P. Battin, Leslie P. Francis, and Bruce M. Landesman. Totowa, N.J.: Rowman & Littlefield.

MEYERS, DIANA T.; KIPNIS, KENNETH; and MURPHY, CORNELIUS F., eds. 1993. *Kindred Matters: Rethinking the Philosophy of the Family.* Ithaca, N.Y.: Cornell University Press.

MOODY, HARRY R. 1992. *Ethics in an Aging Society.* Baltimore: Johns Hopkins University Press.

MURRAY, THOMAS. 1991. "Meaning, Aging, and Public Policy." In *Too Old for Health Care? Controversies in Medicine, Law, Economics, and Ethics,* pp. 164–179. Edited by Robert H. Binstock and Stephen G. Post. Baltimore: Johns Hopkins University Press.

POST, STEPHEN. 1991. "Justice for Elderly People in Jewish and Christian Thought." In *Too Old for Health Care?* pp. 120–137. Edited by Robert H. Binstock and Stephen G. Post. Baltimore: Johns Hopkins University Press.

PRESTON, SAMUEL H. 1984. "Children and the Elderly in the U.S." *Scientific American* 251, no. 6:44–57.

SMEEDING, TIMOTHY M.; BETTIN, MARGARET P.; FRANCIS, LESLIE P.; and LANDESMAN, BRUCE M. eds. 1987. *Should Medical Care Be Rationed by Age?* Totowa, N.J.: Rowman & Littlefield.

IV. HEALTH-CARE AND RESEARCH ISSUES

What is so different about the ethics of health care and research in older people that would render a general discussion of these topics insufficient? Basic principles, such as autonomy, beneficence, and justice, are no different and no less important because the individuals involved in health care or research are older. Many factors associated with aging, however, do alter substantially the facts of clinical and research encounters with older people.

Health care of older people

The nature of illness in older people greatly influences the ethical issues in their health care. Older people have a higher burden of illness than younger people. On average, they are likely to have several chronic medical conditions, be on multiple medications, and have frequent encounters with the health-care system, including more hospitalizations. Because older people are closer to the end of their life expectancy, they have a greater chance of being involved in situations where difficult health-care decisions must be made. Decisions about the appropriate use of life-sustaining medical treatment for older patients are commonplace. These range from Do-Not-Resuscitate (DNR) orders, to decisions to discontinue dialysis, to decisions about withholding or withdrawing artificial nutrition and hydration. Many, if not most, deaths in health-care institutions in the United States are preceded by explicit decisions to limit treatment. These treatment limitation decisions, more properly viewed as decisions to change to a palliative care plan from life-sustaining or death-delaying efforts, are generally more common in the care of older people.

While any individual may become incompetent during a critical illness, older people are at greater risk of impaired decision-making capacity because of either a transient delirium or a chronic dementing illness, such as Alzheimer's disease, that results in permanent cognitive impairment. Thus, older people are not only at risk of having end-of-life decisions made in the health-care setting; they frequently are not capable of making those decisions themselves at the time required. In such situations, physicians routinely turn to the family of an older person to serve as a surrogate decision maker or proxy. Several studies of the treatment preferences of older patients and their potential proxies (spouses, children, and physicians) have uncovered serious discord between the choices that would be made by patients and by their proxies (Seckler et al., 1991). While this raises concerns about the validity of proxy decision making vis-à-vis its accuracy as a substituted judgment, one can argue that family members are still appropriate surrogates and that many older people care more about who makes decisions for them than about the exact decisions being made (High, 1991).

The foreseeability of both serious illness and the loss of competency for older people, as well as questions about proxy decision making, have created a strong interest in the use of advance directives in the care of older people (Danis et al., 1991; Emanuel et al., 1991). Advance directives include instructional documents, such as living wills, and proxy appointment documents, such as the durable power of attorney for health care. Interestingly, most of the empirical studies done on both proxy decision making and advance directives have focused on older people. Advance directives have received increasing attention in the United States with the 1991 enactment of the Patient Self-Determination Act, a federal law requiring health-care institutions to educate patients about the availability and use of these instruments. While it is hoped that these efforts will increase the number of older people giving advance instructions for their health care, it remains to be seen if older people will execute advance directives in significant numbers, and if physicians will respect the preferences outlined in these documents.

Because of its effects on the competency of older individuals, dementia occasions significant ethical dilemmas (Sachs and Cassel, 1989). Dementia affects perhaps as high a proportion as 10.3 percent of individuals over age sixty-five and 47 percent of those over age eighty-five, and raises ethical concerns for several reasons. First, rather than presuming competence and working within the bounds of confidentiality, truth-telling, and patient autonomy expected in the normal doctor–patient dyad, when the patient has dementia, the doctor–patient relationship is altered in a fundamental fashion. A physician caring for an older person with dementia must reassess decision-making capacity frequently, carefully evaluate what the patient says for useful information, weigh what can be shared with the patient, and rely on others for information and assistance in executing a care plan. Second, the progressive and irreversible nature of the most prevalent kinds of dementia alters the goals of medical care of the patient with dementia. While promising research on dementia continues, there is no standard therapy that will improve, let alone cure, most dementias. As with hospice care or rehabilitation medicine, many argue, the medical care of a patient with dementia properly focuses on maximizing function, including socialization, palliation of symptoms, maintaining hygiene, and preserving dignity (Rango, 1985). Third, the family members of an older person with dementia are not only proxies for decision making, they also usually provide the bulk of their relative's daily care needs. The great burden of caregiving places family members at risk of depression and other illness, causing health professionals to consider the psychosocial needs of the family as well as the patient.

While only about 5 percent of people over the age of sixty-five are in a nursing home at any one time, it has been estimated that the lifetime risk of spending time in a nursing home in the United States is as high as 40 percent (Kemper and Murtaugh, 1991). Thus, many older people do receive medical care in a nursing home for some portion of their lives. At least in the United States, nursing home care frequently has been cited more for its deficiencies: unwarranted mechanical restraint of residents, inattention to treatable conditions such as urinary incontinence, and inappropriate and excessive use of psychotropic medications. At least part of the problem of poor nursing home care has been the lack of continuity in medical care of older people once they enter a nursing home. A minority of physicians in the United States visit their older patients once the patients enter a nursing home (as few as 28 percent in one U.S. nationwide study) (Mitchell and Hewes, 1986). Subspecialty care, including psychiatry, is even less available to older people residing in nursing homes.

Problems with access to good medical care for nursing home residents are actually a subset of the larger problem of the level of expertise in the medical care of all older people. While geriatrics is an established specialty in the United Kingdom, a subspecialty certifying exam in geriatric medicine in the United States was offered for the first time only in 1988. Very few physicians enter fellowship programs that provide postresidency training in geriatric medicine.

Research on older people

As with the relationship between health care of older people and health care in general, research involving older people emphasizes different ethical issues because of the history of research on older people and specific health-care attributes of older populations. As geriatrics has been late in being recognized as a specialty in American medicine, so too has serious research on older people been a relatively recent phenomenon in the United States. The National Institute on Aging (NIA) was established within the National Institutes of Health in 1974 to promote research on aging. That the creation of

NIA was necessary is supported by the dearth of research on the problems of older people in earlier years. People over the age of sixty-five were frequently excluded from clinical studies, even from trials examining cancer, heart disease, diabetes, and hypertension, all conditions more prevalent in older populations.

While it is not clear why older people were excluded from research in the past, conducting research on older people *is* more difficult than working with younger subjects (Zimmer et al., 1985). Surveys have shown that older people tend to be less willing than younger people to become research subjects. As noted earlier, they are likely to have multiple medical conditions and to be taking several medications, factors that may cause them to be excluded from research projects that are trying to study single illnesses and the unadulterated effects of single medications. Because of these factors, older people also have a higher attrition rate, necessitating larger numbers of older subjects when the study begins in order to compensate for dropouts over time. Impairments in vision, hearing, or cognition may make efforts to obtain informed consent and enroll older subjects more time-consuming and labor-intensive. These factors together may make research on older people more expensive to complete.

Two additional attributes of older people that most affect research ethics were mentioned in discussing their health care: the prevalence of dementia and the frequent use of nursing homes. Dementing illnesses fundamentally change the investigator–subject relationship, as well as the doctor–patient relationship. Far less is known empirically about issues in the research setting, such as the ability of subjects with dementia to give informed consent, the reliability of proxies in giving consent for experiments, or the practices of investigators in safeguarding vulnerable, cognitively impaired subjects. Serious concerns were raised by one study of relatives who gave proxy consent for their cognitively impaired older family members residing in nursing homes (Warren et al., 1986). Many of these proxies gave consent for a study on urinary catheters despite saying that they thought the older person would not have wanted to participate and that they themselves would not want to be in such a study.

Various organizations and authorities have published guidelines for research involving subjects with dementia (American College of Physicians, 1989; Berg et al., 1991; Melnick and Dubler, 1985). Most endorse the practice of proxy consent, as long as the subject assents when the particular study commences. Some explicitly prohibit the participation of subjects with dementia if it is known that the older person would not have wanted to participate in a study. Others worry, however, that excessive safeguards may end up serving as barriers to research that might benefit people with dementia.

The ethics of research on older people in nursing homes also focuses on consent issues because of the high prevalence of dementia in nursing homes, but there are other ethical concerns (Hofland, 1988). On the one hand, access to research may mean access to improved care and increased socialization for an older nursing home resident. On the other hand, limited freedom and the existence of less than optimal care in many nursing homes may create a coercive environment for enrolling subjects. Another concern is that although much nursing home research is conducted in large, academically affiliated, well-staffed nursing homes, these conditions do not exist in many nursing homes, raising the question of how much one can generalize the research findings to more typical nursing homes.

Additional ethical issues

Unfortunately, many of the issues that affect younger individuals with regard to access to health care and research do not disappear when people get older. While this is not a great concern in countries with a national health service or national health insurance, it remains a major issue in the United States. Many people, including a surprising number of older people, assume that most health-care needs are covered by Medicare, the federal health insurance program for older people. While Medicare pays a substantial portion of hospital and physician fees for acute care, it does not cover the cost of medications, many preventive services, and important items for older people such as eyeglasses and hearing aids; most important, Medicare pays for very few long-term care services. Older people who are poor, female, or minority, especially African-Americans, are disproportionately affected by problems with access to care. In the United States, the difference between African-Americans and whites in terms of access to hospitals and nursing homes narrowed from the 1960s to the 1980s (Smith, 1990). However, studies in the late 1980s and early 1990s continued to uncover less utilization of aggressive and expensive treatments for cardiac disease, for example, in African-Americans and women compared with white men, even when insurance status was taken into account (Goldberg et al., 1992).

GREG A. SACHS

Directly related to this article are the other articles in this entry: THEORIES OF AGING AND LIFE EXTENSION, LIFE EXPECTANCY AND LIFE SPAN, SOCIETAL AGING, *and* OLD AGE. *For a further discussion of topics mentioned in this article, see the entries* CHRONIC CARE; DEATH AND DYING: EUTHANASIA AND SUSTAINING LIFE, *especially the article on* ADVANCE DIRECTIVES; HEALTH-CARE FINANCING; LONG-TERM CARE; MENTALLY DISABLED AND MENTALLY ILL PERSONS; *and* RESEARCH, HUMAN:

Historical Aspects. *For a discussion of related ideas, see the entries* Autonomy; Competency; Family; *and* Informed Consent.

Bibliography

American College of Physicians. 1989. "Cognitively Impaired Subjects [Position Paper]." *Annals of Internal Medicine* 111, no. 10:843–848.

Berg, Joseph; Karlinsky, Harry; and Lowy, Frederick, eds. 1991. *Alzheimer's Disease Research: Ethical and Legal Issues.* Toronto: Carswell.

Danis, Marion; Southerland, Leslie I.; Garret, Joanne M.; Smith, Janet L.; Hielema, Frank; Pickard, C. Glenn; Egner, David M.; and Patrick, Donald L. 1991. "A Prospective Study of Advance Directives for Life-Sustaining Care." *New England Journal of Medicine* 324, no. 13: 882–888.

Emanuel, Linda L.; Barry, Michael J.; Stoeckle, John D.; Ettleson, Lucy M.; and Emanuel, Ezekiel J. 1991. "Advance Directives for Medical Care—A Case for Greater Use." *New England Journal of Medicine* 324, no. 17:889–895.

Goldberg, Kenneth C.; Hartz, Arthur J.; Jacobsen, Steven J.; Krakauer, Henry; and Rimm, Alfred A. 1992. "Racial and Community Factors Influencing Coronary Artery Bypass Graft Surgery Rates for All 1986 Medicare Patients." *Journal of the American Medical Association* 267, no. 11:1473–1477.

High, Dallas M. 1991. "A New Myth About Families of Older People?" *Gerontologist* 31:611–618.

Hofland, Brian, ed. 1988. "Autonomy and Long Term Care." *Gerontologist* (suppl. iss.) 28:2–96.

Jonas, Hans. 1970. "Philosophical Reflections on Experimenting with Human Subjects." In *Experimentation with Human Subjects*, pp. 1–31. Edited by Paul A. Freund. New York: George Braziller.

Kane, Rosalie A., and Caplan, Arthur L., eds. 1990. *Everyday Ethics: Resolving Dilemmas in Nursing Home Life.* New York: Springer.

Kemper, Peter, and Murtaugh, Christopher M. 1991. "Lifetime Use of Nursing Home Care." *New England Journal of Medicine* 324, no. 9:595–600.

Melnick, Vijaya L., and Dubler, Nancy N., eds. 1985. *Alzheimer's Dementia: Dilemmas in Clinical Research.* Clifton, N.J.: Humana.

Mitchell, Janet B., and Hewes, Helene T. 1986. "Why Won't Physicians Make Nursing Home Visits?" *The Gerontologist* 26:650–654.

Rango, Nicholas. 1985. "The Nursing Home Resident with Dementia: Clinical Care, Ethics, and Policy Implications." *Annals of Internal Medicine* 102, no. 6:835–841.

Sachs, Greg A., and Cassel, Christine K. 1989. "Ethical Aspects of Dementia." *Neurologic Clinics* 7, no. 4:845–858.

———. 1990. "Biomedical Research Involving Older Human Subjects." *Law, Medicine, and Health Care* 18, no. 3:234–243.

Seckler, Allison B.; Meier, Diane E.; Mulvihill, Michael; and Paris, Barbara E. Cammer. 1991. "Substituted Judgment: How Accurate Are Proxy Predictions?" *Annals of Internal Medicine* 115, no. 2:92–98.

Smith, David Barton. 1990. "Population Ecology and the Racial Integration of Hospitals and Nursing Homes in the United States." *Milbank Quarterly* 68, no. 4:561–596.

Warren, John W.; Sobal, Jeffrey; Tenney, James H.; Hoopes, J. Michael; Damron, Dorothy; Levenson, Steven; DeForge, Bruce R.; and Muncie, Herbert L., Jr. 1986. "Informed Consent by Proxy: An Issue in Research with Elderly Patients." *New England Journal of Medicine* 315, no. 12:1124–1128.

Zimmer, Anne Wilder; Calkins, Evan; Hadley, Evan; Ostfeld, Adrian M.; Kaye, Janet M.; and Kaye, Donald. 1985. "Conducting Clinical Research in Geriatric Populations." *Annals of Internal Medicine* 103, no. 2: 276–283.

V. OLD AGE

Every generation seems to yearn for some glorious era in a mythic past when older people were honored and suffered little from material deprivation, derision, or debility. In the late twentieth century, the aging society of the United States has many reasons to seek such comforting ideas about the experience of old age in Western history. Growing alarm about the "graying" of an unbalanced federal budget, concern about allocating expensive medical resources, fears of intergenerational conflict, anxiety about prolonged technological dying and medical indigence, all give a strikingly contemporary, secular resonance to the Psalmist's plea: "Do not cast me off in old age, when my strength fails me and my hairs are gray, forsake me not, O God."

Recent historical scholarship (Cole et al., 1992) reveals no grand narrative, and certainly no "golden age," capable of unifying the diverse experiences of aging and old people in the past. Of all previously silenced groups, the elderly—"clothed as they were with official respect and buried, as they often were, in reality"—may prove the greatest challenge to historians (Stearns, 1982, p. 2). Despite the difficulty of generalizing about the historical experience of older people, we can follow the evolution of life in Western history. This article will sketch these themes. It will also highlight research findings about aging and the life course in ancient, medieval, early modern, and modern Western societies and conclude with the problems posed by the end of modernity.

Every society creates symbols, images, and rituals that help people live meaningfully within the limits of human existence. Cultural meanings of aging and old age are linked to these symbolic forms. Western culture has traditionally relied on two archetypal images to represent the wholeness, unity, or meaning of human experience in time: the division of life into ages (or stages), and the metaphor of life as a journey. Classical antiquity first connected the ages of life and the journey of life, weaving them into its beliefs about the nature of human existence and the cosmos to which human life was intimately linked. In the Middle Ages, Christian writers adopted Graeco-Roman ideas about the ages of life and conceived the journey of life as a sacred pilgrimage. Between the sixteenth and the twentieth centuries, secular, scientific, and individualistic tendencies steadily eroded ancient and medieval understandings that aging was a mysterious part of the eternal order of things. Instead it became an individual experience that was best explained scientifically and divorced from larger communal rituals and cosmic meanings. In the late twentieth century, we are living through the search for ideals adequate to contemporary culture, in which the recovery of cosmic and collective sources of meaning may stimulate appreciation of the spiritual and moral aspects of aging without devaluing individual development (Cole, 1992).

All traditions that preceded the modern, scientific effort to master old age share an appreciation of its mystery and complexity. The resulting tendency to view old age as both a blessing and a curse is therefore prominent in Hebrew, Graeco-Roman, and Christian writings, each with its own variation.

Ancient societies

Ancient Hebrew religious literature contained an ambiguous vision of old age. It commanded the young to honor their parents and respect the old for their wisdom, yet it also described the old as "apelike . . . and childlike," loathed by their children and household (Isenberg, 1992, p. 149). Despite the special place Jewish biblical culture reserved for the old, the ancient Hebrews acknowledged that not all old people would be wise, nor would all children support their elders in time of need. The Book of Job specifically challenges the view that old age brings wisdom and asks why God grants long life to the wicked. Later rabbinic law translated the Biblical injunction to honor one's parents as requiring children to provide care, a task that belonged primarily to women.

Greco-Roman literature on old age shares three common themes: the "relationship between wisdom and age; the social and political authority of the elderly; and the care of the aged" (Falkner and de Luce, 1992, pp. 4–5). While the Greeks of the classical era generally portrayed old people more harshly than did the Romans, they also viewed old age as one of life's great mysteries. Plato considered virtue a possibility, rather than a necessary by-product, of old age. Aristotle saw middle age as the peak of human life and considered old men unfit

for political office. Weakness and poor judgment rendered them objects of pity or scorn.

Greek representations of old age also revealed practical worries. In ancient Greece, a son's coming of age did not absolve him of legally enforced filial duties. Greek drama emphasized that every hero's death deprived his father of *threpteria,* or support in old age. "Sons formed the only pension plan available to the elderly" (Falkner and de Luce, 1992, p. 15). While care of older family members also fell to Roman children, the absolute power of the Roman *pater familias,* who retained authority over his children as long as he lived, intensified the fires of intergenerational conflict (Bertman, 1976). Roman comedy, which openly flaunted rules of respect for elders, mercilessly portrayed old men as weak fools or aging lovers as objects of ridicule.

The evidence on attitudes toward and conditions of older women in Graeco-Roman antiquity is scanty yet suggestive. Greek idealization of young men and emphasis on female fertility weighed against cultural appreciation for older women. Yet, postmenopausal women of substance may have experienced unusual freedom in a male-dominated, hierarchical society. Despite the literary contempt that older Roman women received, those with the necessary resources and relations apparently achieved a measure of personal freedom after the constraints of spousal roles and motherhood were removed (Falkner and de Luce, 1992). Roman custom accorded respect and authority to aging women and expected sons to support their older mothers (Banner, 1992). Even prior to menopause, Roman women did not experience the same exclusion from education or power that Greek women suffered.

The ancients divided the cycle of human life into ages or stages, each corresponding to a generation, each possessing its own set of natural characteristics. Aristotle formalized this threefold division in the *Rhetoric.* Hippocrates' four physiologically determined ages was the most common scheme until the late Middle Ages, when Ptolemy's astrologically based system of seven ages was translated into the vernacular and eventually immortalized by Shakespeare's cynical Jaques:

> All the world's a stage,
> And all the men and women merely players.
> They have their exits and entrances;
> And one man in his time plays many parts,
> His acts being seven ages.
>
> (*As You Like It,* Act II, vii)

In *De Senectute* (On Old Age), Cicero identified the philosophical bedrock beneath these ages-of-life schemes, that is, the belief that despite the diversity of size, appearance, ability, and behavior that characterizes the different stages, the human life span constitutes a single natural order. "Life's racecourse is fixed," he wrote, "nature has only a single path and that path is run but once, and to each stage of existence has been allotted its appropriate quality" (cited in Burrow, 1986, p. 1).

Ancient writers such as Aristotle, Galen, Hippocrates, and Cicero, also sought to explain the nature and causes of aging. Associating old age with "dryness" and "coldness," they saw aging as a process of diminution of vital heat or fluids.

Medieval societies

In the Middle Ages, Christian writers took up these explanations and added a supernatural cause—the Fall of Man. According to Saint Augustine, sickness, aging, and death were unknown in the Garden of Eden; they entered the world after the sin of Adam (Post, 1992). While Christian theology considered aging a punishment for original sin, medieval writers also envisioned the journey of life as a sacred pilgrimage to God and eternal judgment. Thus Christian writers fashioned a vision encompassing both physical decline and the possibility of spiritual ascent (Cole, 1992).

For the period after the decline of the Roman Empire and the emergence of a decentralized feudal society in Europe, generalizations about the material conditions of older people become even more perilous. The practical experiences of growing old in the chaotic and often violent Middle Ages are difficult to isolate. Early wills reveal the practice of notarizing contracts by which middle-aged peasants agreed to maintain their parents. This was a sign that loss of property or physical vitality rendered older people vulnerable. Such negotiated retirement practices were apparently most common among urban artisans and merchants (Troyansky, 1992). To date, there is little evidence on the socioeconomic status of older women in the Middle Ages. While old women and widows were cruelly attacked in both high and popular culture, older widows of substance may have often maintained the authority of their late husbands, while poor, single women and widows became even more vulnerable.

Early modern society

Early modern Europe—the age of Montaigne and Shakespeare, of Petrarch and the revival of Ciceronian Stoicism, and later of the Protestant Reformation—was an age of widely disparate images of old age (Troyansky, 1992). It was also the period when quintessentially modern ideas and images of the human lifetime were born (Cole, 1992). During the Reformation, the traditionally circular representations of life's stages were recast iconographically into a rising and falling staircase, a visual map of the life course, complete with virtues and vices for each stage of life. This new iconography encouraged

urban burghers to envision life as a career, a sequence of events over which individuals had some control. Long before longevity became a realistic expectation, Protestant writers and artists urged people to seek a long, orderly, and stable life. They wove together qualifications for salvation with requirements for longevity, thus drawing the cultural cognitive maps for the secular, institutionalized life course of the modern era.

Historians no longer identify the transition to modernity as the key to understanding changes in the lives of older people. In the shift from rural, communal, preindustrial to urban, individualist, industrial society, old people did not simply lose venerated positions of power or security and become scorned outcasts of the past (Stearns, 1982). While historians have spilled considerable ink debating the power and status of older people in North America since the colonial period, we still lack sufficient empirical data to justify strong generalizations (Achenbaum, 1978; Fischer, 1977; Haber, 1983).

It is clear, however, that the experience of growing old in modernizing Western societies was shaped by basic changes in the structure of the life course conceptualized not simply as an aggregate of individuals, but as "a pattern of rules ordering a key dimension of life" (Kohli, 1986, p. 271). Beginning in the late eighteenth century, shifts in demography and family life, as well as by the growth of age-stratified systems of public rights and duties, forged the modern life course. Demographically, age at death was transformed from a pattern of relative randomness to one of predictability (Imhoff, 1986). Average life expectancy rose dramatically, especially after 1900. By the mid-twentieth century, death struck primarily in old age, and with much less variance than in the past. (The AIDS [acquired immunodeficiency syndrome] epidemic that began in the 1980s altered this trend.) Meanwhile, the experience of a modern family cycle (including marriage, children, survival of both spouses to age fifty-five, "empty nest," and widowhood) became increasingly common and standardized (Hareven and Adams, 1982).

Modern society

In the century roughly between 1870 and 1970, the social transition to adulthood (end of school, first job, first marriage) became more abrupt and uniform for a growing segment of the population. At the same time, the spread of universal, age-homogeneous public school and chronologically triggered public pension systems divided the life course into three "boxes": education, work, and retirement. In the modern life course, old age was transformed from a cultural category and a negotiated phase of work and family life into a separate, bureaucratically defined segment of the life course.

The rise of the welfare state facilitated the creation of old age as the capstone of the institutionalized life course. Following the example of Germany (in 1889) and other industrial democracies (e.g., Great Britain, 1908; Austria, 1909; France, 1910; the Netherlands, 1913), the United States instituted a national pension system in 1935 through its Social Security Act (Quadagno, 1988). In linking retirement benefits to a specific age, public pension systems provided the economic basis for a chronologically defined phase of life beyond gainful employment. During the middle third of the twentieth century, this "new" phase of life became a mass phenomenon. Increasing life expectancy, the dramatic growth of the elderly population, the spread of retirement benefits, the emergence (in 1965) of Medicare and Medicaid to help defray medical costs, a booming nursing-home industry, and the rise of gerontology as an area of scientific research and professional service, transformed old age into the final stage of the institutionalized life course.

By the mid-1970s, increasing longevity, economic security, and medical care available to most older people testified to the success of welfare-state policies. Shortly thereafter, however, economic troubles, initially provoked by the 1973 oil crisis, helped undermine the political legitimacy of old age (Minkler, 1990). To a number of critics, an aging society threatened the welfare of other age groups. These critics, who focused on Social Security and Medicare, blamed the deteriorating condition of children and families on the graying of the federal budget, and raised questions of generational equity (Longman, 1987). Heightened awareness of an aging population blended silently with fears of nuclear holocaust, environmental deterioration, economic decline, social conflict, and cultural decadence.

Fears about the economic consequences of an aging society framed in terms of generational equity seemed especially troubling, because modern U.S. culture offered no convincing answers to questions of meaning or purpose in old age. During the long period between the Reformation and the modern welfare state, old age was removed from its ambiguous place in life's journey, rationalized, and redefined as a scientific problem. The triumph of mass longevity was not accompanied by culturally rich notions of what old age could or should mean for individuals or society. Instead, modern old age became a permanent threshold, marked by exit but devoid of entry into a world of shared ideals, a season without a purpose.

In the late twentieth century, which coincides with the end of the modern era, we are living through a search for ideals and roles in later life—a search involving renewed concern about the moral and spiritual dimensions of growing old (Cole, 1992). The outcome of this search that attempts to integrate the ancient value of submission to natural limits with the modern value of unlimited individual development will influence the answers to many pressing ethical questions in our aging society (Moody, 1992).

THOMAS COLE
MARTHA HOLSTEIN

Directly related to this article are the other articles in this entry: THEORIES OF AGING AND LIFE EXTENSION, LIFE EXPECTANCY AND LIFE SPAN, SOCIETAL AGING, *and* HEALTH-CARE AND RESEARCH ISSUES. *For a further discussion of topics mentioned in this article, see the entries* FAMILY; HEALTH-CARE RESOURCES, ALLOCATION OF, *article on* MICROALLOCATION; ROMAN CATHOLICISM; *and* WOMEN, *articles on* HISTORICAL AND CROSS-CULTURAL PERSPECTIVES, *and* HEALTH-CARE ISSUES. *For a discussion of related ideas, see the entries* FIDELITY AND LOYALTY; *and* JUSTICE. *Other relevant material may be found under the entries* ABUSE, INTERPERSONAL, *article on* ELDER ABUSE; CHRONIC CARE; FUTURE GENERATIONS, OBLIGATIONS TO; LIFE, QUALITY OF; *and* LONG-TERM CARE.

Bibliography

ACHENBAUM, W. ANDREW. 1978. *Old Age in the New Land: The American Experience Since 1790.* Baltimore: Johns Hopkins University Press.

ARISTOTLE. 1924. *Rhetoric.* Translated by W. Rhys Roberts. London: Oxford University Press.

BANNER, LOIS W. 1992. *In Full Flower: Aging, Women, Power, and Sexuality: A History.* New York: Alfred A. Knopf.

BERTMAN, STEPHEN. 1976. "The Generation Gap in the Fifth Book of Vergil's *Aeneid.*" In *The Conflict of Generations in Ancient Greece and Rome,* pp. 205–210. Edited by Stephen Bertman. Amsterdam: Grüner.

BURROW, JOHN A. 1986. *The Ages of Man: A Study in Medieval Writing and Thought.* Oxford: At the Clarendon Press.

COLE, THOMAS. 1992. *The Journey of Life: A Cultural History of Aging in America.* Cambridge: At the University Press.

COLE, THOMAS; VAN TASSEL, DAVID; and KASTENBAUM, ROBERT, eds. 1992. *The Handbook of the Humanities and Aging.* New York: Springer.

FALKNER, THOMAS, and DE LUCE, JUDITH. 1992. "A View from Antiquity." In *The Handbook of the Humanities and Aging,* pp. 3–39. Edited by Thomas Cole, David Van Tassel, and Robert Kastenbaum. New York: Springer.

FISCHER, DAVID HACKETT. 1977. *Growing Old in America.* New York: Oxford University Press.

HABER, CAROLE. 1983. *Beyond Sixty-Five: The Dilemma of Old Age in America's Past.* New York: Cambridge University Press.

HAREVEN, TAMARA K., and ADAMS, KATHLEEN, eds. 1982. *Aging and Life Course Transitions: An Interdisciplinary Perspective.* New York: Guilford.

IMHOFF, ARTHUR E. 1986. "Life-Course Patterns of Women and Their Husbands: The 16th to the 20th Century." In

Human Development and the Life Course: Multidisciplinary Perspectives. Edited by Aage Sorensen, Franz Weinert, and Lonnie Sherrod. Hillsdale, N.J.: Erlbaum.

ISENBERG, SHELDON. 1992. "Aging in Judaism: 'Crown of Glory' and 'Days of Sorrow.'" In *The Handbook of the Humanities and Aging*, pp. 147–174. Edited by Thomas Cole, David Van Tassel, and Robert Kastenbaum. New York: Springer.

KOHLI, MARTIN. 1986. "The World We Forgot: A Historical Review of the Life Course." In *Later Life: The Social Psychology of Aging*, pp. 271–303. Edited by Victor Marshall. Beverly Hills, Calif.: Sage.

LONGMAN, PHILIP. 1987. *Born to Pay: The New Politics of Aging in America.* Boston: Houghton Mifflin.

MINKLER, MEREDITH. 1990. "Generational Equity and the Public Policy Debate: Quagmire or Opportunity?" In *A Good Old Age? The Paradox of Setting Limits*, pp. 222–239. Edited by Paul Homer and Martha Holstein. New York: Simon & Schuster.

MOODY, HARRY R. 1992. *Ethics in an Aging Society.* Baltimore: Johns Hopkins University Press.

PLATO. 1968. *The Republic.* Translated by Francis MacDonald Cornford. London: Oxford University Press.

POST, STEPHEN. 1992. "Aging and Meaning: The Christian Tradition." In *The Handbook of the Humanities and Aging*, pp. 127–146. Edited by Thomas Cole, David Van Tassel, and Robert Kastenbaum. New York: Springer.

QUADAGNO, JILL S. 1988. *The Transformation of Old Age Security: Class and Politics in the American Welfare State.* Chicago: University of Chicago Press.

STEARNS, PETER N. 1982. *Old Age in Preindustrial Society.* New York: Holmes & Meier.

TROYANSKY, DAVID. 1992. "The Older Person in the Western World: From the Middle Ages to the Industrial Revolution." In *the Handbook of the Humanities and Aging*, pp. 40–61. Edited by Thomas Cole, David Van Tassel, and David Kastenbaum. New York: Springer.

AGRICULTURE

If bioethics is "the ethics of the life sciences," agriculture is historically, conceptually, and institutionally fundamental to bioethics. Agricultural technologies used in food production contribute as much to sustaining life as do health-profession technologies. The life sciences have their roots in agricultural science and remain embedded in historically agricultural institutions. Public-sector research in the United States had its origins in the agricultural experiment stations created by the Hatch Act of 1887 (Busch and Lacy, 1983; Marcus, 1985). The Darwinian foundation of the life sciences derives from the breeding technology of seventeenth-century British farmers. Twentieth-century genetic theory came from research in agricultural colleges by scientists seeking theoretical foundations for Gregor Mendel's work. Agricultural colleges have contributed to dramatic increases in agricultural production in the United States by a research, development, and extension agenda that has emphasized "production efficiency" through industrializing agricultural practices. This agenda has helped reduce the number of persons engaged in farming in the United States from 85 percent of the population to less than 5 percent.

With fewer farmers to serve, many agricultural colleges began calling themselves "colleges of natural resources and life sciences," reflecting broader concerns than scientific farming, such as food and environmental safety, human health and nutrition, and conservation of resources. Links between these colleges and schools of veterinary medicine and the health sciences have strengthened. Animal scientists commonly conduct National Institutes of Health–sponsored research. These links reveal shared conceptions of applied science and the values it promotes. Some bioethicists find that just as the notion of "health" presupposed by medical research remains relatively unexamined, so does the notion of "agriculture." "What is agriculture?" and "What is health?" are important topics of investigation for bioethics. So are questions about how the life sciences should provide information on how to maintain good health and how to practice good agriculture. The conception of good agriculture supported by the agricultural life sciences and by federal policy in the United States has been fundamentally industrial.

A critique of U.S. industrial agriculture came to the public's attention through books by Rachel Carson (1962), Jim Hightower (1973), and Wendell Berry (1977). These authors challenged the industrial vision of agriculture. Carson questioned the impact of chemical farming on the environment. Hightower viewed highly capitalized farmers as the chief beneficiaries of public agricultural research. Berry saw in industrial agriculture the same fragmentation of modern culture that creates irresponsible specialists ignorant of the impact of their work.

These critiques have stimulated a growing critical and ethical literature about agriculture and the conception of the life sciences that supports industrial practices. Critics question the standard assumptions underlying science-based agriculture and the ways in which the costs and benefits of such practices are distributed. The criticisms are analogous to those raised in other fields of bioethics, but some are unique to agriculture. Literature on the bioethics of the agricultural sciences focuses on four main topics: (1) competing conceptions of agriculture and its goals; (2) the beneficiaries of agricultural research; (3) the notion of sustainable agricultural development; and (4) the biotechnological "revolution." Public-sector agricultural research has been accused of being an "island empire." The bioethical literature in agriculture has helped build bridges to other fields of inquiry and other areas of bioethical concerns. New directions in the research agenda are beginning to emerge.

Competing conceptions of agriculture

If "agriculture," and "medicine" are viewed as technologies or techniques for sustaining life, their *philosophical examination* belongs to the philosophy of technology. If new technologies simply increase human power, ethical questions about their appropriate use are about the responsible use of power. Do these technologies provide appropriate social benefits that justify their social costs? What is the assumed end they are designed to serve? Critics of agricultural research complain that its agenda is driven by "productionism," the only goal of which is to increase productive efficiency: "to make two blades of grass grow where only one grew before" (Burkhardt, 1992; Harding, 1940). Critics of productionism argue that food quality, a fairer distribution of the costs and benefits of the production system, and the safety and health of the nonhuman environment should also be goals. The idea that technologies are morally neutral instruments ignores these other values.

A more fundamental criticism concerns the metaphysical or religious status of the practice of industrial agriculture, which replaces natural systems with intensely managed ones. The goal of re-creating nature, or holding human "dominion" over it, has been critically examined by those concerned about the moral limits of agriculture. There is a similar concern about the moral dimensions of genetic, reproductive, and other interventions into human natural capacities. For example, some forms of human "dominion over nature" are regarded as symptomatic of a patriarchal domination of the nonhuman environment, women, and other victims of oppression.

Dominion theories of the relationship between humans and nature are justified within Western religious traditions by either a stewardship model or a humanistic model. The former regards natural systems as part of creation. They are to be conserved. The latter regards them as the raw material for re-creation. For critics like Berry (1977), who sees the re-creation of natural forms as an inevitable consequence of human interaction with nature, agriculture signifies the margin between nature and culture—between the products of nature and the products of human labor. Agriculture is an experiment in the creation of new forms of the natural; but "science-based agriculture" does not adequately record these new forms of nature and compare them against the old forms that are replaced: "We do not know where we have been."

Science-based agriculture fails to be conscious of itself in other ways. It depends on a mechanistic conception of nature (Merchant, 1989) and a reductionistic conception of science. It views production systems only in terms of component inputs, and it excludes value judgments from the realm of science (Busch and Lacy, 1983). In more "traditional" forms of agriculture, many of the "inputs," such as nitrogen, potassium, phosphate, and water, come from within the production system. Agricultural science has identified these essential inputs so that they can be replaced by those manufactured or mined off-site by industry. And it replaces animal traction and manual labor with motorized tools. Monocropping (the practice of planting only one crop in a large area) has replaced traditional cropping patterns to accommodate the more efficient use of large machinery. These changes, modeled on the way production is organized in modern industry, justify applying the label "industrial agriculture" to science-based systems. The proponents of industrial agriculture do not generally question the goals that set the agricultural research agenda, the conception of scientific inquiry upon which it is based, or the conception of nature that justifies it.

Berry's radical humanism challenges the domination view of the human–nature relationship by stressing the interdependency of humans and other life forms and the need for humans continually to reaffirm their connectedness to "the source of their being" in the way they conduct their practical activities. As humans re-create nature, they remain a part of it, and in the process they also re-create themselves. The domination "paradigm" underlying scientist agriculture (based on the uncritical use of modern science) results in the alienation of the self and the loss of autonomy.

Critical opposition to a "productionistic" conception of agriculture and the distance it produces between producer and consumer, and producer and nature, is part of an agrarian tradition that values farming as a way of life as important as its products (Montmarquet, 1989). In this tradition, criteria for evaluating production systems should include the intrinsic value of the production process to the producer and the producer's community as well as its efficiency. A particular type of practice may provide more fulfilling lives for those who engage in it, or make them more dependable citizens, or create the basis for more stable communities, or increase food security for the producer's immediate community. With these additional criteria, the benefits of production include more than money for the producer and food and fiber for the consumer.

In addition to science-based or industrial farming techniques, the agricultural research agenda has supported the development of new methods to store agricultural products and to distribute them once they leave the farm. These new technologies have led to the industrialization of food processing for better storage, distribution, and marketing. This has led to an enlarged conception of agriculture that replaces the farming conception with one that includes all technologically and economically related activities—including the industries that produce farming inputs (fertilizers, pesticides, farm machinery) and those that process and market farm commodities—as well as related policymaking, administration, government, research, and education. This expanded notion of agriculture broadens the area of agricultural bioethics to include the ethics of business, science and technology, the professions, the environment, and policymaking. What values should this broadened conception of agriculture provide? Whom should agriculture serve, and how?

The question of equity

The question of equity concerns the equitable distribution of the costs and benefits of the agricultural policies and practices that the research agenda has supported. Since this agenda has promoted industrialized, science-based agriculture, how have the costs and benefits from this form of agriculture been distributed? Benefits include access to the goods produced on farms (food and fiber) and the economic benefits derived from agricultural activities. Costs include loss of opportunities to practice agriculture, loss of access to farm products, and loss of nonagricultural resources (such as potable water). Nonhuman animals and natural systems also have received inequitable treatment from agriculture.

Carson's (1962) criticism of "chemical farming"—that it has serious negative environmental consequences—is largely acknowledged (National Research Council of the National Academy of Sciences [NRC], 1989). Industrial agriculture has serious negative impacts both on and beyond the sites of production. The research agenda that supports these practices has not provided adequately for the study of these impacts and how to avoid them (Busch and Lacy, 1983; NRC, 1989). Negative effects include loss of soil fertility; contamination of groundwater by high levels of nitrates from fertilizer runoffs and by pesticides (these endanger wildlife and make the water unfit for human consumption); excessive drawdowns of groundwater levels; destruction of wildlife habitats; and loss of genetic diversity. Agriculture is the largest source of nonpoint (not derived from some single site, like from a sewer pipe that empties into a river) water pollution (NRC, 1989). Pesticides pose threats to on-farm safety and to consumer safety (NRC, 1989). Highly managed agricultural systems reduce genetic diversity and increase ecological vulnerability. Industrial agriculture has social costs external to the production system, and the burdens of these costs are not shared equitably.

Hightower (1973) argues that the benefits are not shared equitably either, since highly capitalized producers benefit more than other groups from industrialized technologies. Access to industrial agriculture has been systematically denied to (1) farmers who lack access to capital, (2) blacks and other oppressed ethnic groups, and (3) women. These groups have been excluded because of their relatively poor access to credit. Capital-intensive technologies provide economic benefits for the early adopters because they increase production efficiency. As others adopt these technologies to keep up, surpluses flood the markets. As the process continues, the "treadmill effect" (Cochrane, 1979) pushes less highly capitalized producers out of production. In addition, women have been excluded from farming as principal operators or farm owners and from the agricultural professions because of male biases against women participating in these practices. In many Third World countries, Western development agents ignore women, who constitute the majority of subsistence producers in many regions. Those excluded lose access to the goods they once produced for themselves, or to income to purchase goods produced by others. Many of the costs and benefits of industrial agriculture, therefore, are not distributed equitably. The failure of some groups to receive an equitable share of the benefits is itself a cost, since the resources used to provide the benefits are appropriated by others.

Certain critics have also charged that the practices of industrial agriculture are unsustainable because they are destroying or using up many of the resources that have thus far sustained them. If we are to secure the continuing production of agricultural goods, these practices must be replaced by more sustainable ones. This criticism has been acknowledged by the publication of a study undertaken by the prestigious National Research Council (NRC, 1989). The study recognizes the need to develop alternative systems of production, systems that are inherently more sustainable. Since industrial agriculture has been used as the model for "developing the agriculture of underdeveloped countries around the globe," the charge that these practices are unsustainable as well as inequitable has led to the search for new models. The critical evaluation of alternative models for agriculture has become part of a growing body of literature focused on the concept of "sustainable agricultural development," now the accepted context for discussions of alternative agriculture.

Sustainable agricultural development

"Agricultural sustainability" refers to the capacity of food, agriculture, and natural-resource systems to meet people's needs over the long run. Agricultural practices become unsustainable when they fail to meet the demands placed on them. Sustainability is thus relative to the extent of these demands. Practices that mine soil fertility must incorporate techniques for replacement. Industrial agriculture has stretched the productivity of farming systems by importing materials no longer generated locally, and by introducing management techniques that substitute for in situ biological relationships. Current practices often depend on the use of diminishing and nonrenewable resources, and on technologies that will become inadequate to perform their needed role. Diminishing resources include soil and water, petro-based chemicals (pesticides and fertilizers), and soil amendments (phosphate and limestone). Inadequate technologies include petroleum-dependent machinery, chemical pesticides, and monocropping. Genetic diversity, a potential resource for new plant varieties, is being threatened as well (NRC, 1989).

Loss of topsoil through soil erosion is a major problem in many parts of the world (NRC, 1989). Edward Hyams (1976) traces the rise and fall of civilizations because of the need to shift production sites due to soil erosion. Since tillage is a primary cause of soil erosion, nontillage forms of agriculture are being developed.

Water resources are threatened by the excessive use of irrigation technology, which in many areas of the United States seriously depletes the water reserves of aquifers (deep-well irrigation agriculture being essentially the mining of fossil water); and the expanding competition for urban water use raises serious doubts about the sustainability of current irrigation practices.

Industrial agriculture's effect on water quality is another serious impediment to sustainability. Soil deposition, nutrient loading, and contamination by pesticides cause major water problems. Environmental and consumer safety concerns also raise doubts about the continued use and effectiveness of pesticides. Contamination of water by pesticides poses threats to wildlife and humans. Pesticide use is a threat to farm workers. Residues negatively affect food safety (NRC, 1989). Pesticide technology is rapidly becoming ineffective, as insects develop resistance faster than new pesticides can be developed (Metcalf, 1987). The use of antibiotics in animal feed is another area of major concern. Antibiotic-resistant bacteria caused by the use of antibiotics in animal feed may be a source of meat contamination (NRC, 1989).

Relatively cheap petroleum since the end of World War II helped create a dependency on petroleum-using machinery and on petroleum-based fertilizers and pesticides. During the oil crisis of the 1970s and 1980s, petroleum prices and farming costs rose significantly. The predicted depletion of global oil reserves may mean that cheap-oil agriculture is unsustainable.

Many of the unsustainable features of conventional agriculture were introduced as replacements in systems that had become unsustainable or "underutilized" for one reason or another. The replacement of one system with another is sometimes referred to as a "revolution," such as the "green revolution" (Danbom, 1979; Merchant, 1989), and sometimes as a "development."

The notion of "agricultural development" has its roots in the rationalization of colonial expansion. During the period of European expansion from the late fifteenth century to the end of World War I, European governments considered many regions of the world underutilized. These regions became both sources of raw materials for manufacturing and new markets for European products. In the process, many indigenous production systems were converted to plantation agriculture by colonizers. These hybrid systems—mixtures of indigenous and imported systems—soon became unsustainable and were replaced by more "progressive" forms of farming (Merchant, 1989). When these former European colonies gained their independence after World War II, "development" became synonymous with nation-building, the creation of urban industrial centers, cheap food for the cities, and marketable export goods to bring in needed capital. "Agricultural development" came to refer to the process of increasing productive efficiency. The classical liberal theory of development assumed that agricultural development would bring rural development; rural producers would benefit from agricultural development through increased incomes and a higher standard of living, or through opportunities in urban labor markets. Frequently, the opposite occurred.

While there is increasing agreement about the need to develop more sustainable production systems, the notion of sustainability means different things to different people (Douglass, 1984; Lockeretz, 1988). Advocates of sustainability variously propose (1) greater use of biotechnology to break dependence on pesticides and nonorganic fertilizers; (2) readoption (with some modern adaptations) of agricultural techniques from earlier local systems (Warren, 1991); (3) adoption of organic or reclamation production techniques; (4) the development of systems that give greater recognition to the environmental and social characteristics of the regions in which production takes place (Altieri, 1989; Harwood, 1992); and (5) the return to more decentralized production systems based on local independent producers who keep capital in their rural communities (Strange, 1988). The use of biotechnology to correct the failures of industrial agriculture has received the greatest amount of attention and of research and development funding.

Agricultural biotechnologies

The development of new life forms through sophisticated biochemical techniques is generally referred to as biotechnology. In agriculture this includes the development of "improved" plant and animal strains, of biological controls for pests, and of biochemicals that stimulate plant and animal growth and productivity.

Equity and sustainability questions arise in regard to the development and use of all of these techniques. Plant improvement is one example. Hybridization is not a new process, but its successful application to seed corn in the 1930s by Henry Wallace (Kirkendall, 1987), to increase corn yields, marked the beginning of research efforts to develop other high-yielding grain varieties. The justification for developing and disseminating these new plants was to help reduce hunger. A geometrically increasing world population requires that yields from farming continue to increase (Borlaug, 1986). However, critics argue that high-yield biotechnology has had only a limited success in alleviating malnutrition. Since it is capital intensive and thus favors highly capitalized farmers, poorer farmers are driven out of production; this diminishes their opportunities for either producing or purchasing food. The higher yields are not distributed equitably and thus rarely benefit malnourished populations. High-yield biotechnology has also often proved ineffective; hybrid varieties that replace more traditional varieties are more vulnerable to adverse growing conditions; more costly to produce, since farmers cannot produce their own seeds; and more dependent on other purchased inputs.

Biotechnology, however, could be used to produce new life forms that tolerate the adverse conditions other developed varieties cannot, by introducing traits from hardy local weeds into unrelated crop species. Through genetic engineering, plants can be "designed" to be resistant to pests, or to use nutrients more efficiently, or to produce their own nutrients, thus eliminating much of the need to depend on fertilizers or pesticides.

Genetic engineering can also be used to develop microorganisms that produce biologically useful materials, such as animal growth hormones that increase yields and lower inputs. But critics raise important equity issues about the technology as well as the products it delivers. For example, bovine growth hormone (bGH) has been the target of some concerns. Many of the newly engineered life forms will be patented by their developers. If they replace more traditional nonpatented varieties, farmers' dependence on the patent holders will increase. And their environmental consequences are unknown. Also, finding suitable traits to introduce into crop plants may mean the mining of the genetic resources of Third World countries (Silva, 1988). Finally, biotechnology may just substitute off-site inputs, not eliminate them. For example, herbicide resistance has been genetically engineered into tobacco. While this allows the use of herbicides to replace tillage, herbicides are another purchased input whose environmental impact is largely unknown.

Critics of the biotechnology "alternative" suggest that this approach is really not very different from the conventional "technical fix" of high-tech global agriculture (Burkhardt, 1992). The technical-fix approach often does not take into account the larger physical and social systems in which agriculture operates. Approaches to sustainable development must take this larger context into account. The systems approach to development appears to represent a more holistic conception of the agricultural sciences than the reductionism that has driven the research agenda in the past. It is reflected in a growing body of agricultural development literature. Whether the adoption of systems analysis incorporates critical reflection about which values are to be included in production systems depends on the extent to which the scientists who design those systems are willing to ask ethical questions about their consequences (Busch, 1989).

New directions

One consequence of adopting systems analysis as a model for agricultural development research is that the research has become more interdisciplinary and includes a wider range of social-science and humanities perspectives. These new perspectives have allowed the introduction of new criteria for evaluating production systems. These criteria incorporate a strong ethical dimension, since they include economic, social, and environmental justice. Environmental justice is a broad concept that includes a reference to the fact that negative environmental impacts of production practices typically weigh more heavily on marginalized groups (Hofrichter, 1993). Justice requires that these burdens be shared more equitably. It also refers to the fact that the burden of preserving global wilderness resources (such as the Amazonian rain forest and the Sundarbans in the Ganges Delta) should not fall inequitably on poorer regions but should be shared by all who benefit from them. For some, the notion also includes a recognition that nonhuman animals and natural ecosystems are entitled to moral consideration in decisions about what to preserve and what to change.

When these ethical criteria are applied to the diversity of human social systems and biological systems found in various regions of the world, and to the often competing values that these systems must serve, it is clear that no single model of sustainable development can satisfy all of them. Given the conflicting demands that will be placed on agriculture in the next century, some critics now argue that "The key to success will be the recognition and structuring of appropriate patterns of diversity. No single pattern is acceptable. No one type can meet the diverse social, economic, and resources availability conditions of even a single country" (Harwood, 1992, p. 29). Included in the social resources of many regions are traditional knowledge systems that do not rely on purchased inputs and that provide more empowerment and less alienation for their users.

Since World War II, agricultural research has broadened its clientele base from producers of food and fiber to the entire agribusiness complex. Until recently it was assumed that by supporting an industrialized system of production and distribution, agricultural research supports the consumers of these products by providing them with a cheap and safe food and fiber supply. The critics of this model have raised serious questions about how adequately this system serves the consumers and how fairly it distributes its costs and benefits. In response, the agricultural sciences in the public sector have attempted to rethink their connections to the broader base of the life sciences to which they belong. One approach is for the public sector to step back from research aimed directly at the development of new technologies in favor of a more basic orientation to biological research, leaving technology development to the private sector. Another approach is to serve consumers more directly by introducing into the research agenda such values as higher standards of food quality, better systems of distribution, more ecologically based systems of production, the preservation of traditional rural landscapes and rural communities, the safety of agricultural workers, and the well-being of nonhuman domestic animals and wildlife.

How these often competing values are to be conceptualized, and how the agricultural life sciences can best serve to integrate them into food and fiber systems, raise important bioethical questions. Public-sector agricultural research continues to be carried out in institutions that are clientele driven and organized chiefly to serve production-oriented values. It is done by scientists whose scientific training is fundamentally reductionistic. The range of problems selected as research goals is determined by the perceived clientele, and the range of considered solutions is determined by the disciplinary matrix. Problem-solving research carried out within this matrix tends to favor a technical-fix conceptualization of the problem. Under these conditions the problem definition is how to integrate production values with consumer values.

Framed in this way, the major question becomes "How can we modify production systems so that they conform better to consumer values?" Included in this new agenda are biological controls of pests to reduce the negative effects of pesticides on the environment, farm workers, and consumers through residues. Some food-science and nutrition research is also beginning to focus on the development of more precise tests to detect the presence of residues and other potentially harmful toxins on food products, on ways to reduce the risk of harmful

bacteria on food products (such as irradiation), and on the development of more environmentally benign packaging materials. Human nutrition research, traditionally carried on either by home economics departments or within the health sciences, rather than the agricultural sciences, continues to be driven by a medical model of health, which focuses more on identifying the negative health factors caused by overconsumption of certain food products. The impact on production research has been to try to develop new food products that contain less of the harmful agents. In some cases this means the production of new kinds of raw materials (such as canola, a new variety of rapeseed with less polyunsaturated fat, or leaner meats); but more frequently it means modifying how raw foods are processed and recombined into value-added products.

A more recent addition to this new research agenda is a concern for increasing the well-being of farm animals. This concern, which is supported by a large segment of the public, coincides with a growing antivivisection movement that is critical of the use of nonhuman animal models in research and testing. Animal-welfare legislation, which was designed to permit the continued use of animals models in research by raising the standards of humane use, does not apply to animals used in agricultural production. But two factors are moving the animal sciences slowly in the direction of more humane treatment of agricultural animals. One is the growing body of public sentiment against "factory animal farming" and the development of a significant vegetarian movement based on both moral and health considerations. The other is the increased use of farm animals as models in research and the development of new connections between the animal sciences and the health sciences.

All of these approaches share in the perpetuation of the industrial division of labor that still depends heavily on the technical fix, and that keeps in the hands of experts the knowledge needed to adequately conceptualize values. Conceptions of safety, health, animal welfare, and nutrition are controlled by the sciences that study them. In order to shift this control to the public domain, critics must show how these conceptions are contaminated by the institutional and organizational matrix in which the scientist works, and are fragmented by the disciplinary character of research. While a systems approach to understanding existing relationships between production, distribution, and human nutrition is essential if we are to understand the ethical consequences of changes in the system, it may be equally important to understand the ethical implications of perpetuating the existing division of labor within systems that require a high degree of technical expertise to maintain them. That this high level of technical knowledge is distributed among specialists places consumers at a considerable disadvantage in assessing both the adequacy of the existing system and the possibility of better alternatives.

As long as needed improvements in production and distribution systems—of food, health care, housing—are addressed in terms of specialists providing service for consumers or clientele, consumers will continue to feel the need to achieve greater control over those aspects of their lives about which they feel most helpless. Patched-up production and distribution systems that do not attend to this need will not end the debate between producers and consumer advocacy groups about the relative safety, cost, and security of the systems on which consumers have come to depend. Experts will continue to be in a position to conceptualize the values that consumers demand they provide. What is needed, some critics argue, is a reduction in the distance between production and consumption that will do a better job of empowering consumers. Research aimed at reducing this distance includes efforts to enlist the help of users in designing systems that do a better job of meeting the users' needs for technological mastery.

RICHARD P. HAYNES

Directly related to this entry are the entries FOOD POLICY; SUSTAINABLE DEVELOPMENT; ENVIRONMENTAL ETHICS, *the* OVERVIEW *and articles on* DEEP ECOLOGY, LAND ETHIC, *and* ECOFEMINISM; ENVIRONMENTAL POLICY AND LAW; BIOTECHNOLOGY; ANIMAL WELFARE AND RIGHTS, *article on* ANIMALS IN AGRICULTURE AND FACTORY FARMING; *and* POPULATION ETHICS, *section on* ELEMENTS OF POPULATIONS ETHICS, *article on* IS THERE A POPULATION PROBLEM? *For a further discussion of topics mentioned in this entry, see the entries* ENVIRONMENT AND RELIGION; FUTURE GENERATIONS, OBLIGATIONS TO; GENETIC ENGINEERING, *article on* ANIMALS AND PLANTS; HAZARDOUS WASTES AND TOXIC SUBSTANCES; JUSTICE; TECHNOLOGY, *articles on* PHILOSOPHY OF TECHNOLOGY, *and* TECHNOLOGY ASSESSMENT; UTILITY; *and* VALUE AND VALUATION. *Other relevant material may be found under the entries* INTERNATIONAL HEALTH; NATIVE AMERICAN RELIGIONS; PUBLIC HEALTH, *article on* DETERMINANTS OF PUBLIC HEALTH; *and* VETERINARY ETHICS. *See also the* APPENDIX (CODES, OATHS, AND DIRECTIVES RELATED TO BIOETHICS), SECTION VI: ETHICAL DIRECTIVES PERTAINING TO THE ENVIRONMENT.

Bibliography

AIKEN, WILLIAM. 1982. "The Goals of Agriculture." In vol. 1 of *Agriculture, Change, and Human Values: Proceedings of a Multidisciplinary Conference*, pp. 29–54. Edited by Richard P. Haynes and Ray Lanier. Gainesville: University of Florida Press.

ALTIERI, MIGUEL A. 1989. "Rethinking the Role of U.S. Development Assistance in Third World Agriculture." *Agriculture and Human Values* 6, no. 3:85–91.

BERRY, WENDELL. 1977. *The Unsettling of America: Culture and Agriculture*. San Francisco: Sierra Club.

"Biologically Based Methods of Pest Control: Contributions to a Sustainable Agriculture." 1988. *American Journal of Alternative Agriculture* 3, nos. 2–3 (special issue).

BLATZ, CHARLES V., ed. 1991. *Ethics and Agriculture. An Anthology on Current Issues in World Context.* Moscow: University of Idaho Press.

BORLAUG, NORMAN E. 1986. "Accelerating Agricultural Research and Production in the Third World: A Scientist's Viewpoint." *Agriculture and Human Values* 3, no. 3: 5–14.

BURKHARDT, JEFFREY. 1992. "On the Ethics of Technical Change: The Case of bST." *Technology in Society* 14, no. 2:221–243.

BUSCH, LAWRENCE. 1989. "Irony, Tragedy, and Temporality in Agricultural Systems; or, How Values and Systems Are Related." *Agriculture and Human Values* 6, no. 4:4–11.

BUSCH, LAWRENCE, and LACY, WILLIAM B. 1983. *Science, Agriculture, and the Politics of Research.* Boulder, Colo.: Westview.

CARSON, RACHEL. 1962. *Silent Spring.* Boston: Houghton Mifflin.

COCHRANE, WILLARD W. 1979. *The Development of American Agriculture: A Historical Analysis.* Minneapolis: University of Minnesota Press.

DAHLBERG, KENNETH A., ed. 1986. *New Directions for Agriculture and Agricultural Research: Neglected Dimensions and Emerging Alternatives.* Totowa, N.J.: Rowman & Allanheld.

DANBOM, DAVID B. 1979. *The Resisted Revolution: Urban America and the Industrialization of Agriculture, 1900–1930.* Ames: Iowa State University Press.

DOUGLASS, GORDON K. 1984. "The Meanings of Sustainability." In *Agricultural Sustainability in a Changing World Order*, pp. 3–29. Edited by Gordon K. Douglass. Boulder, Colo: Westview.

HARDING, T. SWANN. 1940. "Science and Agricultural Policy." In *Farmers in a Changing World.* The Yearbook of Agriculture. Washington, D.C.: U.S. Department of Agriculture.

HARWOOD, RICHARD R. 1992. "The Structure of Biological Diversity at the Agricultural, Environmental, and Social Interface (an Agricultural Perspective)." Keynote address, Diversity in Food, Agriculture, Environment and Health Conference. Michigan State University, June 4–7.

HIGHTOWER, JIM. 1973. *Hard Tomatoes, Hard Times.* Cambridge, Mass.: Schenkman.

HOFRICHTER, RICHARD, ed. 1993. *Toxic Struggles: The Theory and Practice of Environmental Justice.* Philadelphia: New Society.

HYAMS, EDWARD. 1976. *Soil and Civilization.* New York: Harper & Row.

KIRKENDALL, RICHARD S. 1987. "Up to Now: A History of American Agriculture from Jefferson to Revolution to Crisis." *Agriculture and Human Values* 4, no. 1:4–26.

KLOPPENBURG, JACK R., JR. 1988. *First the Seed: The Political Economy of Plant Biotechnology, 1492–2000.* New York: Cambridge University Press.

LAPPÉ, FRANCES MOORE; COLLINS, JOSEPH; and FOWLER, CARY. 1978. *Food First: Beyond the Myth of Scarcity.* Rev. ed. Boston: Ballantine.

LOCKERETZ, WILLIAM. 1988. "Commentary: Open Questions in Sustainable Agriculture." *American Journal of Alternative Agriculture* 3, no. 4:174–181.

MARCUS, ALAN I. 1985. *Agricultural Science and the Quest for Legitimacy: Farmers, Agricultural Colleges, and Experiment Stations, 1870–1890.* Ames: Iowa State University Press.

MERCHANT, CAROLYN. 1989. *Ecological Revolutions: Nature, Gender, and Science in New England.* Chapel Hill: University of North Carolina Press.

METCALF, ROBERT L. 1987. "Benefit/Risk Considerations in the Use of Pesticides." *Agriculture and Human Values* 4, no. 4:15–25.

MONTMARQUET, JAMES A. 1989. *The Idea of Agrarianism: From Hunter-Gatherer to Agrarian Radical in Western Culture.* Moscow: University of Idaho Press.

NATIONAL RESEARCH COUNCIL (NRC). BOARD ON AGRICULTURE. COMMITTEE ON THE ROLE OF ALTERNATIVE FARMING METHODS IN MODERN PRODUCTION AGRICULTURE. 1989. *Alternative Agriculture.* Washington, D.C.: National Academy Press.

PERKINS, JOHN H. 1982. *Insects, Experts and the Insecticide Crisis: The Quest for New Pest Management Strategies.* New York: Plenum.

SILVA, J. SOUSA. 1988. "The Contradictions of the Biorevolution for the Development of Agriculture in the Third World: Biotechnology and Capitalist Interest." *Agriculture and Human Values* 5, no. 3:61–70.

STRANGE, MARTY. 1988. *Family Farming: A New Economic Vision.* Lincoln: University of Nebraska Press.

WARREN, DENNIS M., ed. 1991. *Agriculture and Human Values* 8, nos. 1–2. Special issue, "Indigenous Agricultural Knowledge Systems and Development."

AIDS

I. Public-Health Issues
   Ronald Bayer
II. Health-Care and Research Issues
   Bernard Lo

I. PUBLIC-HEALTH ISSUES

At the conclusion of *Plagues and People,* a magisterial account of epidemics and their impact on history, William McNeill asserts, "Infectious disease, which antedates the emergence of humankind, will last as long as humanity itself and will surely remain, as it has been hitherto, one of the fundamental parameters and determinants of human history" (McNeill, 1976, p. 291). In the mid-1970s, this observation seemed overdrawn, especially in relation to economically advanced societies, where chronic diseases had displaced infectious threats to communal well-being. Yet just five years later, McNeill's comment seemed prescient.

In June 1981, the first cases of what would ultimately be called acquired immunodeficiency syndrome (AIDS) were reported by the U.S. Centers for Disease Control (CDC). Within three years of the first CDC report, human immunodeficiency virus (HIV), the viral agent responsible for AIDS, was identified. Although those who were infected could experience a long disease-free state—50 percent remained symptom-free for up to ten years—in the end the virus attacked the immune system, resulting in a series of ultimately fatal opportunistic disorders. By the beginning of the 1990s, it was estimated that approximately one million Americans and ten million people worldwide were infected. Found on every continent, AIDS had made its most stunning impact on Africa. Projections by the World Health Organization forecast an even grimmer picture. By the year 2000, forty million would be infected worldwide, and the level of infection in Asia would surpass that in Africa.

Although in the first years of the epidemic there was considerable uncertainty about how AIDS was transmitted, the epidemiological picture that emerged indicated that the new disease was transmitted in a limited number of ways: during sexual intercourse—both homosexual and heterosexual; by blood-to-blood contact, for example, transfusions; by the sharing of drug injection equipment; and by pregnant women to their fetuses. Both the distribution of AIDS cases in the population (its epidemiology) and the understanding of how the virus behaved soon made it clear that AIDS was not an airborne disease. HIV could not be transmitted by casual contact.

The epidemiology of AIDS not only gave those concerned with public health an understanding of the nature of the risks posed by the new disease, it also shaped the public response to the epidemic during its formative period. Because gay and bisexual men and intravenous drug users were among those first diagnosed with AIDS in the United States and western Europe, and because they accounted for the vast majority of the cases—in Africa, however, AIDS was in most instances heterosexually acquired—the disease was quickly identified as an affliction of the socially marginal and despised. The stigma associated with all sexually transmitted diseases was thus amplified. Indeed, AIDS became known in the popular culture as the "gay plague" (Sontag, 1990). That stigma extended to those who became infected through blood transfusions or as a result of treatment with clotting factor, and as a result of maternal infection, even though such individuals were viewed as "innocent victims."

Stigma, reinforced by popular fears about casual transmission, was responsible for a pattern of discrimination that soon developed. Parents sought to bar children with AIDS from the classroom; employers attempted to exclude the infected, whether symptomatic or not, from the workplace; landlords sought to evict the sick from their homes. And even within the health-care system, nurses, doctors, hospitals, and nursing homes sought to avoid contact with the "new lepers." Repeated here was a pattern of social response that was no less awful because it was predictable on the basis of the history of epidemic disease.

The emergence of AIDS represented an immediate challenge to public-health officials in the advanced industrial nations, which had begun to focus their attention on chronic diseases. When the term "epidemic" was used in industrial nations, it was typically applied in a figurative manner to describe the pattern of morbidity and mortality associated with poor diet and behaviors such as smoking. Against unhealthy eating habits and smoking, the conventional public-health strategies developed to confront viral and bacteriological conditions—case finding, public-health reporting, and control—seemed inappropriate. For both pragmatic and political reasons, public-health officials instead developed campaigns of mass education designed to encourage changes of behavior.

Confronted with AIDS, a disease at once viral and behavioral, those responsible for the public health had to determine whether the strategies historically used in the face of epidemic disease, or those interventions associated with the control of chronic conditions, would be more effective against the epidemic of HIV infection. Would the strategy of control, with its reliance on the police powers of the state, or the voluntaristic approach of mass persuasion prevail (Bayer, 1991a)?

In the United States, as well as in virtually all other liberal democracies, a determination was made to reject the traditional public-health approach to epidemic control—Sweden, with its strong paternalistic welfare state, was a striking exception (Kirp and Bayer, 1992). AIDS was typically transmitted in intimate settings between consenting adults. An incurable disease, it affected marginalized populations with deeply rooted fears of the state and its agencies. Traditional public-health strategies of control would entail intrusions on privacy and create antagonism among those whose cooperation was required to halt the spread of HIV infection. Since radical modifications in sexual and drug-using behaviors—behaviors that were the source of pleasure—were essential, it would be necessary to create a social context con-

ducive to change. Persuasion rather than coercion was deemed the most effective approach to this daunting challenge. Respect for privacy and the pragmatics of mass behavioral change required a voluntarist approach to AIDS. The determination to reject traditional public-health measures, to embrace a posture of "HIV exceptionalism," was endorsed by public-health officials, gay leaders, proponents of civil liberties, and their generally liberal political allies (Bayer, 1991b).

AIDS education

The controversial centerpiece of the voluntarist approach to AIDS was education. What was to be the content of the education campaign? Those committed to "traditional" moral values believed that the AIDS epidemic was the result of sexual license and a social climate that tolerated drug use. The antidote was a message of conventional sexual morality: abstinence among the unmarried, fidelity within heterosexual marriage, refraining from drug use. Against this perspective, which had strong support among some political conservatives and in the highest councils of the Reagan administration, public-health officials urged a strategy of pragmatism (Shilts, 1987). It was not sexual behavior per se that increased the risk of HIV transmission, they argued, but unprotected sexual behavior. Thus they sought to promote the use of condoms among all sexually active persons. Recognizing the difficulty of discouraging drug use among the addicted, they urged drug injectors not to share syringes and needles.

With homosexual behavior illegal in half the American states—a situation that did not prevail in other liberal democracies—and drug use illicit in all the states, public-health officials were challenged repeatedly by those who interpreted this pragmatic strategy as an endorsement of illegal and immoral behaviors. Messages characterized by great timidity were often the result. Nevertheless, the virulence of the AIDS epidemic and effective leadership by public-health officials, including Surgeon General C. Everett Koop, made possible campaigns for condom use hardly imaginable in the period before the epidemic. The bluntest and most imaginative educational campaigns were undertaken by community-based gay organizations, often with public funding.

One of the most complex ethical questions posed by the educational effort to prevent the spread of HIV infection centered on what to tell infected women of childbearing age. Should they be discouraged from becoming pregnant? If pregnant, should they be encouraged to seek abortion (Arras, 1991)? HIV is transmitted from mother to fetus in 20 to 30 percent of pregnancies. From the perspective of the infected woman, the chance of having a healthy child is thus 70 to 80 percent. From the perspective of those concerned with preventing the transmission of HIV, however, the collective consequence of infected women choosing to become mothers could be many thousands of infected babies (Bayer, 1990).

When the CDC as well as many state health departments adopted a position urging infected women to postpone pregnancy, it provoked a storm of controversy. Critics charged that the recommendation to postpone pregnancy represented a radical departure from the norm of nondirective counseling that had been the ethical standard in reproductive counseling more generally. That the vast majority of infected women were poor and African-American or Hispanic only fueled the sense of outrage on the part of those who viewed the effort to discourage pregnancy as a reflection of the legacy of racism and eugenics in America.

Testing and screening for HIV infection

From 1985, when the HIV antibody test was first developed, it became the focus of controversy. The test was first intended to screen the blood supply in order to prevent the transmission of infection to transfusion recipients and those dependent upon clotting factor. It immediately became apparent that it could be used to identify those who were asymptomatic but could nevertheless transmit HIV during sexual relations, childbearing, or intravenous drug use. To those who believed such identification could play a crucial role in the strategy of prevention, the test represented an opportunity. To those who believed that identification would be used as a basis for discrimination in employment, insurance, housing, access to health care, and the right to travel, the test was viewed as a threat. Furthermore, since counseling and education about the importance of the modification of sexual and drug-use behavior were crucial regardless of one's HIV status, the test was characterized by opponents as unnecessary from the perspective of public health.

These controversies pitted gay rights advocates, proponents of civil liberties and privacy, and their political allies against public-health officials who wanted to foster widespread voluntary testing and some archconservatives who proposed extensive mandatory testing on a traditional public-health model. From among these disparate viewpoints, a consensus emerged (Bayer et al., 1986). Testing was to be undertaken only after individuals gave their specific informed consent. As part of the consent process, individuals were to be informed of the risks and benefits of testing. After testing, extensive counseling was to be given to all who were tested. The extraordinary array of protections built into this process and codified in a number of states as a matter of law was one of the hallmarks of the extent to which HIV was to

be treated differently from other sexually transmitted and communicable diseases. Indeed, the requirement of specific informed consent set the HIV test apart from other blood tests performed as part of diagnostic work in clinical practice.

To encourage individuals to come forward for HIV testing, public-health officials placed great stress on the importance of protecting the confidentiality of the results. Immediately after the test became available, public-health officials in locales with large numbers of AIDS cases sought to encourage testing through the creation of testing sites where individuals could be screened anonymously—they did not provide their names and were identified only by a number.

While the principle of voluntary testing was endorsed by public-health officials, federal authorities responsive to conservative political pressure moved quickly to require HIV tests of all military recruits, Job Corps applicants, and those seeking to enter the foreign service. Those who were infected were to be excluded. Mandatory testing was also initiated in federal prisons. Finally, HIV testing became a condition for immigration into the United States.

For many clinicians, requiring specific informed consent intruded on sound diagnostic practice by creating barriers to the routine testing of those deemed by the physician to be at risk. It also represented a barrier to detecting infection in patients who could be a source of danger in case of accidents involving needle sticks or surgical mishaps. Surreptitious testing—without consent—was reported in a number of hospitals. Physicians pressed for a looser definition of consent, one that would permit routine testing on the presumption of consent. Such pressure intensified as the prospects improved for clinical intervention during the asymptomatic phase of HIV infection.

Nowhere was the pressure for unconsented testing more obvious than in the context of pediatrics (Institute of Medicine, 1991). Newborn testing had long been proposed by some pediatricians, who argued that routine testing of neonates for a host of conditions—for example, PKU—was widely viewed as good public-health practice and ethically acceptable. But until the end of the 1980s, it was possible to resist such proposals for two reasons. First, antibody testing was a poor diagnostic strategy in newborns, since all babies born to infected mothers carried maternal antibodies for up to eighteen months, regardless of whether they were truly infected. Thus, the false-positive rate was 70–80 percent. Second, there was no clinical advantage to identifying asymptomatic newborns, since there was then no therapeutic intervention that could be prescribed to all children who tested positive. Under these circumstances mandatory newborn testing would achieve little for the child. It would, on the other hand, represent mandatory surrogate screening of their mothers. As the importance of early presymptomatic treatment of infants became clear in the early 1990s, and as the capacity to identify infection improved, the case for treating HIV more like PKU became stronger.

In the proposals both for newborn testing and for more routine screening of adults, a move away from the HIV exceptionalism of the epidemic's formative decade could be seen.

Reporting

The shift toward a more traditional public-health practice also became apparent in terms of reporting the names of those with HIV infection to public-health registries. Early in the epidemic AIDS became reportable to all state health departments. Despite concern about confidentiality, this move, which required physicians and hospitals to report the names and addresses of AIDS patients—as they were required to report the names of those diagnosed with a host of other infectious conditions—provoked little controversy. Support for AIDS case reporting reflected the widespread recognition that the public-health authorities needed such information to assist in the characterization of the epidemic's course. The picture was very different with regard to asymptomatic HIV infection. Soon after the initiation of antibody testing, some public-health officials, typically those from states with few AIDS cases, called for the extension of reporting to HIV positives. These proposals provoked a storm of controversy. It was argued that such reporting would represent a profound violation of privacy and discourage individuals from coming forward for voluntary testing. The latter argument persuaded public-health officials in states with large AIDS caseloads to resist the extension of AIDS reporting to HIV. HIV became reportable in only a handful of states with few cases.

By the beginning of the 1990s, the alliance that had resisted HIV reporting had been fractured. The American Medical Association (AMA), the CDC, and increasing numbers of public-health officials had begun to press for HIV reporting. Three arguments for such a move were made. First, whatever foundation for distinguishing between HIV and AIDS had existed early in the epidemic no longer existed. Early clinical intervention in the asymptomatic state had shifted the focus of attention from full-blown AIDS to the spectrum of HIV disease. Second, it was claimed that public-health officials needed to know who had HIV infection in order to assure adequate clinical follow-up, more important in the early 1990s, when large numbers of poor African-American and Hispanic men and women were being diagnosed with HIV. Third, only with HIV reporting would it be possible to develop aggressive partner noti-

fication programs designed to reach individuals exposed to those with HIV infection. By the early 1990s, about half the states had adopted some form of HIV reporting.

Partner notification

In programs designed to treat and control sexually transmitted diseases (STDs), contact tracing has played a central role for more than five decades. Patients diagnosed with STD are urged to reveal the names of their sexual partners so that they may be examined and, if infected, treated. Contact tracing thus serves two functions: case finding and interrupting the chain of transmission. To encourage individuals to provide the names of their partners, a guarantee of absolute anonymity is provided: those who are notified are never informed of the identity of the person who provided their name. In this way, contact tracing has always been voluntary and has always rested on the foundation of confidentiality.

In the early years of the AIDS epidemic, contact tracing programs designed to reach sexual partners who unknowingly may have been placed at risk were greeted with protest. Despite the long history of such programs for STDs, proposals to initiate them were deemed coercive. They were viewed as an intrusion on the privacy of the notified partner. In the absence of a therapy for HIV infection, the information provided by the public-health official was considered an unwelcome burden (Bayer and Toomey, 1992).

By the end of the first decade of the AIDS epidemic, most of the principled opposition to contact tracing had vanished, and public-health departments began to devote greater resources to such programs.

The issues raised by contact tracing are fundamentally different from those posed to the physician faced with an infected patient who makes clear the intention not to inform sexual partners of that fact. Does the duty to protect confidentiality take precedence over the obligation to protect unsuspecting partners? (Dickens, 1990). If a duty to protect exists, it requires that the clinician act despite the preferences of the patient. It may require that the identity of the threatening patient be revealed to the endangered party. Thus, the duty to warn is in all fundamental respects different from voluntary contact tracing.

As clinicians and public-health officials confronted this issue, they were faced with a dilemma that was starkly presented in the landmark *Tarasoff* case, in which the California Supreme Court held that a psychotherapist had a duty to protect or warn the potential victims of a violent patient. If it became known that under some circumstances clinicians would breach confidentiality, would this inhibit patient candor? Would such a reduction in candor, if it occurred, deprive clinicians of the capacity to affect patients' behavior? In short, might the duty to warn ultimately subvert the very good it was de-signed to achieve—enhanced public safety?

Faced with this complex situation in the context of the AIDS epidemic, many state legislatures opted to grant physicians a "privilege to disclose," thus freeing them from Tarasoff-like liability if they did not warn, as well as from liability for breaching confidentiality if they did warn. In a striking reflection of the concerns about privacy provoked by the AIDS epidemic, a number of states have prohibited physicians who do warn third par-ties from revealing the patient's identity to those being notified.

Criminal law and public health law

In the long history of epidemic control, quarantines have played a significant role, though the efficacy of such measures has remained a matter of some contro-versy (Musto, 1988). With the changing pattern of mor-bidity in advanced industrial nations and the availability of effective therapies, the use of quarantine all but vanished in the pre-AIDS era. Because AIDS was not casually transmitted, and because HIV transmission typ-ically involved activities between consenting adults, only those utterly without concern for individual rights have even suggested that all HIV-infected persons be quarantined. Only Cuba has taken such a drastic mea-sure. There, public-health officials argue that since it is impossible to know which individuals will behave re-sponsibly, the communal health requires that all HIV-infected persons be treated as potentially dangerous (Bayer and Healton, 1989). Quarantine in the context of AIDS is thus equivalent to preventive detention.

The question of how to respond to those individuals who know themselves to be infected but who continue to place unsuspecting partners at risk is more complex (Gostin, 1989). In many ways, this was an issue that took on greater salience in the context of heterosexual transmission of HIV, when infected persons failed to in-form their unsuspecting partners of their status, or when men refused to use condoms when asked to do so.

Two approaches to this matter have been consid-ered; one based on the use of public-health law, the other on the use of the criminal law (Field and Sullivan, 1987). From the perspective of the former, an individual who has demonstrated by past acts an unwillingness to behave in a sexually responsible way could be subject to public-health control in order to prevent future harm. As an alternative, some have proposed that individuals who have willfully or recklessly exposed their unsuspect-ing partners to the risk of HIV infection be subject to criminal sanctions.

As the first decade of the AIDS epidemic drew to a close, there had been only a few instances in the United States of efforts to control the behavior of HIV-infected individuals through the use of the public-health law, most commonly by the issuance of cease-and-desist or-ders to those defined as "recalcitrants." More common, although relatively rare, has been the use of the criminal law to punish individuals for such behavior. But in either case, such interventions have been widely viewed as at best marginal to the overall strategy of AIDS pre-vention focused on mass behavioral change through mass persuasion and individual counseling.

From privacy to equity

In the epidemic's first years the central debates focused on questions of the right to privacy and its limits. As the decade progressed, increasing attention was given to as-suring access to care for those in need, both the symp-tomatic and those infected but symptom-free. Not only was the number of individuals large, but the proportion of those who were poor, African-American, and Latino was increasing. Who would pay for such care? Would the poor be deprived of potentially life-prolonging but ex-pensive treatments? Before these issues, early concern about the refusal of some health-care workers to treat AIDS patients (Zuger, 1991) and the discriminatory practices of many private insurers paled (Daniels, 1990). At stake was the fundamental issue of whether Ameri-ca's inequitable health-care system could or would help those with AIDS. As AIDS activists demanded that in-dividuals with HIV be cared for regardless of cost, it was inevitable that questions would be raised about the eq-uity and viability of disease-specific solutions to the cri-sis in American health care.

AIDS and the Third World

This article has focused on issues that have been of cen-tral concern to economically advanced democratic na-tions and, more specifically, to the United States. Yet as the second decade of the AIDS epidemic commences, it is clear that the trauma will be most severe in the Third World. There the incidence of infection remains high, but therapeutic agents now under development in the economically advanced countries move further and fur-ther out of reach. The solidarity born of a common viral threat in the early 1980s, when little could be done for the sick, whether in the United States or Africa, has been shattered. Increasingly we will witness the phe-nomenon of one virus but many epidemic patterns of AIDS. The fundamental moral question posed by this challenge centers on the nature and the extent of the obligations of the rich nations to those that are poor, not only to provide therapies and a vaccine, if one were to become available, but also to make available the re-sources to assist in the efforts to prevent the further spread of infection.

RONALD BAYER

Directly related to this article is the companion article in this entry: HEALTH-CARE AND RESEARCH ISSUES. *Also directly related is the entry* LIFESTYLES AND PUBLIC HEALTH. *For a further discussion of topics mentioned in this article, see the entries* BEHAVIOR CONTROL; BLOOD TRANSFUSION; CONFIDENTIALITY; EPIDEMICS; FREEDOM AND COERCION; HEALTH PROMOTION AND HEALTH EDUCATION; HEALTH SCREENING AND TESTING IN THE PUBLIC-HEALTH CONTEXT; HOMOSEXUALITY; INFANTS, *article on* MEDICAL ASPECTS AND ISSUES IN THE CARE OF INFANTS; INFORMATION DISCLOSURE; INFORMED CONSENT, *articles on* CLINICAL ASPECTS OF CONSENT IN HEALTH CARE, *and* LEGAL AND ETHICAL ISSUES OF CONSENT IN HEALTH CARE (*with its* POSTSCRIPT); PRIVACY IN HEALTH CARE; PRIVILEGED COMMUNICATIONS; *and* SEXUALITY IN SOCIETY. *Other relevant material may be found under the entries* LAW AND MORALITY; OCCUPATIONAL SAFETY AND HEALTH; *and* PUBLIC HEALTH, *articles on* DETERMINANTS OF PUBLIC HEALTH, *and* PHILOSOPHY OF PUBLIC HEALTH.

Bibliography

ARRAS, JOHN D. 1991. "HIV and Childbearing. 2. AIDS and the Reproductive Decisions: Having Children in Fear and Trembling." *Milbank Quarterly* 68, no. 3:353–382.

BAYER, RONALD. 1990. "AIDS and the Future of Reproductive Freedom." *Milbank Quarterly* 68 (supp. 2):179–204.

———. 1991a. *Private Acts, Social Consequences: AIDS and the Politics of Public Health.* New Brunswick, N.J.: Rutgers University Press.

———. 1991b. "Public Health Policy and the AIDS Epidemic: An End to HIV Exceptionalism?" *New England Journal of Medicine* 324, no. 21:1500–1504.

BAYER, RONALD, and HEALTON, CHERYL. 1989. "Controlling AIDS in Cuba: The Logic of Quarantine." *New England Journal of Medicine* 320, no. 15:1022–1024.

BAYER, RONALD; LEVINE, CAROL; and WOLF, SUSAN M. 1986. "HIV Antibody Screening: An Ethical Framework for Evaluating Proposed Programs." *Journal of the American Medical Association* 256, no. 13:1768–1774.

BAYER, RONALD, and TOOMEY, KATHLEEN E. 1992. "HIV Prevention and the Two Faces of Partner Notification." *American Journal of Public Health* 82, no. 8:1158–1164.

DANIELS, NORMAN. 1990. "Insurability and the HIV Epidemic: Ethical Issues in Underwriting." *Milbank Quarterly* 68, no. 4:497–526.

DICKENS, BERNARD M. 1990. "Confidentiality and the Duty to Warn." In *AIDS and the Health Care System,* pp. 98–112. Edited by Lawrence O. Gostin. New Haven, Conn.: Yale University Press.

FIELD, MARTHA A., and SULLIVAN, KATHLEEN M. 1987. "AIDS and the Criminal Law." *Law, Medicine and Health Care* 15, nos. 1–2:46–60.

GOSTIN, LAWRENCE O. 1989. "The Politics of AIDS: Compulsory State Powers, Public Health and Civil Liberties." *Ohio State Law Journal* 49, no. 4:1017–1058.

INSTITUTE OF MEDICINE. COMMITTEE ON PRENATAL AND NEWBORN SCREENING FOR HIV INFECTION. 1990. *HIV Screening of Pregnant Women and Newborns.* Edited by Leslie M. Hardy. Washington, D.C.: National Academy Press.

KIRP, DAVID L., and BAYER, RONALD, eds. 1992. *AIDS in the Industrialized Democracies: Passions, Politics and Policies.* New Brunswick, N.J.: Rutgers University Press.

LEVINE, CAROL. 1991. "AIDS and the Ethics of Human Subjects Research." In *AIDS and Ethics,* pp. 77–104. Edited by Frederic G. Reamer. New York: Columbia University Press.

McNEILL, WILLIAM H. 1976. *Plagues and Peoples.* Garden City, N.Y.: Anchor.

MUSTO, DAVID. 1988. "Quarantine and the Problem of AIDS." In *AIDS: The Burdens of History,* pp. 67–86. Edited by Elizabeth Fee and Daniel M. Fox. Berkeley: University of California Press.

SHILTS, RANDY. 1987. *And the Band Played On: Politics, People, and the AIDS Epidemic.* New York: St. Martin's Press.

SONTAG, SUSAN. 1990. *Illness as Metaphor; and, AIDS and Its Metaphors.* New York: Doubleday.

ZUGER, ABIGAIL. 1991. "AIDS and the Obligations of Health Care Professionals." In *AIDS and Ethics,* pp. 215–239. Edited by Frederic G. Reamer. New York: Columbia University Press.

II. HEALTH-CARE AND RESEARCH ISSUES

This article discusses the duty of health-care workers to treat persons with human immunodeficiency virus (HIV) infection, the risk to patients from health-care workers infected with HIV, insurance coverage for HIV infection, and clinical research regarding HIV infection. HIV infection is a chronic illness that progresses from asymptomatic infection to acquired immunodeficiency syndrome (AIDS), which is defined by opportunistic infections and cancers and end-stage debilitating conditions, such as dementia and a wasting syndrome characterized by severe weight loss.

Duty to treat persons with HIV infection

Health-care workers are most likely to contract HIV infection if they injure themselves with a needle or other sharp instrument contaminated with the blood of a patient who is HIV-positive. Needlesticks are frequent and, fearing for their own safety, many physicians are reluctant to care for HIV-infected patients. The self-interest of health-care workers to avoid occupational HIV infection, however, may conflict with their professional duty and the need such patients have for medical care.

The risk of occupational HIV infection. The risk of occupational HIV infection is small but not zero (Lo and Steinbrook, 1992). The risk of contracting HIV after a single needle-stick exposure to the blood of a seropositive patient is estimated to be 0.3 percent. The cumulative risk of occupational HIV infection depends on the health-care worker's specialty. Surgeons and operating room staff are at highest risk for occupational HIV infection; they sustain skin injuries in 1.7 percent to 6.9 percent of operations (Gerberding et al., 1990).

The magnitude of risk is only one component of a person's perception of risk. People regard familiar and voluntary risks as more acceptable than unfamiliar, involuntary, and uncertain risks, even if the latter are statistically far less likely. The risk of occupational HIV infection seems especially ominous since the progression of HIV is fatal and the virus can be transmitted to loved ones. Physicians do not have complete control over the risk because percutaneous exposure can occur despite precautions.

Strategies for minimizing occupational HIV infection.   Threatened by a currently incurable and fatal illness, health-care workers may respond in several ways. Some advocate testing all hospitalized or surgical patients for HIV infection because it would allow health-care workers to take precautions with patients identified as seropositive. This strategy, however, has several drawbacks: results are not available in emergencies, and HIV antibody tests may be falsely negative, particularly during the early stages of the infection. In addition, mandatory testing of hospitalized or surgical patients is problematic for ethical and political reasons discussed below.

The Centers for Disease Control and Prevention (CDC) recommends universal precautions such as gloves, masks, goggles, and gowns whenever there is a risk that a health-care worker will be exposed to a patient's body fluids (CDC, 1988). Health-care workers should always use infection control procedures. However, universal precautions have some drawbacks. In areas with a low prevalence of HIV and hepatitis, the cost of supplies may be prohibitive compared with the number of cases of HIV their use would prevent. Caregivers find it difficult to be equally vigilant with all patients. Most important, universal precautions do not eliminate the risk of occupational HIV infection: gowns and gloves, even double gloves, do not protect against needlesticks and scalpel cuts.

The most effective way for physicians to reduce their risk of occupational HIV infection is not to care for persons who are infected with or at risk for HIV. Physicians commonly offer several reasons to justify their refusal to care for HIV-infected persons. First, in the absence of an established doctor-patient relationship or contractual obligations, physicians have no legal obligation to care for particular patients (Annas, 1988). The legal right to decline to care for individuals, however, is limited in many important ways, for example, in

emergency situations. Employment contracts with hospitals or health maintenance organizations may oblige physicians to care for all qualified persons who seek treatment. Antidiscrimination laws may also limit the physician's right to decline care for individuals on the basis of disability or illness.

Second, some physicians claim that they should not care for HIV-infected individuals because they lack the necessary expertise. However, caring for patients who are asymptomatic or who have common opportunistic infections are within the scope of expertise of primary-care physicians. In addition, physicians who completed their training before the HIV epidemic began cannot legitimately claim their lack of knowledge as justification for not treating persons with HIV infection. After completing formal training, physicians have a professional obligation to update their knowledge and skills.

Third, some physicians argue that the risks outweigh their duty to treat patients. Being a health-care professional is an inescapable mixture of self-interest and altruism. Financial remuneration, lifestyle, prestige, and personal satisfaction are all factors in career decisions. Virtually all health-care workers also regard personal safety as a pertinent consideration.

Professional societies such as the American College of Physicians have condemned refusals to care for HIV-positive patients (Health and Public Policy Committee, 1988). One physician-philosopher has written, "To refuse to care for AIDS patients, even if the danger were much greater than it actually is, is to abnegate what is essential to being a physician. The physician is no more free to flee from danger in the performance of his or her duties than the fireman, the policeman, or the soldier" (Pellegrino, 1987, p. 1939). Some writers argue that there is a binding precedent for the profession. Throughout history many physicians have provided care to patients during epidemics, even at great personal risk.

Most clinical care does not involve invasive procedures and therefore presents little risk of occupational HIV infection. Physicians should be willing to provide such care as needed. With respect to invasive procedures, how can the patient's need for medical care and the risk to health-care workers be balanced? Health-care workers should be willing to perform invasive procedures in spite of the risk of contracting HIV infection, if the medical benefit to the patient is clearly established, highly probable, and substantial. For example, obstetricians should care for seropositive women, including performing emergency cesarean sections. However, there are some justified exceptions to the physician's moral obligation to treat. If the benefits of intervention for the patient are unproved, uncertain, or marginal, physician safety should be given more weight in management decisions.

HIV-infected health care professionals

In 1990, publicity concerning Kimberly Bergalis, a twenty-three-year-old woman who contracted HIV infection during dental care, caused public alarm about the risk of HIV infection from health-care workers. The patient asserted that she should have been told about the dentist's HIV status: "I'm not asking that we be able to live in a risk-free world. I want people to be able to choose their risks. I didn't have a choice to walk out of the office and seek another dentist" (Lo and Steinbrook, 1992, p. 1100). The Bergalis case posed several questions: What risk do HIV-positive health-care workers present to patients? Do patients have a right to know if their health-care workers are HIV infected? Should the practice of HIV-infected health-care workers be restricted?

The risk of transmitting HIV to patients. The CDC has estimated the risk that a patient will contract HIV from a seropositive surgeon during an operation to be between 1 in 42,000 and 1 in 420,000 (Lo and Steinbrook, 1992). This risk is comparable with the risk of HIV infection after the transfusion of screened blood and less than the risk of mortality due to general anesthesia. As of early 1994, such transmission of HIV to patients has been documented only in the six cases traced to the same dentist who infected Kimberly Bergalis.

The public perceives the risk of contracting HIV infection from health-care workers as much greater than the data would suggest. This risk seems especially ominous, for the reasons previously discussed. In addition, patients have no control over the risk if they do not know that a health-care worker is infected. In contrast, if informed that a surgeon is seropositive, patients can completely avoid the risk by switching care to a seronegative physician. Patients feel betrayed if a physician or dentist places them at any risk beyond that caused by their illness. Furthermore, recalling the Bergalis case, the public distrusts reassurances that patients are unlikely to contract HIV in health-care settings. Dramatic cases, however, may distort policymaking. In general, such cases lead people to overestimate the frequency of unusual events, and to downplay the long-term and indirect consequences of policies.

Strong arguments can be made for restricting the clinical activities of certain HIV-infected health-care workers (Lo and Steinbrook, 1992). The ethical principle of nonmaleficence requires that physicians avoid harming their patients. Physicians also have a duty to act in the best interests of their patients, even if they harm their own interests in the process.

The principle of respect for patient autonomy requires physicians to obtain informed consent for procedures. Physicians must generally disclose to patients information that a reasonable person would find material to the decision at hand. Even a very small risk may need to be disclosed if it is serious or if patients would find it material. Most patients would want to know that their surgeon is infected with HIV. While some patients might proceed with surgery, many would seek another surgeon or decline surgery.

Cogent arguments can also be made against broad restrictions on the clinical activities of HIV-infected health-care workers (Lo and Steinbrook, 1992). Health-care workers, like other individuals, have a right to privacy, and seropositive health-care workers should be protected from discrimination. Several HIV-infected health-care workers have been excluded from practice, even though they did not perform invasive procedures and were qualified to work.

Physicians and public health officials contend that the risk that patients will contract HIV infection is too low to justify restrictions on the work and the livelihood of seropositive health-care workers who follow infection-control precautions. Furthermore, a policy of testing health-care workers for HIV and restricting the clinical work of those who are seropositive would be counterproductive. Thus, to reduce their own risk and protect their livelihood, health-care workers might decide to avoid patients who are seropositive or who are suspected of being so. Public hospitals, which care for large numbers of HIV-infected patients, might find it impossible to recruit workers.

Justice also requires that the resources devoted to reducing the risk of nosocomial infection (an infection acquired during hospitalization) be proportionate to the expected benefits. The cost of testing all health-care workers in the United States once for HIV infection is projected to be $250 million. It would cost an estimated $50 million to prevent a single case of HIV infection (U.S. National Commission, 1992). Opponents of testing health-care workers for HIV contend that it would only divert attention and finances from combating the predominant modes of transmission: unprotected sexual intercourse and injection drug use.

Some argue that it is unfair to require health-care workers to know and disclose their HIV-antibody status to patients without allowing such workers the protection of identifying their seropositive patients. For example, the American Medical Association (AMA) advocated relaxing the requirements for informed consent for HIV-antibody testing, making HIV testing part of a routine lab workup. But such testing is not just a "routine" laboratory test because patients identified as seropositive may face subtle or overt discrimination.

Federal responses to HIV-infected health-care workers have struggled to accommodate sharply divergent interests. In July 1991, the CDC recommended restrictions on HIV-infected health-care workers who perform certain types of "exposure-prone" invasive procedures on patients (CDC, 1991). The CDC recommended voluntary HIV testing of such health-care workers, but rejected mandatory HIV testing. HIV-infected health-care workers should perform exposure-prone invasive procedures only if an expert review panel so advises and if they inform patients that they are seropositive. The CDC posed no restrictions on the clinical activities of seropositive health-care workers who do not perform exposure-prone invasive procedures, provided they comply with infection–control precautions.

The CDC guidelines provoked strong and conflicting responses (Lo and Steinbrook, 1992). Congress required states to adopt the CDC recommendations or their equivalent as a condition of receiving federal Medicare and Medicaid funds. Professional groups strongly opposed the CDC guidelines and none was willing to draw up a list of exposure-prone invasive procedures. According to the American College of Surgeons, such a list would be "irrelevant and counterproductive" because such procedures "cannot be defined in any scientific or rational way" (Lo and Steinbrook, 1992, p. 1102).

In December 1991, faced with strong opposition from health-care professionals, the CDC withdrew its plan to compile a list of exposure-prone invasive procedures. Instead, the CDC recommended that health-care workers who perform "invasive surgical, dental, or obstetric procedures" know their HIV-antibody status (Lo and Steinbrook, 1992). An expert review panel should decide on an individual basis which invasive procedures a seropositive health-care worker may or may not perform and when patients must be told that a health-care worker is infected. The focus shifted from the nature of the procedure to "the skill and technique of the individual infected health care worker and the health care worker's physical condition" (Lo and Steinbrook, 1992, p. 1102). Policies for assessing HIV-positive health-care workers on a case-by-case basis, taking into account their technique, skill, and possible impairment, are considered in compliance with CDC recommendations.

Financial barriers to health care

Financial barriers prevent many persons with HIV infection from receiving optimal medical care. The lifetime cost of care for a person with HIV infection is $119,000, based on 1991 data on charges (Hellinger, 1993).

Coverage of HIV infection by self-insured employers. Employers and insurers may seek to control the soaring cost of health insurance by limiting coverage for HIV infection. John McGann, an employee of a small company, was diagnosed with AIDS and filed a claim under the company's group medical plan. The policy provided lifetime medical benefits of $1 million. Several months later, the company became self-insured and limited benefits for HIV-related illnesses to $5,000, while maintaining coverage for other illnesses. McGann sued, alleging discrimination. In rejecting his suit, an appeals court declared that employers have the "freedom to amend or eliminate employee benefits" in health insurance (*McGann* v. *H & H Music Company*, 1990). The court allowed self-insured employers to reduce or eliminate benefits for any particular illness, even if all other medical conditions are covered.

For employees and patients, the *McGann* ruling, while legally unimpeachable, is deeply disturbing. When people purchase health insurance their purpose is to gain access to medically needed health care. This goal is negated if self-insured employers can restrict benefits after illness strikes and a claim is filed. To some critics, the *McGann* case suggests that the current system of U.S. health insurance is untenable.

Coverage of HIV infection by third-party insurers. Virtually all commercial insurers either deny coverage to individual applicants with HIV infection, or offer more expensive or more limited coverage. Under the U.S. system for health insurance, people who know that they are at high risk for illness try to purchase more coverage, while those who know they are at low risk purchase less coverage. Furthermore, those who know they are at high risk for illness try to take advantage of insurance companies that offer the most favorable rates and coverage. To ensure actuarial accuracy, insurers insist on setting higher rates for those with serious illness. Furthermore, to avoid expensive claims, insurers seek to exclude persons with high-cost conditions such as HIV infection. In a competitive market, companies that do not exclude high-risk persons will be at a disadvantage because they will enroll a disproportionately large number of high-risk applicants.

Critics of such underwriting policies, however, assert that actuarial accuracy must not be confused with moral fairness (Daniels, 1990). In order to avoid violating important social values, society in fact prohibits insurers from using certain factors in setting rates. For example, overt racial discrimination is considered so objectionable that race is not a morally acceptable variable in underwriting, even though it helps to estimate future expenditures on claims.

Shifting to public funds. Ultimately, employers' and insurers' reluctance to insure persons with HIV infection increases the burden on the public sector to provide care through the Medicaid program and at public hospitals. Over one half of hospitalizations for persons with AIDS are financed by Medicaid. The proportion of costs covered by private insurance has decreased during the course of the epidemic (Green and Arno, 1990). Several factors explain this trend. The diagnosis of AIDS makes most persons presumptively eligible for Medicaid. As their disease progresses, previously employed persons cease working and lose their health insurance.

This shift to Medicaid funding causes several problems. Because of low reimbursement levels, many physicians do not accept Medicaid patients. Thus, patients who lose private insurance may also lose access to care. As a result, emergency departments and public hospitals bear a greater burden of care. In addition, because of large budget deficits, many states and counties are finding it increasingly difficult to pay for such indigent care.

The definition of AIDS.   Earlier definitions of AIDS were criticized because the list of indicator diseases, such as opportunistic infections and cancers, did not include some major clinical syndromes, particularly in women. In January 1993, the CDC expanded the list of indicator diseases. During that year, the number of persons classified as having AIDS more than doubled under the new definition, with women, blacks, and injection drug users especially likely to be newly classified as persons with AIDS (CDC, 1994a).

The definition of AIDS has great impact on access to health care and social services. Public funds may be allocated according to the number of AIDS cases in a region. Under the older definition, persons with AIDS were eligible for extended benefits, such as Medicaid, disability, and community-based social services. It is not clear whether such benefits will be extended to persons who are labeled as having AIDS under the new CDC definition.

Clinical research in HIV infection

Compound Q, a drug extracted from Chinese cucumber roots, was found in 1989 to have a strong activity against HIV in the laboratory and was touted as a therapeutic breakthrough. Frustrated by the slow pace of research conducted by the medical establishment, Project Inform, an HIV-activist group, organized its own clinical trials to evaluate Compound Q. Supplies of the drug were smuggled into the United States from China. Several participants in this underground study developed serious side effects, including seizures, coma, and death. As of May 1994, Compound Q had not been shown to be clinically effective, but its story dramatized how the hope for a cure may conflict with the need to evaluate new drugs rigorously (Lo, 1992).

Two types of errors can be made regarding unproven new therapies. On the one hand, delaying the approval of an effective new drug harms patients. On the other hand, releasing a drug that is later shown to be ineffective or unsafe is also harmful. Persons with HIV infection and their advocates may weigh these errors differently than do scientists or governmental officials.

Activists and the scope of the HIV epidemic have forced society in general, and scientists in particular, to reconsider fundamental questions about clinical trials of promising new therapies (Lo, 1992).

First, what is the goal of the clinical trial? To most scientists and to the U.S. Food and Drug Administration (FDA), the goal is to determine the safety and effectiveness of new drugs. Historically, clinical research has been considered dangerous for subjects. Currently, however, many patients consider clinical trials beneficial rather than risky, because they offer promising new treatments, closer medical follow-up, and more sophisticated laboratory monitoring than does standard care (Levine et al., 1991). Participants motivated by the goal of obtaining promising new drugs may feel no obligation to follow the protocol. If they do not receive the active drug, they may drop out of the study or obtain the drug outside the clinical trial. Similarly, subjects may take other drugs not on the protocol. Such deviations from protocol undermine the clinical trial's power to determine if the drug under study is actually effective.

Second, should participants be randomly assigned to treatment and control groups? Randomized clinical trials (RCTs) are more convincing than other research designs, because randomization minimizes baseline differences between the treatment and control groups. Thus if the treatment group fares better than the control group, randomization strengthens the inference that the difference is due to the treatment and not to some confounding factor, chance, or bias. RCTs convincingly showed that HIV infection could be effectively treated with antiviral agents and prophylactic antibiotics (Lo, 1992). These new therapies were adopted as standard practice months before the results of clinical trials were published in peer-reviewed journals and scrutinized by the scientific community. In addition, these RCTs convinced physicians, federal agencies, and advocacy groups to urge that persons at risk be tested for HIV infection. Insurers have provided coverage for these therapies, and drug manufacturers have been pressured to reduce their prices. It is highly unlikely that nonrandomized trials would have been considered so conclusive.

RCTs in HIV infection, however, have been criticized because the disease is considered fatal. Some people consider it unethical to conduct any clinical trials in which some participants receive placebos rather than the promising new drugs. Moreover, they point out that in general most medical interventions have not been subjected to RCTs. In one instance, nonrandomized trials provided sufficient evidence of a drug's effectiveness in HIV infection. A randomized, placebo-controlled trial was originally planned to evaluate the antiviral drug gancyclovir in cytomegalovirus retinitis, an opportunistic infection that usually causes blindness

(Lo, 1992). Advocates for persons with HIV infection complained that the natural history of the infection was so grim it was unnecessary and unethical to give patients RCTs, especially since historical controls had already demonstrated the drug's effectiveness. Furthermore, the proposed protocol would exclude patients taking other drugs. Critics protested that the proposed RCT would be unethical not only because it was unnecessary, but also because it would harm participants by denying them other therapies known to be beneficial. Ultimately, such thinking prevailed and gancyclovir was approved by the FDA without randomized trials.

Third, who should participate in clinical trials? Critics contend that access to clinical trials is inequitable. Many persons are excluded from clinical trials because there are no study sites in their geographic area. In addition, women, children, and people of color are underrepresented in clinical trials. Usually, children are restricted from clinical trials to protect them from the risks of unproven therapies. Unlike adults, children cannot give informed consent to take on such risks. The rationale for excluding women of childbearing age, particularly women who are pregnant, is to protect their developing and future children from possible long-term side effects of unproven drugs. But restricting women and children from clinical trials also harms them. They lack access to potentially beneficial therapies. In the long run, there is no rigorous information about the effectiveness of interventions in women and children.

Finally, what are the appropriate end points of clinical trials? Traditionally, clinical trials employ "hard" end points such as patient death or the development of opportunistic infections. Critics, however, object and say that using such end points needlessly prolongs research and delays the release of beneficial new therapies. Alternatively, using laboratory tests such as CD4 lymphocyte counts as surrogate end points, clinical trials can be conducted more quickly. The development of opportunistic infections is associated with a drop in CD4 counts. Drugs that increase CD4 levels may also prevent opportunistic infections. In July 1991, an FDA expert panel relied on surrogate end points in recommending that the drug didanosine be approved for marketing. Clinical trials showed increases in CD4 lymphocytes, compared with zidovudine. Data regarding the impact of the drug on hard end points were not yet available. While surrogate end points can lead to quicker approval of new drugs, they can be misleading. For example, while zidovudine causes a sustained improvement in CD4 counts, it offers no long-term clinical benefits (Concorde Coordinating Committee, 1994).

Persons with HIV infection and their advocates complain that the testing and release of new drugs have been delayed needlessly. Stirred by compassion for persons with HIV infection, some have urged greater access to unproven drugs. These advocates claim that informed persons with a rapidly fatal illness have a right to choose their treatments, including those of unknown safety and effectiveness. These advocates argue that it makes no sense to talk about protecting such patients from harm because they will die without treatment. Compared with ineffective standard treatment, unproven treatments at least offer patients hope and a sense of control over their illness.

Patients who are denied access to unproven therapies through the medical system may still obtain them through underground channels. In the gay community, newsletters disseminate detailed information about unproven therapies for HIV infection, and buyers' clubs import drugs from other countries. But this underground market has potential risks. The dosage and purity of drugs may be uncertain. Desperate patients may be financially exploited, and self-medication without individualized physician monitoring or advice may be dangerous.

In response to demands for greater access, the National Institutes of Health (NIH) and the FDA have established a "parallel track" to provide unproven therapies to certain persons with HIV infection outside of clinical trials. Eligible persons include those who cannot tolerate standard treatments, who have not responded to them, or who are otherwise not eligible for clinical trials of the therapy. The goal of this approach is to provide earlier access to promising but unproven drugs, while researchers conduct clinical trials. The parallel track, however, has been criticized because it facilitates the use of unproven and possibly dangerous drugs and may hinder recruitment of participants into clinical trials.

HIV infection in women and children

The epidemiology and clinical picture of HIV infection in women may differ from that in men. Among women in the United States, the HIV epidemic is concentrated among women of color in inner cities along the East Coast. As of 1994, AIDS is the leading cause of death among women of reproductive age in New York and New Jersey. Women acquire HIV infection through heterosexual contact and injection drug use (CDC, 1993). The two modes of transmission are linked because heterosexual transmission occurs most commonly in women who are sexual partners of injection drug users. Worldwide, most women contract HIV infection through heterosexual sex. In parts of Africa, 30 percent of women of childbearing age are infected with HIV.

The clinical presentation of AIDS in women differs from that in men. Responding to criticisms that AIDS was being underdiagnosed in women, the CDC modified its case definitions for AIDS in 1993 to include invasive cervical cancer, which commonly occurs in women with HIV infection (CDC, 1992). Many women with HIV infection are poor and lack health insurance. As a result, they find access to care problematic and often present for medical care later in the course of their illness.

In pediatrics, the vast majority of pediatric cases of HIV infection are transmitted vertically, from mother to infant. All infants whose mothers are HIV-infected also have HIV antibodies because of passive transfer of maternal antibodies through the placenta. These maternal antibodies, which persist from fifteen to eighteen months, are detected by HIV testing at birth. However, only a minority of such infants, about 30 percent but perhaps as low as 13 percent, are themselves infected with HIV. Currently there are no additional tests that accurately determine which infants are actually infected with HIV infection and which test positive for HIV infection because antibodies from their mothers have crossed the placenta.

The most difficult issues regarding the care of women with HIV infection occur when pregnant women make choices about their health care that conflict with the well-being of the fetus. Treatment of pregnant women and their newborn children with antiviral agents has been shown to lower the rate of HIV infection in the children, in addition to any medical benefits to the women (CDC, 1994b). Thus it would be desirable to identify pregnant women who are seropositive. However, HIV testing of pregnant women may harm them. Poor pregnant women, once identified as HIV-positive, often find services, such as drug addiction programs, pregnancy care, or abortion services, difficult or impossible to obtain because of discrimination. Most women consent to HIV testing when it is recommended for their own sake or for the sake of their child or fetus. Controversy occurs when they do not consent.

Screening of infants and pregnant women for HIV infection raises several difficult questions (Faden et al., 1991; Hardy, 1991). First, who should be targeted for testing? Most women with HIV infection are black and Latina/Hispanic. While epidemiologically sound, targeting women of color or their infants for HIV testing has been criticized as racist and discriminatory (Faden et al., 1991; Hardy, 1991). Screening programs for sickle-cell anemia in the 1970s illustrate problems with targeting persons according to ethnicity. Mandatory screening programs were criticized as "racist eugenic measures" (U.S. Congress, 1992, p. 259). In addition, these sickle-cell anemia screening programs were flawed because they confused sickle-cell disease with the benign carrier condition, failed to protect confidentiality, and led to job and insurance discrimination.

On the other hand, testing of women or infants at very low risk for HIV infection would not be cost-effective. Currently it is reasonable to recommend voluntary HIV testing to women with risk factors for HIV infection and to all pregnant women in high-risk geographic areas. Second, do women and children identified as seropositive have adequate access to services? Some contend that more widespread testing programs are unwarranted unless better access to services is assured. Third, is mandatory HIV testing ethically acceptable under some circumstances? To the extent that discrimination is eliminated, access to care is improved, and the benefits of treatment are demonstrated to be substantial, the arguments for mandatory HIV testing of pregnant women would be more compelling.

Conclusion

In summary, the HIV epidemic has raised new ethical and policy dilemmas and forced reconsideration of established guidelines and policies that apply to a much broader range of issues. In the future, controversies will likely occur regarding insurance coverage, the approval of promising new therapies, and mandatory HIV testing for pregnant women. In turn, these debates will have important implications for the larger issues of health-care reform, the role of the FDA in regulating new drugs, and compulsory treatment of pregnant women.

BERNARD LO

Directly related to this article is the companion article in this entry: PUBLIC-HEALTH ISSUES. *For a further discussion of topics mentioned in this article, see the entries* BENEFICENCE; CHILDREN, *articles on* RIGHTS OF CHILDREN, *and* HEALTH-CARE AND RESEARCH ISSUES; CHRONIC CARE; CONFLICT OF INTEREST; DENTISTRY; EPIDEMICS; HARM; HEALING; HEALTH-CARE FINANCING; HEALTH SCREENING AND TESTING IN THE PUBLIC-HEALTH CONTEXT; INFORMED CONSENT, *especially the article on* CONSENT ISSUES IN HUMAN RESEARCH; LABORATORY TESTING; MEDICINE, PHILOSOPHY OF; MEDICINE AS A PROFESSION; OBLIGATION AND SUPEREROGATION; OCCUPATIONAL SAFETY AND HEALTH; PLACEBO; PRIVACY AND CONFIDENTIALITY IN RESEARCH; PRIVACY IN HEALTH CARE; RESEARCH METHODOLOGY, *especially the article on* CONTROLLED CLINICAL TRIALS; RESEARCH POLICY; RISK; SURGERY; *and* WOMEN, *articles on* HEALTH-CARE ISSUES, *and* RESEARCH ISSUES. *For a further discussion of related ideas, see the entries* ABORTION; ABUSE, INTERPERSONAL, *article on* CHILD ABUSE; BLOOD TRANSFUSION; CONSCIENCE; FEMINISM; FETUS; FREEDOM AND COERCION; HEALTH PROMOTION AND HEALTH EDUCATION; HOMOSEXUALITY; HOSPITAL, *article on* CONTEMPORARY ETHICAL PROBLEMS; INFANTS, *article on* MEDICAL ASPECTS AND ISSUES IN THE CARE OF INFANTS; MATERNAL–FETAL RELATIONSHIP; MEDICAL INFORMATION SYSTEMS; PATIENTS' RIGHTS; PROSTITUTION; PUBLIC HEALTH, *article on* HISTORY OF PUBLIC HEALTH; RACE

AND RACISM; RESEARCH, UNETHICAL; RESPONSIBILITY; SUBSTANCE ABUSE, *articles on* ADDICTION AND DEPENDENCE, *and* ALCOHOL AND OTHER DRUGS IN A PUBLIC-HEALTH CONTEXT; *and* VIRTUE AND CHARACTER. *Other relevant material may be found under the entries* HOSPICE AND END-OF-LIFE CARE; LIFESTYLES AND PUBLIC HEALTH; LONG-TERM CARE, *article on* HOME CARE; PUBLIC HEALTH AND THE LAW; *and* RESEARCH ETHICS COMMITTEES.

Bibliography

ANNAS, GEORGE J. 1988. "Not Saints, but Healers: The Legal Duties of Health Care Professionals in the AIDS Epidemic." *American Journal of Public Health* 78, no. 7: 844–849.

CENTERS FOR DISEASE CONTROL (CDC). 1988. "Update: Universal Precautions for Prevention of Transmission of Human Immunodeficiency Virus, Hepatitis B Virus, and Other Blood Borne Pathogens in Health-Care Settings." *Morbidity and Mortality Weekly Report* 37, no. 24:377–382, 387–388.

———. 1991. "Recommendations for Preventing Transmission of Human Immunodeficiency Virus and Hepatitis B Virus to Patients During Exposure-Prone Invasive Procedures." *Morbidity and Mortality Weekly Report* 40, no. RR–8:1–9.

CENTERS FOR DISEASE CONTROL AND PREVENTION (CDC). 1992. "1993 Revised Classification System for HIV Infection and Expanded Surveillance Case Definition for AIDS Among Adolescents and Adults." *Morbidity and Mortality Weekly Report* 41, no. RR–17:1–19.

———. 1993. "Update: Acquired Immunodeficiency Syndrome—United States, 1992." *Morbidity and Mortality Weekly Report* 42, no. 28:547–551, 557.

———. 1994a. "Update: Impact of the Expanded AIDS Surveillance Case Definition for Adolescents and Adults on Case Reporting—United States, 1993." *Morbidity and Mortality Weekly Report* 43, no. 16:160–161, 167–170.

———. 1994b. "Zidovudine for the Prevention of HIV Transmission from Mother to Infant." *Morbidity and Mortality Weekly Report* 43:285–287.

CONCORDE COORDINATING COMMITTEE. 1994. "Concorde: MRC/ANRS Randomised Double-Blind Controlled Trial of Immediate and Deferred Zidovudine in Symptom-Free HIV Infection." *Lancet* 343, no. 8902:871–881.

DANIELS, NORMAN. 1990. "Insurability and the HIV Epidemic: Ethical Issues in Underwriting." *Milbank Quarterly* 68, no. 4:497–525.

FADEN, RUTH R.; GELLER, GAIL; and POWERS, MADISON, eds. 1991. *AIDS, Women, and the Next Generation: Towards a Morally Acceptable Public Policy for HIV Testing of Pregnant Women and Newborns.* New York: Oxford University Press.

GERBERDING, JULIE L.; LITTELL, CARY; TARKINGTON, ADA; BROWN, ANDREW; and SCHECTER, WILLIAM P. 1990. "Risk of Exposure of Surgical Personnel to Patients' Blood During Surgery at San Francisco General Hospital." *New England Journal of Medicine* 322, no. 25:1788–1793.

GREEN, J., and ARNO, P. S. 1990. "The Medicaidization of AIDS." *Journal of the American Medical Association* 264: 1261–1266.

HARDY, LESLIE M., ed. 1991. *HIV Screening of Pregnant Women and Newborns.* Washington, D.C.: National Academy Press.

HEALTH AND PUBLIC POLICY COMMITTEE, AMERICAN COLLEGE OF PHYSICIANS, and INFECTIOUS DISEASES SOCIETY OF AMERICA. 1988. "The Acquired Immunodeficiency Syndrome (AIDS) and Infection with the Human Immunodeficiency Virus (HIV)." *Annals of Internal Medicine* 108, no. 3:460–469.

HELLINGER, FRED J. 1993. "The Lifetime Cost of Treating a Person with HIV." *Journal of the American Medical Association* 270, no. 4:474–478.

LEVINE, CAROL; DUBLER, NANCY N.; and LEVINE, ROBERT J. 1991. "Building a New Consensus: Ethical Principles and Policies for Clinical Research on HIV/AIDS." *IRB* 13, no. 1:1–17.

LO, BERNARD. 1992. "Ethical Dilemmas in HIV Infection: What Have We Learned?" *Law, Medicine and Health Care* 20, nos. 1–2:92–103.

LO, BERNARD, and STEINBROOK, ROBERT. 1992. "Health Care Workers Infected with the Human Immunodeficiency Virus: The Next Steps." *Journal of the American Medical Association* 267, no. 8:1100–1105.

McGann v. H & H Music Company. 1990. 742 F. Supp. 392 (S.D. Tex.); 946 F.2d 401 (5th Cir. 1991).

NATIONAL COMMISSION ON ACQUIRED IMMUNODEFICIENCY SYNDROME. 1992. *Preventing HIV Transmission in Health Care Settings.* Washington, D.C.: Author.

PELLEGRINO, EDMUND D. 1987. "Altruism, Self-Interest, and Medical Ethics." *Journal of the American Medical Association* 258, no. 14:1939–1940.

U.S. CONGRESS. OFFICE OF TECHNOLOGY ASSESSMENT. 1992. *Cystic Fibrosis and DNA Tests: Implications of Carrier Screening,* OTA-BA-532, p. 259. Washington, D.C.: U.S. Government Printing Office.

ALCOHOL AND OTHER DRUGS

See SUBSTANCE ABUSE.

ALLIED HEALTH PROFESSIONS

The growth and complexity of medical science and technology in the twentieth century have necessitated a division of labor in health care to include new types of specialized medical and health-care personnel. The term "allied health" emerged in the mid-twentieth century in the United States as a convenient label for the numerous health-related occupations created as a consequence of this growth and complexity. The primary motive for the development of this collective term was to facilitate federal funding legislation for the growing number of health-occupations education programs in the United States. Most definitions of "allied health" are derived from the government definition.

The U.S. Department of Health and Human Services (U.S. Health Resources and Services Administration, 1990) defines an "allied health professional" as one who has received a certificate, academic degree, or post-baccalaureate training in a discipline related to health care. The federal definition also lists those health practitioners who are not classified as allied health: physicians and surgeons, osteopaths, dentists, veterinarians, optometrists, podiatrists, pharmacists, public-health personnel (graduate-degree level), chiropractors, health administrators (graduate-degree level), social workers, and clinical pathologists (doctoral-degree level). Nurses, too, are not considered allied health practitioners. The federal definition, therefore, is arbitrary rather than essential. Whether or not a health-related occupation or profession is included in the allied health category is a result of social or political influence.

In the final decade of the twentieth century, allied health personnel in the United States make up 35 percent of the health-care work force. Allied health personnel include practitioners who are patient-oriented (e.g., occupational therapist) and those who are laboratory- or technology-oriented (e.g., medical technologist). They function at the various levels of health care: primary to tertiary; acute to rehabilitative and chronic. Allied health personnel are involved in every area of the health-care system—entry and processing, evaluation and diagnosis, intervention and treatment, and education and prevention. They practice in all health-care settings, including hospitals, health maintenance organizations, ambulatory care clinics, freestanding specialty laboratories or clinics, and home care. Comparable health-care personnel are found in other parts of the world; however, titles, practice responsibilities, educational requirements, and the like vary.

The level of education and training required for practice in the allied health disciplines ranges from on-the-job-training to completion of a master's degree. Within specific allied health disciplines, such as physical therapy and the clinical laboratory sciences, even greater specialization has occurred, resulting in differentiated levels of responsibility and, hence, of education and training. In 1991, the U.S. Bureau of Health Professions listed eighty-five allied health disciplines, of which 35 percent required an associate degree for entry into practice, 38 percent required a bachelor's degree, and 27 percent a graduate degree (Associated Schools of Allied Health Professions, 1992).

In the United States, most academic allied health education programs have access to professional accreditation through their respective professional associations and/or the Committee on Allied Health Education and Accreditation of the American Medical Association. For some allied health groups, other regulatory mechanisms, such as certification and licensure, are tied to successful completion of an accredited program of study or of a standardized examination. Licensure laws usually define the scope of practice as well as regulate entry into practice. Licensure is traditionally viewed as a mechanism to protect consumers. Other economic and political motivations, however, may play a role.

Because of the differences that exist among the many specialized health personnel and the politically arbitrary nature of the allied health category, a number of health professions have resisted being designated as "allied health" disciplines. A universally accepted definition of "allied health" has not emerged (National Commission on Allied Health Education [NCAHE], 1980; National Academy of Sciences [NAS], 1989).

History of the development of the allied health professions

An examination of the history of the allied health disciplines reveals their relationship to medicine (or dentistry), sets the stage for a discussion of their emerging status as professions, and highlights the bases for their ethical concerns. The generation of most of the allied health disciplines can be linked to the advancement of the science and technology of medicine and its subsequent specialization and success.

Some allied health disciplines sprang from specific scientific or technological discoveries or inventions. For example, with Wilhelm Conrad Roentgen's discovery of X rays in 1895, radiologic technology was born. Although the first wave of X-ray enthusiasts included pharmacists, dentists, photographers, and gadgeteers, in succeeding years, physicians dominated the use of the X ray. These physicians, the pioneers of the new medical specialty of "roentgenology," began to employ and train young men and women apprentices to position patients, and to expose and develop X-ray plates. In 1920, the American Registry of X-ray Technicians was created, and by 1927 there were 432 registered technicians who formed the membership of the American Association of Radiological Technicians. Between 1920 and 1940, more formal training programs for technicians were established in medical schools and hospitals, and in 1944, accreditation of qualified educational programs was begun (Soule, 1974). In 1964 radiation therapy technology was designated as a separate discipline within the field of radiologic technology. Today, community colleges as well as medical schools and hospitals have accredited programs offering associate degrees or certificates in both radiologic technology areas. Many other allied health disciplines grew out of scientific discovery and technological invention, including diagnostic medical sonography, nuclear medicine technology, and cardiovascular technology.

In other instances, the burgeoning of allied health disciplines was related to the growth in the scientific understanding and increased efficacy of medicine. Physiotherapy, or physical therapy, as it is now called in the United States, began to flourish as a field of study after World War I. The recognition of physical therapy as a healing art dates back to ancient times. Prior to World War I, physiotherapists were trained on the job by orthopedic surgeons to assist in the treatment of patients with poliomyelitis. During World War I, military orthopedic surgeons, recognizing the role that physical therapy played in decreasing the convalescence time of the wounded, organized the Reconstruction Aide Corps in the U.S. Army military hospitals. Women nurses and physical educators, because of their training and their availability in wartime, were recruited for the Corps, and the first training program was established at Reed College in Oregon in 1918 (Scully, 1977). Two thousand women had completed their studies in physiotherapy by the end of the war.

The number of formal programs grew in both hospital and college settings as new and greater demands were made for physical therapy service. In 1925, the American Physical Therapy Association (APTA) assumed responsibility for delineating standards for approved physical therapy schools, and by 1928 six such schools had received approval. Between 1936 and 1976, the Committee on Medical Education and Hospitals of the American Medical Association had joint responsibility with APTA for accreditation. Subsequently the APTA, through its Commission on Accreditation of Physical Therapy Education, resumed sole responsibility for accreditation. World War II increased the demand for physical therapists and solidified the role and importance of rehabilitation in health care (Scully, 1977). To meet the growing demands for service, in 1967 the APTA approved the establishment of the physical therapist assistant (Scully, 1977).

As physical therapy grew as a field of study, the educational requirements increased from informal on-the-job training to bachelor's and master's degree completion. In addition, the responsibility and authority of the physical therapist in many states evolved from that of an orthopedic surgeon's apprentice to that of independent practitioner without need for physician referral. The history of physical therapy is a model case of the growth and maturation of an allied health occupation into a profession. Other allied health occupations that began to flourish as our knowledge of medicine grew and became more complex and specialized included occupational therapy, speech pathology and audiology, and respiratory therapy.

The development of the clinical laboratory occupations illustrates the critical political, economic, and social factors that shape the unique division of labor in medical care. Physicians negotiated the division of labor in medicine; their professional interests and values dominated (Starr, 1982). Physicians wanted more than to control competency in these new occupations. Paul Starr asserts, "They wanted to be able to use hospitals and laboratories without being their employees, and consequently they needed technical assistants who would be sufficiently competent to carry on in their absence and yet not threaten their authority" (1982, p. 220). Physicians achieved this outcome by using interns and residents in hospitals along with the new health-care personnel whose work they supervised and in whom they promoted a keen sense of responsible professionalism. While interns and residents were predominantly men, the new health-care workers were primarily women, who although professionally trained, were not likely to challenge the physician's authority or economic position (Starr, 1982).

In the clinical laboratory occupations, the pathologist—a physician—controlled both the practice and the laboratory workers, overseeing the educational process, the certification process, and even the code of ethics for the "profession." Among other stipulations, the early ethical codes of most of the allied health disciplines required that their members show deference to, and work at all times under the supervision of, a qualified physician. So, Starr observes, autonomy did not mean the same thing for the allied health worker as for the physician. The pathologist would have no need to fear competition from the hospital or the medical technologist. The profession of medicine succeeded in shaping the medical system "so that its structure supported professional sovereignty instead of undermining it" (Starr, 1982, p. 232).

Common elements in the histories described above that are relevant to the subsequent discussion of the status of the allied health disciplines as professions and to their special ethical concerns include (1) the subordinate status of and low economic compensation for allied health personnel, most of whom were women; (2) the gradual, at times reluctant, decrease of the dominating influence of medicine in the education and training of allied health personnel and in their specialized practices; (3) the progressively higher levels of education and training required as the professional knowledge and skill base grew; and (4) the concern for the development of practice-specific ethical codes and standards of education (program accreditation) and practice (certification and licensure).

Status as professions

There is no consensus in the literature about the characteristics that unequivocally identify a profession. Generally, in the literature, a descriptive or sociological approach, rather than a philosophical or essential one, is used to define a profession. Much of the sociological literature deals with "developing" professions or occupations undergoing "professionalization." Several authors, representing these two definitional approaches—the sociological and the philosophical—concede that, indeed, some of the allied health occupations are either full or developing professions, but they question the legitimacy of calling all allied health occupations "professions."

Nathan Hershey, who examines several different sociological definitions of the term "profession," concludes that even though most allied health practitioners have formed professional associations, have mastered a specialized body of knowledge or skills, and have developed standards for professional education as well as codes of ethical practice, some do not meet all of the pertinent criteria commonly used to identify a profession, such as licensure or some degree of practice autonomy. Some allied health disciplines do meet all of these criteria (Hershey, 1989).

Nursing professionals, whose experiences provide some precedents for allied health, have identified similar sociological criteria against which they measure nursing's achievement of the status of "full" profession. Lysaught asserts that there are six criteria that are almost universally identified as significant in defining a profession and that should, therefore, be used with regard to nursing. They are (1) a strong level of commitment to the field of practice; (2) a long and disciplined educational process; (3) a unique or specialized body of knowledge and skill; (4) discretionary authority and judgment in practice decisions and in establishing standards of education and of practice; (5) an active and cohesive professional organization; and (6) acknowledged social worth and contribution (Lysaught, 1981). Using the criteria of either Hershey or Lysaught, a number of allied health occupations, such as physical therapy, occupational therapy, and speech/language therapy, would be considered professions. The sociological approach to defining the professions, however, can be criticized precisely because it is sociological, that is, descriptive of what is commonly accepted by society as a "full," "true," "traditional," or "paradigmatic" profession. The difficulty with determining what is "commonly accepted by society" is apparent in the lack of consensus about the definition of a profession.

Edmund D. Pellegrino attempts to provide a philosophical rather than a social definition of the professions. He does not dismiss the sociological criteria but insists that they do not identify the essence of a true profession. What is essential for Pellegrino is the special relationship—the healing relationship—that exists between practitioner and patient. The significant elements of this relationship include the practitioner's promise or declaration to help the ill patient, who is in a special existential state of vulnerability, and to put the patient's interest above her or his own. The needs of the vulnerable patient are of the most personal or intimate kind, and to address these needs the patient must reveal personal confidences and must trust the practitioner's integrity, competency, and beneficence. Only those health occupations that have direct personal contact with the vulnerable patient are true professions.

Pellegrino admits that his criteria define a very limited number of healing professions and that these are bound by obligations that transcend not only self-interest but also general social standards of moral behavior. Although he avoids delineating specialities within medicine or allied health that would not meet his criteria, Pellegrino observes that, based on his criteria, nursing and some allied health occupations are more fully professional than the more technical fields of medicine (Pellegrino, 1983). Pellegrino's philosophical definition of profession might, then, include such occupations as physical therapy, speech/language therapy, and dental hygiene but would exclude medical records and medical technology. Pellegrino can be criticized for focusing too narrowly on the curative or healing facet of health care and thereby relegating some significant areas (such as health promotion, disease prevention, clinical laboratory sciences) to professional limbo. The narrowness of his focus (the phenomenology of illness and healing), however, is necessary if he is to achieve the outcome he seeks—the prescription of moral standards for medical professionals that transcend ordinary standards of moral behavior.

Although all of the approaches described result in identifying a number of the allied health occupations as professions, the criteria described by Lysaught best suit the allied health disciplines. These criteria reflect much of the scholarship regarding the sociological definition of professions, and they avoid the narrowness and exclusivity of Pellegrino's approach. But what of those allied health occupations that do not meet these criteria? Some of these occupations are new and may be professions in process. Others, however, may never be capable of achieving professional status. What of them?

What is overlooked by the various criteria, and by many of the medical and health occupations/professions as well, is the essential interdependence of medical and health-care roles. The growth and success of the science and technology of medicine that necessitated its division and specialization did not essentially change its primary objective. What did change is that a greater number of specialized practitioners, some of whom may not be "full" professionals, are now necessary to achieve that objective. The collective knowledge and skill of an array of practitioners and their collaborative decision making and action have become increasingly necessary in medical/health care. It is, therefore, no longer the individual practitioner who must meet the knowledge, skill, practice, and ethical standards of the professional; it is the collective, the team, that must. If, indeed, the collective or team is the "professional," all those who form the collective participate in both the privileges and the responsibilities of that status. It is past time, perhaps, for the paradigmatic notion of the medical professional, rooted in a simpler intellectual and technological age, to catch up.

Ethical issues

The evolutionary development of allied health personnel from physician apprentices to organized, credentialed specialists who are essential members of the health-care system has generated ethical questions, not all of which have been fully addressed or resolved. These questions relate primarily to the new roles that were created. The roles initially were established as subordinate to the physician or dentist, who took control of the education and training of the health-care worker and supervised her or his practice. Perhaps this control was necessary initially to ensure the quality of practice and to protect patients. However, it worked, as well, to achieve less morally worthy ends: to promote the power, authority, self-interest, and economic position of the physician and the health-care institution. Women were especially vulnerable since they were most frequently hired to fill these subordinate positions because, as Starr observed, they were less likely to challenge the authority of the physician and were willing to work for low wages. The treatment of these women reflected the general lack of status and opportunity for women in American society. As the demand for allied health practitioners, whether women or men, has increased, status and salaries have improved.

In most of the new allied health disciplines, the knowledge and skill base continues to expand. In many fields, the expertise of the supervisory physician has not kept pace with that of the allied health practitioner, exacerbating conflicts over the control of practice judgments and standards. The persistent struggle of many of the allied health occupations to achieve the status of profession reflects the degree to which they have grown beyond and rejected their original, subordinate role. The achievement of the status of profession has not, however, guaranteed allied health practitioners equal respect, power, or economic compensation. Even so, allied health personnel have assumed greater professional responsibility and autonomy in making practice decisions. They have tried to become moral partners rather than subordinates to physicians.

Health practitioner to patient.   Just as moral obligations vary among medical specialities, depending on role or function (for example, pathology in contrast to family medicine), so they vary among allied health occupations (medical technology in contrast to occupational therapy). Moral responsibilities shared by all medical and health-care providers include those to maintain professional competency, respect the person of the patient/client, provide services without discrimination, and guarantee the patient's privacy and confidentiality. The patient-oriented allied health practitioner, such as the nurse, spends considerable time with the patient and, consequently, has more opportunities to exercise these responsibilities than does the physician.

These basic, practice-related obligations usually are incorporated into the codes of ethics of the allied health professions. The obligation to maintain confidentiality has become especially important as the number of health-care providers with access to patients' records has proliferated and as medical records have been computerized (Siegler, 1982). The HIV/AIDS epidemic has compelled allied health professionals, both those providing direct patient care and clinical laboratory technologists, to reexamine their obligation to provide care without discrimination (Sim and Purtilo, 1991). In the laboratory-oriented disciplines (such as medical technology), where the patient seems relatively remote, the health professional's immediate moral obligation to the patient has gradually become fully recognized (Bingold et al., 1988).

Another moral obligation of the patient-oriented health professional is respect for the autonomy and freedom of choice of the patient. Discussion of issues related to informed consent has increased in the allied health literature as allied health professionals have assumed greater authority or autonomy in patient care. With the growth in the population of chronically ill and impaired elderly who require or might profit from treatment, allied health professionals (such as speech pathologists, occupational therapists, and clinical nutritionists) have been drawn into the debate about informed consent (Crabtree and Caron-Parker, 1991; Coy, 1989).

Health team to patient.   To achieve its purpose effectively, health care must pull together the many specialties that have resulted from the division of its labor. The sharing of patient-care responsibility among the various medical and health professionals has given rise to a number of new ethical complexities.

By virtue of their expertise and relationship to the patient, allied health professionals have become significant members of the health-care collective or team. The allied health practitioner has, therefore, been drawn into both the daily practice quandaries over moral agency and responsibility in collective decisions, and into the theoretical and policy debates about such decisions (Hansen et al., 1988; Brody and Noel, 1991). Three of the most basic ethical questions that all health professionals must address in group or collective decision making are, Who is morally responsible—the sum of individuals within the collective or the group as a unit? How are the allied health professional's individual moral responsibility and choice respected within the collective decision-making context; can they ever be denied or abrogated by a physician or the hospital administration? When there are conflicting obligations within the group, what priority of obligations or values should prevail—the patient's, a colleague's (including institutional administration) within the group, or one's own (Pellegrino, 1982)? Although models of group decision making that address these major questions have been described, neither the literature nor allied health and medical school ethics course syllabi evidence any widespread consensus around one model (Ozar, 1982; Thomasma, 1982).

Although reaching group consensus around ethical issues is not an easy task, David T. Ozar observes that collectives such as formally established and specialized health-care teams often do succeed in agreeing on a course of action that all members of the team consider morally acceptable. Agreement is usually achieved when the team and its members hold the life and health of the patient as primary in their collective activity. Where teams share this common primary interest, they also share a strong commitment to succeed together, thereby increasing their chances of doing so (Ozar, 1982).

If, as suggested above, the collective or team should be viewed as the "professional," it is imperative that all members of the collective develop the skills and the dedication to make responsible collective decisions. The commitment to interdisciplinary team education, training, and practice has been evident in the schools and colleges of allied health professions since the late 1960s.

Allied health professional to society. Insofar as allied health personnel aspire to achieve or have achieved the status of professional, they assume both the prerogatives and the obligations traditionally assigned to the professional. They also assume the problems faced by the professions in contemporary society, among them the conflicts between entrepreneurship and professionalism and between building a profitable career and responding to a vocation or calling (Jennings et al., 1987). In some health professions—for example, physical and occupational therapy—the push for private and independent practice and for a better position in the health-care marketplace has forced this conflict to the fore (Faust and Meaker, 1991).

Professional ethics involves more than obligations to individual patients and other appropriate constituencies; it includes obligations to the "public as a whole." The growth in consciousness of the "public duties" of the professions parallels the growth in significance and power of these professions (Jennings et al., 1987). With allied health practitioners, too, professional maturity and growth in political stature have led to an increasing awareness of their social obligations. Many of the emerging issues in the allied health professions will need to be addressed in the context of these social obligations.

One of the significant questions the allied health professions must address is the extent of their obligation for assuring society access to the specialized health care they provide. This obligation requires consideration of their responsibility to control the cost of their services, to maintain (or allow for) an adequate supply of professionals, and to cultivate a professional culture that promotes service to others over self-interest. In addition to considering these and other obligations to serve the "public interest," the allied health professions must reflect and act on their responsibility to the common good, for all health professions have a responsibility in every age to the common good—to assist society in defining the nature of health and its relationship to the other critical dimensions of the common good (Jennings et al., 1987).

Edmund J. McTernan underscores the challenge that must be met by allied health practitioners and educators alike to balance their growing power with their concomitant social obligations in an age of change. The moral challenge to allied health professionals, according to McTernan, is to remember that they exist to serve the health-care needs of the community and that those needs do not exist simply to provide them with opportunities for achieving status or wealth. The difficult two-fold challenge for allied health educators is, first, to educate and motivate students to altruism—a resource that is in scant supply—and, second, to prepare them to practice in a changing, uncertain health-care environment where there may be no assurance that their unique piece of the health-care puzzle will fit or be welcomed (McTernan, 1989).

JANET I. PISANESCHI

Directly related to this entry is the entry TEAMS, HEALTH-CARE. *For a further discussion of topics mentioned in this entry, see the entries* HEALTH-CARE RESOURCES, ALLOCATION OF, *article on* MICROALLOCATION; LICENSING, DISCIPLINE, AND REGULATION IN THE HEALTH PROFESSIONS; MEDICAL CODES AND OATHS; PROFESSION AND PROFESSIONAL ETHICS; TECHNOLOGY, *article on* HISTORY OF MEDICAL TECHNOLOGY; *and* WOMEN, *section on* WOMEN AS HEALTH PROFESSIONALS. *This entry will find application in the entries* DENTISTRY; NURSING AS A PROFESSION; PASTORAL CARE; *and* SOCIAL WORK IN HEALTH CARE. *For a discussion of related ideas, see the entries* AUTHORITY; AUTONOMY; COMPETENCY; CONFIDENTIALITY; *and* PROFESSIONAL–PATIENT RELATIONSHIP.

Bibliography

ASSOCIATED SCHOOLS OF ALLIED HEALTH PROFESSIONS. 1992. Unpublished data.

BINGOLD, JANET M.; MALCHIODI, LYNNE R.; and TERRY, JAMES S. 1988. "Ethical Dilemmas in the Laboratory: The

Not-So-Distant Patient." *Clinical Laboratory Science* 1, no. 4:230–234.

BRODY, HOWARD, and NOEL, MARY B. 1991. "Dieticians' Role in Decisions to Withhold Nutrition and Hydration." *Journal of the American Dietetic Association* 91, no. 5: 580–585.

COY, JANET A. 1989. "Autonomy-Based Informed Consent: Ethical Implications for Patient Noncompliance." *Physical Therapy* 69, no. 10:826–833.

CRABTREE, JEFFREY L., and CARON-PARKER, LAURA M. 1991. "Long-Term Care of the Aged: Ethical Dilemmas and Solutions." *American Journal of Occupational Therapy* 45, no. 7:607–612.

FAUST, LAWRENCE, and MEAKER, MYRA K. 1991. "Private Practice Occupational Therapy in the Skilled Nursing Facility: Creative Alliance or Mutual Exploitation?" *American Journal of Occupational Therapy* 45, no. 7:621–627.

HANSEN, RUTH ANN; KAMP, LINDA; and REITZ, SHARON. 1988. "Two Practitioners' Analyses of Occupational Therapy Practice Dilemmas." *American Journal of Occupational Therapy* 42, no. 5:312–319.

HERSHEY, NATHAN. 1989. "Policy Issues Relevant to Independent Practice of the Health Professions." *Journal of Allied Health* 18, no. 1:33–61.

JENNINGS, BRUCE; CALLAHAN, DANIEL; and WOLF, SUSAN M. 1987. "The Professions: Public Interest and Common Good." *Hastings Center Report* 17 (spec. suppl., February):3–10.

LYSAUGHT, JEROME P. 1981. *Action in Affirmation: Toward an Unambiguous Profession of Nursing.* New York: McGraw-Hill.

McTERNAN, EDMUND J. 1989. "The Impact of Independent Practice upon Allied Health Education." *Journal of Allied Health* 18, no. 1:87–93.

NATIONAL ACADEMY OF SCIENCES. INSTITUTE OF MEDICINE. 1989. "Allied Health Services: Avoiding Crisis: Executive Summary." *Journal of Allied Health* 18, no. 4:335–347.

NATIONAL COMMISSION ON ALLIED HEALTH EDUCATION. 1980. *The Future of Allied Health Education: New Alliances for the 1980s.* San Francisco: Jossey-Bass.

OZAR, DAVID T. 1982. "Three Models of Group Choice." *Journal of Medicine and Philosophy* 7:23–34.

PELLEGRINO, EDMUND D. 1982. "The Ethics of Collective Judgments in Medicine and Health Care: Editorial." *Journal of Medicine and Philosophy* 7, no. 1:3–10.

———. 1983. "What Is a Profession?" *Journal of Allied Health* 12, no. 3:168–176.

SCULLY, ROSEMARY M. 1977. "Physical Therapy Education." In vol. 2 of *Review of Allied Health Education,* pp. 148–159. Edited by Joseph Hamburg, Daniel J. Mase, J. Warren Perry, and Mary Dulmage. Lexington: University of Kentucky Press.

SIEGLER, MARK. 1982. "Confidentiality in Medicine: A Decrepit Concept." *New England Journal of Medicine* 307, no. 24:1513–1521.

SIM, JULIUS, and PURTILO, RUTH B. 1991. "An Ethical Analysis of Physical Therapists' Duty to Treat Persons Who Have AIDS: Homosexual Patients as a Test Case." *Physical Therapy* 71, no. 9:650–655.

SOULE, A. BRADLEY. 1974. "Radiologic Technology: The Birth, Growing Pains and Maturing of a Profession." In vol. 1 of *Review of Allied Health Education,* pp. 136–180. Edited by Joseph Hamburg, Daniel J. Mase, J. Warren Perry, and Mary Dulmage. Lexington: University of Kentucky Press.

STARR, PAUL. 1982. *The Social Transformation of American Medicine.* New York: Basic Books.

THOMASMA, DAVID C. 1982. "Moral Education in Interdisciplinary Terms." *Surgical Technologist* 14 (Jan.–Feb.):15–19.

U.S. HEALTH RESOURCES AND SERVICES ADMINISTRATION. BUREAU OF HEALTH PROFESSIONS. 1990. *Seventh Report to the President and Congress on the Status of Health Personnel in the United States.* Washington, D.C.: U.S. Department of Health and Human Services, Public Health Service, Health Resources and Services Administration, and Bureau of Health Professions.

ALLOCATION OF HEALTH CARE or ALLOCATION OF SCARCE MEDICAL RESOURCES

See HEALTH-CARE RESOURCES, ALLOCATION OF; *and* JUSTICE. *See also* ARTIFICIAL HEARTS AND CARDIAC-ASSIST DEVICES; ARTIFICIAL ORGANS AND LIFE-SUPPORT SYSTEMS; KIDNEY DIALYSIS; LIFE, QUALITY OF, *article on* QUALITY OF LIFE IN HEALTH-CARE ALLOCATION; *and* ORGAN AND TISSUE TRANSPLANTS, *article on* ETHICAL AND LEGAL ISSUES.

ALLOWING TO DIE

See ACTION; DEATH AND DYING: EUTHANASIA AND SUSTAINING LIFE; *and* INFANTS, *articles on* ETHICAL ISSUES, *and* PUBLIC-POLICY AND LEGAL ISSUES.

ALTERNATIVE THERAPIES

I. Social History
        Robert C. Fuller
II. Ethical and Legal Issues
        James F. Drane

I. SOCIAL HISTORY

Healing is a profoundly cultural activity. The very act of labeling a disease and prescribing treatment expresses a healer's commitment to a particular set of assumptions about the nature and structure of reality. These assumptions not only help specify the agents thought to cause disease but also contain implicit understandings of what health optimally or normatively enables humans to do.

Because rival medical systems typically subscribe to differing philosophical and cultural outlooks, the notion of orthodoxy pertains to medicine as surely as it does to religion or politics. What makes a therapy "orthodox" is its adherence to a belief system that, for intellectual and sociological reasons, informs the practice of the dominant members of a culture's medical delivery system. A therapy is therefore "unorthodox" to the extent that its diagnoses and treatments are not deemed legitimate by the dominant belief system.

The philosophical and professional differences that separate orthodox and unorthodox therapies give rise to complex ethical questions. How, for example, are we to understand medical "legitimacy," when this notion is the product of ever-changing philosophical, cultural, and social factors? What does it mean for a medical treatment to be unethical? Must it in some way bring about negative results, or is it unethical even if it is—such as vitamin placebo treatment—merely a harmless fraud? What constitutes a therapeutic benefit? Is it an improvement in physical, mental, or spiritual well-being?

First, the sheer diversity of alternative therapies hampers attempts to generalize about the kinds of ethical issues that unorthodox treatments present. There is an almost bewildering array of alternative therapies, ranging from chiropractic, osteopathy, and acupuncture, to shiatsu, herbal medicine, and religious faith healing. Further complicating this task is the fact that these alternative therapies find themselves labeled unorthodox for quite different reasons. Some, for example, are practiced by healers committed to an alternative belief system or worldview that grants reality to causal forces that differ greatly from those specified by medical orthodoxy. Such is the case with various "faith healing" traditions and New Age medical systems. Religious therapies such as these invoke an overtly metaphysical explanation of the causes of physical illness and depict human health in terms of adherence to specific spiritual or ethical outlooks on life.

Second, healing systems may become unorthodox when they employ therapies that, although predicated upon the consensus worldview, have not yet been validated or confirmed as efficacious by orthodox medical standards. Many of the treatments suggested for combating cancer or acquired immunodeficiency syndrome (AIDS) are considered unorthodox for this reason. Third, healers find themselves outside the medical mainstream when they provide services that are typically ignored or deemed of secondary importance by a culture's dominant medical practitioners. This has been the case, for example, with dentists in the nineteenth century, podiatrists in the early twentieth century, and midwives throughout most of modern history. The case of midwifery is instructive. While never as widespread in

the United States as in other parts of the world, the use of midwives provided the only obstetrical assistance available to many women until early in the twentieth century. As obstetrics became a recognized medical specialty, primarily under the control of male physicians, hospitals equipped with surgical facilities supplanted the home as the normal site for giving birth. Increasingly the last resort of those who could not afford hospital births, midwifery generally fell into disrepute. Midwifery, then, became an "unorthodox" form of medical care not because it employed an alternative worldview or because it could not be validated as a treatment, but because the dominant providers of medical services decided that the home and the assistance of other women at childbirth were not of primary importance. Interestingly, midwifery has witnessed a modest resurgence in recent decades as part of a general cultural trend toward "natural" medicine and woman-centered health care. Nurse-midwives now perform about 2 percent of all deliveries in the United States, and more than a dozen universities currently offer certification programs for midwives.

What alternative therapies have in common is economic, legal, and cultural disenfranchisement from the socially empowered institution of scientific medicine. Any attempt to reflect upon the ethical questions raised by these "alternative" approaches to healing requires sensitivity to the historical and philosophical roots of this disenfranchisement. "Regular" physicians coalesced into state and local medical societies during the nineteenth century, securing an institutional power base for what was to become medical orthodoxy in the United States. This emerging corps of physicians shared a more or less common approach to medical practice and were eventually able to "institutionalize" this approach through the influence they exerted over licensure laws enacted by state and federal governments, the accreditation of medical schools, and access to technologically equipped hospitals. The American Medical Association (founded in 1847, but lacking strong organization and sufficient membership until the early twentieth century) eventually succeeded in organizing and promoting the interests of the nation's dominant medical practitioners on a national level.

Medical orthodoxy aligned itself with the worldview spawned by the Western scientific tradition. Its approach to therapeutic intervention has been firmly rooted in the evolving body of information that has emerged from advances in physiology, chemistry, and pharmacology. Accompanying this reliance upon the Western scientific tradition has been an implicit endorsement of a secularist and rationalist ontology (i.e., a worldview skeptical of claims concerning the supernatural or other unquantifiable influences). What has given scientific medicine its "public" character is its insistence that theories concerning the etiology and treatment of disease specify physical, as opposed to spiritual or metaphysical, causal forces. Its theories and strategies for therapeutic intervention are thus more susceptible to empirical verification, and disputes can at least potentially be resolved by an appeal to observable and quantifiable sets of data. This is also why scientific medicine found itself more amenable than many of its alternative counterparts to the economic and legal institutions of modern Western governments. Rejecting the "private" claims to truth made in religious arguments, Western democracies have required that all civic discourse be advanced according to rational and public grounds of argumentation.

To the extent that scientific medicine's academic and experimental foundations facilitate such "public" argumentation, it has largely merited its enfranchisement within the legal and economic institutions that make judgments about the allocation of medical resources. Any consideration of the ethical status of these judgments and their effect upon the practice of alternative medical systems must take into account the important role that such rational and public discourse has had in the development of Western culture.

Nineteenth-century alternative medicine

The Thomsonian system.   One of the first challenges to the orthodoxy of "regular physicians" occurred in the early 1800s. Samuel Thomson (1769–1843) was a poor New Hampshire farmer whose mother and wife had suffered from the bleedings and mercurial drugs forced upon them by regular physicians. Thomson believed that better treatments must be available, and he began studying the therapeutic value of herbs. He soon developed his own system of botanical medicine predicated upon the assumption that there is only one cause of disease, cold, and one cure, heat. Thomson believed that by restoring heat to his patients' systems, he could cure any ailment. Using botanics such as cayenne pepper, supplemented with steam baths, Thomson sought cures without the incessant bloodletting or mercurial drugs utilized by the era's orthodox physicians.

The Thomsonian system reached the height of its popularity in the 1820s and 1830s. Some estimate that its methods were employed in varying degrees by as many as a million Americans. One obvious reason for its appeal was that its treatments were generally more benign than the aggressive arsenal of bloodletting, alcohol, opium, mercury, arsenic, and strychnine that many regular physicians used to stimulate their patient's systems. Perhaps more important, Thomsonianism could be studied relatively inexpensively (although the official price for the right to use his methods was a substantial $20) and practiced by family members. During the days

of medical professionalization in the United States, Thomsonianism strengthened the role of parents, and especially mothers, in caring for family members. Thomsonianism also fit nicely with the period's moral and religious climate, which urged individuals to take responsibility for their own moral and spiritual regeneration. It endeavored "to make every man his own physician" and encouraged individuals to take responsibility for restoring their rightful relationship to the divinely decreed laws of nature. Of lasting significance is the fact that Thomsonianism was the first system to take on the issue of licensing of medical practitioners, and to assert the public's right to free choice of healers. Thomsonians led the successful campaign to repeal medical licensing legislation in the mid-1800s and drew public attention to the somewhat predatory tactics with which orthodox physicians sought to restrict the right of would-be healers to practice whatever system they wanted.

Homeopathy.   A second form of sectarian medicine, homeopathy, emerged more or less concurrently with the public's gradual loss of enthusiasm for the Thomsonian system. The homeopathic system of medicine was the creation of the German physician Samuel Christian Hahnemann (1755–1843), who grew increasingly critical of the indiscriminate prescription of drugs by contemporary physicians. He coined the term "allopathic" to refer to orthodox medicine's alleged overreliance upon invasive therapeutic treatments (e.g., bloodletting, surgery, or the administration of strong pharmacological agents). In contrast to allopathic medicine, Hahnemann enunciated a medical theory that he thought relied more upon the body's natural powers to bring about recovery. The first principle of homeopathic medicine is "like cured by like." By this Hahnemann meant that physicians should treat symptoms by prescribing drugs that produce similar symptoms in a healthy individual. The second fundamental principle of homeopathic medicine is the doctrine of infinitesimals. It was Hahnemann's conviction that the greatest therapeutic benefit was to be achieved by administering diluted doses of a drug, sometimes only 1/1,000,000 of a gram. Although homeopathic physicians' use of infinitesimal doses undoubtedly negated any therapeutic value their drugs might have had, at least these small doses had the virtue of not assaulting the patient's recuperative powers. It is thus not surprising that many turned to homeopathy as a viable alternative to orthodox medicine.

Homeopathy spread quite rapidly in the United States. It was introduced by Hans Gram, who opened an office in New York after studying the homeopathic system in Europe. By 1835 a homeopathic college had been formed, and in 1844 the American Institute of Homeopathy was organized. Throughout the 1800s,

10 to 12 percent of the country's medical schools and medical school graduates were adherents to homeopathy. In contrast to Thomsonianism, which was practiced by nonprofessionals, homeopathic practitioners were educated professionals who often came from the ranks of regular physicians. Moreover, while those who received Thomsonian treatment tended to be rural and poor, there is evidence to suggest that homeopathy thrived among the urban upper and middle classes. This latter fact led to direct economic competition with the regular system and proved an important catalyst in the formation and success of the American Medical Association as economic motives joined with scientific ones to rally regular physicians in opposition to their irregular competitors. As the most popular of the century's alternative systems, homeopathy raised a number of important ethical questions. For example, could allopathic physicians consult with "unscientific" practitioners? (The AMA's original code of ethics included a consultation clause that prohibited such interactions.) Or should homeopathic physicians be allowed to practice in publicly supported hospitals or in the military? Even today there is some debate about whether pharmacies should be required to stock homeopathic medicines.

Hydropathy and dietary regimens.   In the mid-1840s another alternative therapy, hydropathy (water cure), began to attract a following in the United States. Based on the theories of Vincent Priessnitz of Austria, hydropathy was based on enhancing the body's inherent vitality and purity. Priessnitz believed that pure water could be used to flush out bodily impurities and stimulate the body's inherent tendencies toward health. Water-cure treatments emphasized drinking large amounts of water and applying water externally through baths, showers, or wrapping wet sheets around the body. Most American adherents of water cure advocated an eclectic approach to health based on the curative powers of fresh air, diet, sleep, exercise, and proper clothing. The philosophy of water cure also had a decidedly moral tone. As one anonymous American enthusiast put it, "We regard Man, in his primitive and natural condition as the perfect work of God, and consider his present degenerated physical state as only the natural and inevitable result of thousands of years of debauchery and excess, of constant and wilful perversions of his better nature, and the simple penalty of outraged physical law, which is just and more severe than any other" (*Water-Cure World*, 1860).

Hydropathy thus equated disregard of the laws of healthful living with defiance of God's will. Systematic efforts to promote healthful living were not only the means to physical well-being but also the key to spiritual renovation of Earth. The hydropathic cause naturally attracted many of the period's moral and religious reformers. William Alcott, Lucy Stone, Amelia

Bloomer, Susan B. Anthony, and Horace Greeley visited major hydropathic retreat centers, where they circulated reformist agendas ranging from vegetarianism to utopian socialism. Critical of the alleged superiority of "official" medical authorities, advocates of hydropathy had a natural affinity with the feminist thought of the time. Hydropathy looked to nature, not credentialed male physicians, as the ultimate source of healing, and in so doing, it provided a vehicle for those seeking to redress what they thought were faulty notions of social and political authority.

Another nineteenth-century forebear of contemporary alternative therapy in the United States was Sylvester Graham (1794–1851), who combined conservative religious beliefs with zealous concern for health reform. An ordained Presbyterian minister and itinerant evangelist, Graham believed that human physical, moral, and spiritual well-being required scrupulous adherence to the natural order established by God. Graham admonished his followers that avoiding alcohol and the overstimulation of the sexual organs could help them maintain moral and physical health. His advice for a healthful diet included a coarse bread, later produced in the form of a cracker that still carries his name. Graham's dietary principles, widely circulated throughout the nineteenth century, served the cause of keeping the soul's "bodily temple" free from impurities.

Ellen White (1827–1915) occasionally visited a hydropathic resort in Dansville, New York, where she became a convert to Graham's dietary gospel. White thereafter had a series of mystical visions in which God revealed to her that He expected humans to follow the divinely given laws governing health and diet as faithfully as His moral laws. The Seventh-Day Adventist denomination founded by White has since then adopted Grahamite principles and a vegetarian diet as essential parts of purifying themselves in expectation of the Second Coming of Christ. Seventh-Day Adventists, one of the largest religious groups to originate in the United States, support a number of health sanatoriums and combine their evangelical religious faith with a strong emphasis on healthy dietary practices. This emphasis upon a healthful diet does not in and of itself constitute an alternative medical practice. Their dietary concerns are, however, closely connected with their belief in the efficacy of petitionary prayer.

The rise of mental healing practices

Mesmerism.   The introduction of Franz Anton Mesmer's "science of animal magnetism," commonly known as mesmerism, in the 1830s and 1840s popularized a belief in the power of the unconscious mind to draw upon an invisible healing energy. Mesmer (1734–1815), a Viennese physician, believed that he had detected the existence of an almost ethereal fluid that permeates the universe. This fluid, called animal magnetism, flows continuously into, and is evenly distributed throughout, a healthy human body. If for any reason an individual's supply of animal magnetism is thrown out of equilibrium, one or more bodily organs will begin to falter. Mesmer proclaimed, "There is only one illness and one healing." The science of animal magnetism revolved around the identification of techniques for restoring a patient's inner receptivity to this mysterious, life-giving energy.

Mesmer held magnets in his hands and repeatedly passed them over the heads and bodies of his patients in an effort to induce the flow of animal magnetism into their systems. His followers later dispensed with the magnets, finding that verbal suggestions from the healer could induce patients into a trance, ostensibly heightening their receptivity to the influx of this metaphysical healing agent. Mesmerized patients claimed to feel prickly sensations running up and down their bodies that they attributed to the influx and movement of animal magnetism. Awaking from their sleeplike trance, they reported feeling refreshed, invigorated, and healed of such disorders as arthritis, nervousness, digestive problems, liver ailments, stammering, insomnia, and the abuse of coffee, tea, or alcohol. Some patients even claimed that the mesmerizing process enabled them to open up the mind's latent powers for telepathy, clairvoyance, and precognition. These claims contributed as much, or even more, to mesmerism's growing popularity than its reputation for healing.

A good many of those drawn to mesmerism were middle- and upper-class individuals who styled themselves progressive thinkers and were interested in uniting science and religion in a single philosophical account of human nature. Mesmerism struck them as an important step in this direction. The phenomena surrounding mesmeric trances were thought to provide empirical proof that each human is inwardly connected with higher, metaphysical planes of reality. Adherents of mesmerism believed that under certain conditions of psychological receptivity, humans are able to open themselves to an influx of energy or guidance from these higher realms. American mesmerists borrowed terminology from transcendentalism, spiritualism, and theosophy to provide their middle-class reading audience with a new vocabulary for understanding the interconnection of their physical, mental, and spiritual natures.

Mind cure and Christian Science.   A popular philosophy known as the mind-cure or New Thought movement grew out of the mesmerists' healing practices. Mind-cure writers in the United States published books and pamphlets describing how thought controls the extent to which we are able to become inwardly receptive to spiritual energies. From Phineas P. Quimby and Warren Felt Evans in the late 1800s to Norman Vincent Peale, Norman Cousins, and Bernie Siegel in the late 1900s, Americans have displayed a remarkable enthusiasm for this "power of positive thinking" literature. The mind-cure movement gave rise to a novel form of religious piety based on the belief that the deeper powers of our mind control our access to a metaphysical power that can instantly help us to achieve peace of mind, improved health, and a never-ceasing flow of energy. The holistic health movement of the 1960s and 1970s relied heavily upon this cluster of metaphysical ideas.

Mesmerism was also instrumental in the formation of Christian Science. In 1862 Mary Baker Eddy, in great physical and emotional distress, arrived on the doorstep of the famous mesmerist healer Phineas P. Quimby. Quimby's treatments gradually cured her of her ailments; they also gave her a new outlook on life, based upon the principle that our thoughts determine whether we are inwardly open to, or closed off from, the creative activity of a spiritual energy (animal magnetism). Soon after Quimby's death, Eddy transformed his mesmerist teachings into the foundational principles of Christian Science. Her principal text, *Science and Health with Key to the Scriptures* (1875), reveals her intention to shift the science of mental healing away from the categories of mesmerism to those that bear more resemblance to Christian Scripture, albeit her own unique interpretation of it. The basic theological postulate of Christian Science is that God creates all that is, and all that God creates is good. Sickness, pain, and evil are not creations of God, and therefore they do not truly exist. They are simply the delusions produced in an erring, mortal mind that has lost a firm hold on the belief that only those things created by God have true existence. For Christian Scientists the universe is spiritual. What we call matter (e.g., bacteria, viruses, etc.) consequently does not really exist and therefore has no causal power. Christian Science healers, known as practitioners, help individuals to overcome their faulty thinking and to elevate their mental attitudes above the delusions of the senses. Healing occurs as the individual learns to function on a metaphysical, rather than a physical plane. Healings are understood not as miracles or faith healings but as the lawful consequence of exchanging false conceptions for true ones, which center solely on the higher laws of God's spiritual presence.

Both Christian Science and the "holistic health" philosophies that emerged from the mind-cure tradition teach that our thoughts control the degree to which we avail ourselves of the higher spiritual source from which health proceeds. As a consequence, illness or disease is understood as something the sufferer has brought upon himself or herself through failure to sustain a "correct" mental posture toward life. Any ethical analysis of these forms of alternative therapy must take seriously their built-in skepticism about whether a medical system really needs to attend to material causes of illness (bacteria, viruses, etc.). The issue is not quite so acute for holistic healing practices that teach that the mind can draw upon a higher energy capable of invigorating matter but do not teach that matter itself is unreal. In other words, most holistic health systems do not deny that there are physical and material causes of illness. They simply maintain that mental and spiritual factors are entailed in the etiology of most illnesses and must be taken into account in any comprehensive medical system. And thus, although they insist that a patient's mental outlook often is a significant factor in the creation and cure of illness, they do not espouse a medical theory that puts all the "blame" for illness or "credit" for recovery upon the patient.

Christian Science, by contrast, goes much further in challenging the empirical and rational foundations of Western science. By denying the ontological reality of matter, and hence the causal power of viruses or bacteria, Christian Science is clearly at philosophical loggerheads with both medical orthodoxy and the legal systems of most Western, democratic nations. For example, the Christian Scientists' belief system is opposed to immunization. The courts have understandably become concerned over the medical well-being of the children of Christian Science practitioners, as well as other students with whom they attend school; this has led to legal restrictions on the right of Christian Scientists to practice their form of religious healing. In 1990 the U.S. courts decided that two Christian Science parents were guilty of child neglect when their sole reliance on Christian Science methods was deemed responsible for their child's death (*Hodgeson* v. *Minnesota*, 1990). Such cases draw attention to the important ethical distinction between "private" religious belief and actions that have consequences in the "public" domain regulated by the legal system.

Christian Science healing practices, fundamentalist faith healing, and outright quackery have prompted strong responses from practitioners of orthodox medicine. The American Medical Association, emerging as a powerful national organization early in the twentieth century, set itself the task of prompting state and federal agencies to enact stricter licensing regulations. Its efforts to restrict medical practice to graduates of AMA-accredited medical schools surely furthered the cause of scientific medicine and protected the public from potentially harmful forms of quackery. It also tended, however, to force out of the medical marketplace those whose approaches to healing utilized a nonscientific worldview or whose medical services did not fit with dominant approaches to medical care.

Chiropractic and osteopathic medicine

Osteopathic and chiropractic medicine provide interesting examples of the fate of alternative philosophical, religious, and ethical interpretations of healing in an age dominated by scientific medicine. Osteopathic medicine emerged from the healing philosophy of Andrew Taylor Still (1828–1917). A former spiritualist and mesmeric healer, Still developed techniques for manipulating vertebrae along the spine in ways that he thought removed obstructions to the free flow of "the life-giving current" that promotes health throughout the body. Still explained the healing principles of osteopathy (a term derived from two Greek words meaning "suffering of the bones") in overtly metaphysical terms that described the origin and nature of "the life-giving current" ultimately responsible for human well-being. His followers largely discarded the occult-sounding dimensions of Still's philosophy and instead insisted that osteopathic medical education be grounded in anatomy and scientific physiology. Thus, although osteopaths originally relied only upon manual manipulations of the spine as a means of restoring health, they soon added surgery and eventually drug therapy to their medical practice.

By the 1950s, so few differences existed in the training or practice of osteopaths and M.D.s that their two national organizations agreed to cease the rivalry that had existed for several decades and to cooperate in such matters as access to hospitals, residency programs, and professional recognition. Having jettisoned the alternative worldview of its founder, osteopathy no longer bore any overt signs of unorthodoxy and finally found itself within the medical mainstream. Interestingly, during the 1960s many osteopaths were concerned about being absorbed into allopathic medicine and gave renewed focus to osteopathy's philosophical origins. Their commitment to osteopathy's historical concern with enhancing the body's natural powers for recuperation made them champions of holistic medicine long before the term "holistic" became commonplace among alternative healers. As of 1990, over 24,000 physicians practiced osteopathic medicine, collectively treating over 20 million patients per year.

The case of chiropractic medicine is more complex. Chiropractic originated in the work of Daniel David Palmer (1845–1913), a mesmerism-inspired magnetic healer in Iowa. Palmer, who knew of Still's osteopathic techniques, theorized that dislocations of the spine are able to block the free flow of the life force, which he called Innate (his nomenclature for animal magnetism). Palmer and his son, B. J. Palmer, explained that Innate is a part of the Divine Intelligence that fills the universe, bringing full physical health whenever it flows freely through the human body. Chiropractic medicine represents the Palmers' art and science of adjusting the spine in ways that remove obstructions to the free flow of Innate within the body.

Over the years, chiropractic physicians began downplaying the movement's metaphysical origins and emphasized its scientific approach to the treatment of musculoskeletal disorders. In this way, they minimized their theoretical unorthodoxy and identified an area of medical practice largely ignored by most medical doctors. Chiropractic physicians' sustained attention to this void in the "orthodox" medical system has earned them a viable niche in the medical marketplace; as of 1990, over 19,000 chiropractic physicians were treating more than 3 million patients annually. Even though most medical insurance companies have come to recognize the medical functions performed by chiropractic medicine, M.D.s are still largely wary of chiropractic medicine because it has failed to elucidate an empirically validated theory that would substantiate its therapeutic claims. This professional tension provides a fascinating example of a continuing theme in the history of alternative medicine: the clash between orthodox medicine's rationalism (its insistence on an acceptable scientific explanation for all methods) and alternative medicine's pragmatism (discovery of therapies that produce results regardless of whether they are "proved" with rational theories).

Holistic, new age, and folk medicine

During the last few decades of the twentieth century, the holistic healing movement led a surge of popular interest in therapies based on an explicitly religious, or quasi-religious, interpretation of the healing process. The precise meaning of the term "holistic medicine" varies among healing systems. Among its meanings are emphasis upon "natural" therapies, patient education and responsibility, prevention, and treating patients as "whole" people. Also common to holistic healing is the basic assumption that, as one handbook put it, "every human being is a unique, wholistic, interdependent relationship of body, mind, emotions, and spirit." The term "spirit," alongside "body," "mind," and "emotions," carries holistic healing beyond psychosomatic medical models; it also represents commitment to a belief in the interpenetration of physical and nonphysical spheres of causality. Even holistic healing's exhortations concerning reliance upon the body's own regenerative and reparative processes are typically laden with references to opening individuals up to the inflow of a divine healing energy. Persons who call themselves holistic health practitioners typically operate according to a worldview that is incompatible with the naturalistic framework of the modern Western scientific heritage.

One example of such a holistically oriented healing movement is Alcoholics Anonymous (AA), and its Twelve-Step program, which has influenced many other "self-regenerative" therapies. Founded in the 1930s, Alcoholics Anonymous now has well over one million members, with about 35,000 groups meeting weekly in over ninety countries. The principal founder of the movement, Bill Wilson, was an alcoholic who became acutely aware of his inability to overcome his addiction. A mystical experience of "a great white light" convinced him that a loving Presence surrounds us and is capable of healing our broken inner lives. Wilson maintained that we need only to cease relying upon our own willpower and surrender to this "Higher Power." Wilson was extremely wary of institutional religion, especially the moralism associated with biblical religion. From psychologists such as William James and Carl Jung, he pieced together a form of spirituality based upon opening the unconscious mind to a higher metaphysical reality. AA counsels its members that "in order to recover, they must acquire an immediate and overwhelming 'God-consciousness' followed at once by a vast change in feeling and outlook" (Alcoholics Anonymous, 1955, p. 569). AA's mystical, nonscriptural approach to personal regeneration sets its doctrines apart from most of America's religious establishment; its denunciation of both material and psychological/attitudinal factors in favor of an overtly spiritual view of healing sets its practices apart from the American medical and psychological establishments. But its open-minded and eclectic sense of the presence of spiritual forces in the determination of human well-being makes it one of the most powerful mediators of wholeness in America today.

The various religious and healing groups that comprise the New Age movement endorse a holistic approach to health and medicine; they envision every human being as a unique combination of body, mind, emotions, and spirit. Central to New Age piety is the conviction that each person exists simultaneously in both the physical and the metaphysical (i.e., the astral and etheric) planes of reality. New Age therapies such as the use of crystals, Therapeutic Touch, and psychic healing seek to channel healing energies from higher metaphysical planes into the physical body. New Age crystal healing, for example, maintains that illness in the physical body is frequently caused by a disruption or disharmony of energies in what is called the "etheric body" (the portion of the self that extends into the astral and etheric planes). Healing consequently requires techniques to achieve harmony between the physical and subtle or etheric bodies. Crystals are thought to have unique properties that enable them to serve as receptors and capacitors of energies that emanate from the astral and etheric planes. Used properly, crystals are assumed to be capable of transmitting these energies in ways that bring the individual's physical, moral, and spiritual natures back into harmony. To this extent, New Age adherents do not reject the therapeutic efficacy of established medical science (though they do condemn what they perceive to be an overreliance on drugs and invasive surgical techniques) so much as its secularist and materialistic worldview, which fails to take into account our spiritual nature or potentials. Healing, for New Agers, is a by-product of the more fundamental goal of attaining an expanded spiritual awareness.

New Age healers are especially drawn to Eastern religious systems that involve entering into meditative states that heighten receptivity to the inflow of a higher spiritual energy, variously referred to as *ch'i, prana, kundalini,* animal magnetism, or divine white light. Yoga, t'ai chi ch'uan, Ayurvedic medicine, shiatsu, acupuncture, and various Oriental massage systems are studied for their advocacy of attitudes and lifestyles geared to the renovation of our moral and spiritual lives. Although each of these healing systems has its own philosophical basis and history, Americans tend to approach them with agendas left over from such nineteenth-century movements as mesmerism, spiritualism, and theosophy. Even acupuncture, whose ability to alleviate pain and promote healing is more or less recognized—though poorly understood—by medical science, is embraced by many Americans not only for its obvious physical benefits but also for its connections with Eastern mystical philosophies.

A wide variety of folk and ethnic remedies exist alongside medical science. Botanical and herbal remedies, while ordinarily aimed at promoting health rather than curing illness, represent a noninvasive approach to physical well-being. Rural Pennsylvania Dutch still practice variations of "powwow," an eclectic tradition using charms, prayers, and rituals, to prevent and cure disease. In the American Southwest, *curanderismo* still flourishes in Mexican-American communities, and recent immigration to the continental United States from the Caribbean has rekindled folk medicine practices (e.g., charms, herbs, incantations) peculiar to the Afro-American heritage. Immigration from Southeast Asia has brought Hindu and Buddhist medical practices like Ayurvedic medicine and prayers to the heavenly saints (bodhisattvas), who reward the faithful with their healing powers. Far East Asian immigrants have included dedicated practitioners of such religiomedical systems as t'ai chi ch'uan, shiatsu, and acupuncture. The continued presence of such folk or ethnic medical treatments may represent a form of preserving cultural identity, economic disenfranchisement from the nation's more expensive established medical system, or the seeds of a new era of genuine medical pluralism. In any case, both legal and economic attitudes toward alternative therapies must be philosophically and culturally nuanced.

The challenge to bioethics

Persons with life-threatening diseases who have not been helped by conventional treatments understandably become interested in pursuing alternative therapeutic strategies. The highly publicized debate over the effec-

tiveness of laetrile for retarding cancer, for example, drew attention to the potential risks of the regulation of medicine by the U.S. Food and Drug Administration (FDA). At stake was the unresolved issue of whether a drug should be restricted only when it is known to cause harm or only when laboratory testing has failed to reveal measurable physical benefits. This debate continues in the controversy over various treatments for AIDS. Persons given a bleak prognosis by medical doctors seek immediate access to experimental drugs that have just entered the slow and laborious regulatory processes mandated by U.S. federal law. Although much has been done to try to speed up the evaluation of experimental AIDS-related treatments, a growing number of persons find themselves barred from access to innovative scientific treatment.

The central ethical question raised by alternative therapies is whether genuine medical treatment can be distinguished from various forms of quackery. Except for isolated instances in which individuals engage in deliberate medical fraud, quackery is difficult to identify or prove. Any reliable definition of therapeutic benefit requires being able to define the factors "known" to affect human well-being and what optimal health consists of. The practitioners of many forms of alternative medicine criticize the assumptions they believe underlie contemporary medical science. They argue that alternative therapies better understand human well-being and are cognizant of mental, moral, and spiritual factors that go well beyond the physiological considerations on which scientific medicine relies. To those who say that their practices or those who utilize them are "irrational," they respond that every therapy is rational insofar as its methods of treatment are logically entailed by its fundamental premises or its assumptions about the nature of disease.

Establishing criteria with which to mediate between competing medical systems is complicated by the fact that the plausibility of the beliefs or assumptions that underlie them are every bit as dependent on sociological factors as on intellectual "proofs." What we consider valid evidence, whom we consider expert authorities, and how we should go about separating relevant from irrelevant information turn not on objective, rational criteria but on the ways we were socialized into one belief system or another. Who, then, is in a position to decide what is an "irrational" medical choice? With what degree of confidence or philosophical integrity can orthodox physicians seek to dissuade persons from seeking alternative treatments? Do persons have a right to what seems to be an utterly ineffective therapy simply because it conforms to their personal belief system?

Alternative therapies may reasonably be expected to demonstrate their benefits to patients and to substantiate the claim that their distinctive healing practices directly cause these therapeutic results. Medical ethics is concerned with protecting persons from intended or inadvertent harm. Well-intentioned tolerance of alternative therapies should not preclude their undergoing rigorous scrutiny. Governmental agencies, health-care facilities, and insurance companies are forced to allocate limited resources and to ensure the welfare of the general public. They must be prepared to make reasonable assessments of alternative medical systems that are based upon belief systems at considerable variance with modern Western science.

Because of the inherent threat that quackery poses to both personal and public well-being, ethical and policy-related judgments must exercise caution and strive for the unrelenting application of "public" (openly demonstrable and subject to empirical scrutiny) standards of evidence. The scientific study of psychosomatic interaction (e.g., of the role of psychological variables in the etiology of ulcers) promises to help practitioners of alternative therapies justify their practices in ways that are more amenable to these standards of evidence. Because psychosomatic medicine has expanded scientific appreciation of the roles nonmaterial factors play in the etiology of illness, alternative medicines now have access to a set of medical categories that will potentially enable them to argue for the therapeutic efficacy of treatments that focus on such nonmaterial factors.

Cases involving patients' desire to be permitted to use drugs before they have received FDA approval testify to the conflict between private needs and the regulation of public well-being. Unlike alternative therapies that are based on different belief systems, unvalidated drug therapies are usually discussed using medically orthodox terms and logic. The ethical concerns here are more frequently about the speed with which regulatory agencies arrive at decisions on potentially lifesaving drugs or the possible collusion of powerful pharmaceutical companies with regulatory agencies to keep competitors from the marketplace. Perhaps the most important consideration in assessing unvalidated therapies is that contemporary medicine differs from its predecessors not because we have become more rational but because we have learned to use the controlled trial to determine the relative merits of competing medical treatments.

Medical systems that are labeled unorthodox because their concerns or treatments are at the periphery of mainstream medicine are reminders that dominant professional groups tend over time to employ predatory tactics to ensure their continued supremacy and keep potential competitors at a distance. These "medically peripheral" systems alert us to the fact that medical science has philosophical and institutional blinders that may close off, rather than open, innovative approaches to human health. The presence of alternative health professionals in the wider system of health care helps safeguard against the kinds of complacency and narrowness of vision that frequently creep into economically entrenched professions. By providing a range of services that address both curative and preventive issues typically neglected by allopathic physicians, many of these alternative therapies contribute to a comprehensive understanding of human health and well-being.

ROBERT C. FULLER

Directly related to this article is the companion article in this entry: ETHICAL AND LEGAL ISSUES. *Also directly related are the entries* UNORTHODOXY IN MEDICINE; HEALTH AND DISEASE, *especially the article on* ANTHROPOLOGICAL PERSPECTIVES; SCIENCE, PHILOSOPHY OF; MEDICINE, PHILOSOPHY OF; MEDICINE, ANTHROPOLOGY OF; *and* BIOLOGY, PHILOSOPHY OF. *For a further discussion of topics mentioned in this article, see the entries* HEALTH CARE, QUALITY OF; *and* LAW AND BIOETHICS. *The topics in this article will find application in the entry* AIDS, *article on* HEALTH-CARE AND RESEARCH ISSUES. *For a discussion of related ideas, see the entries* HEALING; HOSPICE AND END-OF-LIFE CARE; LICENSING, DISCIPLINE, AND REGULATION IN THE HEALTH PROFESSIONS; MEDICAL ETHICS, HISTORY OF, *section on* THE AMERICAS, *articles on* COLONIAL NORTH AMERICA *and* NINETEENTH-CENTURY UNITED STATES, *and* UNITED STATES IN THE TWENTIETH CENTURY; PROFESSION AND PROFESSIONAL ETHICS; *and* PROTESTANTISM. *See also the* APPENDIX (CODES, OATHS, AND DIRECTIVES RELATED TO BIOETHICS), SECTION II: ETHICAL DIRECTIVES FOR THE PRACTICE OF MEDICINE, *especially the* CODE OF ETHICS [1847] *of the* AMERICAN MEDICAL ASSOCIATION, *and* CODE OF ETHICS *of the* AMERICAN OSTEOPATHIC ASSOCIATION; *and* SECTION III: ETHICAL DIRECTIVES FOR OTHER HEALTH-CARE PROFESSIONS, *especially the* CODE OF ETHICS *of the* AMERICAN CHIROPRACTIC ASSOCIATION.

Bibliography

ALCOHOLICS ANONYMOUS. 1955. *Alcoholics Anonymous.* 2d ed. New York: Author.

BYNUM, WILLIAM FREDERICK, and PORTER, ROY, eds. 1987. *Medical Fringe and Medical Orthodoxy, 1750–1850.* Wolfeboro, N.H.: Croon Helm.

CAYLEFF, SUSAN E. 1987. *"Wash and Be Healed": The Water-Cure Movement and Women's Health.* Philadelphia: Temple University Press.

FROHOCK, FRED M. 1992. *Healing Powers: Alternative Medicine, Spiritual Communities and the States.* Chicago: University of Chicago Press.

FULLER, ROBERT C. 1989. *Alternative Medicine and American Religious Life.* New York: Oxford University Press.

GEVITZ, NORMAN. 1982. *The D.O.s: Osteopathic Medicine in America.* Baltimore: Johns Hopkins University Press.

———, ed. 1988. *Other Healers: Unorthodox Medicine in America.* Baltimore: Johns Hopkins University Press.

Hodgeson v. Minnesota. 1990. 110 S. Ct. 2926.

HUFFORD, DAVID. 1988. "Contemporary Folk Medicine." In *Other Healers: Unorthodox Medicine in America*, pp. 228–264. Edited by Norman Gevitz. Baltimore: Johns Hopkins University Press.

INGLIS, BRIAN. 1965. *The Case for Unorthodox Medicine*. New York: G. P. Putnam.

KAUFMAN, MARTIN. 1971. *Homeopathy in America: The Rise and Fall of a Medical Heresy*. Baltimore: Johns Hopkins University Press.

NUMBERS, RONALD L. 1976. *Prophetess of Health: A Study of Ellen G. White*. New York: Harper & Row.

PORTER, ROY. 1989. *Health for Sale: Quackery in England, 1680–1850*. Manchester, U.K.: Manchester University Press.

RABOTEAU, ALBERT J. 1986. "The Afro-American Traditions." In *Caring and Curing: Health and Medicine in the Western Religious Traditions*, pp. 539–562. Edited by Ronald L. Numbers and Darrel W. Amundsen. New York: Macmillan.

Water-Cure World. 1860. Unsigned article. April, no. 5.

WHORTON, JAMES C. 1982. *Crusaders for Fitness: The History of American Health Reformers*. Princeton, N.J.: Princeton University Press.

YOUNG, JAMES H. 1967. *The Medical Messiahs: A Social History of Health Quackery in Twentieth-Century America*. Princeton, N.J.: Princeton University Press.

II. ETHICAL AND LEGAL ISSUES

"Alternative medicine" covers a dizzyingly heterogeneous group of medical theories and practices. Alternatives range from the different forms of faith healing, Christian Science, and folk medicine to allegedly scientific systems like homeopathy, chiropractic, and visualization therapy. Also included under the term are acupuncture; herbalism; iridology; the traditional medicines of India, China, Japan, the Philippines, and indigenous peoples; holistic medicine; naturopathy (treatment using agents or elements found in nature); shamanism; yoga; radiesthesia (therapy based on detection of natural waves of force emanating from nature); color healing; aromatherapy; transcendental meditation; crystal therapy; thalassotherapy (treatment based on sea bathing, sea voyages, etc.); massage therapy; midwifery; and many others. Certain shared negative elements justify lumping together such diverse medical theories and practices. They include marginal social standing or fringe status; exclusion from mainline professional journals and public funding for research; exemption from mainline licensing requirements; and opposition to conventional medicine. The essential ethical and legal considerations raised by alternative medicine are veracity and nonmaleficence. Because false claims of healing efficiency can cause direct and indirect harm to patients, any such claims violate the essential ethical standards of all medical practice, whether alternative or conventional practice.

The meaning of "alternative" and "conventional"

"Alternative" implies alternative to orthodox, regular, mainline, or conventional medicine. These latter adjectives refer to a medical theory, based on modern science, that began to emerge in the Renaissance with medical innovators such as Andreas Vesalius (1514–1564) and Paracelsus (1493–1541), and to scientifically validated medical therapies that blossomed in the twentieth century. If alternative medicine is characterized by an enormous variety of different medical theories and practices with little in common either conceptually or culturally, conventional medicine has the appearance of a single powerful system based on a narrowly conceived biology and focused primarily on the organic needs of sick people. Besides being scientific and materialistic, conventional medicine is also rationalistic: a system that relies on hard data, observation, controlled experimentation, logical argument, and a somewhat outdated view of causality. Alternative and conventional medicine actually help to define one another by contrast and opposition.

What is today classified as either "conventional" or "alternative" medicine was not always so designated. Formerly alternative medical theories and practices have moved into conventional standing; for example, the use of antioxidant vitamins and other dietary remedies for both prevention and therapy (Steinberg, 1993; Stampfer et al., 1993; Rimm et al., 1993). Formerly conventional medicine is now in the alternative category; this includes most nineteenth-century therapies like baths, massage, and purgatives. Between the Renaissance beginnings of modern orthodoxy and its dominance in the twentieth century, conventional medicine was practiced by relatively few university-trained physicians. Most sick people during these centuries got along on remedies developed under older theories. Even university physicians used bleedings and purgings, sweating, and vomiting in addition to quinine and digitalis; not much separated scientific orthodoxy from nonscientific alternative practice when it came to therapeutic interventions. In the nineteenth and twentieth centuries, university-educated physicians established their own medical associations, adopted updated ethical standards, reformed their educational systems, proved that microorganisms cause infectious disease, developed vaccines to control them, employed technologies to improve both diagnosis and therapy, and finally gained legal status for their practice, along with monopolistic control of health-care institutions. The line between a unified, socially supported, conventional medicine and separate, alternative medical practices became much more clearly drawn.

Differences between conventional and alternative medicine are accentuated by a continuing polemic. The term "alternative" is still used by conventional physicians as synonymous with quackery, falsehood, uselessness, and dishonesty. "Alternative" is frequently used to mean foreign or antiquated, or to emphasize the different cultural origins and ancient practices of alternative medicine. In literature favoring alternative therapies, conventional medicine is characterized by toxic and addictive drugs, high costs, aggressive procedures, impersonalness, unnecessary surgeries, economic monopoly, and iatrogenic (physician-induced) illnesses. For their part, orthodox critics create the impression that alternative medicines are products of prescientific cultures, but that conventional medicine is purely scientific and transcends historical and cultural influence.

What constitutes disease and illness, however, as well as how they are understood and treated by any medical system, is necessarily historical and cultural. Contemporary culture's medical–industrial complex, for example, has as much influence on mainline medicine as the military–industrial complex has on modern warfare. Indeed, the historical and cultural content of conventional and alternative medicines is an important consideration wherever legal and ethical issues are addressed. What is ethically right cannot simply be reduced to what is culturally dominant. Cultural dominance does not equate with ethical correctness; minority status or identification with another culture does not reduce to moral incorrectness. Only when cultural and historical factors are identified on both sides can ethical and legal questions about alternative medicine be clearly addressed. Then dialogue can be substituted for hostility and common ethical standards can be developed for both types of practice.

Conventional allopathic medicine: Justifying its preferred status

Conventional medicine today is known as allopathy. This term sets it apart from homeopathy, a nineteenth-century theory and practice that treated disease by administration of minute doses of a remedy that would, in healthy persons, produce the same symptoms as the disease being treated (*similis similibus curantur*). Allopathy, in contrast, is a system that counteracts disease by the use of remedies that produce effects different from those produced by the disease (*contraria contrariis curantur*). Allopathic medicine by definition combats, counteracts, and aggressively opposes specified disease entities. Today's conventional allopathic medicine has its own history and is the product of strong cultural influences. The allopathic approach, originating in ancient Greece with the Hippocratics, was reinforced in the nineteenth century by opposition to the homeo-

pathic alternative. Another important historical influence was a high school teacher from Kentucky, Abraham Flexner, who wrote a book on U.S. medical practice that laid the foundations of what today we call medical orthodoxy.

The Flexner Report, published in 1910, not only criticized medical education and practice in North America but also held up a model of ethical medicine grounded on hard laboratory science and universal laws. For Flexner, ethical medicine targeted disease objects rather than patient complaints, and like engineering was founded upon hard science. Under his influence, nineteenth-century German medicine came to be orthodox medicine in the United States, and a new medical school at Johns Hopkins University was held up as the model for the way orthodox medicine should be taught and practiced. Doctors William Welch (1850–1934), William Osler (1847–1919), William S. Halsted (1852–1922), and Howard Kelly (1858–1943) at Johns Hopkins became the architects of mainline orthodoxy, and all four were products of German training (Ackerknecht, 1982). Because Flexner applied the images of war to medical practice, orthodox medicine became an aggressive, hands-on science. Engineering and military science shaped mainline medical attitudes and procedures, while biology, histology, embryology, anatomy, physiology, pathology, and bacteriology provided the substance of orthodox medical understanding. For Flexner all other approaches were both unscientific and unethical.

What over several centuries came to be orthodox medicine enjoys great power and prestige in so-called developed societies because it alone of the classic professions (law, medicine, ministry) wrapped itself in the mantle of hard science. Alternative medicine is alternative because it lacks that mantle. If alternative medicine is ethically suspect, it is because hard science became the ethical as well as the epistemological standard in twentieth-century culture. Being unscientific or deficiently scientific amounts to being irresponsible in medicine. All alternative medicines are not the same in this regard, but in general, alternative medicine's moral weakness can be traced to an absent or weak science.

Some alternative medicines claim to use "a different science." They adopt the stand that modern science is just another cultural variable or another historical belief system. Some defenders of alternative medicine argue that one cultural variable or belief system is as good as another. No rational grounds exist, they claim, to prefer one medical system to another or to assign to one a greater social and ethical standing. From the fact that mainline science is itself cultural and historical, radical advocates for alternative medicine make their basic argument for equal legal and ethical status. Patients, they insist, must be totally free to make their own choices about treatment. Their argument is strengthened by calling attention to the theoretical flaws in modern science.

Karl Popper's work, *The Logic of Scientific Discovery* (1939 German edition; 1959 English edition), on the concepts of verifiability and falsifiability undermined claims about what is proved in science. He argued that the best science can do is demonstrate what is false, not prove what it true. Later, Popper's claims about falsifiability were themselves shown to be flawed. Then Thomas Kuhn (*The Structure of Scientific Revolution*, 1962) showed how what he called a "paradigm" defines what counts as admissible evidence in science, and how these paradigms change. The foundations, then, on which modern medical orthodoxy bases its claims to ethical and social superiority are strongly influenced by cultural-historical factors.

Modern science and mathematics may have rational and conceptual flaws, but all flaws are not equal. Despite the flawed epistemological foundations of science and mathematics, they still can be used to build bridges that work and spacecrafts that arrive at their destinations. Modern medical science too has real explanatory power. The rigor of scientific explanation, however, is often absent in alternative medicines. Mainline scientific research is much more credible than unscientific and unsubstantiated claims. Admittedly, alternative medicines lack the government funding to carry out sound research, which is expensive, but many alternative medicines ignore research and have unrigorous standards for subjecting therapeutic claims to critical review. If a medicine is ethical and earns preferential social status because it bases its claims and practices on publicly confirmable evidence and continuing critical review, then orthodox scientific medicine warrants the ethical and legal priority it enjoys.

Some alternative medicines

Christian Science. All alternative medicines do not have the same relationship to modern science. Christian Science is an alternative to conventional medicine in the most radical sense: denying the existence of matter as well as disease, illness, pain, and death. Mary Baker Eddy (1821–1910) was a sickly person who had a healing experience in 1866, which she understood as the discovery of Christian Science, a religion centered on healing and health. Her book *Science and Health: With Key to the Scriptures* (1875) is read at all Christian Science services along with the Bible, thereby continuing her healing ministry. It contains her metaphysical beliefs about disease, death, matter, spirit, and God, one famous synopsis of which is as follows:

> *Question.* What is the scientific statement of being?
> *Answer.* There is no life, truth, intelligence, nor sub-

stance in matter. All is infinite Mind and its infinite manifestation, for God is All-in-all. Spirit is immortal Truth; matter is mortal error. Spirit is the real and eternal; matter is the unreal and temporal. Spirit is God, and man is His image and likeness. Therefore man is not material; he is spiritual (Eddy, 1903, p. 469).

Christian Science healing is not like the "miracle cures" of faith healers. Ministers who claim to heal acknowledge the existence of disease and evil, but Mary Baker Eddy did not. Her religion trains "practitioners," who devote their energies to healing in a different sense. They are called upon by believers just as non–Christian Scientists seek out physicians when they are ill. The practitioner talks to people on the phone, visits them at home, and heals by restoring patients to the spiritual plane of thinking that according to Christian Science is reality. Healing, then, is actually reeducation, in which the patient is brought to exchange mental errors and delusions for God's truth and God's reality, where evil, illness, disease, and death have no place.

Christian Science is a radical alternative because it is founded upon a worldview at odds with the theoretical base of conventional medicine. According to this metaphysical theory, disease, pain, sickness, and death only seem real because people believe them to be so, and practitioners heal by stripping away these false beliefs. Conventional doctors in this view are engaged in "unchristian and sinful" activities; indeed, they live in an unreal world. And yet a certain civility characterizes the debate between orthodox medicine and Christian Science. The latter belief system may be too bizarre for most mainline physicians to take seriously. Christian Science apologists, however, tend to be middle-class and well educated, and they respond to objections with reasoned discourse.

This civility has been strained by several legal cases involving parents whose children died after being treated by Christian Science practitioners instead of by conventional physicians. Following the court decisions, calls were issued in the *Journal of the American Medical Association* and *New England Journal of Medicine* for stronger child-protection legislation and stronger penalties for "parents who use the pain and anguish of their children to demonstrate the strength of their belief in Christian Science." Conventional physicians warned against child-neglect legislation in Colorado, Texas, and Louisiana that provides religious exemptions for Christian Scientists. In some places Christian Science has become in effect the legal equivalent of conventional medicine. Mainline doctors object to this as well as to the fact that Christian Science practitioners have legal standing comparable to their own. Blue Cross and Blue Shield pay practitioners in some states, as do major insurance companies and Medicare. Practitioners may even sign certificates for sick leave and for disability payments. According to conventional physicians, this policy creates a double standard. Practitioners, they insist, should be required to meet much higher standards if they are to receive comparable medical responsibilities (and benefits).

In 1989 the parents of a seven-year-old girl were convicted of third-degree murder and child abuse in connection with her death from diabetes. A Sarasota, Florida, jury rejected the parents' claim that they had not sought medical treatment for their daughter because of Christian Science belief. This was the first case in the United States since 1967 in which Christian Scientists were held criminally responsible for relying on the practices of their faith alone to cure a child's illness.

In July 1990, a Boston jury convicted Christian Science parents of manslaughter because they relied on the services of practitioners rather than conventional medical care to treat their two-year-old son, who had died of bowel obstruction in 1986. The parents were sentenced to ten years' probation and ordered to take their other children for periodic medical checkups. This case aroused unusual interest because it took place in Boston, the headquarters of the Christian Science Church. Both cases reflect a pattern in U.S. courts, which have ruled that competent adults have a right to refuse treatment—even life-saving treatment—for themselves, but not for their children. The same response was made regarding Jehovah's Witness children whose parents refuse blood for them based on religious belief.

Official Christian Science response to these decisions has been reserved and moderate. In an official publication (First Church of Christ, Scientist, 1989), church officials recognize that the state has an interest in and a responsibility to protect children against abuse, including the possibility of their being used by parents to prove the strength of their faith. They acknowledge that the death of a child treated by practitioners alone is a tragedy, but counter with examples of thousands of children cured from certified illnesses by Christian Science practitioners and many deaths resulting from treatment with conventional medicine. They also recognize the distinction between unrestricted First Amendment freedom of belief, on the one hand, and restrictions on behavior or acting on belief, on the other. Still, church officials argue against any law that would radically restrict Christian Science treatment of children. Like advocates of alternative medicine generally, they argue for a right to unrestricted practice on the basis of the patient's right not to be interfered with in private matters. It would, however, be more ethically responsible for Christian Scientists to make explicit the childhood conditions where practitioners can cooperate with physicians, instead of forcing parents to make an either–or choice. This same solution could apply to other alternative practices; it would require increased communication and cooperation between conventional physicians and alternative practitioners.

Cases involving children put at risk because of parents' religious beliefs pose questions that can be addressed either by ethics or by law. In the language of ethics, these cases create a conflict between a negative individual right—not to be interfered with in private matters like religious belief and health-care decisions—and a positive societal right or obligation: to protect vulnerable people. Put differently, they reflect a conflict between the principle of individual autonomy and the principle of justice. If the principle of autonomy is respected, justice is compromised, and vice versa.

In the history of Western ethics, individual rights and autonomy concerns are late arrivals—dating from the eighteenth-century Enlightenment period. Societal rights to protect life and the duties of citizens to obey societal norms are much older. Dilemmas involving the two types of ethics are worked out by emphasis on the importance of societal rights and justice, but restriction and limitation of their implementation by reference to individual rights and autonomy. Societal rights (justice) in effect are balanced with individual rights (autonomy), and the only justified degree of societal influence is that which is necessary to accomplish basic justice. In ethical language, the state has an interest not only in justice but in the protection of individual autonomy; therefore it has an interest in balancing the two goods. In legal language it is the balancing of negative constitutional rights—founded on the Bill of Rights (freedom of religion)—and a positive legal obligation of *parens patriae*. The particulars of the legal balancing are worked out through common law decisions in Anglo-Saxon systems. Statutory laws and policies that in effect deny a child access to effective treatment for serious illness can be considered both ethically and legally deficient.

Laetrile.   Alternative medicine is used by most patients for prevention and as an adjunct to conventional treatments. Alternative medicine, however, also flourishes where conventional medicine is weak, inattentive, or an outright failure. When conventional medicine has nothing more to offer and the patient faces death, many people look to alternatives. Cancer at certain stages of development provides a case in point. Because of devastating side effects associated with conventional cancer treatment (chemotherapy and radiation), alternative approaches are particularly attractive. Ten billion dollars is spent annually on unproven alternative cancer treatments, in many cases by affluent and well-educated patients. One such alternative that generated great public debate, court cases, and then finally involvement by the federal government was laetrile, a controversial drug derived from apricot pits and held up as the last hope for terminal cancer patients.

In the 1970s this drug, which had been around for decades, received wide publicity not only because of claims made about its effectiveness but also because the U.S. Food and Drug Administration (FDA) had banned its interstate shipment and sale. This created another conflict between an individual negative right not to be interfered with in choosing treatment and the positive social right to protect vulnerable people against exploitation. In 1979, the U.S. Supreme Court ruled that the FDA could legally inhibit the distribution of the drug, based on the agency's powers to establish "safe and effective" standards; this ruling validated the agency's positive social right. In *Rutherford v. United States* (1979), the Supreme Court remanded the case to the U.S. Tenth Circuit Court of Appeals for reconsideration of other arguments. The appeals court held that the FDA ban did not violate the individual negative right to privacy of cancer patients.

Responding to public pressure, the FDA on January 3, 1980, gave approval for the National Cancer Institute to initiate scientific trials to study laetrile. First, animal studies would be conducted, then stage-one toxicity trials on six human patients, and finally a clinical trial involving 200 to 300 advanced cancer patients who volunteered for the laetrile treatment. The studies were delayed by debate over the money and time required to test an allegedly ineffective drug and over who would perform the tests. Although some alternative practitioners were board certified in conventional medicine, most conventional physicians and scientists resisted involvement with an "alternative" therapy.

On April 30, 1981, the National Cancer Institute announced that it had found laetrile, or amygdalin, to be ineffective as a cancer treatment. The announcement was made at a meeting of the American Society of Clinical Oncology. Over half the patients given the alternative therapy had died and the rest had not responded to the treatment. Charles G. Moertel, director of cancer treatment at the Mayo Clinic, who gave the report, added that he hoped the study would end "the exploitation of desperate cancer patients" by doctors prescribing the drug in twenty-three states where its use was legal despite the FDA ban on interstate sale and shipment. (This apparent contradiction is rooted in the fact that federal regulations are often imperfectly coordinated with state statutes, which may allow the use of federally banned drugs.) Laetrile advocates claimed that the test was rigged and that a less than optimum form of laetrile was used. The contemporary debate over alternative therapies—especially for cancer—continues, although one hears little today about laetrile (Cassileth et al., 1984).

Homeopathy.   Homeopathy originated in Germany at the end of the 1700s in the work of Samuel Hahnemann. By the end of the next century, one in every seven physicians in the United States was a homeopath. The nineteenth- and twentieth-century successes of allopathic medicine considerably reduced the influence of homeopathy. As the limits of allopathic medicine have become better recognized, homeopathy has begun to make something of a comeback. Currently, about 1,500 homeopaths practice in the United States, and medical practitioners use homeopathy in Australia, the United Kingdom, Germany, India, Brazil, and Argentina.

Included under conventional allopathic practices are drug therapies in the process of scientific trial but not yet officially approved (unproven or nonvalidated therapies), and fully approved and scientifically validated drugs being used in novel ways (innovative therapies). Homeopathy uses its own special brand of unproven and innovative "drugs." Homeopathic medicines or remedies are available in many health and natural food stores in the United States. Because mainline pharmacy and professional pharmacists are strongly aligned with the allopathic system and conventional physicians, they have few incentives to become involved with homeopathic practices. Licensed conventional pharmacists would have little understanding of homeopathic preparations and little economic motivation to add these to their stock. Homeopathic pharmacists/practitioners prepare their own medications; a large part of the homeopathic doctors' work involves modifications (dilutions) of these remedies for each individual illness or patient.

If interest in alternative medicine continues, mainline drug stores may begin to carry some over-the-counter homeopathic remedies. Then, presumably, mainline pharmacists will learn about homeopathic background theories in order to explain these preparations to customers. Would doing so compromise the scientifically trained pharmacist's belief system because of the appearance of endorsement? Ordinarily not. Pharmacists as a group learn about natural remedies and understand the importance of patient belief in such products for therapeutic effectiveness. Pharmacists have their own professional code (American Pharmaceutical Association, 1981; see the Appendix) and standards of practice. These would be compromised only if an alternative therapy were known to be harmful.

Visualization therapies.   The biological sciences of orthodox medicine are materialistic (i.e., founded on physical realities and quantifiable data) and are ill-equipped to handle many of the problems listed as disease categories in psychiatry's diagnostic manual (American Psychiatric Association, 1994). A narrowly focused conventional psychiatry relies on chemical therapies and restricts practice to drug prescriptions and medication reviews. Beyond this narrow range of orthodoxy, psychological and social theories have added a broad assortment of nonchemical approaches to conventional practice—from classical psychoanalysis (through cognitive, behavioral, and group treatments) to visualization therapies.

Hypnosis, guided imagery, and biofeedback are all forms of visualization therapy often used in orthodox treatment centers. Practitioners may be conventional physicians, psychologists, social workers, or nurses. The conditions addressed by these techniques include everything from mental and emotional illness to immunological disorders, childhood hyperactivity, and cancer and senility. On the theoretical level, practitioners and advocates work to demonstrate just how the mind controls the brain and immune system (the mechanisms of psycho-neuro-immunology). The effect of biofeedback on psyche (stress reduction) and physiology (temperature, heart rate, blood pressure) is well documented. Advocates of visualization therapies argue that they can enhance the functioning of the immune system. Controversy about this last use of visualization therapies has centered on its scientific status. Whether it will be considered an alternative therapy or an extension of conventional medicine, in the sense that it broadens conventional medicine's positivistic base to include psyche, will depend on whether the visualization techniques can generate satisfactory scientific proof of effectiveness in this important area. Advocates of mainline medicine, such as Norman Cousins, Bernie Siegel, and Andrew Weil, testify to the need for a wider theoretical base for mainline practices, one that includes a place for the mind's influence on bodily healing (Cousins, 1979; Siegel, 1986; Weil, 1993).

Chiropractic.   Chiropractic is probably the best-known alternative medicine in the United States. Practitioners call themselves doctors and complain bitterly about being excluded from mainline medical institutions. The effectiveness of manual manipulations, they insist, is based on scientific studies, but it is difficult for hands-on chiropractic manipulation to eliminate placebo effect and to satisfy double-blind requirements. Back pain could be called the chiropractic specialty, and orthopedic physicians the mainline competition. One double-blind scientific study of the effectiveness of chiropractic versus conventional treatment conducted in 1990 strongly favored chiropractic therapy (Mead et al., 1990). Conventional physicians attacked the study's science, attempting to show that the statistics were unreliable because the study's method was not rigorous enough. Most chiropractors feel discomfort about requiring that any claim of effectiveness satisfy a double-blind requirement, because doing so would throw doubt upon many of their own scientific studies of effectiveness, which are statistical but not double-blind. Some chiropractic medical schools have their own research institutes and are continuously involved in effectiveness or

outcome studies; one example is the ongoing research of the Palmer College of Chiropractic Graduate School in Davenport, Iowa. Despite extensive use of chiropractic in certain parts of the United States, serious dialogue and cooperation with mainline practitioners are limited.

Orthodox public health and alternative practices

No practice has been more orthodox since the nineteenth century than public-health medicine. When microscopic technologies aided in the discovery of bacterial causes of infectious diseases, public-health physicians began energetic application of laboratory science on behalf of societal health. Public-health physicians were laboratory science's strongest advocates. They insisted upon strict quantitive standards of proof for what they considered ethical medical practice. Only what could be shown quantitatively to be effective (e.g., vaccine) commanded their respect and endorsement. Laboratory science alone was the ground for real medicine. They used the police power associated with public health (health laws and their enforcement) to support the narrow positivistic foundation of conventional medicine. Medicine for them was narrowly focused on microbes and they tended to leave broader cultural and environmental issues out of consideration. We know now that an adequate science does not leave ecology out of consideration, and it does not ignore sociocultural influences on behaviors that spread disease.

The new public-health practice requires "cultural competence," that is, an understanding of the culture of the people to whom public-health policies are applied. Ethnic ways, which include particular attitudes and practices related to health and disease, have to be taken into consideration in order to provide the most effective public-health services. Cooperation between conventional physicians and alternative practitioners, we now know, may make the difference between compliance and noncompliance in minority populations.

The World Health Organization has strongly advocated cooperation between conventional physicians and alternative practitioners because neither one is likely to disappear. In the United Kingdom, one in seven people currently visits alternative practitioners. In the Netherlands, a survey of 293 conventional generalists showed that many believe in the efficacy of certain alternative practices: manual therapy, yoga, acupuncture, hot baths, and homeopathy. In Germany, a distinction is made between scientifically supported alternatives such as naturopathy, which stimulates the body's own healing resources, and unscientifically based alternatives. The former are covered by some insurance policies and the state plan pays a subsidy to patients using them. In Norway, a group of conventional physicians and alternative practitioners are meeting to promote closer cooperation (Rankin-Box, 1992).

Because the use of alternative treatments continues to increase both in the United States and in Europe, new studies of alternative approaches have been initiated. In 1993, the National Institutes of Health (NIH) created an office of alternative medicine, where alternative approaches are tested; the public will be kept informed of research results. The U.S. Congress mandated the creation of this project and required that NIH spend two million dollars of its annual budget on it. An oversight committee includes both conventional physicians and alternative practice advocates. They have agreed that alternative practices will be evaluated with the same methods and standards as conventional therapies (outcome research, relative efficiency, double-blind where possible). This is an important development because ethical considerations of alternative practices have to start from reliable information about their effectiveness. This project has added ethical importance because the projects funded require cooperation and collaboration between alternative and conventional practitioners wherever possible.

Ethical standards and alternative practice

Alternative medicine is governed by ethical obligations derived from what medical practitioners of any variety publicly profess and what societies have always required of them: to heal, to relieve pain, to restore function, and to comfort and accompany their dying, when patients are beyond treatment. In the Hippocratic tradition this basic ethical standard was encapsulated in the imperative "to help and not to harm." Late twentieth-century medical ethics talks about the same basic ethical obligation in terms of the principles of beneficence and nonmaleficence.

Alternative or conventional interventions that harm patients without providing offsetting benefits are unethical. Alternative treatments that are harmless may not violate either individual or social ethical standards—especially if patients have strong faith in them or if the illnesses for which they are used are self-limiting and conventional treatments are either expensive, have serious side effects, or have proven ineffective. When diseases being treated are more serious, however, harmlessness is not enough to satisfy individual and social ethical standards. If harmless alternative remedies prevent patients from seeking an effective treatment available from conventional medicine, then individual alternative practitioners would actually be preventing patients from being helped, and just social policy would require that such practice be curtailed. Although alternative remedies are most often adjuvant and complementary to mainline remedies, it remains important to respect the social and professional ethical requirement that treatment actually provide some benefit to patients. Patient benefit is a complicated concept that sometimes involves unquantifiable quality of life considerations, but patient benefit cannot be permitted to slip beyond empirical proof entirely. Societies have to make laws that use rigorous empirical standards for approval of treatment modalities. Anecdotal evidence of therapy effectiveness or claims of effectiveness dependent upon depth of commitment to an alternative belief system are not enough to satisfy basic individual and social medical ethical obligations.

Modern medical-ethical standards add another basic obligation derived from patient rights, that is, that the patient has the right to consent to treatment or to refuse consent. Alternative practitioners, like conventional doctors, are ethically obligated to provide patients with information relevant to their decisions and to protect patients against coercion, fraud, or manipulation. If patients are not competent, informed consent or refusal must be provided by surrogates—either family members or, in their absence, a guardian. Even decisions of competent patients, however, must meet professional standards, so that an irrational choice or insistence upon a treatment that is ineffective or futile or economically devastating might not—perhaps should not—be respected. The modern principle of patient autonomy must be balanced with the ageless principle of beneficence/nonmaleficence, which protects patients against irrational or incompetent decisions that involve harm without offsetting benefit. Care must be exercised, however, in judging irrationality so as not to confuse it with decisions based on value systems different from those of the treating physician or practitioner. Patients have their own values, and these cannot be set aside because they differ from what a scientifically focused specialist may think is organically best for a patient. True patient benefit requires consideration of both personal and scientific interests.

A competent adult may refuse an effective conventional treatment associated with real burden and choose instead an unproven or ineffective alternative therapy. Similar choices, made for children or for incompetent adults without advance directives, however, are neither ethically nor legally acceptable. Justice and autonomy, beneficence and nonmaleficence are broad, abstract ethical standards. Agreement about these standards in their abstract form is possible even in pluralistic and heterogeneous societies. But principles can come into conflict with one another. Respect for patient autonomy may mean not providing patient benefit or violating principles of justice and equality. When such conflict occurs, ethics at a more pragmatic level of discourse is required: concrete norms and rules that attempt to offer compromise, or to effect a balance between the conflicting principles. Working out the relationship between mainline conventional medicine and alternative practices involves just this form of concrete ethics. Appeal to abstract principles only in a situation of conflict between conventional and alternative medicine can turn an ethics discussion into an exchange of slogans. One important test of an ethics that addresses the relationship between alternative and conventional medicine is whether it encourages a needed dialogue between different practitioners and whether it can generate concrete norms and public policies to handle interaction between the two traditions (Eisenberg et al., 1993).

Ethics has been intimately associated with mainline medicine since its beginning in Hippocratic times. Hippocratic physicians were distinguished from other healers not only by their emphasis on science but also by their commitment to patient benefit rather than to selfish goals. Medicine of any variety derives its ethics from obligations generated by a doctor–patient relationship in which a healer commits himself or herself to help someone in need by cure or pain relief or function restoration. Unselfishness and altruism are at the core of medicine's professional ethics. Truthfulness traditionally was not part of medical ethics, but recently it has been added in order to fulfill the obligations associated with patient autonomy. This essential and structural medical ethics is applicable to alternative and conventional medicine alike.

Mainline medicine obliges physicians to high ethical standards but has been weak in policing deviant members and sanctioning ethical failures. Alternative practitioners are not as well organized as conventional physicians, and some lack the strong ethical emphasis of the mainline tradition. Both face a daunting challenge: developing and maintaining the character traits without which concrete moral rules and abstract ethical principles are ineffective, in a new economic climate that encourages profit making more than altruism.

JAMES F. DRANE

Directly related to this article is the companion article in this entry: SOCIAL HISTORY. *Also directly related are the entries* UNORTHODOXY IN MEDICINE; MEDICINE, PHILOSOPHY OF; SCIENCE, PHILOSOPHY OF; *and* BIOLOGY, PHILOSOPHY OF. *For a further discussion of topics mentioned in this article, see the entries* AUTONOMY; BENEFICENCE; HEALTH CARE, QUALITY OF; JUSTICE; RESEARCH METHODOLOGY; *and* VALUE AND VALUATION. *The topics in this article will find application in the entry* AIDS, *article on* HEALTH-CARE AND RESEARCH ISSUES. *For a discussion of related ideas, see the entries* HARM; HEALTH AND DISEASE, *especially the article on* ANTHROPOLOGICAL PERSPECTIVES; MEDICAL ETHICS, HISTORY OF, *section on* THE AMERICAS, *articles on* COLONIAL NORTH AMERICA AND NINETEENTH-CENTURY UNITED STATES, *and* UNITED STATES IN THE TWENTIETH CENTURY; PATERNALISM; PSYCHOANALYSIS AND DYNAMIC THERAPIES; PSYCHOPHARMACOLOGY; *and* PUBLIC HEALTH.

Bibliography

ACKERKNECHT, ERWIN H. 1982. *A Short History of Medicine.* Rev. ed. Baltimore: Johns Hopkins University Press.

AMERICAN PSYCHIATRIC ASSOCIATION. 1994. *Diagnostic and Statistical Manual of Mental Disorders: DSM-IV.* Washington, D.C.: Author.

CASSILETH, BARRIE R.; LUSK, EDWARD J.; STROUSE, THOMAS B.; and BODENHEIMER, BRENDA J. 1984. "Contemporary Unorthodox Treatments in Cancer Medicine: A Study of Patients, Treatments, and Practitioners." *Annals of Internal Medicine* 101, no. 1:105–112.

CLOUSER, K. DANNER, and HUFFORD, DAVID J. 1993. "Nonorthodox Healing Systems and Their Claims." *Journal of Medicine and Philosophy* 18, no. 2:101–106.

COUSINS, NORMAN. 1979. *Anatomy of an Illness.* New York: W. W. Norton.

EDDY, MARY BAKER. 1903. *Science and Health: With Key to the Scriptures.* Boston: J. Armstrong.

EISENBERG, DAVID M.; KESSLER, RONALD C.; FOSTER, CINDY; NORLOCK, FRANCIS E.; CALKINS, DAVID R.; and DELBANCO, THOMAS L. 1993. "Unconventional Medicine in the United States: Prevalence, Costs and Patterns of Use." *New England Journal of Medicine* 328, no. 4: 246–252.

FIRST CHURCH OF CHRIST, SCIENTIST. 1989. *Freedom and Responsibility: Christian Science Healing for Children.* Boston: Author.

FLEXNER, ABRAHAM. 1910. *Medical Education in the United States and Canada: A Report to the Carnegie Foundation for the Advancement of Teaching.* Birmingham, Ala.: Classics of Medicine Library.

FROHOCK, FRED M. 1992. *Healing Powers: Alternative Medicine, Spiritual Communities, and the State.* Chicago: University of Chicago Press.

FULLER, ROBERT C. 1992. "The Turn to Alternative Medicine." *Second Opinion* 18:11–31.

GEVITZ, NORMAN C., ed. 1988. *Other Healers: Unorthodox Medicine in America.* Baltimore: Johns Hopkins University Press.

———. 1991. "Christian Science Healing and the Health Care of Children." *Perspectives in Biology and Medicine* 34, no. 3:421–438.

GREENBERG, KURT. 1991. *Challenging Orthodoxy: America's Top Medical Preventives Speak Out!* New Canaan, Conn.: Keats.

HUFFORD, DAVID J. 1993. "Epistemologies in Religious Healing." *Journal of Medicine and Philosophy* 18, no. 2: 175–194.

KOTTOW, MICHAEL H. 1992. "Classical Medicine v. Alternative Medical Practice." *Journal of Medical Ethics* 19, no. 1:51.

MEADE, T. W.; DYER, SANDRA; BROWNE, WENDY; TOWNSEND, JOY; and FRANK, A. O. 1990. "Low Back Pain of Mechanical Origin: Randomised Comparison of Chiropractic and Hospital Outpatient Treatment." *British Medical Journal* 300, no. 6737:1431–1437.

MURRAY, RAYMOND H., and RUBEL, ARTHUR J. 1992. "Physicians and Healers—Unwitting Partners in Health Care." *New England Journal of Medicine* 326, no. 1:61–64.

PATTERSON, ELIZABETH G. 1989. "Health Care Choice and the Constitution: Reconciling Privacy and Public Health." *Rutgers Law Review* 42, no. 1:1–91.

RANKIN-BOX, DENISE. 1992. "European Developments in Complementary Medicine." *British Journal of Nursing* 1, no. 2:103–105.

RIMM, ERIC B.; STAMPFER, MEIR J.; ASCHERIO, ALBERTO; GIOVANNUCCI, EDWARD; COLDITZ, GRAHAM A.; and WILLETT, WALTER C. 1993. "Vitamin E Consumption and the Risk of Coronary Heart Disease in Men." *New England Journal of Medicine* 328, no. 20:1450–1456.

Rutherford v. United States. 1979. 99 S. Ct. 2470.

SAKS, MIKE, ed. 1992. *Alternative Medicine in Britain.* Oxford: Oxford University Press.

SALMON, J. WARREN, ed. 1985. *Alternative Medicines: Popular and Policy Perspectives.* London: Tavistock.

SIEGEL, BERNIE S. 1986. *Love, Medicine, and Miracles: Lessons Learned About Self-Healing from a Surgeon's Experience with Exceptional Patients.* New York: Harper & Row.

STAMPFER, MEIR J.; HENNEKENS, CHARLES H.; MANSON, JOANN E.; COLDITZ, GRAHAM A.; ROSNER, BERNARD; and WILLETT, WALTER C. 1993. "Vitamin E Consumption and the Risk of Coronary Heart Disease in Women." *New England Journal of Medicine* 328, no. 20:1444–1449.

STEINBERG, DANIEL. 1993. "Antioxidant Vitamins and Coronary Heart Disease." *New England Journal of Medicine* 328, no. 20:1487–1489.

TAVOLARO, KAREN B. 1991. "Effectively and Efficiently Protecting Children in Faith Healing Cases: A Proposed Statutory Revision for State Intervention." *Medicine and Law* 10, no. 4:311–325.

WEIL, ANDREW. 1983. *Health and Healing: Understanding Conventional and Alternative Medicine.* Boston: Houghton Mifflin.

AMERICAN INDIANS

See NATIVE AMERICAN RELIGIONS.

AMNIOCENTESIS

See GENETIC TESTING AND SCREENING, *article on* PRENATAL DIAGNOSIS.

ANENCEPHALY

See INFANTS; *and* ORGAN AND TISSUE PROCUREMENT, *article on* ETHICAL AND LEGAL ISSUES REGARDING LIVING DONORS.

ANIMAL EXPERIMENTATION

See ANIMAL RESEARCH.

ANIMAL RESEARCH

I. HISTORICAL ASPECTS

The history of discussion of the ethics of animal experimentation will be examined by considering first the rise of medical research (physiology and pharmacology particularly), then the emergence and consolidation of opposition to research using live animals. Both developments were shaped by the capabilities and goals of science in every era, but also by the philosophical and religious environments within which science functioned.

The history of animal experimentation

Vivisection—the cutting open of living animals to observe their inner structure and functioning—can be dated to Greek antiquity. The physician Alcmaeon of Croton (fl. 500 B.C.E.) was the first to use vivisection to study physiology, severing an animal's optic nerve and noting the resulting blindness. The Alexandrian practitioners Herophilus (ca. 330–250 B.C.E.) and Erasistratus (ca. 305–240 B.C.E.) relied still more heavily on animal investigations in formulating their physiological theories (Herophilus was rumored—probably falsely—to have performed vivisections on human prisoners). These early studies, however, are better characterized as observation than as true experimentation; inferences about physiological mechanisms were drawn from the structure and position of organs, but the hypotheses were not tested by controlled manipulations.

The Greek Galen (129–ca. 210 C.E.), the most renowned physician of the Roman Empire, was the first to carry vivisection into the realm of methodical experimentation. His ligating of the ureters to show they channeled urine from the kidneys to the bladder, for example, and his serial sections of the spinal cord to establish the relations between nerves and the body regions they served, demonstrated that surgical intervention to control specific functions could yield a deeper understanding of physiological phenomena (Rupke, 1987).

Animal research fell into the same desuetude as most other scientific inquiry during the early medieval period. Ancient scientific traditions were preserved and elaborated upon by Arabic scholars, but not until the later Middle Ages did an experimental spirit revive in the European world. Skepticism about the adequacy of the scientific legacy of antiquity built to a head during the 1500s, culminating for the life sciences in the 1543 publication of *De humani corporis fabrica* by Andrea Vesalius (1514–1564). The first anatomy text based on careful dissection of the human body, Vesalius's work sharply revised the long-accepted anatomical system of Galen (which had been derived entirely from animal dissections), and thus encouraged experimental reevaluation of Galenic ideas in physiology. Vesalius carried out some vivisection studies in order to observe the functioning of anatomical structures, as did other sixteenth-century scientists.

It was the English physician William Harvey (1578–1657), however, who used animal experimentation to make a dramatic break with Galen's physiology. His demonstration of the circulatory movement of the blood was based on observations of the contractions of the heart, ligation of the aorta and vena cava, and other vivisection procedures performed on more than eighty species. Harvey's *De motu cordis* (1628) heightened doubt about the validity of other Galenic ideas and confirmed animal experimentation as an invaluable technique for physiological discovery. Vivisection became a commonplace scientific activity by the latter 1600s; it was used over the next century and a half to investigate such varied phenomena as respiration, pancreatic secretion, and blood pressure (Rupke, 1987; Foster, 1970).

Yet as late as 1800, experimentation was still only one of several approaches to elucidating physiological processes. Drawing conclusions about function on the basis of structure—deducing physiology from anatomy—remained popular, as did a priori theorizing in accord with some physical or chemical model; experimentation might be employed in either of those cases, but only to substantiate the preestablished theory. That overly rationalistic orientation to physiology and medicine was already coming under attack, however, by the philosophe-physicians of the Paris School. Their call for a medicine rooted in empiricism was answered most eagerly and effectively by François Magendie (1783–1855), who from 1809 through the 1820s used animal experimentation to clarify such questions as the mode of

action of strychnine, the mechanism of emesis, and the functioning of the nervous system. Magendie insisted on analyzing function without being prejudiced by anatomical structure, and thereby established irrevocably the superiority of the experimental method for physiological inquiry. (Contemporaneously, researchers at French veterinary schools were developing physiology along experimental instead of speculative lines.)

Magendie's pupil Claude Bernard (1813–1878) employed the experimental method with remarkable success, discovering the vasomotor nerves, the glycogenic activity of the liver, the digestive role of pancreatic juice, and the mechanism of curare's effects on neuromuscular function. But Bernard was equally significant for the compelling philosophical analysis of the necessity of animal experimentation presented in his *Introduction à l'étude de la médecine expérimentale* (1865). There he argued that it was unethical to experiment on human beings, no matter how beneficial the findings might prove for others, if the experiment could harm the subject to any extent whatever. Benefit to others did, however, justify experiments, including painful ones, on animals. The fact that many human lives could be saved by a relatively few animal deaths made the practice of vivisection a "right," he concluded, "entirely and absolutely." Bernard's analysis solidified the recognition of experimental research with animals as an essential practice for medical advance (Bernard, 1865, p. 178; Lesch, 1984; Rupke, 1987; Schiller, 1967, 1973).

At the same time, physiology and other experimental medical sciences were achieving the status of distinct, institutionalized professions. Historically, physiology had been pursued by physicians in whatever time they had left after treating patients or giving university lectures (and also, on occasion, by amateurs of means). The French had taken the lead in making physiology an independent discipline, yet it was in Germany that research physiology bloomed as a new professional field. The nineteenth-century reformation of universities in the German states, with its emphasis on research and the uncovering of new knowledge, led to the establishment of research institutes employing full-time physiologists, along with pharmacologists and other biological experimenters (Coleman and Holmes, 1988). The expectation that research would result in practical medical applications useful to humankind attracted both political and philanthropic support, and ultimately that expectation was fulfilled with the flowering of medical microbiology and immunology in the 1880s. The germ theory was built upon laboratory experiments on thousands of animals; applications of the theory quickly made surgery far more effective and safe, and sharply refined programs for the prevention of epidemic disease.

Louis Pasteur's 1885 discovery of a vaccine for rabies was accomplished by infecting numerous dogs and rabbits with the disease; the research leading to the introduction of diphtheria antitoxin in 1891 involved injecting guinea pigs, rats, and other species with diphtheria toxin. Such breakthroughs allowed experimental medicine to grow by feeding on itself, discovery generating support for more laboratories and scientists, leading to further discovery. By 1900, the German research ethos had established itself throughout the western hemisphere, even in the United States (Fye, 1987). During the course of the twentieth century, the use of animals in research has spread beyond the boundaries of physiology and pharmacology into areas such as psychology, the standardization of drug products, and the testing of food additives and cosmetics. The laboratory animal has become a universal tool and a symbol of medical progress and modern civilization.

The history of opposition to animal experimentation

The laboratory animal has also become, in recent years, the chief object of concern of a widespread and energetic animal rights movement (Plous, 1991). There is a seeming irony in that movement's concentration on the immorality of animal experimentation, for unlike other uses of animals as means to human ends—for food, clothing, sport, entertainment—medical research has yielded unquestionable and inestimable benefits (and not just for people, but for animals as well). When examined historically, however, the focus on medical research becomes understandable, as it was the development of vivisection that most forcefully raised the question "Do animals deserve the same moral consideration as humans?"

Initially, the answer was no. The rapid expansion of animal experimentation during the 1600s did provoke objections, but complaints were the exception, and were usually an experimenter's personal expression of revulsion rather than the product of a moral philosophy condemning cruel treatment of animals (anesthetics were not introduced into surgery, or research, until the late 1840s). The absence of significant opposition to animal experimentation in the seventeenth century has often been attributed to the influence of the French philosopher and speculative physiologist René Descartes (1596–1650), who believed animals to be insensitive automata. Yet most experimenters recognized that animals did indeed feel pain; they simply did not regard the infliction of pain in experiments as cruelty. Physiologists accepted, with the rest of society, that humankind had been given dominion over animals to use as they saw fit. As scientists, furthermore, they considered experimentation the noblest of uses, since the unveiling of nature's design was a moral duty whose fulfillment deepened understanding of the Creator (Guerrini, 1989; Ritvo,

1987; Rupke, 1987). Up to the present time, animal research has continued to be justified on those two grounds: that it is a practical good—it benefits people; and an intellectual good—it enlarges understanding of the natural world.

Those justifications were exposed to increasingly hostile fire during the second half of the eighteenth century. The humanitarian turn of mind engendered by the philosophical and religious emphases of the Enlightenment included a greatly heightened sensitivity to suffering that was readily extended beyond fellow humans to the higher animals. William Hogarth's *The Four Stages of Cruelty* (1750–1751), for example, depicted the barbarous treatment of dogs and cats as the first stage of descent into savagery. The French Revolution's declaration of liberty, equality, and fraternity could likewise be interpreted as applicable to the animal creation. To be sure, the great majority of philosophers believed the exercise of natural rights required rational thought and speech, and thus could be granted only to people. The Enlightenment's abhorrence of pain, however, made sentience a primary consideration for some thinkers. Jeremy Bentham (1748–1832) argued that animals' ability to feel and suffer earned them entrance into the sphere of moral consideration; less well-known writers even insisted that kind handling was a "right" to which animals were entitled. And although the most common criticisms of abuse were directed at the use of animals for food, labor, and sport, explicit attention was occasionally given to experimentation. Samuel Johnson (1709–1784), for one, not only denied that any practical benefits had come from animal research, he maintained that even if there had been a payoff, the gain was ill-gotten, tainted by the torture of innocent creatures. Obtaining knowledge through torment, in fact, was repudiated as ultimately hurtful to society as well, for the callous treatment of animals would harden experimenters' hearts toward human suffering. Through assertions of the inutility, immorality, and corrupting influence of experimentation, philosophical argument overtook aesthetic distaste as the basis of opposition to animal research (Passmore, 1975; Stevenson, 1956).

Philosophical argument matured into political action during the nineteenth century, hardening that triad of objections into the spearhead of an organized antivivisectionist movement. At first, the protesting of vivisection lacked an independent identity; rather, it was subsumed under the broader animal welfare movement, largely because the country where animal protectionist sentiment was strongest—England—was the country where experimental physiology was weakest. Despite Harvey's example of two centuries earlier, English physiologists had come to rely primarily on dissection and anatomical reasoning rather than vivisection. There was too little animal experimentation at home to necessitate a distinct campaign; it seemed sufficient to fire occasional shells at less civilized scientists across the Channel.

By the 1850s, however, English physiologists realized that they had fallen behind their continental counterparts, and that animal experimentation was the key to catching up. Since ether and chloroform had been introduced as anesthetics in the 1840s, vivisection was far less harrowing, and it soon became as common in England as in Europe. Medical experimentation involved any number of species, but dogs and cats were especially common. The keeping of domestic pets had assumed an almost sacred place in genteel British culture during the first half of the century, so even with anesthesia, vivisection could be horrifying. (And not all researchers employed anesthetics, for the drugs sometimes interfered with the experiment.) Animal protectionists could thus still equate vivisection with cruelty, and this invasion of British soil by scientific barbarism provoked a counterattack. The redoubtable Frances Power Cobbe (1822–1904) assumed generalship of the antivivisection forces, mobilizing them, in 1875, into the Society for the Protection of Animals Liable to Vivisection—the first organization dedicated to overthrowing animal experimentation. Parliament, meanwhile, had appointed a royal commission to investigate charges of experimental cruelty, and though the commission discovered no significant mistreatment of laboratory animals, it did recommend that vivisection be regulated by the state. The Cruelty to Animals Act of 1876 resulted, bringing experimenters and their laboratories into a system of registration and inspection, and requiring the administration of anesthesia. The 1876 act was replaced in 1986 by the Animals (Scientific Procedures) Act (French, 1975; Ritvo, 1987; Turner, 1980).

Like so many pieces of legislation, the English Cruelty to Animals Act was a compromise that pleased neither side. Scientists regarded it as an insulting interference with their search for truth; antivivisectionists saw it as a skimpy fig leaf for scientists' arrogance. In truth, many proponents of animal welfare were placated by the requirement of anesthesia, but others noted that the law permitted experiments without anesthetics if drugs would interfere with a potentially valuable study, insisted that the inspection system was inadequate to ensure anesthetics would be used in ordinary experiments, and declared that even when anesthesia was employed, the deprivation of freedom and life suffered by the animals was unacceptable cruelty. The 1876 law actually roused antivivisectionists to more vigorous opposition, because it struck them as official hypocrisy—it claimed to rescue animals from suffering when in fact it gave legal blessing to their confinement and killing.

Objections to animal experimentation now came to be broadcast more loudly than ever, and in other European countries and the United States. Antivivisectionist agitation was stronger in northern than in southern European nations; in America, Henry Bergh (1811–1888) launched an antivivisection movement in the 1870s, but there was no federal legislation regulating animal experimentation until 1966 (Rupke, 1987). The arguments raised against vivisection were not essentially new. As in the eighteenth century, the utility of vivisection experiments was denied, corruption of the experimenters' character was alleged, and, most important, the sacrificing of animals' lives for human benefit was condemned as fundamentally immoral. Ultimately, practical benefits from animal experiments were deemed irrelevant, as sinfully earned as if they had been derived from painful experiments on humans.

Yet it was the supposed utility of vivisection that gave experimentation overriding significance in the formulation of a philosophy of animal rights. If one wished to extend animals the same rights as people, treating them as ends in themselves rather than as means to others' ends, animal experimentation was the purest test case. The ends supposedly achieved by vivisection—saving human lives and relieving suffering—were clearly far worthier than the ends obtained by hunting, trapping, bear baiting, or other forms of animal killing. If the principle of equal rights for animals could be shown to obtain in the laboratory, it would necessarily obtain everywhere else. It was vitally important as well that experimentation was the one form of animal abuse practiced exclusively by educated and refined people, by an elite who should serve as models of civilized behavior for the rest of society. If scientists could not be made to recognize the moral claims of fellow creatures, what hope was there for educating drovers and butchers? The very nobility of the ends of medical research made (and makes) it the most attractive target for animal rights marksmen. Thus Henry Salt's 1892 treatise—*Animals' Rights Considered in Relation to Social Progress*—attacked every form of animal abuse, but singled out medical research as "the *ne plus ultra* of iniquity" (Salt, 1892, p. 102).

By 1900, however, the question of the utility of animal experimentation had blown up in the faces of antivivisectionists, for animal research was finally delivering its long-promised benefits. The newfound power over diphtheria, for so long the gruesome slayer of children, was particularly important for eroding public empathy for laboratory animals. Although concern for sparing animals from pain remained high, support for eliminating experimentation altogether dwindled rapidly as medicine began to save lives, and virtually disappeared with the coming of the wonder drug era in the 1930s.

Antivivisectionist agitation made a dramatic return during the last third of the twentieth century. The extraordinary expansion of government funding of medical research in the post–World War II decades markedly increased the number of animals used in the laboratory (nearly twenty-nine million warm-blooded animals were used for research in the United States in 1978). At the same time, the American and European publics were voicing ever greater dissatisfaction with the impersonal, specialized, high-technology style of modern medical care, bringing the whole medical establishment under critical scrutiny. Finally, just as the political and religious trends of the late eighteenth century generated broad social sympathy for the oppressed, which was then extended to animals, so the late-twentieth-century determination to combat racial and sexual discrimination promoted the revival of concern to be just to all creatures and rid society not only of racism and sexism but also of speciesism. Recent philosophical critiques of speciesism—Peter Singer's *Animal Liberation* (1975) most notably—in fact echo Bentham, asserting that the ability to suffer rather than the power to think should be the criterion for granting moral status to creatures. The plight of laboratory animals has once again become the focus of animal-rights activists, who not only employ all the tactics of nineteenth-century antivivisectionists (organizations, periodicals, lectures, demonstrations) but also have turned to harassment of experimenters, vandalism, and violence.

JAMES C. WHORTON

Directly related to this article are the other articles in this entry: PHILOSOPHICAL ISSUES, *and* LAW AND POLICY. *Also directly related is the entry* ANIMAL WELFARE AND RIGHTS. *For a further discussion of topics mentioned in this article, see the entries* MEDICAL ETHICS, HISTORY OF, *section on* EUROPE; PAIN AND SUFFERING; RACE AND RACISM; RESEARCH, HUMAN: HISTORICAL ASPECTS; RESEARCH, UNETHICAL; RESEARCH METHODOLOGY; RIGHTS; SEXISM; *and* UTILITY. *For a discussion of related ideas, see the entries* AGRICULTURE; ENDANGERED SPECIES AND BIODIVERSITY; GENETIC ENGINEERING, *article on* ANIMALS AND PLANTS; JAINISM; RESEARCH BIAS; RESEARCH ETHICS COMMITTEES, RESEARCH POLICY, *and* VETERINARY ETHICS.

Bibliography

BERNARD, CLAUDE. 1865. *Introduction à l'étude de la médecine expérimentale.* Paris: Ballière.

COLEMAN, WILLIAM, and HOLMES, FREDERIC L., eds. 1988. *The Investigative Enterprise: Experimental Physiology in Nineteenth-Century Medicine.* Berkeley: University of California Press.

FOSTER, MICHAEL. 1970. *Lectures on the History of Physiology During the Sixteenth, Seventeenth and Eighteenth Centuries.* New York: Dover.

FRENCH, RICHARD D. 1975. *Antivivisection and Medical Science in Victorian Society.* Princeton: Princeton University Press.

FYE, W. BRUCE. 1987. *The Development of American Physiology: Scientific Medicine in the Nineteenth Century.* Baltimore: Johns Hopkins University Press.

GUERRINI, ANITA. 1989. "The Ethics of Animal Experimentation in Seventeenth-Century England." *Journal of the History of Ideas* 50, no. 3:391–407.

LESCH, JOHN E. 1984. *Science and Medicine in France: The Emergence of Experimental Physiology, 1790–1855.* Cambridge, Mass.: Harvard University Press.

PASSMORE, JOHN. 1975. "The Treatment of Animals." *Journal of the History of Ideas* 36, no. 2:195–218.

PLOUS, S. 1991. "An Attitude Survey of Animal Rights Activists." *Psychological Science* 2, no. 3:194–196.

RITVO, HARRIET. 1987. *The Animal Estate: The English and Other Creatures in the Victorian Age.* Cambridge, Mass.: Harvard University Press.

RUPKE, NICOLAAS A., ed. 1987. *Vivisection in Historical Perspective.* London: Croom Helm. (Text references to Rupke include articles by several authors in this collection.)

SALT, HENRY S. 1892. *Animals' Rights Considered in Relation to Social Progress.* London: George Bell and Sons.

SCHILLER, JOSEPH. 1967. "Claude Bernard and Vivisection." *Journal of the History of Medicine and Allied Sciences* 22, no. 3:246–260.

———. 1973. "The Genesis and Structure of Claude Bernard's Experimental Method." In *Foundations of Scientific Method: The Nineteenth Century,* pp. 133–160. Edited by Ronald N. Giere and Richard S. Westfall. Bloomington: Indiana University Press.

SINGER, PETER. 1975. *Animal Liberation.* New York: Avon.

STEVENSON, LLOYD. 1956. "Religious Elements in the Background of the British Anti-Vivisection Movement." *Yale Journal of Biology and Medicine* 29:125–157.

TURNER, JAMES. 1980. *Reckoning with the Beast: Animals, Pain, and Humanity in the Victorian Mind.* Baltimore: Johns Hopkins University Press.

II. PHILOSOPHICAL ISSUES

Ethical problems about research on nonhuman animals are grounded in the assertion that animals have conscious experiences, and that their lives can go well or badly for them. Particularly central to the issue is the belief that nonhuman animals can experience pain and other unpleasant or distressing mental states. The seventeenth-century philosopher René Descartes denied this (Regan and Singer, 1989). One or two contemporary philosophers continue to deny it (Carruthers, 1989). On the whole, however, popular opinion and the overwhelming majority of contemporary scientists and philosophers agree that animals, especially vertebrate animals, can suffer (Smith and Boyd, 1991). To take a contrary view, one must now refute not just the common sense of everyday owners of animal companions but also the increasing body of empirical evidence, both physiological and behavioral, suggesting close parallels between animal and human behavior (Dawkins, 1980, 1990; Rolling, 1989; Griffin, 1992). Moreover, these behavioral parallels are supported by the known similarities of the nervous systems of all vertebrate animals, and by the fact of our common evolutionary origin (Rachels, 1990). It seems difficult to believe that despite all these similarities, the nervous systems of human and nonhuman animals operate in radically different ways. From this point, therefore, the existence of animal suffering will be taken for granted.

Before we consider the ethical questions arising from the existence of animal suffering, however, some further information is necessary.

Nature and extent of animal experimentation

Some governments provide detailed information on the number of animal experiments carried out each year. In Great Britain, for instance, annual reports during the 1980s showed between 3.5 million and 5 million animals being used each year. An incomplete Japanese survey published in 1988 reported a total in excess of 8 million. There are no comparable figures for the United States, but in 1986 the U.S. Congress Office of Technology Assessment estimated the figure to be "at least 17 million to 22 million" (Office of Technology Assessments, 1986). Many think that this figure is very conservative, and several unofficial estimates indicate a higher figure. Rats and mice are the most common experimental animals, but dogs, cats, primates, guinea pigs, and rabbits are also widely used (Singer, 1990; Rowan, 1984).

Opponents of animal experiments have focused on examples such as those discussed below (Singer, 1990).

Toxicity testing. From about 1950 until the late 1980s, the standard way of assessing the toxicity of any product was the LD50 (Lethal Dose 50 percent) test. Despite mounting criticism, this test is still widely used (Balls, 1992). The object of the test is to find the dose level that will fatally poison 50 percent of a sample of animals. Often more than one species of animal is used. In the process of stepping up the dose until half the animals die, all of them are likely to become ill, experiencing symptoms like nausea, thirst, diarrhea, stomach cramps, and fever. The LD50 test was routinely carried out on most household products, including food colorings, household cleaners, shampoos, and cosmetics. Many of these products, especially cosmetics and shampoos, are also placed in the eyes of conscious, unanesthetized rabbits, in what is known as the Draize Eye Test. In the late 1980s, following a decade of campaigning against this test, some leading cosmetic companies announced that they had found an alternative to the Draize Test and would no longer conduct tests on animals.

Military testing. It is difficult to find out exactly what happens to animals undergoing military experimentation, but in the United States, in experiments carried out in 1984, monkeys were trained with electric shock to run for hours on a treadmill, and then exposed to lethal doses of radiation in order to see how long the sick and dying animals could keep running (when they stopped, they received more electric shocks).

Psychology experiments. In a psychology experiment performed at the University of Pennsylvania in 1968, dogs were placed in cages with wire floors that could be electrified. Subjected to repeated, inescapable electric shock, the dogs at first jumped, ran, attacked the cage, howled, defecated and urinated; but the shocks continued until the dogs ceased to attempt to escape. The experiment was designed to demonstrate the existence of a state known as "learned helplessness," in the belief that this might throw light on some forms of depression in human beings. From 1984 to 1986, researchers at Temple University used rats in similar experiments with inescapable electric shock; at the same time other researchers at the University of Tennessee at Martin were trying to apply inescapable electric shock to goldfish.

Student use of animals. In schools of medicine and the biological sciences, animals are given to students who are instructed to perform crude surgery, such as removing ovaries, to see how this affects the animals' behavior. There are many equally valuable alternatives to the use of animals in education (Smith and Boyd, 1991; Smith, 1992).

In defense of current animal experimentation

Defenders of animal experimentation emphasize the use of animals in medical experimentation, particularly in areas like diabetes and hypertension research, where the use of animals is claimed to have led to important medical breakthroughs (Paton, 1984; OTA, 1986). They assert that statistics on the large numbers of animals used can be misleading because a great deal of animal experimentation is of a relatively harmless nature (like running a rat through a maze with a reward of food as encouragement to good performance rather than an electric shock as punishment for poor performance). They argue that animal experimentation is the only way to advance our basic knowledge of human anatomy and physiology, and that it offers the best hope of finding cures for diseases such as cancer and AIDS. They may also point out that a considerable amount of animal experimentation is carried out in schools of veterinary medicine to find ways of treating diseases that affect animals. The majority of this work is concerned with farm animals, but some is also directed toward companion animals and wild animals.

If experiments now being carried out inflict substantial suffering on animals, how is this practice to be defended? The usual justification offered is that the suffering of animals is outweighed by the benefits to humans of discoveries that can be made only by the use of animals. Sometimes, however, it is said that the goal of increasing our scientific knowledge is an overriding one, and hence sufficient justification for whatever suffering might be inflicted on animals in the process of advancing toward that goal. Since this goal is not said to justify inflicting substantial suffering on nonconsenting human experimental subjects, however, some further justification is needed to account for the alleged difference in moral status of human beings and other animals.

Behind such arguments lie a variety of philosophical positions. For instance, it may be said that, as related in Genesis, God has given human beings "dominion" over the other animals, to use them as we please. Combined with other theological notions, such as the idea that humans, alone of all animals, have immortal souls, this idea has been influential throughout the Christian world. But it can also be turned the other way: As long ago as 1713, Alexander Pope argued against cruel experiments on the grounds that our dominion requires us to play the role of the good shepherd, caring for our flock (Turner, 1992). More recently a number of Christians have suggested that the gift of dominion should be interpreted as one of "stewardship," which makes us responsible for the care of the nonhuman creation (Attfield, 1983; Linzey, 1987). It remains unclear, however, precisely what follows from this reinterpretation. In particular, does it imply that we are not entitled to use animals in harmful experiments? Or only that we need a strong reason for doing so?

It has also been said, by writers as diverse as Thomas Aquinas and Immanuel Kant, that animals are not "ends in themselves" or that they have no rights (Regan and Singer, 1989). In support of this, it is alleged that the status of a being who is an "end in itself" or has rights belongs only to a being who is rational, is capable of autonomous action, or is a moral agent. This position attempts to equate the universe of moral agents—those *to whom* moral judgments or prescriptions can sensibly be addressed—with the universe of moral patients—those *about whom* it matters, morally, what we do. One possible justification for this equation would be a social contract model of ethics: We have a moral obligation to respect the rights or interests only of those who can reciprocally respect our rights or interests (Gauthier, 1986). This position, however, does not provide any grounds for distinguishing between nonhuman animals, on the one hand, and infants and the profoundly intellectually disabled, on the other. It may be true that many people care more about members of their own species, and hence wish to give infants and the intellec-

tually disabled "courtesy status" as members of the moral community. But what if they do not? A social-contract theory of morality then offers no footing for insisting on equal consideration for the interests of these human beings.

A second possible justification claims that all human beings form a moral community, not because of any implicit contract but because of natural feelings for members of our own species. These natural feelings, it is argued, resemble the natural affection of parents for their own children, which we take as a basis for the special moral obligation we think parents have to give preference to the interests of their own children over the greater interests of the children of strangers. The natural ties between members of a species should, the argument continues, serve as the basis for holding that humans have a greater obligation to other humans than they do to members of other species (Midgley, 1984; Gray, 1991a, 1991b).

If this argument were valid, it is not clear how much experimentation on animals it would justify, since we do not think that parents are justified in causing serious harm to the children of strangers in order to benefit their own children. But is the argument valid? Understandably, those who use these arguments are silent about the obvious case that lies in between the family and the species: preference for the interests of members of our own ethnic group, or race, over the greater interests of members of other ethnic groups or races. It would seem that if the argument works for both the narrower circle of the family and the wider sphere of the species, it should also work for the middle case. If we reject the extension from families to ethnic groups, the further extension to the whole of our species looks very dubious (Singer, 1991).

A utilitarian defense of current practice might be based on the idea that the benefits produced outweigh the harm done to the animals (Paton, 1984; OTA, 1986). Prominent among the claimed benefits is a considerable extension of the human life span. The first important question raised by this defense is how much animal experimentation has helped to extend human longevity. In polemical debates, dramatic claims are often made, but the consensus among those who have studied trends in human health from a historical point of view is that almost all of the increase in human longevity that has occurred over the past century is due to improved sanitation, diet, and living conditions rather than to medical research of any kind, whether on animals or not (McKeown, 1979; McKinlay et al., 1989).

It is possible to accept this verdict but to maintain that medical research, including research on animals, has benefited humans. For example, defenders of the value of animal research often point to the development of coronary artery bypass graft surgery as something that was facilitated by research on animals. The contribution of this form of surgery to the prolongation of life is not clear, but it is more effective than conventional medication in relieving angina, a painful condition that results from coronary artery disease (OTA, 1986). Thus it may contribute to a better quality of life rather than to a greater quantity of life. Against this, it might be claimed that the funds spent on this research, and on the surgery itself, would have been more effective if directed to reducing the cause of the disease by promoting healthier diets and lifestyles.

A second important point to note in considering a genuinely utilitarian defense of current practice in animal research is that the classical utilitarian tradition has steadfastly required us to take all suffering—that of humans and of nonhuman animals—into consideration. The leading nineteenth-century utilitarians—Jeremy Bentham, John Stuart Mill, and Henry Sidgwick—are unwavering on this point (Bentham, 1948; Mill, 1963, 1991; Sidgwick, 1962). Modern utilitarians who cast their views in terms of the satisfaction of preferences, rather than of pleasure and pain, are equally comprehensive in the scope of their theories (Singer, 1993; Hare, 1981). This makes it more difficult to claim that a genuinely utilitarian approach favors animal experimentation in general or as an institution. Nevertheless, some individual experiments—those that do not involve any or very much suffering for the animals, and promise major benefits for humans or animals—may be defensible on utilitarian grounds.

Some seek to justify what researchers do to animals by appealing to a human-centered version of utilitarianism. In the extreme version of this view, the conscious experiences of beings who are not members of our own species do not matter at all. In the more moderate version, these experiences do matter, but they do not matter as much as the similar experiences of members of our own species. Both positions frankly endorse an ethic that is limited to, or biased toward, our own species. Once such an ethic is accepted, of course, the justification of animal experimentation becomes much easier. The difficulty of this position lies in defending such a "speciesist" ethic (see below).

Finally, defenders of current practice often accuse their opponents of inconsistency in objecting to the deaths of animals in laboratories while continuing to participate in the practice of rearing and killing animals for food. The rise of the animal liberation movement in the 1980s has made this accusation less effective because most of those actively involved in this movement have been vegetarians as well as opponents of animal experimentation. In any case, the issue of whether animal experimentation is justified cannot be resolved by appealing to the characters of some individuals who object to animal experimentation.

Objections to current animal experimentation

Critics of the present practice of experimenting on animals tend to divide into two groups: abolitionists and reformers. Abolitionists usually rely on the principle that the end does not justify the means. To inflict pain and death on an innocent being is, they maintain, always wrong. They point out that we do not think that the possibility of advancing scientific knowledge justifies us in taking healthy human beings and inflicting painful deaths upon them; similarly, they say, the infliction of suffering on animals cannot be justified by reference to future benefits, either for humans or for other animals (Ryder, 1983; Regan, 1983).

One weakness in the abolitionist position is that when the end is sufficiently important, most people do think that otherwise unacceptable means are justifiable if there is no other way of achieving the end. We do not approve of telling lies, but most of us accept that politicians should tell lies in order to mislead the enemy when our country is fighting a war we believe to be right. Similarly, if the prospects of finding a cure for cancer depended upon a single experiment, most people would probably think that the experiment should be carried out.

In response to objections along these lines, some abolitionists argue that while a single experiment, taken in isolation, might appear justifiable, the benefits of such experiments do not outweigh the suffering inflicted by the institution of animal experimentation as a whole. One must also take into account, these abolitionists would say, two other factors. First, a large (if uncertain) proportion of experiments are quite worthless; and second, even if no pain or distress is caused by the experiments themselves, experimental animals typically have been raised in conditions that constitute a severe deprivation for a being of that species. The common laboratory rat, for instance, is a highly intelligent animal with a strong urge to explore new surroundings. Rats also like to get into small, dark spaces; yet in most laboratories they are kept in bare plastic buckets with a bit of sawdust at the bottom. Such treatment indicates the lack of consideration for the interests of animals that prevails in the world of animal experimentation; and abolitionists doubt that this will ever change while we continue to regard laboratory animals primarily as tools for research.

Reformers believe that a changed practice of experimenting on animals could be defensible. They demand that any benefits believed likely to arise from the experimentation should be sufficiently probable and sufficiently great to offset the costs to the animal subjects; they urge that every experiment should come under close and impartial scrutiny to determine if this is the case. Reformers point out that although during the

1980s several countries (for example, Australia, Sweden, and Switzerland) developed legally obligatory systems of review based on institutional ethics committee review of proposals to carry out experiments on animals, experimenters are usually well represented on such committees, whereas animal welfare advocates either are not represented or are heavily outnumbered by experimenters. An impartial committee that weighed the cost to the animal in the same way that we would weigh a comparable cost to a human would, the reformers maintain, approve at most a small fraction of the experiments now performed. In other countries, such as the United States, institutional ethics committees exist, but they are not always legally required, and their coverage of animal experimentation is incomplete. Moreover, in the United States these committees do not always have the authority to prevent experimenters from going ahead with painful experiments if the experimenters assert that to alleviate the animals' pain would interfere with the purpose of the experiment (Office of Technology Assessment, 1986; Dresser, 1988; Finsen, 1988; Smith and Boyd, 1991; Gavaghan, 1992).

Among opponents of current practices regarding animal experimentation, the line between reformers and abolitionists is not clear-cut, because questions of long-term goals and short-term strategy also intervene. A threefold division might be more appropriate: In the first category one could place those whose long-term goals do not go beyond better regulation and control of animal experiments to eliminate the most painful and trivial experiments. In the next category would be those whose long-term goal is the abolition of all or virtually all animal experiments, but who consider this an ideal rather than a realistic objective for the immediate future. This group therefore seeks reforms in the interim period, and its short-term goals do not differ significantly from those of the first category. The third category consists of those who aim at abolition and are not interested in advocating anything less.

Although members of these three categories disagree sharply among themselves, they all agree that the present situation is indefensible. They also agree on promoting the use of alternatives to animal experimentation. The use of such alternatives by cosmetic companies to replace the Draize Eye Test has already been mentioned. Opponents of animal experimentation suggest that other alternative methods would be developed more rapidly if they were to receive more substantial government support (Ryder, 1983; Rowan, 1984; Balls, 1992).

The ethical stance of those in the first category, who seek only limited reforms, is often of a relatively conventional kind: They can be thought of as following an "animal welfare" line rather than accepting an ethic of "animal rights" or "animal liberation." They accept that animals may be used for human purposes but want safeguards to ensure that the purposes are serious ones, and that no more suffering occurs than is necessary for the purpose to be realized. Those who take an "animal rights" or "animal liberation" stance want to narrow the ethical gulf that now separates humans from other animals in conventional morality. They thus raise a philosophically deep question with implications that go beyond experimentation, to the treatment of animals in general.

The moral status of animals

In examining the case in favor of current practices, we examined some attempts to justify, in ethical terms, the sharp distinction now made between treatment of members of our own species and members of other species. The problems noted there bedevil all attempts to make the boundary of our species coincide with the boundary of our moral obligations. Although it is commonly said that humans are superior to other animals in such respects as rationality, self-awareness, the ability to communicate with others, a sense of justice, and so on, human infants and humans with severe intellectual disabilities fall below many nonhuman animals on any objective test of abilities that could mark humans as superior to other animals. Yet surely these less capable human beings are also "ends in themselves"; and it would not be legitimate to experiment on them in the ways in which we experiment on animals. (For a contrary view, accepting the moral possibility of harmful experimentation on both nonhuman animals and humans at a similar mental level, see Frey, 1983.)

Ryder, Singer, Regan, and other critics of current practices claim that our respect for the interests of these humans, and our comparative neglect of the interests of members of other species with equal or superior capacities, is "speciesism"—a prejudice in favor of "our own kind" that is analogous to, and no more justifiable than, racism. This argument has widely been seen as the most difficult for defenders of animal experimentation to meet—so much so that one leading philosopher has referred to it as a "won argument" (McGinn, 1991). Certainly the view that species is in itself a reason for giving more weight to the interests of one being than another is more often assumed than explicitly defended. Some writers who have claimed to be defending "speciesism" have in fact been defending a very different position: that the morally relevant differences between species—such as differences in mental capacities—entitle us to give more weight to the interests of members of the species with the superior mental capacities (Cohen, 1986; Leahy, 1991). If this argument were successful, it would not justify speciesism, because the claim would not be that species in itself is a reason for giving more weight to the interests of one being than another. The reason would be the difference in mental capacities, which happens to coincide with the difference in species. But in view of the overlap in mental capacities between some members of the species *Homo sapiens* and some members of other species, it is difficult to see how this argument can be used to defend present practices. In other contexts we insist on treating beings as moral individuals rather than lumping them together as members of a group—it is precisely those who practice racism and sexism who treat all members of a group in the same way (for instance, assuming that women cannot perform heavy physical labor as well as men can), without recognizing individual variation.

Defenders of animal experimentation have sometimes portrayed the animal liberation position in an extreme form—for example, as implying that it is as wrong to kill a mosquito as it is to kill a normal human adult. This is, however, a caricature. Animal liberationists do not claim that all animals have the *same* interests, only that interests are not to be given less consideration merely on the grounds of species. Thus it is quite compatible with the animal liberation view to say that the interests of beings with different mental capacities will vary, and that these variations will be morally significant. If we are forced to choose between saving the life of a being who understands the meaning of death and wants to go on living, and a being who is not capable of having desires for the future because the being's mental capacities do not enable it to grasp that it is a "self," a mental entity existing over time, then it is entirely justifiable to choose in favor of the being who wants to go on living. This is a choice based on mental capacity and not on species membership (as we can see by the fact that the former being may be a chimpanzee and the latter a human with profound brain damage) (Singer, 1990).

At least one controversial scientist who experiments on animals has attempted to sweep aside such issues by denying that animal experimentation raises a moral issue at all. Robert J. White, whose own work has involved keeping severed monkeys' heads alive and apparently conscious for as long as possible, has written that "the inclusion of lower animals in our ethical system is philosophically meaningless" (White, 1971, p. 507). Unfortunately, White does not explain why (to take only one example) the clear proposal of utilitarian writers—that pain as such is an evil, whatever the species of the being that suffers it—is devoid of meaning. It may be difficult to compare the suffering of a human and, say, a rabbit; but sometimes rough comparisons can be made. It seems undeniable that to put into the eye of a rabbit a chemical that causes the eye to blister or be-

come ulcerated is to do more harm to the rabbit than we would do to any number of human beings by denying them the possibility of choosing a new type of shampoo that can be marketed only if the chemical is tested in this way. When such rough comparisons can be made, the mere fact that rabbits are "lower animals" is no reason to give less weight to their suffering.

Seen in this light, the argument that restricting experiments on animals interferes with scientific freedom and medical progress also appears less conclusive. We do not grant scientists the freedom to experiment at will on humans, although such experiments would do more to advance our knowledge of human physiology and be more likely to find cures for human diseases than would animal experiments. It would seem, therefore, to be incumbent upon the defenders of experiments on animals to show that there is a relevant difference between *all* humans and other animals that justifies experiments on the latter but not the former; but success at this task still eludes the defenders of animal experimentation.

Conclusion

Controversy over experiments on animals has often been polarized, and—especially in the United States—public exchanges between those who carry out animal experiments and those who oppose them have scarcely risen above the level of abuse. There has been a more serious discussion of the status of animals in the philosophical journals and in books by philosophers, and it can only be hoped that this level of discussion will eventually influence the more popular debate over the use of animals in research.

PETER SINGER

Directly related to this article are the other articles in this entry: HISTORICAL ASPECTS, *and* LAW AND POLICY. *Also directly related is the entry* ANIMAL WELFARE AND RIGHTS. *For a further discussion of topics mentioned in this article, see the entries* AGRICULTURE; AIDS; ETHICS, *article on* RELIGION AND MORALITY; INFANTS; LIFESTYLES AND PUBLIC HEALTH; MEDICAL EDUCATION; PAIN AND SUFFERING; PUBLIC HEALTH, *article on* DETERMINANTS OF PUBLIC HEALTH; RESPONSIBILITY; RIGHTS; UTILITY; *and* VETERINARY ETHICS. *For a discussion of related ideas, see the entries* CONFLICT OF INTEREST; GENETIC ENGINEERING, *article on* ANIMALS AND PLANTS; JAINISM; ORGAN AND TISSUE PROCUREMENT; ORGAN AND TISSUE TRANSPLANTS; *and* XENOGRAFTS.

Bibliography

ATTFIELD, ROBIN. 1983. *The Ethics of Environmental Concern.* Oxford: Basil Blackwell.

BAIRD, ROBERT, and ROSENBAUM, STUART E., eds. 1991. Animal Experimentation: The Moral Issues. Buffalo, N.Y.: Prometheus.

BALLS, MICHAEL. 1992. "Time to Reform Toxic Tests." New Scientist, 2 May, pp. 31–33.

BENTHAM, JEREMY. 1948. [1789]. An Introduction to the Principles of Morals and Legislation. New York: Hafner.

CARRUTHERS, PETER. 1989. "Brute Experience." Journal of Philosophy 86:258–269.

COHEN, CARL. 1986. "The Case for the Use of Animals in Biomedical Research." New England Journal of Medicine 315:865–870.

DAWKINS, MARIAN STAMP. 1980. Animal Suffering: The Science of Animal Welfare. London: Chapman and Hall.

———. 1990. "From an Animal's Point of View: Motivation, Fitness and Animal Welfare." Behavioral and Brain Sciences 13:1–61.

DRESSER, REBECCA. 1988. "Standards for Animal Research: Looking at the Middle." Journal of Medicine and Philosophy 13:123–143.

FINSEN, LAWRENCE. 1988. "Institutional Animal Care and Use Committees: A New Set of Clothes for the Emperor?" Journal of Medicine and Philosophy 13:145–158.

FREY, RAY G. 1983. "Vivisection, Morals and Medicine." Journal of Medical Ethics 9, no. 2:94–97.

GAUTHIER, DAVID. 1986. Morals by Agreement. Oxford: Oxford University Press.

GAVAGHAN, HELEN. 1992. "Animal Experiments the American Way." New Scientist, 16 May, pp. 32–36.

GRAY, JEFFREY. 1991a. "On the Morality of Speciesism." Psychologist 4, no. 5:196–198.

———. 1991b. "On Speciesism and Racism: Reply to Singer and Ryder." Psychologist 4, no. 5:202–203.

GRIFFIN, DONALD. 1992. Animal Minds. Chicago: University of Chicago Press.

HARE, RICHARD M. 1981. Moral Thinking: Its Levels, Method, and Point. Oxford: At the Clarendon Press.

LEAHY, MICHAEL P. T. 1991. Against Liberation: Putting Animals in Perspective. London: Routledge.

LINZEY, ANDREW. 1987. Christianity and the Rights of Animals. London: Society for the Propagation of Christian Knowledge.

MCGINN, COLIN. 1991. "Eating Animals Is Wrong." London Review of Books, 24 January, pp. 14–15.

MCKEOWN, THOMAS. 1979. The Role of Medicine: Dream, Mirage or Nemesis? Oxford: Basil Blackwell.

MCKINLAY, JOHN B.; MCKINLAY, SONIA M.; and BEAGLEHOLE, ROBERT. 1989. "Trends in Death and Disease and the Contribution of Medical Measures." In Handbook of Medical Sociology, pp. 14–15. 4th ed. Edited by Howard E. Freeman and Sol Levine. Englewood Cliffs, N.J.: Prentice-Hall.

MIDGLEY, MARY. 1984. Animals and Why They Matter. Athens: University of Georgia Press.

MILL, JOHN STUART. 1963–1991. Collected Works. Edited by John M. Robinson and Jack Stillinger. 33 vols. Toronto: University of Toronto Press.

PATON, WILLIAM. 1984. Man and Mouse: Animals in Medical Research. Oxford: Oxford University Press.

RACHELS, JAMES. 1990. Created from Animals: The Moral Implications of Darwinism. Oxford: Oxford University Press.

REGAN, TOM. 1983. The Case for Animal Rights. Berkeley: University of California Press.

REGAN, TOM, and SINGER, PETER, eds. 1989. [1976]. Animal Rights and Human Obligations. 2d ed. Englewood Cliffs, N.J.: Prentice-Hall.

ROLLIN, BERNARD. 1989. The Unheeded Cry: Animal Consciousness, Animal Pain, and Science. Oxford: Oxford University Press.

ROWAN, ANDREW. 1984. Of Mice, Models and Men: A Critical Explanation of Animal Research. Albany: State University of New York Press.

RYDER, RICHARD D. 1983. [1975]. Victims of Science: The Use of Animals in Research. London: National Anti-Vivisection Society.

SHARPE, ROBERT. 1988. The Cruel Deception: The Use of Animals in Medical Research. Wellingborough, U.K.: Thorsons.

SIDGWICK, HENRY. 1963. [1907]. The Methods of Ethics. 7th ed. London: Macmillan. First published 1874.

SINGER, PETER. 1990. [1975]. Animal Liberation. 2d ed. New York: New York Review of Books/Random House.

———. 1991. "Speciesism, Morality and Biology: A Response to Jeffrey Gray." Psychologist 4, no. 5:199–200.

———. 1993. [1979]. Practical Ethics. 2d ed. Cambridge: Cambridge University Press.

SMITH, JANE A. 1992. "Dissecting Values in the Classroom." New Scientist, 9 May, pp. 31–35.

SMITH, JANE A., and BOYD, KENNETH M. 1991. Lives in the Balance: The Ethics of Using Animals in Bio-medical Research: The Report of a Working Party of the Institute of Medical Ethics. Oxford: Oxford University Press.

TURNER, ERNEST S. 1992. [1964]. All Heaven in a Rage. Fontwell, U.K.: Centaur Press.

U. S. CONGRESS. OFFICE OF TECHNOLOGY ASSESSMENT(OTA). 1986. Alternatives to Animal Use in Research, Testing and Education. Washington, D.C.: U.S. Government Printing Office.

WHITE, ROBERT J. 1971. "Anti-Vivisection: The Reluctant Hydra." American Scholar 40, no. 3:503–512.

III. LAW AND POLICY

This article describes the laws and policies of the United States governing the care and use of animals in research, education, and testing; the history of these policies and laws since 1966; the issues addressed by these laws; and the lawsuits that have followed publication of regulations implementing these laws. Two federal laws govern the use of animals: the Health Research Extension Act of 1985 (P.L. 99-158), and the Animal Welfare Act, (7 U.S.C. 2131–2159, 1993), as amended. While all states have laws governing the care of animals, research usage is often exempted. Twenty states have simple facility licensure and a few have only very general regulations governing research usage of animals. In reality, nearly all states defer to federal law in this area. Public Health Service Policy on Humane Care and Use of Laboratory Animals (PHS policy) implements P.L. 99-158 for all activities conducted or supported by the PHS involving animals, while regulations implementing the Animal Welfare Act are in 9 CFR, Subchapter A, Parts 1, 2, and 3 (animal-welfare regulations, or AWRs). The PHS includes fourteen health agencies within the Department of Health and Human Services (DHHS).

History of Public Health Service policy

Regulations have been promulgated by the PHS since 1935, originally through one of its constituents, the National Institutes of Health (Whitney, 1987). NIH guidelines have provided direction and recommendations for caring for and using laboratory animals at NIH. Subsequently, in 1963, the *Guide for the Care and Use of Laboratory Animals* (NRC guide) was written by a committee of laboratory scientists assembled by the Institute of Laboratory Animal Resources of the National Research Council and has become the standard guide in the field. The first policy based upon the 1963 NRC Guide came from NIH in 1971. PHS published its first policy on animal care in 1973, with revisions in 1973, 1979, and 1986. Each successive revision increased the specificity and level of responsibility of animal-care committees in the supervision of animal use.

At the outset of NIH policymaking in animal care and use in 1971, all institutions and organizations using warm-blooded animals for the purpose of research or other projects supported by NIH were required to give assurances that facilities for animals met "acceptable standards for the care, use, and treatment of such animals." This assurance could be met either by a recognized professional laboratory-accrediting body (such as the American Association for the Accreditation of Laboratory Animal Care [AAALAC]) or by establishing a committee to evaluate the care and housing of animals used for NIH-sponsored activities. Institutions were also obligated to follow pertinent sections of the Animal Welfare Regulations. In 1973, the 1971 NIH policy was replaced by the first of the PHS policies. Like the NIH policy preceding it, the 1973 PHS policy required institutions either to be fully accredited or to have a standing institutional committee with a minimum of three members including a veterinarian for those institutions using a "significant" number of animals. The charge of these committees was required periodic facility inspection and optional review of applications and proposals involving the use of animals.

The 1979 revision to the PHS policy required all institutions using animals, regardless of numbers used and accreditation status, to have a standing committee whose responsibility was oversight of the institution's animal-care program. In addition to the establishment of a committee of at least five members including one veterinarian, the institution was obligated to establish a mechanism to review its facilities for warm-blooded animals for adherence to the principles contained in the NRC Guide. The PHS policy recommended that AAALAC accreditation was the best means of satisfying this obligation, although periodic committee review of facilities and animals' care would suffice. Absent from the 1979 PHS policy was the requirement for review of individual proposals or projects, although review was encouraged. In 1986, however, the PHS policy was revised again, this time requiring specific organizational and supervisory responsibilities for the animal-care committees of institutions in an effort to strengthen the system of institutional assurance.

History of animal welfare regulations

In 1966, *Life* magazine ("Concentration Camps," 1966) and other publications dramatized poor care and treatment of animals by some dealers who sold animals for biomedical research. This disclosure and the ensuing public outcry resulted in the introduction of twenty-nine bills in Congress relating to the regulation of animal research. The bill that eventually became law was the Laboratory Animal Welfare Act of 1966 (LAWA, shortened after its first amendment to AWA in 1970), which was limited to regulation of the sale and transportation of animals by dealers and the holding of animals by certain research facilities. Although the bill was passed, it was a compromise between far-reaching legislation and none at all; it did not apply to actual research usage of animals. The regulations implementing the LAWA specified that the housing facility provide shelter and protection from temperature extremes, that food and water be provided at least daily, and that cages be of a certain size and cleaned daily. These regulations also specified cage sizes and frequency of feeding and watering during transportation. Passage of amendments to the AWA in 1970, 1976, 1985, and 1989 and passage of a law calling for the PHS policy extended federal regulations into areas covering the appropriate use and humane treatment of laboratory animals.

The 1970 amendments of the AWA broadened the U.S. Department of Agriculture's (USDA) administrative responsibility to cover animal care throughout an animal's stay in research facilities, including the period during which research was being conducted. The 1976 amendments to the AWA brought transportation carriers under the purview of the act, leading to more stringent standards for shipment of animals. The 1985 version of the AWA invested the USDA with responsibility for issuing and enforcing regulations regarding humane care, handling, and treatment of animals. Animals covered under the AWA include warm-blooded animals such as dogs, cats, monkeys, guinea pigs, hamsters, rabbits, marine mammals, and normally wild animals, any of which are being used for research, testing, experimentation, exhibition purposes, or as a pet. Excluded from coverage by the act are birds, rats, mice, and horses and other farm animals intended for use as food or fiber, or for use in improving animal nutrition, breeding, or management. The 1989 changes to the act added college-student work with animals to the list of areas over which a research institution has oversight responsibility.

Public Health Service policy

PHS policy requires that each awardee institution provide a written assurance setting forth how that institution will comply with regulations. This assurance then forms the basis for the care and use of animals in research, education, and testing at that institution and is the basis for judging the adequacy of the institution's compliance with policy. PHS policy calls for the establishment of a program for animal care and use, using the NRC guide as a basis for developing the program. PHS policy requires the creation of an Institutional Animal Care and Use Committee (IACUC), appointed by the chief executive officer of the institution. This committee must have at least five members, including at least one veterinarian experienced in laboratory animal science, one scientist, one lay person, and one person unaffiliated with the institution. Policy then charges this committee with oversight responsibility for semiannual review of the program of animal care and use; for semiannual inspection of facilities; for review of research protocols, or proposals, for the use of animals; for investigation of all concerns raised by anyone regarding the humane use of animals at the institution; for recommendations for personnel training; and for suspension of activities deemed improper.

An institution's program for the care and use of laboratory animals encompasses institutional policies, laboratory-animal husbandry procedures, and veterinary care practices. Institutional policies address such personnel provisions as veterinary qualifications, procedures for handling hazardous agents safely, occupational health and personal hygiene including appropriate clothing and practices, prohibition of smoking and eating in animal rooms, and such special considerations as policy concerning prolonged physical restraint of animals and multiple surgeries on a single animal. Laboratory animal husbandry procedures include housing systems (size of cages and provision for social interaction among animals where appropriate), temperature, humidity, ventilation, lighting control, cage and room sanitation schedules, and methods of animal identification and of clinical recordkeeping. Veterinary care programs address preventive-medicine strategies, methods for detecting and treating diseases, giving investigators advice about appropriate anesthesia, analgesia, surgical and postoperative care, and methods of euthanasia.

Facility inspection covers not only visiting the physical plant but also assessing the health of the animals and reviewing portions of the institutional program for animal care. The physical plant should be properly constructed to house the species being used and to permit sterile surgery to be performed, if necessary. The inspections of the physical plant and the review of the institutional program must be conducted semiannually by the IACUC.

PHS policy sets forth several criteria to be followed by the IACUC in reviewing protocols. These criteria go beyond mere care and housing guidelines. The care and use of animals in proposed research must be consistent with the NRC guide unless acceptable scientific justification is provided for any deviation. The investigator must explain the rationale for using animals at all in the proposed research as well as the appropriateness of the species to be used, the number of animals, and their proposed use. PHS policy stipulates requirements for the use of sedatives, analgesics, and anesthetics if the proposed procedure might cause more than slight pain or distress; it also requires prompt euthanasia at the end of (or, when appropriate, during) a procedure, and imposes methods of euthanasia consistent with American Veterinary Medical Association (AVMA) guidelines (Panel on Euthanasia, 1993). All personnel involved in the use of animals in research must be appropriately trained and qualified in the procedures to be employed in the experiment.

Each IACUC must have procedures for investigating concerns raised about the care and use of animals at the institution. In addition, the IACUC must ensure that the institution has a training program for both animal-care staff (people actually caring for the animals) and research staff; videotapes and training handbooks may be used to satisfy this requirement. The final charge—power to suspend an improperly conducted activity—must come from an official of the institution such as the chief executive officer or the vice president. Without this official support, the IACUC cannot fulfill its duty to ensure compliance with PHS policy.

Several features of PHS policy are of special importance. While its legal force is restricted to awardee institutions, its scope includes all live vertebrates. It was the first U.S. law to call for a consideration of animal welfare during a procedure and to call for the establishment of a committee to review protocols for the appropriateness of design, the importance of knowledge sought (as set forth in U.S. Government Principles for the Utilization and Care of Vertebrate Animals Used in

Testing Research and Training, published in both the PHS policy and the NRC guide), and the competency of personnel. Thus, a committee has been created to review use of animals in research much like committees that review the participation of humans in research.

Animal-welfare regulations

Animal-welfare regulations (AWRs) pertaining to the care and use of laboratory animals were extensively modified and rewritten following the 1985 amendments of the Animal Welfare Act to include provisions for an IACUC, for protocol review, and for more social interaction among the same species and between animals and their caretakers. These regulations are similar to PHS policy provisions since the secretary of USDA was directed to consult with the secretary of DHHS concerning the writing of regulations. An IACUC committee with only slight differences from PHS policy is required (e.g., three members instead of five as a minimum, including an unaffiliated member and a veterinarian). The duties of the committee are very similar to the duties specified by PHS policy; instructions for reviewing protocols, however, are more detailed than is required by PHS policy. AWRs require the investigator to search for alternatives to any procedure that may cause more than slight pain or distress and to assure that the proposed activity does not unnecessarily duplicate previous work. Several aspects of a personnel-training program are specified. In contrast to PHS policy, which requires institutions to develop an animal care and use program based upon the NRC guide, the AWRs have an extensive set of standards specifying the humane handling, care, treatment, and transport of various species of animals. The standards section of the regulations detail facility and operating standards, animal health and husbandry standards, and transportation standards for each regulated species. In addition, detailed specifications are given for marking dogs, cats, and other animals for the purpose of identification. In most, but not all, cases, AWRs standards are the same as those of the PHS policy and, thus, are similar to the guidelines given in the NRC guide.

The AWA calls for the USDA to issue regulations in several areas. These regulations, which have engendered considerable public debate as well as the filing of a lawsuit, require exercise of dogs and the provision of a physical environment adequate to promote the psychological well-being of nonhuman primates. After considerable debate, the final regulations combined performance-based standards (standards that specify the desired outcome and leave the details of achieving that outcome to the regulated party) with design or engineering standards (standards that specify in measurable and objective terms how a particular outcome is to be achieved). It is the choice of performance-based standards that is especially controversial since plaintiffs in a lawsuit (see below) have alleged that they allow too much latitude for compliance by the regulated parties. However, it is generally true that humane care and use of animals can be achieved under a variety of circumstances, making it difficult to use detailed engineering standards or specifications. For example, the regulations call for dry floors for most mammals. This can be accomplished by mopping the floor until dry, by wet-vacuuming the floor, by sloping the floor and letting water run off before placing an animal on the surface, and so on. Thus, there are a number of ways of achieving the desired goal, and it is the outcome itself that is specified rather than the steps needed to reach it. Critics of performance standards state that the goal often is not well described, leaving too much discretion to the regulated parties.

Another controversial aspect of the AWRs is that the regulatory definition of animal excludes birds, rats, and mice that have been bred for use in research; hence, these animals are not protected under the AWRs. The exclusion is a major one because more than 85 percent of animals used in research, education, and testing are rats, mice, and birds. The reason for the exclusion is to limit the scope and cost of annual USDA inspections; there are barely sufficient numbers of inspectors to review facilities and procedures involving larger vertebrate animals, whose use is thought to require more sensitivity and therefore more intense scrutiny. Adding rats, mice, and birds to the mandatory inspection list would exceed the capacity of the USDA, both because of the increased numbers of animals to be inspected and because there would be an increase in the number of registered research facilities requiring inspection. (A number of institutions use only rats and/or mice and therefore are not subject to inspection.) Because PHS policy defines "animal" as any vertebrate (with no exclusions), rats, mice, and birds are covered by PHS policy. In institutions not covered by PHS policy (e.g., industry and colleges not receiving PHS funds), the use of rats and mice remains largely unregulated, a glaring oversight unique to the United States (Orlans, 1993).

Protocol review: Consideration of pain and distress and numbers of animals used

Since both PHS policy and AWRs explicitly require minimization of pain and distress of animals during research, there have been examinations of the implications and possible effectiveness of the IACUC consideration of these issues during protocol review (Dresser, 1988; Brody, 1989). Both regulations attempt to incorporate cost–benefit considerations, utilitarian theory, and some elements of a modified rights-based philosophy

(Dresser, 1988). The success of PHS policy and AWRs depends fundamentally upon the recognition that animals can experience pain and distress that can be alleviated (Institute of Laboratory Animal Resources, 1992). USDA requires an annual report from all registered institutions that lists numbers of animals used in research and testing, classified by the degree of pain and distress: (1) minimal, transient, or no pain or distress; (2) pain and distress relieved by anesthetics, analgesics, or tranquilizers; and (3) pain and distress not treated. A detailed statement on category 3 procedures is required, including scientific justification for withholding drugs. Another classification scheme, developed by Scientists Center for Animal Welfare (SCAW), lists six categories instead of three (Orlans, 1987). Many IACUCs use some classification scheme for pain and distress, applying the three Rs (replacement, reduction, and refinement) of William Russell and Rex Burch (1992), to reduce the number of animals used in research that falls in the higher categories of pain and distress.

Some observers feel that IACUC review does not adequately reduce the number of animals used in research, or the pain and distress of these animals. Mimi Brody (1989) has suggested new legislation that would implement two levels of review, first by a local committee and then by a national committee, to review those uses of animals with "high ethical cost." Gary Francione (1990) has maintained that open IACUC meetings, publicly announced and attended by interested members of the community, would improve the quality of protocol review. The two-committee approach has the disadvantage of delaying approval of certain types of research and has the potential for becoming excessively bureaucratic. The open-meetings approach presumes that the general public could comprehend the scientific details of described procedures and would be able to judge the ethical and social justifications for the proposed procedure.

Lawsuits concerning the animal-welfare regulations

The definition of animals in the AWRs excludes birds, rats, and mice specifically bred for use in research. After parts 1 and 2 of the AWRs became final in 1989, the Animal Legal Defense Fund (ALDF) and the Humane Society of the United States (HSUS) filed a rule-making petition with the USDA to amend the regulations to include rats, mice, and birds in the definition of animals. After the USDA denied the petition in 1990, ALDF and HSUS brought suit in federal court, seeking a declaratory judgment and an injunction preventing the USDA from excluding coverage of rats, mice, and birds. In 1992, ALDF and HSUS were granted summary judgment, and the USDA was ordered to reconsider its denial of plaintiffs' petition in light of the court's opin-

ion holding the exclusion of rats, mice, and birds to be arbitrary and capricious (*Animal Legal Defense Fund* v. *Madigan*, 1992). The USDA appealed, and on May 20, 1994, the court of appeals vacated the district court's decision and directed the lower court to dismiss, holding that none of the petitioners had demonstrated both constitutional standing to sue and a statutory right to judicial review under the Administrative Procedure Act—leaving regulations, and presumably practice, to stand unchanged (*Animal Legal Defense Fund* v. *Espy*, 1994).

The USDA regulations concerning requirements for exercise of dogs and for a physical environment adequate to promote the psychological well-being of nonhuman primates were published in February 1991. ALDF and others sued, alleging that these regulations did not comply with the 1985 amendments of the AWA because they did not provide minimum standards for exercise of dogs and for adequate cage size and environmental enrichment for nonhuman primates as required by the U.S. Congress. The district court granted plaintiffs' motion for summary judgment in February 1993 (*Animal Legal Defense Fund* v. *Secretary of Agriculture*, 1993). It was unclear at the time of this decision whether the federal government would appeal this decision, so the National Association for Biomedical Research (NABR) moved to intervene in the case to ensure an appeal. Although the NABR motion was originally denied, the denial was reversed by the court of appeals. The federal government subsequently decided to pursue an appeal and the consolidated appeal was argued on May 12, 1994. On July 22, 1994, the court of appeals vacated the district court's decision and directed the lower court to dismiss, concluding that the ALDF and the other appellees lacked standing to challenge USDA regulations as argued in the case discussed above, again leaving policy unchanged.

Conclusion

Federal laws and policies regarding the use of animals in research, education, and testing have progressed rapidly from the first enunciation of principles for the care of laboratory animals in the early days of NIH and the first animal-welfare laws passed in 1966. Early policy had limited impact on the use of animals due to generally careful practice standards already in place and to lack of enforcement of new policy. Several U.S. programs and institutions had their funding suspended in the early 1980s, serving as a warning that all animal-care policies must be followed (Rozmiarek, 1987). The evolution of policies for animal care and use shows a trend toward increased responsibility and supervision for IACUCs, with greater emphasis on the level of assurances institutions must give, on IACUC membership, on the process of protocol review, and on the committee's power in matters involving activities using animals. This has resulted in more scrutiny of the care and use of animals in scientific research. The regulations now in effect are comprehensive and, if followed, result in excellent care for animals. The penalties for not adhering to the regulations are great enough to encourage compliance and will assure that the privilege of using animals in research is carried out in a humane and careful manner.

JEFFREY KAHN
RALPH DELL

Directly related to this article are the other articles in this entry: HISTORICAL ASPECTS, *and* PHILOSOPHICAL ISSUES. *Also directly related are the entries* ANIMAL WELFARE AND RIGHTS, *article on* ETHICAL PERSPECTIVES ON THE TREATMENT AND STATUS OF ANIMALS; *and* XENOGRAFTS. *For a further discussion of topics mentioned in this article, see the entries* AGRICULTURE, ANIMAL WELFARE AND RIGHTS, *especially the article on* ANIMALS IN AGRICULTURE AND FACTORY FARMING; ECONOMIC CONCEPTS IN HEALTH CARE; LAW AND BIOETHICS; RESEARCH ETHICS COMMITTEES; *and* RESPONSIBILITY. *For a discussion of related ideas, see the entries* CONFLICT OF INTEREST; ENVIRONMENT AND RELIGION; GENETIC ENGINEERING, *article on* ANIMALS AND PLANTS; JAINISM; PAIN AND SUFFERING; RESPONSIBILITY; *and* RIGHTS, *article on* RIGHTS IN BIOETHICS. *Other relevant material may be found under the entries* BIOETHICS; ENDANGERED SPECIES AND BIODIVERSITY; ENVIRONMENTAL ETHICS; *and* VETERINARY ETHICS. *See also the* APPENDIX (CODES, OATHS, AND DIRECTIVES RELATED TO BIOETHICS), *SECTION V:* ETHICAL DIRECTIVES PERTAINING TO THE WELFARE AND USE OF ANIMALS.

Bibliography

Animal Legal Defense Fund v. Espy. 1994. 23 F. 3d 496 (DC Cir.).

Animal Legal Defense Fund v. Madigan. 1992. 781 F. Supp. 797 (D.D.C.).

Animal Legal Defense Fund v. Secretary of Agriculture. 1993. 813 F. Supp. 882 (D.D.C.).

BRODY, MIMI. 1989. "Animal Research: A Call for Legislative Reform Requiring Ethical Merit Review." *Harvard Environmental Law Review* 13, no. 2:423–484.

"Concentration Camps for Dogs." 1966. *Life,* February 4, pp. 22–29.

DRESSER, REBECCA. 1988. "Assessing Harm and Justification in Animal Research: Federal Policy Opens the Laboratory Door." *Rutgers Law Review* 40, no. 3:723–795.

FRANCIONE, GARY L. 1990. "Access to Animal Care Committees." *Rutgers Law Review* 43, no. 1:1–14.

INSTITUTE OF LABORATORY ANIMAL RESOURCES. COMMITTEE ON EDUCATIONAL PROGRAMS IN LABORATORY ANIMAL SCIENCE. 1991. *Education and Training in the Care and Use of Laboratory Animals: A Guide for Developing Institutional Programs.* Washington, D.C.: National Academy Press.

———. COMMITTEE ON PAIN AND DISTRESS IN LABORATORY ANIMALS. 1992. *Recognition and Alleviation of Pain and Distress in Laboratory Animals.* Washington, D.C.: National Academy Press.

Laboratory Animal Welfare Act (LAWA). 1966. P.L. 89-544 1, Aug. 24, 80 STAT, 350.

ORLANS, F. BARBARA. 1987. "Research Protocol Review for Animal Welfare." *Investigative Radiology* 22, no. 3:253–258.

———. 1993. *In the Name of Science: Issues in Responsible Animal Experimentation.* New York: Oxford University Press.

PANEL ON EUTHANASIA. AMERICAN VETERINARY MEDICAL ASSOCIATION (AVMA). 1993. *Journal of the American Veterinary Medical Association* 202, no. 2:229–249.

ROZMIAREK, HARRY. 1987. "Current and Future Policies Regarding Laboratory Animal Welfare." *Investigative Radiology* 22, no. 2:175–179.

RUSSELL, WILLIAM M. S., and BURCH, REX L. 1992. *The Principles of Humane Experimental Technique.* Potters Bar, U.K.: Universities Federation for Animal Welfare.

WHITNEY, ROBERT A., JR. 1987. "Animal Care and Use Committees: History and Current National Policies in the United States." *Laboratory Animal Science* 37 (suppl.): 18–21.

ANIMAL USE AND CARE COMMITTEES

See ANIMAL RESEARCH, *article on* LAW AND POLICY.

ANIMAL WELFARE AND RIGHTS

I. ETHICAL PERSPECTIVES ON THE TREATMENT AND STATUS OF ANIMALS

Normative ethical theory may be conceived as the systematic inquiry into the moral limits on human freedom. Philosophers and theologians throughout history and across cultures have offered different, often contradictory, answers to the central question of ethics thus conceived. Some have argued, for example, that the only justified limits on human freedom are those grounded in the rational self-interest of the agent, while others have maintained that the foundations of morality, and thus the basis of morally justified limitations on human freedom, are logically distinct from self-interest, though not from the dictates of reason. Still others have alleged that the foundations of morality have nothing to do with either reason or self-interest.

In view of the variety and conflicting nature of answers to the central question of normative ethics, it is hardly surprising that ethical theories sometimes offer strikingly different accounts of the moral status of those nonhuman animals we humans raise or hunt for food and clothing, use as beasts of burden, train to entertain us, and utilize as models for purposes of biomedical research. No philosopher or theologian has gone so far as to say that, from the moral point of view, there are no justified limits on what we may do to these animals. Even René Descartes, much celebrated for his theory that nonhuman animals are automata and thus incapable of feeling either pain or pleasure (Descartes, "Animals Are Machines," in Regan and Singer, 1976; 1989), is said to have treated his dog humanely. At a certain minimal level, then, all normative ethical theories speak with one voice. But at other levels, the differences are both real and deep.

Direct and indirect duties

These differences emerge clearly when we consider how competing theories answer two distinct but related questions. The first asks, What are the grounds for morally limiting human freedom when it comes to human interactions with nonhuman animals? The second asks, How extensive are these moral limits on human freedom? The former inquires as to why human freedom should be limited at all when our actions affect other animals; the latter challenges us to investigate how much our freedom should be limited. Of the two questions, the first is the more basic, for the reasons given in support of views about how much our freedom should be limited ultimately are based on views about why our freedom should be limited in the first place.

Two opposed possibilities present themselves as answers to the first, more basic question. One possibility holds that it is because of how animals themselves are affected or treated by human agents that we should limit our freedom. Viewed from this perspective, nonhuman animals are entitled to a certain kind of consideration or treatment. Because such views stress the idea that something is owed or is due directly to these animals, it is common to refer to them as "direct duty" views.

The second possibility, by contrast, locates the ground of moral constraint in some basis other than the animals. Viewed from this perspective, humans owe nothing to other animals, nor do these animals deserve any sort of treatment or consideration. Rather, human freedom should be limited because, for example, human cruelty to other animals will cause humans to treat one another cruelly. Because such views deny that we have duties directly to other animals, while recognizing that other factors should limit our freedom in our dealings with them, they are commonly referred to as "indirect duty" views.

All normative ethical theories, as they address the moral status of nonhuman animals, fall into one or the other of these two classes. That is, either they affirm that we have direct duties to nonhuman animals, or they deny that we have direct duties. Some of the major theoretical options within each class, as these have been developed by ethicists within the history of Western thought, will be considered in what follows.

Abolition, reform, and status quo

As noted earlier, a second important question asks how much our freedom should be limited in our dealings with other animals. Three sorts of options may be distinguished: abolitionist, reformist, and status quo. An abolitionist position argues on behalf of ending human practices that routinely utilize nonhuman animals (for example, as a source of food or as models in scientific research). A reformist position accepts these institutions in principle but seeks in various ways to improve them in practice (for example, by enlarging the cages for animals used in research). A status quo position, unlike the abolitionist position, accepts these institutions in principle and, unlike the reformist position, does not recognize the need to improve them. Representative examples of each outlook and their logical relationship to competing normative ethical theories will be explained below.

While the heated, sometimes acrimonious, debate among partisans of abolition, reform, and the status quo captures the attention of the media, far less attention has been devoted to the critical assessment of the competing ethical philosophies, whether of the direct or indirect duty variety. This by itself suggests the degree to which the public debate over "animal rights," broadly conceived, has assumed the greater part of what is most in need of informed, critical reflection. For clearly, whether we should favor the goals of supporters of abolition, reform, or the status quo in practice depends on determining the most adequate account of how we should treat nonhuman animals in theory. It is to a consideration of some of the major options in ethical theory that we now turn.

Perfectionism

Aristotle (384–322 B.C.E.) presents the broad outlines of a moral theory that goes by the name "perfectionism." The cornerstone of this theory has a high degree of initial plausibility. Justice, it is claimed, consists in giving to individuals what they are due, and those individuals whose character is morally better (more "perfect") than the character of others prima facie deserve more of what is good in life than do other, less good people. Aristotle's accounts of what makes people morally better and of "the good of man" have helped shape much of Western moral theory. Concerning the latter first, Aristotle accepts the commonplace notion that the good we humans seek is happiness, but he argues that the true happiness we seek is not wealth, fame, or even pleasure in abundance but, rather, the possession and exercise of those virtues (those "excellences") that are uniquely human. Thus happiness, in his view, is characterized as "an activity of the soul in accordance with virtue." Those are happiest who optimally express their humanity in how they live and, in doing so, take pleasure in being the human beings they are.

As for the moral virtues (prudence, justice, courage, and temperance), Aristotle characterizes each as a mean between the extremes of excess and deficiency. A courageous person, for example, is neither foolhardy (an excess) nor cowardly (a deficiency); a courageous person has the right mix of the willingness to take risks and the fear of doing so. Among the intellectual virtues, a detached, contemplative wisdom, wherein one knows eternal truths and in this way shares in that knowledge possessed by the gods, is the highest. In the case of both the moral and the intellectual virtues, finally, the human capacity to reason plays a decisive role. For man is, in Aristotle's view, unique in being "a rational animal," and "the good of man" consists in actualizing, to the fullest extent possible, those unique potentialities that define what it is to be human. Thus, since those are happiest who optimally express their humanity in how they live, those are happiest who exercise their reason optimally.

Because it prescribes the distribution of what is good in life on the basis of one's possessing the favored virtues and, thus, on the basis of degrees of human perfection, perfectionism can—and in Aristotle's hands, does—sanction or require radically inegalitarian treatment of different individuals. In the case of nonhuman animals in particular, perfectionism provides no direct protection. Despite his teaching, in sharp contrast to Descartes's, that these animals share many of the same psychological capacities possessed by humans—including, for example, sensation and desire—Aristotle confidently denies that they share the capacity to reason. Moreover, because in his view the "lesser" exists to serve the interests or purposes of the "greater," Aristotle maintains that nonhuman animals exist for the purpose of advancing the good of human beings. He writes: "Other animals exist for the sake of man, the tame for use and food, the wild, if not all, at least the greater part of them, for food, and for the provision of clothing and various instruments" (Aristotle, "Animals and Slavery," in Regan and Singer, 1976, p. 110; 1989, p. 5). There is no implication here that Aristotle's teachings permit the wanton infliction of pain on nonhuman animals for no good reason. What is clear is that because he recognizes no greater purpose for nonhuman animals than to serve the interests of human beings, Aristotle can recognize only indirect duties in their case. Finally, while many of today's more controversial practices involving human utilization of nonhuman animals, such as factory farming and animal-to-human organ transplants, were unknown in his day, all the available evidence seems to indicate that Aristotle was well disposed to the status quo with respect to the relevant practices current while he was alive.

It is not only nonhuman animals, however, that exist for the sake of those who are more perfect. In general, women do not measure up to Aristotle's standards of "the good of man." "The male is by nature superior, and the female inferior," he writes, "and the one rules, and the other is ruled; this principle, of necessity, extends to all mankind" (ibid.). Moreover, some humans, whether male or female, lack the ability to grasp through reason those truths understood by the more virtuous among us; of such individuals Aristotle writes that they are "slave[s] by nature" (ibid.). And so it is that Aristotle affirms the obvious parallel, given the form perfectionism takes in his hands, between the moral status of human slaves and nonhuman animals: "The use made of slaves and of tame animals is not very different; for both with their bodies minister to the needs of life" (ibid.). Those humans who, because of their superior rationality, are morally more perfect are entitled to make use of those, whether human or not, who lack the virtues defining human perfection.

Few today will publicly embrace Aristotle's perfectionism. Not only does his view of women offend the emancipated gender egalitarianism of our time, but the comfortable elitism and classism that enable him to pronounce some humans "slaves by nature" will find no home among the most basic precepts of contemporary moral, political, and legal thought. The practical implications for humans of the fundamental principle of Aristotelian perfectionism—that those who are lacking in reason exist to serve the interests of those who are most virtuous—is morally offensive. It is one thing to affirm that those people who are more perfect than others prima facie deserve more of what is good in life; it is quite another to maintain that those who are less perfected exist for the sole purpose of ministering to the more virtuous. Moreover, since we cannot rationally defend the exploitation of some humans on the grounds that "by nature" they lack the potential to acquire the virtues possessed by those who exploit them, we cannot rationally defend human exploitation of nonhuman animals by offering an analogous defense—cannot, that is, rationally defend such exploitation by claiming that nonhuman animals "by nature" lack the potential to acquire uniquely human virtues.

Despotism and stewardship

An alternative to Aristotle's philosophy is rooted in the biblical teaching that the God of Judaism and Christianity gives human beings dominion over nature in general and other animals in particular. As so often happens, however, there is more than one way to interpret the biblical message. Two ways in which human dominion can be understood—despotism and stewardship—will be sketched here.

Despotism teaches that nature in general and the other animals in particular are created by God for the sake of humans, and thus are ordained by the divine creator to serve such myriad human purposes as a source of food and clothing. Nothing within the natural order, save humans, has value in and of itself; what value the natural world possesses is entirely dependent on the extent to which it serves human interests. In this sense, human interests *are* the measure of all things, at least all things of value. Various biblical passages are cited to confirm the despotic reading, for example, "Then God said, 'Let us make man in our image, after our likeness; and let them have dominion over the fish of the sea, and over the birds of the air, and over the cattle . . . and over all the earth'" (Gen. 1:26).

Seen in this light, despotism's appeal to what God has ordained provides a reason for human supremacy over nonhuman animals that Aristotle's appeal to what is guaranteed "by nature" seems to lack, and it is a small step from acceptance of the despotic interpretation of human dominion to the conclusion that we owe nothing to nonhuman animals. Thus we find Saint Thomas Aquinas (ca. 1225–1274), for example, urging in words barely distinguishable from those of Aristotle except for their reference to God that it is by "Divine ordinance that the life of animals and plants is preserved not for

themselves but for man" (Thomas Aquinas, "On Killing Living Things and the Duty to Love Irrational Creatures," in Regan and Singer, 1976, p. 119; 1989, p. 11). Mindful, moreover, that some biblical passages prohibit cruelty to nonhuman animals, Aquinas firmly places himself within the indirect duty tradition when he maintains that the import of such prohibitions is, for example, "to remove man's thoughts from being cruel to other men, and lest through being cruel to animals one become cruel to human beings" (Thomas Aquinas, "Differences Between Rational and Other Creatures," in Regan and Singer, 1976, p. 59; 1989, p. 9).

To the extent that Saint Thomas's philosophy is rooted in the Scripture of the Christian tradition, those who stand outside this tradition are unlikely to be persuaded that God established in nature what nature was incapable of establishing by itself. Even granting biblical underpinnings to one's ethic, moreover, questions arise concerning the accuracy of the despotic interpretation of human dominion. While the Hebrew concept of *rada*, translated as "having dominion," often is interpreted to mean human despotism over the nonhuman world—an idea that, according to some early critics (White, 1967; McHarg, 1969), is the root cause of today's environmental crisis—a significantly different interpretation has been proposed by more recent thinkers (Barr, 1974; Linzey, 1987; McDaniel, 1989; Callicott, 1993).

For *rada* can be understood as the idea of human responsibility toward and care for a created order that is good independent of the human presence. According to this latter interpretation, commonly referred to as stewardship, humans are given the task of being as loving within the natural order as God was in creating the natural order in the first place. Humans, that is, are to be the loving caretakers of an independently good creation. Because, viewed from the stewardship perspective, the natural world in general, and those nonhuman animals with whom we share it in particular, are good apart from human interests, our duties with regard to these animals emerge as direct duties owed to them rather than indirect duties owed either to other humans or to their creator.

Although when thus interpreted all of creation is seen as having a kind of value that is independent of human interests, the value of nonhuman animals arguably is especially noteworthy. One might note, first, that these animals were created on the same day—the sixth—as were humans (Gen. 1:24–27); that in the original state of perfection, in Eden, humans did not eat other animals (Gen. 1:29); and that, in God's covenant with Noah after the flood (Gen. 9:8–12), animals (but not plants) are included. Using these images, one can argue that the choice we face today is *either* to continue to move further from the sort of relationship with the animals God hoped would prevail when the world was created *or* to make daily efforts to recapture that relationship—to journey back to Eden, as it were. Given this latter reading, the practical consequences of a stewardship interpretation of dominion would depart significantly from those favored by the status quo position, just as the goals one would hope to achieve would differ from those advanced by reformists. For if our righteous relationship with the other animals, in our capacities as their caretakers and protectors, is one of nonutilization (they are not to be eaten, not to be worn, etc.), then the stewardship interpretation of human dominion would seem to support an abolitionist ideal.

However these matters are to be settled, the biblical grounding of morality characteristic of both despotism and stewardship places these moral perspectives outside the mainstream of normative ethical theory, at least from the Enlightenment forward, where rigorous, imaginative attempts have been made to ground ethics independently of belief in God and the moral authority of the Bible. One such attempt is contractarianism.

Contractarianism

Among the most influential nontheological political and moral theories, contractarianism has a legacy that reaches at least as far back as Thomas Hobbes (1588–1679) and, among our contemporaries, includes such notable philosophers as John Rawls (1971) and Jan Narveson (1988). Like other theorists united by a common outlook, contractarians often disagree on many of the most fundamental points. It will not be possible to do justice to the rich fabric of disagreement that characterizes proponents of the theories under review.

As its name suggests, contractarianism conceives of morality as a kind of contract into which people (the "contractors") enter voluntarily. For contractarians, morality emerges as a set of mutually agreed upon and enforceable constraints on human freedom, constraints that each party to the contract rationally believes to be in his or her own self-interest. There is, then, according to contractarian theory, nothing that by its nature is morally right or wrong, just or unjust; rather, acts or institutions become right or wrong, just or unjust, as a result of the agreements reached by rational, self-interested contractors. In this sense, all of morality is conventional, and none is natural. Morality is created, not discovered, by human beings.

Both the self-interest that motivates and the rationality that guides the contractors are significant. We are not to imagine that people, as they deliberate about what limits on their freedom they will accept, are motivated by a natural sympathy for the misfortune of others or that they are willing altruistically to accept personal loss so that others might gain. Each contractor is motivated exclusively by his or her self-interest. The conception of individual self-interest each contractor has, moreover, is neither whimsical nor uninformed. Each person asks the same basic question: From the point of view of what is best for me, rationally considered, what limitations on my freedom would I be willing to accept? Morality, understood as rational, enforceable constraints on human freedom, arises when all the contractors jointly agree on the same constraints, not out of sympathy for others or because of altruistic motivations, but because each judges the outcome to be in his or her personal self-interest.

Two fundamentally opposed forms of contractarianism may be distinguished. The first permits the contractors to enter into their contractual deliberations equipped with the knowledge of who they are and what they want out of life, given their individual interests, talents, and hopes. This is the form of contractarianism favored by Hobbes and Narveson, for example. The second, favored by Rawls, requires that the contractors imagine that they lack such detailed knowledge of their individual psychology and circumstances, and instead deliberate about the terms of the contract from behind what Rawls calls "a veil of ignorance." Why Rawls would have recourse to this imaginative point of view will be explained momentarily. First, however, the implications of Hobbesian contractarianism for the treatment of nonhuman animals deserve attention.

Judged on the basis of the interests of these animals, the implications are not particularly salutary. In view of their inability to express these interests and to negotiate with others, nonhuman animals obviously are not to be counted among the potential contractors. Moreover, even while it is true that some things are in the interests of pigs and wolves, for example, the idea that these animals can have an informed understanding of what is in their rational self-interest has no clear meaning. Not surprisingly, therefore, what protection these animals are provided by Hobbesian contractarianism necessarily depends on what interests the human contractarians happen to have in them.

Narveson, for one, cheerfully indicates that this need not be very much (Narveson, "A Defense of Meat Eating," in Regan and Singer, 1989). Because many contractors have a special place in their hearts for companion animals ("pets"), these animals will be treated reasonably well, not because they are entitled to such treatment but because we owe it to their human friends not to upset them (these humans) gratuitously. In the case of most other nonhuman animals, however, including those slaughtered for food or used in research, Narveson finds no good reason to cease and desist. Clearly, then, given Hobbesian contractarianism, all our duties with respect to other animals are indirect duties owed to those human beings who help forge the contract. And just as clearly, considered from a political perspective, one finds little within this version of contractarianism that could mount an abolitionist or a far-reaching reformist approach to how other animals are treated; what one finds instead is a theory well disposed to the status quo while remaining open to modest reforms.

Critics of Hobbesian contractarianism have raised various objections (Regan, 1983). One concerns the possibility of arbitrary discrimination between people—for example, discrimination based on race. If we imagine that a large majority of potential contractors (say, 95 percent) are white, and the remainder black, then it is not obviously irrational for those who comprise the majority to exclude members of the minority from negotiating the contract; perhaps the majority might even agree to keep the minority in bondage, as chattel slaves, the better to advance the rational self-interests of those individuals comprising the majority. That such an arrangement would be unjust seems too obvious to need a supporting argument. And (for Hobbesian contractarianism) there's the rub. For since what is just and unjust is created by the agreements reached by the contractors, there is, within this form of contractarianism, no theoretical grounding for the evident injustice involved in excluding the minority from participating. The theory, that is, not only fails to illuminate why such discrimination is unjust, but it also seems to deprive us of the means even to raise this objection. If a moral theory is so fundamentally flawed when it comes to how human beings, given their differences in skin pigmentation, should be treated, it is unclear how it can be any nearer the truth when it comes to how nonhuman beings, given their species differences, should be treated.

Rawls's introduction of the veil of ignorance, mentioned earlier, can be interpreted as his attempt to preserve the spirit of Hobbesian contractarianism while departing importantly from the letter. Rawls invites would-be contractors to imagine themselves in what he calls the "original position," in which, because they deliberate from behind the veil of ignorance, they do not know when they will be born or where, whether they will be rich or poor, of exceptional intelligence or below average, male or female, Caucasian or non-Caucasian. The question now to be asked, by each of the contractors, is what limits on human freedom each would accept, in the face of such profound ignorance concerning such details.

The full scope of Rawls's answer need not concern us. Only two points are of particular importance here. The first concerns how Rawlsian contractarianism improves on Hobbesian contractarianism when it addresses the issue of discrimination based on race. Hobbesian contractors, as noted above, can have a self-interested reason for accepting such discrimination, given that they know they belong to a racial majority. Rawlsian

contractors, in contrast, lack such a reason since, for all they know, they might be one of the minority. In this respect, Rawlsian contractarianism seems to represent a notable improvement over Hobbesian contractarianism.

Despite its apparent strengths in response to issues involving arbitrary discrimination, Rawls's account of the moral status of nonhuman animals seems to fail to live up to its own standards (VanDeVeer, 1979). While the imaginary contractors behind the veil of ignorance are denied detailed knowledge about their individual interests and circumstances, and thus do not know whether, say, they will be male or female, black or white, Rawls does permit them to know that they will be born as human beings. To allow knowledge of this detail, however, seems to prejudice the case against nonhuman animals from the start. Granted, rational, self-interested contractors, making choices from behind the veil of ignorance, will negotiate direct duties to human beings and indirect ones to nonhumans, if they know they will be born human. But this only shows that these contractors will discriminate against these animals if they are provided with an arbitrary reason for doing so. In short, neither Hobbesian nor Rawlsian contractarianism seems to offer a reasonable basis on which to ground the only duties each recognizes in the case of nonhuman animals: indirect duties.

Kantianism

A final example of an indirect duty view is provided by the great Prussian philosopher Immanuel Kant (1724–1804). In some respects Kant's moral philosophy regarding the treatment of nonhuman animals is an amalgam of Aristotle's and, stripped of its appeals to God, Aquinas's. In concert with both, Kant emphasizes rationality as the defining characteristic of being human and, echoing Saint Thomas, objects to cruelty to animals because of the deleterious effect this has on how humans are treated. "He who is cruel to animals," Kant writes, "becomes hard also in his dealings with men," whereas "tender feelings towards dumb animals develop humane feelings towards mankind" (Kant, "Duties in Regard to Animals," in Regan and Singer, 1976, p. 123; 1989, p. 24).

Despite these historical echoes, Kant's moral philosophy is in many ways highly original. Of particular note is his thesis that humanity exists as an "end in itself." Kant does not attempt to prove this thesis by appeal to some more basic principle; rather, it is set forth as a postulate in his system. In this capacity it places humans and other rational, autonomous beings in a unique moral category that distinguishes them, as "persons," from everything else that exists. Like Aristotle and Aquinas before him, Kant views the rest of the natural order as existing to serve human interests. In particular, animals, in his words, exist "merely as a means to an end. That end is man" (ibid.). Thus, whereas in Kant's view we are morally free to use other animals as we wish, subject only to the injunction to avoid cruelty, we are not morally free to treat human beings in a comparable fashion. Because humans exist as ends in themselves, we are never to treat them merely as means, Kant argues, which is what we would be doing if we treated them as we treat other animals (for example, if we raised humans as a food source). An abolitionist, a radical reformist, Kant is not. Provided only that we are not cruel in our treatment of nonhuman animals, we do nothing wrong when we treat them as we do.

A common objection against Kant's position is the argument from marginal cases (Regan, 1983; for criticism of this argument, see Narveson, 1977). All humans, Kant implies, exist as ends in themselves. To restrict this supreme moral value to humans among terrestrial creatures is not arbitrary, Kant believes, because humans, unlike the other animals, are unique in being rational and autonomous. However, not all humans are rational and autonomous. Those who are mentally enfeebled or deranged, for example, lack these capacities. Are these humans nevertheless ends in themselves? If Kant's answer is affirmative, then it is not the presence of rationality and autonomy that ground this supreme moral value; if, on the other hand, Kant's answer is negative, then it follows that these "marginal" human beings do not exist as ends in themselves, in which case it would seem that they, no less than other animals, may be treated as mere means. Because one assumes that this latter consequence would be seen by Kant to be morally grotesque, it seems fair to assume that he would want to avoid it; but he can do so, it seems, only by accepting the view that individuals who are neither rational nor autonomous nevertheless exist as ends in themselves, a view that undermines his confident assertion that nonhuman animals, deficient in reason and autonomy, exist "merely as means to an end," the end being "man."

Utilitarianism

The pioneering work of the nineteenth-century utilitarians Jeremy Bentham (1748–1832) and John Stuart Mill (1806–1873) represents a significant departure from the Aristotelian legacy we find in Kant's moral theory. Bentham, referring to nonhuman animals, writes, "The question is not, Can they *reason?* nor, Can they *talk?* but, Can they *suffer?*" (Bentham, "A Utilitarian View," in Regan and Singer, 1976, p. 130; 1989, p. 26). The possession of sentience (the capacity to experience pleasure and pain), not the possession of rationality, nor autonomy, nor linguistic competence, entitles any individual to direct moral consideration; and it is the possession of this particular capacity, in Bentham's and Mill's view, that creates in humans the direct duty not to cause nonhuman animals to suffer needlessly. We owe it to these animals themselves, not to those humans who might be affected by what we do, to take their (the nonhuman animals') pleasures and pains into account and, having done so, to ensure that we never make them suffer without good reason.

Both Bentham and Mill give a utilitarian interpretation of what such a good reason might be. Utilitarianism, roughly speaking, is the view that our duty is to perform that act that will bring about the best consequences for all those affected by the outcome. For value hedonists like Bentham and Mill, who recognize only one intrinsic good, pleasure, and only one intrinsic evil, pain, the best consequences will be those that include the greatest possible balance of pleasure over pain. A good reason for permitting animal suffering, then, is that such suffering is a necessary price to pay in bringing about the best consequences, all considered. How much of the spirit of reform, abolition, or the status quo happens to characterize individual utilitarians depends on how much animal suffering is judged to be necessary. Bentham opposes hunting, fishing, and the baiting of animals for sport, for example, while Mill's name is to be found among the earliest contributors to England's Royal Society for the Prevention of Cruelty to Animals. But neither Bentham nor Mill aligns himself with the cause of antivivisection, and both are lifelong meat eaters. So reformers they are, but abolitionists they are not. Even so, in their time, and given the broader social context in which they lived, they were seen by many of their contemporaries as radicals, if not extremists.

The degree to which utilitarians can differ over important practical matters is illustrated in our time by Peter Singer and R. G. Frey. Singer is justly famous for his seminal 1975 book, *Animal Liberation,* while Frey has written two books (1980, 1983) and many essays devoted to the issues under review. The two philosophers, while agreeing on some of the most fundamental points in ethical theory, disagree on many of the most important consequences each believes follow from the application of utilitarianism, including how nonhuman animals should be treated. For example, in *Animal Liberation* Singer advocates vegetarianism, on moral grounds; Frey disagrees, appealing to the same grounds in his *Rights, Killing, and Suffering: Moral Vegetarianism and Applied Ethics* (1983). It will be useful to explain how such profound disagreements can arise between partisans of the same moral philosophy.

By its very nature, utilitarianism is a forward-looking moral theory. The consequences of our actions, and the consequences alone, determine the morality of what we do. As such, utilitarians will reach opposing judgments about what is right and wrong if they have opposing views of what the consequences of a given act will be. In the case of vegetarianism in particular, utilitarians like Singer believe that, taking everyone's interests into account, and counting equal interests equally, the consequences that flow from abstaining from animal flesh will be better than if people continue to include animal flesh in their diets; Frey, however, believes that the consequences of a vegetarian diet are not sufficiently better so as to impose an obligation on us to become vegetarians. It is, then, factual disagreements over what the future might hold that underlie the type of moral disagreement separating Singer and Frey on the issue of vegetarianism.

Some critics of utilitarianism (e.g., Clark, 1977) argue that the apparently unresolvable impasse created by Singer's and Frey's application of utilitarian theory to the particular case of vegetarianism illustrates a major weakness in utilitarian theory in general. Because so much—indeed, because everything—depends on our ability to know what will happen in the future, and in view of the limitations of human knowledge in this regard, utilitarianism, these critics maintain, reduces moral judgment to guesswork about what might or might not occur.

Despite this problem, utilitarianism may seem to be a congenial theory for those who utilize nonhuman animals in animal model research. The most common justification of such research consists in appealing to the improvements in human health and longevity to which this research allegedly has led; and while researchers may recognize the need to look for alternatives to the animal model, lest these animals be used unnecessarily, it seems clear that the moral justification they offer is utilitarian. (For dissenting voices regarding the human benefits of such research, from the perspective of the history of medicine, see McKinlay and McKinlay, 1977; for epistemological concerns, see LaFollette and Shanks, 1993). Part of the enduring greatness of *Animal Liberation* lies in Singer's relentless documentation of how much of this research prima facie fails to meet the utilitarian standard favored by researchers themselves. No less important is the way Singer exposes a prejudice that he, following Richard Ryder (1975), denominates "speciesism," and that he characterizes as "an attitude of bias in favor of the interests of members of one's own species and against those of other species" (Singer, 1990, p. 6). Research scientists, Singer believes, frequently offer at best half a utilitarian justification of their work: Human interests are considered; those of nonhuman animals are not. To be consistent, the interests of both must be counted, and counted equitably. It is Singer's considered judgment that few researchers are consistent in this regard.

Frey, too, examines the lack of moral consistency among researchers ("Vivisection, Morals, and Medicine," in Regan and Singer, 1989). Given any reasonable view about the richness and variety of psychological life, it is unquestionably true, Frey believes, that the psychological life of nonhuman primates, or even that of a cat or a dog, is richer and more varied than the psychological life of some human beings (a child born with only the stem of the brain, for example). Thus, if the moral defense of animal model research is supposed to lie in the good results allegedly produced by using these animals, then a similar defense for utilizing marginal humans is at hand. To be consistent in their utilitarianism, therefore, Frey believes that researchers should be willing to conduct their studies on marginal humans—a finding researchers are unlikely to welcome. Frey is unperturbed, insisting that researchers cannot have it both ways, using utilitarian modes of thinking when they believe it justifies their practice of using other than human animals in their studies, only to discard utilitarianism when its implications for the selection of marginal humans as research subjects are made manifest.

Whatever form utilitarianism takes, one of the principal objections its advocates face centers on questions of justice (Lyons, 1965). What limits, if any, can utilitarianism recognize on how future good is to be obtained? The theory seems to imply that good ends justify whatever means are necessary to achieve them, including means that are flagrantly unjust. Classic examples include situations in which the judicial execution of the innocent is sanctioned on the grounds that others will be deterred from committing similar offenses. Here, critics concede, good consequences are brought into being, but the means used to secure them are reprehensible because they are unjust.

Utilitarians have replies to this and similar lines of criticism that go beyond the scope of the present essay (Brandt, 1979). Suffice it to say that among those philosophers who are not utilitarians, many dissociate themselves from utilitarianism because they believe that respect for the rights of the individual is a principle that should not be compromised in the name of achieving some greater good for others. Not surprisingly, perhaps, a position of this kind, one that prohibits the use of nonhuman animals in the name of advancing the general human welfare, has been advanced (Regan, 1983). Though not the only possible theory of animal rights (see, e.g., Rollin, 1981, 1989), this particular theory (the "rights view") can be seen as an attempt to blend certain features of utilitarianism and Kant's theory.

The rights view

Kant, it will be recalled, recognizes only indirect duties to nonhuman animals; we humans are not to be cruel to animals, for example, not because we treat them wrongly by our cruel treatment but because cruelty to animals can lead people to be cruel to one another. By contrast, utilitarians from Bentham to Singer recognize direct duties to nonhuman animals; they believe that there are certain things we owe to these animals, apart from how humans will be effected. On this divisive issue the rights view sides with utilitarians against Kantians: Nonhuman animals are of direct moral significance; we have direct duties in their case.

In a second respect, however, the rights view sides with Kantians against utilitarians. Utilitarians believe that duty is determined by the comparative value of consequences; the right thing to do is what causes the best results. Kant and his followers take a decidedly different view: What is right does not depend on the value of consequences, it depends on the appropriate, respectful treatment of the individual—in particular, whether humans are treated as ends, not merely as means. In this regard, the rights view is cut from Kantian, not utilitarian, cloth. What is right depends not on the value of consequences but on the appropriate, respectful treatment of the individual, including individual nonhuman animals. Thus, the fundamental principle of the rights view (the respect principle) is Kantian in spirit: we are always to treat individuals who exist as ends in themselves (those who have "inherent value") with respect, which means, in part, that we are never to treat them merely as means.

One problem the rights view faces concerns which nonhuman animals possess value of this kind. Like other line-drawing issues ("Exactly how tall do you have to be to be tall?" "Exactly how old do you have to be to be old?"), this one has no precise resolution, in part because the criterion for drawing the line is imprecise. The criterion the rights view proposes is that of being the subject of a life, a criterion that specifies a set of psychological capacities (the capacities to desire, remember, act intentionally, and feel emotions, for example) as jointly sufficient. At least some nonhuman animals (e.g., mammals and birds) arguably possess these capacities, thus are subjects of a life, and thus, given the rights view, are to be treated as ends in themselves. (For criticism, see Frey, 1980).

Such a view, for obvious reasons, has massive political, social, and moral implications concerning how these animals ought to be treated. From an animal rights perspective of this kind, the abolition of human exploitation of these animals, whether on the farm, at the lab, or in the wild—not merely the reform of these practices, and certainly not approval of the status quo—is what duty requires.

Line-drawing issues aside, the rights view faces daunting challenges from other quarters. One concerns the idea of inherent value. Some critics (e.g., Sapontzis, 1987) allege that the idea is "mystifying," meaning that it lacks any clear meaning. Advocates of animal rights reply that the notion of inherent value is no less "mystifying" than Kant's idea of end in itself. As applied to

human beings, Kant's idea of end in itself attempts to articulate the cherished belief that the value or worth of a human being is not reducible to instrumental value—not reducible, that is, to how useful a human being happens to be in forwarding the interests or purposes of other human beings. Neither John Doe nor Jane Doe, in Kant's view, exists as a mere resource relative to what other people want for themselves, and to treat the Does as if their value—their worth or dignity—consists merely in their resource or instrumental value for others is morally wrong. All that the rights view alleges, then, is that to be consistent, the same moral judgment must be made in those cases where nonhuman animals that are subjects of a life are treated in a similar fashion.

Another set of challenges alleges that the philosophy of animal rights, if acted upon, would lead to catastrophic consequences, either to human interests in particular or to the community of life in general. Concerning the former challenge, some critics argue that human health and longevity would be seriously harmed if, as the philosophy of animal rights requires, nonhuman animals ceased to be used as models of human disease (see C. R. Gallistel, "The Case for Unrestricted Research Using Animals," in Regan and Singer, 1989; and Cohen, 1986). Several responses seem apposite.

First, given the massive allocation of public monies that fund such research, it needs to be asked whether abandoning reliance on the whole-animal model really is contrary to what is in the collective best interests of human beings. Some (e.g., Sharpe, 1988) argue that customary reliance on this well-entrenched scientific methodology retards the development of alternative methodologies that would be more useful in understanding and curing major human diseases; in addition, these critics insist that humans would benefit more if the dominant focus of biomedical research were shifted away from curing disease to preventing it, a goal that is more efficiently advanced, these critics allege, by methodologies other than the use of the whole-animal model.

Second, recall one of the fundamental objections raised against utilitarianism: Just as one does not justify the violation of a human being's rights because doing so will benefit others, so one does not justify the violation of the rights of nonhuman animals on similar grounds. More generally, some gains others might obtain may be ill-gotten, and they are ill-gotten if the price of obtaining them involves the violation of another's rights. Thus, even if it is true that humans stand to lose some benefits if animal model research is abandoned, this by itself does not constitute a telling moral objection to the abolitionist implications of the philosophy of animal rights, assuming that these animals, like humans, have the right to be treated as ends in themselves.

Concerning the second line of criticism—the one alleging that acting on the philosophy of animal rights would have catastrophic implications for the community of life in general—the principal objection may be summarized as follows. Predatory animals obviously live off the death and flesh of their prey. Because prey animals have the right to be treated with respect, according to the rights view, critics (e.g., Callicott, 1980; Sagoff, 1984) allege that it follows that we should intervene to stop predatory animals in their natural depredations. However, if we were to do this, there would be no check on the balance that exists in nature between predators and preys; instead, the population of prey animals would explode, and this would have the effect of irreparably damaging the balance and sustainability of life forms within the larger life community.

Advocates of the philosophy of animal rights have a number of possible replies to the predation problem, the principal one of which is the following. Situations can and do arise where the right thing to do is to come to the assistance of another, whether the potential victim is a human or a nonhuman animal. However, in these situations the potential victim not only is at risk of serious injury but also is less than capable of mounting a defense. Thus, an elderly woman who is attacked by a psychotic killer, or a puppy who is being tormented by children, merits our intervention. But the predator–prey relationship seems to bear little resemblance to such cases. Most prey animals, most of the time, are perfectly capable of eluding their predators without anyone's assistance. Thus it would seem to be human arrogance, not informed responsibility, that would lead humans to believe that because animals in the wild have rights, we are duty bound to "police" nature. From an animal rights perspective, we have no general duty to intervene in predator–prey relations; that being so, the catastrophic environmental costs alleged to be implied by acting on the rights view seem to be more in the nature of fiction than of fact. (For a different response to the predation problem, see Sapontzis, 1987.)

Deep ecology

Despite the significant differences separating the philosophy of animal rights and other, more traditional moral theories, such as Kant's, there are important similarities. For example, like Kant's theory, the philosophy of animal rights recognizes the noninstrumental value of the individual; and animal rights philosophy, as is true not only of Kant's theory but of utilitarianism as well, articulates an abstract, universal, and impartial fundamental moral principle—abstract because the respect principle enjoins us to treat others with respect, without regard to time, or place, or circumstance; universal because the respect principle applies to everyone capable of making moral decisions; and impartial because this principle does not favor some individuals (e.g., family members or companion animals) over others. Some contemporary moral philosophers find this approach to ethics archaic;

among these critics, some of those who classify themselves as deep ecologists (see, in particular, Devall and Sessions, 1985) command a growing audience. (For a more systematic and in some ways different version of deep ecology, see Naess, 1989. For importantly different approaches to environmental ethics, see Taylor, 1986; Rolston, 1988; Callicott, 1980.)

Both traditional moral theories and the philosophy of animal rights are doubly to be faulted, according to Devall and Sessions—first, because these moral outlooks offer an overly intellectualized account of the moral life, and second, because they perpetuate the myth of the moral preeminence of the individual. Considering this latter charge first, Devall and Sessions argue that the concept of the isolated, atomistic individual, which arises out of the anthropocentric traditions of Western philosophy, is false to the facts of all life's embeddedness in the larger life community. People are not independent bits of mind existing by themselves; they are enmeshed in networks of relationships that bind them both to their evolutionary past and to their ecological present. Expressed another way, humans do not stand "above" or "apart from" nature; they stand "within" nature. And the natural world does not exist "for us," as a storehouse of renewable human resources (a view that is symptomatic of a "shallow" view of humanity's relationship to nature); we are inseparable from the natural environment (a view that indicates a "deeper" understanding of what it means to be human).

Thus, acceptance of the illusory concept of the isolated individual, existing outside the natural order, has done, and continues to do, incalculable damage to those who seek self-understanding. So long as we carry out this quest with a fundamentally flawed preconception of our place in the larger scheme of things, the longer we search, the less we will understand. As for the charge that traditional moral theories overintellectualize the moral life, Devall and Sessions argue that the moral life should be viewed as primarily experiential, not inferential, a life that is characterized by our coming to experience certain values in the concrete particularities of day-to-day life, rather than by apprehending abstract, universal, impartial moral principles by means of our rational powers.

Among those values to be found in the concrete particularities of day-to-day life, some involve other animals; and although deep ecologists have not written extensively on some of the most pressing practical issues, the general disdain these thinkers display toward reductionist science and industrial societies' technological domination of the natural world suggests that they would be strong reformists, at a minimum, in response to such practices as factory farming and animal model research. In the case of sport and recreational hunting, however, Devall and Sessions not only find nothing wrong, they applaud the practice. In pursuit of their prey, hunters tap into natural means whereby, through the act of killing, they can obtain greater self-understanding. Viewed in this light, Devall and Sessions seem to understand our duties with respect to animals as indirect duties limited by the overarching quest for self-knowledge. While, therefore, deep ecologists like Sessions and Devall can be counted upon to add their voices to those of reformists and abolitionists in some cases, they emerge as defenders of the status quo in others.

Ecofeminism

Ecofeminists, not just advocates of the rights view, are among those contemporary moral philosophers who differ significantly with deep ecologists. Like other isms, ecofeminism is not a monolithic position (see Adams, 1990; Diamond and Orenstein, 1990; Warren, 1990; Gaard, 1993); instead, it represents a number of defining tendencies, including in particular a principled stance that puts its advocates on the side of those who historically have been victims of oppression. For obvious reasons, women are pictured as among the oppressed, but the scope of ecofeminism's concern is not limited to women. The same ideology that sanctions oppression based on gender, ecofeminists maintain, also sanctions oppression based on race, class, and physical abilities, for example; moreover, beyond the boundaries of our species, this same ideology, ecofeminists believe, sanctions the oppression of nature in general and of nonhuman animals in particular.

In a number of fundamental ways, ecofeminism's diagnosis of the ideology of oppression resembles deep ecology's diagnosis of the deficiencies of traditional moral theory. As is true of the latter, ecofeminism challenges the myth of the isolated individual, existing apart from the world, and instead affirms the interconnectedness of all life. Moreover, no less than deep ecologists, ecofeminists abjure the overintellecutalization of the moral life characteristic of traditional moral theories, with their abstract, universal, and impartial fundamental principles. But whereas deep ecologists locate the fundamental cause of moral theory gone awry in anthropocentrism (human-centeredness), ecofeminists argue that it is androcentrism (male-centeredness) that is the real cause.

Nowhere is this difference clearer than in the case of sport or recreational hunting. Devall and Sessions celebrate the value of this practice as a means of bonding ever more closely with the natural world, of discovering "self in Self"; ecofeminists, by contrast, detect in the hunt the vestiges of patriarchy—the male's need to dominate and subdue (Kheel, 1991). More fundamentally, there is the lingering suspicion that deep ecologists continue to view the value of the natural world instrumentally, as a means to greater self-awareness and self-

knowledge. In this respect, and despite appearances to the contrary, deep ecology does not represent a "paradigm shift" away from the anthropocentric worldview it aspires to replace.

Ecofeminists believe they offer a deeper account of the moral life than do deep ecologists, one that goes to the very foundations of Western moral theorizing. The idea of "the rights of the individual" is diagnosed as a symptom of patriarchal thought, rooted in the (male) myth of the isolated individual. Morally, a "paradigm shift" occurs when, in place of assertions of rights, we freely, lovingly choose to take care of and assume responsibility for those who are victims of oppression, both within and beyond the extended human family, other animals included. Writing for the growing number of ecofeminists, Josephine Donovan states:

> Natural rights and utilitarianism present impressive and useful arguments for the ethical treatment of animals. Yet, it is also possible—indeed, necessary—to ground that ethic in an emotional and spiritual conversation with nonhuman life forms. Out of a woman's relational culture of caring and attentive love [there] emerges the basis for a feminist ethic for the treatment of animals. We should not kill, eat, torture, and exploit animals because they do not want to be so treated, and we know that. If we listen, we can hear them. ("Animal Rights and Feminist Theory," in Gaard, 1993, p. 185)

Thus, whereas the grounds for practical action offered by ecofeminists differ fundamentally from those favored by the rights view, and despite the foundational gulf that separates these two theories, both philosophies arguably have the same abolitionist practical implications.

Conclusion

The "animal rights debate," broadly conceived, is more than a contest of wills representing professional, economic, and ethical concerns; it is also a divisive, enduring topic in normative ethical theory (Vance, 1992). Until comparatively recently, discussions of the moral status of nonhuman animals had all but disappeared from the work of moral philosophers. (For a historical overview, see Ryder, 1989.) Beginning in the 1970s (Godlovitch et al., 1972; Singer, 1975; Linzey, 1976; Clark, 1977), however, we have witnessed a historically unprecedented outpouring of philosophical and theological interest in exploring the moral ties that bind humans to other animals, and there is every indication that this interest will intensify in the coming decades. The moral theories of philosophers are not the stuff of politics; still, the contributions philosophers make can help shape the political debate by clarifying the major theoretical options available to an informed public.

Principal among these options are those that have been canvassed here: perfectionism, despotism and stewardship, contractarianism, Kantianism, utilitarianism, the rights view, deep ecology, and ecofeminism. Doubtless other options will evolve as the discussion continues (Garner, 1994). Among these options, two in particular—utilitarianism and the rights view—have offered the most systematic accounts of those duties owed directly to nonhuman animals. It will be instructive, before concluding, to highlight some of the important practical differences, particularly as these pertain to animal model research, that flow from these competing philosophies.

Because utilitarianism is committed to reducing the total amount of suffering in the world, its proponents must be prepared to recognize the moral legitimacy of some research on nonhuman animals. Even Peter Singer, contemporary utilitarianism's most forceful critic of such research, has conceded this possibility (Singer, 1993). Moreover, utilitarians must be similarly well disposed to the activities of animal care and use committees (Singer has served as a member of such a committee), provided that these committees conscientiously work to eliminate unnecessary animal suffering. Legislative attempts to improve the well-being of animals, whether in laboratories or on the farm, find support among utilitarians. Viewed in these respects, utilitarianism offers a philosophical basis for those who would reform the ways in which nonhuman animals are utilized by humans; what it does not offer is a categorical condemnation of this utilization. For this reason utilitarianism is congenial to those individuals and groups working to advance animal welfare—who accept, that is, the morality of human utilization of nonhuman animals in principle but who seek to improve it, by making it more humane, in practice.

The rights view has a different perspective on such matters (Francione and Regan, 1992). This philosophy is opposed to human utilization of nonhuman animals in principle and seeks to end it in practice. Its practical implications are abolitionist, not reformist. Because those nonhuman animals who exist as ends in themselves are never to be treated merely as means, it is wrong to experiment on them in the name of advancing the well-being of others. Moreover, to the extent that animal care and use committees and reformist legislation help to perpetuate social acceptance of human exploitation of these animals, whether on the farm or in the laboratory, advocates of the rights view will—or, to be consistent, should—withhold their support. What animal rights advocates *can* consistently support are incremental steps that put an end to certain practices within the larger context of animal exploitation—for example, legislation that would prohibit the use of nonhuman animals in cosmetic testing and in drug addiction experiments, and the creation of policies that end compulsory vivisection and dissection in the classroom (Francione and Charlton, 1992). When, as can often happen, util-

itarians deem such practices unjustified because they cause gratuitous animal suffering, these two conflicting normative ethical philosophies—utilitarianism and the rights view—can speak with one voice. And when this happens, their potential political power is greater than the sum of its parts.

No one can predict which of the tendencies examined above—reform, abolition, or the status quo—will prevail in the coming years. Some positions (e.g., the rights view and ecofeminism) call for fundamental social change; others (e.g., Aristotelian perfectionism and Kant's view) call for much less. To the extent that people act because of their beliefs, the future of how humans treat other animals depends on what we humans believe the latter to be and how we think they should be treated. Because what we should do in practice depends on understanding what we ought to do in principle, our ability to give an appropriate response to the practical issues constituting the animal rights debate, broadly conceived—from whether we ought to be vegetarians to whether we should continue to use nonhuman animals in biomedical research—depends on our ability to make an informed, rational choice among normative ethical theories. In this respect, while a fair consideration of such theories may not be the end-all, it can make some claim to being at least part of the begin-all of a commitment to seek understanding and truth in these troubled waters.

TOM REGAN

Directly related to this article are the other articles in this entry: VEGETARIANISM, WILDLIFE CONSERVATION AND MANAGEMENT, PET AND COMPANION ANIMALS, ZOOS AND ZOOLOGICAL PARKS, HUNTING, *and* ANIMALS IN AGRICULTURE AND FACTORY FARMING. *Also directly related are the entries* ANIMAL RESEARCH; *and* VETERINARY ETHICS. *For a further discussion of topics mentioned in this article, see the entries* ENVIRONMENTAL ETHICS, *especially the articles on* ECOFEMINISM, *and* DEEP ECOLOGY; ETHICS, *especially the article on* NORMATIVE ETHICAL THEORIES; FEMINISM; JUSTICE; LOVE; OBLIGATION AND SUPEREROGATION; PAIN AND SUFFERING; RACE AND RACISM; RIGHTS; SEXISM; UTILITY; *and* VIRTUE AND CHARACTER. *For a discussion of related ideas, see the entries* AGRICULTURE; CARE; ENDANGERED SPECIES AND BIODIVERSITY; GENETIC ENGINEERING, *article on* PLANTS AND ANIMALS; LIFE; NATURAL LAW; *and* WOMEN, *article on* HISTORICAL AND CROSS-CULTURAL PERSPECTIVES.

Bibliography

ADAMS, CAROL J. 1990. *The Sexual Politics of Meat: A Feminist–Vegetarian Critical Theory.* New York: Continuum. A groundbreaking work in which the oppression of nonhuman animals is viewed as a symptom of patriarchy.

BARR, JAMES. 1974. "Man and Nature: The Ecological Controversy over the Old Testament." In *Ecology and Religion in History*, pp. 58–72. Edited by D. Spring and E. Spring. New York: Harper & Row. One of the first expositions of the stewardship interpretation of human dominion.

BRANDT, R. B. 1979. *A Theory of the Good and the Right*. Oxford: At the Clarendon Press. Among the most sophisticated defenses of utilitarianism.

CALLICOTT, J. BAIRD. 1980. "Animal Liberation: A Triangular Affair." *Environmental Ethics* 2, no. 4:311–328. Reprinted in his *In Defense of the Land Ethic: Essays in Environmental Philosophy*, pp. 15–38. Albany: State University of New York Press, 1989. An important early critique of animal liberation/animal rights.

———. 1993. "The Search for an Environmental Ethic." In *Matters of Life and Death: New Introductory Essays in Moral Philosophy*, pp. 322–382. 3d ed. Edited by Tom L. Beauchamp and Tom Regan. New York: McGraw-Hill. An excellent overview of recent work in environmental ethics, including critical discussions of despotism and stewardship, as well as deep ecology and ecofeminism. Has an excellent bibliography.

CLARK, STEPHEN R. L. 1977. *The Moral Status of Animals*. Oxford: At the Clarendon Press. An erudite exploration of human duties to nonhuman animals.

COHEN, CARL. 1986. "The Case for the Use of Animals in Biomedical Research." *New England Journal of Medicine* 315, no. 14:865–870. Includes a defense of the position that more, rather than fewer, nonhuman animals should be used in research.

DEVALL, BILL, and SESSIONS, GEORGE. 1985. *Deep Ecology: Living as if Nature Mattered*. Salt Lake City: Gibbs Smith. A widely read, accessible introduction to the tendencies informing deep ecology.

DIAMOND, IRENE, and ORENSTEIN, GLORIA FENMAN, eds. 1990. *Reweaving the World: The Emergence of Ecofeminism*. San Francisco: Sierra Club. An important anthology of ecofeminist thought.

FRANCIONE, GARY L., and CHARLTON, ANNA E. 1992. *Vivisection and Dissection in the Classroom: A Guide to Conscientious Objection*. Jenkintown, Pa.: American Anti-Vivisection Society.

FRANCIONE, GARY, and REGAN, TOM. 1992. "A Movement's Means Create Its Ends." *Animals' Agenda* 12, no. 1:40–43. A critical exploration of the theoretical and practical implications of the belief that nonhuman animals have basic moral rights.

FREY, R. G. 1980. *Interests and Rights: The Case Against Animals*. Oxford: At the Clarendon Press. A sustained criticism of the idea of animal rights.

———. 1983. *Rights, Killing, and Suffering: Moral Vegetarianism and Applied Ethics*. Oxford: Basil Blackwell. A sustained defense of the view that vegetarianism is not morally obligatory.

GAARD, GRETA C., ed. 1993. *Ecofeminism: Women, Animals, Nature*. Philadelphia: Temple University Press. An important, timely collection of essays from an ecofeminist perspective.

GARNER, RICHARD. 1994. *Beyond Morality*. Philadelphia: Temple University Press. A pioneering multicultural approach to ethics, emphasizing the importance of the virtue of compassion rather than adherence to abstract, universal, impartial moral principles, with important implications regarding the treatment of nonhuman animals.

GODLOVITCH, STANLEY; GODLOVITCH, ROSLIND; and HARRIS, JOHN. 1972. *Animals, Men, and Morals: An Enquiry into the Maltreatment of Non-Humans*. New York: Taplinger. The book that initiated the modern philosophical interest in animal rights.

KHEEL, MARTI. 1991. "Ecofeminism and Deep Ecology: Reflections on Identity and Difference." *Trumpeter* 8:62–72. An important contribution to ecofeminist scholarship.

LAFOLLETTE, HUGH, and SHANKS, NIALL. 1993. "Animal Models in Biomedical Research: Some Epistemological Worries." *Public Affairs Quarterly* 7, no. 2:113–130. A sophisticated philosophical critique of the human benefits attributed to animal model research.

LINZEY, ANDREW. 1976. *Animal Rights: A Christian Assessment of Man's Treatment of Animals*. Oxford: S.M.C. The first modern consideration of the moral status of nonhuman animals, viewed from a Christian perspective.

———. 1987. *Christianity and the Rights of Animals*. New York: Crossroad. An important theological exploration of the moral status of nonhuman animals.

LINZEY, ANDREW, and REGAN, TOM, eds. 1988. *Animals and Christianity: A Book of Readings*. New York: Crossroad. An anthology of Christian explorations of the relevant issues. Includes an extensive bibliography.

LYONS, DAVID. 1965. *Forms and Limits of Utilitarianism*. Oxford: At the Clarendon Press. A modern classic noteworthy for the depth and breadth of its critical examination of utilitarianism.

MAGEL, CHARLES R. 1981. *A Bibliography on Animal Rights and Related Matters*. Washington, D.C.: University Press of America. The first comprehensive bibliography on topics central to the debate over animal rights.

———. 1989. *Keyguide to Information Sources in Animal Rights*. Jefferson, N.C.: McFarland. Extensive overview of historical and contemporary discussions of animal rights.

MCDANIEL, JAY B. 1989. *Of God and Pelicans: A Theology of Reverence for Life*. Louisville, Ky.: John Knox. Represents a major advance in the systematic exploration of the moral status of nonhuman animals viewed theologically.

MCHARG, IAN L. 1969. *Design with Nature*. Garden City, N.Y.: Natural History Press. An early critique of despotism.

MCKINLAY, JOHN B., and MCKINLAY, S. 1977. *Health and Society*. London: Milbank. An important, lucid examination of the various factors that have contributed to improvements in human health.

MIDGLEY, MARY. 1983. *Animals and Why They Matter*. Harmondsworth, U.K.: Penguin. Includes critical discussions of contractarianism and other ethical theories, as well as a defense of the importance of sentiment or feeling in morality.

NAESS, ARNE. 1989. *Ecology, Community, and Lifestyle: Outline of an Ecosophy*. Edited and translated by David Rothenberg. Cambridge: At the University Press. The most systematic presentation of Naess's widely influential ideas.

NARVESON, JAN. 1977. "Animal Rights." *Canadian Journal of*

Philosophy 7, no. 1:161–178. Contains an early critique of the argument from marginal cases.

———. 1988. *The Libertarian Idea.* Philadelphia: Temple University Press. A bold, imaginative attempt to offer a contemporary contractarian grounding of morality.

RACHELS, JAMES. 1990. *Created from Animals: The Moral Implications of Darwinism.* Oxford: Oxford University Press. Explores the importance of Darwin's theory of evolution for the reconsideration of the moral status of nonhuman animals.

RAWLS, JOHN. 1971. *A Theory of Justice.* Cambridge, Mass.: Harvard University Press. A modern classic in moral and political theory.

REGAN, TOM. 1983. *The Case for Animal Rights.* Berkeley: University of California Press. A scholarly work in systematic ethical theory; includes extensive critical discussions of contractarianism, utilitarianism, and Kant's theory.

———, ed. 1986. *Animal Sacrifices: Religious Perspectives on the Use of Animals in Science.* Philadelphia: Temple University Press. Collected papers by leading scholars that explore the issue of animal research from the perspectives of Judaism, Christianity, Confucianism, Hinduism, and other world religions.

REGAN, TOM, and SINGER, PETER, eds. 1976. *Animal Rights and Human Obligations.* Englewood Cliffs, N.J.: Prentice-Hall. A compilation of major historical sources, including selections from Aristotle, Saint Thomas Aquinas, René Descartes, Voltaire, Immanuel Kant, Arthur Schopenhauer, Jeremy Bentham, and John Stuart Mill.

———. 1989. *Animal Rights and Human Obligations.* 2d ed. Englewood Cliffs, N.J.: Prentice-Hall. Retains some of the major historical sources from the first edition but emphasizes contemporary debates; separate sections on farm animals, the use of nonhuman animals in science, and wildlife issues; includes selections from R. G. Frey, Bernard Rollin, James Rachels, Jan Narveson, and Mary Midgley.

ROLLIN, BERNARD E. 1981. *Animal Rights and Human Morality.* Buffalo, N.Y.: Prometheus. Incorporates Aristotelian ideas about the telos (natural purpose) of nonhuman animals in support of recognition of their rights.

———. 1989. *The Unheeded Cry: Animal Consciousness, Animal Pain, and Science.* New York: Oxford University Press. Especially noteworthy for its discussions of the minds of animals and the ideology of research science.

ROLSTON, HOLMES, III. 1988. *Environmental Ethics: Duties to and Values in the National World.* Philadelphia: Temple University Press.

RYDER, RICHARD D. 1975. *Victims of Science: The Use of Animals in Science.* London: Davis-Poynter. A book that helped launch the modern animal-rights movement.

———. 1989. *Animal Revolution: Changing Attitudes Towards Speciesism.* Oxford: Basil Blackwell. The most complete historical overview of organized efforts to help animals published to date.

SAGOFF, MARK. 1984. "Animal Liberation and Environmental Ethics: Bad Marriage, Quick Divorce." *Osgoode Hall Law Journal* 22, no. 2:297–307. An energetic essay by one of America's leading environmental ethicists.

SAPONTZIS, STEVE F. 1987. *Morals, Reason, and Animals.* Philadelphia: Temple University Press. Includes sustained criticisms of the role of reason in morals and provocative discussions of a range of practical issues, including animal model research and predation.

SHARPE, ROBERT. 1988. *The Cruel Deception: The Use of Animals in Medical Research.* Wellingborough, U.K.: Thorsons. A sustained critique of the scientific basis of animal model research.

SINGER, PETER. 1975. *Animal Liberation: A New Ethics for Our Treatment of Animals.* New York: New York Review. A pioneering examination of the treatment of nonhuman animals.

———. 1990. *Animal Liberation.* 2d ed. New York: New York Review of Books.

———. 1993. "Animals and the Value of Life." In *Matters of Life and Death: New Introductory Essays in Moral Philosophy,* pp. 280–321, 3d ed. Edited by Tom Regan. New York: Random House. Singer here attempts to answer some of the questions not addressed in *Animal Liberation;* includes a useful bibliography.

TAYLOR, PAUL W. 1986. *Respect for Nature: A Theory of Environmental Ethics.* Princeton, N.J.: Princeton University Press. The most systematic environmental ethic available at this time.

VANCE, RICHARD P. 1992. "An Introduction to the Philosophical Presuppositions of the Animal Liberation/Rights Movement." *Journal of the American Medical Association* 288, no. 13:1715–1719. Demythologizes many of the most common misconceptions about animal-rights advocates while criticizing the movement's philosophy.

VANDEVEER, DONALD. 1979. "Of Beasts, Persons, and the Original Position." *Monist* 62, no. 3:368–377. The first work to challenge Rawls's account of the moral status of nonhuman animals.

WARREN, KAREN J. 1990. "The Power and the Promise of Ecological Feminism." *Environmental Ethics* 12, no. 2:125–146. A clear, accessible paper by one of America's leading ecofeminists.

WHITE, LYNN, JR. 1967. "The Historical Roots of Our Ecological Crisis." *Science* 155, no. 3767:1203–1207. A classic examination of the role despotism has played in humanity's abuse of the natural world.

II. VEGETARIANISM

Vegetarianism is traditionally defined as the practice of abstaining from eating animal flesh. Modern vegetarian societies, such as the Vegetarian Society of the United Kingdom, define the practice as abstaining from flesh, fish, and fowl, with or without the addition of dairy produce and eggs. Those who wholly or occasionally abstain from "red meat" but eat fish and/or poultry are described as "demi-" or "semi-" vegetarians. Veganism, or "pure" vegetarianism, is the practice of abstaining as completely as possible from all products and by-products of the slaughterhouse, including products derived from treatment deemed exploitative to animals. Vegans do not consume dairy produce or eggs and also exclude products such as honey on the grounds that animals are used and/or killed in producing such types of human nourishment. Most vegetarians do not wear slaughter-house by-products such as leather, and vegans avoid wearing leather completely.

Health vegetarians

As late as the 1950s, the unwritten consensus among health specialists and dieticians was that animal protein in some form is essential to maintain adequate human health. While this position has not been completely reversed, medical advice from official studies increasingly recommends low-animal-fat diets, some of which eschew animal protein completely. Studies suggest that vegetarians have lower rates of diet-related cancer (Chang-Claude et al., 1992), especially colon and rectal cancer (Phillips, 1975; Willett et al., 1990) and prostate cancer (Giovannucci et al., 1993). Vegetarians experience lower mortality from coronary heart disease than nonvegetarians, possibly due to their lower serum cholesterol levels (Burr and Butland, 1988). One study has shown that mortality from cardiovascular disease among vegetarians was less than half that of the general population (Chang-Claude et al., 1992; see also Snowdon et al., 1984). Vegetarians suffer less from hypertension (Armstrong et al., 1977; Rouse et al., 1983), obesity (Thorogood et al., 1989), and diabetes (Snowdon and Phillips, 1985).

Interpretation of these and other studies has become a source of controversy, with advocates for each side citing evidence in their favor (Frey, 1983; Robbins, 1987). Increasingly, however, health specialists seem to favor vegetarian diets on medical grounds alone. According to present knowledge, a balanced vegetarian diet poses no health problems and offers some indisputable advantages.

"Green" vegetarians

Green political parties in Europe (i.e., those parties committed to programs that give priority to ecological sustainability) increasingly advocate a vegetarian diet or, at least, reduced meat consumption for environmental reasons. For example, the policy of the Green Party of the United Kingdom "encourage[s] a reduction in consumption of animal produce and promote[s] the development and use of foods which are more healthy and humane" (Green Party, 1993, p. 15). They offer two arguments. The first is that if enough Westerners become vegetarians, worldwide food distribution will become more equitable. It is calculated that "if we all had a vegetarian diet and shared our food equally, the biosphere could support around six billion people; if 15 percent of our calories came from animal products (and again food were shared equally), the figure would come down to

four billion people; if 25 percent of our calories came from animal products, then it would fall to three billion; and if 35 percent of our calories came from animal products, as in North America today, then it would fall to 2.5 billion" (Myers, 1990, discussed in Tickell, 1992, p. 67). The second argument is that the present system of intensive farming, while cost-efficient, will prove inefficient in the long run in terms of energy and environmental costs (Porritt, 1984). Hence, Greens argue that the "expanding livestock industry contributes to . . . the destruction and pollution of the planet" by being "energy intensive rather than labour intensive" and contributes to "world starvation" (Green Party, 1993, p. 15).

Assessing these arguments is problematic. While intensive farming is energy inefficient and environmentally damaging—apart from concerns it raises about animal welfare—any measurement of food resources must take into account not only the quantity of food available but also the way in which complex systems of supply and demand militate against egalitarian food distribution. Again, while animal farming is not always an efficient use of food resources, it is not clear that the political will exists to adopt alternative economic policies. Those who are sympathetic to vegetarianism on environmental grounds believe that widespread and increasing vegetarianism can and will affect worldwide trade. Despite the evident increase in the number of vegetarians in the West, it is as yet unclear how far, if at all, such minorities will have lasting economic impact.

In response to the "Green" argument against vegetarianism, some environmental ethicists, while sympathetic to the view that modern industrial agriculture is environmentally damaging, hold that since nature is a predatory system, it is natural for humans as well as animals to consume sentient life forms. Frederick Ferré argues, "From the broadest biotic perspective, life is cannibalistic upon itself; an ecological ethic must begin with the affirmation of the nutrient cycle" (Ferré, 1986, p. 392; see also Birch and Cobb, 1981). This view is reinforced by Holmes Rolston III, who states that "humans in their eating habits follow nature; they can and ought to do so." Rolston's argument is dependent upon a distinction between nature and culture: "Humans, then, can model their dietary habits on their ecosystems, but they cannot and should not model their interpersonal justice or charity on ecosystems" (Rolston, 1988, p. 81).

Both arguments presuppose to some degree that what should be must be modeled on what is. Only faintly, if at all, do ethical considerations fundamentally apply to the human act of killing sentient animals even when it is unnecessary. Ferré and Rolston do not sufficiently consider that what is "given in nature" is as much a social construct as what may be presupposed in "human nature." No perception of nature is value-free. What we judge to be "given in nature" often turns out to be what we ourselves judge on other criteria should be the case. In sum: There is no ecological shortcut to avoiding the question of whether the human killing of sentient animals is a moral issue. Since not all ethicists, especially theological ethicists, are convinced that the natural order exists as God intended, arguments based on what is "natural" beg metaphysical questions about the justice of what is (see Linzey, 1987, 1994; Clark, 1994).

Ethical vegetarians

Of three main arguments for vegetarianism on ethical grounds, the first is based on the value of animal life. Even if we grant animal life secondary or even minimal value, it is difficult to see how human taste preference alone can justify killing. In general, killing for food when it is not required for human health or survival fails the test of moral necessity. Consuming flesh when we could do otherwise is "empty gluttony" (Clark, 1977, p. 183). Some philosophers have argued that it is not justifiable to kill animals even painlessly, asserting that it is logically inconsistent to care whether animals suffer without also valuing animal life itself (Godlovitch, 1971).

Other philosophers perceive gradations of value. Ferré, for example, argues against the assertion that all beings with inherent value possess that value equally. "There is no reason to suppose that the quality and intensity of the mental life—and with it its value for itself—of an oyster is on a par with that of a pheasant; but there is likewise no reason to suppose that the quality and intensity of the mental life of the pheasant is on a par with that of a human child" (Ferré, 1986, p. 396). Ferré argues that "there is no 'line.' . . . All living beings have some degree of inherent value . . . but different organisms call for different forms of respect" (Ferré, 1986, pp. 397–398). But even if such gradations are admitted, the case of mammals, as distinct from plants, calls for greater ethical justification. We still need to know how the killing of animals—which are sentient beings with inherent value superior to that of plants—without strict necessity is compatible with appropriate "respect" for their lives. The logic of Ferré's position is inclusive. Even the killing of plants requires strong ethical justification.

The second argument derives from considerations of animal welfare. If animals should be spared unnecessary suffering, then eating meat should be avoided, since the rearing, transport, and slaughter of farm animals invariably—and in some cases, necessarily—involves suffering, sometimes of a severe and prolonged kind (see Singer, 1976; and Frey, 1983, in response). This argu-

ment gains credibility in light of modern farming methods and the recognized fallibility of slaughtering techniques (Harrison, 1964; Mason and Singer, 1980; Johnson, 1991).

Ferré accepts that many modern farming practices are cruel but argues that "moderate" meat eating is justifiable if "nearly painless methods" of slaughter are adhered to (Ferré, 1986, p. 400). If such a goal were to be achieved, fundamental changes would be required at all levels of livestock management. Minimally, slaughtering techniques would have to be indisputably humane (i.e., render the animal instantaneously unconscious), slaughterhouses would have to be regularly inspected, and regulations would need to be enforced by law. Animals would need to be killed as close as possible to their point of origin to avoid suffering in transit. Handling of animals on farms would have to be subject to a new range of welfare criteria. Conscientious meat eaters could justify eating meat only in specific circumstances when all such conditions have been met. The current failure to secure humane farm management and slaughter renders "moderate" meat eating ethically problematic. While in theory this second argument justifies only provisional vegetarianism in most, perhaps all, circumstances as a protest against animal abuse, it is difficult to envisage a time when conditions will universally prevail so as to preclude animal suffering in agriculture.

The third argument appeals to notions of animal rights. Sentient beings, or beings that can be classed as "subjects of a life," have a right to live that is equal to, or analogous with, human beings' right to live. Vegetarianism, according to the rights view, is obligatory in principle, and entails the end of commercial animal agriculture in practice. However, even this animal right not to be harmed is viewed as "a prima facie, not an absolute right" (Regan, 1983, p. 330).

The precise implications of this argument are not always clear. Do animals have in each and every case an equal right with humans to life? To what extent may individual rights be overridden in particular crisis situations? Commercial nonanimal agriculture also depends to some degree upon the control of competing species. Some animal rightists defend a stricter definition of avoidability or necessity than others. For example, some would concede that meat eating may be justified in those limited situations were alternative resources are inadequate (Linzey, 1987).

Discussion has sometimes centered on the cultural survival of the Inuit peoples, for example, and the question of whether their cultural rights should override the rights of the animals they hunt for food and clothing. Some animal rightists would accept the legitimacy of a limited human-preference approach in such circumstances. George Woodcock maintains that there is not "a single responsible person in the animal rights movement who would object to the Indian or Inuit, where he can, following a partly subsistence life of hunting for food" (Woodcock, 1989, p. 5). Other animal rightists, however, would question whether cultural considerations should be paramount when considering the exploitation of animals. Both "moderate" and "strong" animal-rights positions would, however, concur with Woodcock's judgment that both indigenous peoples, as well as fur-bearing animals, "have always been the victims of the fur trade" (Woodcock, 1989, p. 5). The rights position may be described as the strong welfare position, more uncompromising in its insistence upon the correctness of not harming animals as a prima facie duty. The rights view may not always require absolute (as distinct from obligatory) vegetarianism, but it would contend that vegetarianism should be the ethical and social norm.

Religious vegetarians

Two primary motifs, ascetic and mystical, have informed an ethico-religious awareness. Vegetarianism has an established place in some Indian religious traditions, especially Jainism and, to some degree, Buddhism and Hinduism. The ascetic motif, particularly within Jainism, is based on the doctrines of nonviolence and nonpossessiveness. The goals of the spiritual life are, among other things, the renunciation of aggressive and possessive urges and following the path of purification (Jaini, 1979).

While Christianity has not formally endorsed vegetarianism, some strands of its tradition have affirmed that abstaining from meat can have value as a spiritual discipline. Some religious orders—for example, the Benedictines—eschewed meat as part of their ascetic regime (Sorrell, 1988). Self-denial as part of striving toward moral perfection has sometimes formed the basis for vegetarian lifestyles (Tolstoy, 1961). Ascetic practices may involve a vegetarian diet as a conscientious ecological response to wasteful consumerism and affluence (Lappé, 1982).

Allied to asceticism has been a mystical appreciation of other creatures as valuable beyond human calculations of utility because of their divine creation. The origins of this outlook are clear in the early and medieval periods (Sorrell, 1988). Only in modern times has this viewpoint received systematic expression in notions of reverence for life or in life-centered ethics (Schweitzer, 1967; McDaniel, 1989; Linzey, 1994). Historical Christianity has not fostered these insights, mainly because of its continuing anthropocentric theology. However, theological affirmations that animals are humans' fellow creatures, whose life or spirit belongs to God—and that they are therefore worthy of respect—undergird an ethical impulse to minimize injury and harm to them. Because of the rights of their Creator, animals can be

said to bear "theos-rights," or God-rights (Linzey, 1987, p. 68).

The "modern vegetarian movement"—in the sense of organized societies specifically founded to advance ethical or religious vegetarianism—can be traced to the emergence of humanitarian sensibility from the nineteenth century onward. The Bible Christian Church, founded in 1809 by an Anglican priest, William Cowherd, made vegetarianism compulsory among its members and heralded the later growth of specifically vegetarian societies in the United Kingdom and the United States. The Bible Christian Church found its inspiration in the biblical command, recorded in Genesis 1:29, to be herbivores. Later commands to eat flesh (for example, in Gen. 9:3) were understood as permission given to humankind only after the fall and the flood (for a discussion of Judaism and vegetarianism, see Schwartz, 1988).

The Bible is, however, ambivalent about meat eating. While carnivorousness may be construed as a divine concession to human sinfulness (Baker, 1975), almost all biblical writers accepted the practice as ethically justifiable. Moreover, Jesus Christ was not a "pure" vegetarian; the gospel accounts record that he ate fish. There were various sects advocating vegetarianism in early Jewish and Christian circles, but none of their practices became normative within Judaism or Christianity (Beckwith, 1988). Carnivorousness has seldom been theologically challenged within mainstream religious traditions and only comparatively recently has ethical vegetarianism emerged as a serious option. Some modern Jewish vegetarians (see, e.g., Kook, 1979) argue that abstaining from meat is one step toward realizing the biblical vision of universal peace as described by prophets such as Isaiah (11:6f). Some Christian theologians hold that contemporary vegetarianism constitutes a more Christlike response to the evil of animal exploitation (Linzey, 1994).

The best defense of meat eating is based not only on a denial that animals have rights (Frey, 1980, 1983; Leahy, 1991; Carruthers, 1992) but also a denial that they have any moral status. According to this view, the gastronomic pleasures humans experience by consuming flesh far outweigh the value of animal life and suffering. "By comparison with animals, our lives are of an incomparably greater texture and richness, and when we say of a dying man that he has led a rich, full life we allude to something incomparably beyond to what we would allude, were we to say the same of a dying chicken, cat or chimpanzee" (Frey, 1983, p. 110).

It is difficult to see how such a position can be sustained without putting at risk the moral status of some classes of humans, for example, the mentally handicapped, the comatose, or newborns. Furthermore, it follows from the denial of animal status that a species superior to humans—as some humans now regard themselves in relation to animals—would not be morally obligated to respect human lives and suffering. The hope that "our aliens' nobility will match the quality of their imagined mentality" (Ferré, 1986, p. 406) and that therefore they will spare us unnecessary suffering and death, sadly cannot be deduced from humans' own moral record in relation to sentient nonhumans.

What has given contemporary secular and theological arguments for vegetarianism their strength and cogency is the realization that meat is not generally essential for human health and well-being. Consuming meat may have been necessary at certain times in the past; it may sometimes be necessary in the present. But eating a balanced vegetarian diet carries with it no medical or nutritional handicap. And, more important, it respects the ethical injunction to avoid killing sentient beings whenever possible.

ANDREW LINZEY

Directly related to this article are the other articles in this entry, especially the articles on ETHICAL PERSPECTIVES ON THE TREATMENT AND STATUS OF ANIMALS, *and* ANIMALS IN AGRICULTURE AND FACTORY FARMING. *Also directly related are the entries* AGRICULTURE; ANIMAL RESEARCH, *article on* PHILOSOPHICAL ISSUES; FOOD POLICY; JAINISM; *and* JUSTICE. *Other relevant material may be found under the entries* BIOTECHNOLOGY; ENVIRONMENTAL ETHICS; ENVIRONMENT AND RELIGION; GENETIC ENGINEERING, *article on* ANIMALS AND PLANTS; POPULATION ETHICS, *section on* ELEMENTS OF POPULATION ETHICS, *article on* IS THERE A POPULATION PROBLEM?; RIGHTS, *article on* RIGHTS IN BIOETHICS; *and* VETERINARY ETHICS.

Bibliography

ADAMS, CAROL J. 1990. *The Sexual Politics of Meat: A Feminist-Vegetarian Critical Theory.* New York: Continuum.

ARMSTRONG, BRUCE K.; VAN MERWYCK, ANTHONY J.; and COATES, HARVEY 1977. "Blood Pressure in Seventh-Day Adventist Vegetarians." *American Journal of Epidemiology* 105, no. 5:444–449.

BAKER, JOHN AUSTIN. 1975. "Biblical Attitudes to Nature." In *Man and Nature,* pp. 87–109. Edited by Hugh Montefiore. London: Collins.

BECKWITH, ROGER T. 1988. "The Vegetarianism of the Therapeutae, and the Motives for Vegetarianism in Early Jewish and Christian Circles." *Revue de Qumran* 13, nos. 49–52:407–410.

BIRCH, CHARLES, and COBB, JOHN B., JR. 1981. *The Liberation of Life: From Cell to Community.* Cambridge: At the University Press.

BURR, MICHAEL L., and BUTLAND, BARBARA K. 1988. "Heart Disease in British Vegetarians." *American Journal of Clinical Nutrition* 48, no. 3(suppl.):830–832.

CARRUTHERS, PETER. 1992. *The Animals Issue: Moral Theory in Practice.* Cambridge: At the University Press.

CHANG-CLAUDE, JENNY; FRENTZEL-BEYME, RAINER; and EILBER, URSULA 1992. "Mortality Pattern of German Vegetarians After 11 Years of Follow-up." *Epidemiology* 3, no. 5:395–401.

CLARK, STEPHEN R. L. 1977. *The Moral Status of Animals.* Oxford: At the Clarendon Press.

———. 1994. *How to Think About the Earth: The Philosophical and Theological Models for Ecology.* London: Mowbray.

FERRÉ, FREDERICK. 1986. "Moderation, Morals and Meat." *Inquiry* 29:391–406.

FIDDES, NICK. 1991. *Meat: A Natural Symbol.* London: Routledge.

FOX, MICHAEL W., and WISWALL, NANCY E. 1989. *The Hidden Costs of Beef.* Washington, D.C.: Humane Society of the United States.

FREY, RAYMOND G. 1980. *Interests and Rights: The Case Against Animals.* Oxford: At the Clarendon Press.

———. 1983. *Rights, Killing and Suffering: Moral Vegetarianism and Applied Ethics.* Oxford: Basil Blackwell.

GIOVANNUCCI, EDWARD; RIMM, ERIC B.; COLDITZ, GRAHAM A.; STAMPFER, MEIR J.; ASCHERIO, ALBERTO; CHUTE, CHRIS C.; and WILLETT, WALTER C. 1993. "A Prospective Study of Dietary Fat and Risk of Prostate Cancer." *Journal of the National Cancer Institute* 85, no. 19:1571–1579.

GODLOVITCH, ROSLIND. 1971. "Animals and Morals." In *Animals, Men and Morals: An Inquiry into the Maltreatment of the Non-Human,* pp. 156–172, by Stanley Godlovitch, Roslind Godlovitch, and John Harris. London: Victor Gollancz.

GREEN PARTY. 1993. "Animal Rights." In *Green Party MfSS,* 15–16. London: Author.

HARRISON, RUTH. 1964. *Animal Machines: The New Factory Farming Industry.* London: Vincent Stuart.

JAINI, PADMANABH S. 1979. *The Jaina Path of Purification.* Berkeley: University of California Press.

JOHNSON, ANDREW. 1991. *Factory Farming.* Oxford: Basil Blackwell.

KOOK, ABRAHAM ISAAC. 1979. "Fragments of Light: A View as to the Reasons for the Commandments." In *The Lights of Penitence; The Moral Principles; Lights of Holiness: Essays, Letters, and Poems,* pp. 303–323. Translated by Ben Zion Bokser. London: SPCK.

LAPPÉ, FRANCES M. 1982. *Diet for a Small Planet.* 2d rev. ed. New York: Ballantine.

LEAHY, MICHAEL. 1991. *Against Liberation: Putting Animals in Perspective.* London: Routledge.

LINZEY, ANDREW. 1976. *Animal Rights: A Christian Assessment of Man's Treatment of Animals.* London: SCM.

———. 1987. *Christianity and the Rights of Animals.* London.

———. 1994. *Animal Theology.* London: SCM.

MASON, JIM, and SINGER, PETER, eds. 1980. *Animal Factories.* New York: Crown.

McDANIEL, JAY B. 1989. *Of God and Pelicans: A Theology of Reverence for Life.* Louisville, Ky.: Westminster/John Knox.

MYERS, NORMAN. 1990. *Mass Extinctions: Palaeogeography, Palaeoclimatology, Palaeoecology.* Amsterdam: Elsevier Science Publishers.

PHILLIPS, ROLAND L. 1975. "Role of Life-Style and Dietary Habits in Risk of Cancer Among Seventh-Day Adventists." *Cancer Research* 35, no. 11:3513–3522.

PORRITT, JONATHON. 1984. *Seeing Green: The Politics of Ecology Explained.* Oxford: Basil Blackwell.

REGAN, TOM. 1983. *The Case for Animal Rights.* London: Routledge & Kegan Paul.

ROBBINS, JOHN. 1987. *Diet for a New America: How Your Food Choices Affect Your Health.* 2d rev. ed. Walpole, N.H.: Stillpoint.

ROLSTON, HOLMES, III. 1988. *Environmental Ethics: Duties to and Values in the Natural World.* Philadelphia: Temple University Press.

ROUSE, IAN L.; ARMSTRONG, BRUCE K.; and BEILIN, LAWRENCE J. 1983. "The Relationship of Blood Pressure to Diet and Lifestyle in Two Religious Populations." *Journal of Hypertension* 1 no. 1:65–71.

SCHWARTZ, RICHARD H. 1988. *Judaism and Vegetarianism.* Marblehead, Mass.: Micah.

SCHWEITZER, ALBERT. 1967. *Civilization and Ethics.* Translated by C. T. Campion. 2d ed. London: Unwin.

SINGER, PETER. 1976. *Animal Liberation: A New Ethics for Our Treatment of Animals.* London: Jonathan Cape.

SNOWDON, DAVID A., and PHILLIPS, ROLAND L. 1985. "Does a Vegetarian Diet Reduce the Occurrence of Diabetes?" *American Journal of Public Health* 75, no. 5:507–512.

SNOWDON, DAVID A.; PHILLIPS, ROLAND L.; and FRASER, GARY E. 1984. "Meat Consumption and Fatal Ischemic Heart Disease." *Preventive Medicine* 13, no. 5:490–500.

SORRELL, ROGER D. 1988. *St. Francis of Assisi and Nature: Tradition and Innovation in Western Christian Attitudes Toward the Environment.* New York: Oxford University Press.

THOROGOOD, MARGARET; McPHERSON, KLIM; and MANN, JIM 1989. "Relationship of Body Mass Index, Weight and Height to Plasma Lipid Levels in People with Different Diets in Britain." *Community Medicine* 11, no. 3: 230–233.

TICKELL, CRISPIN. 1992. "The Quality of Life: What Quality? Whose Life?" *Interdisciplinary Science Reviews* 17, no. 1:19–25.

TOLSTOY, LEO. 1961. "The First Step." In *Recollections and Essays,* 4th ed., pp. 123–134. Translated by Aylmer Maude. London: Oxford University Press.

WILLETT, WALTER C.; STAMPFER, MEIR J.; COLDITZ, GRAHAM A.; ROSNER, BERNARD A.; and SPEIZER, FRANK E. 1990. "Relation of Meat, Fat and Fiber Intake to the Risk of Colon Cancer in a Prospective Study Among Women." *New England Journal of Medicine* 323, no. 24:1664–1672.

WOODCOCK, GEORGE. 1989. "A Briefing on the Fur Trade and Aboriginal Cultures." In *Skinned,* pp. 1–5. Nottingham, U.K.: Lynx.

III. WILDLIFE CONSERVATION AND MANAGEMENT

Wildlife management may be thought a contradiction in terms. The logic of "wild" precludes "managed." Wildlife lived for millions of years, unmanaged by humans. Part of what humans value in wildlife is animals that can look out for themselves. Wildlife that is managed is not wild; it is managed life. So there is logical difficulty in the idea. There is also ethical difficulty. Perhaps humans are not responsible for wildlife; wild lives are on their own. But then again, human activities affect wildlife quite adversely. Have we no duty to care for it, either because of what humans have at stake or because of what wildlife is in itself?

This article outlines some main issues: the contemporary crisis of conserving historically evolved wildlife populations on rapidly developing human landscapes; ownership, control, management, and stewardship responsibilities for wildlife; conservation of endangered wildlife species; fishes and fisheries as managed wildlife populations; wildlife as game for hunting and trapping, including hunting as a conservation strategy; "hands-on" versus "hands-off" management; and feral animals. These are issues of management, but there are ethical questions at every point.

Wildlife and human populations: An emerging crisis

There are more species on Earth today than there have ever been in the 2.5-billion-year history of life. Estimates run from five to thirty million species; ten million is a typical figure. Most of the vertebrate wildlife and birds are known; most unknowns are in the invertebrate animal, insect, and plant species. During evolutionary history, there was no wildlife management; wildlife conservation takes care of itself if no humans intervene. On statistical average, more species have been produced than have become extinct; diversity has gradually increased.

Some five catastrophic extinctions have been followed by rather swift regeneration of the lost species. On landscapes that have grown colder or drier, species may become fewer. Some groups of species were more numerous in the past, such as dinosaurs in the Cretaceous period, or birds in the Pleistocene. Nevertheless, diversity is at an all-time high. In one sense, all biology is conservation biology (biology that conserves life), whether or not humans are involved.

There are many more humans on Earth today than ever, and the expansion of human habitat, coupled with pollution, hunting, and trade in wildlife, threatens populations of wild animals and their habitats. Humans now threaten the biological processes that have been creating and conserving life for billions of years. Hardly an American landscape has not been impoverished of its native fauna. The larger once-dominant animals—such as eagles, wolves, cougars, grizzly bears, wolverines, bison, otters, crocodiles—are especially depleted. The New World depletion in both hemispheres is a result of Europeans entering a relatively empty continent and engaging in explosive development over recent centuries.

The Amerindians had coexisted with wildlife for ten to fifteen thousand years.

Long-settled continents do not escape the problem either. Humans have inhabited Africa since evolving there over a hundred thousand years ago. Only in the twentieth century, as contemporary nations have grown rapidly, has African megafauna or avifauna been seriously threatened. Wildlife in China, India, and Tibet, among the oldest settled areas in the world, has been greatly depleted in this century. The crisis is as serious in the Old World as in the New.

The crisis is now potentially more urgent than at any previous time in the history of the planet. This generates unprecedented responsibilities because humans previously did not have much effect on wildlife, which took care of itself; unprecedented demands for trade-offs between human values and the welfare of wildlife; and unprecedented implications because of its global and irreversible scale.

Wildlife conservation is now challenged to mix human values with wildlife values. Fortunately, wildlife is valuable to humans and, so far, can be included among the human values. Humans wish to hunt and fish; they enjoy watchable wildlife; wildlife art is the most popular American art form. If backyard bird feeding is included, almost one in four Americans spends some time birdwatching. Animals are chosen as state animals; sports teams and automobiles are named for animals. Many animals serve useful roles in ecosystems; hawks catch mice, birds control insect populations. Wildlife can indicate the health of an ecosystem. Unfortunately, many human values conflict with wildlife on landscapes, as shown by the massive depletion of wildlife. Here human interests seem contrary to wildlife's flourishing. And what if wildlife is not valuable to humans? Have we some responsibilities for the values of wild things for what they are in themselves?

The Wildlife Society, the principal professional organization of management and conservation, affirms that "Wildlife, in its myriad forms, is basic to the maintenance of a human culture that provides quality living." The society seeks "to develop and promote sound stewardship of wildlife resources and of the environments upon which wildlife and humans depend; to undertake an active role in preventing human-induced environmental degradation; to increase awareness and appreciation of wildlife values." It also urges "ethical restraints in the use of living natural resources" (Wildlife Society, 1990).

Ownership, control, management, and stewardship responsibilities for wildlife

According to long legal tradition in the United Kingdom, Canada, the United States, and many other nations, individual persons do not own vertebrate wildlife.

Animals and birds do not belong to the landowner on whose property they are found. They move around, with dens and nests in particular places, but the larger animals and the birds can range over hundreds or thousands of square miles. They sometimes live on public land, sometimes on different tracts of private land. Continental European nations, by contrast, sometimes hold that property owners own wildlife resident on their lands.

In the Anglo-American tradition, landowners have the right to control access to their property; they control who, for instance, may hunt there. But the state determines whether and how much game may be taken. Permitted by the state, individuals can "take" wildlife—capture or kill it—at which point the animal enters their possession. State control of wildlife was long understood as state ownership, but wildlife paid no more attention to state lines than to local property boundaries; indeed, migratory birds resided in various nations. The U.S. federal government has often regulated wildlife, since much wildlife crosses state lines and much inhabits federal lands. In recent court decisions, the state ownership doctrine has been rejected as based on a flawed characterization of wildlife, which should be regulated like other natural resources considered commons, not so much owned as held in trust. State ownership of wildlife has been subsumed under the state and federal power to regulate all natural resources, an expanding public trust doctrine. Wildlife is a public good held in trust by the state for the benefit of the people (Bean, 1983).

The general idea is that there is a corporate responsibility for wildlife, a duty to persons concerning wildlife in which they have an interest, and a duty of individual persons to relate to wildlife, caring for it, tolerating it, perhaps hunting it, all within the context of a larger public interest and stewardship. Animal welfare was long subsumed under this rubric, since maintaining this public good required healthy wildlife populations. But animal welfare has increasingly become a concern in its own right, independent of human benefits. This is called the intrinsic value of wildlife, a value also held in trust. This concern becomes evident in concern for endangered species as well as in shifting attitudes toward hunting.

Conservation of endangered wildlife species

The legal tradition arose with regard to individual animals, but protecting endangered species has increasingly figured in regulations covering both game and nongame species. State departments, once of "Game and Fish," have largely been renamed departments of "Wildlife"; though hunting and fishing remain a large part of their assignments, their interest in threatened wildlife has dramatically increased. If the government can regulate individual animals, by the same logic it can regulate species. In the fall of 1981, when black-footed ferrets were discovered on private ranches near Meeteetse, Wyoming, the ranchers were legally obligated to protect them. Furthermore, the federal government can designate critical habitat on private land.

Landowners ought not to shoot the bald eagles that fly over their property or cut the trees in which they nest. In compliance with the Endangered Species Act, in order to protect eighty bald eagle nesting sites, the Weyerhaeuser Company in the early 1980s set aside more than nine hundred acres in Washington and Oregon, representing over nine million dollars in unharvested timber. Lest it be supposed that the bald eagle, the national symbol, is a unique public good, Weyerhaeuser also, complying with the act, set aside 155 acres in southern states to protect 22 colonies of the endangered red-cockaded woodpecker. These woodpeckers prefer to nest in prime timber, eighty-year-old pine forests; loggers would rather cut these lands more often than that. Though these landowners cannot use the land as they once intended, costing them that opportunity, it does so lest they destroy, at the species level, eagles and woodpeckers that, though on their land, do not belong to them but are a common good.

The Endangered Species Act of 1973 is the most far-reaching wildlife statute adopted by any nation. The U.S. Fish and Wildlife Service is charged by the act to list both domestic and foreign wildlife species threatened with extinction. No government agency may undertake projects likely to jeopardize listed species, at home or abroad, except under authority of a high-level committee that has granted few exemptions. Jeopardizing species includes disrupting their habitat. Neither can persons take listed wildlife species on private lands. In evaluating whether to list a species, economic considerations may not be considered, a point of repeated contention but one that the U.S. Congress has reaffirmed several times. Importing species on the worldwide list into the United States is illegal except under specific conditions.

Generally this concern, enacted into legislation, reveals an increasing sense of human duty toward wildlife that comes to special focus when a species becomes endangered. Game managers who may once have thought of their responsibility as the production of an annual crop of game to shoot now see themselves as wildlife managers whose responsibility is to provide for a diverse native fauna on the landscape, both for the benefits such wildlife brings to humans and out of respect for what all species of wildlife, not just the game species, are in themselves.

Fish and fisheries as managed wildlife populations

Analogous changes have taken place with regard to fishes. Once, what one wanted was fish to catch; and fishing remains a popular recreation. But there is an increasing concern with native fish populations, now including all species.

The native fish fauna of North America has been tampered with possibly as extensively as, and certainly more rapidly than, the fish on any other continent. Managers have introduced "game" and eliminated "trash" fish; humans have made dams and water developments for domestic, industrial, and agricultural uses; polluted; caused erosional sedimentation; and accidentally introduced parasites and diseases. Of the endangered fishes of the world, about 70 percent are in North America; 56 percent are receiving some degree of protection. The fishes in the United States have been as disturbed as any other wildlife, more so in the West than in the East, most of all in the Southwest. The Endangered Species Committee of the Desert Fishes Council identifies 164 fishes in North American deserts as endangered, vulnerable, rare, or warranting various degrees of concern.

Concern for these fishes has modified or stopped water development projects. On the Virgin River and its tributaries in Utah in 1980, for example, water authorities abandoned the Warner Valley project lest it jeopardize the woundfin, and built the Quail Creek project instead. Water release from dams may be adjusted in time and volume for the benefit of endangered fish and bird species (Minckley and Deacon, 1991).

Coming to focus again in endangered species legislation, what humans think they ought to manage for is shifting from game species to native fishery populations. There is an increasing sense of duty, represented in wildlife managers, to ensure the presence of fishes as an integral part of the wildlife community, not just for the human benefits involved but out of respect for what these fishes are in themselves, as well as for their roles in the riparian ecosystems.

Hunting and trapping: Hunting as a conservation strategy

Wildlife management has traditionally meant game management. Hunting both for meat and for sport is an ancient practice. Humans evolved as omnivores; meat has been important in human nutrition, although it is quite possible for humans to be well nourished as vegetarians. The character of hunting has accentuated sport hunting in modern times; few hunters today are primarily meat hunters, although in most cases the carcass will be eaten. Most hunters have a code of ethics. They think it unethical to waste the meat. Hunters also seek a fair chase, a clean kill, minimal suffering, and respect for the animal; and hunters have long been among the most effective conservationists. Predators, especially wolves, were often eliminated as competitive hunters.

Since the mid-1960s, a strong antihunting movement has emerged, on the ground that shooting animals for sport is unethical, even if the hunter's ethic is observed. Such persons regard wildlife management for the purposes of maintaining hunting as morally wrong. A further problem is that much funding for wildlife conservation comes from hunting and fishing licenses, and if these activities are curtailed, alternative funding sources will have to be found. Hunters also argue that properly managed hunting can ensure conservation, since this activity makes wildlife valuable both to the hunter and to others who profit from the hunter's presence.

Such an argument is especially used for African wildlife. In Africa, although much hunting is legal, poaching has also been rampant, resulting in an international ban on skins, hides, horns, tusks, and other parts of various species. Wildlife managers may argue that whereas such bans may discourage poachers, they also prevent legal hunting, which can be quite profitable; this makes wildlife worthless to native peoples, who can neither hunt for food nor sell wildlife products. Even the products from culled animals (shot to reduce excess populations) cannot be sold. Ivory has been a case in point. Most world ivory trade is now illegal, but some authorities argue that the sale of legal ivory could greatly benefit elephant conservation.

Trapping has been a traditional use of wildlife, largely for the pelts and hides made into mink coats, beaver hats, alligator-skin purses and shoes, and so on. Given available substitutes, many people object to such use of animals, on grounds that this trapping involves needless cruelty. Furs on fashion models simply flatter female vanities, somewhat as trophy animals mounted in sportsmen's dens flatter male vanities. The leghold trap is especially objectionable to opponents of trapping. A counterargument is that a high value on animal skins, with effective management, can ensure conservation. Most of the world's crocodile species are endangered; crocodiles are dangerous and often frequent rivers where humans are present. Only if the crocodiles are of considerable value to local peoples are they likely to be tolerated and saved.

"Hands-on" versus "hands-off" management

Although there is a growing consensus that humans have an urgent responsibility actively to conserve wildlife, many argue that the less wildlife is managed, the better. So far as wild animals are managed, their wildness is compromised—the paradox of wildlife management. The animals become artifacts, more like pets. This leads to a debate between "hands-on management," which favors active intervention, habitat enhancement, supplemental feeding, breeding, radio-collared monitoring, and so on, versus "hands-off management," which favors as little management as possible consistent with animal welfare.

From a medical point of view, there is contention whether veterinarians ought to treat wildlife diseases. Like all physicians, veterinarians seek good health. Colorado veterinarians treated a lungworm disease in bighorn sheep successfully. By contrast, when an epidemic of pinkeye ravaged the bighorn sheep of Yellowstone Park, authorities refused to let Wyoming veterinarians treat the disease. The welfare of the sheep, they said, required letting the disease take its course; disease-resistant sheep would survive and the genetic fitness of the herd would improve. Whether the disease is introduced by humans is a factor. The *Chlamydia* parasite producing pinkeye was not thought to be introduced; some said that the lungworm was introduced from domestic sheep, or at least that the sheep were weakened due to human disruptions, especially of their winter range. Although over half the Yellowstone herd perished by starvation and injury following partial blindness, the herd has recovered, although not yet to its former numbers.

Many argue that although hands-off management is an ideal for animals that inhabit extensive ranges, owing to development and human needs there remains insufficient habitat for hands-off management. With elephants in Africa, they say, only hands-on management is possible. Given the elephant's destructiveness and its tendencies to migrate, herds must be fenced, water holes provided, herds culled, and so on. This strikes a balance between responsibilities for elephants and for humans. A controversial case in the United States involved supplemental feeding for grizzly bears in Yellowstone Park, where, after such feeding went on for decades, park officials, preferring a wild bear over a managed bear, elected to risk letting the endangered species survive on its own.

Feral animals

Feral animals are those introduced by humans, not native to landscapes, that have managed to survive on their own. Management of such animals is disputed, especially of mustangs and burros in the western United States. Although not now living in their native ecosystems, such animals may have been living wild for centuries. Management policy is typically to eliminate them, on grounds that they are not authentic wildlife, although the U.S. Congress has mandated preserving mustangs in some localities. Animal-welfare advocates have protested eliminating the mustangs and burros. Other cases involve feral hogs and goats. On San Clemente Island, off the coast of California, nearly thirty thousand goats were eliminated, about half of them shot, the other half captured and relocated with poor survival rates, in order to protect endangered species of plants, as well as to prevent further degradation of the island ecosystem. The goats had been left there by the Spanish in earlier centuries. The argument here is that we have a greater responsibility to native wildlife and plants than to feral species.

HOLMES ROLSTON, III

Directly related to this article are the other articles in this entry, especially the articles on ETHICAL PERSPECTIVES ON THE TREATMENT AND STATUS OF ANIMALS, HUNTING, *and* ZOOS AND ZOOLOGICAL PARKS. *For a further discussion of topics mentioned in this article, see the entry* ENDANGERED SPECIES AND BIODIVERSITY. *Other relevant material may be found under the entry* ENVIRONMENTAL ETHICS. *See also the* APPENDIX (CODES, OATHS, AND DIRECTIVES RELATED TO BIOETHICS), SECTION VI: ETHICAL DIRECTIVES PERTAINING TO THE ENVIRONMENT.

Bibliography

BAILEY, JAMES A. 1984. *Principles of Wildlife Management.* New York: John Wiley.

BEAN, MICHAEL J. 1983. *The Evolution of National Wildlife Law.* Rev. ed. New York: Praeger.

Endangered Species Act of 1973. 1973. Publ. L. no. 93-205, 87 Stat. 884.

HARGROVE, EUGENE C., ed. 1992. *The Animal Rights, Environmental Ethics Debate: The Environmental Perspective.* Albany: State University of New York Press.

MINCKLEY, WENDELL L., and DEACON, JAMES E., eds. 1991. *Battle Against Extinction: Native Fish Management in the American West.* Tucson: University of Arizona Press.

WILDLIFE SOCIETY. 1990. *Conservation Policies of the Wildlife Society.* Bethesda, Md.: Author.

IV. PET AND COMPANION ANIMALS

The term "companion animals" refers to those animals human beings keep for purposes of control, companionship, and comfort. The word "pet," which suggests the indulgent use of animals (Shell, 1986), is being increasingly replaced by the term "companion animals." However, the term "pet animal" seems indispensable in conveying the relationship of intimacy between some humans and selected domesticated species.

The emergence of pet keeping

The precise origins of pet keeping are obscure. There appear always to have been symbiotic relationships both between species and within species (see, for example, Kropotkin, 1939), although some argue that "almost alone among animals, humans domesticate and dwell with other animals" (Clark, 1982, p. 110). Keeping animals as companions may have been a by-product of both killing and domesticating them. Stephen Clark argues that "[p]eople who cared for their animals [kept for food] left more descendants than those who used them

carelessly" and that "it 'paid' our ancestors to love what wasn't human" (Clark, 1982, p. 111).

Some animals were undoubtedly kept for their own value as sources of fascination or as mediators of unusual benefits. For example, cats, although domesticated for a much briefer time than other species, have frequently been associated with the supernatural, as agents either of benign or malign forces (Clutton-Brock, 1993).

English society in the eighteenth and nineteenth centuries saw the emergence of widespread pet keeping, especially among the upper classes. Keith Thomas writes of how, as early as 1700, "symptoms of obsessive pet-keeping were in evidence," especially in the keeping of horses, cats, dogs, and pet birds (Thomas, 1983, p. 117). These species were clearly "privileged" in comparison with food animals, which were still reared and killed with hideous cruelty. Although the "idea of a pedigree did not originate in the nineteenth century," Harriet Ritvo shows how the notion of purity of species through selective breeding became widespread among the middle and upper classes, for whom particular companion animals were themselves indicators of social class and good breeding (Ritvo, 1986).

Since the nineteenth century, the phenomenon of pet keeping has increased not only among all English classes but also within European and U.S. societies. Although reliable estimates of animal populations are very difficult to obtain (partly because of nonexistent or unenforced licensing laws), one conservative estimate is that the total annual U.S. turnover in owned dogs in 1991 was 7.71 million, 4 million of which were handled by animal shelters and 2.1 million of which were euthanized (Patronek and Glickman, 1994). The current situation in the Western world of millions of animals being kept for purposes of companionship extends far beyond any reasonable interpretation of symbiosis and is historically without parallel.

Quite apart from the personal and psychological factors involved, one obvious reason accounts for this development. Pet owning has become an established part of consumer-oriented cultures in which animals are bought and sold like any other commodity. The pet industry itself, not to mention the allied supply (including veterinary) services, benefit directly or indirectly from the trade, management, and treatment of companion animals. In 1991, in the state of Washington alone, it is estimated that the number of dogs available from pet stores amounted to 11,442, and through breeders, 37,523 (Patronek and Glickman, 1994).

The benefits of pet keeping

These may be classed under three broad headings:

Psychological benefits to humans.   It seems impossible to doubt that some human–animal bonds can contribute significantly to human flourishing. Relationships with pets seem to help prevent two sources of emotional disorder: deprivation and frustration. They enable nongenital physical contact, provide tactile comfort, improve self-esteem, enhance emotional security, boost personal prowess (as when a beautiful or socially appealing animal is owned), and engender loving relationships that are sometimes seemingly impossible with other humans (Ryder, 1973; Levinson, 1978; Fogle, 1981; see also Serpell, 1986).

Potential or actual benefits for pet owners specifically include lower blood pressure (Baun et al., 1984), lower heart rates (DeShriver and Riddick, 1990; Wilson and Nettling, 1987), reduced anxiety (Wilson, 1991), and reduced depression (Bolin, 1987). However, Cindy Wilson argues that although "much has been made over the potential benefits of a pet," it is also true that a large amount of such research "remains anecdotal, nongeneralizable, and scientifically flawed" and that a new methodology should be based on assessable "quality of life measurements" (Wilson, 1994, pp. 4–8).

In the absence of large amounts of data based on objective evidence, interpretation of the psychological effects of pet keeping turns on whether interspecies relations are natural and commendable. Richard Ryder warns against the view that such interspecies relationships are "unnatural or cranky" (Ryder, 1973, p. 5); but that accepted, it is still questionable to what extent legitimate psychological needs are met through pet keeping and whether these needs can or should be met through relationships with members of our own species.

Benefits to human society. It has long been thought that pet keeping can help sensitize children, even train them in attitudes of care and respect (Rothschild, 1986). One study goes so far as to claim that "companion animals are a vital part of the healthy emotional development of children" (Robin and Bensel, 1991, p. 174). Studies have also suggested that relationships with pets can contribute to the psychological and social well-being of adult humans, especially elderly people who live alone (Connell and Lago, 1991). Animal-assisted therapy is sometimes utilized for patients in psychiatric hospitals and for individuals with special needs, such as people with the human immunodeficiency virus (HIV) or aquired immunodeficiency syndrome (AIDS) (Gorczyca, 1991) and those suffering from chronic schizophrenia (Bauman et al., 1991).

Benefits to pet animals. The benefits of pet keeping to the animals themselves are difficult to quantify. Leaving aside the wider ethical question of whether animals should be domesticated at all, the impact on the individual pet depends on how well it is kept and to what degree its owners understand and meet its emotional and environmental needs. For example, although pet keeping can provide a stimulus to sensitize children, it can also conversely provide an opportunity for cruelty by abused or disturbed children or by children who lack

parental supervision. Some commentators see something psychologically, even politically, perverse about indulging pet animals (see, for example, Shell, 1986), and, as discussed below, it is not clear that such indulgence is always beneficial to the animals' welfare.

The disadvantages of pet keeping

Formidable ethical and welfare problems are associated with pet keeping (Carpenter et al., 1980). These may be classified under three headings:

Abuse. Recorded acts of cruelty against pets appear to be increasing in both the United States and the United Kingdom. Living in close proximity to animals, whatever the benefits to both parties, substantially increases the risk of abuse. Apart from deliberate acts of cruelty, even sadism, unsuitable environmental conditions can cause unacceptably high levels of stress for animals. Few owners fully understand the complex psychological and physiological needs of the animals they keep. Cruelty sometimes arises through ignorance and misunderstanding rather than deliberate neglect, especially when the subjects are exotic animals. Abuse or neglect does occur despite the many and various pet-care programs available.

Overpopulation. Present high levels of pet populations inevitably mean death, and sometimes suffering, for other animals. In order to sustain high populations of species such as cats and dogs, for example, other species such as whales, kangaroos, and horses must be killed in order to feed them. Few pet animals of any size can be sustained without meat, though it now appears that dogs can live well on an appropriately balanced vegetarian diet. The commercial production of pet food has also been criticized as a waste of resources. The average cost of feeding an eighty-pound dog has been estimated at $8,353 for its lifetime (Shell, 1986).

High pet populations also raise other problems for humans. These include possible health hazards, nuisance, and social control. Dogs can communicate diseases such as *Toxicara canis*, which can cause blindness in children. Fortunately, such cases are rare, but an awareness of this hazard in the United Kingdom has recently led to local councils outlawing dogs from public parks, particularly children's parks. Animal organizations, such as the United Kingdom's Royal Society for the Prevention of Cruelty to Animals (RSPCA), have argued the case for compulsory registration of dogs as a means of ensuring responsible ownership; so far, such schemes have operated only on a voluntary or local basis. In 1992, the Dangerous Dogs Act was introduced in the United Kingdom to deal with the threat posed by aggressive dogs after some distressing incidents in which children were attacked by uncontrolled dogs.

Commercial usage. Since domestic animals have almost everywhere only the legal status of property

(Sandys-Winsch, 1984; Sweeney, 1990), the breeding and sale of pets is subject to few legal constraints, save principally that direct and "unnecessary" cruelty must be avoided. The view that pets are merely human property has inevitably led, as with other consumer items, to the refashioning of pets. Nonveterinary mutilation of pets (e.g., tail docking, ear cropping, declawing, and removal of a dog's larynx to prevent barking) is not uncommon, though in the United Kingdom the British Veterinary Association now refuses to authorize all nonveterinary procedures; performance of such procedures can lead to revocation of a veterinarian's license. The RSPCA opposes all "selective breeding of animals which produces changes in bodily form and/or function," in addition to the commercial sale of puppies and kittens in pet shops (RSPCA, 1984, pp. 7–8).

Animal protectionists argue that the commercial trade in animals leads inevitably to overbreeding and the consequent abandonment and disposal of millions of unwanted animals. In the United Kingdom, the RSPCA estimates that it destroys on average about 1,000 unwanted dogs every week. In the United States, estimates vary from 2.1 million to 9.1 million for dogs alone (Patronek and Glickman, 1994). Such a wide discrepancy in the figures indicates, among other things, the difficulty in collecting uniform data from the estimated 1,800 to 3,000 animal shelters in the United States. Current widespread euthanasia suggests a prima facie disregard for the worth of pet animals (for a discussion of the ethical problems surrounding large-scale euthanasia, see Kay et al., 1988).

Is pet keeping immoral?

Despite the emergence of a strong animal-rights movement over the last twenty years, the ethics of pet keeping is seldom questioned. The major works in animal ethics (Singer, 1976; Clark, 1977; Regan, 1983; Rodd, 1990) largely or entirely bypass this question, and only lone voices are raised in critical opposition (Linzey, 1976; Bryant, 1982). Animal-rights philosophy has evolved without offering any critical analysis of the pet trade, though some argue that abuse of pet animals is a "human breach of contract" (Rollin, 1992, p. 219). Since so many animal-rights thinkers oppose a purely utilitarian justification for animal exploitation, this omission is surely anomalous.

Part of the reason may be that, historically speaking, sensibility to animal suffering seems to have arisen as a necessary corollary to the practice of keeping pets (Thomas, 1983; Tester, 1991). The physical inclusion of animals into the human community seems to have signified a moral inclusiveness also. It may be no accident that the first country to found a society for the prevention of cruelty to animals—England—was also the coun-

try renowned for its love of pet animals. Moreover, one cannot but be struck by the way in which anecdotes about animal behavior, especially that of pet animals, have formed the basis for a whole string of pioneering humanitarian books appealing for greater kindness to animals and a fundamental recognition of their rights (see, for example, Youatt, 1839; Wood, 1874; Nicholson, 1879; Thomas, 1993; Lessing, 1991).

Yet questions must be asked about the ethical appropriateness of the psychological needs that pet animals apparently meet. Ryder accepts that some of these are "selfish" (Ryder, 1973, p. 8). One early critique argued that "we need to distinguish between a kind of love which respects animals for what they are and allows them to pursue their own lives according to their own natural instincts, and another selfish form of love which seeks to condition animal lives in accordance with our own human desires." Pet keeping, it is argued, represents a "false anthropomorphism" in which we seek to "humanise" animals and "regard them as extensions of our own egos" (Linzey, 1976, p. 68). This view was subsequently modified on the grounds that "all loving is in practice a subtle blend of altruism and self-seeking," although "where the interests of animals are entirely subordinated to human emotional needs, we need to beware that we are not involved in a self-deceiving tyranny" (Linzey, 1987, p. 137). According to this perspective, at least some forms of pet keeping are wrong because they are insufficiently symbiotic and fail to recognize the right of animals to their own natural life.

ANDREW LINZEY

Directly related to this article are the other articles in this entry: ETHICAL PERSPECTIVES ON THE TREATMENT AND STATUS OF ANIMALS, VEGETARIANISM, WILDLIFE CONSERVATION AND MANAGEMENT, ZOOS AND ZOOLOGICAL PARKS, HUNTING, *and* ANIMALS IN AGRICULTURE AND FACTORY FARMING. *For a discussion of related ideas, see the entries on* FAMILY; *and* LOVE. *Other relevant material may be found under the entries* LIFESTYLES AND PUBLIC HEALTH; *and* VETERINARY ETHICS. *See also the* APPENDIX (CODES, OATHS, AND DIRECTIVES RELATED TO BIOETHICS), SECTION V: ETHICAL DIRECTIVES PERTAINING TO THE WELFARE AND USE OF ANIMALS, *especially the* VETERINARIAN'S OATH *and* PRINCIPLES OF VETERINARY MEDICINE *of the* AMERICAN VETERINARY MEDICAL ASSOCIATION.

Bibliography

ANDERSON, ROBERT S., ed. 1975. *Pets, Animals and Society.* London: Bailliere Tindall.
BAUMAN, LAWRENCE; POSNER, MONTE; SACHS, KARL; and

Szita, Robert. 1991. "Effects of Animal-Assisted Therapy on Communications Patterns with Chronic Schizophrenics." In *Universal Kinship: The Bond Between All Living Things*, pp. 21–48. Edited by the Latham Foundation Staff. Saratoga, Calif.: R & E.

Baun, Mara M.; Bergstrom, Nancy; Langston, Nancy F.; and Thoma, Linda. 1984. "Physiological Effects of Human/Companion Animal Bonding." *Nursing Research* 33, no. 3:126–129.

Bolin, S. E. 1987. "The Effects of Companion Animals During Conjugal Bereavement." *Anthrozoos* 1:26–35.

Bryant, John. 1982. [1978, privately published]. *Fettered Kingdoms: An Examination of a Changing Ethic.* Rev. ed. Winchester, U.K.: Fox.

Carpenter, Edward; Bates, Angela; Beeson, Trevor; Brambell, Michael; Carpenter, Kenneth; Carpenter, Lillian; Coffey, David; Harrison, Ruth; Jennings, Sydney; Linzey, Andrew; Montefiore, Hugh; and Thorpe, William H. 1980. *Animals and Ethics.* London: Watkins.

Clark, Stephen R. L. 1977. *The Moral Status of Animals.* Oxford: At the Clarendon Press.

———. 1982. *The Nature of the Beast: Are Animals Moral?* Oxford: Oxford University Press.

Clutton-Brock, Juliet. 1993. *Cats, Ancient and Modern.* Cambridge, Mass.: Harvard University Press.

Connell, Cathleen M., and Lago, Daniel J. 1991. "Effects of Pets on the Well-Being of the Elderly." In *Universal Kinship: The Bond Between All Living Things*, pp. 51–62. Edited by the Latham Foundation Staff. Saratoga, Calif.: R & E.

Dawkins, Marian Stamp. 1993. *Through Our Eyes Only? The Search for Animal Consciousness.* Oxford: W. H. Freeman.

Deshriver, M. M., and Riddick, C. C. 1990. "Effects of Watching Aquariums on Elders' Stress." *Anthrozoos* 4: 44–48.

Fogle, Bruce, ed. 1981. *Interrelations Between People and Pets.* Springfield, Ill.: Charles C. Thomas.

Gorczyca, Ken. 1991. "Special Needs for the Pet Owner with AIDS/HIV." In *Universal Kinship: The Bond Between All Living Things*, pp. 13–20. Edited by the Latham Foundation Staff. Saratoga, Calif.: R & E.

Kay, William J.; Cohen, Susan P.; Nieburg, Herbert A.; Fudin, Carole E.; Grey, Ross E.; Kutscher, Austin H.; and Osman, Mohamed M., eds. 1988. *Euthanasia of the Companion Animal: The Impact on Pet Owners, Veterinarians and Society.* Philadelphia: Charles.

Kropotkin, Petr Alekseevich. 1939. *Mutual Aid: A Factor in Evolution.* Harmondsworth, U.K.: Penguin.

Lessing, Doris. 1991. *Particularly Cats—and Rufus.* Rev. ed. New York: Alfred A. Knopf.

Levinson, Boris M. 1978. "Pets and Personality Development." *Psychological Reports* 42, no. 3, pt. 2:1031–1038.

Linzey, Andrew. 1976. *Animal Rights: A Christian Assessment of Man's Treatment of Animals.* London: SCM.

———. 1987. *Christianity and the Rights of Animals.* London: SPCK.

———. 1994. *Animal Theology.* London: SCM.

Nicholson, Edward W. B. 1879. *The Rights of an Animal: A New Essay in Ethics.* London: C. Kegan Paul.

Patronek, Gary J., and Glickman, Lawrence T. 1994. "Development of a Model for Estimating the Size and Dynamics of the Pet Dog Population." *Anthrozoos* 7, no. 1:25–41.

Regan, Tom. 1983. *The Case for Animal Rights.* Berkeley: University of California Press.

Ritvo, Harriet. 1986. "Pride and Pedigree: The Evolution of the Victorian Dog Fancy." *Victorian Studies* 29, no. 2: 227–253.

———. 1994. "A Dog's Life." *New York Review of Books*, January 13, pp. 3–6.

Robin, Michael, and Bensel, Robert ten. 1991. "Pets and the Socialization of Children." In *Universal Kinship: The Bond Between All Living Things*, pp. 173–196. Edited by the Latham Foundation Staff. Saratoga, Calif.: R & E.

Rodd, Rosemary. 1990. *Biology, Ethics, and Animals.* Oxford: At the Clarendon Press.

Rollin, Bernard E. 1992. *Animal Rights and Human Morality.* Rev. ed. Buffalo, N.Y.: Prometheus.

Rothschild, Miriam. 1986. *Animals and Man.* Oxford: Oxford University Press.

Royal Society for the Prevention of Cruelty to Animals (RSPCA). 1984. *Policies on Animal Welfare.* Rev. ed. Horsham, Sussex: Author.

Ryder, Richard D. 1973. *Pets Are Good for People.* London: Pet Manufacturers' Association.

Sandys-Winsch, Godfrey. 1984. *Animal Law.* 2d ed. London: Shaw.

Serpell, James. 1986. *In the Company of Animals: A Study of Human-Animal Relationships.* Oxford: Basil Blackwell.

Shell, Marc. 1986. "The Family Pet." *Representations* 15:121–153.

Singer, Peter. 1976. *Animal Liberation: A New Ethics for Our Treatment of Animals.* London: Jonathan Cape.

Stallones, Lorann. 1994. "Pet Loss and Mental Health." *Anthrozoos* 7, no. 1:43–54.

Sweeney, Noel. 1990. *Animals and Cruelty and Law.* Bristol, U.K.: Alibi Books.

Tester, Keith. 1991. *Animals and Society: The Humanity of Animal Rights.* London: Routledge.

Thomas, Elizabeth Marshall. 1993. *The Hidden Life of Dogs.* Boston: Houghton Mifflin.

Thomas, Keith. 1983. *Man and the Natural World: A History of the Modern Sensibility.* New York: Pantheon.

Wilson, Cindy C. 1991. "The Pet as an Anxiolytic Intervention." *Journal of Nervous and Mental Disease* 179, no. 8:482–489.

———. 1994. "Commentary: A Conceptual Framework for Human-Animal Interaction Research: The Challenge Revisited." *Anthrozoos* 7, no. 1:4–12.

Wilson, Cindy C., and Nettling, F. E. 1987. "New Directions: Challenges for Human-Animal Bond Research and the Elderly." *Journal of Applied Gerontology* 7, no. 2: 51–57.

Wood, John George. 1874. *Man and Beast: Here and Hereafter. Illustrated by More Than Three Hundred Original Anecdotes.* London: Daldy, Isbister.

Youatt, William. 1839. *The Obligation and Extent of Humanity to Brutes, Principally Considered with Reference to Domesticated Animals.* London: Longman.

V. ZOOS AND ZOOLOGICAL PARKS

Wild animals have been displayed in captivity for millennia (Luoma, 1987). The first known large collections were assembled in Egypt around 2500 B.C.E. Early rulers displayed their exotic menageries, captured during campaigns or expeditions, for personal amusement and as symbols of wealth and political power. Romans later maintained menageries for bloody public spectacles, sending elephants, lions, bears, and other wildlife into battle in arenas throughout Europe. Urban zoos appeared in sixteenth-century Europe and North Africa; visitors ogled strange creatures captured on colonial adventures. In 1828, the first zoo dedicated to the scientific study of captive wildlife opened in London, and in 1889, the U.S. Congress established the National Zoo for the purpose of breeding native wildlife. As zoos continued to evolve in the twentieth century, they developed a broad mission that included research, conservation, education, and entertainment.

Zoos, aquariums, safari parks, and wildlife theme parks are popular worldwide. Approximately 400 professionally managed zoos exist in the world, in addition to thousands of roadside menageries and petting zoos (Chiszar et al., 1990). Annual zoo attendance in the United States alone exceeds one hundred million (Nelson, 1990). According to studies conducted in the United States and Canada, one-third of the public has visited a zoo within the last twelve months, and 98 percent of adults have visited a zoo in their lifetimes (Nelson, 1990).

Despite their broad popularity, zoos are increasingly criticized on ethical grounds. As the public has grown more sensitive to animal-welfare and conservation issues, animal advocates have begun to question whether or not the benefits of zoos justify the incarceration of live, and often rare, wild animals. (Although the term "zoo" may refer to a broad range of animal facilities, for the purposes of this article it will refer only to zoos and aquariums that meet at least minimum professional standards. These minimum standards are defined by the American Association for Zoological Parks and Aquariums [AAZPA] in the United States.)

The ethics of captivity

Many zoo opponents hold that wild animals should not be kept in captivity for human benefit. Dale Jamieson (1985) argues that animals taken from the wild are deprived of the opportunity to behave naturally. They are removed from their natural habitats, separated from family and social groups, and prevented from performing natural behaviors such as gathering food. Most important, the animals lose the freedom to pursue their own lives. Therefore, even under the best zoo conditions, Ja-

mieson believes there exists a moral presumption against keeping animals in captivity.

Critics also focus on the possibility of physical or psychological suffering caused by captive conditions. Despite improvements in exhibit design, many animals remain confined in dirty, cramped, and isolated cages. Indoor facilities often lack fresh air and natural light, while outdoor enclosures may expose animals to extreme weather conditions to which they are not adapted. Without social or environmental stimulation, captive wildlife may become listless, self-abusive, or develop stereotypical behaviors such as the pacing often observed in big cats (Fox, 1990). When elephants or other potentially dangerous animals display aggression, zookeepers may respond with harsh discipline or physical restraints. The capture of animals in the wild, their transportation to zoos, and the handling required for veterinary care are other sources of stress.

Perhaps the most controversial source of potential suffering is the disposition of "surplus" animals. The zoo surplus includes aged adults and excess offspring of breeding programs. Animal activists assert that many surplus animals suffer inhumane treatment when zoos sell them to animal dealers who, in turn, sell them to research laboratories, private collectors, roadside menageries, and hunting parks (Clifton, 1988). An equally controversial disposal method is "culling," or mercy killing for management purposes. Critics decry this killing of healthy animals, especially when the surplus results from careless management. Animal advocates stress that zoos have a moral obligation to care for all zoo animals, regardless of their utility for breeding and other zoo goals.

Zoo advocates agree that culling is ethically problematic. However, they contend that responsible zoo directors manage breeding programs to avoid surpluses through contraception and segregation of sexes (Bostock, 1993). When contraception fails or a zoo's needs change, the director is expected to follow the AAZPA's code of ethics for distributing surplus animals to other qualified zoos or dealers. Euthanasia is seen as a last, though sometimes unavoidable, resort. To sustain viable captive populations of endangered species, zoo scientists must carefully balance age and sex ratios to maintain genetic diversity. Animals that are old, infertile, or genetically undesirable become surplus because zoos have limited space and financial resources. Zoo proponents defend culling these individuals as a necessary evil. Euthanasia and other disposal methods, proponents claim, allow zoos to conserve populations and species, although some individual animals must be sacrificed.

Animal welfare, according to zoo advocates, remains a high priority (Hutchins and Fascione, 1991). While recognizing that inferior enclosures still exist, they applaud the revolution in naturalistic exhibit design. At many zoos, for example, primates have been moved from isolated, tiled cells to family groupings in outdoor facsimiles of their native habitat. Tropical birds have flown from their cages into reproductions of rain forests. In addition, animal behaviorists are studying ways to stimulate animals' physical and mental activity, and veterinarians are investigating how to improve their nutrition and health. Through advances in captive breeding, zoos have also been able to reduce their demand for animals captured in the wild. Zoo advocates point proudly to these improvements, arguing that mortality and morbidity rates at zoos do not support claims that the animals are miserable (Chiszar et al., 1990).

Furthermore, zoo proponents object to claims, such as Jamieson's, that captive animals suffer as humans would from the loss of liberty. Animals, they believe, may be happier in an enclosure free from predation and hunger than they are in the wild. Expecting animals to have the same needs and desires as humans do—an attitude called anthropomorphism—is viewed as a reflection of animal activists' sentimentality and biological ignorance (Robinson, 1989).

Justifications of zoos

Another approach to the zoo debate is to examine the reasons for keeping animals in captivity. If the benefits of zoos are negligible, animal advocates contend, then keeping wildlife captive cannot be justified. However, if significant benefits can be shown, captivity for at least some animals might be defensible.

Entertainment. Historically, the predominant function of zoos has been entertainment. Studies of zoo visitors show that most people continue to see these facilities as parklike settings for casual family socializing (Kellert, 1987). To zoo opponents, public amusement is a trivial reason for holding animals in confinement (Jamieson, 1985). Opponents especially attack circuslike events, such as sea lion shows, that use trained animals to draw large crowds. Similarly, zoos that import animals such as giant pandas to boost attendance and revenues have been condemned. Such events are seen as denigrating the animals by exploiting them as public spectacles.

Although zoo directors vaunt high attendance rates, many now deemphasize entertainment as a zoo goal (Luoma, 1987). Baby elephant rides and similar amusements are gradually disappearing as zoos try to develop a more serious image. However, zoo educators claim that entertainment is necessary to keep visitors interested in learning. Also, zoo administrators assert that animal shows, special events, and traveling exhibits are sometimes essential to raise the funds needed to pay for research and other zoo missions (Cohn, 1992).

Research. Few visitors are familiar with the scientific efforts of zoos. Although a handful of zoos sponsor field research, most studies are conducted on site by zoo staff or affiliated researchers. Common topics include animal behavior, nutrition, reproductive biology, genetics, and pathology (Hutchins and Fascione, 1991). Animal activists challenge both the quality and usefulness of this research (Jamieson, 1985). According to critics, the experimental design of most zoo research lacks scientific rigor, rarely qualifying for publication in peer-reviewed journals. In a nutrition study, for example, a small sample size or the absence of a control group may obscure study results. Some critics also say that much of the research is aimed at improving captive husbandry and exhibit design—unnecessary benefits if wildlife were not confined in the first place. Regardless of any benefits, some animal-rights advocates oppose all animal research. Tom Regan (1983) argues that the utility of research, whether to gain practical information of basic knowledge, is no justification for violating an individual animal's basic rights.

Zoo scientists reject the position that animal research is intrinsically wrong. They emphasize that most zoo research is noninvasive, nonterminal, and aimed at benefiting captive and wild populations (Hutchins, 1988). While acknowledging weaknesses in past studies, zoo proponents see a growing commitment to quality research at many institutions. Zoos are hiring research staff, cooperating with university faculties, and investing in major research facilities such as the U.S. National Zoo's 3,000-acre Conservation and Research Center. Much current research employs sophisticated, controversial techniques, such as embryo transfers, in efforts to improve captive breeding success. Although the experimental techniques may harm individual animals, zoo scientists contend that the long-term benefits for species conservation outweigh the costs to individual animals.

Conservation. Animal advocates doubt that zoos can make a significant contribution to conservation (Fox, 1990). Although many recognize the biodiversity crisis, critics hold that zoos can do little to resolve the primary cause of extinction: habitat destruction. Nor can zoos protect more than an insignificant portion of the estimated five to thirty million species on the planet. Further, zoo conservation efforts are biased toward the charismatic large mammals preferred by zoo visitors, nearly ignoring disliked organisms such as bats and invertebrates (Kellert, 1987). When zoos do have success in maintaining a captive population, critics worry that the animals suffer from inbreeding and loss of natural behavioral characteristics. Are zoo animals and their wild relatives equivalent organisms? Could animals bred in zoos for generations be successfully reintroduced into the wild? If reintroduction is never possible, how long should the species be perpetuated in zoos? Extinction, to some zoo opponents, is more respectful of individual animals than endless confinement.

Yet conservation is viewed by many as the preeminent function of modern zoos. Zoo advocates liken the zoo to a crowded ark, struggling to accommodate as many threatened species as possible. Advocates remind critics that several organisms have already been saved from extinction by zoos, including the European bison and Mongolian wild horses (Tudge, 1991). Increasing resources are devoted to captive breeding through programs such as the AAZPA's Species Survival Plans (SSP) (Wiese and Hutchins, 1993). SSPs manage rare animal populations at zoos throughout the country, asking zoos to cooperate in breeding plans that promote genetic variability and demographic stability. SSP organizers hope that as such programs grow, world zoos will eventually be able to protect 500 to 900 endangered species (Luoma, 1987).

Zoos are also expanding efforts to reintroduce animals born in captivity to the wild, using some reintroduction projects to study techniques for managing small, isolated populations in the wild and to encourage habitat protection in developing countries. While they agree that zoos cannot directly save the majority of endangered species, zoo advocates proclaim that saving any species keeps options open for the future.

Education.   The educational benefits of zoos are also viewed skeptically by animal advocates. Visitor studies indicate that relatively few people are interested in learning about animals or conservation, and there is little evidence that the zoo experience improves knowledge of biological facts or conservation issues (Kellert, 1987; Kellert and Dunlap, 1989). Given zoos' poor record of educational effectiveness, critics suggest that films, lectures, books, and nature centers may offer superior learning benefits without the ethical costs of confining wildlife. Most important, critics charge that zoos may be presenting harmful information and values (Sommer, 1972). Seeing rare animals in captivity, for example, may give visitors an inaccurate impression of human abilities to combat extinction. In addition, witnessing listless creatures in sterile cages may diminish respect for animals or concern for conservation.

Zoo advocates respond by describing the diversity of education programs and a growing commitment to educational progress (Chiszar et al., 1990). Zoos attempt to teach casual visitors through signs, demonstrations, learning laboratories, and interactive computer technologies. Part of the revolution in exhibit design aims at enhancing learning by immersing visitors in natural environments. To extend their educational impact, zoos are developing curricula for primary and secondary students, holding workshops for teachers, visiting community centers, and organizing public lecture series. Michael Robinson (1989) promotes such changes as part of an educational revolution committed to teaching visitors about the interactions between wild animals, plants, and humans. Zoo proponents believe that, in our urbanized society, the zoo may be the only institution capable of demonstrating these vital links to the public.

Education, in fact, may offer zoos their best hope of effecting long-term, large-scale benefits (Kellert and Dunlap, 1989). If zoo educators could demonstrate positive program impacts, they could defuse criticisms and justify program expansion. Zoos should embark on a coordinated program of systematic educational evaluation and implement their findings through innovative programs dedicated to further progress. Given the wide popularity of zoos, it is doubtful that the ethical debate will result in their abolition. If zoos can learn how to teach the public scientific information and humane and conservation values, animal advocates, zoo proponents, and wildlife will all benefit.

JULIE DUNLAP
STEPHEN R. KELLERT

Directly related to this article are the other articles in this entry, especially the articles on ETHICAL PERSPECTIVES ON THE TREATMENT AND STATUS OF ANIMALS, WILDLIFE CONSERVATION AND MANAGEMENT, *and* PET AND COMPANION ANIMALS. *Also directly related are the entries* ANIMAL RESEARCH; ENDANGERED SPECIES AND BIODIVERSITY; *and* VETERINARY ETHICS. *Other relevant material may be found under the entries* ENVIRONMENTAL ETHICS; ENVIRONMENTAL POLICY AND LAW; *and* RESEARCH BIAS. *See also the* APPENDIX (CODES, OATHS, AND DIRECTIVES RELATED TO BIOETHICS), SECTION V: ETHICAL DIRECTIVES PERTAINING TO THE WELFARE AND USE OF ANIMALS.

Bibliography

BOSTOK, STEPHEN. 1993. *Zoos and Animal Rights: The Ethics of Keeping Animals.* New York: Routledge.

CHISZAR, DAVID; MURPHY, JAMES B.; and ILIFF, WARREN. 1990. "For Zoos." *Psychological Record* 40, no. 1:3–13.

CLIFTON, MERRITT. 1988. "Chucking Zoo Animals Overboard: How and Why Noah Culls the Ark." *Animals Agenda* 8, no. 2:14–22, 53–54.

COHN, JEFFREY P. 1992. "Decisions at the Zoo." *BioScience* 42, no. 9:654–659.

FOX, MICHAEL W. 1990. "The Zoo: A Cruel and Outmoded Institution?" In his *Inhumane Society: The American Way of Exploiting Animals*, pp. 145–155. New York: St. Martin's Press.

HUTCHINS, MICHAEL. 1988. "On the Design of Zoo Research Programmes." *International Zoo Yearbook* 27:9–19.

HUTCHINS, MICHAEL, and FASCIONE, NINA. 1991. "Ethical Issues Facing Modern Zoos." In *Proceedings—American Association of Zoo Veterinarians.* Edited by Randall Junge. Wheeling, W. Va.: American Association for Zoological Parks and Aquariums.

JAMIESON, DALE. 1985. "Against Zoos." In *In Defence of Animals*, pp. 108–117. Edited by Peter Singer. Oxford: Basil Blackwell.

KELLERT, STEPHEN R. 1987. "The Educational Potential of the Zoo and Its Visitor." *Philadelphia Zoo Review* 3, no. 1: 7–13.

KELLERT, STEPHEN R., and DUNLAP, JULIE. 1989. *Informal Learning at the Zoo: A Study of Attitude and Knowledge Impacts.* A report to the Zoological Society of Philadelphia.

LUOMA, JON R. 1987. *A Crowded Ark: The Role of Zoos in Wildlife Conservation.* Boston: Houghton Mifflin.

NELSON, ANDREW J. 1990. "Going Wild." *American Demographics* 12, no. 2:34–37, 50.

REGAN, TOM. 1983. *The Case for Animal Rights.* Berkeley: University of California Press.

ROBINSON, MICHAEL. 1989. "Zoos Today and Tomorrow." *Anthrozoos* 2:10–14.

SOMMER, ROBERT. 1972. "What Do We Learn at the Zoo?" *Natural History* 81, no. 7:26–29, 84–85.

TUDGE, COLIN. 1991. *Last Animals at the Zoo.* London: Hutchinson Radius.

WIESE, ROBERT, and HUTCHINS, MICHAEL. 1993. "The Role of Captive Breeding and Reintroduction in Wildlife Conservation." In *Proceedings of the AAZPA Regional Conferences.* Wheeling, W. Va.: American Association for Zoological Parks and Aquariums.

VI. HUNTING

Hunting, the pursuit of wild animals for food, adornment, or sport, is one of the most ancient human activities. Nevertheless, today it is viewed by some as one of humankind's most ethically problematic enterprises. How has the practice of hunting evolved from human necessity to moral quandary? This article explores this most interesting transformation and attempts to flesh out some of the meatier ethical issues in the debate.

Then

Humans have always hunted. Stone projectile points dating from the Paleolithic period (which includes Neanderthal and Cro-Magnon man) have been found embedded in the skeletons of animals, some now extinct, in many parts of the world. Since heavy tools are of relatively little use to arboreal vegetarians, some anthropologists hold the view that the increased use of stone tools by early hominids was associated with a shift from a largely vegetarian diet to one including a greater proportion of meat.

The social organization necessary for the hunt may have played an important role in human evolution, as well as in that of other intelligent, cooperative primates that are not especially well equipped with tooth and claw. Because meat provides a highly concentrated form of caloric energy, a diet high in flesh freed early humans from the need to eat almost continuously—as other primates, such as the lowland gorilla, must. An omnivorous way of life may have given humans greater leisure to develop new tools and new skills and to increase their control over the environment. If this theory is correct, even in broad outline, hunting has made humans what they are today (Oakley, 1961; for a contrasting view see Tanner, 1981).

The ancient roots of hunting, and its obvious cultural importance to early humans, have long been the basis for one of the classical arguments in favor of hunting as a moral activity. According to this argument, hunting is an atavistic or foundational activity that keeps humans in touch with their deepest roots and can be ignored only at the price of neglecting what is most quintessentially human (Shepard, 1973; Causey, 1989). More recently some theorists have attributed a praiseworthy environmental ethic to preliterate hunting cultures. It must be noted, however, that although preliterate hunting-and-gathering cultures lived in harmony with their environment, it is not clear whether the restraints involved were moral or simply technological.

Later, with the advent of agriculture, hunting became, for the first time, a form of recreation. Egyptian tomb paintings, for example, provide evidence that hunting was a favorite pastime of that ancient people. In highly stratified societies, hunting became an important means of displaying social prestige and power.

In the fourth century B.C.E. Xenophon (1925) argued that hunting is an important part of the moral education of a virtuous (male) citizen. He advised young men to take up hunting as the first part of education because hunting keeps the body healthy, improves sight and hearing, prevents aging, and promotes good character.

With the rise of feudalism in medieval Europe, the nobility protected forests for the express purpose of hunting. Charlemagne, for instance, promulgated laws prohibiting poaching in 802. By the thirteenth century, royal forests covered a quarter of England. Like Xenophon, medieval Europeans argued that hunting was a path to virtue. The *Livre de chasse* (Book of Hunting) of Gaston III, count of Foix, written about 1387, clearly expresses this belief. Aside from offering practical advice, the book argues that hunting is an excellent way to avoid sin (e.g., sloth) and to acquire virtue and good health. In the Middle Ages, hunting began to be associated with sexuality. The Latin term *venera* can mean either hunting or sexual activity. And many medieval poems and tales that are ostensibly about hunting are obvious metaphors for sexual pursuit.

And now

In the modern context any discussion of hunting must first make distinctions between subsistence hunting, sport hunting, and market hunting. Subsistence hunting generally refers to full-time hunting by small groups of indigenous peoples, usually in remote parts of the world. Although these are not the only people who depend on the surrounding fauna to sustain their lives—given, for example, that people in inner-city slums may catch and eat rats—subsistence hunters make hunting an integral part of their cultural and spiritual life. As such, subsistence hunting seems to maintain a certain ethical priority over other forms of hunting.

This is not to say, however, that such hunting is automatically viewed as ethically justified. Not all standards and practices indigenous to even the most primitive cultures should be given carte blanche in terms of moral permissibility—for example, the keeping of slaves or the amputation of female genitalia. Further, some ethicists have reservations about subsistence hunting by indigenous peoples when nonindigenous methods—modern firearms, motor vehicles, and other forms of modern technology—are used in hunting. The point is that in the case of subsistence hunting—where the rights of animals to life or avoidance of pain are weighed against the fundamental rights of persons to gain food, to maintain their heritage, and to articulate their spiritual beliefs—the question of its rightness becomes much more complicated than in the case of sport or market hunting. (See below for further discussion.)

Sport hunting, discussed earlier, still exists. And with the advance of technology we now have market, or commercial, hunting as well. Commercial hunting (excluding trapping and fishing) is now illegal in the United States, but is still practiced in many parts of the world, including Europe. Commercial hunters are not the same as subsistence hunters, for they hunt in order to make a living, not merely to live. Although these two objectives clearly overlap, commercial hunters are not granted the same moral imprimatur that subsistence hunters are. Given that the main objective of market hunting is to make a profit, the hunter has every incentive to take as many animals as possible with as little effort as possible. The unregulated commercial hunter is caught in a "tragedy of the commons" situation (Hardin, 1968); for instance, it is not irrational for the market hunter to kill even the last animal, since if one market hunter does not, another one will.

Critique

The modern moral critique of hunting—most specifically sport and market hunting—is based on a general belief that hunting is killing for fun and destroys a life of value without sufficient justification. This belief involves several components. Among them are that hunting is *cruel to animals*, hunting has a *negative influence on the character of the hunter*, hunting is a form of *male domination*, hunting furthers an attitude of *exploitation toward*

the natural world, and, most fundamentally, hunting violates the *rights of animals*. We will look at each in turn.

Hunters argue, first, that while hunting may be cruel to animals, especially those unintentionally crippled and not recovered, it is no more cruel than nature itself; and secondly, but along the same lines, that humans are the top animals in the food chain and have every right to partake in the natural order of things, even if this includes the infliction of pain. Hunters are participating in a natural ecology that includes animal suffering.

A response to the first part of this argument would be difficult if all the animal advocate had to go on was the "fact of the matter" of the animal's pain, for it may be impossible to test this empirically. It may be that animals cannot feel pain at all, or at least not entirely as humans do. Or it may be that they can feel pain, but that we could never be certain that they do, given their behavior. Or they may feel pain, but in different and more subdued ways than humans, since they have different anatomies and neural structures, and are adapted to their wilder ways of life.

The second part of this argument, however, may be easier to defeat. It may be true that the hunter, like any other animal in the natural order, is justified in causing pain in the same way that every other animal is justified. But it may be completely misguided to consider an animal that can shop at grocery stores, and has the power to destroy the entire planet with the push of a button, as just another member of the food chain. Humans are not just another species of predator. Human hunters kill for sport.

The allegation that hunting animals has a detrimental effect on the character of the hunter has little, if any, empirical support. The same is true of the claim that hunters are more likely than nonhunters to engage in violence toward other humans. The centers of human violence are largely urban, and the hunting of animals is a rural activity. In the United States people living in rural areas are four times more likely to be hunters than those living in the central city.

It is just as natural to be hunted as to hunt. Here one can imagine that the search for the most challenging hunt may lead one to consider that humans are not only hunters but also a uniquely intelligent species of big game. This idea of humans as game has been toyed with in stories and screenplays, and there is some evidence to suggest that the sport hunting of humans has actually occurred.

An argument championed by many feminists is that hunting is a leading example of the quintessential male activity—domination (Warren, 1990). They maintain that men, believing that their needs and wants always override those of every other being, including animals, simply authorize the chasing, terrorizing, and killing of whatever animal they see fit. Hunting, some feminists argue, is an act of domination (Gaard, 1993) and, like all acts of domination, is morally wrong.

Unfortunately, this response is both sexist and philosophically naive. It is sexist for two reasons: first, not all hunters are male; and second, not all killings of animals are acts of domination (e.g., the euthanasia of pets). It is philosophically naive because it assumes that we can label all relationships of dominance as morally wrong. Is the parent/child relationship morally reprehensible? Or the student/teacher? This line of attack on hunting seems to create more problems than it solves.

In response to the charge that hunting fosters the exploitation of the natural environment, many hunters have claimed once again that the human hunter is no different from the natural predator. They also point out, however, that hunted animals are typically replaced by others of the same species. According to this "replaceability principle," one nonhuman animal is a fully adequate replacement for another of the same species, so it is morally justifiable to kill one animal if such replacement will occur. Hunters have often been active conservationists, but it is important to note at this point that this principle would be reprehensible if applied to humans, opening up the question of possible species chauvinism.

In addition, hunters often use the argument that hunting is actually beneficial to a species, insofar as the hunter fills the role formerly occupied by disappearing natural predators. (Of course it must be recognized that many such niches are empty because of human interference, usually habitat destruction, but at times overhunting.) According to this argument, game animals will overpopulate and place undue stress on the environment unless their numbers are controlled by regulated hunting. Hunting, like predation, is thus said to aid the process of natural selection by culling animals.

While these arguments are valid in some limited contexts, they are often misapplied. Most game animals will not overpopulate and place stress on their habitat (though some, such as ungulates, will). Also, hunting does not cull the herd in the same way that natural predation does. Natural predators kill the prey that are easiest to take: the old, weak, young, sick, or wounded. Hunters, on the other hand, often select the most fit animals, such as the largest individual or the stag with the most impressive rack.

It may seem at first blush that if animals have rights at all, then hunting clearly violates them. But this is not true. Animals may have only limited rights, such as the right to be free from gratuitous pain and suffering, or the right to live to reproductive maturity. In either case, hunting could be made consistent with such limited animal rights. But full-blown rights, including the unqualified right to life, will need to be established by sustained argument. This is the difficulty faced by the animal advocate. The establishing of rights for animals requires complex philosophical analysis that must begin with a deep understanding of the nature of rights along with the reasons why we believe that most humans—possibly excluding, for example, comatose patients, fetuses, and criminals—have rights. Next, careful moves must be made to show that animals are appropriately similar to humans in relevant ways. Animal rights, if such there are, are likely not to be entirely parallel with human rights, and hunting animals may be consistent with their limited rights.

Finally, some objections must be addressed. With respect to the issue of hunting, one fundamental objection may simply be the belief held by many hunters that even if animals have a right not to be hunted, it is part of the hunters' human rights to hunt. Given a conflict of rights, and given that the rights of animals seem to be weaker than the rights of humans, the burden of proof is always on the animal advocate. The creation of prima facie animal rights has yet to be presented in the literature.

Of course, if the rights of other humans—for example, of those working for the preservation of natural areas (Loftin, 1984)—conflict with the rights of those who like to hunt, another problem in adjudication arises. The outcome of this argument, however, does not turn on the question of animal rights.

Conclusion

Hunting has existed as long as humans have been a species, and it will probably be part of (some) human culture for a long time to come. One can certainly imagine a world in which hunting is impossible: when there are no animals left to kill. One can even imagine a world where hunting becomes unnecessary: when everyone has enough to eat and wear, when the sporting desires or the atavistic needs become passé, or when holographic images or robotics fill the hunters' domain. However, one cannot imagine a world in which the serious ethical issues permeating the question of the moral justifiability of hunting will become extinct.

ROBERT W. LOFTIN
ELLEN R. KLEIN

Directly related to this article are the other articles in this entry: ETHICAL PERSPECTIVES ON THE TREATMENT AND STATUS OF ANIMALS, VEGETARIANISM, WILDLIFE CONSERVATION AND MANAGEMENT, PET AND COMPANION ANIMALS, ZOOS AND ZOOLOGICAL PARKS, *and* ANIMALS IN AGRICULTURE AND FACTORY FARMING. *For a further discussion of topics mentioned in this article, see the entries* ENDANGERED SPECIES AND BIODIVERSITY; ENVIRONMENTAL ETHICS; LIFE; *and* RIGHTS. *For a discussion of related ideas, see the entries* HARM; *and* PAIN AND SUFFERING. *Other relevant material may be found under the entries* AGRICULTURE; CARE; ENVIRONMENTAL POLICY

AND LAW; ENVIRONMENT AND RELIGION; EVOLUTION; FEMINISM; SUSTAINABLE DEVELOPMENT; *and* VETERINARY ETHICS.

Bibliography

ADAMS, CAROL J. 1990. *The Sexual Politics of Meat: A Feminist–Vegetarian Critical Theory.* New York: Continuum.

CARTMILL, MATT. 1993. *A View to a Death in the Morning: Hunting and Nature Through History.* Cambridge, Mass.: Harvard University Press.

CAUSEY, ANN S. 1989. "On the Morality of Hunting." *Environmental Ethics* 11, no. 4:327–343.

GAARD, GRETA C., ed. 1993. *Ecofeminism: Women, Animals and Nature.* Philadelphia: Temple University Press.

HARDIN, GARRETT. 1968. "The Tragedy of the Commons." *Science* 162, no. 3859:1243–1248.

KRUTCH, JOSEPH W. 1957. "A Damnable Pleasure." *Saturday Review,* August 17, pp. 8–9, 39–40.

LEE, RICHARD B., and DEVORE, IRVEN, eds. 1968. *Symposium on Man the Hunter.* Chicago: Aldine.

LOFTIN, ROBERT W. 1984. "The Morality of Hunting." *Environmental Ethics* 6, no. 3:241–250.

OAKLEY, KENNETH P. 1961. "On Man's Use of Fire, with Comments on Tool-making and Hunting." In *Social Life of Early Man,* pp. 176–193. Edited by Sherwood L. Washburn. Chicago: Aldine.

OLSON, STORRS, and JAMES, HELEN. 1991. "Lost and Found—Avian Life in Hawaii." *American Birds* 45:1036.

REIGER, JOHN F. 1975. *American Sportsmen and the Origins of Conservation.* New York: Winchester.

SCHEFFER, VICTOR B. 1974. *A Voice for Wildlife.* New York: Charles Scribner's Sons.

SHEPARD, PAUL. 1973. *The Tender Carnivore and the Sacred Game.* New York: Charles Scribner's Sons.

TANNER, NANCY M. 1981. *On Becoming Human.* Cambridge: At the University Press.

THIEBAUX, MARCELLE. 1974. *The Stag of Love: The Chase in Medieval Literature.* Ithaca, N.Y.: Cornell University Press.

U.S. DEPARTMENT OF THE INTERIOR. NATIONAL PARK SERVICE. 1986. *1982–1983 Nationwide Recreational Survey.* Washington, D.C.: U.S. Government Printing Office.

WARREN, KAREN J. 1990. "The Power and the Promise of Ecological Feminism." *Environmental Ethics* 12, no. 2: 125–146.

XENOPHON. 1925. *Cynegiticus (On Hunting).* In *Xenophon, VII, Scripta minora,* pp. 365–456. Translated by Edgar C. Marchant. Loeb Classical Library. Cambridge, Mass.: Harvard University Press.

VII. ANIMALS IN AGRICULTURE AND FACTORY FARMING

For almost all of human history, animal agriculture has involved human management of animals under living conditions for which the animals were biologically and evolutionarily adapted. Human intervention has consisted largely in ensuring the animals' health, nutrition, and reproduction by providing supplementary rations when forage was scarce, medical assistance, shelter from harsh elements, and so on. The symbiotic relationship between human and animal has been strongly reinforced by the cultural values of animal agricultural societies. To this day, for example, among ranchers in the American West, who are primarily traditional agriculturists and raise animals on open ranges, one finds a doctrine passed from generation to generation: "We take care of the animals, and the animals take care of us."

Factory farming

Intensive agriculture, also known as confinement agriculture or factory farming, differs dramatically from traditional animal agriculture. The key notion behind confinement agriculture is the application of industrial methods to producing animals or animal products. This way of thinking about agriculture emerged in the middle of the twentieth century; before that, neither the technology nor the social conditions existed to make confinement agriculture possible. After World War II, various technological developments and changing social conditions combined to alter radically the face of animal agriculture, and to model farms on factories. At about the same time, departments of "animal husbandry" in agricultural universities began to change their names to departments of "animal science." Increasingly, agriculture became a business, not merely a way of life combined with a way of making a living.

The conditions that generated confinement or intensive agriculture are relatively clear. After World War II, increasing numbers of workers moved from rural, agricultural regions into urban localities, where wages were higher and economic opportunities were perceived to be greater. At the same time, urban centers grew, encroaching onto traditional farmland, so that rising land prices and higher taxes militated against keeping that land for agricultural use. Inevitably the land was developed. Thus fewer and fewer people were directly involved in production agriculture.

With less land and fewer workers (as of 1993, 1.7 percent of Americans were engaged in production agriculture), it was difficult to keep animals under far-ranging, open, extensive conditions. With fewer people caring for them, animals were brought into closer and closer confinement, both outdoor and indoor, so that effects of temperature, rain, snow, and so on could be minimized. Instead of depending on human labor, farmers began to rely on machinery to feed, clean, water, milk, collect eggs, and so forth. Animal agricultural operations became capital-intensive rather than labor-intensive.

Animals began to be crowded together in an attempt to get as many as possible into the expensive production unit. Laying hens, for example, are typically placed 5 to 6 birds in a 12-inch-by-18-inch cage, and up to 100,000 birds may be kept in one building. Broiler chickens are raised in huge open sheds at a density of approximately two birds per square foot. Beef cattle, traditionally raised on range grass, are moved for the latter portion of their lives into feedlots, where they are fed grain diets, thus producing both increased weight gain and an outlet for U.S. grain surplus. Hogs are increasingly raised in confinement buildings where they never see the light of day—buildings holding 500 to 1000 sows are not uncommon. Most notoriously, veal calves are raised in small crates in order to restrict movement and keep their flesh tender, and are also kept anemic or near-anemic to keep the meat "white."

Thus animals are forced into environments for which they are not biologically suited. Because the operations are so expensive, producers are motivated to crowd as many animals as possible into the systems, since profit per animal is small. Thus, even though it is well known that chickens will lay more eggs if given more space, it is more profitable to crowd as many birds as possible into cages, yielding fewer eggs per bird but more eggs for the operation as a whole. Such methods would be impossible without recent technology. In the absence of antibiotics and vaccines, the spread of disease would decimate the animals in weeks. Without growth promoters, the animals could not be processed quickly enough to be profitable—broiler chickens for instance, reach full growth in eight weeks. The rise of confinement agriculture has, according to its proponents, provided cheap and plentiful food. For example, the price of chicken has remained virtually the same for more than twenty years, even in the face of inflation. Advocates of intensive agriculture also argue that confinement provides animals with shelter from extremes of weather, protection from predators, and a consistent nutritional regimen.

Harms of confinement

But there are hidden costs offsetting these benefits, the most important of which is the cost to the animals. The animals being produced in confinement are still essentially the animals that were genetically adapted to extensive conditions. Their fundamental biological interests are systematically violated in confinement. Thus animals that are built to move about are unable to do so. Social animals may be deprived of companionship. Air laden with dust and ammonia in confinement chicken, egg, and swine barns is execrable; in some swine operations, workers must wear respirators. Diets designed to maximize growth may lead to metabolic disease for some of the animals, even though this loss is balanced by economic gain in the other animals. In chicken and swine barns, unnatural floor surfaces such as wire and concrete slats may lead to leg, foot, and joint

problems. With the advent of confinement agriculture, there has arisen a class of diseases, known as "production diseases," that result from the systems of production. Since intensive systems have a low profit margin, they are often understaffed, and care of sick or injured animals is impossible for workers whose other duties stretch them to their limit.

As a result of such systematic violation of their physical and psychological (animal scientists prefer the word "behavioral") needs, animals suffer psychologically as well as physically. Many animals in confinement show chronic signs of long- and short-term stress, which can lead to both disease and behavioral problems. Cannibalism among chickens increases in the absence of either space to flee or small enough numbers to establish a pecking order; to prevent cannibalism, producers "debeak" chickens with a hot blade and without anesthesia, sometimes producing chronic pain. Similarly, pigs are tail-docked to prevent tail-biting, a stress-induced result of confinement. Confined animals also show many bizarre, stereotypical behaviors that seem to result from the thwarting of natural inclinations and from boring, austere environments.

Confinement agriculture also exacts other social costs. In an industry requiring large amounts of capital, small operators cannot compete effectively, and large, well-capitalized corporations inevitably drive out small "family farmers." Young people cannot afford to enter agriculture. Efficiency and productivity eclipse other values traditionally maintained in small farm communities, such as independence, self-sufficiency, and husbandry. Environmental problems such as waste disposal and water and energy consumption also arise from intensive agriculture. Lack of pasturing of animals contributes to soil erosion when land no longer used for pasture is tilled for grain. Drug residues in animal products may pose human health problems, and widespread use of antibiotics essentially breeds for resistant pathogens by eliminating microbes susceptible to the drugs. *Salmonella* and *Campylobacter* bacterial contamination are significant problems in chickens, turkeys, and eggs, since they can cause severe enteric disease in humans who consume these products.

Toward reform

Agriculturists have recognized that the welfare of animals in confinement represents one of the three major challenges to agriculture in the next century, the other two being food safety and environmental concerns. When the British public became aware of factory farms in the 1960s as a result of Ruth Harrison's pioneering book *Animal Machines,* the outcry generated a royal commission, the Brambell Commission, that was highly critical of confinement agriculture as violating the animals' natures. In the face of confinement agriculture,

European society is moving toward legal protection for farm animals. Laws in Britain, Denmark, Germany, and Switzerland have restricted certain aspects of confinement agriculture, and Sweden has essentially abolished such agriculture and guaranteed certain rights for farm animals, in a law that has been called a "bill of rights" for farm animals because it aims at protecting their fundamental interests. In the United States, public attention was first directed toward animals in research, and certain basic protections for such animals have been legally encoded in two federal laws passed in 1985. Public attention is now beginning to focus on the treatment of farm animals as well as on the environmental consequences of confinement agriculture, and articles in agricultural journals show that agriculture is starting to pay more attention to these concerns.

Until very recently, U.S. confinement agriculturists (in contrast to their counterparts in Europe and Canada) tended to deny that there were any problems of animal welfare intrinsically related to confinement agriculture, and acknowledged only occasional "bad management." This was further exacerbated by widespread skepticism in the scientific community about the existence and knowability of animal consciousness, pain, and suffering. Since the early 1990s, however, there have been indications that at least some parts of the industry and government are engaging such issues as animal deprivation, boredom, and inability to move in confinement, primarily by inaugurating research into improving animal welfare.

While it is unlikely that industrialized agriculture will ever revert to being fully or even largely extensive, it is possible to make intensive agriculture much more "animal-welfare friendly," and perhaps to change certain systems from full to partial confinement. For example, it is possible to raise swine profitably without keeping sows confined in small gestation crates for their entire lives. In addition, concern about sustainable agriculture may well result in a concerted social effort to return to less industrialized systems guided by husbandry. On the other hand, confinement agricultural systems are being introduced into Third World countries as a shortcut to rapid economic growth and as a way of adding animal products to the diets of these countries. This has generated a variety of ethical concerns, including fear of environmental despoliation, concern that successful indigenous agriculture will be lost, worries about importing Western health problems to these countries, and concern about proliferating animal suffering.

Growing social concern

Animal agriculture raises other animal welfare issues beyond confinement. Although cattle ranching is highly extensive and in fact presupposes a good fit between animal and environment, management techniques such as castration without anesthesia, hot-iron branding, and dehorning without anesthesia produce pain and suffering in these animals. Transportation of agricultural animals over long distances, for example to slaughter, is very stressful, and can cause disease and injury. Handling of farm animals by people ignorant of their behavior is an extremely widespread problem that creates high levels of stress and significant injury. Slaughter of food animals raises the issue of whether these animals can be provided with a death free of pain, suffering, and fear. This problem is particularly acute in the area of Jewish and Muslim religious slaughter, where preslaughter stunning has been considered incompatible with religious demands. Genetic engineering of farm animals for traits that are desirable to producers for reasons of efficiency and productivity may well exact costs in welfare from the animals' perspective. For example, swine and chickens engineered for greater size have suffered from a variety of diseases, including foot and leg problems. A cow engineered for double muscling was unable to stand on its own and required euthanasia. On the other hand, genetic engineering can also work to the benefit of farm animals, for example, by engineering for disease resistance.

Other branches of animal agriculture rear animals for uses other than food. Raising traditionally "wild" animals for various purposes has generated concerns about the well-being of these animals—pheasants for hunting, mink for fur, and deer for antler velvet (which is considered an aphrodisiac in the Orient) provide salient examples. Numerous welfare concerns have also been raised by the production of horses for human purposes—breakdown and injury in racehorses; injury in endurance horses (those used in long, grueling, competitive rides over difficult terrain); heat, water deprivation, and poor air for urban carriage horses. Indeed, no branch of animal agriculture is being ignored by growing social concern about animal welfare.

BERNARD E. ROLLIN

Directly related to this article are the other articles in this entry, especially the articles on ETHICAL PERSPECTIVES ON THE TREATMENT AND STATUS OF ANIMALS, *and* VEGETARIANISM. *Also directly related are the entries* AGRICULTURE; FOOD POLICY; BIOTECHNOLOGY; *and* GENETIC ENGINEERING, *article on* ANIMALS AND PLANTS. *Other relevant material may be found under the entries* ANIMAL RESEARCH, *article on* PHILOSOPHICAL ISSUES; ENDANGERED SPECIES AND BIODIVERSITY; JAINISM; VETERINARY ETHICS; *and* XENOGRAFTS.

Bibliography

DAWKINS, MARIAN S. 1980. *Animal Suffering: The Science of Animal Welfare.* London: Chapman and Hall.

Fox, Michael W. 1984. *Farm Animals: Husbandry, Behavior, and Veterinary Practice: Viewpoints of a Critic.* Baltimore: University Park Press.

Harrison, Ruth. 1964. *Animal Machines: The New Factory Farming Industry.* London: Vincent Stuart.

Lohr, Steve. "Swedish Farm Animals Get a Bill of Right." *New York Times,* October 25, pp. A1, A8.

Martin, Jerome, ed. 1991. *High Technology and Animal Welfare: Proceedings of the 1991 High Technology and Animal Welfare Symposium.* Edmonton: University of Alberta Press.

Mason, Jim, and Singer, Peter. 1990. *Animal Factories.* Rev. ed. New York: Harmony.

Rollin, Bernard E. 1981. *Animal Rights and Human Morality.* Buffalo, N.Y.: Prometheus.

———. 1989. *The Unheeded Cry: Animal Consciousness, Animal Pain, and Science.* Oxford: Oxford University Press.

———. 1990. "Animal Welfare, Animal Rights and Agriculture." *Journal of Animal Science* 68:3456–3462.

———. 1993. *Social, Bioethical, and Researchable Issues Pertaining to Farm Animal Welfare* (USDA-CSRS Contract Research).

ANTHROPOLOGY OF MEDICINE

See Medicine, Anthropology of.

ANTIVIVISECTION

See Animal Research, *articles on* historical aspects, *and* philosophical issues.

ARAB NATIONS

See Medical Ethics, History of, *section on* near and middle east, *article on* contemporary arab world. *See also* Islam.

ARGENTINA

See Medical Ethics, History of, *section on* the americas, *article on* latin america.

ARS MORIENDI

See Death: Art of Dying.

ART OF DYING

See Death: Art of Dying.

ARTIFICIAL HEARTS AND CARDIAC-ASSIST DEVICES

In 1964, the U.S. Congress budgeted $581,000 to establish an artificial heart program at the National Institutes of Health (NIH). This was the first large-scale effort by any nation to support systematic research into the development of an artificial heart. As of 1994, the effort to build a reliable, totally implantable artificial heart had still not succeeded. But even though an effective device does not exist, the artificial heart has, since the 1960s, been at the center of a heated ethical, economic, and policy debate. The debate over the wisdom of building and testing an artificial heart has also served as a paradigm for debating the future of expensive technologies in the U.S. health-care system.

Scientists and physicians in many countries have dreamed for centuries of curing fatal heart diseases by creating a mechanical substitute. As recently as the 1950s, most physicians and engineers thought there were too many technical and design problems to undertake the creation of an implantable mechanical heart. But technological advances during the 1960s in engineering fields such as metallurgy, fluid dynamics, electronics, and computer modeling made some scientists think that it might be possible to actually construct such a device. The emergence of the kidney dialysis machine, which could mimic the functions of a human kidney, created a fundamental change in attitude in medicine about the feasibility of building an artificial heart.

The total artificial heart

Constructing an artificial heart requires materials such as metals, ceramics, plastics, and polymers that are lightweight and durable. At the same time, these materials must be biologically inert. They must not trigger attacks by the body's natural system of immune defenses that would lead to the disruption of the circulatory system and, ultimately, death. An artificial heart also requires sufficiently smooth surfaces so as not to disrupt blood flow through the heart or to damage fragile blood cells. A total artificial heart (TAH) needs a power source that can maintain a steady stream of energy for long periods of time while being small enough to fit completely inside the body. Both the pump and the power source must be capable of responding to changes in position, temperature, and pressure associated with the needs of the person using the machine.

The decision to launch a program to build a totally implantable heart had its roots in a series of exploratory meetings held during the 1950s at the NIH (Shaw, 1984). Enthusiasm for undertaking the research accelerated in the 1960s as physicians and engineers began to build and successfully use the first heart-lung machines, external pumps that could be used to support blood circulation in the body. After a few hours, these machines damaged the blood cells. Still, the heart-lung machine was a crude, partial artificial heart that inspired physicians to think that perhaps a permanent device was not beyond reach.

Moreover, as the U.S. space program began to enjoy success, optimism grew in both scientific and government circles about the feasibility of taking on large-scale technological challenges. Many in government were impressed with the productive results being secured in the space program and the military from centrally funded, programmatic research. U.S. physicians and biomedical scientists saw themselves as being able to overcome the many technical obstacles through hard work, directed budgets, and targeted programs. The space program had as its goal putting a man on the moon before the end of the 1960s. The artificial heart program launched at the NIH in 1964 set as its goal the testing of a total artificial heart in a human being by Valentine's Day, February 14, 1970 (Bernstein, 1984). Every year since, there has been funding for an artificial heart program at the NIH as a part of what became the National Heart, Lung, and Blood Institute, with a budget of about $10 million per year.

The goal of implanting an artificial heart by the end of the 1960s was not attained. A major hurdle was the development of an energy source capable of providing long-term power to an artificial heart and of fitting inside the body. Not only was progress slow but, during the time artificial heart researchers were trying to overcome the large number of technical challenges that confronted them, an alternative to the mechanical heart appeared—cardiac transplantation.

On December 3, 1967, Christiaan N. Barnard, using an organ obtained from a cadaver, performed the first heart transplant in a human being at Groote Schuur Hospital in Cape Town, South Africa. Although Barnard's patient survived for only eighteen days, the prospect of transplanting hearts from cadavers somewhat diminished interest in medical and government circles in the artificial heart.

While Denton Cooley did implant a crude mechanical heart in a human recipient at Baylor University College of Medicine in 1969, most of the device, including the power source, remained outside the body. Cooley explicitly stated that his sole motive for using this primitive, untested device was the desperate hope that it might help an imminently dying patient live long enough for a donor heart to become available for transplant. He did not believe the device he implanted was a permanent replacement for his patient's heart.

This attempt to use an artificial heart as a "bridge" to keep a patient alive in the hope a transplant could be done was done without the approval of Cooley's superiors or any government agency. The recipient, Haskell Karp, died shortly after the implant. Cooley's decision set off a storm of controversy within his medical center. Karp's wife later filed suit against Cooley for failure to obtain proper informed consent to the experiment. Texas courts held that since the procedure was experimental, there were no agreed-upon informed-consent standards that governed artificial heart implant surgery, and dismissed the suit.

Some researchers in the late 1960s believed that the problem of how to power a TAH could be solved by using a small, implantable capsule of plutonium. In 1972 a specially convened NIH panel, the Artificial Heart Assessment Panel, conducted the first governmental review of such technology. It concluded in 1973 that while the "advent of the totally implantable artificial heart" would be "an earthshaking event," the use of atomic power to drive a mechanical heart posed unacceptable radiation-exposure risks to the public health (National Heart, Lung, and Blood Institute, 1973).

Continuing problems with materials and limited success in animal studies spawned more doubts about the feasibility of the project. James Shannon, then director of the NIH, decided in 1973 to change the mission of the federal government's artificial heart program. Instead of trying to fund research aimed at the construction of a TAH, federal funds would be directed toward the design, construction, and testing of a partial artificial heart—the left-ventricular assist device (LVAD).

The left-ventricular assist device

The left chamber, or ventricle, of the human heart does the greatest share of the work of circulating blood throughout the body. Heart attacks and other forms of heart disease frequently damage this portion of the heart. An LVAD is a pump capable of supplementing the function of the left ventricle, thus allowing a weakened or damaged heart to support life. It does not require an implantable power source and its design can be simpler since it does not have to duplicate all the functions of a heart for prolonged periods of time.

Starting in 1973, the NIH spent approximately $10 million per year over the next decade and a half on research on LVADs for damaged hearts. By the early 1990s, a number of universities and private companies were undertaking clinical trials of LVADs in many countries. Some work on the TAH continued outside of the United States but, as in the United States, support for this research came almost entirely from private funds.

The artificial heart goes private

In 1967, Willem Kolff, the inventor of an early prototype of an artificial kidney dialysis machine built in

Holland during the Nazi occupation, moved to the University of Utah in Salt Lake City. His work on the dialysis machine led him to believe that it might be possible to build a mechanical heart. Over the next ten years he assembled a large, interdisciplinary team of medical, veterinary, and engineering researchers, among whom were the physicians Clifford Kwan-Gett and Robert Jarvik.

In the early 1970s, Kwan-Gett, and later Jarvik, began testing mechanical hearts in sheep and calves. These hearts fit inside the body of the animal but used an external air compressor powered by electricity from a wall outlet to create the force necessary to circulate blood. The Kwan-Gett artificial heart was made of plastic with carefully designed internal surfaces to minimize the danger of damage to blood cells caused by the machine's pumping action. In 1974, what had become known as the Jarvik-3 model kept a calf alive for three months.

In 1976, Kolff and some of his Utah colleagues formed a private company, Kolff Medical Associates, to attract venture capital to support their research. In order to interest private investors they had to create a marketing program for their mechanical heart. The decision to proceed with a private company constituted a first step into the emerging and often ethically controversial world of public–private partnerships intended to advance medical research.

After further testing and redesign of the Jarvik heart, Kolff's research team managed to use a Jarvik-7 to keep some animals alive for as long as eight months. In 1980, Kolff Medical Associates applied for permission from the institutional review board (IRB) of the University of Utah Medical Center to try the device on a human being. They also sought permission from the U.S. Food and Drug Administration (FDA), which, since 1976, had authority to regulate the testing and marketing of medical devices. While awaiting approval, members of the Utah artificial heart group traveled to Philadelphia and conducted a series of three practice implants of a Jarvik-7 heart on brain-dead patients at Temple University Medical Center. Permission from family members to use the cadavers was obtained by Jack Kolff, Willem Kolff's son, then a surgeon at Temple.

After many weeks of resubmissions and revisions the IRB at Utah and the FDA granted approval to undertake a series of seven implants of a Jarvik-7 heart in human beings at the University of Utah. Kolff and Jarvik, who had renamed their company Symbion, selected a young surgeon, William DeVries, to perform the first implant in a human recipient.

Initially the Utah group thought they would try the device on patients who encountered life-threatening problems while undergoing heart surgery. Sometimes during a heart operation, surgeons find that their patient's heart is so severely damaged that they cannot "wean" or remove the patient from a heart-lung machine without causing the patient's immediate death. The Symbion researchers argued and the IRB accepted the view that since persons who could not be weaned from heart-lung machines were doomed to die they constituted a reasonable pool of people to approach for permission to try out the Jarvik-7 device. A few patients who had severe heart disease were asked about their willingness to be put on a Jarvik heart if they could not be weaned from life support during surgery. A few patients agreed to an implant if life-threatening problems developed during their heart operations. Since all were successfully taken off life support after surgery, DeVries and his colleagues revised their research protocol to expand the pool of possible subjects. These subjects now included patients with very severe, life-threatening congestive heart failure resulting from cardiomyopathy, a poorly understood condition that causes irreversible, fatal damage to the muscle of the heart. This change was approved by the IRB in May 1982.

The experiment on Barney Clark.   Barney B. Clark, a retired dentist who had been admitted to the University of Utah Medical Center on November 29, 1982, with cardiomyopathy, was deemed to be an "ideal candidate" for the first implant of the Jarvik heart (Fox and Swazey, 1992) as he was educated, enthusiastic, and had a very supportive family. He signed the eighteen-page consent form the night he was admitted to the hospital. When his heart began to fail on December 1, he was taken to the operating room, and after a nine-hour operation, he became the first human being to receive an artificial heart as a permanent replacement for his own.

The Clark experiment was certainly the most intensively publicized medical experiment in the history of human experimentation. Jarvik and DeVries as well as other University of Utah officials spent many hours speaking with the media about the operation, the device, and their patient's health status. In the days after the implant, the health-care team made many optimistic pronouncements to the media about Clark's chances for survival. But Clark followed a very rocky course during the 112 days he lived with the Jarvik-7 device. He suffered a wide range of complications that required three additional surgical procedures. After a few weeks on the machine, his emotional and cognitive state deteriorated severely, and on more than one occasion, he asked that the artificial heart be turned off. This was not done. After his death, more than 1,300 people, including political figures, members of the governing council of the Latter-Day Saints (Mormon) Church, of which Clark was a member, many of his doctors, and media representatives from around the world, attended his funeral in Seattle, Washington.

DeVries and the Utah group pronounced the Clark experiment a success. They had kept alive a man in the final stages of heart failure for well over three months. But the IRB at Utah, troubled by the many complications that had arisen during the experiment, asked for many changes and clarifications in the research protocol before giving DeVries permission to try another implant. Among other things, the Clark experiment raised questions about the adequacy of informed consent of potential recipients. Could those facing certain death really be said to choose? And were those conducting the research so enthusiastic and hopeful about its prospects that they could not provide a realistic picture of the risks and dangers inherent in the experiment (Fox and Swazey, 1992)?

Controversies also swirled around the issues of stock ownership of Symbion, of how best to find sources to pay for the next implant (Barney Clark's bill exceeded $250,000), and of financial sources for the support of the research team. On July 31, 1984, DeVries abruptly brought all these controversies to a halt. He announced at a press conference that he and the artificial heart program were leaving Salt Lake City and would begin work immediately at the Humana Hospital-Audubon in Louisville, Kentucky.

The artificial heart at Louisville. Humana-Audubon was part of a corporation that was trying to establish itself as a national leader in the for-profit health-care sector. One of the principal owners of the company, David Jones, pledged to DeVries that the company was willing to underwrite the costs of "up to a hundred implants" if he would move his artificial heart program to Louisville.

Between 1984 and 1987, four more implants were done using artificial hearts as permanent replacements for the human heart. William J. Schroeder received his implant of a Jarvik heart on November 29, 1984, less than two months after the IRB at Humana-Audubon gave its approval. Schroeder initially did well on the heart, but within nineteen days he suffered a stroke. During the course of the next 620 days he spent on the device, he had three more strokes; the last brought about his death. The other recipients of total artificial hearts—two at Louisville, one in Sweden, and one in Arizona—all experienced similar difficulties and ultimately died. It became clear from these experiments that the Jarvik-7 was not suitable for use as a permanent replacement device. In 1987 Humana commissioned its own review of the ethics of its artificial heart program. Three outside reviewers were critical of the consent process and the scientific design of the research. To some extent, this probably contributed to Humana's discontinuation of the program and DeVries's leaving.

In January of 1988, the new director of the National Heart, Lung, and Blood Institute, Claude Lenfant, de-

cided to cancel the NIH program to build a total artificial heart. The recent experience with artificial hearts, he believed, clearly indicated that such devices could be best used to assist failing hearts or for temporary use until a transplant could be found. Lenfant argued that a totally implantable artificial heart was still at least ten years away and might well wind up benefiting a relatively small number of patients at great cost. The threat of shutting down research on the TAH created a whirlwind of political protest in Congress. Legislators from states such as Utah and Massachusetts, where heart research was being conducted, fought to block Lenfant's plan. By the end of 1988, $20 million had been awarded to four centers to continue this research.

On January 11, 1990, the FDA cited concerns about the safety of the device and the quality control of the manufacturer, Symbion, and withdrew its approval for the clinical testing of Jarvik-7 devices in human beings. In July of 1991, the National Academy of Sciences' Institute of Medicine issued a study in which they recommended continued federal funding for both LVADs and TAHs. They predicted that a reliable LVAD should become available in the late 1990s and a TAH by around 2005 (Institute of Medicine, 1991). Federal funding for research on both permanent and temporary artificial hearts continued.

Ethics and mechanical hearts

The history of artificial heart research and use raises many ethical issues. Three issues stand out as especially important. These issues are both specific to the artificial heart and also apply more generally to all forms of new and expensive high-technology health care.

Human experimentation. The existing protections for persons who participate in medical research are informed consent and review by local committees of scientists (IRBs) of research proposals. The history of artificial heart research has called into question the adequacy of both protections.

Patients asked to serve as subjects in the use of artificial hearts were extremely vulnerable. They faced certain death if the device was not used. Often, their heart failure came about suddenly and unexpectedly. For many of the subjects, the complexities of the research and the rigorous postimplant monitoring of the device were extremely intimidating. Moreover, subjects may hear the risks and benefits of participation only from researchers who themselves have a powerful interest in wanting their work to proceed. Those who have sought subjects to receive artificial hearts have acted as both clinician and researcher to the recipients of the device, generating a strong conflict of interest.

The threat of imminent death tends to coerce subjects to make particular choices; furthermore, those charged with reviewing requests to use artificial hearts have faced serious moral challenges. There has been a great deal of pressure associated with the race to be the first medical center to use a mechanical heart or to be the first to use one successfully. Considerable financial and publicity stakes are involved for the researcher, the institution, and any companies in which the institution or researcher might have an interest. Local IRBs may not have the requisite expertise or independence to evaluate exactly what sorts of criteria to use to govern subject selection, consent forms, or the methods for accumulating data on subjects over long periods of time.

Bridge and temporary use. As it became clear in the 1980s that the devices then available could not safely support long-term heart function in human beings, enthusiasm for artificial hearts turned to their temporary use. Here, too, tough ethical questions must be confronted.

If artificial hearts are to be used on a temporary basis, is it permissible to implant them without the explicit consent of a person who has undergone a sudden, unexpected heart failure? Which patients would constitute the best patient population for testing devices intended for temporary use only—those nearest death (i.e., those who made up the population of subjects for permanent implants of Jarvik hearts), or those not quite as sick, who are most likely to recover if given a "respite" by an LVAD or temporary use of an artificial heart? It is not clear that those who are given artificial hearts or LVADs on a temporary basis understand what their rights are to turn off these devices. Nor is it clear that the use of these devices will contribute overall to an increase in the number of lives saved (Annas, 1993). When cadaver hearts are scarce, the use of artificial hearts or bridge devices as a prelude to transplant means only that the identity of those getting a chance at a transplant may change while the overall number of transplants done remains the same (Caplan, 1992). Assist devices will not save more lives since there are only a small number of cadaver hearts available for transplant.

The societal impact of the artificial heart. One of the obvious moral questions raised by research to develop an artificial heart is whether developing this device is the best way to spend limited research dollars in meeting the health-care needs of Americans or of the world's population as a whole. Artificial heart research is expensive. The costs of doing the first TAH implants ran into the hundreds of thousands of dollars. Does it make more sense to pursue other options for the treatment of heart disease or even the prevention of heart disease?

Many experts note that a fully perfected artificial heart would probably cost billions of dollars. Those most likely to benefit from access to such a device would likely be those who could afford insurance to pay for me-

chanical hearts. There are obvious problems of equity and justice in asking all to bear the cost of research for a device that would only be available to some. Questions of fairness also exist in deciding to build a machine that may add years of life to those at the end of the life span, when tens of millions of persons around the globe die before reaching adolescence from diseases and injuries that can be prevented. Explicit debates about fairness have not been very much in evidence in terms of how best to allocate resources to perfect new therapies in American health-care policy. If the pursuit of a TAH is to continue, it would seem prudent to make considerations of fairness a more central part of the policy debate.

ARTHUR L. CAPLAN

Directly related to this entry are the entries ARTIFICIAL ORGANS AND LIFE-SUPPORT SYSTEMS; INFORMED CONSENT, *article on* CONSENT ISSUES IN HUMAN RESEARCH; RESEARCH, HUMAN: HISTORICAL ASPECTS; *and* TECHNOLOGY, *article on* HISTORY OF MEDICAL TECHNOLOGY. *For a further discussion of topics mentioned in this entry, see the entries* COMMUNICATION, BIOMEDICAL, *article on* MEDIA AND MEDICINE; FUTURE GENERATIONS, OBLIGATIONS TO; HEALTH-CARE RESOURCES, ALLOCATION OF; *and* RESEARCH POLICY, *articles on* GENERAL GUIDELINES, *and* RISK AND VULNERABLE GROUPS. *For a discussion of heart transplants, see the entry* ORGAN AND TISSUE TRANSPLANTS, *article on* MEDICAL OVERVIEW. *Other relevant material may be found under the entries* BIOMEDICAL ENGINEERING; KIDNEY DIALYSIS; *and* MEDICAL ETHICS, HISTORY OF, *section on* THE AMERICAS, *article on* UNITED STATES IN THE TWENTIETH CENTURY. *See also the* APPENDIX (CODES, OATHS, AND DIRECTIVES RELATED TO BIOETHICS), SECTION IV: ETHICAL DIRECTIVES FOR HUMAN RESEARCH.

Bibliography

ANNAS, GEORGE J. 1994. *Standard of Care: The Law of American Bioethics.* New York: Oxford University Press.

BERNSTEIN, BARTON. 1984. "The Misguided Quest for the Artificial Heart." *Technology Review* 87, no. 6:12–17.

BLAKESLEE, SANDRA, ed. 1986. *Human Heart Replacement: A New Challenge for Physicians and Reporters.* Los Angeles: Foundation for American Communications.

CAPLAN, ARTHUR L. 1992. *If I Were a Rich Man Could I Buy a Pancreas? and Other Essays on the Ethics of Health Care.* Bloomington: Indiana University Press.

DEVRIES, WILLIAM C.; ANDERSON, JEFFREY L.; JOYCE, LYLE D.; ANDERSON, FRED L.; HAMMOND, ELIZABETH H; JARIK, ROBERT K.; and KOLFF, WILLEM J. 1984. "Clinical Use of the Total Artificial Heart." *New England Journal of Medicine* 310, no. 5:273–278.

Fox, Renée C., and Swazey, Judith P. 1992. *Spare Parts: Organ Replacement in America.* New York: Oxford University Press.

Gil, Gideon. 1989. "The Artificial Heart Juggernaut." *Hastings Center Report* 19, no. 2:24–31.

Institute of Medicine. Committee to Evaluate the Artificial Heart Program of the National Heart, Lung, and Blood Institute. 1991. *The Artificial Heart: Prototypes, Policies and Patients.* Edited by John R. Hogness and Malin Van Antwerp. Washington, D.C.: National Academy Press.

Jonsen, Albert R. 1973. "The Totally Implantable Artificial Heart." *Hastings Center Report* 3 (November):1–4.

———. 1986. "The Artificial Heart's Threat to Others." *Hastings Center Report* 16, no. 1:9–11.

Miles, Stephen; Siegler, Mark; Schiedermayer, David L.; Lantos, John D.; and La Puma, John. 1988. "The Total Artificial Heart: An Ethics Perspective on Current Clinical Research and Deployment." *Chest* 94, no. 2: 409–413.

National Heart, Lung, and Blood Institute. Artificial Heart Assessment Panel. 1973. *The Totally Implantable Artificial Heart: Economic, Ethical, Legal, Medical, Psychiatric, and Social Implications: A Report.* Bethesda, Md.: National Institutes of Health.

———. Working Group on Mechanical Circulatory Support. 1985. *Artificial Heart and Assist Devices: Directions, Needs, Costs, Societal and Ethical Issues.* Bethesda, Md.: Author.

Shaw, Margery W., ed. 1984. *After Barney Clark: Reflections on the Utah Artificial Heart Program.* Austin: University of Texas Press.

ARTIFICIAL INSEMINATION

See Reproductive Technologies, *articles on* artificial insemination, ethical issues, *and* legal and regulatory issues.

ARTIFICIAL ORGANS AND LIFE-SUPPORT SYSTEMS

The life-support systems of the modern intensive-care unit are designed to support the function of vital organs long enough for them to recover from infection or injury. Their role is to maintain the body's physiological homeostasis in as near a normal state as possible, and to monitor their success in doing so. Respiration can be assisted or controlled by artificial ventilation; the rate of the heart can be controlled by electrically driven pacemakers and and its mechanical function supported by an intra-aortic balloon pump; metabolic needs can be met by intravenously administered total parenteral nutrition; the function of the heart and lungs can be taken over by cardiopulmonary bypass (the "heart-lung machine")

for periods long enough to perform open-heart surgery; and the function of the lungs of premature infants with pulmonary hypertension can be assumed by a similar device, the extracorporeal membrane oxygenator, for four or more days to allow immature lungs to develop sufficiently to assume their natural function. Adaptation of the artificial kidney to provide continuous cleansing of the blood and regulation of fluid volume by hemofiltration in patients in septic shock and acute kidney failure is in an early stage of clinical evaluation. An artificial liver, designed to take over the function of an injured liver long enough to allow it to recover naturally, is in an even earlier stage of development and clinical trial.

Evolution of the modern intensive-care unit

The modern intensive-care unit, fully equipped to carry out the functions mentioned above, and staffed by trained professionals known as "intensivists," is the product of years of physiological research and technical ingenuity. The development of artificial organs to substitute for the functions of the natural organs responded to urgent medical needs at a time when basic medical science had progressed sufficiently for their practical application.

Respiration was the first of the body's vital functions for which the problem of artificial substitution was solved. The problem for which a solution was initially sought was surgical: how to breathe for anesthetized patients in order to allow the chest to be opened for lung surgery. The solution was the use of positive-pressure ventilation by anesthesiologists (and later by automatic ventilators). The earliest successful intrathoracic operations, made possible by controlled ventilation, took place in the mid-1930s.

The control of ventilation by manually applying positive pressure to force gases into the lungs, simulating natural breathing, was a new skill that anesthesiologists needed to learn in response to surgical needs. World War II presented an even more challenging set of needs: to resuscitate severely injured soldiers, who were often in shock, while providing anesthesia to allow urgent surgery that often was a lifesaving component of the resuscitative process. The physician, who may or may not have been trained in anesthesia, now had the responsibility for the functions of the heart and circulation, as well as that of breathing. From the war emerged a new generation of physicians armed with life-support skills to meet the needs of surgical anesthesia and ready to tackle the life-threatening medical problems of civilian life. These skills were soon turned to the needs of patients suffering from bulbar poliomyelitis and dying from respiratory failure.

Between July and December 1952, more than two thousand patients were admitted to the Blegdam Hospital, Copenhagen's infectious disease hospital, for the treatment of poliomyelitis. In more than three hundred the brain stem was affected to a degree requiring assistance to respiration, as many as seventy patients at one time. Up to this time the standard treatment for the respiratory insufficiency of poliomyelitis involving the brain stem ("bulbar" poliomyelitis) had been the iron lung, a large tank or chamber encasing the entire body except the head, in which negative pressure was induced rhythmically to assist the patient's respiration. Nearly entirely encased, the patient was almost completely inaccessible for essential nursing care. An alternative was a device encompassing only the chest, the cuirass respirator, which facilitated nursing but supported respiration less effectively.

At the beginning of the epidemic in Copenhagen, the Blegdam Hospital had one iron lung and six cuirass respirators. After twenty-seven of the first thirty-one respirator patients had died, a senior anesthetist, Bjorn Ibsen, was asked "to determine whether positive-pressure breathing as used in modern anesthesia might be of value." Responding in the affirmative, Ibsen recruited medical students, nurses, and interns to provide around-the-clock manual assistance or complete control of their patients' breathing. Thirty percent of the patients so managed survived (see Hilberman, 1975; Snider, 1989; and Bryan-Brown, 1992, for historical review).

The principles for the management of respiratory failure established during the Copenhagen poliomyelitis epidemic were immediately adopted in the similar epidemics that rapidly followed elsewhere. It had been learned that positive-pressure ventilation applied directly through the patient's airway provided more effective gas exchange than could be achieved with the iron lung. A mechanical, rather than manual, source of positive pressure was urgently needed, however, and the manufacturers of respiratory equipment quickly converted to the manufacture of mechanical respirators that could deliver positive pressure. Poliomyelitis virtually disappeared in developed countries following the introduction of polio vaccine in 1956, but the lessons learned and the ventilators developed laid the foundation for the respiratory-care units that rapidly developed to care for patients suffering from other causes of respiratory depression.

Procedures and equipment with which to manage respiratory depression were developed hand in hand with advances in the anesthetic management of patients undergoing surgery. In a somewhat similar way, the management of cardiac emergencies, and ultimately the development of cardiac-care units, emerged from the operating room experience. During surgery the function of the heart may be depressed or fail entirely as a result of inadequate ventilation, of surgical blood loss, or of the cardiac depressant effect of anesthetic agents. When this occurred, the proper procedure was to open the chest

wall immediately and to restore function by massaging the heart manually, under direct vision. The same procedure was employed when a patient's heart stopped elsewhere in the hospital. Such a major surgical procedure performed outside the operating room had little likelihood of success, however, and efforts to resuscitate patients suffering from myocardial infarct and cardiac arrest were largely futile.

Prospects for the successful resuscitation of such patients were markedly enhanced by reports in 1960 and 1961 that cardiac function can be restored by rhythmically and forcefully pressing the sternum against the heart, thereby achieving closed-chest cardiac massage and eliminating the need to open the chest. The most common cause of loss of cardiac function following myocardial infarct is ventricular fibrillation, a disturbance in cardiac rhythm. It had already been shown in 1956 that ventricular fibrillation could be converted to the heart's normal rhythm by externally applied electrical countershock. The combination of external cardiac massage and external defibrillation now gave the opportunity for effective management of patients suffering ventricular fibrillation. The next step was to collect patients believed to be at high risk in a single hospital unit or ward where it would be possible to monitor cardiac function continuously by electrocardiogram and with facilities immediately at hand with which to respond to arrhythmias and other cardiac emergencies. For this to succeed, highly trained personnel were (and are) needed in constant attendance, a need now filled by specially trained coronary-care nurses working in collaboration with the cardiologists who rapidly assumed their new responsibilities as a second generation of intensivists.

Since the early respiratory and coronary care units of the 1950s and 1960s there has been an unbroken period of extraordinary technological achievement in the capability to maintain physiologic homeostasis over longer and longer periods of time. The rapid development of support systems in collaboration with industry has been the result of a broad international effort, although the clinical introduction and use of the products of this effort have varied widely from country to country. There are few precise data by which to document each country's investment in life-support systems, but the United States almost certainly has incorporated such systems into respiratory-care units, intensive-care nurseries, and coronary-care units in much greater numbers than any other country. There are an estimated sixty thousand intensive-care beds in acute-care hospitals in the United States, with a total cost estimated to be approximately 10 percent of the country's total medical expenditures, slightly more than 1 percent of its gross national product (Raffin et al., 1989).

Following the virtual disappearance of poliomyelitis, the newly developed external respirators began to be

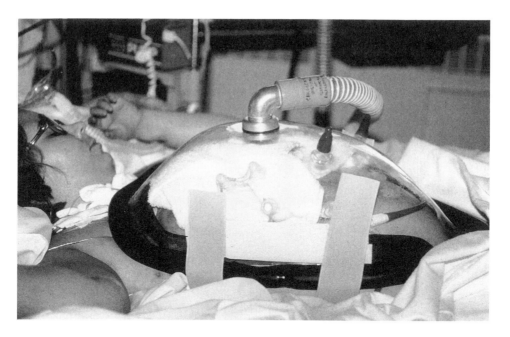

FIGURE 1 Postoperative patient suffering from multiple organ failure. Respiration is being assisted by cuirass respirator to avoid need for endotracheal intubation. *Courtesy* Department of Visual Arts, Stanford Medical Center, Stanford University.

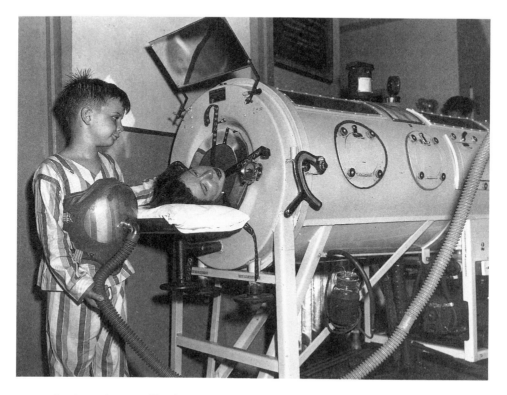

FIGURE 2 An eight-year-old polio victim wears a "Monaghan" one-pound "iron lung." A model shows the use of an older-type iron lung. Photograph by Dennis Burke, June 22, 1949. Reprinted by permission of The Bettmann Archive.

used in the care of patients suffering from other types of respiratory depression. The indications for ventilatory support grew rapidly. In 1958, sixty-six patients were ventilated for twenty-four hours or longer in the respiratory intensive-care unit at Massachusetts General Hospital. "By 1964 the number had grown to 400, by 1968 to almost 900, and by 1982 to almost 2,000" (Snider, 1989).

Improved life-support skills and technology in the operating room, and postoperatively in intensive care, allowed sicker patients to be operated on. And if seriously ill patients could be brought through surgery with relative safety, seriously ill medical patients should be able to benefit from similar intensive care. These included patients with heart failure, liver failure, kidney failure, and stroke and other intracranial catastrophes, many with two or more organ system failures. Improved instruments for the monitoring of physiological function markedly improved the success in fine-tuning life-support devices in their goal of maintaining homeostasis.

Benefits of life-support systems

What has been achieved? Many patients in imminent danger of death have been rescued: Treatment of patients with drug overdose, of patients unable to resume normal respiratory or cardiac function immediately following surgery, and of some premature infants can be predicted with confidence to have a favorable outcome. The prognosis for many others, however, is grave. The in-hospital mortality of mechanically ventilated patients suffering from pneumonia, septic shock, respiratory failure as a complication of cancer, intracranial hemorrhage, and congestive heart failure ranges from 40 percent to over 80 percent. When more than one organ system fails, there is a progressively increasing mortality with each successive day of failure. For example, the anticipated mortality of patients on the first day of the failure of a single organ system is estimated to be 22 percent, rising to 41 percent at the end of a week. By contrast, the estimated mortalities of patients presenting on the first day with two or three organs in failure are 52 percent and 80 percent, respectively, rising to 68 percent and 100 percent at the end of a week (Knaus et al., 1985).

Some of the sickest patients gain only a few additional months of life, months often of questionable quality. The mortality reported in 1989 for patients suffering from AIDS complicated by pneumocystis pneumonia was approximately 85 percent; with new and presumably improved treatment the mortality fell over the next two years to 60 percent, but all of the AIDS patients surviving intensive care and mechanical ventilation were dead at the end of a year (Wachter et al., 1991). How valuable are the few additional months of life? The doubts

that doctors harbor are reflected in the higher percentage of mechanically ventilated AIDS patients for whom "do not resuscitate" orders are given. Patients also have their doubts. In a survey of 118 homosexual men with AIDS, only slightly more than half indicated that they would want to be admitted to the intensive-care unit and to receive mechanical ventilation in the event of pneumocystis pneumonia (Steinbrook et al., 1986).

The benefits of life support for very-low-birthweight, premature infants (weight 500–750 grams) are little better. One of three will survive if provided intensive care, but many of these will have serious pulmonary and central nervous system disabilities. Some eight thousand of these babies are born each year in the United States, and the care of those who survive is estimated to cost $250 million. The policy of most U.S. pediatricians and neonatologists caring for such infants has been characterized as vigorous treatment for as long as there is any hope of survival. In Britain attempts are made to save far fewer of these infants, and fewer still in Sweden (Young and Stevenson, 1990). Ernle Young and David Stevenson attribute the aggressive approach in the United States at least in part to the legacy of the "Baby Doe regulations" implemented in 1984 by the federal government following the death of a baby born with Down syndrome and birth defects for which the baby's parents refused corrective surgery. Although the Baby Doe regulations were later struck down by the Supreme Court, the Child Abuse and Neglect and the Discrimination Against the Handicapped statutes, amended to strengthen the Baby Doe regulations, have served much of the government's intended pro-life purpose (Caplan et al., 1992). The legacy of this policy is reflected in the results of intensive care of these extremely small infants: an overall survival rate of 33 percent; 31 percent of survivors left with significant neurodevelopmental handicaps; a mean cost of $158,800 for the initial care per infant, not including the lifelong costs of those with handicaps (Hack and Fanaroff, 1989).

Procedures for the protection of individuals and the public

The list of ethical concerns in life support is a long one: issues of distributive and social justice, notably the development and clinical introduction of advanced life-support technology, often at great cost, with benefits potentially great but often unmeasured and unknown, accompanied by the potential for harm; the ethics of subjecting a patient, when death appears imminent or highly likely, to procedures with small likelihood of benefit—procedures that may, in fact, contribute to an increase in suffering; the justification of very large expenditures for providing life-support devices to a small number of individuals with potential for only small ben-

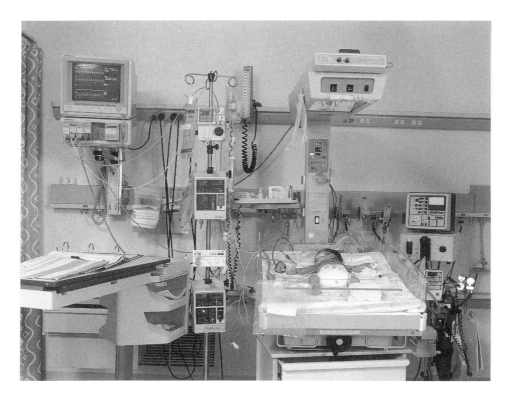

FIGURE 3   Three-and-a-half-month-old infant, born ten weeks prematurely. Respiratory distress syndrome required assistance to respiration via an endotracheal tube for three and a half weeks. The photograph was taken 24 hours following surgical removal of a subglottal cyst that obstructed airway. Infant is again receiving endotracheal assistance to respiration; heart rate, blood pressure, and arterial blood oxygenation are being monitored continuously. *Courtesy* Department of Visual Arts, Stanford Medical Center, Stanford University.

efits when many individuals do not receive basic medical care that is known to provide large (but less dramatic) benefits; the equitable distribution of life-support systems among potential beneficiaries; the ethics of subjecting patients, even very sick patients, to treatment with new and untested life-support devices; and how to obtain informed consent from a patient who may be too ill to understand or to respond.

When mechanical ventilators were introduced to save the lives of patients, most of them young, suffering from bulbar poliomyelitis, there was no basis for ethical concern. Without life support most such patients died; with it many survived and could look forward to lives of good quality. The treatment clearly worked, and the cost was relatively modest. The introduction of closed-chest cardiac massage and electrical defibrillation for the resuscitation of patients in whom ventricular fibrillation complicated myocardial infarction similarly presented little concern. Death invariably follows ventricular fibrillation unless it is treated immediately; with treatment many survive and return to useful lives. When the effect of treatment is as large as for each of these two conditions, no formal experiments are necessary to establish its efficacy. Indeed, it would be unethical to sub-

mit patients to a clinical trial in which treatment is withheld from a control group.

When, on the other hand, the effectiveness of new treatment is uncertain, it is now generally considered unethical not to evaluate the treatment through a properly controlled experiment, preferably a randomized clinical trial. There are, however, a number of obstacles to randomization, both ethical and practical, and it may be particularly difficult to implement in the treatment of life-threatening conditions. On ethical grounds it is often argued that seriously ill patients should not be denied any treatment, whether or not of proven efficacy, that might possibly help them. This has been repeatedly invoked in arguments for relaxation of restrictions on the use of new drugs for the treatment of AIDS, and is an argument implicit in the widespread application of life-support systems. From a practical viewpoint, it is argued that when a condition is usually fatal, the success of a new treatment will be obvious without resorting to the statistical formality of a randomized trial.

The introduction of extracorporeal membrane oxygenation (ECMO) provides an example of such a life-threatening condition and a proposed treatment of great but uncertain potential. ECMO was introduced in the early 1970s for the care of newborn infants suffering from a then almost invariably fatal combination of pulmonary hypertension and inadequate uptake of oxygen by the lungs. It was proposed to provide oxygen to the infant long enough for the lungs to develop and assume their natural function. Any improvement in survival could be assumed to establish the efficacy of treatment. Nine of the first thirteen patients treated with ECMO died, and although there was subsequent improvement in survival, a randomized trial was ultimately considered necessary to dispel growing doubts. Two trials were carried out, the second of which demonstrated fewer deaths in the group of infants treated with ECMO than in those receiving "standard" conservative treatment (O'Rourke et al., 1989). The degree of improvement was large enough to be considered statistically significant—but just barely—and some considered the trial an insufficient basis on which to establish ECMO as standard therapy (Pocock, 1992). Further to complicate the assessment of ECMO, and hardly before completion of the trials, an improvement in conservative treatment, with results as good as those reported with ECMO, was reported (Dworetz et al., 1989), leaving unresolved the question of the ultimate value of ECMO to newborn infants suffering from pulmonary hypertension and inadequate oxygenation.

Although randomized clinical trials of new drugs are almost always required by the U.S. Food and Drug Administration (FDA), they are not required for devices and therefore would not have been required of the manufacturers of the equipment used in ECMO. ECMO was first used prior to any regulation of devices and therefore has been largely, though not entirely, exempt from FDA controls. Newer life-support devices, such as an experimental instrument designed to facilitate oxygenation and avoid the need for ventilatory support—called the intravenous oxygenator (IVOX)—and the artificial liver, just beginning clinical trials in 1992, must comply with FDA device regulations. How rigorously they will be enforced in life-threatening situations remains to be seen, in view of the growing willingness to relax regulations for the use of unproven drugs and biologicals for the critically ill.

Regulation of the development and introduction into clinical practice of medical devices vary greatly among Western countries. In the United States, regulation of devices became law in 1976 with the passage of the Medical Device Amendments (Public Law 94-295) to the Food and Drug Act. The law categorizes devices on the basis of risk and safety, with those "that are life supporting or sustaining, that are of substantial importance in preventing impairment of health, or that have a potential for causing risk of injury or illness" constituting the class subject to the closest regulation.

The requirements of the device amendments are in many ways similar to those for drugs. Devices that are accepted as "substantially equivalent" to a previously approved device—about 90 percent of all new devices—are exempted from further requirements. For those not exempted, marketing approval entails presentation of "valid scientific evidence" or "well-controlled scientific studies" based on institutional review, but not randomized clinical trials. If a device is deemed to present a significant risk, a request for an investigational device exemption must be submitted to the FDA. A major difference between most new devices and new drugs is that the device usually is modified over time and its efficacy needs continual reassessment. In practice this process is optimally carried out in close collaboration between the FDA, the institutional review board, the investigator, and the manufacturer. This is, in fact, what has happened with the introduction of IVOX, the artificial liver, and ECMO, though the latter does not automatically come under FDA regulation.

In the past, regulation of medical devices in Great Britain relied on a voluntary system of manufacturer registration, product approval, and reporting of adverse events. The adoption of more formal regulations was initiated in collaboration with other members of the European Community in 1990, to be implemented in a series of directives over a several-year period beginning in January 1993. The first directive will cover high-risk medical devices designed to be implanted within the human body, such as cardiac pacemakers, automatic defibrillators, and most or all of the medical devices for use in intensive care.

The institutional review boards in the United States and the medical research ethics committees in Great Britain provide a second and important set of ethical controls over the introduction of life-support devices. Their principal responsibility is to protect subjects of research from undue risk and to ensure that their informed consent is secured. There is considerable variation among both types of committees in how they interpret and carry out their responsibilities (Goldman and Katz, 1982; Royal College of Physicians, 1990). A major shortcoming of committees in both countries is that they have no jurisdiction over innovative therapies that are introduced clinically but not classified as research.

A third mechanism of control of innovative therapy is reimbursement. In the United States many medical insurance companies will not reimburse physicians for new procedures unless and until they have been clearly demonstrated to be efficacious. Total parenteral nutrition provides a good example of the problems confronted by the insurer in the implementation of such a policy. It is used in a wide variety of circumstances, some indicated and some not, and it is not apt to be possible, based on claims submitted for reimbursement, to distinguish one from the other.

Total parenteral nutrition is an expensive therapy, costing an estimated $200 a day for the average patient; approximately $6 billion is spent on it per year in the

United States (Pillar and Perry, 1990). How it is used is an ethical as well as an economic problem. While evidence of its efficacy may not be adequate to ensure its appropriate and ethical use (it has been reported to result in worse outcomes when used in patients suffering from cancer), purely economic considerations will raise increasing obstacles to its overutilization. Under health systems in which total funding is fixed and limited, such as the British National Health Service, expensive treatment can be provided only if other, equally expensive uses of medical resources are forgone. The United States is moving toward similar forms of global funding. The "diagnosis-related group" system of payment for the care of Medicare patients provides a specific, limited amount for a given diagnostic category. In so doing, it introduces a strong economic motive to limit treatment to procedures that are known to be cost-effective. Many health insurance companies have adopted capitation schemes of payment that incorporate similar disincentives.

The final level of control in the clinical adoption of new medical technology, including life-support devices, is exercised by patients and doctors themselves. Some argue that the ultimate decision must belong to patients or their families (Angell, 1991), and some argue that doctors are the only ones equipped with sufficient knowledge and judgment to make life-support decisions, with the final choice made jointly by doctor and patient or the patient's surrogate (Young and Stevenson, 1990). In addition to the inherent difficulties in assigning autonomy to patient or doctor, there are special difficulties when life-support systems are at issue.

Patients are often too ill to make decisions, and family members or other proxies may not be sufficiently aware of the patient's wishes or of the medical issues to make appropriate decisions. An advance directive, living will, or durable power of attorney, if prepared on a previous occasion by the patient, can be critically useful in the event; but even such a document may not be sufficiently specific to cover the exact circumstances that are actually encountered (Schneiderman et al., 1992). In practice, however, they have been infrequently executed by patients in the United States. When the patient is a child or incompetent adult, an appropriate decision by parents or family members may be difficult to obtain.

In the absence of an advance directive, however, the doctor must turn to the family for direction, and while there are often doubts that members of the patient's family are able to know what the patient's wishes would have been, doctors and families in most instances have been able to arrive at a decision that was consistent with the family's values and the doctor's medical judgment. The medical and legal grounds for withdrawing ventilation once brain death has been diagnosed are now well established in most developed countries. The patient in a persistent vegetative state (PVS) presents a more difficult problem because ventilator support is not needed, and the persistent nonsentient patient can live for years if tube feeding is continued.

The problem in withdrawing tube feeding to allow such patients to die is that they are not suffering, they are not terminally ill, and there are no reliable diagnostic tests such as those for brain death. Nevertheless, in the United States a consensus has emerged on the medical, ethical, and legal basis for withdrawing tube feeding. Medical groups have agreed upon guidelines, and many cases have come before the courts including one to the U.S. Supreme Court. According to the Court, such decisions should now be made informally by doctors and families, without court intervention.

The first such case in Great Britain came to court in November 1992 and resulted in a unanimous decision by nine judges in the High Court and two levels of appeal to allow withdrawal of tube feeding (Jennett, 1992). The judges also ruled that future cases should continue to come for judicial review, pending the deliberations of a committee set up to discuss this and other issues associated with withholding and withdrawing treatment.

The Medical Council of New Zealand, by contrast, in 1993 recommended that such a decision should not come to court, but that hospital ethics committees should adjudicate if there are disagreements to resolve. In the Netherlands, it is considered appropriate for doctors to discuss life termination by active euthanasia or withdrawal of tube feeding, once the vegetative state is declared permanent. All countries emphasize the need to wait long enough to rule out the prospect of useful recovery (usually one year) before deciding to withdraw life support, and they recommend having more than one opinion. (See "Advance Directives," 1992; and Jennett, 1992, for summary and discussion of advance directives and the PVS.)

Difficulties have arisen in the infrequent instances when a family or one of its members insists on the continuation of life support when such action is deemed medically futile and is opposed by the doctors in charge. Two such instances deserve mention. In one, "Baby L," semiconscious since birth, required mechanical ventilation and cardiovascular support, and had suffered multiple episodes of cardiac arrest requiring resuscitation. The baby's doctors urged that life support be stopped, but the mother insisted that life support be continued. The hospital asked court intervention to allow care to be terminated, but before a judgment could be made, the baby was transferred to another hospital and the care of another doctor willing to continue life support, leaving the legal issue unresolved (Paris et al., 1990).

In the case of Helga Wanglie (Miles, 1991; Angell, 1991), an eighty-six-year-old woman had been in PVS for over a year. The controversy pitted the patient's husband and children, who wanted respiratory support continued, against her doctors, who wished to discontinue it on the grounds that it was medically inappropriate. The court, asked for a judgment, found in favor of the family, and the patient died still supported by respirator. As Angell (1991) points out, the case differed "in a crucial way from earlier right-to-die cases," in which families wished to terminate life support contrary to the institution's opinion that continued support was medically indicated. While expressing sympathy for the doctors' judgment that the further life support of Mrs. Wanglie could not be justified on medical grounds (Miles, 1991), Angell in an accompanying editorial agreed with the court decision according priority to self-determination as reflected in Mrs. Wanglie's family's wishes.

Difficulties have also arisen, again only occasionally, when hospitals have continued tube feeding in defiance of an advance directive supported by the family, thereby prolonging the vegetative state. A number of families have successfully sued in U.S. Courts for wrongful extension of life (Weir and Gostin, 1990).

Conclusion

The clinical use of life-support systems presents few ethical problems when the patient is otherwise healthy, is relatively young, has an expectation of future years of good quality, and requires life support with artificial organs for discrete periods of time to allow a natural organ to recover from infection or injury and to resume its natural function. Investment in research and development of new artificial organs and of technology to monitor their performance for use in the care of such patients similarly presents few ethical problems.

Life support for the terminally or near terminally ill, or for those with a very poor prognosis (such as extremely-low-birth-weight infants), presents very difficult ethical problems for both the individual and society. For such individuals or their surrogates and their doctors, the ethical issues are whether to intervene when intervention may be fruitless—indeed, may cause more harm than good—or whether to withhold intervention and forgo even a remote possibility of return to health or reasonable well-being and function.

For society the ethical issues are ones of distributive justice: the fair distribution of a particular life-support technology to all who might benefit, and the cost-effective distribution of social resources between life-support technologies and other medical and social needs. Response to these ethical problems will require investment in research and development of improved life-support technology, in better methods of evaluating such technology, in better methods of determining the values placed by patients on life-support intervention, in involving them or their surrogates in the decision whether to intervene, and in information systems that will make reliable, relevant data available to doctor, patient, and society.

JOHN P. BUNKER

For a further discussion of topics mentioned in this entry, see the entries DEATH AND DYING: EUTHANASIA AND SUSTAINING LIFE, *article on* ETHICAL ISSUES; INFANTS, *articles on* MEDICAL ASPECTS AND ISSUES IN THE CARE OF INFANTS, *and* PUBLIC-POLICY AND LEGAL ISSUES; LIFE, QUALITY OF; RESEARCH ETHICS COMMITTEES; *and* RESEARCH METHODOLOGY. *For a discussion of related issues, see the entries* ARTIFICIAL HEARTS AND CARDIAC-ASSIST DEVICES; DEATH, DEFINITION AND DETERMINATION OF, *article on* CRITERIA FOR DEATH; HEALTH-CARE FINANCING; HEALTH-CARE RESOURCES, ALLOCATION OF; *and* INFORMED CONSENT, *articles on* CLINICAL ASPECTS OF CONSENT IN HEALTH CARE, *and* LEGAL AND ETHICAL ISSUES OF CONSENT IN HEALTH CARE (*with its* POSTSCRIPT). *Other relevant material may be found under the entries* HARM; IATROGENIC ILLNESS AND INJURY; PAIN AND SUFFERING; *and* RISK.

Bibliography

"Advance Directives." 1992. *Lancet* 340:1321–1322.
ANGELL, MARCIA. 1991. "The Case of Helga Wanglie: A New Kind of 'Right to Die' Case." *New England Journal of Medicine* 325, no. 7:511–512.
ANONYMOUS. 1992. "Advance Directives." *Lancet* 340: 1321–1322.
BRYAN-BROWN, CHRISTOPHER W. 1992. "Pathway to the Present: A Personal View of Critical Care." In *Critical Care*, 2d ed., pp. 5–12. Edited by Joseph M. Civetta, Robert W. Taylor, and Robert R. Kirby. Philadelphia: J. B. Lippincott.
CAPLAN, ARTHUR L.; BLANK, ROBERT H.; and MERRICK, JANNA C., eds. 1992. *Compelled Compassion: Government Intervention in the Treatment of Critically Ill Newborns*. Totowa, N.J.: Humana Press.
DWORETZ, APRIL R.; MOYA, FERNANDO R.; SABO, BARBARA; GLADSTONE, IGOR; and GROSS, IAN. 1989. "Survival of Infants with Persistent Pulmonary Hypertension Without Extracorporeal Membrane Oxygenation." *Pediatrics* 84, no.1:1-6.
GOLDMAN, JERRY, and KATZ, MARTIN D. 1982. "Inconsistency and Institutional Review Boards." *Journal of the American Medical Association* 248, no. 2:197–202.
HACK, MAUREEN, and FANAROFF, AVROY A. 1989. "Outcomes of Extremely-Low-Birth-Weight Infants Between 1982 and 1988." *New England Journal of Medicine* 321, no. 24:1642–1647.
HILBERMAN, MARK. 1975. "The Evolution of Intensive Care Units." *Critical Care Medicine* 3, no. 4:159–165.

JENNETT, BRYAN. 1992. "Letting Vegetative Patients Die." *British Medical Journal* 305:1305–1306.

KNAUS, WILLIAM A.; DRAPER, ELIZABETH A.; WAGNER, DOUGLAS P.; and ZIMMERMAN, JACK E. 1985. "Prognosis in Acute Organ-System Failure." *Annals of Surgery* 302, no.6:685–693.

MILES, STEVEN H. 1991. "Informed Demand for 'Non-Beneficial' Medical Treatment." *New England Journal of Medicine* 325, no.7:512–515.

O'ROURKE, P. PEARL; CRONE, ROBERT K.; VACANTI, JOSEPH P.; WARE, JAMES H.; LILLEHEI, CRAIG W.; PARAD, RICHARD B.; and EPSTEIN, MICHAEL F. 1989. "Extracorporeal Membrane Oxygenation and Conventional Medical Therapy in Neonates with Persistent Pulmonary Hypertension of the Newborn: A Prospective Randomized Study." *Pediatrics* 84, no. 6:957–963.

PARIS, JOHN J.; CRONE, ROBERT K.; and REARDON, FRANK. 1990. "Physicians' Refusal of Requested Treatment: The Case of Baby L." *New England Journal of Medicine* 322, no.14:1012–1015.

PILLAR, BARBARA, and PERRY, SEYMOUR. 1990. "Evaluating Total Parenteral Nutrition: Final Report and Core Statement of the Technology Assessment and Practice Guidelines Forum." Washington, D.C.: Program of Technology and Health Care, Department of Community and Family Medicine, Georgetown University School of Medicine. Mimeo.

POCOCK, STUART J. 1992. "When to Stop a Clinical Trial." *British Medical Journal* 305:235–240.

RAFFIN, THOMAS A.; SHURKIN, JOEL N.; and SINKLER, WHARTON. 1989. *Intensive Care: Facing the Critical Choices.* New York: W. H. Freeman.

ROYAL COLLEGE OF PHYSICIANS. 1990. "Guidelines on the Practice of Ethics Committees in Medical Research." London: Royal College of Physicians. Mimeo.

SCHNEIDERMAN, LAWRENCE J.; PEARLMAN, ROBERT A.; KAPLAN, ROBERT M.; ANDERSON, JOHN P.; and ROSENBERG, ESTHER M. 1992. "Relationship of General Advance Directive Instructions to Specific Life-Sustaining Treatment Preferences in Patients with Serious Illness." *Archives of Internal Medicine* 152, no. 10:2114–2122.

SNIDER, GORDON L. 1989. "Historical Perspective on Mechanical Ventilation: From Simple Life Support System to Ethical Dilemma." *American Review of Respiratory Disease* 140, no. 2, pt. 2:S2–S7.

STEINBROOK, ROBERT; LO, BERNARD; MOULTON, JEFFREY; SAIKA, GLENN; HOLLANDER, HARRY; and VOLBERDING, PAUL A. 1986. "Preferences of Homosexual Men with AIDS for Life-Sustaining Treatment." *New England Journal of Medicine* 314, no. 17:457–460.

WACHTER, ROBERT M.; RUSSI, MARK B.; BLOCH, DANIEL A.; HOPEWELL, PHILIP C.; and LUCE, JOHN M. 1991. "Pneumocystis carinii Pneumonia and Respiratory Failure in AIDS." *American Review of Respiratory Disease* 143, no. 2:251–256.

WEIR, ROBERT F., and GOSTIN, LARRY. 1990. "Decisions to Abate Life-Sustaining Treatment for Nonautonomous Patients: Ethical Standards and Legal Liability for Patients after Cruzan." *Journal of the American Medical Association* 284, no. 14:1846–1853.

YOUNG, ERNLE W. D., and STEVENSON, DAVID K. 1990. "Limiting Treatment for Extremely Premature, Low-Birth-Weight Infants (500 to 750 g)." *American Journal of Diseases of Children* 144, no. 5:549–552.

ART OF MEDICINE

See MEDICINE, ART OF.

ASIA

See MEDICAL ETHICS, HISTORY OF, *section on* SOUTH AND EAST ASIA.

ASSISTED SUICIDE

See DEATH AND DYING: EUTHANASIA AND SUSTAINING LIFE; *and* SUICIDE.

AUSTRALIA

See MEDICAL ETHICS, HISTORY OF, *section on* AUSTRALIA AND NEW ZEALAND.

AUSTRIA

See MEDICAL ETHICS, HISTORY OF, *section on* EUROPE, *subsection on the* CONTEMPORARY PERIOD, *article on* GERMAN-SPEAKING COUNTRIES AND SWITZERLAND.

AUTHORITY

The primary purpose of this entry is to trace the relationship between authority and morality. The task is complicated by two factors. First, the concept of authority is used in many different ways; those usages have evolved over time, and they differ in their relevance to morality. Second, in the twentieth century, authority, especially in its political context, has come to be associated with its cognate "authoritarian," and thus linked to the cruelties inflicted by despotic, totalitarian regimes.

For some people, indeed, authority might appear to stand in contrast to morality. Two possible answers to the question, "Why should I do this?" are first, that it is the right thing to do (ethics) and second, that someone in authority commands it. There is a problem with this disjunction, however. It conflates authority with power.

Authority and power

The Romans, whose concept *auctoritas* is the predecessor of the English word, distinguished authority from power, or *potestas*. One scholar describes the *auctoritas* of the Republic's Senate as "more than a counsel and less than a command; rather a counsel with which one could not properly avoid compliance" (Mommsen, 1874). Compliance to *auctoritas* should come, not because of any threat of force but for other factors deemed important; for the Romans, such factors included honor, influence, old age, family lineage, moral character, and wisdom.

Power, in one of its core meanings, is the ability to direct another's action by implied or express threat of force. Authority has no necessary linkage to coercion and force. Though authority may have force at its disposal, the reliance on coercion substitutes power for authority. Bertrand de Jouvenal wrote: "Authority is the faculty of inducing assent. To follow an authority is a voluntary act. Authority ends where voluntary assent ends. There is in every state a margin of obedience which is won only by the use of force or the threat of force: it is this margin which breaches liberty and demonstrates the failure of authority" (Jouvenal, 1957, p. 33). The conflation of authority with power is eminently understandable: It has long been advantageous to those in power to claim that they also possess authority, or indeed exercise their coercive power in the name of authority, at least since the transformation of the Roman Republic into the Roman Empire (Krieger, 1973). R. S. Peters contrasts authority with power: "The concept of authority is necessary to bring out the ways in which behavior is regulated *without* recourse to power" (Peters, 1958, p. 220). Another way of seeing the difference between power and authority is to note that if one were to disobey power, one's concern would be to avoid getting caught. If one did not follow the counsels of authority, one would feel that he or she had erred in some way.

Authority and morality

Rescuing the concept of authority from its near—and morally suspect—relative power, does not tell much about its relation to morality. As the attributes the Romans associated with *auctoritas* clearly show, there are aspects of authority that have no direct connection with morality, such as influence and family lineage. Today as well there are quite common and sensible uses of the concept of authority with little relation to morality. A person wishing to learn to speak a language would be wise to enlist the aid of an authority on that language. This example illustrates several points about authority. First, authority may rest on some personal attribute such as expertise. Second, it need not be narrowly held, as

any skilled speaker of a particular language is, in a genuine sense, an authority on it. Third, authority is a relational concept: One entity is an authority with respect to another. It is relative in another sense as well. The skilled native speaker of Italian, who is an authority on that language, must give way where appropriate to another, higher authority, for example a grammarian of the same language. Fourth, authority is context-specific. The student of Italian might serve as an authority on basketball, for example, for the same person who serves as an authority on Italian for him or her. Fifth, under some circumstances, refusal to comply with an authority—to insist on using, for example, incorrect vocabulary, grammar, and pronunciation in attempting to speak Italian—may identify a person as stubborn, stupid, or foolish, but not necessarily as immoral.

We do speak of "moral authority," but the ability to persuade someone to accept a particular moral belief or perform a particular morally relevant act is not synonymous with possessing personal moral authority. It is quite possible for people who have never seemed to possess moral wisdom or moral authority to convince us, by force of argument, to accept certain beliefs or to perform specific acts. Their arguments carry a kind of authority that the persons themselves do not (although if they continued to show a facility in making persuasive moral arguments—and exemplifying them in their own lives—in time we might describe them as moral authorities).

Authority, then, is related to but distinct from both power and morality. Peters describes authority's place as lying between the other two. Authority, he writes, "is a manner of regulating human behavior which is an intermediary between moral argument and the use of force, incentives and propaganda" (Peters, 1958, p. 218). The relationship of the three concepts may be even closer than implied by the quote from Peters: Authority resorts to power, if at all, when its appeal to morality fails. The appeal to morality may fail because a party cannot understand or fails to accept that the authority is justified in what is asked in a particular instance. We speak of legitimate authority in such cases. Or, the appeal to morality may fail because the authority is not justified in asking for this particular act, or in asking this particular party, or because it has no jurisdiction over such actions or persons, or because it lacks legitimacy in general. We describe such cases as the illegitimate exercise of authority, or as illegitimate authority.

There are, it appears, two important but distinct issues in the relation of morality and authority. There are questions about authority in morality, about what authorizes or warrants moral belief. And there are questions about the morality of authority, about what makes authorities and their requests legitimate or illegitimate, about when authorities ought to be obeyed, defied, or overthrown, and, more broadly, about the relation between morality and an authority's requests for compliance.

These two issues appear to be rooted in two alternative conceptions of authority, both of which appeared as early as Roman times. *Auctus* means an increasing or augmentation. It reflects the weight authority adds to the considerations for accepting a belief or engaging in an act. Whatever reasons we have for accepting or rejecting a proposition or an action, the fact that an authority on such issues supports such a belief or action adds to, or augments, the case for accepting it. Authority in this sense is relevant to moral deliberation and choice of beliefs and actions.

Auctor means one who enlarges, confirms, or gives to a thing its complete form. It also identifies one who has originated a thing—who is, in the modern sense, its author. This sense of authority has been attractive to political theorists. For example, in 1651 Thomas Hobbes explained the authority of the sovereign as a case where each man as the author of his own acts commissions a representative to act on his behalf and, thus, authorizes the sovereign to "use the strength and means of them all" (Hobbes, 1958, p. 143). The moral appeal of such notions of political authority is based probably on the centrality of consent in the stories constructed by the theorist about the origins or basis of the political community.

These two meanings of authority—to augment as to enhance, and to "author-ize" as to consent—may be useful in understanding the role the concept plays in, respectively, understanding authority in morality, and the morality of authority.

Varieties of authority

Max Weber's sociological analysis of authority has been very influential. Weber distinguished three types of authority: charismatic, traditional, and legal-rational. Charismatic authority rested on "devotion to the specific and exceptional sanctity, heroism, or exemplary character of an individual person, and of the normative patterns or order revealed or ordained by him" (Weber, 1947, p. 300). Traditional authority for Weber rested "on an established belief in the sanctity of immemorial traditions and the legitimacy of the status of those exercising authority under them" (Weber, 1947, p. 300). Legal-rational authority's legitimacy was based on "a belief in the 'legality' of patterns of normative rules and the right of those elevated to authority under such rules to issue commands" (Weber, 1947, pp. 300–301).

Weber distinguished sharply between power and authority, seeing the former as the ability to impose one's will on others, and the latter as the ability to secure their obedience. He believed that the legal-rational type of authority was displacing the other types, which he regarded as socially more primitive, their activity in modern societies a survival of past, outmoded forms.

Peters offers a different categorization of authority, into de jure and de facto types. Peters argues that a person can be in authority, and yet in another perfectly plausible sense, lack authority (Peters, 1958). The building inspector who determines that a building does not meet the city's fire safety code may have the de jure authority to insist that the unsafe building be closed immediately. If the building at that moment is occupied by a thousand young people who are screaming and dancing to the music of a popular heavy metal rock band, he may well lack the de facto authority to accomplish his goal.

De facto authority rests on effectiveness, not on any moral justification either in terms of the rightness of the particular request made by the putative authority or of a position held within a legitimate normative hierarchy. De jure authority rests on a claim of legitimacy in which social position is an important but not sufficient criterion. Timo Airaksinen argues that what he calls normative de jure authority, in its full sense, "requires that the superior agent has consensual support and that his status rests on some good normative reasons for his claim to power and to be respected and obeyed" (Airaksinen, 1988, p. 131). Weber's charismatic authority requires de facto authority, or it would be no authority at all. The notion of a de jure charismatic authority per se seems unintelligible, although a person might use his or her charismatic authority in order to gain positions of de jure authority. Traditional and legal-rational authority are both forms of de jure authority, although they differ in what entitles individuals to hold the social positions that confer de jure authority.

As descriptive categories, Weber's triad of charismatic, traditional, and legal-rational authority, and the additional de jure and de facto types, provide some useful distinctions. Although the focus might be on political authority—on the morality of authority, there are also implications for moral authority—authority in morality. We have the charismatic, de facto authority of the prophet whose message may not be welcomed by his listeners, but that carries a moral force they cannot ignore (Walzer, 1987). The prophet's authority may be both political and moral. It is interesting that even someone as mistrustful of authority as John Stuart Mill should find some need for prophets of a sort.

Authority and liberty

In his essay *On Liberty* (1975), Mill identified authority, along with power and coercion, as the enemies of liberty. Mill found no room for the notions of authority as counsel that one somehow could not reject, or as a defensible intermediary between persuasion and compulsion. Modern history was a "struggle between Liberty and Authority" and liberty deserved to be the victor. Mill had a problem, though. The majority was capable not only of political tyranny, against which one could build certain protections, but also of intellectual tyranny. That is, by its suspicion of originality in thought, the majority might prevent progress: "No government by a democracy or a numerous aristocracy . . . ever did or could rise above mediocrity, except insofar as the sovereign Many have let themselves be guided . . . by the counsels and influence of a more highly gifted and instructed One or Few" (Mill, 1975, pp. 62–63). This "One or Few" would have to be, it appears, just the kind of uncoercive authority Mill seemed to find no place for earlier.

Modern political theorists must confront the apparent antinomy between authority and freedom, as those are principal terms of the debate left by the tradition of liberal and antiliberal social thought. Some twentieth-century thinkers have tried to simplify matters. As Leonard Krieger describes it: "Where nineteenth-century political thinkers had defended the superiority of authority or liberty respectively but admitted the autonomy and subordinate validity of the opposite principle, their twentieth-century sociopolitical successors asserted the exclusive validity of authority or liberty respectively, and categorically worked out the entire absorption or denial of the opposite principle" (Krieger, 1973, p. 158). Fascists and other totalitarians exalted authority; anarchists and other radical antitotalitarians exalted liberty.

Morality of authority

Questions about the morality of authority are generally of two kinds: questions about the morality of obeying or tolerating the particular commands of an authority; and questions about the general moral legitimacy of a particular authority. Under the former come such questions as civil disobedience; under the latter arise questions of political theory, especially theories of just action by a state. The two types of questions affect one another. A state or other authority that lacks legitimacy would also seem to lack the moral authority to command obedience. It may have the power to command, but it cannot legitimately claim the authority to do so. An otherwise legitimate authority that persistently requested or commanded its members to perform immoral acts would, by that reason alone, undermine its own legitimacy.

Some theorists have endeavored to rescue authority by examining its place in collective action. Yves Simon considered whether authority should be seen exclusively as a response to deficiency, such that the need for authority disappears when defects in virtue, judgment, and organization are overcome. He argues that authority is needed, even in communities characterized by excellence. The good for a community may be pursued in

many ways, and choices must be made. Simon concludes, "An ideally enlightened and virtuous community needs authority to unify its action" (Simon, 1962, p. 50). Robert Nisbet describes periods he calls "twilight" ages, in which institutions decline, values decay, and military or paramilitary power occupies the vacuum left by the loss of social and moral authority. He argues that "the greatest need in our age is that of somehow redressing the balance between political-military power on the one hand and the structure of authority that lies in human groups such as neighborhood, family, labor union, profession, and voluntary association" (Nisbet, 1975, p. 276). Authority, in his view, belongs to the smaller-scale institutions, within the nation-state, that provide the bulwark against raw power.

Authority in morality

We can put the question about authority in morality several ways: What gives authority to moral propositions—statements of moral belief or judgment? What sorts of considerations are authoritative in morality? What warrants particular moral beliefs or judgments, and what justifies particular actions?

One set of answers given in the twentieth century would deny any authority to moral judgments. Metaethical theories that see moral statements as equivalent to commands or to grunts of approval or disapproval appear to deny any authority to morality that would be worth having. An answer more broadly accepted among scholars in ethics is that the authority of any particular moral proposition depends on the solidity of its foundation and the logical validity with which the particular proposition is derived from its foundational premises. This view—that ethics gains its authority from indubitable premises and errorless reason—has characterized ethics since René Descartes. As a view of authority in morality, it was created in response to a crisis in authority.

To a medieval thinker such as Thomas Aquinas, knowledge belonged to one or the other Aristotelian category, *scientia* or *opinio*. *Scientia* was the province of knowledge that could be demonstrated—the product, that is, of the sort of deductive reasoning characteristic of geometry. *Opinio* included all knowledge that could not be demonstrated in a comparable way. To establish the plausibility of some statement that was *opinio* rather than *scientia*, a medieval thinker would examine the views of learned and distinguished authorities. Jeffrey Stout argues that the realm of *scientia* had been severely narrowed by contemporary skeptics and the rediscovery of the work of ancient skeptics, placing an increasingly heavy burden on *opinio*. *Opinio* in turn was undermined by what he calls the "problem of many authorities" (Stout, 1981, p. 41). When authorities disagreed among themselves, what should one believe?

An answer provided by the Reformation, in the early sixteenth century, was divine authority as revealed through Scripture. Scripture, however, is silent on some issues, ambiguous on others, and requires in all instances interpretation. Because human authorities such as the Church were to be bypassed as all too fallible, the Reformation placed its confidence in each individual's capacity to interpret scripture for himself or herself—the inner light present in all believers. This strategy may have been successful in depriving existing institutions of their claims to legitimate authority in matters of faith and morals, but it reproduced the problem of many authorities, enlarged by several orders of magnitude. Now there was not merely a small group of quarreling authorities, but "ten authorities in every pew" (Stout, 1981, p. 44).

Descartes was exposed to these failures, and to the concurrent political strife and war that they engendered. It seems reasonable to suppose that his interest in discovering indubitable, firm foundations for belief was in part a response to the chaos and violence around him (Toulmin, 1990). He had good reason at that time to doubt the usefulness of *opinio* for resolving disagreements; his strategy then was to try to show that *scientia* would yield the sort of undeniable proof the world so desperately needed. By insisting on absolute certainty before he would accept anything as true, Descartes yielded a great deal of ground to the skeptics, who argued that any knowledge short of absolute certainty was essentially worthless.

The Cartesian program, with its quest for knowledge that is completely certain, and its devaluation of merely probable truths, set the terms for discussion of authority in ethics until the present day. If the only moral propositions having any authority are those derived as necessary conclusions from indisputable premises, then we are in desperate straits indeed. If those are the minimal hallmarks of moral knowledge, it is doubtful that there is any statement we might make that would both fulfill these requirements and be generally convincing, given the unending dispute over what the foundations of ethics might be, if they can be found at all. The rebirth of practical reasoning or practical ethics is forcing a reconsideration of the debate about the place of foundations in morality, the usefulness of a deductive approach to ethics for reasoning about practical moral problems, and the nature of probable moral knowledge.

Moral authority in practical reasoning

There are many good reasons not to wax nostalgic for a return to the days of Aquinas, the learned doctors, and the medieval notion of probable opinion. Nonetheless, there is also good reason to believe that Descartes and his heirs have framed the problem in a manner that gives away too much to skeptics. Workers in bioethics and other realms of practical ethics do not have the luxury of waiting until the foundations of ethics are firmly and finally established before they offer moral analyses and judgments. Nor can they treat practical moral problems as only interesting tests for one or another foundational theory. They are often called on to make judgments and to give reasons for those judgments. What if anything gives authority to moral judgment in the absence of universally accepted foundations?

The issue of authority in morality is crucial for all practical moral reasoning. The debate on it has been greatly enlivened by bioethics, which has underscored both the inadequacy of the foundationalist-skeptic framing of the problem, and its enormous practical consequences. One approach is to recover the middle ground of moral knowledge, looking for the sorts of considerations that make a moral judgment more or less reasonable—that, in one of the original senses of authority, augment or add to our reasons for accepting a proposition. It may well be that the "learned doctors" of today, like their medieval counterparts, should carry some authority. But our concepts of evidence and of probability have changed so dramatically that an "authority" per se carries little weight other than her or his ability to provide cogent analyses of problems in terms of the kinds of circumstances and arguments that can persuade disputing parties.

If we accept that even in the absence of foundations, there are better and worse moral judgments, more and less sound and defensible morally relevant actions, then the search for what provides authority for moral beliefs, judgments, and actions is both sensible and necessary. Of concern to bioethics, authority is exercized regularly by those with expertise and power.

Authority in health care

Howard Brody's work *The Healer's Power* (1992), despite its title, offers distinctions useful for understanding authority in contemporary health care. Brody distinguishes among three types of power physicians may have by virtue of their role. Though his focus is on the power held by physicians, his analysis can readily be extended to encompass other health professionals, and to extend to authority as well as power. Indeed, Brody takes authority to be socially legitimated power, and uses the words interchangeably.

Brody describes three types of power or authority wielded by physicians. Aesculapian power resides in the healer's specialized and often obscure knowledge and skills. It is a craft or art, realized in its practical applications. Aesculapian power is impersonal, may be transferred to other healers, and does not depend upon social class or status. Charismatic power, as in Weber, is rooted in the healer's personality. As such it cannot be transferred or institutionalized. Social power derives from the status and roles entrusted to healers. For example, physicians are delegated the authority to determine who may enter the social classifications "sick" and "well," "disabled" and "able-bodied." Such classifications can have profound social consequences, determining whether a person must work or may remain home, as well as whether or not one is eligible for certain social benefits contingent upon illness or disability (Brody, 1992).

It is possible to see the early history of bioethics as an effort to strip physicians of some of the enormous power they wielded over patients. The struggles over truth-telling, informed consent, the nature of physicians' expertise, and patient autonomy attempted to transfer control from physician to patient. Autonomy became the rallying cry against the evil of physician paternalism, which can be taken as a synonym in this instance for illegitimate authority. The revolt against illegitimate uses of authority by physicians brought many benefits. But that same revolt may have directed attention away from authentic and legitimate uses of authority by healers. The tendency to oversimplify, indeed to demonize, authority may have blinded us to its nuances and to the very real significance of authority—and power—in health care.

Authority, properly understood, is a supple and subtle concept, well suited not only for understanding the complexities of relationships between physicians and patients, but also for illuminating relationships and tensions among health professionals, including physicians as well as nurses, physician assistants, and others engaged in healing. Distinguishing among the kinds of authority, understanding the sources of authority, and elaborating the circumstances that make authority legitimate or illegitimate may enhance our comprehension of many pressing problems, from the physician–patient relationship to the proper locus for decisional authority within large health-care systems. The concept of authority in health care deserves a thorough rehabilitation.

THOMAS H. MURRAY

Directly related to this entry are the entries FREEDOM AND COERCION; BEHAVIOR CONTROL; RESPONSIBILITY; TRUST; *and* PROFESSIONAL–PATIENT RELATIONSHIP, *articles on* SOCIOLOGICAL PERSPECTIVES, *and* ETHICAL ISSUES. *For a discussion of related ideas, see the entries* AUTONOMY; BENEFICENCE; CARE; *and* COMPETENCY. *Other relevant material may be found under the entry* CIVIL DISOBEDIENCE AND HEALTH CARE.

Bibliography

AIRAKSINEN, TIMO. 1988. *Ethics of Coercion and Authority: A Philosophical Study of Social Life.* Pittsburgh, Pa.: University of Pittsburgh Press.

BRODY, HOWARD. 1992. *The Healer's Power.* New Haven, Conn.: Yale University Press.

HOBBES, THOMAS. 1958. [1651]. *Leviathan.* New York: Bobbs-Merrill.

JOUVENAL, BERTRAND DE. 1957. [1955]. *Sovereignty: An Inquiry into the Political Good.* Translated by J. F. Huntington. Chicago: University of Chicago Press.

KRIEGER, LEONARD. 1973. "Authority." In vol. 1 of *Dictionary of the History of Ideas: Selected Pivotal Ideas,* pp. 141–162. Edited by Philip P. Wiener. New York: Scribner.

MILL, JOHN STUART. 1975. [1859]. *On Liberty.* Edited by David Spitz. New York: W. W. Norton.

MOMMSEN, THEODOR. 1874. *Römisches Staatsrecht.* Leipzig: Hirzel.

NISBET, ROBERT A. 1975. *Twilight of Authority.* New York: Oxford University Press.

PETERS, R. S. 1958. "Authority." *Proceedings of the Aristotelian Society* 32:207–224.

SIMON, YVES. 1962. *A General Theory of Authority.* Notre Dame, Ind.: University of Notre Dame Press.

STOUT, JEFFREY. 1981. *The Flight from Authority: Religion, Morality, and the Quest for Autonomy.* Notre Dame, Ind.: University of Notre Dame Press.

TOULMIN, STEPHEN E. 1990. *Cosmopolis: The Hidden Agenda of Modernity.* New York: Free Press.

WALZER, MICHAEL. 1987. *Interpretation and Social Criticism.* Cambridge, Mass.: Harvard University Press.

WEBER, MAX. 1947. [1925]. *Theory of Social and Economic Organization.* Translated from the German by Alexander M. Henderson and Talcott Parsons. Edited by Talcott Parsons. New York: Oxford University Press.

AUTOEXPERIMENTATION

Autoexperimentation, which refers to the practice of intentionally utilizing oneself as an experimental subject, is not a rare event. Over the past four centuries, more than 135 examples have been documented, and the true incidence is undoubtedly much higher (Altman, 1972; Franklin and Sutherland, 1984). Although the preponderance of recorded autoexperimentation has been conducted in the name of biomedical research, investigators in the physical and social sciences have also engaged in this practice. Their exploits, on the whole, though less well known, are no less significant.

Autoexperimentation has long enjoyed a measure of romantic appeal in the scientific and popular tradition. "The experimenter," wrote Sir George Pickering, "has one golden rule to guide him as to whether the experiment is justifiable. Is he prepared to submit himself to the procedure? If he is, and if the experiment is actually carried out on himself, then it is probably justifiable. If he is not, then the experiment should not be done" (Pickering, 1949, p. 229). Beecher suggested that any scientist wishing to engage in human experimentation ought to experiment on himself "as evidence of good faith" (Beecher, 1959).

Despite a reputation for nobility of purpose, the practice of autoexperimentation has become the focus of substantial scientific and ethical debate. The scientific controversy concerns the methodological limitations of autoexperimentation and its capacity to yield useful data. The ethical debate is more complicated. Superficially, it concerns the extent to which autoexperimentation ought to be regulated. At its heart, however, lies a fundamental conflict between two opposing views of scientific research. The libertarian view considers the attainment of scientific knowledge a superior good. On this basis, it advocates a relatively laissez-faire policy toward all forms of scientific inquiry, including autoexperimentation. The paternalistic view, in contrast, emphasizes the importance of protecting experimental subjects from risk, whether self-imposed or imposed by others. It does not distinguish autoexperimentation from other studies involving human beings. As a result, it demands strict regulation of autoexperimentation and scrupulously consistent standards for the conduct of human experimentation.

May autoexperimentation be treated any differently from other forms of human experimentation? Must it be subject to the same regulation? May it be construed simply as an expression of personal autonomy on the part of the scientist? Is autoexperimentation ethically privileged in any way?

Neither the methodological nor the ethical aspects of this debate can be fully understood without examining the historical and cultural context in which autoexperimentation developed.

Historical perspectives

Why do scientists turn to autoexperimentation? What forces figured in the emergence of autoexperimentation as a respected tradition?

One important factor, upon which many investigators have remarked, is the existence of an extremely powerful and deeply rooted obligation to pursue scientific knowledge regardless of personal risk. A good example is John Hunter's unfortunate experiment with venereal disease. Throughout the eighteenth century, physicians debated whether gonorrhea and syphilis were two separate entities or different manifestations of the same disease. Hunter, a prominent surgeon, anatomist, and fellow of the Royal Society, believed they were the same. In 1770, to prove the point, he inoculated his own penis with the fresh urethral discharge of a man with gonorrhea. When syphilitic chancres developed at the site of inoculation, Hunter erroneously concluded that his theory was correct. Even though he thought he had contracted gonorrhea, Hunter eventually died of syphilis (Hunter, 1837; Franklin and Sutherland, 1984). It is clear, in retrospect, that the discharge most probably transmitted both diseases.

Closely related is the idea that the true scientist must always be prepared to engage in resolute acts of personal daring (including, though not necessarily limited to, autoexperimentation) to overcome impediments to research. There are two famous cases in point. In 1929, despite the direct prohibition of his department chief, Werner Forssmann surreptitiously passed an intravenous catheter into his own heart to prove the feasibility of cardiac catheterization in humans. He later shared the Nobel Prize for these experiments (Altman 1972). The second case pertains to the thymidine experiments of Beppino Giovanella during the late 1970s. Thymidine had been shown to be a promising cancer drug in animals, but the U.S. Food and Drug administration (FDA) refused to authorize clinical trials on the grounds that its safety had not been established. Giovanella proceeded to ingest huge doses of thymidine, thereby proving its safety and overcoming the objections of the FDA (Franklin and Sutherland, 1984).

A third factor has to do with the problem of justifying human experimentation before the safety of an experiment has been established. Experimenting on oneself or one's colleagues signals the conviction that the experiment is at least worthwhile, if not necessarily safe (see Beecher, 1959; Pickering, 1949; Leake, 1967; Bok, 1978). In addition, autoexperimentation offers a mechanism to ensure the willing participation of motivated subjects and, simultaneously, a concession to Article 5 of the Nuremberg Code, which prohibits perilous research in man "except, perhaps, in those experiments where the experimental physicians also serve as subjects" (Germany [Territory Under Allied Occupation], 1949).

A fourth factor derives from the observation that autoexperimentation is usually the best, and sometimes the only, way to ensure absolute adherence to an exacting research protocol. In 1962, for example, Victor Herbert undertook an investigation to explore a possible link between nutritional folic acid deficiency and megaloblastic anemia. To deplete the body of folic acid reserves, he subsisted for eighteen weeks upon an extraordinarily insipid and unpalatable diet (Altman, 1972). Herbert commented that the experiment would probably have failed had he not experimented upon himself (Herbert, 1962).

Finally, autoexperimentation has often been fostered when it appeared that certain researchers, by virtue of special training and experience, might extract significantly more from an experiment by participating than by observing. The histories of military and of aviation medicine are replete with examples of this sort. Data obtained uniquely through autoexperimentation proved critical, for example, in the development of protective clothing for ultrahigh-altitude airplane ejection, in studies of extreme acceleration and deceleration, in investigations of decompression sickness, and in studies of human physiology in space (Gibson and Harrison, 1984; Dille, 1984; Franklin and Sutherland, 1984).

From a historical perspective, the pursuit of autoexperimentation cannot be separated from the pursuit of certain ideals, including the attainment of knowledge, the realization of moral improvement, and the achievement of personal and professional virtue. It must be noted, however, that the exact nature of these ideals has changed over time and place (Leake, 1967; Schaumburg and Byck, 1968; Jonas, 1977; Dagi and Dagi, 1988).

Criticisms of autoexperimentation

Methodological issues. The worth of an experiment depends upon its scientific merit, upon its permissibility from ethical and legal perspectives, and upon its advisability on other grounds. Before any experiment is carried out, each of these elements must be assessed. Autoexperimentation suffers from three major methodological problems. First, there is an inherent difficulty in observing oneself dispassionately. This difficulty often leads to the confusion of objective and subjective data. Second, it is virtually impossible to establish adequate controls, particularly because autoexperiments tend to involve serial observations of one individual. Third, it is very difficult to extract statistically valid information because of the typically very small numbers of subjects and experiments. As a general rule, the likelihood that useful data will result from experiments on very small groups is determined by the likelihood that the data would not be materially affected by iterations (repetitions of the experiment) on larger groups.

Because of these weaknesses, autoexperimentation rarely proves to be a wholly satisfactory experimental method. There may be two important exceptions, however: pilot studies to establish the feasibility of a procedure or the safety of a pharmacological agent in normal subjects; and studies in which the scientist consents to be treated as an ordinary research subject and to remain under the supervision of other investigators for the duration of the experiment. It is worth noting that the second exception complies with the provisions of the Declaration of Helsinki stipulating that "the responsibility for the human subject must always rest with a medically qualified person and never rest on the subject of the research" (World Medical Association, 1989, I. Basic Principles, §3).

Ethical issues. The principle that scientists ought to be willing to participate as subjects in their own experiments does not always outweigh the problems that

arise when they do. The fundamental issue is whether any of the precautions required to protect the subject in other forms of human experimentation may be legitimately suspended in the case of voluntary autoexperimentation.

The four basic arguments that have been brought to bear on this question are not easily reconciled: (1) Individuals are entitled to assume voluntarily risks they may never impose on others; (2) under proper circumstances, both self-sacrifice (martyrdom) or assumption of high risk for good reason (heroism) are universally lauded; (3) societies have a vested interest in protecting the welfare of their members; (4) some degree of regulation in recognition of this interest is required or, at the very least, ought to be permissible.

Part of what makes these arguments so hard to reconcile is the fact that they echo the broader debate between proponents of absolute experimental freedom and advocates of strict social regulation of scientific inquiry (Bok, 1978). Libertarians argue that the principle of autonomy grants scientists the right to engage voluntarily in risky behavior. On this basis, they refute the applicability of regulations for the protection of human subjects in autoexperimentation. Champions of a more paternalistic approach, in contrast, oppose unlimited risk taking in any experimental context because of the following concerns: (1) Many risks have been undertaken for unimportant goals; (2) habitual risk takers might turn to self-experimentation even when other, more desirable forms of investigation exist; (3) investigator-subjects may be at greater risk than other potential subjects because curiosity, enthusiasm, and other intangible factors may induce them to ignore risks that would otherwise deter a prudent individual from participation (Bok, 1978); (4) certain levels of risk are, or ought to be, beyond consent (Bok, 1978; Patullo, 1982); (5) investigators reckless with respect to their own safety are wont to become reckless in other aspects of their investigations; (6) the autonomy of investigator-subjects might be tainted by various levels of institutional or peer coercion, or even by self-imposed psychological pressures (Dagi and Dagi, 1988); and (7) large-scale, unregulated self-experimentation might subvert accepted guidelines for the protection of human subjects under other experimental conditions. The apparent contradiction between concerns (3) and (4) and the respect and admiration traditionally accorded to martyrs and heroes in Western society is not easily reconciled.

Existing policies and regulations

While it is generally agreed that institutions are ultimately responsible for the regulation of all forms of experimentation carried out within their jurisdiction, there is no consensus regarding how—or even whether—autoexperimentation should be regulated. The Nuremberg

Code tacitly encourages autoexperimentation through the provisions of Article 5: Perilous human experimentation is prohibited "except, perhaps, in those experiments where the experimental physicians also serve as subjects" (Germany [Territory Under Allied Occupation], 1949). The Declaration of Helsinki seems to exclude autoexperimentation by stipulating that "The responsibility for the human subject must . . . never rest on the subject of the research" (World Medical Association, 1989, *I. Basic Principles*, §3). Massachusetts General Hospital (1981) simply recommends that investigators "not take undue or unusual risk with themselves in self-experimentation, but . . . exercise the same prudence and judgment as they would in studies of others." The National Institutes of Health promulgated a code for self-experimentation "to provide the same safeguards for physician–subjects as for the normal volunteer" (Altman, 1972). The Office for Protection of Research Risks of the Department of Health and Human Services has ruled that autoexperimentation *is* subject to the same regulations as other human research, including review by institutional review boards.

Policy trends and recommendations

There is a clear tendency toward increasing paternalism in policies governing autoexperimentation. This trend reflects a growing hesitation to equate risks undertaken in the course of scientific experimentation with risks assumed by private parties for their individual benefit and amusement. Virtually no serious scientific investigation, including autoexperimentation, is pursued outside an institutional setting. Acts of autoexperimentation may have untoward consequences that far exceed those assumed or foreseen by the experimenter. For these reasons, no act of autoexperimentation, no matter how worthy or well intentioned, should be sanctioned until three conditions are fulfilled: (1) The proposed experiment has been fully described; (2) potential sources of coercion influencing the experimenter have been investigated and excluded; (3) the institutional and social consequences of the experiment have been thoroughly explored, particularly with respect to risks such as the appearance of condoning inconsistent standards for the protection of human subjects. In most cases, fulfillment of these conditions will result in autoexperimentation being held to the same standard of review as any other forms of human investigation. These conditions are expressly designed to protect both the experimenter–subject *and* the institution, in equal measure.

Summary and conclusion

Despite the methodological and ethical concerns raised by critics of autoexperimentation, there have been circumstances in which autoexperimentation has resulted in unique and invaluable contributions, and there is every reason to think that such circumstances will continue to occur. But even if the willingness to subject oneself to experimentation serves as a minimal condition for demonstrating the worth of an experiment, it must by no means be construed as sufficient (see Beecher, 1959; Pickering, 1949; Leake, 1967; Bok, 1978; Dagi and Dagi, 1988). The worth of an experiment depends upon its scientific merit, upon its permissibility from ethical and legal perspectives, and upon its advisability on other grounds. When an experiment is to be carried out within an established institution, each of these elements must be weighed. From an organizational and institutional standpoint, the process of judging these elements is no less important than the ultimate outcome, and arguably more open to criticism. The inherent ambiguity of existing codes allows for a wide range of nuanced interpretations in many circumstances, but matters of procedure are typically held to a higher standard of consistency. The decision-making process, therefore, should involve peer review, and it should accord with established criteria for determining the acceptability of experimental protocols. At the very least, judgments about the permissibility of autoexperimentation must weigh questions of risk, benefit, voluntariness, and scientific significance, as well as the more elusive issues comprehended by the term "institutional interests." While the requirement for institutional review may induce some scientists to experiment on themselves outside the scientific mainstream, this effect is unlikely to prevail and, as a practical matter, is virtually impossible to repress.

TEODORO FORCHT DAGI

For a further discussion of topics mentioned in this entry, see the entries RESEARCH, HUMAN: HISTORICAL ASPECTS; RESEARCH BIAS; RESEARCH ETHICS COMMITTEES; RESEARCH METHODOLOGY; *and* RESEARCH POLICY, *especially the article on* SUBJECT SELECTION. *For a discussion of related ideas, see the entries* AUTONOMY; PATERNALISM; RISK; *and* VALUE AND VALUATION. *See also the* APPENDIX (CODES, OATHS, AND DIRECTIVES RELATED TO BIOETHICS), SECTION IV: ETHICAL DIRECTIVES FOR HUMAN RESEARCH.

Bibliography

ALTMAN, LAWRENCE K. 1972. "Auto-experimentation: An Unappreciated Tradition in Medical Science." *New England Journal of Medicine* 286, no. 7:346–352. Reprinted in *Hippocrates Revisited: A Search for Meaning*, pp. 193–210. Edited by Roger J. Bulger. New York: MEDCOM Press, 1973.
———. 1987. *Who Goes First? The Story of Self-Experimentation in Medicine.* New York: Random House.
BEECHER, HENRY K. 1959. "The Experimentation in Man."

Journal of the American Medical Association 169, no. 5:461–478.

BOK, SISSELA. 1978. "Freedom and Risk." *Daedalus* 107, no. 2:115–127.

DAGI, T. FORCHT, and DAGI, LINDA RABINOWITZ. 1988. "Physicians Experimenting on Themselves: Some Ethical and Philosophical Considerations." In *The Use of Human Beings in Research with Special Reference to Clinical Trials*, pp. 249–260. Edited by Stuart F. Spicker, Ilai Alon, André de Vries, and H. Tristram Engelhardt, Jr. Dordrecht, Netherlands: Kluwer.

DILLE, J. ROBERT. 1984. "Introduction to the First of Two Aerial Voyages of Dr. Jeffires and Mons. Blanchard." *Aviation, Space, and Environmental Medicine* 55, no. 11:993–999.

FORSSMANN, WERNER. 1964. "The Role of Heart Catheterization and Angiocardiography in the Development of Modern Medicine." In *Physiology or Medicine, 1942–1962*, pp. 506–510. Vol. 3 of *Nobel Lectures*. Amsterdam: Elsevier.

FRANKLIN, JON, and SUTHERLAND, JOHN. 1984. *Guinea Pig Doctors: The Drama of Medical Research Through Self-Experimentation.* New York: Morrow.

GERMANY (TERRITORY UNDER ALLIED OCCUPATION, 1945–1955: U.S. ZONE) MILITARY TRIBUNALS. 1947. "Permissible Medical Experiments." In Vol. 2 of *Trials of War Criminals Before the Nuernberg Tribunals Under Control Law No. 10*, pp. 181–183. Washington, D.C.: U.S. Government Printing Office. Reprinted in *Ethics in Medicine: Historical Perspectives and Contemporary Concerns*, pp. 272–273. Edited by Stanley J. Reiser, Arthur J. Dyck, and William J. Curran. Cambridge, Mass.: MIT Press, 1977.

GIBSON, T. MIKE, and HARRISON, MIKE H. 1984. *Into Thin Air: A History of Aviation Medicine in the RAF.* London: Robert Hale.

HERBERT, VICTOR. 1962. "Experimental Nutritional Folate Deficiency in Man." *Transactions of the Association of American Physicians* 75:307–320.

HUNTER, JOHN. 1837. A Treatise on the Venereal Disease. In vol. 2 of *The Works of John Hunter, F.R.S., with Notes.* Edited by James F. Palmer. London: Longman.

IVY, A. C. 1948. "The History and Ethics of the Use of Human Subjects in Medical Experiments." *Science* 108, no. 2792:1–5.

JONAS, HANS. 1977. "Philosophical Reflections on Experimenting with Human Subjects." In *Ethics in Medicine: Historical Perspectives and Contemporary Concerns*, pp. 304–315. Edited by Stanley J. Reiser, Arthur J. Dyck, and William J. Curran. Cambridge, Mass.: MIT Press.

LEAKE, CHAUNCEY D. 1967. "'Technical Triumphs and Moral Muddles' and 'Discussion.'" *Annals of Internal Medicine* 67 (Supp. 7):43–56.

MASSACHUSETTS GENERAL HOSPITAL. 1981. "Guiding Principles for Human Studies." Internal publication.

PATULLO, E. L. 1982. "Institutional Review Boards and the Freedom to Take Risks." *New England Journal of Medicine* 307, no. 18:1156–1159.

PICKERING, GEORGE W. 1949. "The Place of Experimental Method in Medicine." *Proceedings of the Royal Society of Medicine* 42, pt. 1:229–234.

SCHAUMBURG, HERBERT H., and BYCK, ROBERT. 1968. "Sin Gib Syn: Accent on Glutamate." *New England Journal of Medicine* 279, no. 2:105.

WORLD MEDICAL ASSOCIATION. 1989. "Declaration of Helsinki." *Law, Medicine, and Health Care* 19, nos. 3–4: 264–265.

AUTONOMY

The concept of autonomy in moral philosophy and bioethics recognizes the human capacity for self-determination, and puts forward a principle that the autonomy of persons ought to be respected. At this level of generality, there is not much with which to take issue; a full account of autonomy must further define self-determination and state how and to what extent autonomy should be respected. Autonomy as a capacity of persons must be distinguished from autonomy as a property of actions and decisions, for a person with the capacity for autonomy may act nonautonomously on particular occasions, for example, a person who is coerced to do something. Autonomy as a fundamental value and a basic right is part of the moral and political theory of liberal individualism. According to this view, autonomous individuals are the ultimate source of value: The basis for an action, social practice, or government policy to be right or good is in the values, preferences, or choices of autonomous individuals. In social philosophy, individual autonomy as a basic value and a fundamental right is in tension with community values, such as caring for others, promoting the good of society, and preserving and enhancing the moral practices of society. In clinical bioethics, the right to autonomy of individual patients is in tension with health-care professionals' obligations to benefit patients. These conflicts will be examined in what follows.

Autonomy as capacity

There are three elements to the psychological capacity of autonomy: agency, independence, and rationality. Agency is awareness of oneself as having desires and intentions and of acting on them. (Desire includes inclinations, aversions, wants, and similar terms.) When people have a desire for some state of affairs, they form an intention to do what they believe will bring about the desired state of affairs; further, they want their desire to determine their action (Benn, 1988; Haworth, 1986).

The capacity for agency distinguishes persons from inanimate objects and from nonhuman animals. Inanimate objects can be affected by objects and conditions external to them, as can persons, but unlike persons, inanimate objects cannot be said to act on desires. Nonhuman animals have desires, but there is no (noncontroversial) reason to believe that they have the capacity for self-consciousness that is manifest in having an awareness of desires and wanting them to be effective in action. Agency does not imply that persons are never influenced by external forces or that persons never act impulsively. It is an account of how persons are able to act and not how they always act.

Independence is the absence of influences that so control what a person does that it cannot be said that he or she wants to do it. This may seem a feature of an autonomous action rather than an element of psychological capacity. However, there are cases in which a person's course of life is under constant threat of violence from others, and the person acts always to avoid harm: war, poverty, abusive relationships, police states. When the whole of a person's beliefs, plans, self-image, and ways of relating to others are the result of unrelenting coercion and manipulation, then that person has little or no capacity for autonomy.

Autonomy also requires that persons have an adequate range of options. Coercion and manipulation limit options, but options are also limited by social and physical environments. If a person's options are numerous and noncoerced but are trivial in relation to what is valued by the person, then there is no capacity for autonomy in a significant sense (Raz, 1986). This would be the case in a totalitarian, caste, or slave society where a combination of coercion and ideology suppress the aspirations and real options of a segment of the members of the society. A full account of the conception of autonomy must distinguish external influences that defeat autonomy from external influences that are consistent with being autonomous. The former includes coercion and manipulation, and the latter includes persuasion and the normal limitations of physical and social environments.

The third element of the capacity for autonomy is "means–end rationality," or "rational decision making." In addition to the self-consciousness of agency, the capacity for rational decision making requires a person: (1) whose beliefs are subject to standards of truth and evidence; (2) with ability to recognize commitments and to act on them; (3) who can construct and evaluate alternative decisions; (4) whose changes in beliefs and values can change decisions and actions; and (5) whose beliefs and values yield rankings of action commitments. Another way to understand rationality as an element of the capacity for autonomy is as the capacity for reflection on desires. A rational person can have a desire for or fear of something, such as a desire for food or a fear of surgery, and also have the wish that he or she not have that desire or not be moved by that fear (Dworkin, 1976, 1988; Childress, 1990). Persons who lack the psychological capacity for rational decision making are those

who are severely mentally ill—paranoiacs, compulsive neurotics, schizophrenics, and psychopaths. Such persons have the capacity for agency, that is, they are aware of acting on their desires, but they fail to meet one or more of the above conditions. For example, a paranoid patient who persists in a delusion that the health-care professionals are Martians attempting to capture him is unable to adjust beliefs and actions to a reality confirmed by evidence (Benn, 1988).

Principle of respect for autonomy

Principles that support autonomy can be directed at the everyday relationships and encounters between persons; at the constitution, laws, and regulations of a nation-state; and at the policies of institutions such as hospitals, insurance companies, schools, and corporations. What ought to be done to respect autonomy will not be the same at all these levels and will be a function of a broad social ideology.

The minimal content for a principle of respect for autonomy is that persons ought to have independence, that is, be free from coercion and other similar interferences. John Stuart Mill made this the main principle in *On Liberty* (1947): No one should interfere with the liberty of action of another except to prevent harm to others. This obligation not to coerce others is defensible as an obligation binding on individuals, private organizations, and governments. Mill defended his principle of liberty, not because he believed that there is a fundamental right to autonomy nor that autonomy is valuable in itself, but because the recognition of liberty is supported by the principle of utility. This principle is that an action or policy is right to the extent that it promotes the greater happiness for the greater number. However, securing negative liberty does not establish autonomy as fundamental in moral theory. Other philosophers have gone further than Mill in their defense of autonomy.

The most widely quoted principle of respect for autonomy is one of Immanuel Kant's versions of the categorical imperative: "Treat others and oneself, never merely as a means, but always at the same time as an end in himself" (Kant, 1956, p. 101). This is frequently expressed as treating others as persons, and its distinctive Kantian claim is that others should be treated as rational beings who have their own ends. A further explanation of this principle is that persons should be seen as having interests in two senses. First, interests in those things that are a benefit to nearly everyone, for example, being free of pain, not being killed, being saved from dying. A physician can treat a patient without that person's consent and still protect these interests. Second, autonomous persons "take an interest" in things, that is, have preferences, projects, and plans. Acting only with concern to serve interests in the first sense, as is sometimes alleged against uses of the principle of utility, is not sufficient for respecting another's autonomy; we must also discover and take into account the individual's values and objectives (Benn, 1988). For example, a physician may believe that a surgical procedure is an effective treatment to relieve the pain of a patient's ulcer, but the patient may have a greater aversion to the risks of surgery than the physician does, and would prefer a restricted diet and medication. To not solicit, or to ignore, the patient's preferences in this matter would not respect his or her autonomy.

Autonomy, rights, and liberty

The concept of rights presupposes that right-holders are beings who have the capacity for autonomy, who make choices and can use discretion to exercise a right or not. Basic liberties in a liberal democracy are protected by constitutional and other legal rights. The idea of a right has three elements: the right-holder (the person who has the right); the object of the right (the activity or thing that the right-holder has a right to); and the duty-bearer (the person or institution who must do what the right requires). Negative rights are rights not to be interfered with; for example, everyone has the right not to be given medical treatment without consent, and all health-care providers must respect this right. Positive rights are rights that a person be provided with something—for example, the right of all senior citizens in the United States to Medicare payment for health care, a right that is binding on government agencies and health-care providers.

Recognizing the negative right to autonomy imposes on everyone the obligation not to coerce or otherwise interfere with the action of another. This protection of autonomy is not as costly to social institutions as recognizing positive rights to autonomy. If there is a positive right to X, this means that someone is under an obligation to provide X to the right-holder(s). For example, if every citizen has a fundamental positive right to the best-quality medical care, then the state must provide full access to medical care to all citizens. While there cannot be a positive right to autonomy per se—for autonomy as capacity is not something that can simply be given to persons who do not have it—there can be rights to other things that are required for, or supportive of, autonomy. Among them are rights to a decent minimum of health care, education, a decent standard of living, political participation, freedom of inquiry and expression, and equal opportunity to compete for positions in society. These goods contribute to autonomy in two ways: First, they make possible the development of the capacity for autonomy; second, they make autonomy meaningful by establishing the personal and social powers and range of options for autonomously chosen projects and plans. Discrimination against minorities and women decreases their autonomy by explicitly excluding them from desirable positions in society and by implicitly agreeing to the limited range of options offered to minorities and women.

Autonomy as an ideal

There is no sharp line separating accounts of autonomy as an ideal from autonomy as an actual capacity of persons. Autonomy can be described as a high level of self-determination that few persons will actually achieve, and yet it can still be regarded as a capacity for all persons, if it is believed that all persons under suitable conditions could acquire it and use it to direct their lives. Views that describe autonomy at a level that nearly all normal adult persons can and do exercise are views of autonomy as capacity, and views that describe it at a higher level are accounts of autonomy as an ideal.

Autonomy as an ideal will center on a person's use of the capacity for deliberation and reflection. The person who realizes the ideal of autonomy is, first, one who is consciously aware of having the capacity, someone who believes that he or she can use it to shape his or her life. Second, the autonomous person will make particular decisions with a sense of control—creating and evaluating options. That person will also reflect on how values, preferences, attitudes, and beliefs received in the socialization process function in his or her own decision making, examine the kind of person this makes him or her, consider alternatives, and make a commitment to accept or try to alter who he or she is. This is of course a matter of degree; like every virtue, it can be realized well and thoroughly or in some small measure. The ideal of autonomy does not require individuals to make conscious, deliberated decisions before every action. A person who has accepted a set of preferences, beliefs, and attitudes can respond without much thinking to common situations that fall into recognized patterns.

Autonomy of actions

In a clinical setting, it is often important to determine whether a patient's decision regarding treatment, or the decision of a proxy in the case of an incompetent patient, is autonomous. A person who has the capacity for autonomy may, for a variety of reasons, not act autonomously on a particular occasion. Determining whether a particular action or decision is autonomous is a matter of how the three elements of the capacity for autonomy (agency, independence, and rationality) are involved in the process of deciding. The autonomy of actions is a matter of degree because independence and rationality are matters of degree, though agency is not.

Ruth Faden and her colleagues describe the three elements of autonomy as intentionality, freedom from controlling influence, and understanding (Faden et al., 1986). They point out that controlling influences and understanding can be seen on two independent continua. An action can be performed within the range of full understanding to full ignorance, and within the range of completely uncontrolled to completely controlled.

Bruce Miller views the autonomy of actions and decisions on four levels: (1) as free action (agency and independence); (2) as authenticity (the decision is consistent with what is known about the person's values, preferences, and plans); (3) as effective deliberation (rationality); and (4) as moral reflection (deliberation about one's values, preferences, and plans) (Miller, 1981). The decision of a patient may be autonomous at one or more, but not all levels. For example, a patient who accepts a recommended treatment without reflecting much about the decision, acted autonomously at the level of free action, and perhaps authenticity, but not at the levels of rationality and moral reflection.

The legal concept of competence is closely related to the concept of autonomy. A competent person is one who has the capacity for autonomy, and a competent decision is one that is autonomously made.

David Jackson and Stuart Youngner present six cases of decision making in an intensive-care unit that "illustrate specific situations in which superficial preoccupation with the issues of patient autonomy and death with dignity could have led to inappropriate clinical and ethical decisions . . ." (Jackson and Youngner, 1979, p. 407). In one of the cases, a patient with multiple sclerosis appeared to autonomously refuse further lifesaving treatment following a suicide attempt. However, psychiatric evaluation showed that the patient had become depressed and withdrawn at the time his wife and sons began spending time with his mother-in-law who had been diagnosed with inoperable cancer.

Jay Katz has said that insufficient attention has been given to the unconscious and irrational motivations of behavior. It is not only patients' motivations that should be examined, but physicians' as well, for example, their denial of uncertainty. Whether a patient's decision to consent to or refuse treatment is autonomous depends on more than the patient's statement of decision and reasons. Physicians and patients must engage in conversations; physicians are obligated to facilitate patients' opportunities for reflection to prevent ill-considered decisions, and patients are obligated to participate in the process of thinking about their choices (Katz, 1984). The U.S. President's Commission (1982) echoes this view in its discussion of the importance of communication between patient and health professional to attain shared decision making based on mutual trust.

Privacy, informed consent, and paternalism

Autonomy as a fundamental right is used to justify rights to privacy, confidentiality, refusal of treatment, informed consent, and a decent minimum of health care. The legal right to privacy has two components. The right to control information about oneself is protected in medicine as the patient's right to confidentiality of information gained by health professionals. The right not to be interfered with and to make one's own decisions is protected in medicine as a competent patient's right to refuse recommended treatment and as the obligation of health professionals to obtain a patient's informed consent to treatment. Informed consent requires that a patient be informed of a recommended treatment and of the options for treatment and their likely consequences, and that the patient give express permission for a treatment (often in writing). The right to autonomy also requires that patients be told the truth about their medical status and prognosis, that their questions be answered, and that they receive assistance from health-care providers in making rational decisions. Meaningful exercise of the right to autonomy in living requires that individuals possess physical and psychological capacities within the normal, human range. So the positive right to autonomy supports a right to a level of health care that will return and maintain a person to the normal range of functioning. This includes acute care, for example, repair of a broken bone; chronic care, for example, treatment of diabetes or heart disease; and supportive care for permanent disability, for example, wheelchairs for paraplegics.

Paternalism in health care is treating a patient against his or her wishes on the grounds that the health-care provider is professionally obligated to provide care that will benefit patients, and that the health-care provider knows better than the patient what is good for the patient. When paternalism is justified, it overrides patient autonomy, at least partially. An example of justified paternalism could be when a physician does not accede to a patient's refusal of emergency treatment because the patient believes he or she will surely die.

Criticisms of autonomy

Some authors (Clements and Sider, 1983; Callahan, 1984; Thomasma, 1984) have criticized the centrality of autonomy in medical decision making. Their argument states that the primary obligation of health-care providers is to maintain and restore health. There are two aspects to this claim. First, if patient autonomy is given primacy over the obligations of health professionals, physicians and other providers may violate their obligation to maintain and restore the health of patients; for example, a patient may refuse a treatment that will save his or her life or prevent a serious illness. These conflicts between autonomy and patient benefit have often been decided by courts, usually in the form of a request by a terminally ill patient's family member, or other agent, that life-preserving treatments such as respirators be withdrawn, a request denied by physicians who cite their obligation to preserve life.

A second aspect of the criticism of autonomy recognizes the centrality of patients' values and wishes in cases of deciding whether to forgo life-preserving treatment for a terminally ill patient, but other sorts of medical-care decisions depend less on respecting patients' rights to autonomy and more on the value of restoring and maintaining the capacity for living a meaningful life. In this sort of case, autonomy is secondary to principles of beneficence, compassion, and caring.

Defenders of autonomy can make several replies to this critique. (1) Some of the attacks on autonomy wrongly assume that it is simply a principle of negative freedom, that is, the right not to be interfered with. (2) The claim of the centrality of patient autonomy in medicine does not imply that it is the only value. The principles of beneficence or nonmaleficence may, in some circumstances, justify paternalism. (3) Autonomy cannot be ignored in medical decision making. Knowing what will be most beneficial for a patient often requires input from the patient on values, objectives, and preferences. This is true not only in morally difficult situations that call for a decision about preserving the life of a terminally ill patient, but in less dramatic cases as well, for example, whether a patient should have surgery for a condition that causes minor discomfort and dysfunction but will not develop into something more threatening to health, or whether the patient should simply "live with" the condition. In cases of acute and severe injury or illness where there is a clearly best treatment that will almost certainly restore the patient to health, it can usually be safely assumed that whatever else the patient values, he or she will value the restoration of health, and hence, discussion of the relative value of options and their consequences is not required to respect the autonomy of the patient.

Criticisms of autonomy have also been launched from a broader, communitarian perspective (MacIntyre, 1981; Sandel, 1982; Callahan, 1984). Communitarians charge that the political theory of liberal individualism states that individuals are fully self-determining and that rights to autonomy are the primary or sole standard for individual behavior, institutional practices, and government policy. Communitarians object to liberal individualism on several grounds. First, the socialization process determines, or shapes, the values and preferences of individuals, hence, the idea of autonomously chosen values is factually incorrect. Second, an individual's actions, desires, and objectives are comprehensible

only within the context of social conventions and institutions. For example, a person cannot report that he or she is thinking about depositing a check without the conventions of language and the institution of banking. Third, the view that an autonomous individual chooses his or her own values, preferences, and desires presupposes a self that does the choosing. This self will have to have a core of values with which to choose, in which case either there are values not autonomously chosen, or it is inexplicable how individuals come to have a set of values. Communitarians also claim that liberal individualism regards persons as separate from others in the sense that individuals have no obligations to others or society that are not voluntarily assumed, other than the obligation to respect the individual rights of others. A society that respects only the autonomy rights of all its members is not morally complete. A good society must recognize obligations to help others; its members must have virtues such as compassion, caring, and love, and they should recognize a commitment to society to maintain social practices and institutions that establish and promote these obligations and virtues (Callahan, 1984).

There may be theories of autonomy that are susceptible to these criticisms, but the fundamental value of autonomy can be defended without embracing such versions of liberal individualism (Sher, 1989; Taylor, 1985). The conceptions of autonomy presented above recognize that persons are social beings whose values and preferences are shaped by society and that the capacity for autonomy is itself socially determined. Being autonomous requires language and reason, and these abilities are not possible without socially given practices and standards. Reflecting on socially given values and preferences and either accepting them as one's own or changing them in some measure, which is a feature of autonomous persons, cannot be done unless there is a social environment that encourages autonomy. A free society makes autonomy possible.

However, a society in which no one does more or less than respect everyone else's liberal rights, in which there is no caring, love, or friendship and no neighborhood associations, political parties, or civic groups, is not one we would want, though it may be a liberal society (Gutmann, 1985). On the other hand, a society organized to promote civic virtues and obligations such as beneficence, caring, and compassion, but which does not recognize a right of individuals to be different, to make their own decisions about matters of importance to them or to find a style of life that makes them happy, is also not one we would want. Love and care can be stifling if they do not recognize an individual's own view of what his or her good is. Finally, a defensible theory of the nature and value of individual autonomy will fall between radical individualism and extreme collectivism. It must explain the obligations to create and maintain social and political institutions that support the exercise and flourishing of autonomy. It must explain how the exercise of autonomy depends upon the opportunity range and values given in the traditions and structure of society. It will also recognize other fundamental values and explain their place in decision making.

In the early period of contemporary medical ethics, much attention was on medical paternalism in cases of life-and-death decision making for terminally ill patients and on what can be called "medical opportunism" in research on human subjects. Critics of these practices brought the rights of patients and subjects to the forefront of medical ethics. In a climate of concern for allocation of health-care resources and other issues of social policy, autonomy appears less frequently in medical ethics literature than do moral concepts such as justice, fairness, equality, economic efficiency, and cost-containment. This shift in issues should not lead to the view that autonomy has lost its importance in moral and social theory and in bioethics.

BRUCE MILLER

For a further discussion of topics mentioned in this entry, see the entries ACTION; BEHAVIOR CONTROL; BENEFICENCE; ETHICS, *article on* SOCIAL AND POLITICAL THEORIES; FREEDOM AND COERCION; HARM; MENTAL ILLNESS; OBLIGATION AND SUPEREROGATION; PATERNALISM; PERSON; PRIVACY IN HEALTH CARE; RIGHTS; UTILITY; *and* VALUE AND VALUATION. *This entry will find application in the entries* INFORMATION DISCLOSURE; INFORMED CONSENT; *and* SUICIDE. *For a further discussion of related ideas, see the entries* ARTIFICIAL ORGANS AND LIFE-SUPPORT SYSTEMS; CARE; COMPASSION; FRIENDSHIP; JUSTICE; LOVE; RACE AND RACISM; *and* SEXISM. *Other relevant material may be found under the entry* CONFIDENTIALITY.

Bibliography

BENN, STANLEY I. 1988. *A Theory of Freedom.* Cambridge: At the University Press.

CALLAHAN, DANIEL. 1984. "Autonomy: A Moral Good, Not a Moral Obsession." *Hastings Center Report* 14, no. 5: 40–42.

CHILDRESS, JAMES F. 1990. "The Place of Autonomy in Bioethics." *Hastings Center Report* 20, no. 1:12–17.

CLEMENTS, COLLEEN D., and SIDER, ROGER C. 1983. "Medical Ethics' Assault on Medical Values." *Journal of the American Medical Association* 250, no. 15:2011–2015.

DWORKIN, GERALD. 1976. "Autonomy and Behavior Control." *Hastings Center Report* 6, no. 1:23–28.

———. 1988. *The Theory and Practice of Autonomy.* Cambridge: At the University Press.

FADEN, RUTH R.; BEAUCHAMP, TOM L.; and KING, NANCY M. P. 1986. *A History and Theory of Informed Consent.* New York: Oxford University Press.

GUTMANN, AMY. 1985. "Communitarian Critics of Liberalism." *Philosophy and Public Affairs* 14, no. 3:308–322.

HAWORTH, LAWRENCE. 1986. *Autonomy: An Essay in Philosophical Psychology and Ethics.* New Haven, Conn.: Yale University Press.

KANT, IMMANUEL. 1956. *Groundwork of the Metaphysics of Morals.* Translated and edited by Herbert James Paton. New York: Harper & Row.

KATZ, JAY. 1984. *The Silent World of Doctor and Patient.* New York: Free Press.

JACKSON, DAVID L., and YOUNGNER, STUART. 1979. "Patient Autonomy and 'Death with Dignity.'" *New England Journal of Medicine* 301, no. 8:404–408.

MACINTYRE, ALASDAIR C. 1981. *After Virtue: A Study in Moral Theory.* Notre Dame, Ind.: University of Notre Dame Press.

MILL, JOHN STUART. 1947. *On Liberty.* Edited by Aubrey Castell. New York: Appleton-Century-Crofts.

MILLER, BRUCE L. 1981. "Autonomy and the Refusal of Life-saving Treatment." *Hastings Center Report* 11, no. 4: 22–28.

RAZ, JOSEPH. 1986. *The Morality of Freedom.* Oxford: At the Clarendon Press.

SANDEL, MICHAEL J. 1982. *Liberalism and the Limits of Justice.* Cambridge: At the University Press.

SHER, GEORGE. 1989. "Three Grades of Social Involvement." *Philosophy and Public Affairs* 18, no. 2:133–157.

TAYLOR, CHARLES. 1985. "Atomism." In *Philosophical Papers,* vol. 2 of his *Philosophy and the Human Sciences.* Cambridge: At the University Press.

———. 1991. *The Ethics of Authenticity.* Cambridge, Mass.: Harvard University Press.

THOMASMA, DAVID C. 1984. "Freedom, Dependency, and the Care of the Very Old." *Journal of the American Geriatrics Society* 32, no. 12:906–914.

U.S. PRESIDENT'S COMMISSION FOR THE STUDY OF ETHICAL PROBLEMS IN MEDICINE AND BIOMEDICAL AND BEHAVIORAL RESEARCH. 1982. *Making Health Care Decisions: A Report on the Ethical and Legal Implications of Informed Consent in the Patient-Practitioner Relationship.* Washington, D.C.: Author.

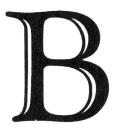

BABY DOE REGULATIONS

See INFANTS, *articles on* PUBLIC-POLICY AND LEGAL ISSUES, *and* ETHICAL ISSUES.

BALTIC COUNTRIES

See MEDICAL ETHICS, HISTORY OF, *section on* EUROPE, *subsection on* CONTEMPORARY PERIOD, *article on* CENTRAL AND EASTERN EUROPE.

BEHAVIORAL RESEARCH

For a discussion of behavioral and biomedical research, see INFORMED CONSENT, *article on* CONSENT ISSUES IN HUMAN RESEARCH; RESEARCH, HUMAN: HISTORICAL ASPECTS; RESEARCH METHODOLOGY; *and* RESEARCH POLICY. *See also* BEHAVIOR CONTROL; BEHAVIORISM; *and* BEHAVIOR MODIFICATION THERAPIES.

BEHAVIOR CONTROL

Behavior control and health care

The term "behavior control" may elicit images of neurosurgical techniques that transform a person into a robot subject to the whim of the controller. In ordinary usage, however, to control is "to exercise restraining or directing influence over." "Behavior control" refers broadly to systematic attempts by an agent or institution to influence behavior. Although health-care providers and institutions routinely influence the decisions and conduct of their patients, important ethical concerns arise when they do so through methods that endanger the morally acceptable relationships between them and their patients. Thus, moral evaluation of various methods of influence requires a theory of acceptable relationships.

Advocates of various moral theories might differ regarding the defensible purposes and parameters of health-care relationships. Utilitarians, for example, endorse relationships and decision making expected to maximize happiness. Communitarians identify a community standard of the common good and promote health-care relationships expected to conform to and promote that common good. Virtue theorists advance an account of the virtuous person, endorsing health-care relationships that exemplify and promote the identified virtues.

This article adopts the patient-centered approach to health care in order to illustrate the manner in which one mainstream theory generates standards of acceptable influence. Competing theories might produce different conclusions about certain forms of influence, but they share a common structure of analysis. Each theory provides an account of acceptable relationships between patients and providers or institutions and evaluates various modes of influence for consistency with these relationships. The patient-centered approach contemplates a process of shared decision making in which competent patients retain authority over their treatment. Providers diagnose disorders and recommend treatment, explaining the advantages and disadvantages of the available alternatives. Patients exercise a right to informed consent and the concomitant right to refuse treatment by selecting from among the options (Buchanan and Brock, 1989; *Cruzan v. Director, Missouri Department of Health,* 1990; Prosser and Keeton, 1984).

Patient-centered health care ordinarily promotes respect for autonomy as a right to self-determination within a sphere of personal sovereignty and conforms to the principle of beneficence, requiring that the provider actively promote the patient's well-being (Beauchamp and Childress, 1989; Feinberg, 1986). It supports autonomy because under the appropriate conditions, either informed consent or treatment refusal constitutes an exercise of personal sovereignty. It promotes well-being because fully informed patients are usually in the best position to make treatment decisions that are likely to promote their interests (Buchanan and Brock, 1989). This approach encounters a variety of difficult issues including the relative priority and weight of autonomy and well-being, the appropriate conception and criteria of informed consent, and the theory and implementation of surrogate decision making (Buchanan and Brock, 1989).

Important moral questions regarding behavior control also arise outside of the health-care system. The criminal and juvenile justice systems, advertising, and research in the life and social sciences, for example, raise important concerns about morally acceptable methods of social influence on human behavior. This discussion directly addresses only behavior control in health care, while acknowledging that the underlying principles apply to the broader contexts of behavior control.

Some attempts by health-care providers to influence the decisions or behavior of their patients threaten the underlying value of autonomy, raising apparent conflicts between the duties to respect autonomy and to promote well-being. Ethical assessment of these practices requires examination of their significance for the two values underlying patient-centered health care.

Persuasion, coercion, and manipulation in health care

Some methods by which providers influence their patients' behavior are clearly ethical. For example, providers routinely influence their patients' decisions and conduct regarding diet, exercise, and treatment through rational persuasion by explaining the probable benefits and costs of the available alternatives. Rational persuasion facilitates patients' exercise of informed consent, enhancing their ability to exercise autonomy and pursue well-being in most circumstances.

The morally troubling instances of behavior control in health care include those in which patients are coercively confined and subjected to intrusive forms of treatment such as surgery or medication despite their express objection. Recent legal cases have addressed the control of psychotic or severely retarded residents of state institutions who engaged in violent behavior, thus endangering themselves and others. These residents challenged various aspects of their treatment, including physical restraint, medication, and training programs, methods intended to alter their dangerous behavior. The courts were called upon to evaluate the legality of administering these methods of behavior control in these circumstances without voluntary consent (*Washington v. Harper,* 1990; *Youngberg v. Romeo,* 1982).

According to one view, subjective irresistibility is central to the relevant conceptions of coercion and control. Coercion completely undercuts individual sovereignty, as the will of the coercing agent controls that of the subjugated patient through a subjectively irresistible threat. Persuasive influences, in contrast, never control the patient because persuasion does not involve subjectively irresistible threats (Faden et al., 1986). The involuntarily committed patient who accepts treatment in response to threats of restraint and unwanted medication, for example, cannot effectively resist this mode of influence.

Emphasis on subjective irresistibility encounters at least three types of difficulty. First, no one has identified a practical criterion of subjective irresistibility (Faden et al., 1986). Second, and perhaps more important, no one has provided any clear interpretation of this notion of "subjective irresistibility." Notions such as "irresistible influence," "unable to resist," "overborne will," or "unable to do otherwise" have proven notoriously difficult to explain in a manner that supports the moral significance often attributed to them (Frankfurt, 1988; Schopp, 1991). Third, irresistibility does not capture the moral quality of some interventions.

Consider, for example, patient Anderson. Mr. Anderson rejects provider Cook's recommendation of outpatient therapy for chronic depression. Ms. Cook threatens to initiate legal proceedings in order to have Anderson involuntarily committed and medicated. Both Ms. Cook and Mr. Anderson doubt Ms. Cook's ability to carry out this threat because Mr. Anderson represents a borderline case under the state's civil commitment law as interpreted and applied by the courts. He suffers chronic depression with episodic exacerbation and remission and has been subject to several previous petitions for commitment with variable results depending on the circumstances. In addition, during one previous commitment, Mr. Anderson refused medication, and the court refused to order it administered involuntarily.

In a second case, provider Davis knows that patient Baker is deeply committed to a set of moral and religious principles vesting fundamental value in protecting human life and maintaining traditional families. Mr. Davis recommends a course of treatment that Mr. Baker rejects due to certain aversive side effects. Mr. Davis confronts Mr. Baker with irrefutable logic and overwhelming empirical evidence demonstrating that Mr. Baker's commitments to maintaining his family as an intact unit and to protecting human life, including his own, mandate his participation in this treatment.

It seems clear that the first case, but not the second, involves coercive pressure. Yet, in an important sense, the influence exerted in the first case is resistible while the influence brought to bear in the second is not. Mr. Anderson has resisted such pressure previously, sometimes prevailing at the commitment hearings. If he decides to accept the prescribed treatment, there is no apparent reason to think that he is unable to resist rather than that he simply decides not to. If he resists the threat, Ms. Cook does not successfully control Mr. Anderson. It seems more accurate to say that Mr. Anderson resists coercive pressure than to say that this particular threat is not coercive. That is, Ms. Cook exerts coercive pressure but does not successfully coerce Mr. Anderson (Feinberg, 1986). Although Mr. Davis's persuasive influence toward Mr. Baker would not usually be considered coercive, Mr. Baker may explain his decision to accept the treatment by stating that in the face of Mr. Davis's reasoning, he "has no choice" or "can do nothing else," suggesting that Mr. Baker finds Mr. Davis's argument subjectively irresistible.

Coercive influence qualifies as coercive and morally troubling, although not necessarily wrong, due to the manner in which it affects the choices and behavior of the subject. The coercive influence brought to bear on Mr. Anderson differs from the persuasive influence exerted on Mr. Baker in that a qualitatively different type of influence is used. The former involves the threat of force, the latter appeals to reason and the patient's values.

Some theorists explain coercion as a psychological concept, while others interpret it as inherently normative, classifying only wrongful interventions as coercive. On the psychological conception, a coercing agent exerts coercive pressure against an individual when the agent threatens the individual with some unwanted state of affairs unless he or she complies with the agent's demand. The coercive pressure constitutes coercion proper when the agent successfully elicits compliance by rendering it less aversive than resistance. Any particular case of coercion may or may not be morally objectionable. The normative conception, in contrast, classifies influence as coercive only when the coercing agent limits the subject's alternatives in a manner that wrongs him or her (compare Feinberg, 1986, with Wertheimer, 1987). In either interpretation, however, coercive influence raises at least prima facie moral concerns under the patient-centered theory that requires informed consent, because the coercive influence raises doubts about the voluntariness of that consent.

Although manipulation does not rely on coercive threats, it also raises a prima facie moral reservation under the patient-centered approach. Manipulative influences appeal to psychological processes in a manner not limited to rational persuasion. Perhaps deception provides the most widely cited example of manipulation. Others include exploitation of vulnerability and appeal to desires the individual experiences but does not endorse, does not want to be motivated by, or does not accept as part of the person he or she wants to be (Faden et al., 1986; Feinberg, 1978; Rudinow, 1978).

Providers can manipulate patients by deceiving them about the likely costs, benefits, or side effects of particular options, particularly when that deception is calculated to circumvent the values or priorities of the patient. Suppose, for example, that Mr. Davis persuades Mr. Baker to accept the treatment by concealing a potential side effect rather than by providing relevant information and rational argument. Mr. Davis would undermine Mr. Baker's values rather than respect them.

Providers can manipulate without deception through arguments, evidence, or appeals to authority that are calculated to overwhelm, confuse, or intimidate the patient rather than to explain to and rationally convince the patient. Providing accurate information in circumstances that prevent careful reflection due to inadequate time or, for example, to the presence of family members who are likely to exhort the patient to accept the treatment, can undermine independent judgment.

Providers who are familiar with a patient can exploit the patient's vulnerability by appealing to motives such as vanity or jealousy, or to ideas that the individual considers foreign or immoral, or of which he or she is ashamed. A plastic surgeon might secure consent for cosmetic surgery, for example, by exploiting the patient's fear that his wife is losing interest in him. Some forms of behavior control combine coercive and manipulative elements. When the patient is physically restrained and involuntarily administered psychotropic medication, for example, the provider coercively overrides the patient's decision not to accept the drugs. The chemical effect on the patient constitutes a manipulative influence in that it alters the psychological processes in a manner other than through rational persuasion.

Although many people ordinarily think of coercion as a more severe infringement than manipulation, manipulative influence can inflict injury that is in one sense deeper than that inflicted by coercion. Coercion relies in some manner on force or threats, but manipulation sometimes harnesses one's own vulnerabilities in order to turn one against oneself, often striking at an intimate level of one's psychology.

Though different theorists may define the parameters of rational persuasion, manipulation, and coercion somewhat differently, each constitutes a method of influencing behavior. Each might prove more or less effective in some circumstances. They differ primarily by virtue of the mechanisms through which they influence an individual's decisions and conduct. Under a patient-centered approach to health care that grants primary authority to the patient's informed consent and the concomitant right to refuse treatment, coercion and manipulation raise prima facie moral concerns, but rational persuasion does not. These concerns arise due to the relationship between these methods of influence and the underlying values of autonomy and well-being.

Autonomy, well-being, and behavior control in health care

Autonomy, liberty, and freedom.   Although autonomy is widely accepted as a core value in contemporary health-care ethics, the precise conception of autonomy at issue often remains vague. Joel Feinberg distinguishes four senses of autonomy as a right, a condition, an ideal, and a set of capacities. Autonomy as a right takes the form of a right to self-determination within a sphere of personal sovereignty. Theorists differ as to the proper boundaries of this sphere, but it generally encompasses central self-regarding life decisions regarding one's body, work, family, privacy, and property (Feinberg, 1986).

Autonomy as a condition is a set of virtues derived from the conception of a person as self-governing. These include self-reflection, direction, reliance, and control; moral authenticity and independence; and responsibility for self (Feinberg, 1986). Feinberg's set of autonomous virtues corresponds roughly to Gerald Dworkin's conception of autonomous persons as those who critically reflect upon and endorse or alter their own motives and values. Dworkin's autonomous persons develop integrated lives by reviewing and shaping projects, motives, and conduct according to higher-order values. They define their lives and make them their own through this process of self-evaluation and development (Dworkin, 1988a, 1988b). Individuals approach autonomy as an ideal to the extent that they develop autonomous virtues and exercise self-determination in defining and pursuing a life in a manner compatible with their membership in communities (Feinberg, 1986).

In order to exercise sovereign self-determination and develop the autonomous virtues, individuals need autonomous capacities. These are the psychological capacities such as consciousness, understanding, and reasoning used in critical self-reflection, deliberation, and decision making (Feinberg, 1986; Dworkin, 1988a, 1988b). For the sake of clarity, the term "autonomy" is reserved for the comprehensive value embracing all four senses in which the term is used. "Autonomous virtues" is used for the virtues that comprise autonomy as a condition, the optimal development of which constitutes autonomy as an ideal. Autonomy as a right is referred to as "sovereignty." Autonomy as capacity is referred to as "autonomous capacities." Autonomous capacities serve as necessary conditions for sovereignty and autonomous virtues. As sovereignty is a threshold concept that applies dichotomously rather than by degree, the autonomous capacities necessary to support personal sovereignty also serve as a threshold concept. Capacities beyond the minimal level required for sovereignty cannot increase the degree to which one is sovereign, although they might improve one's ability to exercise the right. Individuals manifest autonomous virtues in various degrees, however, and the extent to which they develop these virtues depends in part on the degree of autonomous capacities they possess (Feinberg, 1986).

Liberty and freedom are closely related to sovereignty, although not identical to it. Liberty is the absence of rule-imposed limitations on action within a political system, and freedom is the presence of open options. One has an open option if one lacks external personal constraints, so that one can either perform an action or refrain from performing it. The more options one has open, the more freedom one has. Some people might be at liberty to move into a particular neighborhood, for example, because no law forbids such a move. Yet they might not be free to do so if owners refuse to rent available housing to them. Sovereignty is a moral right that constitutes part of autonomy. A political system that respects autonomy must protect individual liberty of action within the domain of sovereignty. A corresponding degree of freedom is necessary to give this sphere of sovereignty and liberty practical effect.

Social and economic conditions can also limit a patient's effective exercise of autonomy. If poverty precludes access to the health-care system, for example, the individual's right to informed consent has little practical value. Similarly, those who lack the education needed to enable them to ask pertinent questions, understand the answers, or negotiate the unfamiliar structure and procedures of health-care institutions suffer disadvantage in their ability to exercise sovereignty. Legal or social discrimination leading to secondary status in the eyes of health-care providers or institutions can generate patterns of interaction that burden participation in a system ostensibly grounded in the patient-centered ethic. Thus, the practical implementation of the patient-centered ethic requires social commitment to effect the opportunity and ability to exercise sovereignty.

One can exercise one's sovereignty in such a manner as to decrease one's freedom. Some people voluntarily decide, for example, to participate in Antabuse therapy that effectively closes their option to drink alcohol during the period of participation. Others voluntarily undergo surgical sterilization, closing the option of having children. By taking action that decreases freedom, people limit the range within which they can exercise their sovereignty, but they do not become "less sovereign." They retain discretionary control within their sphere of sovereignty.

Behavior control, autonomy, and well-being. The patient-centered model of health care protects individual sovereignty by requiring informed consent. Autonomous acts must involve the exercise of autonomous capacities; that is, the actor must act intentionally, voluntarily, and with understanding of important relevant information. By granting informed consent for health care, patients exercise their sovereignty through an autonomous act, authorizing the treatment and accepting responsibility for the decision (Buchanan and Brock, 1989; Faden et al., 1986).

In ordinary circumstances, the requirement of informed consent promotes well-being. Some theorists identify individual well-being with some form of preference satisfaction, while others endorse an objective criterion of well-being such as happiness or self-fulfillment. According to either type of theory, people have welfare interests in certain states of affairs that allow them to pursue their ultimate good. These welfare interests include some minimal level of tangible goods, health, psychological functioning, and freedom to act as they see fit. Attainment of most plausible conceptions of individual well-being will be very difficult or impossible unless these welfare interests are met (Buchanan and Brock, 1989; Feinberg, 1984). The right to informed consent ordinarily allows patients the opportunity to select health care that is expected to promote their welfare interests and their ultimate good.

The significance of informed consent for autonomy and well-being explains the prima facie moral objections to coercive and manipulative methods of behavior control. Under ordinary conditions, rational persuasion facilitates informed consent, influencing behavior in a manner consistent with both values, but coercion and manipulation distort informed consent, undermining both values. Rational persuasion appeals to the autono-

mous capacities that serve as a necessary condition for sovereignty and autonomous virtues. Thus, those who respond to persuasion in a manner appropriate to that mode of influence exercise their autonomous capacities within their sphere of sovereignty. By appealing to autonomous capacities in order to elicit an exercise of sovereignty, rational persuasion respects sovereignty and, insofar as exercising these capacities promotes their development and that of autonomous virtues, it encourages that development.

Manipulation and coercion, in contrast, distort or override the exercise of autonomous capacities. These processes undermine sovereignty, depriving patients of the opportunity to exercise their autonomous capacities and develop autonomous virtues. To the extent that the individual is in the best position to make accurate decisions regarding his or her own well-being, these methods interfere with the ability to pursue it.

In some circumstances, however, particularly those in which the individual lacks autonomous capacities, individual decision making neither constitutes an exercise of sovereignty nor promotes well-being. Incompetent patients suffer impairment of autonomous capacities. A thorough discussion of incompetence would require careful examination of traditionally difficult psychological, legal, and philosophic issues including competing theories of responsibility, moral agency, and free will (Buchanan and Brock, 1989). It is sufficient to say here that certain types of psychological dysfunction undermine the autonomous capacities required to meet the threshold for sovereignty, although most individuals who suffer these disorders possess autonomous capacities and virtues to some degree. Also, most have the potential to develop further these traits.

Respect for the comprehensive value of autonomy demands both deontological and consequentialist components (Beauchamp and Childress, 1989). The deontological value of autonomy requires respect for competent self-regarding choice as an exercise of sovereignty, although it allows temporary intervention to ascertain whether the choice is competent, informed, and voluntary (Feinberg, 1986). It vests significance in the intrinsic nature of the choice as an exercise of sovereignty by a competent moral agent. The consequentialist aspect of autonomy, in contrast, emphasizes the expected consequences of any decision or action on the development of autonomous capacities and virtues. Those who recognize the consequentialist value of autonomy evaluate an act positively insofar as it promotes development of these traits and negatively insofar as the act undermines them. Encouraging development of autonomous capacities increases the probability that certain individuals will qualify for sovereignty.

Competence and behavior control in health care

Incompetence and well-being. Ordinarily, coercive and manipulative but not persuasive methods of influence raise moral concerns from the perspective of the patient-centered approach because the former but not the latter infringe on sovereignty and circumvent autonomous capacities. In certain circumstances, however, these three modes of influence interact with the underlying values of well-being and the deontological and consequentialist aspects of autonomy in a different manner. Incompetent individuals lack the capacities needed to qualify for sovereignty, reducing the importance of autonomy and thus, increasing the relative significance of well-being for them. Some severely impaired patients lack the potential to develop further their autonomous capacities and virtues. In such circumstances, providers adhering to the patient-centered approach can only maximize other aspects of well-being. The severely retarded resident in *Youngberg v. Romeo* (1982), for example, lacked the capacity to significantly improve his cognitive functions. Thus, providers were limited to promoting other aspects of his well-being by training him in a manner intended to reduce his violent behavior, decreasing the probability of injury and increasing freedom from restraint.

Autonomy remains a fundamental value, however, for those patients who possess some degree of autonomous capacities or virtues or the potential to develop these traits. The consequentialist aspect of autonomy commands weight both in itself and as a component of the patient's well-being. It commands independent weight because autonomous capacities and virtues constitute part of the comprehensive value for autonomy. Concern for patients' well-being demands concern for their autonomous capacities because they retain a welfare interest in maintaining these psychological capacities that enable them to pursue their ultimate interests effectively. Finally, self-fulfillment as development of the autonomous virtues constitutes at least part of a person's well-being in a moral system vesting fundamental value in autonomy.

In some cases, autonomy and well-being converge in that promoting the consequentialist aspect of autonomy also promotes well-being without violating sovereignty because the patient in question lacks the capacities necessary to qualify for sovereignty. Medicating grossly psychotic and assaultive patients without their consent, for example, may improve their cognitive functioning and reduce assaultive behavior, allowing more freedom from restraint, decreasing risk of injury, and improving autonomous capacities. The *Harper* Court, for example, allowed the involuntary administration of antipsychotic drugs to seriously mentally ill pris-

oners who are dangerous to themselves or to others when the treatment is in their medical interests as determined by the clinical review procedure provided by statute (*Harper*, 1990). If "serious mental illness" is sufficient to undermine the capacities necessary for sovereignty, *Harper* allows manipulative influence of prisoners' behavior in a manner that improves well-being by promoting safety from injury, freedom of motion, and autonomous capacities without violating sovereignty.

In different circumstances, however, it may be possible to influence incompetent patients through several different methods, each of which will address different aspects of well-being, requiring a choice regarding the most important component to pursue. For example, medication might reduce a severely disturbed patient's injurious behavior by sedating him or her in a manner that further reduces an already impaired alertness, comprehension, and capacity to make conscious choices, thus undermining already impoverished autonomous capacities. A strictly applied behavioral program involving both positive and aversive consequences for the patient's behavior, in contrast, might avoid reducing autonomous capacities at the cost of inflicting the aversive consequences.

Ms. Jones, for example, is a severely disturbed patient who engages in repetitive self-injurious behavior such as severely biting her hands and wrists as well as banging her head against the walls and floor. Psychotropic medication might reduce her injurious behavior, but it would do so at the expense of sedating her and slowing her already impaired mental processes. A behavioral treatment program including contingent electric shock might reduce her injurious behavior without sedating her, but she would experience the aversive shock.

Priorities among values

Decision makers who encounter these cases must establish priorities between autonomy and well-being as well as among various components of these basic values. Some writers advocate a categorical priority for sovereignty over well-being, rejecting any paternalistic intervention concerning voluntary self-regarding decisions. Others balance sovereignty against well-being in each case (Buchanan and Brock, 1989; Feinberg, 1986). Certain aspects of contemporary U.S. law appear consistent with each school of thought. The common law right of competent individuals to control their body is often interpreted to include the right to refuse all treatment, including life-sustaining procedures. In constitutional analysis, however, courts balance the liberty interest in being free from unwanted treatment against countervailing state interests, including the protection of human life and well-being (*Conroy*, 1985; *Cruzan v. Director, Missouri Department of Health*, 1990).

Theorists from both schools can accept intervention in the case of an incompetent patient in order to promote well-being, but they may differ regarding which aspect of well-being to emphasize. Those who endorse a comprehensive priority for autonomy opt to maximize autonomous virtues and capacities at the expense of other components of well-being. Those who balance autonomy and well-being as well as some who advocate a priority for sovereignty balance the consequentialist value for autonomous virtues and capacities against other aspects of well-being. Some theorists might endorse the priority of sovereignty over well-being but balance the consequentialist aspects of autonomy against other components of well-being.

Consider, for example, the following cases. Mr. Johnson is an elderly widower with serious coronary disease. He knows smoking and drinking markedly increase his probability of suffering a fatal heart attack. He continues to smoke regularly and meets with three old friends to share a bottle of bourbon twice a week, explaining that these activities provide the only real enjoyment in his life.

Ms. Bell is a moderately retarded adult who suffers a painful form of cancer. The only effective treatment for the pain is medication that significantly sedates her, decreasing her alertness and mental acuity, reducing her already impaired autonomous capacities and virtues. Due to Ms. Bell's incompetence, a surrogate must decide either to administer the medication, reducing the pain and her already impoverished autonomous capacities and virtues or to withhold the treatment, maximizing her autonomous capacities and virtues but leaving the pain unabated. In short, the surrogate must choose between the physical comfort that constitutes one aspect of Ms. Bell's well-being and the autonomous capacities and virtues that constitute the consequentialist aspect of autonomy and another component of her well-being.

Ordinary practice and contemporary law would respect Mr. Johnson's sovereign choice but call upon a surrogate to decide for Ms. Bell. Some might accept the intuitive judgments that Mr. Johnson's sovereignty ought to prevail over his well-being as evaluated from an external perspective and that the surrogate ought to opt for the medication, weighing Ms. Bell's physical comfort more heavily than the marginal cost to her autonomous capacities and virtues. Can one consistently advocate a priority for the deontic aspect of the value of autonomy over well-being by endorsing respect for Mr. Johnson's sovereignty, yet sacrifice the consequentialist aspect of the value for autonomy to other aspects of Ms. Bell's well-being? What justifies a priority for the deontic aspect of the value for autonomy but allows balancing of the consequentialist aspect?

Two arguments support a priority for sovereignty over well-being. The first is conceptual. State authority to monitor and intervene in the individual's domain of "sovereignty" undermines the claim of discretionary control, even if the state never exercises this power. The mere fact that some external source retains the authority to review and reverse decisions renders the person less than sovereign regarding these choices. Thus, one cannot consistently endorse individual sovereignty and state authority to intervene in that domain in order to promote well-being.

The second argument develops from the ramifications of the first. Individuals merit praise or blame and define their lives and the principles they live by through the exercise of sovereign discretion. Each individual creates his or her own life as an extended project uniquely his or her own by exercising sovereign choice regarding the central self-defining decisions. Certain interests, including food, shelter, and safety, form part of virtually everyone's well-being. Only by exercising sovereignty, however, can one define one's life and embrace one's own well-being (Dworkin, 1988b; Feinberg, 1986; Rachels and Ruddick, 1988). Thus, others can act to promote various states of affairs that would be good for Mr. Johnson, but only by exercising sovereignty can he render them part of his good. Sovereignty takes priority because it enables Mr. Johnson to define his own life and embrace various aspects of well-being as his well-being.

Increases in autonomous capacities that qualify an individual for sovereignty take priority over other aspects of well-being for similar reasons. Such increases provide persons with the opportunity to exercise sovereignty and define their lives. Merely incremental increases in autonomous capacities below the threshold that qualifies one for sovereignty do not have this effect. Thus, one can advocate a priority for sovereignty but balance these consequentialist aspects of the value for autonomy because the latter lack the special significance of the former in enabling the individual to define his or her life.

Other cases require choices between the deontological and consequentialist aspects of autonomy. Mr. Michaels is chronically moderately depressed, but he suffers no major cognitive dysfunction. He remains civilly competent and understands his condition, its pattern of periodic exacerbation and partial remission, and the proposed treatments. Mr. Michaels endangers neither his own life nor others' well-being, but he fails to develop his talents, pursue any interests or projects, or enrich his life. Mr. Michaels refuses offers of voluntary treatment. His history of responsiveness to structured treatment and his fear of civil commitment suggest that threats to initiate commitment proceedings would probably motivate his participation in an outpatient program and that doing so would likely improve his well-being, including his autonomous capacities and virtues. When a competent patient refuses treatment that is likely to improve well-being by promoting autonomous capacities or virtues, the deontological value for autonomy conflicts with the consequentialist aspect of the same value.

The reasoning that supports the priority for sovereignty over well-being but allows balancing of the consequentialist aspect of autonomy against other components of well-being also supports the priority for the deontological value of autonomy over the consequentialist aspect. To promote Mr. Michaels's good is to promote the human good that he chooses, pursues, and endorses as his own (Frankfurt, 1988). To violate sovereignty, and thus the deontological value of autonomy, in favor of the consequentialist aspect of autonomy that constitutes part of his well-being, is to alienate that good from this person, undermining both the values for autonomy and for well-being. Doing so severs the well-being from Mr. Michaels, rendering its attainment no longer attributable to him.

Conclusion

Behavior control in health care raises ethical concern when it threatens the morally acceptable relationship between the provider and the patient. Ordinarily, coercive and manipulative but not rationally persuasive influences undermine this relationship. Ethical evaluation of any specific application of behavior control requires examination of the method used in light of the circumstances and the underlying values of health care. The search for the most defensible account of the values underlying health care and the patient-provider relationship continues. The patient-centered theory is one viable candidate that converges reasonably well with current practice and law.

The debate between those who would grant priority to autonomy over well-being and those who would balance the two values remains active. The patient-centered approach to health care and the legal right to informed consent suggest that some legal and ethical institutions favor the priority for sovereignty. The moral reasoning that supports the priority for sovereignty rejects coercive and manipulative forms of influence intended to promote the competent patient's well-being, including those components of well-being that also constitute the consequentialist aspects of autonomy. When incompetence justifies the use of coercive influence in order to protect the incompetent patient's well-being, however, this reasoning does not demand a priority for promoting autonomous capacities and virtues over other components of well-being unless the improved autonomous capacities would be sufficient to qualify the individual for sovereignty. Many plausible circumstances that justify resorting to modes of influence other than

persuasive ones apparently justify coercion rather than manipulation.

ROBERT F. SCHOPP

Directly related to this entry is the entry BEHAVIOR MODIFICATION THERAPIES. *For a further discussion of topics mentioned in this entry, see the entries* ACTION; AUTONOMY; FREEDOM AND COERCION; INFORMED CONSENT; LAW AND BIOETHICS; PROFESSIONAL–PATIENT RELATIONSHIP; RIGHTS, *article on* RIGHTS IN BIOETHICS; VALUE AND VALUATION; *and* VIRTUE AND CHARACTER. *This entry will find application in the entries* COMMITMENT TO MENTAL INSTITUTIONS; HEALTH PROMOTION AND HEALTH EDUCATION; INJURY AND INJURY CONTROL; MENTALLY DISABLED AND MENTALLY ILL PERSONS; MENTAL-HEALTH THERAPIES; PSYCHOPHARMACOLOGY; RACE AND RACISM; *and* SEXISM. *For a discussion of related ideas, see the entries* AUTHORITY; BENEFICENCE; ETHICS, *article on* NORMATIVE ETHICAL THEORIES; LIFESTYLES AND PUBLIC HEALTH; RESPONSIBILITY; *and* UTILITY.

Bibliography

BEAUCHAMP, TOM L., and CHILDRESS, JAMES F. 1989. *Principles of Biomedical Ethics.* 3d ed. New York: Oxford University Press.

BUCHANAN, ALLEN E., and BROCK, DAN W. 1989. *Deciding for Others: The Ethics of Surrogate Decisionmaking.* Cambridge: At the University Press.

Conroy, in re. 1985. 486 A.2d 1209 (N.J.).

Cruzan v. Director, Missouri Department of Health. 1990. 110 S.Ct. 2841.

DWORKIN, GERALD. 1988a. "The Concept of Autonomy." In *The Inner Citadel: Essays on Individual Autonomy,* pp. 54–62. Edited by John P. Christman. New York: Oxford University Press.

———. 1988b. *The Theory and Practice of Autonomy.* Cambridge: At the University Press.

FADEN, RUTH R.; BEAUCHAMP, TOM L. and KING, NANCY M. P. 1986. *A History and Theory of Informed Consent.* New York: Oxford University Press.

FEINBERG, JOEL. 1978. "Behavior Control: II. Freedom and Behavior Control." In vol. 1 of *Encyclopedia of Bioethics,* pp. 93–101. Edited by Warren T. Reich. New York: Free Press.

———. 1984. *Harm to Others.* New York: Oxford University Press.

———. 1986. *Harm to Self.* New York: Oxford University Press.

FRANKFURT, HARRY G. 1988. *The Importance of What We Care About: Philosophical Essays.* Cambridge: At the University Press.

PROSSER, WILLIAM L., and KEETON, W. PAGE. 1984. *Prosser and Keeton on the Law of Torts*. 5th ed. St. Paul, Minn.: West.

RACHELS, JAMES, and RUDDICK, WILLIAM. 1988. "Lives and Liberty." In *The Inner Citadel: Essays on Individual Autonomy*, pp. 221–233. Edited by John P. Christman. New York: Oxford University Press.

RUDINOW, JOEL. 1978. "Manipulation." *Ethics* 88, no. 4:338–347.

SCHOPP, ROBERT F. 1991. *Automatism, Insanity, and the Psychology of Criminal Responsibility: A Philosophical Inquiry*. Cambridge: At the University Press.

Washington v. Harper. 1990. 110 S.Ct. 1028.

WERTHEIMER, ALAN. 1987. *Coercion*. Princeton, N.J.: Princeton University Press.

———. 1993. "A Philosophical Examination of Coercion for Mental Health Issues." *Behavioral Sciences and the Law* 11, no. 3:239–258.

Youngberg v. Romeo. 1982. 102 S.Ct. 2452.

BEHAVIOR AND GENETICS

See GENETICS AND HUMAN BEHAVIOR.

BEHAVIORISM

I. History of Behavioral Psychology
   Daniel N. Robinson
II. Philosophical Issues
   Rem B. Edwards

I. HISTORY OF BEHAVIORAL PSYCHOLOGY

That the systematic application of rewards and punishments provides an effective means by which to control behavior was undoubtedly appreciated by the earliest human communities. The domestication of animals throughout prehistory and the numerous early historical references to the proficiency of animal trainers further establish a form of "behavioral psychology" as the most venerable of the folk psychologies. Thus, if the term "behavioral psychology" is taken to mean only a set of techniques useful for the prediction and control of behavior, then its history is coeval with human history.

As generally understood, however, behavioral psychology is not merely a collection of methods but a more or less developed position on the nature of psychology itself: a position informed by identifiable traditions within philosophy and philosophy of science, as well as by the larger scientific context within which psychology seeks a proper place.

Understood in this light, the subject has its origins in the first great age of modern science, the seventeenth century: the century of Francis Bacon, Johannes Kepler, Galileo, Thomas Hobbes, René Descartes, and Isaac Newton, to mention only several of the more celebrated figures. Setting aside the many and fundamental conceptual and scientific disagreements hosted by this era, a coherent theme is found: namely, that an unprejudiced and objective inquiry into the operations of the natural world will yield lawful and useful knowledge. The older world of logical analysis, occult powers, hidden forces, revealed truths, and scriptural authority was now to be replaced by the more modest but more solid discoveries of direct experience. The knowable cosmos, on this understanding, is just the observable cosmos.

The two divisions of science most fully developed in the seventeenth century were mechanics and optics, and both of these served as models and metaphors for phenomena only poor understood. The well-ordered Hobbesian state, the clockwork precision of the Newtonian heavens, and Descartes's stimulus–response psychology are based upon the metaphor of the machine, and upon the conviction that fuller explanations in these areas will be drawn from the science of mechanics. Descartes's (1596–1650) psychology of animal behavior, which he extended to include those aspects of human psychology not dependent upon language and abstract thought, is entirely mechanistic and behavioristic, even in the more modern senses of the terms. His explanations of all animal and most human behavior are grounded in what would now be called instinctual reflex mechanisms and acquired but still reflexive habits. On this account, the nervous system is an elaborate input–output system organized in such a way that specific patterns of stimulation lead to organized and adaptive patterns of behavior. The tendency to focus on Descartes's famous dualistic solution to the mind/body problem and his emphasis upon the cognitive, rational, and linguistic uniqueness of human beings should not obscure the essentially behavioristic content of his overall psychology.

Criticized in Descartes's own time by Thomas Hobbes and Pierre Gassendi, among others, Cartesian psychology was stripped of its introspective features in the eighteenth century, where it survived within progressive circles as a primitive biological psychology. In British philosophy, David Hartley (1705–1757) stands out in the movement to adapt Newtonian and Cartesian mechanistic principles to the needs of an emerging mental science. His *Observations on Man* (1749) provides a richly argued and illustrated defense of a behavioristic psychology grounded in (Humean) associationistic principles operating within the sort of reflex-framework advocated by Descartes. In France, Julien de La Mettrie's *L'Homme machine* (1748) was an uncompromisingly materialistic psychology: antispiritual, reductionistic, behavioristic. The circle of French philosophes included stridently mechanistic theorists (e.g., Paul, Baron d'Holbach) but also those of radically environmentalistic orientation (e.g., Claude-Adrien Helvétius) who insisted that social and familial pressures were totally responsible for human psychological development.

As the philosophes and natural philosophers of the eighteenth century were assembling strong rhetorical arguments in behalf of a fully naturalistic psychology, the medical and scientific communities were broadening and deepening the empirical foundations. Robert Whytt's (1714–1766) pioneering studies of spinal reflexes are illustrative. These were accomplished while La Mettrie was offering little more than polemical defenses of psychological materialism. Whytt's research exemplified the steady, modest, and entirely experimental approach of scientists loyal to what they took to be the methods of Newton and Bacon. Early in the nineteenth century programmatic research of this sort had unearthed the distinct sensory and motor functions of the spinal cord—the Bell-Magendie Law—and had put the mechanistic-behavioristic perspective on firm anatomical foundations. By the 1830s Marshall Hall (1790–1857), in a tradition of Scottish medical science that includes Whytt and Charles Bell, would put the concept of *reflex* function at the very center of a nascent biological psychology that would influence the ultimate character of modern behaviorism.

It should be noted that it was in this same period (1750–1850) that the so-called animal model became accepted such that, in the early decades of the nineteenth century, a single laboratory might perform vivisection on *thousands* of animals, none of them anesthetized. Again, "Cartesianism" in still another sense was the gray eminence here, fortifying the scientific community in the belief that nonhuman animals were merely a species of machinery. This perspective, shorn of its horrific surgical practices, would survive in the confident anti-mentalism of twentieth-century behaviorism.

By the middle of the eighteenth century, the medical clinic, too, was yielding an ever more coherent account of the causal efficacy of the nervous system in human sensory and behavioral functions. By the end of the century, and as a result of his own original and exhaustive studies, including post mortem examinations of exceptional as well as feeble and felonious persons, Franz Joseph Gall (1758–1828) would offer the "science" of *phrenology* as a developed and systematic psychology—a psychology grounded in the principle that all sensory, motor, affective, and cognitive functions are brought about by conditions in the brain and in its numerous subsystems. Once again, the evidence all pointed to a quasi-mechanistic system, complex though law-governed, and functioning in such a manner as to adjust (or fail to adjust) behavior to the demand-features of the environment.

The evolutionary perspective

By the time Darwin published his *On the Origin of Species* (1859), the "Darwinian" perspective was already dominant in scientific and progressive circles. Adam Smith's *The Wealth of Nations*, Jacques Turgot and his party of "physiocrats," and the writings of any number of philosophes point to a more or less settled Enlightenment position: The free movement of ideas, goods, and persons—constrained by no more than "natural" forces—produces an ever more refined, successful, and robust stock.

But Darwin's monumental contribution went beyond this general perspective and reached the level of a developed and richly integrative theory. Its implications for psychology were clear: As there is no sharp line dividing places along the broad evolutionary continuum that humanity shares with the balance of the animal economy, there is no reason to confine inquiries into complex psychological functions to studies of human beings.

Antecedents in psychology

Evolutionary theory in Darwin's hands emphasized differences in *degree*, not in essence. Thus, the most complex human psychological attributes could, in principle, be examined in a more systematic fashion by studying their simpler but kindred manifestations in nonhuman animals. Studies of this sort, it was assumed, would establish psychology's own independent scientific status. As Herbert Spencer (1820–1903) declared:

> The claims of Psychology to rank as a distinct science . . . are not smaller but greater than those of any other science. If its phenomena are contemplated objectively, merely as nervo-muscular adjustments by which the higher organisms from moment to moment adapt their actions to environing coexistences and sequences, its degree of specialty, even then, entitles it to a separate place. (*Principles of Psychology*, 1896, p. 141)

In the patrimony of Darwin, and influenced chiefly by his *The Descent of Man* (1871), specialists in animal psychology appeared before the end of the nineteenth century and made their own contributions toward a behavioral science. George Romanes (1848–1894), in his *Animal Intelligence* (1882) and *Mental Evolution in Animals* (1883)—for all his anthropomorphic tendencies—put the study of animal behavior on the map of the new psychology. All that was needed to prepare this Darwinian psychology for adoption by the forthcoming generations of behaviorists was to strip it of just this anthropomorphism. C. Lloyd Morgan, in his *Introduction to Comparative Psychology* (1893), delivered his famous canon:

> In no case may we interpret an action as the outcome of the exercise of a higher psychic faculty, if it can be interpreted as the outcome of the exercise of one which stands lower in the psychological scale. (p. 53)

Thus, with this insistence on explanatory parsimony, did the "ism" in behaviorism begin to take shape.

It is customary, if misleading, to date the birth of experimental psychology itself with Wilhelm Wundt's founding of the discipline's first university laboratory at Leipzig in 1878–1879. Wundt (1832–1920) was perhaps the discipline's most prolific writer. His texts, which were wide-ranging and immensely influential at the time psychology departments were being formed in Europe, England, and the United States, emphasized experimental over ethological (naturalistic) modes of inquiry. But the reading of Wundt was rather selective. In his less consulted multivolume *Völkerpsychologie* (best rendered as "anthropological psychology") he developed and defended the nonexperimental and essentially historical–anthropological mission of psychology, drawing attention to the limits of reductionistic strategies and explanations. Even with this broadened perspective, Wundt remained loyal to the scientific views of his age, acquired in his medical education and as he assisted the great Hermann von Helmholtz. In these respects he was representative of an entire generation of thinkers committed to the scientific study of psychology and the abandonment of purely philosophical modes of analysis wherever the scientific and experimental alternative was practicable.

In the Wundtian tradition, however, the subjects of scientific inquiry were taken to be mental processes and functions: those now generally dubbed "cognitive." Moreover, although he did much to advance comparative psychology in his textbooks, the bulk of his theoretical writings and all of the research undertaken in the Leipzig laboratory focused on *human* psychology and the development of a *science of mental life*. To this extent, Wundtian psychology formed a path distinct from that so heavily trod by the neurophysiologists, anatomists, and clinicians, a path more readily associated with the introspective philosophical psychologists (e.g., John Locke and David Hume). Nor was it clear that Wundtian psychology had a place within the larger naturalistic context of Darwinian science.

Labels offer useful shortcuts but can be misleading. It may be said, with ample qualifications, that the Wundtian perspective, at least in the hands of his most influential students (e.g., Edward B. Titchener), was

structuralist. Any number of passages and entire chapters in books by Wundt are devoted to the (hypothetical) constituents or components of thought. And, if *structuralism* and *functionalism* are to be understood in essentially dialectical terms, it is also the case that Wundt's major works are not beholden to the idiom of functionalism. But his attention to the workings of the nervous system, his attempts to provide a loosely evolutionary framework for both human and animal psychology, and his problem-centered cognitive psychology are all anticipations of the functionalist psychology so explicit in the works of William James (1842–1910).

What is relevant here in the tension (real or apparent) between structuralism and functionalism in the history of modern psychology is the claim later made by John B. Watson (1878–1958) that behaviorism was to replace both. In significant respects, it may be said to have replaced both by merging the two rather than by fully rejecting either. Structuralism, which was never a central feature of Wundt's own agenda for the discipline, has this much in common with behaviorism: a reductionistic theory or strategy according to which complex and psychologically significant ensembles can be analyzed into more elementary components; further, that the only valid evidence is the observable and repeatable evidence gleaned by laboratory investigations. For all their differences, then, behaviorism and structuralism, in their mechanistic and reductive commitments, were faithful to that "religion of science" launched in the seventeenth century.

Functionalism, of course, is the immediate precursor to behaviorism and even a version of it, depending on how the term is to be understood. One account of it is defended by Alexander Bain (1818–1903), founder of the journal *Mind* and intimate friend of John Stuart Mill. In *The Senses and the Intellect* (1855) and *The Emotions and the Will* (1859), Bain argued that the discipline of psychology is to be advanced by merging its issues and findings with the science of physiology in such a way as to ground psychological processes in the functions of the nervous system. "Functionalism" in this sense is a function-based psychology whose general laws are derived from neurophysiology. On still another but quite compatible account, such as that defended by William James, the question to ask of any psychological process or phenomenon is what *function* it serves in the larger context of the organism's (person's) overall and long-term interests. The psychological event is explained when the functions it serves are delineated. These, in the most general sense, are *adaptive* functions, rendering the organism more successful in its transactions with the environment. In the writings of William James, this orientation is tied to a *pragmatism* which itself would anticipate central tenets of modern behaviorism.

Modern behavioral psychology

The Nobel Prize–winning research of Ivan Pavlov (1849–1936) was addressed to gastric physiology and the chemistry of digestion. But in the process of studying the formation and secretion of digestive enzymes, Pavlov discovered that initially automatic or innate reflex-mechanisms could be controlled externally by associating them with specific events in the environment. His theories of "classical conditioning" were grounded in neurophysiology and were intended to replace the mentalistic terms of traditional psychology. In this aim he was joined by the American psychologist John B. Watson, widely regarded as the father of behaviorism.

In his influential essay in the *Psychological Review* (1913), "Psychology as the Behaviorist Views It," and his widely read and cited *Psychology from the Standpoint of a Behaviorist* (1919), Watson waged relentless war on introspective psychology, structuralism, "folk" psychology, and the entire tradition of philosophical speculation regarding the nature of human nature. He insisted that the proper (only) subject matter of any science is directly observable events, which for psychology means observable *behavior*. In tying his recommendations to a version of the Pavlovian theory, Watson failed to produce the sort of behavioral psychology compatible with the functionalistic and pragmatic bent already dominant in America. But his writing did much to put mentalistic psychologies on notice and to promote a seemingly objective, scientific, and descriptive discipline, practical in its aims and stridently antimetaphysical.

This much of the Watsonian legacy was accepted by the most influential figure in the history of behavioral psychology, B. F. Skinner (1904–1991). In numerous books and articles, in scores of laboratory demonstrations, and through a veritable legion of students and co-workers, B. F. Skinner dominated psychology in the United States and, indeed, much of psychology around the world, for a quarter of a century. From 1950 until the 1970s, specialists in a wide variety of psychological employments came to regard themselves as "behavioral scientists"; came to adopt the idiom and perspective of "Skinnerian" psychology; came to fashion methods and measurements akin to those of the "Skinner box" and the cumulative recorder.

As early as 1938, in *The Behavior of Organisms*, Skinner had argued for the independence of *behavioral* science from physiology or other (even if somehow related) sciences. The facts of observed behavior, he insisted, remain what they are, no matter what the nervous system is found to be doing; no matter what the genetic composition of the organism proves to be; no matter what theory is invented or adopted to account for these facts. Taking his lead from the research of Edward L. Thorndike (1874–1949), Skinner devoted himself to the study of *operant* or instrumental behavior, the behavior that is instrumental in securing positive reinforcers or in avoiding aversive stimulation. Unlike Pavlovian reflexes (or "respondents," in Skinner's terminology), operant behaviors actually operate on and alter the animal's environment. The behavior that results in positive reinforcement (for example, food) becomes statistically more probable. Nonreinforced behavior—behavior that has no systematic effect on the environment—simply drops out. Thus, behavior within an environment containing reinforcing contingencies is not unlike the evolutionary arena itself. Those behaviors survive that result in more successful adaptations; those that do not are extinguished.

As developed by Skinner, behavioral psychology is a descriptive, empirical science—more akin to engineering, perhaps, than to physics—able to identify the conditions under which behavior is rendered more or less probable. Useless to this enterprise are theories laden with hypothetical processes, hidden variables, private "states." Perhaps the most concise philosophical defense of the perspective was provided by Gilbert Ryle in *The Concept of Mind* (1949), in which the Cartesian "ghost in the machine" was analytically exorcised, leaving in its wake a collection of psychological attributes uniquely specified by observable behavioral events and dispositions.

Skinner's version of behavioral psychology, though the most influential, is but one of several developed in the twentieth century. The main points of division among various schools or types are three: first, the level of explanation to be attained by a behavioral psychology; second, the room within such a psychology for nonobservable ("mental") events and processes; third, the proper place of such a psychology within the larger context of the natural (biological) sciences. On each of these points major and self-proclaimed behaviorists have taken positions at variance with Skinner's.

Clark Hull (1884–1952), for example, adopted the nomological-deductive model of scientific explanation and attempted to develop a formal theory of behavior based on a number of hypothetical constructs (for example, "habit-strength") and intervening variables (for example, fatigue-substances generated by muscular activity). Hullian behavioral psychology is characterized by pages of mathematical equations expressing such relationships as that obtaining between learning and practice, or between strength of response and magnitude of reward, or between speed of response and hours of food-deprivation, and so forth.

E. C. Tolman (1886–1959) defended a form of *cognitive* behavioral psychology that grounded explanations of problem-solving on the part of nonhuman animals in such notions as "cognitive maps." Rats, for example, who learn the various turns in a maze and who are later placed on top of the maze-box will run directly toward the goal rather than retracing the successful maze-paths. What the rats have, in Tolman's theory, is a map or representation of the situation such that very different patterns of behavior can be arranged to achieve the same results.

Yet other behavioristic psychologists, notably Karl Lashley (1890–1958), retained their commitment to study observable behavior, but insisted that a science of behavior had to be fully integrated into the brain sciences, and had to make contact with the well-established cognitive dimensions of human and animal psychology. In this the influences and criticisms of such Gestalt psychologists as Wolfgang Köhler (1887–1968) wrought changes on the behavioristic outlook, or otherwise rendered the outlook itself dubious.

Ethical implications

From the first, the Darwinian, reductionistic, and positivistic character of behaviorism targeted it for criticism from expected (humanistic) quarters. Yet, unlike the value-neutral orientation of much of modern science, behaviorists have tended to defend their perspective on ethical grounds. Both Watson and Skinner were explicit in this regard. Skinner's *Beyond Freedom and Dignity*, though dismissive of traditional moral theories and their supporting "folk" psychologies, contended nonetheless that a behaviorally engineered society would achieve the most precious of the ends envisaged by ethical theorists. His work inspired the formation of several small communities organized around principles of operant conditioning, with desired behavior brought about without the moral tags of "praise" and "blame." His work also provided the theoretical and technical foundations for various "behavior therapies" applied to disturbances ranging from bed-wetting to catatonic withdrawal. Considered ethically, these methods would seem to be neither more nor less coercive than those arising within other theoretical contexts and employed for the benefit of consenting patients.

In taking human nature to be part of nature at large, and impelled by the same evolutionary pressures faced by the balance of the animal kingdom, behavioral psychology is neither more nor less "humanistic" than, say, psychoanalytic theory or, for that matter, the contemporary neurocognitive psychologies that have all but replaced behaviorism. Skinner rejected moral theories grounded in deontological or transcendental arguments, but accepted the proposition that complex societies require the imposition of constraints, and that the coercive principles and practices must be justified in ways conducive to a flourishing and productive life within such societies.

This much granted, it must also be noted that the overall sketch of life depicted by Watson and Skinner, and otherwise implicit in the very language of behavioral psychology, matches up poorly with the life actually lived by most human beings and many other species. In ignoring or depreciating the richly social, self-moving, self-conscious dimensions of life—and, thus, the irreducibly moral terms that rational beings must invoke if they would live together in a principled way—the architects and defenders of radical versions of behavioral psychology have more or less resigned from the domain of ethical discourse.

DANIEL N. ROBINSON

Directly related to this article is the companion article in this entry: PHILOSOPHICAL ISSUES. *Also directly related are the entries* BEHAVIOR CONTROL; *and* HUMAN NATURE. *For a further discussion of topics mentioned in this article, see the entries* ANIMAL RESEARCH, *article on* HISTORICAL ASPECTS; *and* EVOLUTION. *Other relevant material may be found under* BEHAVIOR MODIFICATION THERAPIES; *and* BIOLOGY, PHILOSOPHY OF.

Bibliography

MORGAN, C. LLOYD. [1893] 1978. *Introduction to Comparative Psychology: The Limits of Animal Intelligence.* Reprinted in serr. D, vol. 2, *Significant Contributions to the History of Psychology.* Edited by Daniel N. Robinson. Westport, Conn.: Greenwood Press.

ROBINSON, DANIEL N. 1986. *An Intellectual History of Psychology.* Madison: University of Wisconsin Press.

RYLE, GILBERT. 1949. *The Concept of Mind.* London: Hutchinson.

SKINNER, B. F. 1971. *Beyond Freedom and Dignity.* New York: Alfred Knopf.

SPENCER, HERBERT. 1896. *The Principles of Psychology.* 3d ed. New York: Appleton.

TOLMAN, EDWARD C. 1948. "Cognitive Maps in Rats and Man." *Psychological Review* 55, no. 4:189–208.

WATSON, JOHN B. 1919. *Psychology from the Standpoint of a Behaviorist.* Philadelphia: J. B. Lippincott.

II. PHILOSOPHICAL ISSUES

Behaviorism is the view that the proper subject matter of psychology is the behavior of persons and animals. There are many forms of behaviorism, and they evoke varied philosophical responses. Behaviorism arose in psychology out of frustration with older introspective approaches to mind and consciousness that appeal to direct awareness of mental states and processes, and out of the desire to turn psychology into a proper natural science with an empirical methodology and subject matter, one that makes claims that are publicly verifiable or falsifiable in repeatable sensory experience.

Methodological and metaphysical behaviorism

Methodological behaviorism does not deny the existence of mind and consciousness. It holds merely that such things are irrelevant in psychology, which, to become scientific, must adopt an empirical, scientific methodology applied to the empirical subject matter of observable human behavior.

Metaphysical behaviorism of the sort espoused by J. B. Watson (1878–1958) and his followers makes a much stronger claim. It denies the existence of mind and consciousness, and proposes that all mentalistic concepts can be properly defined (or redefined) in terms of observable behavior. Watson maintained that behavior can be explained entirely in terms of stimulus and response, without the intervention of mental or conscious events and activities. For Watson, all behavior is environmentally derived and cannot be explained by appeals to heredity, instincts, the unconscious, human nature, or internal predispositions.

Some behaviorists recognize two different kinds of observable behavior: external behavior that is sometimes called overt, external, or molar (pertaining to the whole), and internal behavior that is alternatively called covert, deep, or central behavior. If "thinking" is defined as "talking" or "speaking," an account must be given of what transpires when we are thinking silently "to ourselves." The wife of a philosopher once complained that she could never tell whether he was working or loafing. Many psychological processes and activities seem, at times, to involve no external behavior. Behaviorists may either deny the reality of those processes and activities or affirm that they involve internal behaviors or processes. Thus, silent thinking becomes "motion in the head," as Thomas Hobbes earlier put it, or "sub-vocal speech," as Watson suggested—that is, subtle and externally undetectable motions of vocal cords and/or electrical activity in the brain and nervous system.

Where internal behavior consists of neurophysiological activity, behaviorism becomes central state materialism, according to which the reality of mental states and processes is identical with that of physical states and processes in the brain and central nervous system. This theory identifies mental processes with "motion in the head"—that is, electrical and chemical processes within the central nervous system. Modern medical brain scanning devices give indirect sensory access to these neurophysiological motions and processes, though not to the mental processes that are supposedly embodied in them. Brain scans can picture structures and electrochemical changes within the brain, but an enormous and highly controversial conceptual leap is necessary if these are designated as thoughts, feelings, volitions, emotions, and so on.

Central state materialism deserves a separate treatment elsewhere, and little will be said about it here. This article will concentrate on the behaviorism of Watson, B. F. Skinner, and those philosophers of language who focus on externally observable acts and/or dispositions to behavior in externally observable ways. It will also raise questions about whether behaviorism is or is not incompatible with presuppositions that are commonplace in ethical theory and bioethics.

Logical or linguistic behaviorism

Many philosophers are attracted to behaviorism's emphasis on observable external behavior for metaphysical or methodological reasons, or both. Some want to escape from the Cartesian mind/body dualism, from "the ghost in the machine," as Gilbert Ryle put it, though this may be done without resorting to behaviorism. Members of the positivistic Vienna Circle, an influential group of scientifically oriented philosophers who flourished in Vienna from the early 1920s to the mid-1930s, wanted to avoid introspective methodology, and so do those influenced by them. They are attracted to the behavioristic methodological program of redefining mentalistic language in terms of external, overt, publicly observable behavior because of its compatibility with the empiricist criterion of meaning: that meaning consists in sensory reference.

Logical or linguistic positivism attempts to analyze the meanings of concepts and beliefs in terms of sensory reference and verifiability. Many recent and contemporary philosophers with a bent toward this form of positivism have tried to analyze in observable behavioral terms the meanings of such psychological concepts as thought, understanding, intelligence, conception, doubt, belief, imagination, memory, choice, decision, will, attention, and the classes and manifold subclasses of feelings, sensations, pleasures, pains, emotions, desires, purposes, and so on.

Gilbert Ryle (1900–1976), a prominent British linguistic philosopher, was convinced that ordinary language is a behavioristic language, that ordinary meanings of psychological terms are behavioral meanings. Without denying the existence of inner mental events, he believed that the ordinary meanings of mental concepts can be captured by reference to observable behaviors or the dispositions to manifest them, without appeal to private or privileged access. Most philosophers and psychologists since Ryle believe that psychological concepts in ordinary language and "folk psychology" cannot be analyzed purely behaviorally without important loss of significance. Many see this as a reason for abandoning familiar psychological terminology for a technically or theoretically constructed and redefined psychological vocabulary. Others, who find self-awareness to be too evident and significant to be abandoned, are persuaded that a purely behavioral outlook only fosters trivialities and ignores the obvious.

Although Ludwig Wittgenstein (1889–1951), a highly influential linguistic philosopher, did not deny the existence of consciousness and its contents, features of his philosophy of mind can be interpreted to support a behavioristic outlook. He argued convincingly against private languages and purely private experience. He contended that human infants originally learn to use psychological concepts by reference to behavioral criteria in a social setting, and that the criteria are themselves integral aspects of the meaning of such concepts. Few philosophers today would deny this intimate connection between mental concepts and behavior. Nevertheless, "How do we learn mentalistic concepts?" and "To what do mentalistic concepts refer?" seem to be very different questions, one not being answered by replies to the other. Wittgenstein would have agreed.

Wittgenstein's position was easily converted to behaviorism by some of his interpreters through dropping his conviction that psychological concepts point to something internal and mental, and by adopting the view that the meanings or references of psychological concepts consist entirely in behavioral criteria. Thus, the meaning of "pain" consists solely in pain behaviors like screaming, crying, moaning, writhing, withdrawing, fleeing, gnashing teeth, or holding one's side or jaw. Internal states do not stand in need of external criteria, for there are no internal states. Psychological concepts are identical in meaning with their external criteria, just as a good Watsonian behaviorist would contend.

Objections to behaviorism

Behaviorism has been criticized from many philosophical perspectives. The new technical psychological language that behaviorism generates is certainly not ordinary language, the language of everyday life and common sense, for that language has not lost sight of consciousness and its manifold contents. Noam Chomsky is convinced that psychological conditioning and associationist learning theory, according to which learning occurs solely through repeated exposures that form connecting links, are too weak to account for the pre-structured dispositions of human infants to learn human languages. Abraham Maslow (1971) reports that having a child of his own made behavioristic views of conditioned associationist learning look so foolish that he could not stomach them anymore. To Maslow, the presence of an inner conscious, creative processing of information in his own children was too obvious to be denied. Further, the teleological (purposive) and the intentional (consciously focused on an object) features of much psychological discourse cannot be accounted for

by a new language having the elimination of teleology and intentionality as a primary objective. Purposive acts cannot be redescribed as nonpurposive behaviors without loss of essential meaning, and no behaviorist has successfully translated one into the other. There can be thought without speech (silent thought) and speech without thought (parrot's speech). Any act of denying the existence of consciousness, purpose, or intentionality is refuted by that very act; it is a conscious, purposive, intentional event. The stipulation that psychological processes and events are identical with behavioral processes and events is self-contradictory, for two different things cannot be numerically identical. The retort that the psychological and the behavioral are only one thing, not two, begs the question. Critics suspect that the identity of the mental and the behavioral (or the mental and the neurophysiological in central state materialism) is established by decree, not by observation or scientific method. Finally, Watsonian behaviorists solve the problem of other minds with the assurance that no problem exists because there are no minds at all; and for Skinner's behaviorism, minds do not matter.

Some philosophers regard first-person self-knowledge based on direct introspective experience as a great obstacle to the acceptance of behaviorism. To be sure, introspection is not always reliable and is often confused; but direct self-awareness is often quite clear and reliable. We know that we are not always mistaken about what we think, how we feel, what we select, and so on. Critics of behaviorism contend that we know many things about ourselves before, not after, they receive overt expression. For example, authors must solve many conceptual problems before they express their ideas in writing. Most persons can tell whether they are feeling well or ill before they look into the mirror in the morning or bounce their countenances off the countenances of others. They can deceive others about their mental states and processes by playing public roles that do not match their private self-awareness. They can know that they are in great pain while they resolutely sit passively and unresponsively in a dentist's chair. They can make short- and long-range plans for their futures without overtly expressing their purposes. They can change their minds about many things, and no one will ever know.

Nonbehaviorists are convinced that persons frequently know many things directly about their psychological states and processes that are not identical with, and find no expression in, overt behavior. Doubtless, all of these things can be expressed overtly, but often they are not; and self-awareness is not diminished thereby. Also, attempts to establish the identity of mentalistic concepts with behaviors or with internal neurophysiological processes must rely initially upon the self-reports of individual experimental subjects.

Behaviorism, ethical theory, and bioethics.
Other objections to behaviorism arise from its incompatibility with concepts and beliefs that are presupposed in most ethical theories, the moral life, and the practice of bioethics. Apparently, one must either give up behaviorism or abandon much that ethics takes with utmost seriousness, such as consciousness, pleasure and pain, agency or autonomy, freedom, and human dignity, just as Skinner has suggested. In his view, we must move beyond such things.

Consciousness.   Ethics asks questions about right and wrong, good and evil. The notions of intrinsic goodness—that which is desirable or valuable in itself or for its own sake—and intrinsic evil—that which is undesirable and to be avoided for its own nasty sake—are of central importance to ethical theory. In teleological theories of right and wrong, right acts result in intrinsic goodness; wrong acts fail to do so or produce intrinsic evil. Doing good and avoiding or preventing evil are momentous moral duties even in deontological theories, except for Immanuel Kant's. Doing one's duty usually, if not always, involves internal and conscious understanding of and deliberate acting in accord with moral rules. Although ethicists disagree about answers to questions like "What acts are right, or wrong?" or "What things are good, or evil?" there is nevertheless massive agreement that there would be no moral obligation and no intrinsic good or evil in a world without consciousness, that moral right and wrong and intrinsic good and evil exist only in and for conscious beings.

John Stuart Mill, Henry Sidgwick, William James, G. E. Moore (in 1912), Hastings Rashdall, Sir David Ross, Brand Blanshard, William Frankena—almost all philosophers who consider the question—agree that ethics would have no point in a world devoid of conscious beings. Yet Watsonian metaphysical behaviorism gives us just such a world in which all behavior is caused by external or environmental stimuli, and no behavior is caused by inner conscious mental states and processes (such as desires, beliefs, pleasures, pains, and so on). Skinner's radical behaviorism affirms that many activities are spontaneous rather than environmentally caused, but these behaviors are repeated only if their consequences are positively reinforcing. Occasionally, Skinner admits the existence of inner mental states and processes, but he denies their causal efficacy in explaining behavior and their relevance to the science of psychology. They are always the effects of stimuli, never the causes of behavior; and they exist only epiphenomenally, that is, as ineffective appearances. Scientific psychology can disregard them, for the scientific control and prediction of behavior do not require them. If behaviorism is true, however, psychologists can adopt it only because of their social conditioning, never because they are rationally persuaded by the evidence that supports it.

Instead of giving up the notion of consciousness, some behaviorists retain and redefine it in purely behavioral terms—as overt wakeful behavior, as opposed to sleep behavior. Most ethicists, however, are convinced that ethics is concerned with wakefulness itself as directly experienced by conscious subjects, not merely with wakeful behavior as experienced by external observers.

Medical professionals also are concerned with wakeful consciousness itself, not solely with its public expressions. They often prescribe analgesics or other pain management strategies for suffering patients. During invasive medical procedures, general anesthesia is administered not merely to prevent external pain behaviors but also to prevent conscious pains. After a lapse of consciousness, a patient's return to awareness is eagerly awaited. Lost consciousness is the tragedy of comatose patients; and, if it is irreversible, hard decisions must be made about prolonging their survival. Death involves the irreversible loss of embodied consciousness and its necessary physiological conditions. The seriousness of these medical interests seems to be quite incompatible with concern only for overt behavior.

Pleasures and pains.   Philosophical ethicists are keenly interested in consciously experienced pleasures and pains, and medical professionals give considerable attention to conscious pains, if not to pleasures. Most ethicists believe that pointless pains, those that are not necessary for the achievement of goals knowingly and freely accepted, are to be avoided for their own sakes if possible; and most have recognized that happiness, conceived as a surplus of conscious pleasures over pains for extended periods of time, is one of the great goods of life, even if not the only good, as hedonists have held. Medical professionals accept the duties of relieving and not inflicting unnecessary conscious pains as serious professional obligations. Patients want relief from pains, not merely the elimination of pain behaviors. "Pleasures" usually means "conscious qualities of inner feeling that persons or other sentient beings normally wish to cultivate and sustain for their own sake," and "pains" means "conscious qualities of inner feeling which persons or other sentient beings normally wish to avoid and eliminate for their own sake" (Edwards, 1979, pp. 74, 92–96).

Although pain behaviors are indispensable for describing or communicating inner sufferings to others, most ethicists and bioethicists do not believe that overt pain behaviors, completely divorced from conscious sufferings, are intrinsically bad, or that they are duty bound to relieve and not induce pain behavior as such. Reflex responses to pain stimuli may be evoked from irreversibly comatose patients with only brain stem but no upper brain functioning; but no one believes that these patients are thereby subjected to intrinsic evil, or that moral duties are being shirked. No one believes that happiness consists merely of overt manifestations of pleasure. Neither pain behavior nor pleasure behavior is of significance to ethics unless it is indicative of inner conscious pains or pleasures themselves. Skinner maintains that only positive and negative reinforcers, not conscious pleasures and pains, are relevant to a correct theory of good and evil. Primarily, good things are nothing but positive reinforcers, and bad things are nothing more than negative reinforcers. Secondarily, good things may be those stimuli, responses, or consequences that promote cultural survival; and evil things are those that threaten cultural survival. The words "good" and "bad" may also be used to reinforce other behaviors, positively or negatively. Positive reinforcers are stimuli that strengthen the behaviors that produce them, and negative reinforcers are stimuli that reduce or terminate the behaviors that produce them. Just why some stimuli reinforce positively and others negatively is obscure, for Skinner cannot maintain that inner pleasures or pains are the mechanisms that induce or inhibit behaviors. Things that are not causes cannot be causes. Skinner maintains that the identification of values with reinforcers results in a purely descriptive, empirical, scientific ethics that overcomes the "is–ought" gap acknowledged in traditional ethical theory.

Although some philosophers accept Skinner's behaviorist ethics (Hocutt, 1977), others are unconvinced. The latter hold that Moore's "open question" ("Granted that x possesses some descriptive property, but is x good?") is not a senseless or self-answering question when the x is a positive reinforcer. Skinner's position would be immune to this objection, however, if he is interpreted to be answering Moore's question "What things are good?" rather than "What is the meaning of 'good'?"

Skinner's theory contains no purely empirical or descriptive method for resolving value conflicts. When suffering patients beg Stoic physicians for pain medication, the latter may refuse to give it because they believe that patients should be allowed to suffer for their own good, in order to strengthen their characters and powers of resolution. This value conflict is not eliminated by the insight that the patients find pain-relieving behavior to be positively reinforcing, whereas the Stoic physicians find it to be negatively reinforcing. Whether any other theory of the good can resolve value conflicts is another matter, but other theories generally do not claim to offer purely descriptive solutions to value problems. A recommendation by Skinner to give pain medication because doing so has survival value would be a prescriptive, not a descriptive, resolution.

Skinner often prescribes norms. He cannot resolve value disagreements about "good" and "ought" merely by describing what is positively reinforcing to individuals or to their communities of value, those groups of individuals who find similar things to be reinforcing. Skin-

ner's contention that psychology should be a strictly behavioral science does not describe the beliefs and practices of all professional psychologists. It is a value prescription, which, if analyzed in Skinner's own terms, means merely that he and those psychologists who belong to his community of value find it positively reinforcing to do psychology behavioristically. Many psychologists and philosophers are unconverted and cannot accept his narrow strictures on psychological inquiry. Skinner's program, which purports to eliminate purposes and prescriptive norms, can be advanced only purposively and as a prescriptive norm.

Agency, freedom, and dignity. Most philosophical ethicists believe that moral obligation and responsibility presuppose internal autonomous agency or choice, that the denial of the existence or efficacy of conscious informed choice in bringing about moral action is fundamentally incompatible with morality. Ethicists disagree about whether autonomous choice is compatible or incompatible with rigid metaphysical determinism. Some maintain that autonomous choice must be creative and spontaneous, while others hold that conscious choice is sufficient for autonomy even if it is strictly caused. However, ethicists have seldom doubted that consciousness is essential for the enterprise of morality.

Human agency or autonomy is also a central value for most theoretical and practicing bioethicists. Informed voluntary consent is a cardinal ethical principle in modern bioethics. This principle affirms that no diagnostic, therapeutic, or experimental medical procedures should be performed on patients unless they have knowingly and voluntarily consented to them. The principle affirms that the rational agency or autonomy of patients—the capacity of conscious patients to make informed choices—is of paramount importance in the medical setting. When behaviorism affirms that all behaviors result from external or environmental stimuli alone, it denies the reality, or at least the efficacy, of all inner mental processes and activities, including inner understandings and decisions. People are controlled entirely by their circumstances. They never control themselves or their circumstances through their conscious knowledge or efforts. Thus, behaviorism seems to be incompatible with the ideal of informed voluntary consent as it functions in applied bioethics.

Skinner makes only an epiphenomenal (causally ineffective) place for inner self-control, choice, agency, or autonomy. He recognizes that freedom of behavior— that is, behavior minus external constraints—is of some importance because it allows individuals to avoid aversive or negatively reinforcing stimuli. However, in his utopia, *Walden Two*, most important decisions would be made by psychological experts (like himself), not by ordinary individuals. In Skinner's view, human dignity consists in behaviors that cultivate the positive reinforcement of praise or credit from others for behaving well. Again, without denying the importance of both escaping aversive stimuli and cultivating social credit, most moral philosophers would balk at Skinner's behavioral reduction of freedom and dignity to solicitous activity. Behavioral freedom means little without personal autonomy, they would maintain; and human dignity, however difficult to define, is something that persons have as persons. We have it all the time, and it makes us all equals, they insist. Dignity is not just something that we possess during those rare moments when others credit us for behaving ourselves.

In sum, it seems that one must give up either behaviorism or bioethics.

REM B. EDWARDS

Directly related to this article is the companion article in this entry: HISTORY OF BEHAVIORAL PSYCHOLOGY. *Also directly related is the entry* HUMAN NATURE. *For a further discussion of topics mentioned in this article, see the entries* DEATH, DEFINITION AND DETERMINATION OF, *article on* PHILOSOPHICAL AND THEOLOGICAL PERSPECTIVES; *and* INFORMED CONSENT, *article on* MEANING AND ELEMENTS OF INFORMED CONSENT. *For a discussion of agency and freedom, see the entries* AUTONOMY; *and* FREEDOM AND COERCION.

Bibliography

BLANSHARD, BRAND. 1955. *The Nature of Thought,* vol. 1, ch. 9. New York: Macmillan.

BLANSHARD, BRAND, and SKINNER, BURRHUS FREDERIC. 1967. "The Problem of Consciousness—A Debate." *Philosophy and Phenomenological Research* 27:317–337.

CHOMSKY, NOAM. 1964. "A Review of B. F. Skinner's *Verbal Behavior.*" In *The Structure of Language: Readings in the Philosophy of Language,* pp. 547–578. Edited by Jerry A. Fodor and Jerrold J. Katz. Englewood Cliffs, N.J.: Prentice-Hall.

DENNETT, DANIEL CLEMENT. 1978. *Brainstorms: Philosophical Essays on Mind and Psychology.* Montgomery, Vt.: Bradford Books.

EDWARDS, REM BLANCHARD. 1979. *Pleasures and Pains: A Theory of Qualitative Hedonism.* Ithaca, N.Y.: Cornell University Press.

HOCUTT, MAX. 1977. "Skinner on the Word 'Good': A Naturalistic Semantics for Ethics." *Ethics* 87, no. 4:319–338.

MALCOLM, NORMAN. 1964. "Behaviorism as a Philosophy of Psychology." In *Behaviorism and Phenomenology: Contrasting Bases for Modern Psychology,* pp. 141–155. Edited by Trenton W. Wann. Chicago: University of Chicago Press.

MASLOW, ABRAHAM. 1971. *The Farther Reaches of Human Nature.* New York: Viking Press.

MODGIL, SOHAN, and MODGIL, CELIA, eds. 1987. *B. F. Skinner: Consensus and Controversy.* New York: Falmer Press.

RYLE, GILBERT. 1949. *The Concept of Mind.* New York: Barnes and Noble.

SCRIVEN, MICHAEL. 1956. "A Study of Radical Behaviorism." In *The Foundations of Science and the Concepts of Psychology and Psychoanalysis,* pp. 88–130. Edited by Herbert Feigl and Michael Scriven. Minnesota Studies in the Philosophy of Science vol. 1. Minneapolis: University of Minnesota Press.

SKINNER, BURRHUS FREDERIC. 1948. *Walden Two.* New York: Macmillan.

———. 1953. *Science and Human Behavior.* New York: Free Press.

———. 1972. *Beyond Freedom and Dignity.* New York: Alfred A. Knopf.

———. 1974. *About Behaviorism.* New York: Alfred A. Knopf.

TAYLOR, CHARLES. 1964. *The Explanation of Behaviour.* New York: Humanities Press.

WATSON, JOHN BROADUS. 1913. "Psychology as the Behaviorist Views It." *Psychological Review.* 20:158–177.

———. 1914. *Behavior: An Introduction to Comparative Psychology.* New York: Henry Holt.

———. 1930. *Behaviorism.* 2d ed. New York: W. W. Norton.

WITTGENSTEIN, LUDWIG. 1953. *Philosophical Investigations.* New York: Macmillan.

BEHAVIOR MODIFICATION THERAPIES

Since the 1960s and 1970s numerous developments have occurred in both the theory and the practice of behavior therapy. There has been a significant shift away from reliance on models of classical and operant conditioning, derived largely from animal studies, as the theoretical basis for behavior therapy, and toward a more cognitive approach in both theory and practice. These two developments have "humanized" behavior therapy to a great extent. In addition, radical or metaphysical behaviorism has reemerged in a gradual, limited way as a basis for new therapeutic technologies and conceptual formulations. These changes imply a growing recognition by behavior therapists that human behavior is the result of a complex interaction of environmental, social, cognitive, genetic, physiological, and emotional factors (Fishman and Franks, 1992).

Criticisms of early behavior therapy

Behavior therapy, prior to 1970, was strongly criticized by proponents of other therapeutic schools, typically humanistic or psychodynamic, as being mechanistic and authoritarian. It was alleged, for example, that terms such as "behavior control" carried with them the implicit and sometimes explicit message that irrevocable, often involuntary, behavioral changes could be induced by the selective application of conditioning techniques. The protestations of behavior therapists notwithstanding, psychosurgery, electroconvulsive therapy, and the enforced ingestion of psychotropic medications were lumped together with mainstream behavior therapy as further examples of this authoritarian approach to behavior change.

The behavior therapy of this era was also accused of attempting to impose therapist goals on unwilling or unaware clients, and of utilizing punishment and other aversion procedures to bring this about. Behavior therapists, it was believed, had the power to impose their wills upon a hapless society by a sinister manipulation of environmental responses to behavior in the form of carefully chosen rewards and punishments.

Finally, early behavior therapy was viewed by its most extreme critics as a nefarious attempt to maintain an unjust status quo, an imposition of majority demands upon a socially deviant minority (e.g., prisoners, the developmentally disabled, chronic psychiatric patients) helpless to resist the behavioral juggernaut. Behavior therapists were viewed as willing agents of a ruling class unable to tolerate any deviation from the prevailing ethos.

While a small proportion of early behavior-therapy practice did reflect these values to some extent, most behavior therapists eschewed such methods of coercive behavior change, preferring a much more egalitarian approach to therapeutic goal setting and behavior change. Then as now, most behavior therapy techniques lacked the potency to bring about involuntary behavior change. Most behavior therapists, then as now, considered it unethical to "enforce" behavior changes against a client's wishes even when such changes appeared, from the therapist's perspective, to carry with them potential client benefits. Regardless of theoretical basis, the "humanization" of behavior therapy referred to above has resulted in an increasing emphasis on teaching clients "self-control."

Cognitive approaches in behavior therapy

In the early 1970s, behavior therapists began to explore the possibility of integrating cognition and self-guided behavior change (e.g., Bandura, 1977; Beck, 1976; Lazarus, 1981; Mahoney, 1974). With the exception of those who espouse a radical perspective, most cognitive behavior therapists implicitly assume that human behavior is guided in part by an internal "self," which consists of cognitive structures called schemas. Schemas comprise learned patterns of information processing that guide both immediate behavior and general perceptions of the world. These perceptions in turn have a significant impact on affective states. Cognitively oriented behavior therapists believe that, to change behavior, one must change the schemas through which the environmental information is processed. By helping the client

to alter maladaptive schemas, the therapist enables the client to engage in broader, more effective information processing, thereby producing changes in attributions that ultimately lead to changes in both behavior and affect.

Most cognitive approaches to behavior therapy still reflect a primarily linear, mechanistic view of behavior. For example, the rational emotive therapy (RET) of Albert Ellis (1962), one of the earliest attempts at integration of cognitive and behavioral approaches, affirms that emotional states occur as the result of an information-processing sequence in which an external event triggers a set of beliefs (a schema) that in turn triggers an emotional response. Thus, a rational emotive therapist would view the emotion of anger as being triggered by the patient's thoughts about the event to which the patient responded with anger rather than by the event itself. In the view of RET, to paraphrase Shakespeare, nothing is good or bad but thinking makes it so. Effective treatment enables the client to alter irrational beliefs that lead to negative emotional states or other maladaptive behaviors. This is accomplished by directly challenging irrational beliefs in a Socratic fashion and by devising behavioral exercises to assist the client in learning that irrational beliefs are in fact incorrect. For example, in order to combat irrational feelings of shame and self-consciousness, which are presumably based on an irrational fear of sanction or ridicule for particular types of behavior, a rational emotive therapist might assign a client to perform the behavioral exercise of boarding a commuter train and loudly announcing each stop to the other passengers. The objective is to demonstrate that such behavior, absurd and inappropriate though it may seem to the client, does not necessarily evoke public sanction or ridicule, and that even if it does, those responses from others are not catastrophic.

In one form or another, this combination of restructured irrational beliefs and behavioral exercises is the hallmark of most cognitive approaches to behavior therapy. Albert Bandura's (1977) social learning theory, for example, aims at altering specific cognitive structures called "self-efficacy expectations" through teaching clients new behavioral skills and helping these clients practice them both in the therapist's office and in the daily world. Self-efficacy is assumed to determine in part whether or not a given set of environmental contingencies will be responded to with a particular behavior by the client. Therapy consists in part of designing graded behavioral exercises leading to both new behavior and a revision of self-efficacy expectations. Accomplishing these goals is presumed to facilitate a change in client behavior in previously problematic situations.

Research has consistently demonstrated that, in spite of the heavy emphasis by many theorists on the "cognitive" component of "cognitive behavior therapy," the most effective means of promoting both cognitive and behavioral changes is through performance-based treatments—that is, by actively engaging in new behaviors that are incompatible with older, problematic ones (e.g., Rachman and Wilson, 1980). Engaging in new behavior, under the guidance of a therapist seems to be an effective approach to the treatment of a variety of emotional and behavioral disorders. For example, a client who suffers from a fear of cats might be encouraged, with the therapist's assistance, to engage in closer and closer contacts with cats, from merely approaching a cat to actually holding one, until the fear subsides.

Radical behaviorist approaches to behavior therapy

In contrast to cognitively oriented behavior therapists, radical behaviorists reject outright the concept of "self." They view cognition as simply a form of behavior that occurs in correlation to the person's responses to environmental contingencies but is not a cause of those responses. All behavior is presumed to be "caused" by a relationship between external events (contingencies) and behavior. According to radical behavior therapists (cf. Hayes, 1987, 1989; Kohlenberg and Tsai, 1991), people learn sets of "rules" that guide their behavior through the experience of being rewarded or punished for particular behaviors in specific situations. Rules, considered to be verbal representations of environmental contingencies (the relationship between behavior and reward or punishment), are largely determined by the individual's cultural and linguistic milieu and prior learning history. According to radical behaviorists, rules and the linguistic milieu constitute a context that forms the causal matrix within which behavior is produced. Emotional disorders result from rigid adherence to "rules" of behavior that do not apply in a particular context or to misattributing the causes of one's behavior to emotions rather than environmental contingencies. Thus, rules themselves are potential causes of emotional or behavioral problems. A similar situation can arise from responding to inappropriately formed environmental contingencies, usually those derived from the structure of the individual's language. These inappropriately formed contingencies reinforce aspects of a person's subjective experience (e.g., association of emotions with events) in a way that leads the person concerned to misattribute behavior to emotions rather than to the external contingencies that, in the radical behaviorist view, actually cause behavior.

Radical behaviorist approaches to treatment place strong emphasis on the role of an individual's linguistic community and language structure in guiding behavior. Cognition per se is irrelevant except to the degree that thought is a part of the client's use of language. Behavior

change is brought about by teaching new linguistic structures that lead to less affective upset. This is accomplished by attempting to alter the way in which clients use language to form attributions about the causes and meanings of their emotional experience. Most often, this involves teaching clients that emotions are not experiences that can or should be avoided. Rather, they are natural accompaniments to the process of living. Clients are taught to accept and utilize in a positive fashion affective and other inner experiences that their linguistic community has taught them should be avoided or eliminated (e.g., anxiety). Clients are also shown how to alter the contexts (contingencies) that control their behavior. Curiously, in some ways radical behaviorist approaches to behavior therapy are philosophically more similar to psychoanalysis than they are to traditional behavioral or cognitive-behavior therapy, in that clients are taught that negative emotions are a natural part of life and cannot be eliminated. Eschewing mechanistic, linear views, radical behavior therapists prefer to view behavior as the product of an interaction between person and context.

Although formally rejecting any direct consideration of cognition, in other ways radical behaviorist and cognitive approaches to behavior therapy are consistent. For example, radical behavior therapists view the person as an active influencer of an environment that, in turn, influences the person. This is similar to Bandura's notion of reciprocal determinism (1982), a key concept in social learning theory. In addition, both radical and cognitive behavior therapists adopt as a treatment goal empowerment of the client to control aspects of behavior or experience that are presumed to be at the root of his or her problems. While the pathways to change are different, direct attempts to alter thoughts and behavior by cognitively oriented behavior therapists and alteration of environmental or personal contingencies by radical behavior therapists are predicated upon the same goal: enabling people to exert more control over the causes of the problems that brought them to treatment in the first place.

Therapist–client relationships in behavior therapy

From the beginning, most behavior therapists have been intensely concerned with the ethical aspects of the application of behavior therapy, the ethical implications of the relationship between therapist and client, and the role of each in treatment. In contrast to other psychotherapeutic approaches, behavior therapy is characterized by heavy emphasis on the responsibility of the therapist for successful treatment outcome. In behavior therapy, failure to achieve treatment goals is presumed to be the result of therapist errors or environmental hazards beyond the therapist's control rather than of client resistance. The therapist is viewed as an "expert" guide who brings to the situation a body of teachable knowledge. In collegial fashion, as a mutual collaborative process, the patient is shown how to use this knowledge to bring about desired change. In this view, therapeutic failures result from several sources of therapist error: (1) errors in selection of therapeutic goals due to inadequate assessment; (2) errors in the selection, teaching, or application of techniques; (3) failure to consider client values in the selection of therapeutic goals, or the placing of societal or therapist values above those of the client in the process of goal selection; and (4) variables beyond the therapist's control.

While early behavior therapists tended to neglect the importance of a workable therapeutic relationship with the client, as the field has evolved, such issues have become increasingly important in behavior therapy (cf. Wilson and Evans, 1977). Most behavior therapists now recognize that without a therapeutic relationship characterized by mutual respect, empathy, trust, and equality, the first three types of therapist error noted above cannot be avoided, and treatment is unlikely to be successful. An increasing emphasis on thought and feeling leads to recognition that an adequate therapeutic relationship is essential to assessment and treatment. Changes in thoughts and emotions can, in and of themselves, be appropriate outcomes of treatment, as can changes in overt behavior. These changes can be facilitated by the establishment of a good therapeutic relationship.

Ongoing ethical concerns in the practice of behavior therapy

The ethical application of behavior-therapy techniques rests in part on the adequacy of the therapist's relationship to the client and on the therapist's sensitivity to complex social and political values and concerns. Particularly in cases where, at least potentially, the application of a technique can inflict pain, or where clients are relatively powerless or are involuntarily the subject of treatment, areas of ethical concern still remain.

Use of aversion procedures. The use of aversion procedures—the application of subjectively unpleasant stimulation contingent upon performance of an undesirable behavior—has been and remains a source of criticism of behavior therapists. Particularly when procedures such as low-level electric shocks are applied to clients who lack the ability to offer informed consent to the use of those procedures, behavior therapists face a dilemma in which the desirability of treatment outcome goals has to be weighed against the rights of the client. Even when aversion therapy seems to be the best, most rapid means of suppressing other, perhaps more inju-

rious, behavior, such as self-destructive behaviors in clients suffering from pervasive developmental disorders, behavior therapists are ethically bound to attempt to reduce the target behavior through other, nonaversive means before considering an aversion procedure. Only when the target behavior has been conclusively shown to be impervious to other means should aversion therapy be used.

The use of aversion techniques with clients for whom rapid, permanent behavior change is not essential, or for whom there may be some question as to the desire or willingness to change, raises significant ethical concerns. Application of aversion procedures to clients in powerless positions, or where the goals of the agent of behavior change seem directly counter to those of the client, requires careful assessment of the interests of all involved parties, with extra weight perhaps being given to the client's right to be free from external influence over his or her behavior. Practices such as those reported to have occurred in the former Soviet Union, including the use of aversion procedures or drugs for the subjugation of prisoners and psychiatric patients, are clearly not in keeping with the ethical application of behavior therapy or any other form of therapy. When aversion procedures are used, clear guidelines need to be established. Review by an institutional ethics board, to set up extensive safeguards of client rights, has to precede treatment.

Token economies in institutional settings. Token economies are based on the notion that behavior can be changed by systematically rewarding desired behaviors contingent upon performance. Token economies set up a micro economy in which desired behaviors are "rewarded" by contingent distribution of tokens or "points" that later can be exchanged for rewards, often food or privileges. Early proponents of token economies in institutional settings frequently sought to enhance the effects of this process by withholding basic needs, which could be regained only by compliance with token-reinforced behavioral contingencies imposed by therapist fiat. This practice is now judged to be legally as well as ethically unacceptable. Clients forced to reside in facilities where token economies are in effect are entitled to have basic needs for food, shelter, clothing, and social companionship met, regardless of ability to earn token reinforcers. As with the application of aversion procedures, the legitimate parameters of reinforcers need to be clearly spelled out and the application of contingencies monitored through continuing and independent peer review. It is the obligation of the therapist to develop effective reinforcers that are consistent with these values.

Token economies present another ethical and theoretical dilemma: the degree to which behavior changes effected through a token economy either will or should generalize to other settings in which the client may be placed in the future. Much research suggests that the sort of reinforcement contingencies that prevail in most token-economy programs do not characterize most naturally occurring reinforcers. When a client who has learned a new behavior under conditions of monitored and controlled reinforcement in a token economy moves to a setting in which different contingencies apply, there is substantial risk that the new behavior may disappear, leaving the client bereft of adequate, meaningful reinforcers. The consequences of both client and society of such a failure of generalization can be significant. For example, psychiatric patients who acquire workplace social skills in a consistent and regulated token-economy program and then enter a "real world" workplace where reinforcement is inconsistent, may not be able to respond adequately to the new contingencies, and therefore be unable to cope with the new setting even though they functioned well under the token-economy conditions. This may lead to financial inability to live independently, and even to homelessness and the need for welfare benefits that might not have been required had attention been paid to the generalization of token-economy-acquired skills to the world outside. This possibility makes it essential for behavior therapists to address the issues of generalization and maintenance of behavior change across settings.

The image of behavior therapy.   As noted, the image of early behavior therapy among nonbehavioral professionals and the lay public was often extremely negative. Grossly inaccurate notions about the nature of behavior therapy were commonplace, and behavior therapy was lumped with such alien procedures as psychosurgery and Erhard Seminar Training. Such misconceptions are now infrequent. This is due largely to the incorporation of behavior therapy into the mental-health mainstream, to increased sophistication and greater acceptance of behavior therapy by the general public, and, perhaps above all, to the concerted attempts of behavior therapists, both as individuals and as members of professional organizations, to correct these misconceptions and thereby improve the image of behavior therapy.

There is a continuing need to modify misconceptions through well-planned public education. Behavior therapists also need continuing formal training in the maintenance of good ethical practice. Measures of consumer satisfaction are now the rule rather than the exception in both clinical research and treatment. Behavior therapists think increasingly in terms of public relations and the necessity for keeping patients informed at all stages of the intervention process. For example, behavior therapists in private practice are now beginning to make available written descriptions of the treatment procedures and policies for discussion and review before treatment begins (Franks, 1994).

Concluding remarks

Contemporary behavior therapy is characterized by emphasis on client participation in therapeutic goal setting and a balancing of client rights—particularly when the client is relatively powerless—against societal needs, values, and expectations. Even in institutional settings the application of techniques is much less mechanistic and intrusive, and behavior therapists are now trained to apply their techniques only with stringent safeguards of client rights.

An increasing awareness of the roles of thoughts and feelings in the production and maintenance of behavior has led to behavior therapists' becoming more client-centered and humanistic in their approaches to behavior change. This awareness has also produced an increasing emphasis on teaching clients "self"-control techniques rather than "applying techniques to clients" without consideration of the active role the client should play in the process of changing behavior.

By virtue of the inclusion of cognitive and contextual variables in theory and application, contemporary behavior therapy is a considerable advance over early behavior therapy, which was based largely on animal models of learning. Behavior therapy is unique among current psychotherapeutic schools in that practitioners rely on repeated, data-based, objective assessments of client behaviors, thoughts, and feelings to aid in the establishment of therapeutic goals and the continuous assessment of therapeutic progress. Contemporary behavior therapy is a diverse field in which theoretical progress and practice are based on demonstrable advances in scientific knowledge rather than on the pronouncements of authorities or "gurus." Although not yet fully integrated into behavior-therapy practice, developments in basic psychology, human rule-governed behavior (Hayes, 1989), cognitive sciences, and computer science all hold promise for enhancing both treatment efficacy and sensitivity to ethical constraints. As practitioners of a discipline and through organizations such as the Association for Advancement of Behavior Therapy, behavior therapists are learning how to apply these rigorous standards to themselves and their personal interaction with clients, colleagues, students, and society at large.

FREDERICK ROTGERS
CYRIL M. FRANKS

Directly related to this entry are the entries BEHAVIOR CONTROL; *and* MENTAL-HEALTH THERAPIES. *For a further discussion of topics mentioned in this entry, see the entries* ELECTROCONVULSIVE THERAPY; EMOTIONS; PATIENTS' RIGHTS; PSYCHOPHARMACOLOGY; *and* RIGHTS, *article on* RIGHTS IN BIOETHICS. *This entry will find application in the entries* MENTALLY DISABLED AND MENTALLY ILL PERSONS; MENTAL HEALTH; MENTAL-HEALTH SERVICES; *and* MENTAL ILLNESS. *For a discussion of related ideas, see the entries* BEHAVIORISM; FREEDOM AND COERCION; INFORMED CONSENT; PROFESSIONAL–PATIENT RELATIONSHIP; *and* TRUST.

Bibliography

BANDURA, ALBERT. 1977. *Social Learning Theory.* Englewood Cliffs, N.J.: Prentice-Hall.
———. 1982. "Self-Efficacy Mechanism in Human Agency." *American Psychologist* 37, no. 2:122–147.
BECK, AARON T. 1976. *Cognitive Therapy and Emotional Disorders.* New York: International Universities Press.
ELLIS, ALBERT. 1962. *Reason and Emotion in Psychotherapy.* Secaucus, N.J.: Citadel.
FISHMAN, DANIEL B., and FRANKS, CYRIL M. 1992. "Evolution and Differentiation Within Behavior Therapy: A Theoretical and Epistemological Review." In *History of Psychotherapy: A Century of Change,* pp. 159–196. Edited by Donald K. Freedheim. Washington, D.C.: American Psychological Association.
FRANKS, CYRIL M. 1994. "Basic Concepts and Models: Behavioral Model." In *Advanced Abnormal Psychology.* Edited by Vincent B. Van Hasselt and Michel Hersen. New York: Plenum.
HAYES, STEVEN C. 1987. "A Contextual Approach to Therapeutic Change." In *Psychotherapists in Clinical Practice: Cognitive and Behavioral Perspectives,* pp. 327–387. Edited by Neil S. Jacobson. New York: Guilford.
———, ed. 1989. *Rule-Governed Behavior: Cognition, Contingencies, and Instructional Control.* New York: Plenum.
KOHLENBERG, ROBERT J., and TSAI, MAVIS. 1991. *Functional Analytic Psychotherapy: Creating Intense and Curative Therapeutic Relationships.* New York: Plenum.
LAZARUS, ARNOLD A. 1981. *The Practice of Multimodal Therapy: Systematic, Comprehensive, and Effective Psychotherapy.* New York: McGraw-Hill.
MAHONEY, MICHAEL J. 1974. *Cognition and Behavior Modification.* Cambridge, Mass.: Ballinger.
RACHMAN, STANLEY J., and WILSON, G. TERENCE. 1980. *The Effects of Psychological Therapy.* 2d ed. Oxford: Pergamon.
WILSON, G. TERENCE, and EVANS, IAN M. 1977. "The Therapist–Client Relationship in Behavior Therapy." In *Effective Psychotherapy: A Handbook of Research,* pp. 544–565. Edited by Alan S. Gurman and Andrew M. Razin. New York: Pergamon.

BELGIUM

See MEDICAL ETHICS, HISTORY OF, *section on* EUROPE, *subsection on* CONTEMPORARY PERIOD, *article on* THE BENELUX COUNTRIES.

BENEFICENCE

"Beneficence" denotes the practice of good deeds. In contemporary ethics, the principle of beneficence usually signifies an obligation to benefit others or to seek their good. It is a principle of major importance in bioethics and has been prominent in the codes of physicians since antiquity.

Beneficence and benevolence

Beneficence as a principle that guides decisions should be distinguished from the virtue that motivates actors. The *Oxford English Dictionary* defines "beneficence" as "doing good, the *manifestation* of benevolence, or kindly feeling" (emphasis added). This definition bespeaks the etymology of both terms. "Beneficence" is derived from the Latin *bene* (well; from *bonus,* good) and *facere* (to do), whereas "benevolence" is rooted in *bene* and *volens* (a strong wish or intention) (Partridge, 1983). Philosophers who emphasize a more rationalist approach, calculated to guide principled choices, tend to endorse beneficence. Those who see ethics as primarily concerned with virtue, character, and the psychological dimensions of the moral life emphasize benevolence.

David Hume, for example, conceived of benevolence as one of the instincts originally implanted in human nature. Like Joseph Butler, Francis Hutcheson, Adam Smith, and other eighteenth-century English-speaking philosophers, Hume was not so much concerned with ethical problem solving as with describing the role and place of benevolence in the moral topography of human beings. Adam Smith used the term "beneficence," but employed it to describe the virtue of goodwill, and saw it as a moral passion rather than a principle. Of concern to all these philosophers was a task set for them by Thomas Hobbes a century earlier.

Hobbes set the modern polemical context for discussions not only of beneficence and benevolence but also of ethics more generally. His moral philosophy was determinist, denying any capacity for choice based on values, and relativist, denying any independent reference for the terms "good" and "evil": Liberty he saw as merely the ability to enact one's desires, not freedom to deliberate and choose. "Good" and "evil" simply denoted human appetites and aversions. "Will" was just another desire, not a distinctive moral capacity (Hobbes, 1947). Obviously such a philosophy was no place for beneficence as a principle of choice or benevolence as a motivation for the good of others. Ethics devolves into a deterministic egoism. Butler, Hutcheson, Hume, and Smith, in a variety of ways, took as their task a survey of the moral psyche, with special regard for the place of benevolence as something innate or natural to human life.

Unless Hobbes's egoistic portrait is correct, any well-rounded view of ethics will include ways of describing and evaluating both the motivational and character-laden aspects, and the decisional, action-oriented elements of ethics—that is, both benevolence and beneficence.

A principle of beneficence can be broadly or narrowly defined. William Frankena views beneficence as an inclusive principle involving elements of refraining from inflicting harm and preventing or removing evil, as well as an obligation actively to promote good (Frankena, 1973). James Childress adopts Frankena's elements but reclassifies them according to two distinct principles: nonmaleficence, the obligation not to inflict harm; and beneficence, the obligations to prevent harm, to remove harm or evil, and positively to promote good (Childress, 1982). This refinement has the merit of following an intuitive division between refraining and active doing. It elucidates why refraining from harm is usually seen as a universal duty to others, while actively promoting good or helping others is typically seen as a less stringent obligation and often as resulting from specific role obligations (being a parent or a doctor) or contractual agreements. A broader-ranging sense of beneficence is, nevertheless, endorsed by some philosophers. For example, in *The Right and the Good*, W. D. Ross claimed that duties of beneficence are incurred because of "the mere fact that there are other human beings in the world whose condition we can make better . . ." (Ross, 1930, p. 21).

Relation to utility

Beneficence has natural affinities with a principle of utility. Tom Beauchamp and James Childress, for example, claim that promoting good always involves a calculation of what harms might also be incurred (Beauchamp and Childress, 1989). A principle of utility is a way to assess harms and benefits. In his *Utilitarianism*, John Stuart Mill asserted in 1863 that the measure of "good" by which all actions are to be judged is whether they promote the greatest happiness for the greatest number. Mill saw his principle of utility as a systematic expression of the teaching of Jesus, for example, as embodied in the Golden Rule (Mill, 1979).

When defined through Mill's utility principle, beneficence becomes vulnerable to two criticisms frequently leveled at utilitarianism. The first is the problem of adequacy. A focus on beneficence as the promotion of happiness, to the exclusion of other kinds of goods and obligations, seems too narrow. People value things other than happiness, however broadly defined. Promoting the happiness of others can conflict with treating them fairly or respecting them as persons. The second problem is idealism. For Mill at least, utilitarianism presented a stringent requirement. "As between his own happiness and that of others utilitarianism requires him to be as strictly impartial as a disinterested and benevolent spectator" (Mill, 1979, p. 16). To count the good of strangers equally with our own good, or that of our families or friends, seems saintly and perhaps impossible to achieve.

These problems have led some philosophers to question utilitarianism as a system but also to see beneficence as only one principle among others, and as usually (if not always) an imperfect or supererogatory duty. While some principle of utility is necessary to enact beneficence, it need not be Mill's rendition. A utility principle that recognized a variety of goods would at least moderate the force of the criticisms above.

Beneficence and autonomy

How beneficence is put into practice depends on how it is modified by other principles. Especially important in this regard is respect for autonomy or self-determination. Another way to put this is to ask whose notion of "good" will be definitive. Respect for autonomy means that "good" will be defined by the recipient of the action rather than the agent. Beneficence not so defined leads to paternalism, in which the beneficent actor overrides or ignores the recipient's ideas of good and imposes his or her own. The history of medical ethics is largely (but not entirely) a history of paternalistic beneficence. In the mid-twentieth century, consistent challenges arose to beneficent paternalism through assertions of patient rights. Defenders of simple paternalism in health-care relationships are now rare, and most ethicists would agree with Erich Loewy that paternalistic actions generally represent a "caricature" rather than a natural extension of beneficence (Loewy, 1991).

Autonomy as a moral principle is historically rooted in freedom as a political principle, to which John Locke's *Second Treatise of Government* (1690) gave definitive expression. Freedom, Locke asserted, is not license "but a *liberty* to dispose, and order as he lists, his person, actions, possessions, and his whole property, within the allowance of those laws under which he is, and therein not to be subject to the arbitrary rule of another, but freely follow his own" (Locke, 1980, p. 32). The eighteenth-century monument to autonomy is the work of the German philosopher Immanuel Kant. Whereas Locke was concerned to protect individuals from the power of the state, Kant focused on freedom of the will. His "practical imperative" requires that others be treated as ends in themselves and never only as a means (Kant, 1959). For Kant this respect for the moral freedom of others was grounded in a recognition of their rational nature. In bioethics this raises the difficult issue of when and to what extent the rational capacities of patients are compromised and in which cases autonomy should give way to medical beneficence.

The grounds for limiting beneficence through respect for autonomy were most powerfully stated by John Stuart Mill. In *On Liberty* (first published in 1859) he cautioned against supposing that the principle of liberty necessitates a "selfish indifference." Indeed, he asserted, "there is need of a great increase of disinterested exertion to promote the good of others." But, he continued, "disinterested benevolence can find other instruments to persuade people to their good than whips and scourges, either of the literal or of the metaphorical sort" (Mill, 1978, p. 74).

While advocacy for autonomy as the preeminent principle of medical ethics was powerful during the 1970s and 1980s, there are still substantial voices for a beneficence-based theory. Edmund Pellegrino and David Thomasma argue that "medicine as a human activity is of necessity a form of beneficence" (Pellegrino and Thomasma, 1988, p. 32). Rather than espousing the older traditions of paternalism, however, they argue for an enlarged beneficence, "beneficence-in-trust"—a non-rights-based approach that includes respect for autonomy but emphasizes a fiduciary grounding for doctor–patient encounters (Pellegrino and Thomasma, 1988). This approach has an advantage over single-principle approaches that ground medical obligations in simple beneficence or simple autonomy, conceived as monolithic norms. Beneficence, unleavened by respect for autonomy, can lead to paternalism, while autonomy alone obviates trust and often deteriorates into indifference. Still the feasibility of trust depends upon shared values and goals, or at least stable role expectations between providers and patients. The greater the pluralism in a society, the less likely it is that the trust Pellegrino and Thomasma commend can be established.

Health professional codes

While beneficence is important to many philosophical and religious systems of ethics, it is central to the health professions. The Hippocratic Oath clearly states that the physician's actions are "for the benefit of the sick" (see Appendix for this and other codes and oaths). The Declaration of Geneva begins with a pledge to "consecrate" one's life to "the service of humanity." The 1980 "Principles" of the American Medical Association opens with the declaration that these principles are established "primarily for the benefit of the patient." The International Code for Nurses devised in 1973 begins with a broad-ranging assertion of beneficence. The "fundamental" responsibility of the nurse, it states, is to promote and restore health, alleviate suffering, and prevent illness.

While duties to specific persons are recognized, the obligation to perform beneficent actions is seen as universal, because the need for nursing services is universal.

The U.S. Code for Nurses of 1976 differs from all physician codes in recognizing that services not only should promote good but also should be guided by the values of those served. The first principle in this formulation asserts the "self-determination of clients." As noted above, self-determination, or autonomy, is frequently seen as a limiting factor in gauging the extent of beneficence, yet this factor is rarely mentioned in the ethical formulations of health professionals. For example, the practice of soliciting consent from patients was evident in medical practices in the United States in the eighteenth century. Yet these solicitations were not commensurate with today's notion of informed consent. Consent was sought in the eighteenth century primarily to enhance therapy rather than to encourage independent decision making by patients (Faden et al., 1986). Jay Katz presses this point by asserting that consent is largely "alien" to medical thinking, which prefers "custody" over "liberty" (Katz, 1984).

Still, claims for the modern uniqueness of informed consent should be viewed with caution, especially when they tend to valorize an "autonomy model" over a "beneficence model" (Faden et al., 1986). It would be anachronistic to believe that eighteenth-century physicians worked with the mid-twentieth-century concept of consent. Yet it is too sweeping and dualistic to believe that, by default, they were under the sway of a "beneficence model." Medical practices, or moral practices more generally, do not lend themselves to easy encapsulation into models, just as beneficence as a practice is not identical with the philosophical principle of beneficence.

While all versions of professional ethics agree that the acceptance of a patient or a client creates a specific obligation of beneficence, some codes go further and talk of a general duty to seek the public good in matters of health. Here the 1847 Code of the American Medical Association is notable. Chapter III of that code enumerates "Duties of the Profession to the Public." Among those listed are vigilance for the welfare of the community, counsel to the public on health matters, and advice about epidemics, contagion, and public hygiene. Twentieth-century medical codes tend to be more parsimonious in their interpretations of what beneficence entails.

Not even the more generous beneficence in the 1847 AMA Code, however, takes it to cover what Charles Fried calls "the duty to work for and comply with just institutions" (Fried, 1978, p. 129). Fried here follows and extends the thinking of Kant, who saw beneficence in terms of a duty of mutual aid (Kant, 1959). Such aid is required because all persons (including ourselves) will at some time need the help of others, so to neglect aiding others would be self-defeating. The societal and public policy implications of beneficence in health care are poorly worked out at present. The issues that require attention include general programs of prevention, medical assistance to specific groups (such as AIDS patients), and health care for the indigent and uninsured. Most proposals for a more equitable healthcare system in the United States build on notions of justice as an independent principle rather than deriving their justifications from an extension of duties of beneficence.

Limits

If beneficent duties are more than supererogatory, or optional, a persistent issue is how to discern their proper scope. Where do obligations to benefit others end? Are we morally required to give away all our surplus income and, beyond that, to chasten ourselves to more modest patterns of consumption? Are physicians obligated never to say "no" to patients so long as any thread of hope for improvement exists? Would beneficence require acceptance of higher taxes to fund universal health coverage, or does acting for my fellow citizens' good require me to die cheaply and forgo expensive treatments with low probability of benefit?

Beneficent duties may be limited in two ways. The first limiting force is duties to oneself. Self-respect, and an appropriate attention to one's own well-being, will of necessity restrict activities for the good of others, unless beneficence is given a preemptive place and is conflated with saintliness. Hume, for example, believed persons can be "too good," carrying "attention for others beyond the proper bounds," blunting a due sense of pride and the self-assertive virtues (Hume, 1966, p. 93). A second kind of limit involves our psychological capacity for identification of and sympathy with those who could use our help. The press of human suffering that could be alleviated by our actions is immense. To conceive of this larger and seemingly inexhaustible world of suffering as our charge would likely be debilitating. Jonathan Glover has suggested that a restricted but feasible beneficence may be the price we pay for our sanity (Glover, 1977). Limits to the duty to promote good restrict us, but also orient and direct our finite capacities. But perhaps the greater risk is that we will draw a circle around duties in a niggardly fashion, that our imagination will not be too large, risking paralysis, but too stingy and self-serving. It is this narrow and parochial tendency that concerns the advocates of a robust and extensive beneficence.

Relational selves

The recent challenges to ethical theory from psychological studies of moral experience have profound implications for beneficence. In 1982 Carol Gilligan published her research on the moral development of women, entitled *In a Different Voice*. She claimed that females tend to see moral problems in terms of relationships. They are prone to think of their choices in problem solving as issues of care and responsibility for those relationships. By contrast, males tend to see moral problems in terms of rules and principles, and are prone to think of their choices as logical adjudications. Women's moral orientations tend toward valuing and preserving ties among persons, while men's tend toward abstract thinking by an agent largely removed from and impartial to the parties involved (Gilligan, 1982). Gilligan's claim is not that there are precise gender types for moral experience but that the model of the moral self as an abstract, isolated, principled, and hierarchical thinker is insufficient.

Consider the case of Jake and Amy, two eleven-year-olds, who discuss the question "When responsibility to oneself and responsibility to others conflict, how should one choose?" (Gilligan, 1982, pp. 35ff.). While Jake adjudicates these responsibilities as if it were a problem of rule application, Amy's response is pragmatic and assumes a relational self. Jake seeks fairness in the manner of a judge; Amy is concerned to see that others' needs are met and relationships are nurtured. The point is not so much that Jake and Amy offer different answers but that they see different issues, and see themselves in different ways.

The implications for a principle of beneficence in bioethics, and in the ethical codes of health professionals, are substantial. Gilligan's research directly challenges the adequacy of thinking of beneficence simply as a principle to be applied to cases, and recommends a notion of beneficence grounded in complex, relational understandings of the self. Hence, the issues of beneficence can no longer be formulated as if the agent were essentially solitary and could contemplate the scope of his or her duties from afar. The self is already, and essentially, immersed in a web of convivial responsibilities. The ethical formulations of most health professions exhibit precisely the hierarchical distancing and the assumption of optional relationships depicted in the "male" model. Attending to the second voice in moral experience would mean moving bioethics beyond an exhaustive reliance on applying beneficence, as a principle, to problem cases. It would also mean taking the ethical codes of health professionals beyond the contract model and into a recognition of a deeper and more integral bond between healers and the sick, and between health professionals and society.

LARRY R. CHURCHILL

Directly related to this entry are the entries AUTONOMY; BIOETHICS; PATERNALISM; PROFESSIONAL–PATIENT RE-

LATIONSHIP; *and* ETHICS, *article on* NORMATIVE ETHICAL THEORIES. *For a further discussion of topics mentioned in this entry, see the entries* CARE; COMPASSION; HARM; JUSTICE; *and* UTILITY. *The topics in this entry will find application in the entries* CLINICAL ETHICS, *article on* ELEMENTS AND METHODOLOGIES; MEDICINE, ART OF: MENTAL-HEALTH SERVICES; MENTALLY DISABLED AND MENTALLY ILL PERSONS; NURSING, THEORIES AND PHILOSOPHIES OF; RESEARCH METHODOLOGY; *and* RESEARCH POLICY. *For a discussion of benevolent character, see* VIRTUE AND CHARACTER. *See also the* APPENDIX (CODES, OATHS, AND DIRECTIVES RELATED TO BIOETHICS), SECTION II: ETHICAL DIRECTIVES FOR THE PRACTICE OF MEDICINE, OATH OF HIPPOCRATES, *and* CODE OF ETHICS (1847) *of the* AMERICAN MEDICAL ASSOCIATION; *and* SECTION III: ETHICAL DIRECTIVES FOR OTHER HEALTH-CARE PROFESSIONS, CODE FOR NURSES *of the* INTERNATIONAL COUNCIL FOR NURSES.

Bibliography

BEAUCHAMP, TOM, and CHILDRESS, JAMES. 1989. *Principles of Biomedical Ethics.* 3d ed. New York: Oxford University Press.

BEAUCHAMP, TOM, and MCCULLOUGH, LAWRENCE. 1984. *Medical Ethics: The Moral Responsibilities of Physicians.* Englewood Cliffs, N.J.: Prentice-Hall.

CHILDRESS, JAMES F. 1982. *Who Should Decide?: Paternalism in Health Care.* New York: Oxford University Press.

FADEN, RUTH, and BEAUCHAMP, TOM, with NANCY KING. 1986. *A History and Theory of Informed Consent.* New York: Oxford University Press.

FRANKENA, WILLIAM. 1973. *Ethics.* 2d ed. Englewood Cliffs, N.J.: Prentice-Hall.

FRIED, CHARLES. 1978. *Right and Wrong.* Cambridge, Mass.: Harvard University Press.

GILLIGAN, CAROL. 1982. *In a Different Voice: Psychological Theory and Women's Development.* Cambridge, Mass.: Harvard University Press.

GLOVER, JONATHAN. 1977. *Causing Death and Saving Lives.* London: Penguin.

HOBBES, THOMAS. 1947. *Leviathan.* Edited by Michael Oakeshott. New York: Oxford University Press.

HUME, DAVID. 1966. [1777]. *An Enquiry Concerning the Principles of Morals.* 2d ed. La Salle, Ill.: Open Court.

KANT, IMMANUEL. 1959. *Foundations of the Metaphysics of Morals.* Translated by Lewis White Beck. New York: Macmillan.

KATZ, JAY. 1984. *The Silent World of Doctor and Patient.* New York: Free Press.

LOCKE, JOHN. 1980. [1690]. *Second Treatise of Government.* Edited by Crawford B. MacPherson. Indianapolis: Hackett.

LOEWY, ERICH. 1991. *Suffering and the Beneficent Community: Beyond Libertarianism.* Albany: State University of New York Press.

MILL, JOHN STUART. 1978. [1859]. *On Liberty.* Indianapolis: Hackett.

———. 1979. [1863]. *Utilitarianism.* Indianapolis: Hackett.

PARTRIDGE, ERIC. 1983. *Origins: A Short Etymological Dictionary of Modern English.* New York: Greenwich House.

PELLEGRINO, EDMUND D., and THOMASMA, DAVID C. 1988. *For the Patient's Good: The Restoration of Beneficence in Health Care.* New York: Oxford University Press.

ROSS, W. D. 1930. *The Right and the Good.* Oxford: At the Clarendon Press.

BENEFIT–COST

See ECONOMIC CONCEPTS IN HEALTH CARE; *and* HEALTH-CARE RESOURCES, ALLOCATION OF, *article on* MACROALLOCATION. *See also* TECHNOLOGY, *article on* TECHNOLOGY ASSESSMENT; *and* UTILITY.

BENEFIT–HARM

See HARM. *See also* TECHNOLOGY, *article on* TECHNOLOGY ASSESSMENT.

BENEFIT–RISK

See RISK. *See also* ECONOMIC CONCEPTS IN HEALTH CARE; *and* TECHNOLOGY, *article on* TECHNOLOGY ASSESSMENT.

BENELUX COUNTRIES

See MEDICAL ETHICS, HISTORY OF, *section on* EUROPE, *subsection on* CONTEMPORARY PERIOD, *article on* THE BENELUX COUNTRIES.

BEREAVEMENT

See DEATH; DEATH, ATTITUDES TOWARD; DEATH EDUCATION; *and* PASTORAL CARE.

BIODIVERSITY

See ENDANGERED SPECIES AND BIODIVERSITY.

BIOETHICS

"There is," says the biblical book of Ecclesiastes, "no new thing under the sun." Those words are worth pondering in light of the emergence of the field of bioethics since the 1950s and 1960s. From one perspective it is a wholly modern field, a child of the remarkable advances in the biomedical, environmental, and social sciences. Those advances have brought a new world of expanded scientific understanding and technological innovation, seeming to alter forever what can be done about the vulnerabilities of nature and of the human body and mind, and about saving, improving, and extending human lives. Yet from another perspective, the kinds of questions raised by these advances are among the oldest that human beings have asked themselves.

They turn on the meaning of life and death, the bearing of pain and suffering, the right and power to control one's life, and our common duties to each other and to nature in the face of grave threats to our health and well-being. Bioethics represents a radical transformation of the older, more traditional domain of medical ethics; yet it is also true that, since the dawn of history, healers have been forced to wrestle with the human fear of illness and death, and with the limits imposed by human finitude.

It is wholly fitting that an encyclopedia of bioethics devote some of its space to defining and understanding the field that it would examine in both breadth and depth. Yet that is not an easy task with a field that is still evolving and whose borders are hazy. The word "bioethics," of recent vintage, has come to denote not just a particular field of human inquiry—the intersection of ethics and the life sciences—but also an academic discipline; a political force in medicine, biology, and environmental studies; and a cultural perspective of some consequence. Understood narrowly, bioethics is simply one more new field that has emerged in the face of great scientific and technological changes. Understood more broadly, however, it is a field that has spread into, and in many places has changed, other far older fields. It has reached into law and public policy; into literary, cultural, and historical studies; into the popular media; into the disciplines of philosophy, religion, and literature; and into the scientific fields of medicine, biology, ecology and environment, demography, and the social sciences.

The focus here will be on the broader meaning, place, and significance of bioethics. The aim will be to determine not only what the field means for specific ethical problems in the life sciences, but also what it has to say about the interaction of ethics and human life, and of science and human values. Bioethics is a field that ranges from the anguished private and individual dilemmas faced by physicians or other health-care workers at the bedside of a dying patient, to the terrible public and societal choices faced by citizens and legislators as they try to devise equitable health or environmental policies. Its problems can be highly individual and personal—what should I do here and now?—and highly communal and political—what should we together do as citizens and fellow human beings?

While the primary focus of this entry will be on medicine and health care, the scope of bioethics—as the encyclopedia as a whole makes clear—has come to encompass a number of fields and disciplines broadly grouped under the rubric "the life sciences." They encompass all those perspectives that seek to understand human nature and behavior, characteristically the domain of the social sciences, and the natural world that provides the habitat of human and animal life, primarily the population and environmental sciences. Yet it is the medical and biological sciences in which bioethics found its initial impetus, and in which it has seen the most intense activity. It thus seems appropriate to make that activity the center of attention here.

Historical background

An understanding of the emergence of bioethics will help to capture the panoramic breadth and complexity of the field. The 1960s is a pertinent point of departure, even though there were portents of the new field and issues in earlier decades. That decade brought into confluence two important developments, one scientific and the other cultural. In biomedicine, the 1960s was an era of extraordinary technological progress. It saw the advent of kidney dialysis, organ transplantation, medically safe abortions, the contraceptive pill, prenatal diagnosis, the widespread use of intensive-care units and artificial respirators, a dramatic shift from death at home to death in hospitals or other institutions, and the first glimmerings of genetic engineering. Here was a truly remarkable array of technological developments, the palpable outcome of the great surge in basic biomedical research and application that followed World War II. At the same time, stimulated by Rachel Carson's book *Silent Spring,* there was a gradual awakening to the environmental hazards posed by the human appetite for economic progress and the domination of nature (Carson, 1962). Taken together, these developments posed a staggering range of difficult, and seemingly new, moral problems.

Bioethics as a field might not have emerged so strongly or insistently had it not been for parallel cultural developments. The decade was the spawning ground for a dazzling array of social and cultural reform efforts. It saw a rebirth, within the discipline of moral philosophy, of an interest in normative and applied ethics, both out of a dissatisfaction with the prevailing academic emphasis on theoretical issues and in response to cultural upheavals. It was the era of the civil-rights movement, which gave African-Americans and other people of color new rights and possibilities. It was the era that saw the rebirth of feminism as a potent social movement, and the extension to women of rights often previously denied them. It was the era that saw a fresh surge of individualism—a by-product in many ways of postwar affluence and mobility—and the transformation of many traditional institutions, including the family, the churches, and the schools. It was an era that came to see the enormous possibilities the life sciences offer to combat disease, illness, and death—and no less to see science's possibilities for changing the way human beings could live their lives.

Some of these possibilities had been foreseen in the important book *Medicine and Morals,* written by Joseph Fletcher, an Episcopal theologian who eventually came to reject religious beliefs (Fletcher, 1954). He celebrated the power of modern medicine to liberate human beings from the iron grip of nature, putting instead in their hands the power to shape lives of their own choosing. This vision began to be lived out in the 1960s. That decade brought together the medical advances that seemed to foreshadow the eventual conquest of nature and the cultural changes that would empower newly liberated individuals to assume full control of their own destinies. There was in this development both great hope and ambition, and perhaps great hubris, the prideful belief that humans could radically transcend their natural condition.

The advances of the biomedical sciences and their technological application had three great outcomes that came clearly into full view by the 1960s. They transformed first many traditional ideas about the nature and domain of medicine, then the scope and meaning of human health, and, finally, cultural and societal views of what it means to live a human life. Medicine was transformed from a diagnostic and palliative discipline into a potent agent able to cure disease and effectively forestall death. Human "health" more and more encompassed the 1947 World Health Organization definition with its broad emphasis on health as "a state of complete physical, mental, and social well-being and not merely the absence of disease or infirmity." Traditional notions of the living of a life were changed by longer life expectancies, the control of procreation, and powerful pharmacological agents able to modify mood and thought.

The advent of bioethics can be seen as the principal social response to these great changes. If there was any single, overarching question, it might have been this: How were human beings wisely to confront the moral puzzles, perplexities, and challenges posed by the confluence of the great scientific and cultural changes? But this large question concealed an intimidating range of more specific issues. Who should have control over the newly emergent technologies? Who should have the right or privilege to make the crucial moral decisions? How could individuals be assisted in taking advantage of the new medical possibilities or, if need be, protected from being harmed by them? How could the fruits of the medical advances be most fairly distributed? What kind

of character or human virtues would be most conducive to a wise use of the new technologies? What kind of institutions, or laws, or regulations would be needed to manage the coming changes in a moral fashion?

Facts and values

It soon became evident that such questions required more than a casual response. Two important tasks emerged. One of them, logically the first, was to distinguish the domain of science from that of ethics and values. As a consequence of the triumphalist positivism that during the late nineteenth and the first half of the twentieth century had come to dominate the general understanding of science, matters of ethics and values had been all but banished from serious intellectual discussion. A sharp line could be drawn, it was widely believed, between scientific facts and moral values (MacIntyre, 1981b). The former were solid, authoritative, impersonally true, while the latter were understood to be "soft," relativistic, and highly, even idiosyncratically, personal. Moreover, doctors should make the moral decisions no less than the medical decisions; indeed, a good medical decision was tantamount to a good moral decision. The first task of bioethics, then, was to erase the supposedly clear line that could be drawn between facts and values, and then to challenge the belief that those well trained in science and medicine were as capable of making the moral decisions as the medical decisions.

The second important task was to find or develop the methodologies necessary to come to grips with the new moral problems. If there is no sharp line between facts and values, how should their relationship be understood? If there is a significant difference between making a medical (or scientific) decision and making a moral decision, how are those decisions different and what kinds of skills are needed to make the one or the other? Who has a right to make the different kinds of decisions? If it is neither sensible nor fair to think of moral and value matters as soft and capriciously personal, hardly more than a matter of taste, then how can rigor and objectivity be brought to bear on them?

As the scope and complexity of these two large tasks became more obvious, the field of bioethics began to emerge. From the first, there was a widespread recognition that the moral problems would have to be approached in an interdisciplinary way (Callahan, 1973). Philosophy and religion, long the characteristic arenas for moral insight, analysis, and traditions, should have an important place, as should the historical moral traditions and practices of medicine and biology. Ample room would also have to be made for the law and for the social and policy sciences. Moral problems have important legal, social, political, and policy implications; and moral choices would often be expressed through court decisions, legislative mandates, and assorted regulatory devices. Hardly less important was the problem of which moral decisions should be left to private choice and which required some public standards. While there was a strong trend to remove procreational choices from public scrutiny, and thus to move toward the legal use of contraception and abortion, environmental choices were being moved from private choice to governmental regulation. Debates of this kind require the participation of many disciplines.

While the importance of an interdisciplinary approach was early recognized, three other matters were more troublesome. First, what should be the scope of the field? The term "bioethics," as it was first used by the biologist Van Rensselaer Potter, referred to a new field devoted to human survival and an improved quality of life, not necessarily or particularly medical in character (Potter, 1971). The term soon was used differently, however, particularly to distinguish it from the much older field of medical ethics. The latter had traditionally been marked by a heavy, almost exclusive emphasis on the moral obligations of physicians and on the doctor–patient relationship. Yet that emphasis, while still important, was not capacious enough to embrace the huge range of emerging issues and perspectives. "Bioethics" came to refer to the broad terrain of the moral problems of the life sciences, ordinarily taken to encompass medicine, biology, and some important aspects of the environmental, population, and social sciences. The traditional domain of medical ethics would be included within this array, accompanied now by many other topics and problems.

Second, if the new bioethics was to be interdisciplinary, how would it relate to the long-standing disciplines of moral theology and moral philosophy? While those disciplines are able to encompass some interdisciplinary perspectives, they also have their own methodologies, developed over the years to be tight and rigorous. For the most part, moreover, their methodologies are broad, aimed at moral problems in general, not just at biomedical issues. Can they, in their broad, abstract generality, do justice to the particularities of medical or environmental issues?

Another problem becomes apparent. An interdisciplinary field is not necessarily well served by a tight, narrow methodology. Its very purpose is to be open to different perspectives and the different methodologies of different disciplines. Does this mean, then, that although parts of bioethics might be rigorous—the philosophical parts taken by themselves or the legal parts—the field as a whole may be doomed to a pervasive vagueness, never as strong as a whole as its individual parts? This is a charge sometimes leveled against the field, and it has not been easy for its practitioners to find the right balance of breadth, complexity, and analytical rigor.

Varieties of bioethics

As the field has developed, it has become clear that because of the range of diversity of bioethics issues, more than one methodology is needed; by the same token, no single discipline can claim a commanding role. At least four general areas of inquiry can be distinguished, even though in practice they often overlap and cannot clearly be separated.

Theoretical bioethics.   Theoretical bioethics deals with the intellectual foundations of the field. What are its moral roots and what ethical warrant can be found for the moral judgments made in the name of bioethics? Part of the debate turns on whether its foundations should be looked for within the practices and traditions of the life sciences, or whether they have philosophical or theological starting points. Philosophers and theologians have a central place in this enterprise, but draw strongly upon the history and practices of the life sciences to grasp the aims and developments of these fields.

Clinical ethics.   Clinical ethics refers to the day-to-day moral decision making of those caring for patients. Because of that context, it typically focuses on the individual case, seeking to determine what is to be done here and now with a patient. Should a respirator be turned off? Is this patient competent to make a decision? Should the full truth be disclosed to a fearful cancer patient? Individual cases often give rise to great medical and moral uncertainty, and they evoke powerful emotions among those with a role in the decisions. Decision-making procedures, as well as the melding of theory and practice—what Aristotle called "practical reason"—come sharply into play. It is the concreteness of the judgment that is central here: What is to be done for *this* patient at *this* time? The experience of practicing physicians, other health-care workers, and patients themselves takes a prominent place, yet on occasion can require a collaborative interplay with those trained more specifically in ethics.

Regulatory and policy bioethics.   The aim of regulatory and policy bioethics is to fashion legal or clinical rules and procedures designed to apply to types of cases or general practices; this area of bioethics does not focus on individual cases. The effort in the early 1970s to fashion a new legal definition of clinical death (from a heart–lung to a brain-death definition), the development of guidelines for the use of human subjects in medical research, and hospital rules for do-not-resuscitate (DNR) orders are examples of regulatory ethics. It can also encompass policies designed to allocate scarce health-care resources or to protect the environment. Regulatory ethics ordinarily seeks laws, rules, policies, and regulations that will command a wide consensus, and its aim is practical rather than theoretical. The law and the policy sciences are highly important in this kind of bioethics work; but it also requires a rich, on-going dialogue among those concerned with theoretical bioethics, on the one hand, and clinical ethics and political realities, on the other. Regulatory bioethics seeks legal and policy solutions to pressing societal problems that are ethically defensible and clinically sensible and feasible.

Cultural bioethics. Cultural bioethics refers to the effort systematically to relate bioethics to the historical, ideological, cultural, and social context in which it is expressed. How do the trends within bioethics reflect the larger culture of which they are a part? What ideological leanings do the moral theories undergirding bioethics openly or implicitly manifest? A heavy emphasis on the moral principle of autonomy or self-determination can, for example, be said to display the political and ideological bias of culturally individualistic societies, notably the United States. Other nations—those in central and eastern Europe, for instance—give societal rather than individual concerns a more pronounced priority (Fox, 1990). Solidarity rather than autonomy would be their highest value.

The social sciences, as well as history and the humanities, have a central place in this interpretive effort (Marshall, 1992). If done well, the insights and analysis they provide can help everyone to a better understanding of the larger cultural and social dynamic that underlies the ethical problems. Those problems will usually have a social history that reflects the influence of the culture of which they are a part. Even the definition of what constitutes an ethical "problem" will show the force of cultural differences. Countries with strong paternalistic traditions may not consider it necessary to consult with patients about some kinds of decisions; they will not see the issue of patient choice or informed consent as a moral issue at all—yet they may have a far livelier dedication to equality of access to health care.

General questions of bioethics

While bioethics as a field may be understood in different ways and be enriched by different perspectives, at its heart lie some basic human questions. Three of them are paramount. What kind of a person ought I to be in order to live a moral life and to make good ethical decisions? What are my duties and obligations to other individuals whose life and well-being may be affected by my actions? What do I owe to the common good, or the public interest, in my life as a member of society? The first question bears on what is often called an ethic of virtue, whose focus is that of personal character and the shaping of those values and goals necessary to be a good and decent person. The second question recognizes that what we do can affect, for good or ill, the lives of others, and tries to understand how we should see our individual human relationships—what we ought to do for others

and what we have a right to expect from them. The third question takes our social relationships a step further, recognizing that we are citizens of a nation and members of larger social and political communities. We are citizens and neighbors, sometimes acquaintances, and often people who will and must live together in relatively impersonal, but mutually interdependent, ways.

These are general questions of ethics that can be posed independently of the making of biomedical decisions. They can be asked of people in almost any moral situation or context. Here we encounter an important debate within bioethics. If one asks the general question "What kind of person ought I to be in order to make good moral decisions?" is this different from asking the same question with one change—that of making "good moral decisions in medicine"? One common view holds that a moral decision in medicine ought to be understood as the application of good moral thinking in general to the specific domain of medicine (Clouser, 1978). The fact that the decision has a medical component, it is argued, does not make it a different kind of moral problem altogether, but an application of more general moral values or principles. A dutiful doctor is simply a dutiful person who has refined his or her personal character to respond to and care for the sick. He or she is empathic to suffering, steadfast in devotion to patients, and zealous in seeking their welfare.

Another, somewhat older, more traditional view within medicine is that an ethical decision in medicine is different, precisely because the domain of medicine is different from other areas of human life and because medicine has its own, historically developed, moral approaches and traditions. At the least, it is argued, making a decision within medicine requires a detailed and sensitive appreciation of the characteristic practices of medicine and of the art of medicine, and of the unique features of sick and dying persons. Even more, it requires a recognition of some moral principles, such as *primum non nocere* (first, do no harm) and beneficence, that have a special salience in the doctor–patient relationship (Pellegrino and Thomasma, 1981). The argument is not that the ethical principles and virtues of medical practice find no counterpart elsewhere, or do not draw upon more general principles; it is their combination and context that give them their special bite.

The foundations of bioethics

There may not be a definitive resolution to the puzzle of whether bioethics should find its animating moral foundations within or outside medicine and biology. In any case, with time these two sources become mixed, and it seems clear that both can make valuable contributions (Brody, 1987). Perhaps more important is the problem of which moral theories or perspectives offer the most help in responding to moral issues and dilemmas.

Does an ethic of virtue or an ethic of duty offer the best point of departure? In approaching moral decisions, is it more important to have a certain kind of character, disposed to act in certain virtuous ways, or to have at hand moral principles that facilitate making wise or correct choices? The traditions of medicine, emphasizing the complexity and individuality of particular moral decisions at the bedside, have been prone to emphasize those virtues thought to be most important in physicians. They include dedication to the welfare of the patient and empathy for those in pain. Some philosophical traditions, by contrast, have placed the emphasis on principlism—the value of particular moral principles that help in the actual making of decisions (Childress, 1989; Beauchamp and Childress, 1989). These include the principle of respect for persons, and most notably respect for the autonomy of patients; the principle of beneficence, which emphasizes the pursuit of the good and the welfare of the patient; the principle of nonmaleficence, which looks to the avoidance of harm to the patient; and the principle of justice, which stresses treating persons fairly and equitably.

The advantage of principles of this kind is that, in varying ways and to different degrees, they can be used to protect patients against being harmed by medical practitioners and to identify the good of patients that decent medical and health care should serve. Yet how are such principles to be grounded, and how are we to determine which of the principles is more or less important when they conflict? Moral principles have typically been grounded in broad theories of ethics—utilitarianism, for example, which justifies acts as moral on the basis of the consequences of those acts (sometimes called consequentialism). Utilitarian approaches ask which consequences of a choice or an action or a policy would promote the best possible outcome. That outcome might be understood as maximizing the widest range of individual preferences, or promoting the greatest predominance of good over evil, or the greatest good of the greatest number. Just what one should judge as a "good" outcome is a source of debate within utilitarian theory, and a source of criticism of that theory. Such an approach to health-care rationing, for instance, would look for the collective social benefit rather than advantages to individuals.

A competing theory, deontology, focuses on determining which choices most respect the worth and value of the individual, and particularly the fundamental rights of individuals. The question of our basic obligations to other individuals is central. From a deontological perspective, good consequences may on occasion have to be set aside to respect inalienable human rights. It would be wrong, for instance, to subject a human being to dangerous medical research without the person's consent even if the consequences of doing so might

be to save the lives of many others. Our transcendent obligation is toward the potential research subject.

Not all debates about moral theory come down to struggles between utilitarianism and deontology, though that struggle has been central to much of the moral philosophy that influenced bioethics in its first decades. Other moral theories, such as that of Aristotle, stress neither principles nor consequences but see a combination of virtuous character and seasoned practical reason as the most likely source of good moral judgment. For that matter, a morality centering on principles raises the problems of the kind of theory necessary to ground those principles, and of how a determination of priorities is to be made when the principles conflict (Clouser and Gert, 1990). A respect for patient autonomy, stressing the right of competent patients to make their own choices, can conflict with the principle of beneficence if the choice to be made by the patient may actually be harmful. And autonomy can also conflict with the principle of nonmaleficence if the patient's choice would seem to require that the physician be the person who directly brings harm to the patient.

Another classical struggle turns on the dilemma that arises when respect for individual freedom of choice poses a threat to justice, particularly when an equitable distribution of resources requires limiting individual choice. Autonomy and justice are brought into direct conflict. Recent debates on health-care rationing, or setting priorities, have made that tension prominent.

Even if principles—like autonomy and justice—are themselves helpful, their value declines sharply when they are pitted against each other. What are we supposed to do when one important moral principle conflicts with another? The approach to ethics through moral principles—often called "applied ethics"—has emphasized drawing those principles from still broader ethical theory, whose role it is to ground the principles. Moral analysis, then, works from the top down, from theory to principles to case application. An alternative way to understand the relationship between principles and their application, far more dialectical in its approach, is the method of "wide reflective equilibrium." It espouses a constant movement back and forth between principles and human experience, letting each correct and tutor the other (Daniels, 1979).

Still another approach is that of casuistry, drawn from methods commonly used in the Middle Ages. In contrast with principlism, it works from the bottom up, focusing on the practical solving of moral problems by a careful analysis of individual cases (Jonsen and Toulmin, 1988). A casuistical strategy does not reject the use of principles but sees them as emerging over time, much like the common law that has emerged in the Anglo-American legal tradition. Moral principles derive from actual practices, refined by reflection and experience.

Those principles are always open to further revision and reinterpretation in light of new cases. At the same time, a casuistical analysis makes prominent use of analogies, employing older cases to help solve newer ones. If, for instance, general agreement has been reached that it is morally acceptable to turn off the respirator of a dying patient, does this provide a good precedent for withdrawing artificially provided hydration and nutrition? Is the latter form of care morally equivalent to the former, so that the precedent of the former can serve to legitimate the latter? Those are the kinds of questions that a casuistical analysis would ask. At the same time, a casuistical analysis runs the risk of being too bound to past cases and precedents. It can seem to lack the capacity to signal the need for a change of moral direction (Arras, 1991).

Still another principle-oriented approach proposes a new social contract between medicine and society (Veatch, 1981). Such a contract would be threefold. It comprises basic ethical principles for society as a whole, a contract between society and the medical profession about the latter's social role, and a contract between professionals and laypersons that spells out the rights and prerogatives of each. This strategy is designed both to place the ethics of medicine squarely within the ethical values of the larger society and to make sure that laypeople have sufficient choice and power to determine the kind of care they, and not paternalistic physicians, choose. Still another approach, more skeptical about finding any strong consensus on ethical foundations, stresses an ethic of secular pluralism and social peace, devising a minimal ethic for the community as a whole but allowing great play to the values and choices of different religious and value subcommunities (Engelhardt, 1986).

Contemporary feminist approaches to bioethics, like casuistry, reject the top-down rationalistic and deductivist model of an ethic of principles (Baier, 1992; Sherwin, 1992). They reject even more adamantly what is seen as the tendency of an ethic of principles to universalize and rationalize. Feminist ethics lays a far heavier emphasis on the context of moral decisions, on the human relationships of those caught in the web of moral problems, and on the importance of feeling and emotion in the making of moral decisions. Feminist approaches, rooted in ways of thinking about morality that long predate the feminist movement of recent decades, also reflect a communitarian bias, reacting against the individualism that has been associated with a principle-oriented approach. Feminist thinkers commonly argue that those who lack power and status in society are often well placed to see the biases even of those societies that pride themselves on equality. While feminism has gained considerable prominence in recent years, it is only one of a number of efforts to find fresh methods and strategies for ethical analysis and understanding. These include phenomenological analyses, narrative-based strategies, and hermeneutical, interpretive perspectives (Zaner, 1988; Brody, 1987).

How important is moral theory?

There can be little doubt that the quest for the foundations of bioethics can be difficult and frustrating, no less so than the broader quest for the foundations of ethics in general (MacIntyre, 1981a). Yet how important for bioethics are moral theory and the quest for a grounding and comprehensive theory? Even the answers to that question are disputed. At one extreme are those who believe that bioethics as a discipline cannot expect intellectual respect, much less legitimately affect moral behavior, unless it can show itself to be grounded in solid theory justifying its proposed virtues, principles, and rules. At the other extreme are those who contend that even if there is no consensus on theory, social, political, and legal agreement of a kind sufficient to allow reasonable moral decisions to be made and policy to be set can be achieved. The President's Commission for the Study of Ethical Problems in Medicine and Biomedical and Behavioral Research of the early 1980s, and the National Commission for the Protection of Human Subjects in the mid-1970s, were able to achieve considerable agreement and gain general public and professional respect even though individual members disagreed profoundly on the underlying principles of the consensus. There is of course nothing new in that experience. The American tradition of freedom of religion, for instance, has been justified for very different reasons, both theological and secular—reasons that in principle are in fundamental conflict with each other, yet are serviceable for making policy acceptable to believers and nonbelievers alike.

What kind of authority can a field so full of theoretical and practical disputes have? Why should anyone take it seriously? All important fields, whether scientific or humanistic, argue about their foundations and their findings. Bioethics is hardly unique in that respect. In all fields, moreover, agreement can be achieved on many important practical points and principles even without theoretical consensus. Bridges can be built well even if theoretical physicists disagree about the ultimate nature of matter. But perhaps most important, one way or another, moral decisions will have to be made, and they will have to made whether they are well grounded in theory or not. People must do the best they can with the material at hand. Even in the absence of a full theory, better and worse choices can be made, and more or less adequate justification can be offered. As the field progresses, even the debates on theory can be refined, offering greater insight and guidance even if the theories are still disputable.

Where, then, lies the expertise and authority of bioethics (Noble, 1982)? It lies, in the end, in the plausible insight and persuasive rationality of those who can reflect thoughtfully and carefully on moral problems. The first task of bioethics—whether the issues are clinical, touching on the decisions that must be made by individuals, or policy-oriented, touching on the collective decisions of citizens, legislators, or administrators—is to help clarify *what* should be argued about. A closely related task will be to suggest *how* these issues should be argued so that sensible, moral decisions can be made. Finally, there will be the more advanced, difficult business of finding and justifying the deepest theories and principles. There can, and will, be contention and argument at each of these stages, and it well may appear at first that no resolution or agreement can be found. Endless, unresolved disagreement in fact rarely occurs in practice, and that is why, if one looks at bioethics over a period of decades, achieved agreement and greater depth can be found, signs of progress in the field. The almost complete acceptance of such concepts as "patient rights," "informed consent," and "brain death," for instance—all at one time heatedly disputed concepts—shows clearly enough how progress in bioethics is and can be made.

Making good moral decisions

Good individual decision making encompasses three elements: self-knowledge, knowledge of moral theories and traditions, and cultural perception. Self-knowledge is fundamental because feelings, motives, inclinations, and interests both enlighten and obscure moral understanding. In the end, individual selves, alone with their thoughts and private lives, must wrestle with moral problems. This sort of struggle often forces one to confront the kind of person one is, to face one's character and integrity and one's ability to transcend narrow self-interest to make good moral decisions. And once a decision is made, it must be acted upon. A decision of conscience blends moral judgment and the will to act upon that judgment (Callahan, 1991). A complementary kind of knowledge, not easy to achieve, is also needed. Even as individuals we are social creatures, reflecting the times in which we live, embodied in a particular society at a particular time. Our social embeddedness will shape the way we understand ourselves, the moral problems we encounter, and what we take to be plausible and feasible responses to them. Moral theory by itself is hardly likely to be able to give us all the ingredients needed for an informed, thoughtful moral judgment. Only if it is complemented by self-understanding and reflectiveness about the societal and cultural context of our decisions, can moral theory be fleshed out sufficiently to be helpful and illuminating.

Good moral judgment requires us to move back and forth among the necessary elements: the reflective self, the interpreted culture, and the contributions of moral theory. No one element is privileged; each has an indispensable part to play.

Yet something else is needed as well: a vision of the human good, both individual and collective. The biomedical, social, and environmental sciences produce apparently endless volumes of new knowledge about human nature and its social and natural setting. However, for that knowledge to be useful or meaningful, it must be seen in light of some notions of what constitutes the good of human life. What should human beings seek in their lives? What constitute good and worthy human ends? Proponents of the technological advances that emerge from the life sciences claim they can enhance human happiness and welfare. But that is likely to be possible only to the extent we have some decent idea of just what we need to bring us happiness and an enhanced welfare.

Bioethics must pay sustained attention to such issues. It cannot long and successfully attend only to questions of procedure, or legal rules and regulations, without asking as well about the ends and goals of human life and activity. Ethical principles, rules, and virtues are in part a function of different notions of what enhances human life. Implicitly or explicitly, a picture of human life provides the frame for different theories and moral strategies of bioethics. This picture should animate living a life of our own, in which we develop our own understanding of how we want to live our individual lives, given the vast array of medical and biological possibilities; living our life with other human beings, which calls up ideas of rights and obligations, bonds of interdependency, and the creation of a life in common; and living our life with the rest of nature, which has its own dynamics and ends but provides us with the nurturing and natural context of our human lives.

Is there such a thing as *the* human good, either individually or collectively? Is there something we can, in an environmental context, call *the* good of nature? There is no agreement on *the* answer to those questions; on the contrary, there is fundamental disagreement. Some would argue that ethics can proceed with a relatively thin notion of the human good, placing the emphasis on developing those moral perspectives that would make it most possible to live with our differences about the meaning and ends of life. Others stress the importance of the substantive issues and reflect some basic doubt about whether ethics can proceed very far, or have sufficient substance, without trying to gain some insight into, and agreement upon, those basic matters (Kass, 1985; Callahan, 1993). Those debates must continue.

The greatest power of the biomedical, social, and environmental sciences is their capacity to shape the way we as human beings understand ourselves and the world in which we live. At one level—the most apparent—they give us new choices and thus new moral dilemmas. At another level, however, they force us to confront established views of our human nature, and thus to ask what we should be seeking: What kind of people do we want to be? A choice about artificial reproduction, say surrogate motherhood, is surely a moral choice. But it is also a way into the question of how we should understand the place of procreation in our private lives and in society. To see that is to appreciate profound challenges to our understanding of sexual and familial roles and purposes. The boundaries of bioethics cannot readily be constrained. The expanding boundaries force us to take up larger and deeper problems, much as a small stone tossed into the water creates larger and larger ripples.

Summary

In its early days, contemporary bioethics was generally seen as an activity on the fringes of research and practice in the life sciences; it had no place within environmental analysis. The dominant view was that the life sciences were a strictly scientific endeavor, with questions of morality and values arising only now and then in the interstices. That view has gradually changed. The life sciences are increasingly understood as, at their core, no less a moral endeavor than a scientific one. Ethics lies at the very heart of the enterprise, if only because facts and values can no longer be clearly separated—any more than the ends of the life sciences can be separated from the means chosen to pursue them.

No less important, questions of the moral means and ends of the life sciences cannot be long distinguished from the moral means and ends of the cultures and societies that pursue and deploy them. Here, fundamental questions must be asked. First, what kind of medicine and health care, what kind of stance toward nature and our environment, do we need for the kind of society we want? Such a question presupposes that we have some end in view for our society, though that may not be all that clear. What *is* clear, however, is that it is almost impossible to think for long about bioethics without being forced to think even more broadly about the society in which it will exist and whose ends—for better or worse—it will serve.

The second question reverses the first: What kind of a society ought we to want in order that the life sciences will be encouraged and helped to make their best contribution to human welfare? The contribution bioethics makes will in great part be a function of the goals sought by the life sciences, and those in turn will be stimulated or formed by society's goals. The life sciences shape the way we think about our lives, and thus they increasingly provide some key ingredients in society's vision of itself and in the lives of the citizens who comprise society.

Understood in terms of these two broad questions, bioethics takes its place at the heart of the enterprise of the life sciences. Only a part of its work will bear on dealing with the daily moral dilemmas and ethical puzzles that are part of contemporary health care and environmental protection. A no less substantial part will be to help shape the social context in which those dilemmas and puzzles play themselves out. At its best, bioethics will move back and forth between the concreteness of necessary individual and policy decisions and the broad notions and dynamic of the human situation. It is still a new field, seeking to better define itself and to refine its methods. It has made a start in shaping its direction and possible contribution, but only a start.

DANIEL CALLAHAN

Directly related to this entry is the entry MEDICAL ETHICS, HISTORY OF. *For a further discussion of topics mentioned in this entry, see the entries* ANIMAL WELFARE AND RIGHTS; CARE; CASUISTRY; CLINICAL ETHICS; ENVIRONMENTAL ETHICS; ETHICS; TECHNOLOGY; UTILITY; *and* VIRTUE AND CHARACTER. *This entry will find application in the entries* ANIMAL RESEARCH; BIOETHICS EDUCATION; LAW AND BIOETHICS; MEDICINE, ANTHROPOLOGY OF; MEDICINE, SOCIOLOGY OF; PUBLIC POLICY AND BIOETHICS; *and* RESEARCH, HUMAN: HISTORICAL ASPECTS. *For a discussion of related ideas, see the entries* HUMAN NATURE; INTERPRETATION; *and* VALUE AND VALUATION. *See also the* APPENDIX (CODES, OATHS, AND DIRECTIVES RELATED TO BIOETHICS).

Bibliography

ARRAS, JOHN D. 1991. "Getting Down to Cases: The Revival of Casuistry in Bioethics." *Journal of Medicine and Philosophy* 16, no. 1:29–51.

BAIER, ANNETTE C. 1992. "Alternative Offerings to Asclepius?" *Medical Humanities Review* 6, no. 1:9–19.

BEAUCHAMP, TOM L., and CHILDRESS, JAMES F. 1989. *Principles of Biomedical Ethics.* 3d ed. New York: Oxford University Press.

BRODY, BARUCH A. 1988. *Life and Death Decision Making.* New York: Oxford University Press.

BRODY, HOWARD. 1987. *Stories of Sickness.* New Haven, Conn.: Yale University Press.

CALLAHAN, DANIEL. 1973. "Bioethics as a Discipline." *Hastings Center Studies* 1, no. 1:66–73.

———. 1993. *The Troubled Dream of Life: Living with Mortality.* New York: Simon & Schuster.

CALLAHAN, SIDNEY CORNELIA. 1991. *In Good Conscience: Reason and Emotion in Moral Decision Making.* San Francisco: HarperSanFrancisco.

CARSON, RACHEL. 1962. *Silent Spring.* Boston: Houghton Mifflin.

CHILDRESS, JAMES F. 1989. "The Normative Principles of Medical Ethics." In *Medical Ethics,* pp. 27–48. Edited by Robert M. Veatch. Boston: Jones & Bartlett.

CLOUSER, K. DANNER. 1978. "Bioethics." In vol. 1 of *Encyclopedia of Bioethics,* pp. 115–127. Edited by Warren T. Reich. New York: Free Press.

CLOUSER, K. DANNER, and GERT, BERNARD. 1990. "A Critique of Principlism." *Journal of Medicine and Philosophy* 15, no. 2:219–236.

DANIELS, NORMAN. 1979. "Wide Reflective Equilibrium and Theory Acceptance in Ethics." *Journal of Philosophy* 76, no. 5:256–282.

ENGELHARDT, H. TRISTRAM, JR. 1986. *The Foundations of Bioethics.* New York: Oxford University Press.

FLETCHER, JOSEPH F. 1954. *Morals and Medicine: The Moral Problems of: The Patient's Right to Know the Truth, Contraception, Artificial Insemination, Sterilization, Euthanasia.* Boston: Beacon.

FOX, RENÉE C. 1990. "The Evolution of American Bioethics: A Sociological Perspective." In *Social Science Perspectives on Medical Ethics,* pp. 201–217. Edited by George Weisz. Philadelphia: University of Pennsylvania Press.

HOFFMASTER, BARRY. 1991. "The Theory and Practice of Applied Ethics." *Dialogue* 30, no. 2:213–234.

JONSEN, ALBERT R., and TOULMIN, STEPHEN E. 1988. *The Abuse of Casuistry: A History of Moral Reasoning.* Berkeley: University of California Press.

KASS, LEON R. 1985. *Toward a More Natural Science: Biology and Human Affairs.* New York: Free Press.

MACINTYRE, ALASDAIR. 1981a. "A Crisis in Moral Philosophy: Why Is the Search for the Foundations of Ethics So Frustrating?" In *The Roots of Ethics: Science, Religion, and Values,* pp. 3–20. Edited by Daniel Callahan and H. Tristram Engelhardt, Jr. New York: Plenum.

———. 1981b. *After Virtue.* Notre Dame, Ind.: University of Notre Dame Press.

MARSHALL, PATRICIA A. 1992. "Anthropology and Bioethics." *Medical Anthropology Quarterly* 6, no. 1:49–73.

NOBLE, CHERYL N. 1982. "Ethics and Experts." *Hastings Center Report* 12, no. 3:7–9.

PELLEGRINO, EDMUND D., and THOMASMA, DAVID C. 1981. *A Philosophical Basis of Medical Practice: Toward a Philosophy and Ethic of the Healing Professions.* New York: Oxford University Press.

POTTER, VAN RENSSELAER. 1971. *Bioethics: Bridge to the Future.* Englewood Cliffs, N.J.: Prentice-Hall.

SHERWIN, SUSAN. 1992. *No Longer Patient: Feminist Ethics and Health Care.* Philadelphia: Temple University Press.

TOULMIN, STEPHEN. 1981. "The Tyranny of Principles." *Hastings Center Report* 11, no. 6:31–39.

VEATCH, ROBERT M. 1981. *A Theory of Medical Ethics.* New York: Basic Books.

ZANER, RICHARD M. 1988. *Ethics and the Clinical Encounter.* Englewood Cliffs, N.J.: Prentice-Hall.

BIOETHICS EDUCATION

I. Introduction
    Stephen G. Post
II. Medicine
    Lachlan Forrow and Robert Arnold
III. Nursing
    Mila A. Aroskar and Anne J. Davis
IV. Other Health Professions
    Ruth B. Purtilo
V. Secondary and Postsecondary Education
    Drew Lader

I. INTRODUCTION

Bioethics interests everyone concerned with the interface of technology, nature, and human nature; as a result, it has been a highly successful addition to educational curricula. This article introduces the goals and conceptual components of bioethics education. The articles that follow focus on the teaching of bioethics at different educational levels and in various professional contexts.

Bioethics is present in curricula from secondary to postgraduate education. While codes of ethics have had a perennial place in the education of health professionals, bioethics as an interdisciplinary field of wide educational appeal emerged in the early 1970s as the social and ethical implications of advances in biological science and health care became matters of public concern and sometimes consternation. This field encompasses the full spectrum of ethical issues in the life sciences, health, and health care.

The "biological revolution" of the late twentieth century forces a confrontation with such basic questions as the genetic malleability of humankind, what it means to be human, what our relations with other species and with nature in general have been and ought to be, and how medical technology can best serve rather than oppress us. Because the questions bioethics responds to are of the highest significance, they must not be left to an intellectual or professional elite, but must be considered by the wider society that is regularly challenged by new developments in the life sciences and health care.

Goals of bioethics education

Bioethics education is designed to sensitize students to the range of issues that the life sciences, health, and health care present. One of the first summaries of the issues for the bioethics curriculum, written under the auspices of the American Association for the Advancement of Science, included genetics, reproductive technologies, human and animal experimentation, behavior control, health care, death and dying, population control, environmental ethics, scientific research, and the physician–patient relationship (Kieffer, 1975). Thus bioethics was conceived to encompass both medical and nonmedical issues. Since the early 1970s, courses in bioethics have varied with respect to emphasis, but a thorough introductory course includes a wide range of issues similar to the above list. The basic content of the field was most clearly defined for an international audience with the 1978 publication of the *Encyclopedia of Bioethics*. This work included articles on such diverse topics as the therapeutic relationship, codes of professional ethics, health-care justice and systems, biomedical and behavioral research, mental-health and behavioral issues, sexuality, contraception, sterilization, abortion, genetic issues, reproductive technologies, organ and tissue transplantation, death and dying, population ethics, and environmental ethics.

A second goal of bioethics education is to aid students in developing skills in ethical analysis, drawing on tools of logic and ethical theory, sociology, literature, religious ethics, history, and anthropology. Because many of the questions bioethics raises challenge cherished beliefs or address areas people—especially young people—have not grappled with before, reasonable discussion can be difficult to establish and is sometimes supplanted by acrimony. Bioethics courses must insist on an environment of mutual respect and tolerance for disparate viewpoints. Many of the standard texts in the field present a spectrum of positions on each issue, reprinting seminal articles by numerous authors (e.g., Beauchamp and Walters, 1994). Such texts expose students to differing perspectives, and press students to clarify their own presuppositions. Rigorous attention to the canons of logical argument and a readiness to consider all coherent positions with seriousness are expected. Bioethics courses require students to go beyond merely making free assertions of moral beliefs or judgments; reasons must be based in a set of basic principles and their interpretation.

A general course in bioethics challenges students to reflect on the appropriate balance between moral universalism and moral relativism in ethics. While the understanding and tolerance of diverse moral viewpoints is important, no one can coherently claim to be a pure moral relativist, for we all condemn certain harmful actions as wrong. Most people can agree on a basic principle such as "do no harm," but this does not indicate consensus on when a developing fetus comes under the protective umbrella of this principle or on when someone is considered dead and therefore beyond harm or on whether nonhuman animals have moral rights. However, such areas of accepted disagreement should not obscure basic areas of moral consensus.

While some issues in bioethics such as abortion or mercy killing admit no obvious solution, other issues do. For example, most people condemn the murderous Nazi experiments conducted during the Holocaust that resulted in the formulation of the Nuremburg Code, or the racism that pervaded the notorious Tuskegee Syphilis Study (1932–1972) in the United States. Teachers of bioethics must assert shared universal moral condemnations while at the same time challenging students to seriously consider differences in culture and world view. Some critics of philosophically shaped bioethics teaching have emphasized the importance of introducing into bioethics courses more cross-cultural perspectives (Marshall, 1992; Weisz, 1990).

Health-care ethics

Health-care ethics is that part of bioethics focused on the delivery of health care, on patient obligations and rights, and on the ethics of the providing professions, including medicine, nursing, and dentistry. Among the major topics considered in courses are refusal or withdrawal of treatment, quality of life, definitions of death, definitions of health and disease, paternalism, informed consent, confidentiality, truth-telling, conflict of interest, professional codes, advance directives such as living wills, research ethics, and analysis of specific clinical cases (Anderson and Glesnes-Anderson, 1987).

In the medical ethics courses offered in most U.S. medical schools, curriculum goes beyond the goal of sensitizing students to issues (Clouser, 1980). According to the Dartmouth Report, a consensus statement prepared by leaders in the field, these courses should also provide medical students and physicians "with the conceptual, moral-reasoning, and interactional abilities to deal successfully with most of the moral issues they confront in their practice" (Culver et al., 1985). While medical ethics as a cognitive discipline can be taught, the influence it has on behavior depends largely on integrating it into the clinical training years and on the example set by clinical faculty (Arnold et al., 1988). Inattention to medical ethics in the later years of medical education suggests to students that ethics is unimportant, despite their earlier exposure to lectures (Pellegrino, 1989).

Teaching medical ethics.   Teaching medical ethics is an international concern. The British Institute of Medical Ethics task force on the teaching of medical ethics emphasized that instruction should occur at regular intervals throughout medical training (Boyd, 1987). A 1990 study of ethics teaching in London-area medical schools indicated that attendance was low in optional courses (Burling et al., 1990). A 1989 study in Germany found a need for more systematic curricula and required courses (Heister and Seidler, 1989).

The goals of ethics teaching for nurses in the United States include the examining of professional values in relation to the care of patients, engaging in ethical reflection, developing skill in moral judgment, and reflecting on issues having policy implications (Fry, 1989). In the early twentieth century, the teaching of courses combining ethics and etiquette in nursing schools was common, but this began to change during the 1950s. In the 1970s, ethics teaching experienced a renaissance; it is now a significant part of the curriculum in 85 percent of nursing schools (Fry, 1989). Ethics courses also exist in schools of pharmacy, occupational therapy, dentistry, and other health-care professions (American Association of Dental Schools, 1989).

In contrast to general bioethics education in a philosophy, psychology, biology, or religion department, courses in professional health-care ethics do, to some extent, certify the student as meeting standards of knowledge and behavior for professional practice. In some cases, state boards have required remedial courses in ethics for professionals against whom complaints of unethical conduct have arisen (Waithe and Ozar, 1990). But the student who lacks basic appreciation for central moral principles—for example, nonmaleficence, confidentiality, veracity, respect for persons—does not have the essential moral consciousness or commitments in which good professional behavior must be grounded. Therefore, the teacher of ethics cannot certify that increased knowledge implies behavioral reform. While courses in professional ethics do much to refine reflective powers and assist in the understanding of moral dilemmas, they cannot be expected to remedy serious flaws in moral character (Waithe and Ozar, 1990). Exemplary mentoring may be of some benefit in such cases.

Building a curriculum.   Courses in health-care ethics, even though present in some form in most U.S. schools of medicine and nursing, struggle to maintain sufficient time in the curriculum. The constant pressure to accommodate more rote memorization in the basic biomedical sciences can relegate ethics lectures and courses to the margins of the schedule. In the late 1980s, Steven H. Miles argued convincingly that medical ethics, while accepted in the medical curriculum, was not yet mature, and that its future contours remained unclear (Miles et al., 1989).

While teaching should be case-based and draw on student experiences when possible, it must simultaneously convey the basic principles of ethics under which cases can be meaningfully analyzed, and it must provide students with significant appreciation for the history of abuse in areas such as human experimentation, health-care access, psychosurgery, behavior control, and genetic screening. Students must understand their profession at its very best and at its very worst.

Every health-care professional in training should have an understanding of basic ethical principles, an appreciation for the past, including paradigm clinical and legal cases to enunciate the significance of these principles, and the ability to recognize and articulate the ethical aspects of his or her everyday clinical experience.

Teaching methodologies vary (Coutts, 1991a). A significant number of useful videos are available (Coutts, 1991b). Effective teachers can be health-care professionals with a deep knowledge of the clinical ethics literature, or they can be trained in the humanities and have a significant knowledge of the clinical environment (Fletcher, 1973). Some teachers use literature effectively, while others succeed with ethics readings from clinical journals and philosophy (Brock and Ratzan, 1988; Coles, 1989). Outside the classroom or the clinical ethics consultation, hospital ethics committees have a major role in educating health-care professionals and other staff on issues in ethics (Barlotta and Scheirton, 1989).

While debates over methodology will continue in the field of bioethics as they do in all other fields, bioethics education is a firmly established and widely accepted part of curricula. As rapid changes emerge in the life sciences and in health care, we must ask where these changes are taking us, and if they add to or detract from the good. Charting a wise future requires investment in education and the involvement of thoughtful teachers from myriad professions and disciplines.

STEPHEN G. POST

Directly related to this article are the other articles in this entry, which discuss bioethics education in MEDICINE, NURSING, OTHER HEALTH PROFESSIONS, *and* SECONDARY AND POSTSECONDARY EDUCATION. *For a further discussion of topics mentioned in this article, see the entries* ALLIED HEALTH PROFESSIONS; BIOETHICS; DENTISTRY; MEDICAL CODES AND OATHS, *especially the article on* HISTORY; NURSING ETHICS; PHARMACY; RACE AND RACISM; REHABILITATION MEDICINE; RESEARCH, UNETHICAL; *and* SOCIAL WORK IN HEALTH CARE. *For a further discussion of related ideas, see the entries* CASUISTRY; CLINICAL ETHICS, *article on* ELEMENTS AND METHODOLOGIES; EMOTIONS; *and* PASTORAL CARE. *Other relevant material may be found under the entries* DEATH EDUCATION; ETHICS, *article on* RELIGION AND MORALITY; IMPAIRED PROFESSIONALS; INFORMED CONSENT, *article on* HISTORY OF INFORMED CONSENT; LITERATURE; MEDICAL EDUCATION; PRISONERS, *article on* TORTURE AND THE HEALTH PROFESSIONAL; *and* PROFESSION AND PROFESSIONAL ETHICS. *See also the* APPENDIX (CODES, OATHS, AND DIRECTIVES RELATED TO BIOETHICS), *introductory article on* THE NATURE AND ROLE OF CODES

AND OATHS; SECTION II: ETHICAL DIRECTIVES FOR THE PRACTICE OF MEDICINE; *and* SECTION III: ETHICAL DIRECTIVES FOR OTHER HEALTH-CARE PROFESSIONS.

Bibliography

AMERICAN ASSOCIATION OF DENTAL SCHOOLS. 1989. "Curriculum Guidelines on Ethics and Professionalism in Dentistry." *Journal of Dental Education* 53, no. 2:144–148.

ANDERSON, GARY R., and GLESNES-ANDERSON, VALERIE A., eds. 1987. *Health Care Ethics: A Guide for Decision Makers.* Rockville, Md.: Aspen Publication.

ARNOLD, ROBERT M.; FORROW, LACHLAN; WARTMAN, STEVEN A.; and TENO, JOAN. 1988. "Teaching Clinical Medical Ethics: A Model Programme for Primary Care Residency." *Journal of Medical Ethics* 14, no. 2:91–96.

ARRAS, JOHN D. 1991. "Getting Down to Cases: The Revival of Casuistry in Bioethics." *Journal of Medicine and Philosophy* 16, no. 1:29–51.

BARLOTTA, FLORA M., and SCHEIRTON, LINDA S. 1989. "The Role of the Hospital Ethics Committee in Educating Members of the Medical Staff." *HEC Forum* 1, no. 3:151–158.

BEAUCHAMP, TOM L., and WALTERS, LEROY. 1994. *Contemporary Issues in Bioethics.* 4th ed. Belmont, Calif.: Wadsworth.

BOYD, KENNETH M., ed. 1987. *Report of a Working Party on the Teaching of Medical Ethics.* London: Institute of Medical Ethics.

BROCK, D. HEYWARD, and RATZAN, RICHARD M., eds. 1988. *Literature and Bioethics.* Baltimore: Johns Hopkins University Press.

BURLING, S. J.; LUMLEY, J. S. P.; MCCARTHY, L. S. L.; MYTTON, J. A.; NOLAN, J. A.; SISSOU, P.; WILLIAMS, D. G.; and WRIGHT, L .J. 1990. "Review of the Teaching of Medical Ethics in London Medical Schools." *Journal of Medical Ethics* 16, no. 4:206–209.

CAELLEIGH, ADDEANE S., ed. 1989. *Academic Medicine* 64, no. 12:699–788. Special issue, "Teaching Medical Ethics."

CLOUSER, K. DANNER. 1980. *Teaching Bioethics: Strategies, Problems and Resources.* New York: The Hastings Center.

COLES, ROBERT. 1989. *The Call of Stories: Teaching and the Moral Imagination.* Boston: Houghton Mifflin Co.

COUTTS, MARY CARRINGTON. 1991a. "Teaching Ethics in the Health Care Setting, Part I: Survey of the Literature." *Kennedy Institute of Ethics Journal* 1, no. 2:171–185.

————. 1991b. "Teaching Ethics in the Health Care Setting, Part II: Sample Syllabus." *Kennedy Institute of Ethics Journal* 1, no. 3:263–273.

CULVER, CHARLES M.; CLOUSER, K. DANNER; GERT, BERNARD; BRODY, HOWARD; FLETCHER, JOHN; JONSEN, ALBERT; KOPELMAN, LORETTA; LYNN, JOANNE; SIEGLER, MARK; and WIKLER, DANIEL. 1985. "Basic Curricular Goals in Medical Ethics." *New England Journal of Medicine* 312, no. 4:253–256.

FLETCHER, JOHN C. 1973. "Who Should Teach Medical Ethics?" *Hastings Center Report* 3, no. 6:4–6.

FRY, SARA T. 1989. "Teaching Ethics in Nursing Curricula: Traditional and Contemporary Models." *Nursing Clinics of North America* 24, no. 2:485–497.

HEISTER, ELISABETH, and SEIDLER, EDUARD. 1989. "Ethik in der ärztlichen Ausbildung an den Hochschulen der Bundesrepublik Deutschland." *Ethik in der Medizin* 1:13–23.

JONSEN, ALBERT R. 1991. "American Moralism and the Origin of Bioethics in the United States." *Journal of Medicine and Philosophy* 16, no. 1:113–130.

KIEFFER, GEORGE H. 1975. *Ethical Issues and the Life Sciences.* Washington, D.C.: American Association for the Advancement of Science.

MARSHALL, PATRICIA A. 1992. "Anthropology and Bioethics." *Medical Anthropology Quarterly* 6, no. 1:49–73.

MILES, STEVEN H.; LANE, LAURA W.; BICKEL, JANET; WALKER, ROBERT M.; and CASSELL, CHRISTINE K. 1989. "Medical Ethics Education: Coming of Age." *Academic Medicine* 64, no. 12:705–714.

PELLEGRINO, EDMUND D. 1989. "Can Ethics Be Taught? An Essay." *Mt. Sinai Journal of Medicine* 56, no. 6:490–494.

WAITHE, MARY ELLEN, and OZAR, DAVID T. 1990. "The Ethics of Teaching Ethics." *Hastings Center Report* 20, no. 4:17–21.

WEISZ, GEORGE, ed. 1990. *Social Science Perspectives on Medical Ethics.* Philadelphia: University of Pennsylvania Press.

II. MEDICINE

Education in medical ethics is as old as medical education itself. The Hippocratic school of medicine of fourth-century Greece is best remembered for the Hippocratic oath, which has provided moral guidance to students of medicine for more than two millennia.

For most of medicine's history, efforts to inculcate ethical precepts relied on the apprenticeship model, through which medical students are guided in the simultaneous development of their knowledge, technical skill and judgment, and evolving sense of proper professional conduct (Bosk, 1979). Direct observation and emulation were the primary methods apprentices used to develop clinical judgment regarding right action.

However, in the second half of the twentieth century, the emerging field of biomedical ethics catalyzed a radical reexamination of the ways in which students learn to understand and manage ethical issues that arise in professional medical practice. Initially, this effort was led by nonphysician humanists—philosophers, theologians, and others, who developed interests in applied ethics and the medical humanities. In the early 1970s, medical schools, led by Penn State University, hired these humanists and began to offer first elective, then required, ethics courses for medical students. Rather than concentrating on the importance of mentorship and role modeling, these courses were rooted in a philosophical model, stressing ethical concepts such as autonomy and the importance of learning to apply ethical principles to discern the proper course of action. Lectures and seminars became the dominant method used to teach these cognitive skills. The differences in goals and methods between an apprenticeship model and philosophical model of teaching medical ethics have continued to arise in current debates over medical ethics education.

The growth of medical ethics education

A series of empirical studies in the 1970s and 1980s documented the rapid growth of teaching programs. In a 1974 survey, ninety-seven of 107 responding medical schools reported teaching medical ethics (Veatch and Solitto, 1976). Only six of these schools, however, reported a required exposure to medical ethics. In 1982, a majority of physicians reported that they had never received formal education in clinical ethics, and many felt inadequately prepared for common ethical problems in medicine (Pellegrino et al., 1985). A 1985 study found that 84 percent of U.S. medical schools had some form of human values curricula during the first two years (Bickel, 1986). By 1989, forty-three of 127 U.S. medical schools reported separate required courses in medical ethics (Miles et al., 1989).

It was not until the latter part of the 1980s that educators began to advocate explicit teaching in medical ethics during residency training, a critical formative period, since it is during their residency that physicians first acquire decision-making responsibilities, and thus can fully appreciate the relevance of medical ethics to patient care. In 1984, researchers found that residents in 40 percent of internal medicine residencies had no formal exposure to clinical ethics teaching (Povar and Keith, 1984). Two reports by influential specialty organizations in the 1980s provided strong impetus to the development of teaching programs during the residency years. In 1983, the American Board of Internal Medicine published a statement on "Evaluation of Humanistic Qualities in the Internist" (American Board of Internal Medicine, 1983). In 1987, the Medical Ethics Subcommittee of the American Board of Pediatrics published "Teaching and Evaluation of Interpersonal Skills and Ethical Decisionmaking in Pediatrics" (American Board of Pediatrics, 1987). Since then, a growing number of other boards have issued recommendations regarding the teaching of medical ethics during residency.

There was a long tradition of teaching medical deontology (study of moral obligation) in both Europe and Latin America, particularly in Catholic medical schools. The 1980s, however, saw in these countries, as in North America, a steady expansion of the number and scope of medical ethics programs. In Great Britain, the General Medical Council created a committee in 1984 to study the teaching of medical ethics in British medical schools and make recommendations. The resulting 1987 Pond Report recommended that the teaching of medical ethics be encouraged in medical school, but no specific guidelines were advocated (Institute of Medical Ethics, 1987). A later study evaluating the effects of the Pond Report found that twelve responding medical schools all reported teaching medical ethics, but with optional attendance at all but two schools (Burling et al., 1990). As a result, only those students who had a prior interest in ethical issues were likely to attend courses, and the majority of students continued to lack any formal training in ethics.

A 1991 study in Canada found that fifteen of the sixteen Canadian medical schools provided medical ethics education and some sort of examination, with the number of required hours ranging from 10.5 to 45 (Baylis and Downie, 1991). Almost all of the schools used physicians as instructors and focused on specific ethical issues (e.g., euthanasia), as opposed to ethical theory or professional codes of ethics.

In numerous other countries, medical schools have developed curricula in medical ethics. As early as 1977, the University of Nijmegen in the Netherlands reported having a strong medical ethics component in every year of medical training (DeWachter, 1978). At Lagos University in Nigeria, two-day workshops were initiated in 1982 for fourth-year students, at which lawyers, doctors, and patients all participated in lectures and discussions of issues in medical ethics (Olukoya, 1984).

During this period of rapid growth in formal medical ethics education, a wide variety of activities were subsumed under the general heading of "ethics programs." There was great variability in the establishment of explicit curricular goals, the identification and support of teaching faculty, the teaching methods that were employed, and the attempts (if any) at evaluation of educational success. Although a degree of consensus evolved for some areas, important areas of controversy remain.

Goals

Ambitious and diverse goals have been proposed for medical ethics education, including increased awareness of ethical issues; a cultivation of basic ethical commitments; more humane medical practice; tolerance toward conflicting views; development of analytic skill in moral reasoning; enhanced intellectual development in ethics and the humanities; positive attitudes toward patients; less paternalism in clinical practice; higher professional conduct; and improved clinical decision making (Callahan, 1980; Miles et al., 1989).

Despite this dauntingly heterogeneous list, a consensus developed regarding some core objectives. First, the primary goal of clinical ethics education is to prepare physicians to deal effectively with ethical issues in clinical practice. Accomplishing this requires that students learn to: (1) recognize ethical issues as they arise in clinical care and identify hidden values and unacknowledged conflicts; (2) think clearly and critically about ethical issues in ways that lead to an ethically justifiable course of action; and (3) apply the practical skills needed to implement an ethically justifiable course of action. Each of these objectives in turn requires that the students possess specific knowledge, attitudes, and skills.

To recognize ethical issues as they appear in clinical care usually requires a positive attitude concerning the importance of the humanistic and value-laden aspects of medical care. For example, a physician's decision regarding chemotherapy for a woman with breast cancer involves his or her awareness of the biomedical issues and morbidity and mortality, as well as of the patient's own views regarding continued life, her body image, and the morbidity of treatment. Recognizing the presence of an ethical issue also requires knowledge of the nature of common ethical issues and how they arise in clinical practice. Finally, proficiency in recognizing these issues requires students to learn certain behaviors. A highly motivated student who understands the importance of autonomy and recognizes the ways in which patients' values are frequently ignored or overridden will still have difficulty incorporating respect for autonomy into care unless he or she becomes skilled in eliciting his or her patients' personal values, concerns, and goals.

A general consensus was also developed in the 1980s regarding most of the core content areas for medical ethics education. In the 1985 report of the DeCamp Conference (Culver et al., 1985), leading physicians and ethicists proposed "basic curricular goals in medical ethics," stressing knowledge and ability as the primary targets of medical ethics education in medical schools. Among the seven items in the "minimal basic curriculum" are the ability to obtain a valid consent or a valid refusal of treatment, knowledge of how to proceed if a patient refuses treatment, and knowledge of the moral aspects of the care of patients with a poor prognosis, including patients who are terminally ill. Notably absent from this "core list," due to a lack of consensus, were issues related to financial aspects of medical care (including distributive justice and access to health care) and questions related to abortion.

Building on these earlier reports, subsequent teaching programs increasingly stressed the importance of ensuring that educational goals are appropriate to students' specific level of training and future career choices. Courses for first- and second-year medical students, who

have limited clinical experience, generally focused on developing an awareness of the complex moral issues that arise in contemporary medicine, and on developing skill in moral reasoning. In contrast, teaching programs for physicians in subspecialty residency programs tended to focus on the specific issues that those physicians were already encountering in their fields of practice, and the specific knowledge, attitudes, and skills needed to address those problems.

Methods

Given the diverse objectives of ethics education, it is no surprise that a variety of methods have been developed to help students develop the knowledge, attitudes, and skills needed to become proficient in dealing with ethical issues in clinical practice. Teaching methods ranged from large group lectures providing conceptual and historical overviews of issues in medical ethics, to seminar room discussions of "paper cases," to participation in discussions of actual cases encountered during clinical rotations, to participation in ethics consultation programs, with each of these supplemented by readings and in some cases videotapes or films. Particularly during the clinical years and the years of residency training, there has been a slow but steady increase in the use of practical teaching exercises, with an emphasis on the communication skills deemed necessary for the identification and resolution of ethical problems. Achieving a thorough conceptual understanding of the doctrine of informed consent, for example, was increasingly understood to be of limited value if physicians were not able to explain information clearly to patients.

By the early 1990s, there was widespread agreement that in almost all settings instruction should be primarily case-based, since using real or detailed hypothetical cases emphasizes the difference that clinical ethics can make in actual patient care. In addition, case discussions allow for integrating moral reasoning with the other tasks of patient care.

Some educators, such as David Barnard and Leon Kass, however, have raised concerns about overreliance on the use of the case method in teaching medical ethics (Barnard, 1988; Kass, 1990). Case discussions typically emphasize problem solving and ethical dilemmas, and may ignore essential issues of clinical ethics, such as what constitutes informed consent in routine office care. In addition, by concentrating on what should be done in a specific case, participants often ignore the institutional or interpersonal factors that may have led to the problem. Analyzing the institutional factors that lead to family–physician conflict regarding life-sustaining treatment may be more important in improving ethical care than teaching house staff about when it is ethically justifiable to override surrogate decision makers. Institutional factors play an important and frequently overlooked role in influencing ethical decisions and behavior; discussion of institutional reforms may constitute an essential part of medical ethics education.

In general, mirroring debates in moral philosophy, considerable disagreement has remained about the importance of theory to ethical analysis. Tom L. Beauchamp and James F. Childress, authors of one of the most widely used texts in medical schools, emphasize the important role of the principles of respect for autonomy, nonmaleficence, beneficence, and justice, both as a framework for identifying moral issues and as a structure for moral justification (Beauchamp and Childress, 1989). Others, such as K. Danner Clouser, argue against a primary stress on principles, for both theoretical and pedagogical reasons (Clouser, 1989). In addition to intellectual concerns about the nature of proper moral justification, Clouser and others stress the importance of training students to attend to the highly specific biotechnical, psychological, and social complexities of individual cases in their moral reasoning, reporting that through a series of case discussions, students often arrived inductively at general precepts that they could then apply to other cases.

For different reasons, feminist theorists (Carse, 1991), virtue theorists (Drane, 1988), and casuists also have argued for less emphasis on theoretical principles. Rather than viewing cases as ways to illustrate principles, for example, casuists argue that they are the primary locus of moral meaning (Arras, 1991). Rather than using short, theoretically driven hypothetical cases, casuists encourage the use of real cases that illustrate the complexities and uncertainties of clinical practice. These cases "display the sort of moral complexities and untidiness that demand the (nondeductive) weighing and balancing of competing moral considerations and the casuistical virtues of discernment and practical judgment (phronesis)" (Arras, 1991). Feminists have argued for greater attention to social, economic, and political factors and their effect on the nature and dynamics of health care (Sherwin, 1992). Finally, virtue theorists and feminist theorists "suggest that bioethical discussions should be addressed not only to the question 'What kind of person ought I be?' and 'What traits and capacities ought I to develop?'" (Carse, 1991). In an attempt to enhance students' moral imagination and empathy, and to stress the narrative aspects of medical ethics, some educators have also begun to include literature and films.

Faculty and program development

As in other areas of medical education, the evolution of teaching in medical ethics was heavily shaped by the availability (or, for many programs, scarcity) of qualified faculty. Throughout the 1970s and early 1980s, a central debate involved the question of whether medical ethics teaching should be done primarily by physicians, or by those trained in the humanities, such as philosophy or religious studies. Mark Siegler, for example, stressed the ways in which the knowledge and professional experience of clinicians was central to an understanding of the true complexities and realities of clinical-ethical problems and their possible solutions (Siegler, 1978). He therefore urged that primary teaching responsibility should lie with the physician-ethicist. Respected clinical teachers who emphasize the importance of medical ethics can be important role models who can help shape students' ethical sensibilities. On the other hand, strong reasons for utilizing nonphysicians to teach medical ethics have been offered. First, many important aspects of the identification, analysis, and resolution of ethical problems in medicine do not fall within a physician's own specialized training or expertise, but depend instead on the intellectual background and analytic skills of individuals trained in other disciplines. Second, involving nonphysicians in teaching medical ethics can help sensitize students to the importance of other viewpoints and improve physicians' ability to communicate with nonphysicians—two primary educational goals. This controversy regarding who should teach has largely been replaced by a consensus that a variety of disciplines have important and distinct contributions to make.

The limited number of trained faculty, more than disputes regarding the academic background of those faculty, limited the growth of ethics education. Many programs depended on faculty who, despite an interest in medical ethics, had little formal background in the field. In part to address this shortcoming, the Kennedy Institute of Ethics at Georgetown University developed both an annual "intensive bioethics" week and a Ph.D. program in philosophy with a concentration in medical ethics. By the early 1990s, a number of schools, including the University of Tennessee, the University of Chicago, Harvard University, the University of Pittsburgh, and others, offered year-long fellowship programs or degree programs in medical ethics. In Great Britain, Kings College and the University of Manchester both established postgraduate master's-level courses in medical ethics in 1987, with nurses, doctors, lawyers, and ministers among the students.

A major constraint on the supply of qualified faculty during this period continued to be the limited financial resources available in many medical schools for this teaching. Teaching in the first two years of medical school has traditionally been underwritten by departments' sizable research budgets as well as students' tuition. In addition, these departments generally had an ample supply of more junior instructors, including doctoral and postdoctoral students. During clinical rotations, and also during the residency years, faculty time was also traditionally supported in part by monies raised when faculty see patients. Although all aspects of the medical school and residency program budget were burdened by increasing financial constraints in the 1980s, few institutions ever had funding from research programs or revenues from clinical service that could help support teaching activities in medical ethics. Therefore, such activities primarily depended upon direct financial support from the office of the Dean, from extramural grants, or from the donated time of highly committed faculty.

In their attempts to develop ethics curricula, medical ethics faculty have encountered a number of other barriers, among them time constraints, students' attitudes toward medical ethics, and the lack of reinforcement by other faculty (Strong et al., 1992). Ethics teaching programs occupy a tenuous position in most medical schools; even when present, they are rarely viewed as central to the education of physicians in the way that the "basic sciences" and traditional biotechnical clinical training are.

Evaluation

Evaluation, both of teaching programs themselves and of individual students, is still in its infancy. Most formal courses have included a pass–fail grading system based on class participation and written exercises, usually either papers or in-class essay examinations. These efforts convey to students the importance of medical ethics in the medical school (as has the addition of questions to the National Boards and many of the specialty boards).

Efforts to develop formal and valid evaluation techniques have remained hampered, however, by uncertainty about what specific teaching goals are most important, about how best to measure whether any of those goals have in fact been accomplished, and about what it is realistic to expect from ethics courses. Underlying the challenge to evaluate the impact of teaching medical ethics is a deeper debate regarding what teaching ethics does. Ethics as an academic discipline can be taught; one can evaluate a student's knowledge of ethical concepts and cognitive skills. Philosophers in undergraduate ethics courses have done this for centuries. Most attempts at evaluation in medical school have tried to measure this aspect of the ethics curriculum using essay or short-answer tests.

In arguing for the importance of formal ethics education, teachers of medical ethics typically have emphasized more ambitious goals, such as improving students' ability to address ethical issues in clinical practice or promoting humanistic qualities such as integrity. Efforts at evaluation, however, have not always distinguished among residents' attitudes, knowledge, or behavior.

Moreover, there are numerous methodological problems, particularly in evaluating ethical behavior or character, problems that are compounded if one tries to determine whether improvements are attributable to formal ethics teaching. Some faculty involved in ethics programs question whether stricter standards of evaluation should be required of their curricula, arguing that courses in the traditional areas of anatomy, biochemistry, and physiology have rarely, if ever, been required to prove their ultimate effectiveness.

Attempts to develop innovative methods of evaluation have included measuring students' moral reasoning, evaluating students' behavior by nonphysicians (such as nurses or patients), and using formal tools such as the Objective Standardized Clinical Exercise. These exercises have attempted to move beyond merely evaluating cognitive skills to analyzing students' actual behavior. They remain at an early stage of development as educators debate the conceptual and empirical merits of this and other evaluation methodologies.

Conclusion

While formal teaching programs in medical ethics were practically nonexistent in 1970, by the early 1990s there was extraordinary diversity both in the United States and elsewhere in formal teaching activities from the undergraduate to the postgraduate level. Today bioethics education is an accepted part of education for students in almost all medical schools, and for residents in many programs.

However, despite this growth and an evolving consensus that began in the 1980s regarding some core goals and teaching methods, many questions remain only partially answered. What should the primary goals of such teaching be? How should those goals vary according to the developmental stage of the health professional and according to his or her specific field of practice within medicine? Who are the most appropriate faculty members to lead teaching efforts in various settings? How can the number of qualified faculty be increased? How can financial and institutional support for their work be strengthened? What teaching methods are most effective and efficient in accomplishing curricular goals in each of the various settings? Finally, what is the proper role of formal evaluation efforts, both of individual students and of overall teaching programs? What methods of evaluation are both valid and feasible?

The difficulty in finding answers to these questions ensures that designing and implementing effective medical ethics education will remain challenging well into the next century.

LACHLAN FORROW
ROBERT ARNOLD

Directly related to this article are the INTRODUCTION *and other articles in this entry, which discuss bioethics education in* NURSING, OTHER HEALTH PROFESSIONS, *and* SECONDARY AND POSTSECONDARY EDUCATION. *For a further discussion of topics mentioned in this article, see the entries* BIOETHICS; CLINICAL ETHICS; INFORMED CONSENT, *article on* MEANING AND ELEMENTS OF INFORMED CONSENT; MEDICAL CODES AND OATHS, *article on* HISTORY; *and* MEDICAL EDUCATION. *For a discussion of theories and principles of ethics, see the entries* AUTONOMY; BENEFICENCE; CARE; CASUISTRY; ETHICS, *articles on* TASK OF ETHICS, *and* NORMATIVE ETHICAL THEORIES; JUSTICE; NARRATIVE; NATURAL LAW; *and* UTILITY. *For a discussion of related ideas, see the entry* PROFESSION AND PROFESSIONAL ETHICS. *See also the* APPENDIX (CODES, OATHS, AND DIRECTIVES RELATED TO BIOETHICS), SECTION II: ETHICAL DIRECTIVES FOR THE PRACTICE OF MEDICINE.

Bibliography

AMERICAN BOARD OF INTERNAL MEDICINE, SUBCOMMITTEE ON EVALUATION OF HUMANISTIC QUALITIES IN THE INTERNIST. 1983. "Evaluation of Humanistic Qualities in the Internist." *Annals of Internal Medicine* 99, no. 5:720–724.

AMERICAN BOARD OF PEDIATRICS, MEDICAL ETHICS SUBCOMMITTEE. 1987. "Teaching and Evaluation of Interpersonal Skills and Ethical Decisionmaking in Pediatrics." *Pediatrics* 79, no. 5:829–834.

ARRAS, JOHN D. 1991. "Getting Down to Cases: The Revival of Casuistry in Bioethics." *Journal of Medical Philosophy* 16, no. 1:29–51.

BARNARD, DAVID. 1988. "Residency Ethics Teaching: A Critique of Current Trends." *Archives of Internal Medicine* 148, no. 8:1836–1838.

BAYLIS, FRANÇOISE, and DOWNIE, JOCELYN. 1991. "Ethics Education for Canadian Medical Students." *Academic Medicine* 66, no. 7:413–414.

BEAUCHAMP, TOM L., and CHILDRESS, JAMES F. 1989. *Principles of Biomedical Ethics.* 3d ed. New York: Oxford University Press.

BICKEL, JANET W. 1986. *Integrating Human Values Teaching Programs into Medical Students' Clinical Education.* Washington, D.C.: Association of American Medical Colleges.

BOSK, CHARLES L. 1979. *Forgive and Remember: Managing Medical Failure.* Chicago: University of Chicago Press.

BURLING, S. J.; LUMLEY, J. S. P.; McCARTHY, L. S. L.; MYTTON, J. A.; NOLAN, J. A.; SISSOU, P.; WILLIAMS D. G.; and WRIGHT, L. J. 1990. "Review of the Teaching of Medical Ethics in London Medical Schools." *Journal of Medical Ethics* 16, no. 4:206–209.

CALLAHAN, DANIEL. 1980. "Goals in the Teaching of Ethics." In *Ethics Teaching in Higher Education,* pp. 61–80. Edited by Daniel Callahan and Sissela Bok. New York: Plenum.

CARSE, ALISA L. 1991. "The 'Voice of Care': Implications for Bioethical Education." *Journal of Medicine and Philosophy* 16, no. 1:5–28.

CLOUSER, K. DANNER. 1989. "Ethical Theory and Applied Ethics: Reflections on Connections." In *Clinical Ethics: Theory and Practice,* pp. 161–181. Edited by Barry Hoffmaster, Benjamin Freedman, and Gwen Fraser. Clifton, N.J.: Humana.

CULVER, CHARLES M.; CLOUSER, K. DANNER; GERT, BERNARD; BRODY, HOWARD; FLETCHER, JOHN; JONSEN, ALBERT; KOPELMAN, LORETTA; LYNN, JOANNE; SIEGLER, MARK; and WIKLER, DANIEL. 1985. "Basic Curricular Goals in Medical Ethics." *New England Journal of Medicine* 312, no. 4:253–256.

DRANE, JAMES F. 1988. *Becoming a Good Doctor: The Place of Virtue and Character in Medical Ethics.* Kansas City, Mo.: Sheed and Ward.

DEWACHTER, MAURICE A. M. 1978. "Teaching Medical Ethics: University of Nijmegen, The Netherlands." *Journal of Medical Ethics* 4, no. 2:84–88.

INSTITUTE OF MEDICAL ETHICS (GREAT BRITAIN). WORKING PARTY ON THE TEACHING OF MEDICAL ETHICS. 1987. *Report of a Working Party on the Teaching of Medical Ethics.* Edited by Kenneth M. Boyd. London: IME.

KASS, LEON. 1990. "Practicing Ethics: Where's the Action?" *Hastings Center Report* 20, no. 1:5–12.

MILES, STEVEN H.; LANE, LAURA WEISS; BICKEL, JANET; WALKER, ROBERT M.; and CASSEL, CHRISTINE K. 1989. "Medical Ethics Education: Coming of Age." *Academic Medicine* 64, no. 12:705–714.

OLUKOYA, A. A. 1984. "A Workshop on Medical Ethics at the College of Medicine, Lagos University." *Journal of Medical Ethics* 10, no. 4:199–200.

PELLEGRINO, EDMUND D.; HART, RICHARD J., JR.; HENDERSON, SHARON R.; LOEB, STEPHEN E.; and EDWARDS, GARY. 1985. "Relevance and Utility of Courses in Medical Ethics: A Survey of Physicians' Perceptions." *Journal of the American Medical Association* 253, no. 1:49–53.

POVAR, GAIL J., and KEITH, KARLA J. 1984. "The Teaching of Liberal Arts in Internal Medicine Residency Training." *Journal of Medical Education* 59, no. 9:714–721.

SHERWIN, SUSAN. 1992. *No Longer Patient: Feminist Ethics and Health Care.* Philadelphia: Temple University Press.

SIEGLER, MARK. 1978. "A Legacy of Osler. Teaching Clinical Ethics at the Bedside." *Journal of the American Medical Association* 239, no. 10:251–256.

STRONG, CARSON; CONNELLY, JULIA E.; and FORROW, LACHLAN. 1992. "Teachers' Perceptions of Difficulties in Teaching Ethics in Residencies." *Academic Medicine* 67, no. 6:398–402.

VEATCH, ROBERT M., and SOLITTO, SHARMON. 1976. "Medical Ethics Teaching: Report of a National Medical School Survey." *Journal of the American Medical Association* 235, no. 10:1030–1033.

III. NURSING

Ethics has received renewed attention in nursing education programs. This article provides an overview of nursing ethics education in the United States and in other countries.

Nursing ethics education in the United States

Nursing ethics has been incorporated to some degree in nursing education since the early twentieth century. In the early 1900s, ethics was taught as a science necessary to the education of the competent nurse who put patient safety and welfare first (Robb, 1909). Ethics teaching, reflecting religious and military influences, focused on the character and ethics of the nurse, the virtues required of nurses (e.g., loyalty and obedience), the duties and obligations nurses owed physicians and the hospitals that employed them, and proper etiquette for nurses. Obligations that nurses have as citizens of the community to participate in public policy and political areas to achieve health-care goals emerged in the *Code of Ethics* proposed by the American Nurses' Association (1976) and in the nursing literature of the first half of the twentieth century (Goodrich, 1932; Densford and Everett, 1946; Fowler, 1984). These wider obligations of nurses as citizens continue to be a very minor theme in nursing ethics education. Ethics as a distinct part of the nursing curriculum almost disappeared in the 1950s and 1960s, except in programs affiliated with religious traditions and institutions.

The 1970s brought renewed attention to nursing ethics education, partly because of the resurgence of medical ethics and the appearance of bioethics in the professional and academic worlds. These were responses to challenges emerging from medical technologies, abuses in research, and changes in the health-care environment, challenges for which no ready-made responses were available. Some nurse educators and philosophers recognized, however, that nurses faced ethical issues and challenges different from those faced by physicians, largely because of nurses' positions as employees rather than as independent professionals in health-care organizations. The National Student Nurses' Association and the American Nurses' Association passed resolutions calling for more attention to ethics in nursing education programs.

A survey conducted to assess the status of ethics teaching in accredited baccalaureate and graduate nursing programs (Aroskar, 1977) disclosed that most schools offered limited opportunities for study of ethical aspects of nursing and that these opportunities were often integrated into other nursing courses. Only 7 percent of the programs required work in ethics or medical ethics. Codes of ethics such as the *Code for Nurses* (American Nurses' Association, 1976) were identified as priority content in ethics courses, followed by patients' rights and obligations. No nursing faculty had primary responsibilities for teaching ethics.

Beginning in the late 1970s and early 1980s, nursing ethics education that incorporates values clarification and a more philosophical, principled approach to ethical issues received increased attention in nursing programs. This continuing development depends on administrative support, faculty priorities, interests, and expertise, and varies greatly from school to school. A few nursing programs have full-time faculty in teaching and research activities devoted to ethics in nursing. Usually these are schools with master's and doctoral programs in nursing that offer studies in ethics, bioethics, and philosophy as electives or as a minor field. Teaching resources such as textbooks and nursing journal articles on ethics have increased significantly. Since 1975, activities to enhance the teaching of ethics in nursing have been supported by the Joseph P. Kennedy, Jr., Foundation, the National Endowment for the Humanities, The Hastings Center, the Fund for the Improvement of Post Secondary Education (FIPSE), and other institutions.

Baccalaureate education provides the foundations for professional nursing practice that requires knowledge of ethical obligations of the profession and ethical decision-making skills for the practitioner. Not all baccalaureate nursing programs have required or elective courses in ethics. Ethics education has not been required for program accreditation. Where ethics is a required curriculum component, content may be offered through separate courses or modules (Payton, 1980); integrated throughout the curriculum in existing courses (Ryden et al., 1989); or presented in some combination of separate courses and integrated into classroom and clinical experiences. An overall goal is to develop morally accountable practitioners who have a clear conceptual framework and the skills for ethical decision making in practice (Cassells and Redman, 1989; Fry, 1989).

Sara T. Fry (1989) identified four models of ethics teaching used in undergraduate and graduate nursing programs and clinical settings. (1) The "moral-concepts model" incorporates three general areas: historical foundations of the nursing ethic, including codes of ethics and medical versus nursing ethics; the value dimensions of nursing, such as advocacy, loyalty, and moral obligations; and the skills needed for ethical decision making. (2) The "moral-issues model" focuses on common moral problems in health-care relationships, such as confidentiality and informed consent, and issues of moral concern in health care, such as abortion, termination of treatment, and allocation of health-care resources. Course content includes historical and contemporary legal cases that illustrate the legal and ethical aspects of specific issues in patient care. (3) The "clinical-practice model," developed by bioethicists and nurse ethicists, incorporates clinical conferences on moral issues in patient care usually specific to a clinical area, case-study presentations, and ethics rounds that focus on ethical issues pertaining to a patient's care rather than to a patient's clinical condition. (4) The "ethics-inquiry model," found primarily at the graduate level, incorporates the forms of traditional philosophical inquiry such as descriptive, normative, and metaethics; explores diverse methods of ethical inquiry; and looks at the relationship of ethical inquiry to other forms of inquiry in science and nursing. Additional topics in ethics education include the role of the nurse as a moral agent; roles of gender and ethnicity in nursing ethics; major ethical theories and principles and their application in nursing practice; the ethics of nursing research; and caring as a foundation of nursing ethics.

Examples of specific outcome objectives for nursing ethics education include: identification of ethical dilemmas in the delivery of nursing care; identification of the components of an ethical decision-making framework; participation in ethical decision making in client care; leadership participation in ethics rounds and institutional ethics committees; analysis of impediments to the ethical practice of nursing; distinguishing the ethical elements of nursing practice from medical or technical elements; and analysis of nursing codes as they relate to client advocacy.

There are underlying tensions and ongoing debates in nursing ethics education. Argument continues over the question of whether nursing ethics does or should exist as a separate field of inquiry. Differences have arisen between those who teach ethics based on cognitive-moral-development theory and those who teach ethics based on moral philosophy and ethical theory. Evaluation of the effectiveness of ethics teaching has been a continuing challenge. Although research on ethics in nursing education has been expanding, it needs to be developed more systematically if it is to contribute to effective curriculum change (Silva and Sorrell, 1991). A shortage of adequately prepared faculty and overcrowded nursing curricula impede ethics teaching in nursing programs. These debates, questions, and tensions contribute to the uneven development of nursing ethics education in the United States and other countries.

Nursing ethics education in other countries

The fact that nursing ethics education in the international arena varies so greatly reflects the state of nursing and nursing education, as well as the priority of health-care problems and issues, in many different countries. The lack of systematic, international information about nursing ethics education creates problems in providing a general overview of the topic.

The International Council of Nursing (ICN), headquartered in Geneva, in an effort to address the uneven development of nursing ethics education, has provided ethics education through publications, programs, and conferences. The ICN's code of ethics serves as the nursing code in many countries. Since these countries have different histories, cultures, and priorities, the question arises as to whether or not all countries have common ethical values and principles regarding nursing and nursing education. In addition, much of nursing ethics education in the United States focuses on the issues that arise from advanced medical technology, whereas the main issue in many other countries is primary health care.

In the United Kingdom nursing education is well developed, and higher education has been available to nurses for many years. In some colleges or departments of nursing, ethics is either taught as a separate course or integrated into other courses. During the last few decades of the twentieth century, the Royal College of Nursing has been active in the articulation of nursing ethics. In addition, nurse educators and others have published numerous papers, research reports, and books focused on nursing ethics. A major British nursing journal includes an ethics column that deals with clinical ethical problems. The first journal devoted solely to nursing began publishing in 1994 in London. The Center for Midwifery and Nursing Ethics in London publishes a newsletter, runs educational programs, and serves as a clearinghouse for ethics materials. In 1990, Swansee University in Wales sponsored the first national conference on nursing ethics and nursing ethics education.

In Canada, numerous conferences have focused on nursing ethics and ethics education. An annual conference to discuss philosophy and nursing touches on many ethical themes. Several schools of nursing have invited visiting professors to teach ethics. The Ministry of Health Chief Nurse coauthored a textbook on nursing ethics that has been widely used in education programs in Canada and in other countries (Curtin and Flaherty, 1982). Canada has its own nursing code of ethics.

The ethics committee of the Swiss Nursing Association wrote a code of ethics in the 1980s and has been instrumental in increasing nurses' awareness of the need for more systematic approaches to teaching ethics in nursing programs. In 1986, the association focused its annual conference on ethics and ethical reasoning in curriculum content and clinical practice. For some years, one nurse educator has taught courses both in Switzerland and France on ethical issues in dying and death with a special focus on suffering.

Nurse educators in Finland have offered seminars around the country on nursing ethics. One nurse educator has published a book on the topic. Several nurse educators in Finland and other Nordic countries have conducted research on ethical questions and have participated in a multinational research project examining selected ethical issues that are used in teaching (Davidson et al., 1990; Davis et al., 1993).

The board of directors of the Center for Medical Ethics at the University of Oslo, Norway, consists of people from diverse health-related professions, including nursing. In 1985, this center sponsored a conference on nursing ethics; it has continued to work with nurse educators and nurse researchers in developing educational programs and research focused on ethical issues.

Both Norway and Sweden have invited nurse educators from overseas to lecture on nursing ethics. The annual, week-long seminar held in Sweden for doctoral students in nursing, which has either a primary or secondary focus on nursing ethics, has been of special interest because of its potential impact on nursing education. Extensive research on the ethics of force-feeding or not feeding senile elderly patients has been conducted by a Swedish nurse educator who has worked with doctoral students (Åkerlund and Norberg, 1985).

One nurse educator in Budapest has developed an ethics course for nursing students (Blasszauer and Rozsos, 1991), and another nurse educator has taught an ethics class at the Academy of Medicine in Lublin, Poland. In the Baltic states and eastern Europe, physicians often have been the only faculty teaching in nursing schools. For example, Estonia has had a shortage of nurses prepared to teach nursing. In this context, emphasis has been placed on the medical model and little, if any, ethics has been included because the teachers have had limited exposure to ethics content.

Throughout Latin America, Colombia has been the most active in nursing ethics education. The National Association of Nursing Schools has had an ethics committee working with schools of nursing, the Ministry of Health, and the Nursing Association to increase ethical content in nursing education. The ethics committee sponsored two workshops on nursing ethics and has been involved in the design of a research project on nursing ethics. Chile has had a nurse who has dealt with ethical issues working in the national nursing association. Much of this work has been limited to issues that arise in situations of torture, disappearance, and the general historical lack of democratic institutions. Such a nursing ethics presence has influenced nursing education.

Australian nursing education throughout the country has supported conferences, seminars, and consultation in nursing ethics. One nurse ethicist in Melbourne has taught in a nursing program and has published a book in the field. In 1986, the Center for Human Bioethics in Melbourne examined the state of nursing ethics in Australia and has continued to work with nurses seeking education in ethics. In Western Australia, a nurse educator completed her doctorate with a dissertation on nursing ethics. In Queensland, the head of a university nursing department served as a member of the research ethics committee at her institution. Sensitivity to ethical issues extended to and influenced her teaching and administrative styles.

New Zealand's National Nursing Association used its visiting scholars program to invite a nurse ethicist to present seminars in several cities on both islands. Some research on ethical issues has been conducted in the nursing department at Massey University.

Numerous nurse educators presented papers at two international conferences on nursing law and ethics held in Israel planned by the chief nurse in the Ministry of Health and Israeli nurse educators. Proceedings of these conferences have been published and used in teaching. Jewish ethics have been taught throughout the nursing curricula.

The School of Nursing, University of Alexandria, Egypt, held a nursing ethics conference in 1993 on ethics in education and practice.

In Asia, the People's Republic of China has developed eleven bachelor of science in nursing programs. The curriculum has included an ethics course that combines Confucian and Maoist ethics. The political slogan, "Serve the people," translates in nursing into respect for patients as persons (Davis et al., 1990). Korean nursing has developed an interest in ethics that manifests the influences of Christian missionary work. In 1992, at Japan's first international nursing research conference, one of the keynote papers discussed international perspectives on ethics for nursing. In addition, nurses presented papers focused on nursing ethics from a clinical and an educational perspective. Japan has held numerous other conferences addressing ethical issues in nursing. The National Center of Bioethics in Kyoto included nurses as speakers and participants in its conferences.

This discussion reflects great differences and many activities in nursing ethics education on the international scene. The lack of teachers and resources to teach nursing ethics remains a serious problem in many countries.

Conclusion

The last two decades of the twentieth century have seen a significant, worldwide resurgence and expansion of nursing ethics education activities and programs. These efforts have varied greatly. Many serious challenges remain for the twenty-first century, including a lack of formal ethics teaching in many programs, inadequate resources such as prepared nursing faculty to teach ethics, and the need for evaluation of the impact of existing nursing ethics education courses and programs on nursing practice.

MILA A. AROSKAR
ANNE J. DAVIS

Directly related to this article are the INTRODUCTION *and other articles in this entry, which discuss bioethics education in* MEDICINE, OTHER HEALTH PROFESSIONS, *and* SECONDARY AND POSTSECONDARY EDUCATION. *Also directly related to this article is the entry* NURSING ETHICS. *For a further discussion of topics mentioned in this article, see the entries* BIOETHICS; CONFUCIANISM; NURSING AS A PROFESSION; VIRTUE AND CHARACTER; *and* WOMEN, *section on* WOMEN AS HEALTH PROFESSIONALS. *For a discussion of related ideas, see the entries* CLINICAL ETHICS, *article on* ELEMENTS AND METHODOLOGIES; EMOTIONS; ETHICS, *article on* TASK OF ETHICS; FEMINISM; PRISONERS, *article on* TORTURE AND THE HEALTH PROFESSIONAL; SEXISM; TEAMS, HEALTH-CARE; *and* WOMEN, *article on* HISTORICAL AND CROSS-CULTURAL PERSPECTIVES. *Other relevant material may be found in the entries* CARE; COMPASSION; DEATH EDUCATION; INTERNATIONAL HEALTH; NURSING, THEORIES AND PHILOSOPHY OF; *and* PROFESSION AND PROFESSIONAL ETHICS. *See also the* APPENDIX (CODES, OATHS, AND DIRECTIVES RELATED TO BIOETHICS), *introductory article on* THE NATURE AND ROLE OF CODES ·AND OATHS, *and* SECTION III: ETHICAL DIRECTIVES FOR OTHER HEALTH-CARE PROFESSIONS.

Bibliography

ÅKERLUND, BRITT MARI, and NORBERG, ASTRID. 1985. "An Ethical Analysis of Double Bind Conflicts as Experienced by Core Workers Feeding Severely Demented Patients." *International Journal of Nursing Studies* 22, no. 3:207–216.

AMERICAN ASSOCIATION OF COLLEGES OF NURSING. 1986. *Essentials of College and University Education for Professional Nursing: Final Report.* Washington, D.C.: Author.

AMERICAN NURSES' ASSOCIATION. 1976. *Code for Nurses with Interpretive Statements.* Kansas City, Mo.: Author.

———. 1985. *Codes for Nurses with Interpretive Statements.* Kansas City, Mo.: Author.

AROSKAR, MILA A. 1977. "Ethics in the Nursing Curriculum." *Nursing Outlook* 25, no. 4:260–264.

BLASSZAUER, ROBERT, and BOZSOS, ELIZABETH. 1991. "Ethics Teaching for Hungarian Nurses." *Bulletin of Medical Ethics* no. 69 (June):22–23.

CASSELLS, JUDITH M., and REDMAN, BARBARA K. 1989. "Preparing Students to Be Moral Agents in Clinical Nursing Practice: Report of a National Study." *Nursing Clinics of North America* 24, no. 2:463–473.

CURTIN, LEAH, and FLAHERTY, M. JOSEPHINE. 1982. *Nursing Ethics: Theories and Pragmatics.* Bowie, Md.: Robert J. Brady.

DAVIDSON, BONNIE; VANDER LAAN, RIKA; DAVIS, ANNE; HIRSCHFELD, MIRIAM; LAURI, SIRKKA; LIN, JU YING; NORBERG, ASTRID; PHILLIPS, LINDA; PITTMAN, ELIZABETH; ZIV, LIORA; and LIN, JU YING. 1990. "Ethical Reasoning Associated with the Feeding of Terminally Ill Elderly Cancer Patients: An International Perspective." *Cancer Nursing* 13, no. 5:286–292.

DAVIS, ANNE J.; DAVIDSON, BONNIE; HIRSCHFELD, MIRIAM; LAURI, SIRKKA; LIN, JU YING; NORBERG, ASTRID; PHILLIPS, LINDA; PITTMAN, ELIZABETH; SHEN, CHANG HUI; VANDER LAAN, RIKA; ZHANG, HUI LAN; and ZIV, LIORA. 1993. "An International Perspective of Active Euthanasia: Attitudes of Nurses in Seven Countries." *International Journal of Nursing Studies* 30, no. 4:301–310.

DAVIS, ANNE J.; HERSHBERGER, ANN; GHAN, LAN CHUN; and LIN, JU YING. 1990. "The Good Nurse: Description from the People's Republic of China." *Journal of Advanced Nursing* 15, no. 7:829–834.

DENSFORD, KATHARINE J., and EVERETT, MILLARD S. 1946. *Ethics for Modern Nurses.* Philadelphia: W. B. Saunders.

FOWLER, MARSHA D. M. 1984. "Ethics and Nursing, 1893–1984: The Ideal of Service, the Reality of History." Ph.D. Diss., University of Southern California, Los Angeles.

FRY, SARA T. 1989. "Teaching Ethics in Nursing Curricula: Traditional and Contemporary Models." *Nursing Clinics of North America* 24, no. 2:485–497.

GOODRICH, ANNIE W. 1932. *The Social and Ethical Significance of Nursing: A Series of Addresses.* New York: Macmillan.

PAYTON, RITA J. 1980. "A Bioethical Program for Baccalaureate Nursing Students." In *Ethics in Nursing Practice and Education,* pp. 53–65. Kansas City, Mo.: American Nurses' Association.

ROBB, ISABEL H. 1909. *Nursing Ethics: For Hospital and Private Use.* Cleveland, Ohio: E. C. Koeckert.

RYDEN, MURIEL B.; DUCKETT, LAURA; CRISHAM, PATRICIA; CAPLAN, ARTHUR L.; and SCHMITZ, KATHY. 1989. "Multi-Course Sequential Learning as a Model for Content Integration: Ethics as a Prototype." *Journal of Nursing Education* 28, no. 3:102–106.

SILVA, MARY C., and SORRELL, JEANNE MERKLE. 1991. *Research on Ethics in Nursing Education: An Integrative Review and Critique.* New York: National League for Nursing.

IV. OTHER HEALTH PROFESSIONS

Bioethics education in health professions other than medicine and nursing takes place both in professional schools and in continuing-education settings. The group to which "other health professions" refers is so diverse that no generalizations embrace all of the professions equally. Some major groups include therapists (e.g., occupational, recreational, respiratory, physical), technologists (e.g., radiologic, medical laboratory), physician assistants, pharmacists, dietitians, dentists, and medical social workers. This entry emphasizes major common themes that have emerged in the content and pedagogy of their educational offerings; it also describes common factors that have led to the introduction of bioethics teaching in these fields.

Common themes in content and pedagogy

A set of guidelines for professional conduct has been one of the first types of documents produced when a new health field emerges. Up until the 1960s the documents often were called codes of ethics, but focused on dress codes and the importance of good manners and a cheerful disposition. They also emphasized the importance of keeping one's proper place in the bureaucracy, so that all documents except those for dentistry stressed deference to the physician's authority. Dedication to one's profession was considered essential. This list served as a foundation for teaching "ethics" to students in that field. The predictable result was that early ethics education was a presentation of a list of dos and don'ts that detailed a professional etiquette and morality punctuated by loyalty to one's group.

Today the educational emphasis has changed, as a result of changes in the focus of ethics documents and developments in the field of bioethics. There is also a growing consensus about the pedagogical methods that should be employed for bioethics education.

Current codes of ethics reflect basic ethical principles and virtues relevant to professional practice. For instance, the Code of Ethics of the National Association of Social Workers is designed around the central notion of ethical responsibility. The American Academy of Physician Assistants followed the model of several others by delineating its major types of interactions and specifying principles for each. Many groups provide accompanying guides for professional conduct that attempt to elaborate behaviors consistent with those principles and virtues. For example, the American Dental Association includes "advisory opinions" for most of its principles, and the American Physical Therapy Association issues a separate guide detailing each of its eight principles. Faculty have adopted these documents as a basis for education, with the predictable result that there is less focus on simply indoctrinating students into behaviors and attitudes and more on urging them to think about the ethical principles and virtues that underpin professional roles and responsibilities.

The development of bioethics as a field also has influenced education in these fields. Teachers focus on basic bioethics theory and methods of ethical analysis. Students are taught to think critically, recognize ethical issues, and reflect on them. Character traits or virtues are not simply declared essential; rather, students are encouraged to understand the significance of behaviors and attitudes that express compassion, honesty, and integrity (to name some). Materials introduced from the social sciences highlight how ethnic, religious, age, sex, class, and other differences among individuals and groups influence situations in which bioethical problems arise. In short, the teaching of ethics has evolved to foster analysis of and reflection on practical issues.

There is a growing consensus about pedagogical methods that should be utilized to teach bioethics. Educational programs actively promote the integration of theoretical content with case examples. The case method is especially effective in allowing students readily to recognize key ethical issues as they arise in everyday practice and to grasp the relevance of bioethics to their chosen professions. A larger proportion of bioethics instruction is taking place in small group discussions during the clinical period of professional preparation, so that challenging cases can be highlighted in discussion. Some programs utilize real or simulated patients with the goal of integrating ethical aspects of a patient's situation into the diagnostic, treatment, and social aspects.

There is less consensus about who should teach bioethics. Some schools of thought favor a stronger emphasis on theory, so that persons formally trained in philosophical ethics or moral theology are thought to be ideal. Others argue that an understanding of the clinical peculiarities and "facts" is most important, so clinicians are favored, especially if they have taken advanced work (or even a short course) in bioethics. Another alternative is a teaching team composed of a bioethicist and clinician working together. Preferences for one or another of these approaches seem less profession-specific than idiosyncratic of particular regions or institutions. In spite of the differences of opinion, the debates revolve around the common goal of effectively integrating theoretical and practical dimensions of bioethics.

Common factors leading to the necessity of bioethics education

At least three major factors have led to the need for bioethics teaching, with its current focus on thoughtful deliberation about complex ethical issues.

The issue of professional autonomy in relation to physicians is the crucial distinguishing feature of bioethics education in the groups being discussed. Their predicament is shared with nurses, and nursing ethics has provided valuable insights into the dilemma that is created. Such groups must gain understanding of their peculiar situation: having moral authority without ultimate decision-making authority. In some states groups such as physician assistants, physical therapists, and social workers have legal license to evaluate or practice independently. But this does not resolve the thorny questions of how to coordinate care for patients in a system largely centered on physician autonomy. The different levels of progress toward full professional status among the groups compound the issue.

A second factor distinguishing bioethics education for the groups under discussion is that many claim, as the rationale for their very existence, the mastery of a particular technology. Reliance on technology may drastically alter the complexion of the traditional health professional–patient relationship. First, technology may create a detrimental distance between health professionals and patients. Patients and health professionals alike may place unrealistic expectations on technologies to bring about "miracles," creating dissent and distrust when they fail to do so. And the high cost of many technologies may add undue burdens on patients and families.

Since the professional–patient relationship is at the heart of professional ethics, germane bioethics education is crucial so that health professionals can respond well to the larger human dilemmas created by technology. The types of technology the various professions employ will differ, but the generic challenges are similar for all. A list of dos and don'ts will not suffice. The concepts and methods of ethics are needed for thinking through and acting on technology-related challenges.

A third factor is the presence of inequities in health care. The tools of bioethics enable students to understand why inequities are morally unacceptable in the health-care system. They also provide an opportunity to encourage reflection on how professionals can contribute to the advancement of just and fair policies.

Since bioethics education in the professions under discussion in this article encourages critical thinking, considered action, and the exercise of ethically appropriate character traits, it will continue to be a powerful resource as new developments in health care and society give rise to ethical issues.

RUTH B. PURTILO

Directly related to this article are the INTRODUCTION *and other articles in this entry, which discuss bioethics education in* MEDICINE, NURSING, *and* SECONDARY AND POSTSECONDARY EDUCATION. *For a further discussion of topics mentioned in this article, see the entries* ALLIED HEALTH PROFESSIONS; BIOETHICS; CASUISTRY; CONSCIENCE; DENTISTRY; EMOTIONS; ETHICS, *article on* TASK OF ETHICS; MEDICAL CODES AND OATHS; MEDICINE AS A PROFESSION; NURSING AS A PROFESSION; PASTORAL CARE; PHARMACY; REHABILITATION MEDICINE; SOCIAL WORK IN HEALTH CARE; TEAMS, HEALTH-CARE; *and* TECHNOLOGY, *article on* HISTORY OF MEDICAL TECHNOLOGY. *For a discussion of related ideas, see the entries* ETHICS, *article on* NORMATIVE ETHICAL THEORIES; HEALTH-CARE RESOURCES, ALLOCATION OF; INTERNATIONAL HEALTH; PROFESSION AND PROFESSIONAL ETHICS; *and* VIRTUE AND CHARACTER. *Other relevant material may be found in the entries* CARE; COMPASSION; *and* LICENSING, DISCIPLINE, AND REGULATION IN THE HEALTH PROFESSIONS. *See also the* APPENDIX (CODES, OATHS, AND DIRECTIVES RELATED TO BIOETHICS), *introductory article on* THE NATURE AND ROLE OF CODES AND OATHS, *and* SECTION III: ETHICAL DIRECTIVES FOR OTHER HEALTH PROFESSIONS.

Bibliography

GOLDEN, DAVID G. 1991. "Medical Ethics Courses for Student Technologists." *Radiologic Technology* 62, no. 6:452–457.

HADDAD, AMY M. 1988. "Teaching Ethical Analysis in Occupational Therapy." *American Journal of Occupational Therapy* 42, no. 5:300–304.

HADDAD, AMY M., and BECKER, EVELYN S., eds. 1992. *Teaching and Learning Strategies in Pharmacy Ethics.* Omaha, Neb.: Creighton University Biomedical Communications.

OZAR, DAVID T. 1985. "Formal Instruction in Dental Professional Ethics." *Journal of Dental Education* 49, no. 10:696–701.

PURTILO, RUTH B. 1990. *Health Professional and Patient Interaction.* 4th ed. Philadelphia: W. B. Saunders.

PURTILO, RUTH B., and CASSEL, CHRISTINE K. 1993. *Ethical Dimensions in the Health Professions.* 2d ed. Philadelphia: W. B. Saunders.

ROGERS, JOAN C. 1983. "Clinical Reasoning: The Ethics, Science and Art." *American Journal of Occupational Therapy* 37, no. 9:601–616.

V. SECONDARY AND POSTSECONDARY EDUCATION

Since 1970 there has been a marked increase in bioethical reflection within the secondary and postsecondary curricula. On the high school level there is a growing movement to incorporate questions concerning social policy and values into science teaching. Many colleges and universities offer courses in bioethics that are popular with both students bound for the health professions and others simply interested in the topical issues raised. There has also been a proliferation of postgraduate programs offering advanced degrees in bioethics, which has become an autonomous and accredited discipline.

It is a rare high school that offers its students a specialized course in bioethics. More commonly, bioethical reflection is embedded within the standard science offerings. To some degree this is an outcome of what has been called the "STS" movement. The acronym stands for Science, Technology, and Society, and reflects an attempt by U.S. secondary schools to include within the science curriculum the profound ethical and policy issues raised by developments in science and technology. This movement is not without its obstacles; for example, the training of science teachers, shaped by the traditional division of science from the humanities, has often placed little emphasis on developing teaching skills for ethical reflection. However, the integrative movement has made inroads.

Most typically, bioethics issues are raised in high school biology courses, often in the context of issues in genetics or, increasingly, ecology and environmental science. The treatment of such topics may be limited to brief case presentations, or to discussions designed to help students with values clarification. However, there is a growing body of opinion that such strategies can be insufficient; not all opinions are of equal value, and students need to develop the critical reasoning skills to evaluate their stances in the light of scientific evidence, material implications, and logical consistency. This approach may eventually prove most appealing to science educators, for it dovetails well with aspects of the scientific method they are trying to transmit.

The move to introduce ethics into the high school biology curriculum has been furthered by the work of a number of foundations and centers. Notable in this regard is Ball State University's Project Genethics, which since 1978 has directly and indirectly trained thousands of biology teachers interested in incorporating ethics into their courses. The Biological Sciences Curriculum Study (BSCS), affiliated with the Colorado College, has developed biology textbooks, programs, and teaching modules that focus on ethical and policy issues. Ethical issues have also featured prominently in the teacher-training workshops and curriculum development projects funded by the National Center for Human Genome Research, a branch of the National Institutes of Health.

On the college level, offerings in bioethics are by now a well-established feature of the curriculum. Certain institutions, such as Brown University, permit students to construct an interdisciplinary major in bioethics. More often, a college or university will offer a course or a small number of courses in bioethics, usually through the philosophy department or, less frequently, through the religion department or an interdisciplinary arrangement. A typical course might utilize one of the standard textbooks of bioethics, either authored from a unitary perspective or offering an edited collection of canonical "pro" and "con" articles on bioethical issues. The instructor may choose to supplement this with a collection of cases or to replace it with an assembled course packet of his or her choice.

A number of didactic approaches may be used to help students become experientially involved with the topics. Most popular is the case analysis mode where students grapple with the dilemmas raised by actual or constructed cases. Class debates can help provoke spirited dialogue, and a growing library of films and videotapes vividly portrays for students the human impact of these issues. Some professors may bring in or team-teach with health-care professionals, or ask students to visit a health-care setting as part of the course.

Most bioethics textbooks and many instructors begin from a framework of ethical theories and principles that are then applied to specific issues: informed consent, abortion, and euthanasia, to name a few. However, this "standard approach"—and indeed the "standard issues" of bioethics—has been criticized by professionals associated with fields such as phenomenology, pragmatism, hermeneutics, feminism, casuistry, virtue ethics, and narrative theory. Critics argue, for example, that to base ethical analysis on high-level theory may obscure the richness of particular cases and the complex modes of interpretation real-life decision makers employ. Moreover, simply to stick to recognized "ethical quandaries" is to risk overlooking the sociopolitical biases and the metaphysics of self and body that have shaped our medical systems in ethically significant ways.

Instructors may therefore choose to supplement the medical ethics textbook with other kinds of resources. For example, a brief selection from René Descartes might be used to reflect on the model of body-as-machine that has powerfully influenced the doctor-patient relationship. A literary work such as Leo Tolstoy's *Death of Ivan Ilych* can render vivid and lucid the experience of illness, the significance of truth-telling, and the dilemmas surrounding death and dying. A work of social critique, such as a feminist history of women and medicine, can raise issues concerning the power relations embodied in medical practice and disease categories. The growing diversity of methodologies used within professional bioethics can thus "filter down" to diversify the methods and materials used in college-level teaching.

On the postgraduate level, a number of centers and universities around the country offer advanced degree programs specializing in bioethics. One popular model is the master's or Ph.D. program, often in philosophy, less frequently in religion, with a bioethics concentration. The program may include a series of courses focused on bioethical issues, some exposure to a clinical setting, and a thesis written on a topic relevant to bioethics. Such programs may attract individuals looking to pursue this field as a primary academic career. Alternatively, health-care professionals may enter such programs, usually for the master's degree, in preparation for teaching and/or service on ethics committees, or out of personal interest. Then, too, certain programs are designed to offer joint degrees through collaborative arrangements, allowing students to complete a medical or a legal degree along with an M.A., M.P.H., or Ph.D. degree. While most degree programs focus on bioethics or medical ethics as such, others define themselves more broadly as teaching the medical humanities, and thus may incorporate diverse disciplines such as history, sociology, anthropology, and literature.

In addition to degree programs, there are many options for those seeking more limited preparation in bioethics. A number of centers, for example, offer intensive courses in bioethics of one to four weeks' duration, or that involve sessions spread out over a longer period of time. Special bioethics fellowships are also available, often directed toward those already engaged in clinical practice.

Much of what this article details concerning bioethics teaching on the high school, college, and postgraduate level has become available since 1978, when the first edition of the *Encyclopedia of Bioethics* appeared. Academic interest in bioethics has been growing apace. With the continued expansion of the health-care industry, the constant development of new and troubling biomedical technologies, and the daily bioethics headlines in the popular press, it is likely that this interest will continue unabated.

DREW LEDER

Directly related to this article are the INTRODUCTION *and other articles in this entry, which discuss bioethics education in* MEDICINE, NURSING, *and* OTHER HEALTH PROFESSIONS. *For a further discussion of topics mentioned in this article, see the entries* BIOETHICS; CARE; CASUISTRY; COMPASSION; EMOTIONS; ETHICS, *article on* TASK OF ETHICS; FEMINISM; LAW AND BIOETHICS; LITERATURE; NARRATIVE; *and* WOMEN, *article on* HEALTH-CARE ISSUES, *and section on* WOMEN AS HEALTH PROFESSIONALS. *For a discussion of related ideas, see the entries* ETHICS, *article on* NORMATIVE ETHICAL THEORIES; *and* WOMEN, *articles on* HISTORICAL AND CROSS-CULTURAL PERSPECTIVES, *and* RESEARCH ISSUES.

Bibliography

"Biomedical Ethics Degree Programs." 1992. Kennedy Institute of Ethics, Georgetown University, National Reference Center for Bioethics Literature, Washington, D.C.

COUTTS, MARY. 1991a. *Basic Resources in Bioethics.* Scope Note no. 15. Washington, D.C.: Kennedy Institute of Ethics, National Reference Center for Bioethics Literature.

———. 1991b. *Teaching Ethics in the Health Care Setting.* Scope Note no. 16. Washington, D.C.: Kennedy Institute of Ethics, National Reference Center for Bioethics Literature.

CUTTER, MARY ANN. 1992. *Mapping and Sequencing the Human Genome: Science, Ethics, and Public Policy.* Colorado Springs, Colo.: Biological Sciences Curriculum Study and American Medical Association.

JENNINGS, BRUCE; NOLAN, KATHLEEN; CAMPBELL, COURTNEY; and DONNELLEY, STRACHAN. 1991. *New Choices, New Responsibilities: Ethical Issues in the Life Sciences: A Teaching Resource on Bioethics for High School Biology Courses.* Briarcliff Manor, N.Y.: Hastings Center.

JUSSIM, DANIEL. 1991. *Medical Ethics: Moral and Legal Conflicts in Health Care.* Englewood Cliffs, N.J.: Julian Messner.

LEVINE, CAROL, ed. 1989. *Cases in Bioethics: Selections from the Hastings Center Report.* Rev. ed. New York: St. Martin's Press.

———., ed. 1991. *Taking Sides: Clashing Views on Controversial Bioethical Issues.* 4th ed. Guilford, Conn.: Dushkin.

McCARRICK, PAT M. 1988. *Bioethics Audiovisuals: 1982 to Present.* Scope Note no. 9. Washington, D.C.: Kennedy Institute of Ethics, National Reference Center for Bioethics Literature.

"Syllabus Exchange Catalog." Kennedy Institute of Ethics, National Reference Center for Bioethics Literature, Washington, D.C. Georgetown University.

THORNTON, BARBARA C., and CALLAHAN, DANIEL. 1993. *Bioethics Education: Expanding Circle of Participants.* Briarcliff Manor, N.Y.: Hastings Center.

BIOETHICS AND LAW

See LAW AND BIOETHICS.

BIOETHICS AND PUBLIC POLICY

See PUBLIC POLICY AND BIOETHICS.

BIOLOGICAL AND CHEMICAL WARFARE

See WARFARE, *article on* CHEMICAL AND BIOLOGICAL WARFARE.

BIOLOGY, PHILOSOPHY OF

Biology is the science of organisms. Some areas, like ecology, deal only with living organisms, looking especially at their behaviors in natural surroundings. Some areas, like physiology, move organisms into the laboratory, often dividing them in an attempt to understand how the parts work. Yet other areas, like paleontology, delve into the past. Looking at the fossil record, paleontologists try to reconstruct and explain life's history.

Philosophers are not scientists. They do not cut up animals or search rocks for traces of pollen. They look at the work and the results of science, considering problems that grow out of such efforts. Philosophers of biology therefore look at the work and claims of biologists, and they find three major areas of interest. First, there is a cluster of questions about the science of biology itself. Second, there are questions about the broader implications of biology for the practical problems of human living. Third, there are questions about biology and the societies or cultures in which it is produced. From the viewpoint of bioethics, the second set of questions is most pressing. But all three areas say things of interest.

(A comprehensive review can be found in Ruse, 1988a; and a collection of articles in Ruse, 1988b.)

Vitalism

The first group of questions opens with the most basic of all: Is there something about life itself that demands a special kind of understanding beyond the grasp of sciences like physics and chemistry? Philosophers and biologists, as far back as the Greek philosopher Aristotle, have thought that there is. They have claimed that there is some kind of life force (the early twentieth-century French philosopher Henri Bergson [1913] called it the *élan vital*) that makes living things living, as it were. A plant or an animal is by its very nature more than a collection of molecules, and as such cannot be understood by the laws and concepts of the physical sciences.

The technical term for the issue around which this controversy swirls is "reduction." Those who defend the special nature of organisms claim that biology cannot be "reduced" to physics and chemistry. The precise meaning of this claim has been a matter of much debate. At one level, the claim might be—and often has been—that the life force is some kind of event or thing. It is visualized as rather like a gas or a liquid, although clearly it has to be a peculiar kind of gas or liquid. This view, which is known as vitalism, is not easy to refute. Many suspect that the difficulty for the critic indicates a weakness in the position itself. Whatever properties the life force may have, it is not visible or tangible. It cannot be located in the same way that normal physical substances are located. Cut open a cabbage, and the life force cannot be seen oozing out of it. Nor would a microscope help to make the life force visible.

On close examination, the life force proves to be elusive. Perhaps it is so difficult to locate because it is nonexistent. Might it be that, incredible though it may seem at first, organisms—even humans—are no more than fantastically complicated pieces of machinery?

Life's organization

At this point, the antireductionists often fall back on a second level of argument: that no one thinks there is an actual force. It is more of a metaphor, acknowledging that the structure and the mechanisms of organisms are different from those of inanimate objects. It is less a matter of substance and more a question of organization. The average plant or animal is put together in a way that defies physicochemical understanding.

It is not so easy to counter this antireductionist position; philosophers warn that the argument must be approached with caution. Indeed, there are obvious apparent counterexamples. The greatest triumph of modern biology came in 1953, when James Watson and Francis Crick discovered the "double helix," the structure of DNA, the ultimate threads of heredity. It thus became possible to decipher the "genetic code," which showed how the information needed for building each new generation of organisms was simply a matter of putting together relatively simple molecules in a special order.

The body of research and findings on DNA is thoroughly molecular and physicochemical. The DNA molecule, though very complex, is not mysterious. And it reveals the most basic information about organisms. Through DNA research the essence of biological organization is being captured more successfully by the physical sciences than it ever was by the biological sciences. This seems to be a very neat case of "reduction." (For more on this point, see Schaffner, 1980.)

Teleology

The case against the distinctive nature of biology is closing fast. Yet there is still something about biology as a science, a result of the distinctive nature of organisms, that marks it off from the physical sciences. Consider one of the most numerous of the dinosaurs, the stegosaurus. It had a double row of diagonal plates or fins along its back. Why did it have these? This is the pressing question for the paleontologist. What purpose or function did the plates serve? What was their "end"? Why was the beast as it was?

A good and satisfactory answer is that the plates or fins served to cool the animal on hot days, just as similar plates cool the water in hydroelectric plants. By contrast, in physics, no one would dream of asking what purpose the moon serves. Such forward-looking questions and explanations, thinking in terms of ends or final causes, rather than of prior causes, are not appropriate in the physical sciences. Apparently, however, they have their place in the biological sciences.

This kind of thinking is called teleological (Wright, 1976). Most modern philosophers are very wary of it, especially if it is linked either with life forces striving to achieve goals or with causes somehow acting from the future to affect the present. Consider an exercise in imagination. Suppose the stegosaurus is still living. It is a cold day at the end of winter. Obviously the stegosaurus does not have fins so that it can be cool today. Rather, it has them in anticipation of hot days next summer, when it will need cooling. But suppose that before next June, a comet hits the earth and wipes out all of the dinosaurs. It can hardly be that the stegosaurus has its plates today for next summer's heat wave, for that heat wave never comes. Or, if it does come, the stegosaurus is dead. Thus the cause was not only in the future but also nonexistent.

Nevertheless, even granting the truth of the teleological argument, perhaps the antireductionist critic does have a point. There may not be anything peculiar about organisms in respect to their composition or even their underlying organization (although this latter is very complex). Nor is there anything distinctive about the causal workings of organisms. Yet they are different from inanimate objects, like rocks and moons. They do seem "as if" designed—the stegosaurus's plates seem "as if" they were made (by a conscious being) for cooling.

This is why teleological language is appropriate. When human-made artifacts are considered, it is in terms of purposes or ends. "What is the purpose of this strange-looking knife?" "What end does this part play in the engine's functioning?" And so it is in biology. (See Kass, 1985, for more on this point.)

Darwinism

A consideration of teleology leads to the most-debated issue in the philosophy of biology. There is no puzzle today about why organisms seem as if designed. It is known why the stegosaurus, for instance, had plates. These characters are called adaptations. They are the end result of evolution, the long, slow process of development that produced all organisms from the original primitive beginnings. (Biologists today think that the earth is 4.5 billion years old, and that life arose naturally over 3.5 billion years ago.)

What drives evolution? In 1859, in *On the Origin of Species*, Charles Darwin revealed the major mechanism: natural selection. More organisms are born than can possibly survive. This leads to a "struggle for existence." Only a few live to maturity and—more important—to reproduce. Those that are successful will, on average, be different from those that are not. There will thus be a kind of differential breeding, akin to the artificial selection practiced by farmers and plant and animal fanciers. This is natural selection and, as Darwin stressed, it leads to the production of ever better adaptations.

There is nothing conceptually or causally odd about natural selection. It needs no life forces or causes working out of the future. The stegosaurus had its fins because those of its ancestors that had finlike protuberances survived and reproduced. And those that did not, did not. Yet evolutionary theory—especially natural selection—has been philosophically controversial from its first days. The best-known criticism was made by the distinguished Austrian-British philosopher Karl Popper (1974). He complains that "Darwinism" fails the acid test of genuine science. It cannot, even in principle, be shown wrong by empirical evidence. It is "unfalsifiable" (Popper, 1959, 1963).

According to Popper, the trouble with evolution is that its predictions—the things one would use to test a theory—tend to be very long-range, and thus beyond our scope. Who knows how the elephant's trunk will evolve a million years hence? And if it is not long-range, things are still too slippery for Darwinism to count as genuine science. Suppose someone shows that the stegosaurus's fins could not possibly be used for cooling. Will the Darwinian be abashed? Not one whit! Another pseudo explanation will be invented: that the stegosaurus needed the fins to attract the opposite sex, or some such thing. Hence, Popper concludes that Darwinism is best considered a "metaphysical research programme"— a kind of world philosophy—rather than hard science.

This is not a conclusion that biologists much like, nor do many philosophers of biology. They argue that Popper is ignorant of much of modern evolutionary biology, and that when it is properly understood, it can be seen as fully testable or falsifiable. Most Darwinian studies, far from being long-range, center on immediate effects and are fully testable. For instance, today there is (as there was by Darwin himself) much interest in mimicry (one animal or plant camouflages itself by pretending to be another organism or thing). Butterflies pretend to be other butterflies, and insects pretend to be leaves. In testing a claim here, a claim that will be based on the power of natural selection, Darwinism opens itself to check and refutation no less than does any theory of physics or chemistry. That a theory is not in fact refuted does not mean that it is unfalsifiable. It may indeed be true. (Gould, 1977, contains many articles dealing with criticisms of natural selection. Some of his more pertinent discussions are reprinted in Ruse, 1986. The best technical treatment of natural selection by a philosopher is Sober, 1984.)

Even if Popper's basic criticism is not well founded, he is hinting at something important. Theories of biology, evolutionary biology in particular, do seem to have a looseness of logical argument—critics would say "flabbiness"—alien to the products of the physical sciences. Whatever the soundness of the overall framework, the biologist working on a particular problem frequently fails to achieve the tight logical control evidenced by the best of physics and chemistry. One mark of this is that much biology stays at the level of description. People working in biology are often unable to bring to bear the formal tools of logic and mathematics, so powerful and so pervasive in the physical sciences.

There are reasons why the biological sciences are as they are in these respects. The most obvious is that such sciences have lagged behind the physical sciences. Their problems are bigger and more challenging, and hence their finished products are incomplete. But perhaps there are other reasons—reasons that bring us toward problems of concern to the bioethicist. Science is made up of laws bound together into theories. For these laws to exist, the world must be analyzable into reasonably uniform sets or groups of entities. Johannes Kepler's laws about planets presuppose that there are readily identifiable groups of things properly called planets. Likewise, the biology of the DNA molecule presupposes that the components will be more or less like another. The completed molecules may be unique, but the parts are as alike as are the blocks in a child's Lego set.

As the net of biology spreads out to organisms, identifiability and uniformity become highly problematic. It is true that biologists divide the living world into groups. The basic class is the species, the group within which organisms breed with and only with themselves. Thus there is a set of fruit flies called *Drosophila melanogaster,* and a set of mammals called *Homo sapiens.* But even in these most basic groups, there is massive variation from one member to another. There must be, if Darwinism be true, for natural selection can work only if there is difference, with one type or form being successful over another.

How, then, can there possibly be generally applicable laws and theories? If the essence of the biological world is variation and difference, then it seems that the tight generality and rigor of the physical sciences (where one can readily pick out repeated instances) is unobtainable. Perhaps this is so. There are indeed genuine laws and theories of biology, but they come at a higher level of generality than particular species. There can be a law about genes, where there is repeatability. There cannot be a law about organisms in a species, for there is no such repeatability. Therefore, there are biological laws about genes—Mendel's law, for instance. However, for all that philosophers like to use such examples, in biology there are never laws like "All swans are white." All swans are never white.

All of this seems to mean that a species is not really like the set or class of the mathematician, for which there are precise membership criteria. Perhaps, especially since species members are bound by blood ties, species are more like supraorganisms. They are biological individuals in their own right. To use the language of the mathematicians, therefore, a particular organism like Michael Ruse or Julius Caesar is a part of the whole, the species *Homo sapiens,* just as a hand is part of a person. Humans are not members of the set *Homo sapiens,* analogous to the way in which a square is a member of the set of quadrilaterals. (Hull, 1989, discusses these questions authoritatively.)

If species really are biological individuals, that seems to be another factor separating biology from physics. There are bioethical implications also. Minorities have often been judged inadequate because they do not measure up to the supposed criteria for inclusion in the set *Homo sapiens.* Those with Down syndrome are judged inadequate because they do not have the standard number of chromosomes. Homosexuals are judged immoral because they do not have a typical sexual orientation, or because they are not part of the breeding pool. However, if species themselves are thought of as individuals, then such judgments are not simply unkind but conceptually flawed. Diversity is part of life, and in itself being heterosexual or homosexual is no more a species matter than being blue-eyed or brown-eyed. (This is not to swing to another extreme and deny the existence of genetic disease. The point is that one judges a genetic disease as one judges all disease, in terms of quality of life, and not by biological class membership.)

There is another point at which highlighting the variation within species has major repercussions. A major biotechnological enterprise is the Human Genome Project (HGP), which involves trying to map (that is, decipher) the total molecular underpinning of human heredity. If variation is the rule rather than the exception, then crude, one-and-for-all readings are doomed to failure or inadequacy. Human nature at the molecular level is far too varied to hope for one archive, wherein all pertinent information must be sorted. To be really useful, there must be a range of readings, telling all of the possible variants. (For more on some of the technical issues of evolutionary theory, see Rosenberg, 1985; and Sober, 1993. For more on the HGP, see Kevles and Hood, 1992.)

Recombinant DNA

The second set of questions of interest to the philosopher of biology comprises the questions that deal with the implications of biology for matters of moral, political, and social concern. What happens, for example, when biologists devise new techniques of inquiry that promise powerful insights into the nature of living beings, yet pose possible threats to the well-being of society?

The obvious example of a tension of this kind came in the 1970s, with the advent of recombinant DNA (r-DNA) techniques for investigating the nature and composition of the basic molecular building blocks of organisms. Here was a powerful new tool—more precisely, a range of tools—that promised ready insights into the functioning of the inner parts of the cell, as well as ways of fabricating new organic forms. Many of these forms could have direct value to humans in medicine, in agriculture, and the like. Yet this set of tools held the threat of potentially dangerous new forms of life that could wreak havoc on humankind and the environment.

Philosophers played a significant role in this debate and in its resolution, drawing up guidelines for the sensible prosecution of r-DNA research. They were able to disentangle some of the moral issues that arise in a conflict between individual rights and interests and the common good and welfare. A simple but important point was showing that many moral conflicts arise not because people differ about the ultimate principles of right and wrong but because the empirical facts of the case are unclear or disputed. In the r-DNA case, it soon became clear that the real problem was that those who devised the new technology were abysmally ignorant of the basic facts of epidemiology, the branch of medicine that treats organisms dangerous to humankind. As soon as some essential empirical information about the spread of disease was brought forward, many of the fears about the dangers of r-DNA research were seen to be ill-founded. (See Jackson, 1979.)

Ecology

Another area of ongoing interest is the threat posed to the environment by population growth, by the profligate use of limited natural resources, by the indifference to the effects of the use of synthetic substances, and by many other factors. Here the science of ecology has a major role to play, as life scientists try to understand the fragile and volatile relations between the living components of this planet. And here, philosophers of biology have a major role to play as they try to discover and assess the moral and social implications of the ecologists' findings.

This becomes clearest through consideration of one of the major theoretical branches of modern ecology, the MacArthur/Wilson theory of "island biogeography." With elegant simplicity, this theory relates two groups of factors. The size of an island and its distance from the mainland are linked with the carrying capacity of the island, which means not just the number of inhabitants the island can hold but also the overall number of species on the island. Essentially, the claim is that a kind of equilibrium is achieved, with the number of species leaving the island or becoming extinct being balanced by the number of new arrivals.

The broader implications of this theory are obvious. Given sufficient time, accidental or intentional cases of island denudation will be righted naturally. It is true that the theory talks only of numbers of species on or off an island, without specifying actual kinds of organisms. It might involve replacement of indigenous flora and fauna by the Norwegian rat. But the bottom line is that nature has a way of righting itself.

Unfortunately, as critics have been able to show, if ever a theory came close to failing Popper's falsifiability criterion, it is the MacArthur/Wilson theory. The direct evidence is slight (and, incidentally, raises questions of its own, for it entails the poisoning of entire populations of small islets). It is not clear what types of evidence actually support the MacArthur/Wilson theory and what types only appear to provide such support. One of the first things that philosophy teaches is to question the use of words—their meaning and their application. Never was such wisdom more needed than at this point, for

ecologists are deeply divided over their terms. When is an island an island, and when is an island not an island? Does it have to be surrounded by water? If so, does it matter if there is a connection to the mainland at low tide? Can there be substitutes for water—desert? jungle? Or simply something inhospitable to a certain species, as savanna might be to a tree-dwelling monkey?

Decisions on questions such as these can influence profoundly the conclusions drawn about whether nature can restock itself naturally, or whether, once disturbed, nature can ever truly regain equilibrium. The trouble is that evidence becomes almost irrelevant as words are expanded and contracted to give the right answers. What appeared to be solid science is exposed as environmental expediency masquerading as genuine knowledge. (More on these points can be found in Haila and Jarrinen, 1982.)

Human sociobiology

Ecology is controversial, but it pales beside the fury in the 1970s and 1980s over sociobiology (pro: Wilson, 1975; Dawkins, 1976; con: Lewontin et al., 1984). This is the attempt to look at animal social behavior from an evolutionary perspective, seeing it as something caused and maintained by natural selection. What has made sociobiology such a "hot" topic is the fact that today's evolutionists have been able to give convincing reasons for the evolution of the most famous case of social behavior: those sterile worker insects who spend their whole lives working for the good of their nests, apparently without any thought for themselves.

What makes sociobiology controversial is that its practitioners, led by Harvard biologist Edward O. Wilson (the Wilson of the ecological equilibrium theory), have applied their science to the human species (Lumsden and Wilson, 1981). But humans are not ants—although some people have suggested that perhaps homosexuals are analogous to sterile workers, and they have looked for evidence that such people do aid their close relatives. The human sociobiologists argue that perhaps humans are controlled in much that they do by their biology, because natural selection favors such control. Perhaps, for instance, the Victorian anthropologist Edward Westermarck was right in suggesting that people do not generally want to have sex with close relatives because biology has provided contrary emotions. It is an established fact that such close interbreeding leads to biologically handicapped offspring. (See Wilson, 1978.)

Wilson certainly has no hidden motives in pushing his science. Yet the history of the twentieth century shows only too well how, in the hands of fanatics, biological determinism can lead to dreadful consequences. Philosophers have therefore been at the front of those who have looked long and skeptically at human sociobiology and its claims. As in the ecology case, they are keenly aware of how easy it is to slide from supposed science to social prescriptions. Even the most moderate of sociobiologists are liable to harbor beliefs about teaching, for instance, and about the degrees to which children are biologically capable of learning. More controversially, they may hold views about the variations between learning capacities, and the futility of expecting some people ever to achieve the heights of others.

For a start, philosophers realize that although analogies and metaphors are invaluable, they should be approached with extreme caution. Take the claim that human homosexuals are akin to sterile worker ants. Humans are not ants, even of a peculiar mammalian variety. Nor is there any evidence whatsoever that gay men and lesbians have reduced fertility. Indeed, even though it is probable that homosexuals have fewer offspring than do heterosexuals, at best this is a matter of averages and by no means a universal truth. In many societies, including those of North America, there is strong social pressure on people (especially females) to marry and have families—no matter who their desired sex partners may be.

This does not mean that the science of human sociobiology necessarily collapses. Some of the greatest moves in science have come through innovative metaphors. Perhaps it is ultimately fruitful to compare people to worker ants. However, when people want to draw social conclusions from science, they should carefully scrutinize the science itself and its links to the conclusions. (For very different assessments of human sociobiology, see Ruse, 1979a, 1986, 1989 [pro]; and Kitcher, 1985 [contra].)

Creationism

The third set of issues that has engaged today's philosophers of biology has to do with a broad spectrum of matters about biology and the culture(s) within which biologists think and work. The most visible is religion. Darwin's *Origin* upset religious sensibilities, and into the twentieth century in America there were strenuous moves to keep the teaching of evolution out of schools. Nor has such opposition subsided, although most Christians and Jews today accept evolution fully. The Fundamentalists, who take the early chapters of the Bible (six days of creation, six-thousand-year earth span, a universal flood) literally, have had considerable success in recent years in influencing educators and others. They have even been able to influence legislative bodies, most notoriously in 1981, when the state of Arkansas mandated the teaching of "creation science" alongside evolution in publicly funded schools.

Philosophers have long been at the forefront of showing why it is reasonable to accept evolution as a fact. Indeed, it was a philosopher who showed Darwin the way. How do you persuade someone of the plausibility of a position when (as in the case of evolution) there is no direct evidence, no eyewitness? The answer, identical to that used by lawyers attempting to determine guilt without such testimony, is to work through circumstantial evidence, showing how many pieces of information point unambiguously to one cause that validates the separate pieces. The English philosopher of science William Whewell (1840) called this procedure a "consilience of inductions," and he taught it to Darwin, who strove (successfully) to show how all the areas of biology—ecology, physiology, paleontology, and more—are unified and explained by evolution through selection. Things like the fossil record are the clues of evolution.

Thus, it is misleading to say "Evolution is just a theory and not a fact." It is both. It is a scientific theory about natural selection. It is an established fact that evolution occurs. It shows also how disastrous it would be if religious enthusiasts dislodged evolution's place in biology teaching. As the geneticist Theodosius Dobzhansky once said, "Nothing in biology makes sense except in the light of evolution." Or, to modify another remark, teaching biology while questioning evolution would be like teaching French while querying the significance of the irregular verbs.

The Arkansas law on teaching "creation science" was overturned. In this case, and in the subsequent and ongoing fight against the pressure of the biblical literalists, philosophy of biology played a crucial role. At the heart of the issue are the relative statuses of evolution and of "creation science." Are they genuine science, or are they religion masquerading as science? No one is denying the right of creationists to believe as they do. The question is whether creationism is truly religion. If it is, then it cannot legally be taught in public schools. The Arkansas court (and other legal bodies, up to the U.S. Supreme Court) have agreed that "creation science" is truly not genuine science. Most crucially, it fails the test of being falsifiable. And no matter what evidence arises, its proponents simply refuse to allow that it could impinge negatively on their central beliefs. (Ruse, 1988c, collects articles dealing with philosophical aspects of the creationism controversy.)

Is biology sexist?

The cries of the creationists may be misguided, but they are heartfelt. Evolution may not be atheistic secular humanism, as they claim, but their fears should lead to consideration of science in its own right and as a reflection of the culture from which it emerges. There is no sharp distinction between a science and its society. Darwinism, for instance, reveals its beginnings both in the central role given to struggle—an idea taken from the influential socioeconomic writings of Thomas Robert Malthus—and in the key place accorded to adaptation—which highlights the designlike nature of organisms, and was taken by Darwin from the natural theology of his day. (See Ruse, 1979b.)

Feminist critics of science are very sensitive to the links between science and society, and they have had some very severe things to say about biology (Harding, 1986; Birke, 1986; Hubbard, 1983; Keller, 1984; but also see Hrdy, 1981). They claim that the biological sciences are tainted by the inherently sexist values of Western society. Darwin is highlighted as a persistent offender, for (particularly in the *Descent of Man*) he was much given to portraying women as men's intellectual and physical inferiors. At present, Wilson is the feminists' favorite bête noire, for he supposedly tends to see women as having a natural (that is, biological) propensity for second-class status.

Some of these criticisms are unfair—or at least unbalanced. Alfred Russel Wallace, the codiscoverer with Darwin of natural selection, was an ardent feminist, arguing that the future of the human race lies in the hands of young women, who can be trusted to breed only with the best young men. (He derived this somewhat optimistic idea from Edward Bellamy's novel *Looking Backward*.) Nor does one often hear that Wilson's student, the primatologist Sarah Hrdy, has argued that because human females have concealed ovulation (they do not come into heat), biology has ensured that females are the major driving force in the species today. Males have to be present in the home and be involved in child care; otherwise, in their absence, females could cheat on them and they would never know that their supposed children are their real children.

Nevertheless, sexist and other offensive ideologies do seep into biology. Ongoing caution is demanded, and here philosophers can, and do, have a significant part to play. This is not to say that the philosopher has to smooth everything to a uniformly gray surface, satisfying only to the politically correct. Rather, as always, the philosopher has to play the gadfly, making people examine their most cherished beliefs. If and when a science makes unwarranted judgments about people, it is the philosopher who must blow the whistle. (Haraway, 1989, is a good place to start with the feminist critique of biology.)

Biological education

That science tends to reflect culture is not a cause for concern. It is a cause for caution. Consider, for example, an aspect of evolutionary thought that has repeatedly been highlighted by the well-known biologist Stephen Jay Gould (1989). From its beginnings in the eighteenth century, evolutionary thought has been infected with "progressionism." The history of life has been portrayed as a more or less uniform succession from the simplest forms to the sophisticated end point, *Homo sapiens*. But, as Gould insists, this interpretation has been a vehicle not just for speciesism but also for racism. What more natural than to assume that there is biological progress among humans, with blacks at the bottom and Anglo-Saxons at the top?

Philosophers of biology have thought about and worked extensively on this very point. They have tried to document the extent to which every evolutionist has espoused progressionism; what senses of progressionism have been favored; whether a progress-free evolutionism is attainable; and whether one can separate the scientific from the social. Nor is this inquiry merely some academic exercise. Survey after survey shows that when evolution is taught, it is taught in a progressionist manner. The myth is being perpetuated.

It might be countered that Gould's fears are exaggerated, and that no one today would use biology in the way of the imperialists of old. Perhaps this is true, although if the threat has diminished, it is certainly a break with history. Or it might be countered that it is better that evolution of some sort be taught than none at all. Again, perhaps this is true, although it is hard to see why things should not be put right at once. It is enough to conclude by saying that if science is a glorious product of the human imagination, and perhaps the salvation of the future, it must be taught and taught well. This being so, the philosophy of biology has its role to play here, as it has a role to play in so many other areas. (See Nitecki, 1988, for more on evolutionary biology and progress.)

MICHAEL RUSE

Directly related to this entry are the entries EVOLUTION; HUMAN NATURE; LIFE; NATURE; *and* SCIENCE, PHILOSOPHY OF. *For a discussion of related ideas, see the entries* GENETICS AND HUMAN BEHAVIOR; *and* GENETICS AND HUMAN SELF-UNDERSTANDING. *For a further discussion of topics mentioned in this entry, see the entries* EUGENICS; GENOME MAPPING AND SEQUENCING; HEALTH AND DISEASE; MEDICINE, PHILOSOPHY OF; *and* RACE AND RACISM.

Bibliography

BERGSON, HENRI. 1913. *Creative Evolution.* London: Macmillan.

BIRKE, LYNDA I. A. 1986. *Women, Feminism and Biology: The Feminist Challenge.* Brighton, Sussex: Wheatsheaf.

DAWKINS, RICHARD. 1976. *The Selfish Gene.* Oxford: Oxford University Press.

GOULD, STEPHEN JAY. 1977. *Ever Since Darwin: Reflections in Natural History*. New York: W. W. Norton.

———. 1989. *Wonderful Life: The Burgess Shale and the Nature of History*. New York: W. W. Norton.

HAILA, Y., and JARRINEN, O. 1982. "The Role of Theoretical Concepts in Understanding the Ecological Theatre: A Case Study on Island Biogeography." In *Conceptual Issues in Ecology*, pp. 261–278. Edited by Esa Saarinen. Dordrecht, Netherlands: D. Reidel.

HARAWAY, DONNA JEANNE. 1989. *Primate Visions: Gender, Race, and Nature in the World of Modern Science*. New York: Routledge.

HARDING, SANDRA G. 1986. *The Science Question in Feminism*. Ithaca, N.Y.: Cornell University Press.

HRDY, SARAH BLAFFER. 1981. *The Woman That Never Evolved*. Cambridge, Mass.: Harvard University Press.

HUBBARD, RUTH. 1983. "Have Only Men Evolved?" In *Discovering Reality: Feminist Perspectives on Epistemology, Methodology, and Philosophy of Science*, pp. 45–69. Edited by Sandra G. Harding and Merrill B. Hintikka. Dordrecht, Netherlands: D. Reidel.

HULL, DAVID L. 1989. *The Metaphysics of Evolution*. Albany: State University of New York Press.

JACKSON, DAVID A., and STICH, STEPHEN P., eds. 1979. *The Recombinant DNA Debate*. Englewood Cliffs, N.J.: Prentice-Hall.

KASS, LEON. 1985. *Toward More Natural Science: Biology and Human Affairs*. New York: Free Press.

KELLER, EVELYN FOX. 1985. *Reflections on Gender and Science*. New Haven, Conn.: Yale University Press.

KEVLES, DANIEL J., and HOOD, LEROY E., eds. 1992. *The Code of Codes: Scientific and Social Issues in the Human Genome Project*. Cambridge, Mass.: Harvard University Press.

KITCHER, PHILIP. 1985. *Vaulting Ambition: Sociobiology and the Quest for Human Nature*. Cambridge: M.I.T. Press.

LEWONTIN, RICHARD C.; ROSE, STEVEN P.R.; and KAMIN, LEON J. 1984. *Not in Our Genes: Biology, Ideology, and Human Nature*. New York: Pantheon.

LUMSDEN, CHARLES J., and WILSON, EDWARD O. 1981. *Genes, Mind, and Culture: The Coevolutionary Process*. Cambridge, Mass.: Harvard University Press.

NITECKI, MATTHEW H., ed. 1988. *Evolutionary Progress*. Chicago: University of Chicago Press.

POPPER, KARL R. 1959. *The Logic of Scientific Discovery*. London: Hutchinson.

———. 1963. *Conjectures and Refutations: The Growth of Scientific Knowledge*. London: Routledge & Kegan Paul.

———. 1972. *Objective Knowledge: An Evolutionary Approach*. Oxford: Clarendon Press.

ROSENBERG, ALEXANDER. 1985. *The Structure of Biological Science*. Cambridge: At the University Press.

RUSE, MICHAEL. 1979a. *Sociobiology: Sense or Nonsense?* Dordrecht, Netherlands: D. Reidel.

———. 1979b. *The Darwinian Revolution: Science Red in Tooth and Claw*. Chicago: University of Chicago Press.

———. 1986. *Taking Darwin Seriously: A Naturalistic Approach to Philosophy*. Oxford: Basil Blackwell.

———. 1988a. *Philosophy of Biology Today*. Albany: State University of New York Press.

———. 1988b. *Philosophy of Biology*. Edited by Paul Edwards. New York: Macmillan.

———, ed. 1988c. *But Is It Science? The Philosophical Question in the Creation/Evolution Controversy*. Buffalo, N.Y.: Prometheus.

———, ed. 1989a. *Readings in the Philosophy of Biology*. New York: Macmillan.

———. 1989b. *The Darwinian Paradigm: Essays on Its History, Philosophy, and Religious Implications*. London: Routledge.

SCHAFFNER, KENNETH F. 1980. "Theory Structure in the Biomedical Sciences." *Journal of Medicine and Philosophy* 5, no. 1:57–97.

SOBER, ELLIOTT. 1984. *The Nature of Selection: Evolutionary Theory in Philosophical Focus*. Cambridge: M.I.T. Press.

———. 1993. *Philosophy of Biology*. Boulder, Colo.: Westview.

WHEWELL, WILLIAM. 1840. *The Philosophy of the Inductive Sciences Founded Upon Their History*. London: J.W. Parker.

WILSON, EDWARD O. 1975. *Sociobiology: The New Synthesis*. Cambridge: Harvard University Press.

———. 1978. *On Human Nature*. Cambridge: Harvard University Press.

WRIGHT, LARRY. 1976. *Teleological Explanations: An Eteological Analysis of Goals and Functions*. Berkeley: University of California Press.

BIOMEDICAL ENGINEERING

Since the early 1960s, biomedical engineering has transformed health care in industrialized countries, confronting both health care professionals and the lay public with new problems, decisions, and possibilities. The need to understand these new problems, decisions, and possibilities has contributed to the rise of bioethics during the same period.

Biomedical engineers and biomedical engineering

Biomedical engineering research uses engineering methods to study normal and pathological physiology. For example, biomedical engineers use engineering methods to study the stresses and pressures that occur in human joints, or the mechanisms that contribute to the thickening of the liquid layer in the lung that causes airway closure in respiratory diseases. Biomedical engineers may also collaborate on the design, development, testing, or refinement of medical devices and procedures to prevent, diagnose, and treat trauma and disease. They may even develop and oversee the manufacture or maintenance of these devices. Biomedical engineers collaborate not only with researchers and providers of health care but also with other mechanical, electrical, chemical, aero/astro, or nuclear engineers, who are not themselves biomedical engineers. The devices that biomedical engineering makes possible range from clinical thermometers for home use to multimillion-dollar imaging equipment. Some biomedical devices come into direct contact with patients, becoming "the machine at the bedside" (Reiser and Anbar, 1984) or even the machine that is part of one's body—new elements in the public's experience of health care.

Although there are more than three million engineers in the United States, engineering work is not well understood by the public, which often confuses the engineer who designs or develops a device with the technician who operates it or the skilled worker who assembles it. The most common (and mistaken) view of engineering in general and biomedical engineering in particular is that it is simply the application of science. This "applied science" model of engineering disregards the central place of design and synthetic or creative thinking. Engineers invent, design, develop, and adapt devices, constructions, materials, and processes in response to human needs and wants. Their concern is the actual behavior of the objects and systems they study, behavior that is the result of many simultaneous influences, only some of which are the object of study in the natural sciences. Biomedical engineers, like other engineers, often extend and enhance scientific theory.

Biomedical engineers are most likely to have backgrounds in the more established fields of mechanical, chemical, electrical, or nuclear engineering, or in computer science. Biomedical engineering has a somewhat different character within each of those established engineering fields. Electrical engineers investigate bioelectric phenomena in nerve and muscle function and in the designs of devices, such as pain-blocking stimulators or implanted electrodes to aid hearing. Biomechanical engineers investigate biomechanics, that is, the large- and small-scale solid and fluid mechanics of the living body. Biomechanical engineers design such devices as artificial joints and limb prostheses and address problems in orthopedic surgery, physical therapy, rehabilitative medicine, and other empirical areas of health care. Although research in biomechanics includes investigation of cartilage at the cellular and subcellular levels, neither biomechanics nor bioelectrics draws heavily on molecular biology. In contrast, biochemical engineering has been transformed by recent work in molecular biology, which provides the theoretical and experimental basis for predicting how the human body interacts with nonhuman materials. Advances in molecular biology have informed the design of devices in which there is dynamic exchange between human and nonhuman systems, such as that found in dialysis machines, heart-lung machines, artificial organs, or implants for sustained delivery of medications. Molecular biology also informs therapeutic protein research and lends important techniques to tis-

sue engineering, the use of engineering theory and methods to develop cell-based artificial organs—a liver, for example. New skin for burn patients is the first of many therapeutic innovations expected from tissue engineering.

Most biomedical engineers are employed outside of health care facilities. However, there is also a small but growing number of "clinical engineers" who work in health care facilities and oversee the use, adaptation, integration, maintenance, and repair of an increasingly sophisticated array of devices. In rehabilitation technology, for example, "rehabilitation" engineers often collaborate in prescribing appropriate devices or in designing unique devices for individuals.

The proportion of biomedical engineers in the United States who are women is high compared with other engineering fields, perhaps because they choose bioengineering over the military, another major source of opportunities to work with devices on the cutting edge of technology. The high proportion of women may also be explained by women's traditional involvement in the helping professions, the relative openness of new scientific fields to women, and the higher representation of women in the life sciences as compared with the physical sciences.

Collaborations between engineers and physicians in the United States tend to be dominated by physicians, highlighting the cultural differences between these professions. Although sometimes constrained by corporate management or "the market," engineers usually work by thoroughly discussing and "brainstorming" about how best to satisfy all criteria to achieve the best design. Physicians, on the other hand, especially surgeons and those who must make critical decisions quickly, are accustomed to unilateral decision making, which engineers often consider shortsighted. The naming of devices illustrates the dominance of medicine over engineering in collaborations on medical devices. Medical devices that are named for individuals (e.g., in orthopedic surgery, the Harris hip and the Galante hip) bear the name of a physician who collaborated on them or brought them into clinical use, even when the design is largely the work of a single biomedical engineer. The influence of physicians on biomedical engineering in the United States is further demonstrated by the fact that in the United States, the market for medical technologies, especially those used in health-care facilities, is driven by physicians and health-care facility administrators. Even when U.S. physicians do not actually collaborate in design and development, their demands as major customers have a much greater effect on the design of biomedical engineering devices than do those of other health professionals. In contrast, in Sweden, where the health-care system is government sponsored, all the health-care workers expected to use the device will be involved in setting the requirements for the device to be designed or purchased.

Biomedical engineering, medical technology, and issues in bioethics

One reason for the growing public interest in bioethics is the rapid change in health-care practice due to biomedical innovation. The resulting technology has both desirable and undesirable effects as well as many effects that, while not clearly negative or positive, alter the responsibilities of professionals and laity regarding birth and death, illness and injury. As people confront new information and new possibilities, they are faced with difficult decisions that were unknown to previous generations. New biomedical technology requires that people become "moral pioneers" (Rapp, 1987).

There are several major categories of medical technology with important implications for the definition of decisions and responsibilities. One is medical information systems, computer-based systems that store patient information and assist in clinical problem solving. Rehabilitation devices often enable patients to experience greater independence, comfort, and dignity. Drug delivery systems often alter patient participation in administering medications, as well as affecting the safety, reliability, and efficacy with which medications are administered. Still another category of medical technology is teaching devices that enable students to learn and practice clinical skills, often reducing patient suffering and lessening guilt and stress in student-practitioners during clinical training. Finally, there are technologies that improve the use of health-care technology. For example, assessment systems help clinicians appropriately match rehabilitation technology to an individual patient's needs and abilities.

New technologies also change responsibilities by altering the health-care labor force. Devices that require special skills to operate or to interpret their output have created new health-care occupations with new responsibilities. Other devices have reduced or eliminated the need for other kinds of work. Some devices, like imaging technologies or therapeutic X ray, have tended to centralize care in large university or urban centers because of the expense or massiveness of such equipment or requirements for its installation and maintenance (Reiser, 1978). For example, the powerful magnets used in magnetic resonance imaging require extensive shielding so as not to affect metal objects in the vicinity. Other kinds of technology, like information technology, have fostered decentralization by enabling practitioners in less populated areas to have ready access to both specialized medical knowledge and patient information (Reiser, 1978).

Often new medical technology has made health care more effective. However, some devices have become deeply entrenched in practice before their clinical value, or lack thereof, has been established. This pattern is illustrated by the example of the electronic fetal heart monitor used in childbirth. After its introduction, this monitor was quickly adopted in hospital obstetrics units, but was later shown not to improve birth outcome even for high-risk births (see Luthy et al., 1987).

Medical technology has had a variety of profound effects on familial as well as health-care practice. For example, some have criticized intensive-care technology's intrusiveness in view of the relatively high frequency with which people die in intensive-care units. The unit isolates the critically ill patient from family members, making it impossible for them to care for and comfort the patient in his or her final hours and disrupting the grieving process.

Engineering innovations often change "standards of care" when the use of a particular device becomes required in order for care to qualify as competent. For example, a physician who does not order a diagnostic X ray in certain cases may be liable for negligence. Lasers, fiber-optic and endoscopic technology, and ultrasound irradiation have made some surgery less invasive. Other areas of surgery, notably invasive neonatal surgery, have grown dramatically as new devices for surgery and new intensive-care technology for postsurgical recovery have been introduced. The outcome of these surgeries is sometimes problematic. In 1987 the U.S. Congress Office of Technology Assessment reported that largely as a result of such heroic interventions, there were 17,000 "technologically dependent" children chronically dependent on respirators, intravenous nutrition, and other medical devices for life support.

Although bioethics has devoted much attention to effective, but sometimes harrowing, new therapies and means of life support, diagnostic and monitoring devices have received less discussion. Diagnostic and monitoring technology often changes the character of medical decisions, the basis for them, and the parties to them. For example, when a pregnancy can be terminated if prenatal testing shows an abnormality, a test such as amniocentesis that is done halfway through pregnancy transforms the pregnancy into a "tentative pregnancy," even if the test results are normal (Rothman, 1986).

Some of the effects of technological change are at least in part the responsibility of the engineers who design them. The engineering profession recognizes that engineers are responsible for both the safety and the performance of their products. For diagnostic, monitoring, and life-critical devices, the safety issue is especially prominent because a failure is often life-threatening. The scope of the biomedical engineer's responsibility for how devices are used has only recently begun to be widely discussed among biomedical engineers. That discussion has considered whether engineers bear some guilt for the suffering caused by the use of respirators on patients who have no hope of recovery (Lewis, 1988). This suggestion proposes a particularly stringent standard of professional responsibility for engineers, since respirators perform their intended function very well and often enable people to resume active lives. However, when they are used on terminally ill patients, respirators may only prolong suffering for patients and families while using precious health-care resources. This kind of misuse must be distinguished from, for example, use of a device in a wet environment. Devices in the home or in a hospital are frequently used in areas that become wet, thus presenting the risk of electrocution. This risk is eliminated through the installation of ground-fault-interrupt circuit breakers. There are no similar engineering measures to ensure that respirators be used only with patients who have some hope of recovery. In recent years, state and national legislation has strengthened the legal standing of patients' advance directives, such as living wills and health-care proxy statements, about their care. These measures have had some success in addressing problems concerning the use of life-support technology, but no final consensus has been reached regarding the propriety of indefinitely prolonging life using medical technology. It is clear that control of medical technology to ensure that it furthers human welfare is only in part the responsibility of the engineers who design and develop it.

CAROLINE WHITBECK

Directly related to this entry are the entries ALLIED HEALTH PROFESSIONS; *and* TECHNOLOGY, *articles on* HISTORY OF MEDICAL TECHNOLOGY, *and* TECHNOLOGY ASSESSMENT. *Other relevant material may be found under the entries* KIDNEY DIALYSIS; MEDICAL INFORMATION SYSTEMS; *and* PHARMACEUTICS, *article on* PHARMACEUTICAL INDUSTRY. *For a discussion of some of the advanced technologies with which biomedical engineers work, see the entries* ARTIFICIAL HEARTS AND CARDIAC-ASSIST DEVICES; ARTIFICIAL ORGANS AND LIFE-SUPPORT SYSTEMS; BIOTECHNOLOGY; CRYONICS; DNA TYPING; GENETIC ENGINEERING; GENOME MAPPING AND SEQUENCING; LABORATORY TESTING; *and* ORGAN AND TISSUE TRANSPLANTS, *article on* MEDICAL OVERVIEW.

Bibliography

BENNER, PATRICIA E., and WRUBEL, JUDITH. 1989. *The Primacy of Caring: Stress and Coping in Health and Illness.* Reading, Mass.: Addison-Wesley.

CRAVALHO, ERNEST G., and McNEIL, BARBARA J., eds. 1982. *Critical Issues in Medical Technology.* Boston: Auburn House.

FOX, RENÉE C., and SWAZEY, JUDITH P. 1978. *The Courage to Fail: A Social View of Organ Transplants and Dialysis.* 2d ed. Chicago: University of Chicago Press.

LEWIS, STEVEN M. 1988. "A Sense of Sin." *Biomedical Engineering Society Bulletin,* 12, 1:1–2.

LUTHY, DAVID A.; SNY, KIRKWOOD K.; VAN BELLE, GERALD; LARSON, ERIC B.; HUGHES, JAMES P.; BENDETTI, THOMAS J.; BROWN, ZANE A.; EFFER, SIDNEY; KING, JAMES F.; and STENCHEVER, MORTON A. 1987. "A Randomized Trial of Electronic Fetal Monitoring in Preterm Labor." *Obstetrics and Gynecology* 69, no. 5:687–695.

MANN, ROBERT W. 1985. "Biomedical Engineering, A Cornucopia of Challenging Engineering Tasks—All of Direct Human Significance." *IEEE Engineering in Medicine and Biology Magazine* 4, no. 3:43–45.

RAPP, RAYNA. 1987. "Moral Pioneers: Women, Men, and Fetuses on a Frontier of Reproductive Technology." *Women and Health* 13, nos. 1 and 2:101–117.

REISER, STANLEY. 1978. *Medicine and the Reign of Technology.* Cambridge: At the University Press.

REISER, STANLEY J., and ANBAR, MICHAEL, eds. 1984. *Machine at the Bedside: Strategies for Using Technology in Patient Care.* Cambridge: At the University Press.

ROTHMAN, BARBARA KATZ. 1986. *The Tentative Pregnancy: Prenatal Diagnosis and the Future of Motherhood.* New York: Viking.

SHAFFER, MICHAEL J., and SHAFFER, MICHAEL D. 1989. "The Professionalization of Clinical Engineering." *Biomedical Instrumentation and Technology* 23, no. 5:370–374.

U.S. CONGRESS. OFFICE OF TECHNOLOGY ASSESSMENT. 1987. *New Developments in Biotechnology.* 5 vols. Washington, D.C.: Author.

WHITBECK, CAROLINE. 1991. "Ethical Issues Raised by New Medical Technologies." In *The New Reproductive Technologies: Medical, Psychosocial, Legal, and Ethical Dilemmas,* pp. 49–64. Edited by Judith Rodin and Aila Collins. Hillsdale, N.J.: Lawrence Erlbaum.

———. 1995. *Understanding Moral Problems in Engineering Practice and Research.* Cambridge: At the University Press.

WHITBECK, CAROLINE, and PRIEST, W. CURTISS. 1986. "Alternative Designs for Medical Information Systems—Consequences for Health and Human Values." Center for Technology, Policy and Industrial Development, Massachusetts Institute of Technology, Cambridge, Mass.

BIOMEDICAL ETHICS

See BIOETHICS; CLINICAL ETHICS; *and* MEDICAL ETHICS, HISTORY OF.

BIOMEDICAL RESEARCH

For a discussion of biomedical and behavioral research, see INFORMED CONSENT, *article on* CONSENT ISSUES IN HUMAN RESEARCH; RESEARCH, HUMAN: HISTORICAL ASPECTS; RESEARCH METHODOLOGY; *and* RESEARCH POLICY.

BIOSTATISTICS AND EPIDEMIOLOGY

See PUBLIC HEALTH, *article on* PUBLIC-HEALTH METHODS: EPIDEMIOLOGY AND BIOSTATISTICS.

BIOTECHNOLOGY

"Biotechnology" includes any technique that uses living organisms to make or modify products, to improve plants or animals, or to develop microorganisms for specific uses. Biotechnology has made it possible to expand knowledge about life. It has been used to make new pharmaceuticals, vaccines, and foods; to develop organisms to destroy toxic waste; to make agriculture more productive; to correct genetic defects in humans; and to help stem the destruction of biological diversity.

Humans have used living organisms in agriculture and food production since early history and have derived important pharmaceuticals from them for decades. Controversies over biotechnology began to arise after the development in the mid-1970s of novel and powerful techniques that allow dramatically increased control over the design of living organisms. Recombinant DNA (rDNA) technology, which allows specific pieces of genetic information to be moved between species, has raised most of the ethical concerns.

Do humans have the knowledge and judgment to use the technology in a responsible way? Are humans "playing God" when they move bits of genetic information between species? Since the mid-1970s, biotechnology's applications and potential risks have been debated in numerous public forums. The development of the technology proceeded more slowly, in order to allow society's opinions and concerns to be presented and discussed (Krimsky, 1982). This tradition is continuing as research progress produces more social questions.

Health-care issues

Pharmaceuticals. Drugs derived from biotechnology have substantially improved patient outcome and quality of life. Most of these drugs have been developed by companies established since the emergence of biotechnology in the 1970s. Because they have no cash flow from product sales for many years, these companies require large infusions of capital to move their drugs from the laboratory to the marketplace. To realize a return on this invested capital, these companies charge substantial prices for the drugs, even though the development and regulatory costs are generally about half of those of traditional pharmaceuticals. For instance, a dose of tissue plasminogen activator for heart attack victims is $2,500; a year's supply of erythropoietin (EPO) for end-stage renal disease is $8,000; human growth hormone costs $30,000 per year; a course of treatment with interleukin-2 for cancer is $9,000; and the treatment for Gaucher's disease is $130,000 per year. In comparison, the more traditional pharmaceutical Mevacor, used for controlling high cholesterol, is $700 per year (Winslow, 1991).

As the United States moves toward more centralized health care, drug pricing is a critical issue. If pricing formulas or caps are imposed on new drugs, their development will slow and biotechnology's contribution to health care will decrease.

Some of these drugs may be misused. Human growth hormone (hGH), used to treat certain cases of dwarfism, was once in short supply, and batches could be contaminated with a deadly neurological virus. Pure hGH is now made through the use of biotechnology, and there is enough to treat valid medical cases. There is also enough to give to children to make them a little taller or more athletic than average. Groups representing society have agreed that modification of genetic traits for enhancement of human capabilities is wrong (Walters, 1991), but it is difficult to control this sort of drug prescribing.

EPO, used to treat end-stage renal disease, can be used to promote athletic performance. It stimulates the production of red blood cells, which in turn allows a body to carry more oxygen to its tissues, thus increasing muscle performance. In contrast to performance-stimulating drugs like anabolic steroids, EPO is a naturally occurring substance and cannot be detected in drug tests. Given the fame and fortune associated with athletic excellence, the potential for misuse is high, not least because policing its distribution and use is very difficult.

Vaccines are one of the most cost-effective ways to prevent disease. Unfortunately, a very small fraction of vaccinated people will get the disease the vaccine is intended to prevent. Because of major liability problems for vaccine producers, only a few companies still make and market vaccines. Biotechnology is being used to develop vaccines that do not produce the disease as a result of vaccination because the disease-causing genes are deleted. However, partly because of continuing liability issues, few companies are pursuing vaccine research. In addition, the rDNA vaccines are generally more expensive. For example, the hepatitis B vaccine costs about $100, putting it out of reach of many people in areas where the disease is endemic.

Gene therapy.   Biotechnology makes it possible to change the genetic makeup of humans. Because of serious potential social and ethical consequences, this issue is widely studied and discussed in the bioethics community. In 1984, a committee was formed within the U.S. National Institutes of Health to help guide the medical profession in determining the appropriateness of gene therapy in humans. This committee, composed of scientists, clinicians, lawyers, and ethicists, developed a list of questions that must be answered satisfactorily before a particular gene therapy experiment can be undertaken. The questions not only ask about the safety and efficacy of the procedure, but also raise questions about fairness in selection of subjects, informed consent, and confidentiality. The committee has final say over whether any human gene-therapy experiment can be performed in the United States.

There are two general kinds of gene-therapy approaches, somatic and germ line (U.S. Congress, Office of Technology Assessment [OTA], 1984). In somatic gene therapy, some of a patient's cells receive a new gene, which functions for the life of the patient but is not passed on to any of the patient's offspring. In general, there has been little or no resistance to somatic gene therapy when it is used to treat serious medical disease (Walters, 1991; Murray, 1991). Most philosophical analyses argue that the somatic therapy is perceived to be like any other medical intervention: It does more good than harm and relieves human suffering.

Germ-line gene therapy, on the other hand, involves a permanent genetic change that is passed on to offspring because every cell, including the sex cells, is genetically changed. Germ-line gene therapy presents more serious ethical questions because the genetic change that is made can be permanent; it may be carried by a fraction of the offspring of the treated individual and subsequently through their lineage. The principle of informed consent cannot apply in any simple way to these descendants. Moreover, the only way we now know to change every cell in a person is to change all of the very few cells of an early embryo. Since the embryo cannot give informed consent, concerns arise about the respect for the individual.

Germ-line gene therapy, which is technically more difficult than somatic gene therapy, is currently being done with experimental animals. As such therapy becomes technically feasible for humans, legitimate needs can be imagined. For instance, if a genetic diagnosis is made prior to implantation of an in vitro fertilized embryo, the parents could choose germ-line gene therapy rather than disposal of the embryo.

Serious debate on germ-line gene therapy in humans would focus on issues including the effects of changing the gene mix in human populations, depletion of diversity in the gene pool, and the philosophical consequences of introducing nonhuman genes into humans, as well as access to this therapy and its cost.

A final issue applicable to both types of gene therapy is what constitutes serious disease. Most people who have studied the ethics of gene therapy agree that it should be used to treat disease and in no way used to enhance normal human characteristics (Anderson, 1990; Walters, 1991). Currently, gene therapy is used only to treat serious diseases that produce significant suffering and premature death. However, as we achieve technical competency in gene insertion, it may be tempting to use the therapy for less serious problems. Parents may increasingly demand "perfect" children. If this happens, there may be a trend toward using gene therapy to affect nondisease traits, such as intelligence and physical traits. This progression must be monitored so that society's degree of concern with manipulating the genetic makeup of offspring can be assessed.

Mapping the human genome.   In the mid-1980s, the U.S. government began funding a project to locate and sequence all the human genes. The human genome contains about 3 billion nucleotide base pairs (building blocks of genes) and an estimated 50,000–100,000 genes. The effort, now international, has mapped out 2,500 genes.

Deciphering the complete sequence of the human genome will not allow scientists to construct a human being, at least not with their current understanding of genetics. It will, however, help identify genes that are responsible for or contribute to disease. Relative vulnerabilities to diseases, such as cancer or heart disease, will be able to be identified, making preventive medicine more effective. The knowledge gained from the identification of human genes can be used to diagnose genetic diseases in utero or postnatally. It will also identify genes that are responsible for human characteristics such as eye color and height and, eventually, the genetic components underlying intelligence and behavior.

The first issue to consider is that of cost. With current technology, the cost of mapping and sequencing the human genome is estimated at $3 billion. The U.S. government's current expenditure is over $160 million a year. There is some concern that this expense is diverting money from research that could more directly benefit the treatment of human disease (Beckwith, 1991). And some think that in the course of scientific research, all the "important" genes will be mapped and sequenced anyway. Therefore, there is concern as to whether the expense of the mapping project is justified.

As the project continues, increasing knowledge of the genome raises other issues (Annas, 1989; "The Human Genome Initiative," 1991; Yesley, 1991). The first is that of control over and privacy of genetic information. Employers and insurers, it is argued, could require the results of genetic tests, and it might be difficult for an individual who needs a job or insurance to refuse access to the information. An employer, for instance, could deny employment to a person with a genetic susceptibility to disease caused by particular chemicals in the workplace; alternatively, the employer could make sure that the workplace is clean enough for the most sensitive person. Although the latter is the ideal solution, it often is not technically or economically feasible. Even though society does not believe that people should be discriminated against on the basis of their genetic makeup, is there an obligation to identify particularly susceptible people and match them with appropriate jobs if the technology is available? The use of genetic information in the workplace could have both positive and negative consequences for a person's employment and health. It is the consensus of medical geneticists and ethicists, however, that the results of genetic tests should be confidential, should respect individual liberty and choice, and should not be accessible for purposes of possible discrimination (Wertz et al., 1990; Murray, 1991).

Genetic information can be used to identify (and eliminate) people with "defective" or "inferior" genes, or to increase "desirable" traits in offspring. Given the history of the involuntary sterilization campaign in the United States in the early part of the twentieth century and the Nazi eugenic program, anything so dramatic in the near future is unlikely. Instead, more and more prepregnancy counseling and in utero diagnosis of defective genes will be done—and, possibly, more abortions. With spiraling health-care costs, insurers could put pressure on women not to have children with potentially deleterious genes. Thus, offspring may be engineered to conform to some societal norm. What will society define as a "normal" set of genes, and how much deviation will be permitted before a genome is determined to be "diseased"?

DNA fingerprinting. Without needing to understand the whole human genome, it is possible to generate maps, somewhat analogous to bar codes, that are specific for each individual (Debenham, 1991). These maps, or DNA fingerprints, rely on repeated hypervariable regions in DNA that vary dramatically in different individuals. If enough of these regions are identified and studied, it is possible to generate a pattern that has a negligible probability of being like anyone else's pattern. This technology is commercially available for identification of crime suspects by comparing the suspect's DNA fingerprint against DNA fingerprints from evidence (blood, hair, semen, etc.) found at the scene of the crime. It can also be used for determining paternity

and for following the course of certain therapies, such as bone marrow transplants.

If the tests are performed properly, there are no inherent disadvantages to the technology and many advantages. National or international standards and quality assurance protocols have not yet been established, however, and DNA evidence is occasionally dismissed because of poor test quality. In addition, some concerns relating to population subcultures need to be investigated before some fingerprints can unequivocally be called unique.

If DNA fingerprints are kept in government data bases, privacy concerns arise. Since DNA fingerprints can be used only for identification and not for determining disease or predisposition to disease, however, the privacy concerns are relatively less significant than those associated with other genetic information.

Ownership of life

Human cells and tissues. With biotechnology, it is now possible to immortalize and modify human cells and tissues and their components, and use them commercially to make diagnostic and therapeutic products, sometimes at great economic gain. Should patients or volunteers who donate tissue for scientific research that leads to these products share in the profits that may result?

In the United States, organs can only be donated, not sold, for transplantation. A market in organs, it is thought, would foster inequities and promote injustice. On the other hand, one can sell one's blood, a replenishable resource. The use of cells and tissues is different in that the tissues do not necessarily go from one person to another, but can be used to make products for a large number of people. It can be argued that donors are not entitled to the value of their donations because they do nothing to develop the materials into the valuable product. This reasoning was used in a landmark ruling, *Moore* v. *Regents of Univ. of Cal.*, 793 P.2d 479, 15 USPQ 2d 1753 (Cal. 1990), involving a patient's cells that were used to produce a commercially useful product. Many institutions currently pay a one-time fee for biological tissue to avoid liability at a later date.

Before donating cells and tissues, subjects, including patients, should be clearly advised that the tissues may be used for research and possible economic gain, and the subject's informed consent should be secured. The latter point is not routinely made in current informed-consent agreements. Advised of possible economic gain, a patient may not make the best decision for his or her health, or may have unreasonable financial expectations.

Ethical and religious traditions do not provide clear guidelines regarding the sale of body parts. However, some questions can be considered. First, is the basic dignity of humans preserved? Second, would more people benefit if the tissues were commercialized? And third, would a commercial market be equitable to all members of society? Overall, the current approach leans toward the donation of tissue or the payment of a reasonably small, one-time fee (U.S. Congress, OTA, 1987).

Plants and animals.   Since the dawn of agriculture, humans have controlled plants and animals. Crop breeding produced seed that was more productive than its wild relatives and, thus, became a product of commerce. The domestication of animals as both food sources and pets, and their subsequent ownership by humans, is well established in history. Yet biotechnology raises new issues about ownership of higher organisms (Karny, 1989; U.S. Congress, OTA, 1989).

The tools of biotechnology can enhance traditional breeding techniques for plants and animals. For instance, gene mapping can track the inheritance of particular characteristics, and new genes for important traits can be inserted into useful plants and animals. These advances have caused inventors of these new organisms to seek patent protection. The U.S. Patent and Trademark Office (PTO) declared that they are in fact patentable. But is it appropriate to patent higher organisms created through biotechnology?

The arguments for and against patenting higher life forms have revolved solely around animals, but the same arguments apply to plants. Plants evoke fewer ethical concerns than animals for two reasons: first, humans feel more evolutionary kinship to animals than they do to plants; and second, many forms of novel plants have been patented by U.S. laws since the 1930s.

The arguments for patenting animals are mostly economic. Patents promote inventiveness and new products. They inspire competition in the marketplace and promote national competitiveness. Finally, patenting greatly reduces reliance on trade secrets, which slows the dissemination of new information and the introduction of useful and important products.

The arguments against patenting animals involve evolutionary kin and economics. The first argument is that patenting involves an improper amount of human control over animal life, an underestimation of the value of nonhuman life, and the first step toward a decline in the belief in the sanctity and dignity of (animal) life. This argument really addresses ownership in general and is not very convincing to people who use animals as food. There is also the recognition that animals, especially higher mammals, are closely related to humans and may exhibit some sentience—and, therefore, should not be owned.

A second argument is that the act of inserting novel genetic information into animals and creating new animals causes more animal suffering than does traditional breeding. This issue better belongs in a discussion of animal rights, not of ownership—or patenting—of animals.

Third, animal patents may force farmers to pay more for patented animals. This economic concern is likely to be addressed in the marketplace, where farmers will be willing to pay more for animals only if the additional cost can be recovered through better performance. However, the question remains whether farmers have to pay a royalty to the patent holder for every birth from a patented animal. In the area of seeds, the government solved this problem by mandating that farmers have a royalty-free, compulsory license for the offspring of the seed they buy.

Fourth, patent offices outside the United States have not completely formed their policies on plant and animal patents, thus leaving the United States open to criticism. The European Patent Office rejected a patent application on a recombinant DNA mouse, the subject of the first U.S. animal patent.

The fact of animal patents suggests the theoretical possibility that a human being who has experienced genetic engineering—through gene therapy, for instance—could be patented. The PTO has expressly stated that claims to animals must be limited to nonhuman animals. More important, the Thirteenth Amendment of the U.S. Constitution can be interpreted to prohibit the ownership of engineered human beings.

Environmental issues

Agriculture.   Biotechnology health-care products have raised little controversy in that they are often the best alternative for treatment of life-threatening diseases. Agricultural products produced using biotechnology, on the other hand, are viewed by some as expensive alternatives to an already very successful agricultural system. Their cost, not only in terms of dollars but also in terms of pollution, and their potential impact on the future of family farms are issues of concern.

Industrial agricultural biotechnology programs have developed herbicide-tolerant crop plants. Herbicides are well known to enhance agricultural productivity and keep food prices low, but they have detrimental environmental and health effects. Herbicide tolerance—crop plants are not affected but weeds are destroyed when the herbicide is applied—is an important part of current agricultural practices. It is also a relatively easy genetic manipulation to perform, compared with drought resistance or improved nutritional quality. The proponents of herbicide-tolerant plants claim that their new varieties will minimize the use of herbicides, thus reducing environmental and health concerns. Some environmental groups claim, on the other hand, that herbicide tolerance will promote the use of pesticides, just when there should be a movement in the other direction, toward sustainable agriculture. Herbicide-tolerant plants will soon be in the marketplace, and their effect on the quantity of pesticide use will be apparent after that. It is worth noting that many of the companies developing herbicide-tolerant plants also produce herbicides.

Opponents of biotechnology claim that agricultural biotechnology will cause severe economic and social dislocations, because the products of biotechnology will favor farming operations that can take advantage of economies of scale. Proponents claim that biotechnology products are mostly "scale neutral," affecting large and small farms alike. The most controversial biotechnology product in this context is bovine somatotropin (BST), which increases milk production 10 to 25 percent in cows with only a small increase in feed consumption. Some think that this product will be more effectively used on large dairy farms, putting small farms out of business. In fact, the consensus is that BST will separate good from bad managers, not large from small farms (U.S. Congress, OTA, 1991). However, BST is often attacked in the context of a trend toward larger farms that has been under way for decades. This trend entails the general demise of the family farm. The larger farm results not only from emerging technology, of which biotechnology is a growing part, but also from industry economics and government policy.

Ecological issues. With the first recombinant DNA experiment, a concern arose that an organism would be produced whose actions were unpredictable and potentially harmful when released into the environment (U.S. Congress, OTA, 1988; National Research Council, 1989). Kudzu and the gypsy moth were mentioned as examples of introduced nonindigenous species gone awry. This ecological concern is set against the potential good of numerous proposed genetically engineered organisms, among them crops with increased productivity and microorganisms that degrade toxic chemicals, enhance agricultural productivity, treat wastewater, extract metals in mining operations, and increase the efficiency of oil recovery.

During the 1980s, numerous genetically engineered organisms were introduced into the environment in carefully controlled studies. On the basis of the results of these experiments and other scientific information, the international scientific community reached the following conclusions in 1987 (National Research Council, 1987):

1. There is no evidence that unique hazards exist either in the use of recombinant DNA techniques or in the transfer of genes between unrelated organisms.
2. The risks associated with the introduction of recombinant DNA–engineered organisms are the same in kind as those associated with the introduction into the environment of unmodified organisms and organisms modified by other genetic techniques.

In assessing risk, a number of factors are taken into account, including our familiarity with the organism being modified, methods to control the organism, and the probable effects on the environment. Although knowledge about the environment is incomplete, we have enough knowledge to guide the safe use of novel organisms and to identify the most problematic introductions. Some modifications, such as increasing the virulence of a known pathogen, should not be permitted.

The issue of comparison with introduced exotic organisms deserves additional clarification. A genetically engineered organism contains one or several genetic modifications of an organism already found in the ecosystem in which it will be placed. The addition of the new genetic information in all likelihood imposes an evolutionary burden on the new organism that makes it less compatible with its environment. This situation is very different from that of exotic organisms, which bring an entirely new, evolutionarily tuned genome to a very foreign environment. The introduction of the exotic organism is quite different from that of the recombinant DNA organism and, thus, not an adequate comparison. In addition, because the genetic changes in a recombinant DNA organism are known, potential risks can be much more accurately predicted.

The international community, through the United Nations Industrial Development Organization and the Organization for Economic Cooperation and Development, has been trying to harmonize regulations concerning the deliberate introduction of genetically engineered organisms into the environment. The conflicting political influences of advocates for industry and for the environment in various countries have led to mixed results. Regulatory regimes in the United Kingdom, China, France, Italy, New Zealand, and Australia are less burdensome than they are in the United States, while in Germany, Denmark, and Japan, they are more stringent (Balter, 1991; Brill, 1988).

Biological diversity. Biological diversity is generated through genetic mutation and the consequent ability of an organism to reproduce in a particular ecosystem. A species becomes extinct when an ecosystem is no longer available to support it. Humans, with their ability to change ecosystems dramatically and rapidly, have caused the extinction of species at much increased rates, especially in the past several decades. Tropical deforestation alone is estimated to be responsible for the extinction of 4,000 species a year. Some fear that we may, in fact, be destroying our ability to survive on the planet.

The preservation of biodiversity is important for at least three reasons. First, it can be argued that all living organisms have an intrinsic value and that society has a moral responsibility to protect its only known living companions in the universe. Second, people derive direct economic benefits from other living organisms in the form of food and numerous industrial products and medicines. Third, diverse ecosystems are responsible for maintaining gases in the atmosphere, recycling rainfall, maintaining the climate, disposing of wastes, and cycling of nutrients—in other words, the systems that maintain life.

Preservation of biological diversity can be achieved by protection of populations in nature or by preservation of samples in gene banks. This latter method, ex situ preservation, can be greatly aided by biotechnology. Advances in biotechnology allow us to preserve cells, ova, embryos, sperm, and tissues in reliable and economically feasible ways. Biotechnology will also help us decide what to store. Ultimately, the genetic information of species could be preserved in DNA data banks. As our knowledge of life increases through biotechnology, we may be able to pick and choose particular organisms or their genes for distinct uses, such as a drug with certain properties or a crop that is disease resistant (Ehrlich and Wilson, 1991; Colwell, 1989).

University–industry relationships

Advances in biotechnology move rapidly from basic research developments to the commercial arena. The speed of this development, as well as the increasing difficulty in obtaining federal research funds, led to greatly increased interactions between industry and university biology laboratories during the 1980s. On several occasions, industries made very large donations, often more than $10 million, to individual university departments.

Universities are characterized by their open environment and free exchange of ideas and information. Industry, on the other hand, is profit-driven and focuses on proprietary product development. If industry funds academic research, universities may lose some of their freedom. Even if universities insist that all industry-funded research be done openly and that the results be published, there is concern that industry will increasingly be able to determine the direction of university research (Government-University-Industry, 1989).

Another concern is industrial funding from foreign sources for domestic university research. Some governments control the access to their university science, but most, including the United States, have no review mechanisms for accepting foreign industrial money for biotechnology research. As the contracts are usually written, the funding group receives an exclusive license to the results of the funded research. Thus, a foreign company can leverage U.S. taxpayers' dollars into prod-

ucts sold at substantial profits (National Academy of Sciences, 1990).

Conclusion

Biotechnology has made great strides since the emergence of rDNA technology in the early 1970s. There are numerous health-care and agricultural products on the market, and scientists have a greatly increased understanding of life itself. During this time, the societal issues associated with advances in biotechnology have been debated in many public forums, sometimes quite contentiously. As a consequence, society is adjusting to the use of the technology, and the users of the technology have become more sensitive to the concerns of society. As the next century approaches, the most important ethical issues to debate include privacy and appropriate use of genetic information, pricing of pharmaceuticals, and germ-line gene therapy.

NANETTE NEWELL

Directly related to this entry are the entries AGRICULTURE; COMMERCIALISM IN SCIENTIFIC RESEARCH; ENVIRONMENTAL POLICY AND LAW; GENE THERAPY; GENETIC ENGINEERING, *article on* ANIMALS AND PLANTS; GENETICS AND THE LAW; PATENTING ORGANISMS; *and* TECHNOLOGY, *article on* TECHNOLOGY ASSESSMENT. *For a further discussion of topics mentioned in this entry, see the entries* ANIMAL RESEARCH; ANIMAL WELFARE AND RIGHTS, *articles on* ETHICAL PERSPECTIVES ON THE TREATMENT AND STATUS OF ANIMALS, WILDLIFE CONSERVATION AND MANAGEMENT, *and* ANIMALS IN AGRICULTURE AND FACTORY FARMING; DNA TYPING; ENDANGERED SPECIES AND BIODIVERSITY; EUGENICS; FOOD POLICY; GENETIC TESTING AND SCREENING; GENOME MAPPING AND SEQUENCING; ORGAN AND TISSUE PROCUREMENT; PHARMACEUTICS, *article on* PHARMACEUTICAL INDUSTRY; *and* XENOGRAFTS.

Bibliography

ANDERSON, W. FRENCH. 1990. "Genetics and Human Malleability." *Hastings Center Report* 20, no. 1:21–24.

ANNAS, GEORGE, J. 1989. "Who's Afraid of the Human Genome?" *Hastings Center Report* 19, no. 4:19–21.

BALTER, MICHAEL. 1991. "How Europe Regulates Its Genes." *Science* 252, no. 5011:1366–1368.

BECKWITH, JON. 1991. "The Human Genome Initiative: Genetics' Lightning Rod." *American Journal of Law and Medicine* 17, nos. 1–2:1–13.

BRILL, WINSTON J. 1988. "Why Engineered Organisms Are Safe." *Issues in Science and Technology* 4, no. 3:44–50.

COLWELL, ROBERT K. 1989. "Natural and Unnatural History:

Biological Diversity and Genetic Engineering." In *Scientists and Their Responsibility*, pp. 1–40. Edited by William R. Shea and Beat Sitter. Canton, Mass.: Watson.

DEBENHAM, PAUL G. 1991. "DNA Fingerprinting." *Journal of Pathology* 164, no. 2:101–106.

EHRLICH, PAUL R., and WILSON, EDWARD O. 1991. "Biodiversity Studies: Science and Policy." *Science* 253, no. 5021:758–762.

GOVERNMENT–UNIVERSITY–INDUSTRY RESEARCH ROUNDTABLE. 1989. *Science and Technology in the Academic Enterprise: Status, Trends, and Issues*. Washington, D.C.: National Academy Press.

"The Human Genome Initiative and the Impact of Genetic and Screening Technologies." 1991. *American Journal of Law and Medicine* 17, nos. 1–2. Special issue devoted to issues surrounding the Human Genome Project.

KARNY, GEOFFREY M. 1989. "Intellectual Property in the 1990s: Patenting Higher Life Forms." In *Biotechnology Law for the 1990s: Analysis and Perspective*. Washington, D.C.: Bureau of National Affairs.

KRIMSKY, SHELDON. 1982. *Genetic Alchemy: The Social History of the Recombinant DNA Controversy*. Cambridge, Mass.: MIT Press.

Moore v. Regents of Univ. of Cal. 1990. 793 P.2d 479, 15 USPQ 2d 1753 (Cal. 1990).

MURRAY, THOMAS H. 1991. "Ethical Issues in Human Genome Research." *FASEB Journal* 5, no. 1:55–60.

NATIONAL ACADEMY OF SCIENCES. 1990. *The Academic Research Enterprise Within the Industrialized Nations: Comparative Perspectives*. Washington, D.C.: National Academy Press.

NATIONAL RESEARCH COUNCIL (U.S.). 1987. *Introduction of Recombinant DNA–Engineered Organisms into the Environment: Key Issues*. Washington, D.C.: National Academy Press.

———. 1989. *Field Testing of Genetically Modified Organisms: Framework for Decisions*. Washington, D.C.: National Academy Press.

U.S. CONGRESS. OFFICE OF TECHNOLOGY ASSESSMENT (OTA). 1984. *Human Gene Therapy*. Washington, D.C.: U.S. Government Printing Office.

———. 1987. *Ownership of Human Tissues and Cells*. Washington, D.C.: U.S. Government Printing Office.

———. 1988. *Field Testing Engineered Organisms: Genetic and Ecological Issues*. Washington, D.C.: U.S. Government Printing Office.

———. 1989. *Patenting Life*. Washington, D.C.: U.S. Government Printing Office.

———. 1991. *U.S. Dairy Industry at a Crossroad: Biotechnology and Policy Choices*. Washington, D.C.: U.S. Government Printing Office.

WALTERS, LEROY. 1991. "Human Gene Therapy: Ethics and Public Policy." *Human Gene Therapy* 2, no. 2:115–122.

WERTZ, DOROTHY C.; FLETCHER, JOHN C.; and MULVIHILL, JOHN J. 1990. "Medical Geneticists Confront Ethical Dilemmas: Cross-Cultural Comparisons Among 18 Nations." *American Journal of Human Genetics* 46, no. 6:1200–1213.

WINSLOW, RON. 1991. "Dose of Reality: Costly Biotech Drugs Will Pose Hard Choices for U.S. Health Care." *Wall Street Journal*, November 5, p. A1.

YESLEY, MICHAEL S. 1991. *Bibliography: Ethical, Legal, and Social Implications of the Human Genome Project*. Los Alamos, N. Mex.: Los Alamos National Laboratory.

BIRTH CONTROL

See FERTILITY CONTROL. *See also* ABORTION.

BIRTH DEFECTS

See INFANTS. *Also see* GENE THERAPY; GENETIC COUNSELING; GENETIC TESTING AND SCREENING; *and* MATERNAL–FETAL RELATIONSHIP.

BLOOD TRANSFUSION

Blood transfusion is one of the essentials of preserving life and maintaining health. Transfusion is required to replace red cell or whole blood loss as a result of chronic illnesses such as hemophilia or thalassemia, or blood loss through acute trauma or surgery. The process of transfusion involves removing blood from one individual (the donor) and giving it to another (the recipient). Defined in such simple terms, it would seem to pose few problems. Yet the collection and distribution of blood require a complex medical technology and raise a set of ethical and legal issues pitting confidentiality and the privacy rights of individuals against the equally compelling public-health demands for a safe blood supply. The onset of acquired immunodeficiency syndrome (AIDS) has exacerbated these concerns.

The symbolic, historical, and religious meaning of blood makes its exchange a metaphor for community. Blood relatives are family; blood feuds indicate disagreement between rival families or clans. The central act of Christian observance, as defined by the New Testament, is the real or symbolic changing of wine into the blood of Christ, thus delineating the community of Christians from outsiders (Murray, 1991). Blood donation has been similarly used to delineate community boundaries. As late as 1968 in Louisiana and Alabama, blood was labeled by the race of the donor and transfusions limited to recipients of the donor's race (Titmuss, 1971). In contemporary society, where the link between blood and the human immunodeficiency virus (HIV) has been documented, exclusion from the ability to participate in this gift-giving relationship results not from external characteristics of individuals but from characteristics of the individuals' blood, unseen but potentially fatal.

The collection and distribution of blood

One significant ethical question with respect to the blood supply relates to the method of collection and distribution of blood. The essential issue is whether blood is to be considered a commodity or a social resource (Titmuss, 1971). Both cash payments, in which individuals are compensated for giving blood, and insurance (credit) systems, in which blood is donated in exchange for the recipient's agreement to supply blood when needed, treat the collection and distribution of blood as commercial transactions. In contrast, voluntary systems are based on the implicit assumption that blood is a social resource. From the late 1940s until the early 1980s, all three systems existed simultaneously in the United States, with some regions utilizing one of the systems exclusively and others relying on a mixture of all three systems.

Because blood is such a vital commodity, commercial approaches to its supply raise questions of social justice. For example, under systems of cash payment, the poor and low-income segments of the population (and thus racial and ethnic minorities, because of their high correlation with poverty) are most likely to participate in the selling of blood yet do not always have the means to pay for blood when it is needed.

The seminal work of the British sociologist Richard Titmuss (1971) characterized the donation of blood as a measure of social connectedness, fulfilling an essential need in persons to act for the benefit of community. He strongly criticized the commercial approach to the blood supply in the United States. Comparing the United States with England and Wales, Titmuss argued that the all-voluntary system in the latter countries assisted in maintaining the sense of community, while the predominantly commercial donor recruitment efforts in the United States threatened the fragile fabric of society. He stated that the use of payment and "blood insurance" as incentives for donation in the United States produced a traffic in blood that reflected this nation's dominant commitment to capitalism. It was Titmuss's view that the commercialization of blood in the United States denied its inhabitants the opportunity to see themselves as participating in a voluntary act of giving and resulted in an inadequate and unsafe supply.

In contrast to Titmuss, Alvin Drake, Stan Finkelstein, and Harvey Sapolsky (1982) found that regardless of the presence of credit systems, the American donors were in fact similar to British donors in that they came if the message was clear and collection agencies made donating simple in an easily accessible place. So, they argued, despite the underlying economic system that might be attached to the collection agency, the American donor approached the act of giving with a desire to participate in providing something needed by another.

The formation of a national blood policy was influenced by Titmuss's argument that however small the percentage of commercial donors, their participation led to a greater risk to the blood supply because of the relationship between a paid donor and infection, particularly with hepatitis B. Thus the adoption of the national blood policy in 1974 began a shift toward a volunteer model for the collection of whole blood, and by the late 1980s nearly all whole blood was collected from voluntary donors.

Whole blood includes red cells, plasma, platelets, and other components. It is increasingly common today for patients to receive only the particular blood component most desirable for their required therapy. This practice, known as component therapy, allows for more efficient utilization of the whole-blood supply and minimizes the risk to recipients that comes from exposure to unneeded substances in the blood (Drake et al., 1982).

Although commercial whole-blood collection has been effectively eliminated in the United States, the plasma fractionation industry, which is the domain of the private pharmaceutical firms, continues to obtain most of its products from paid donors. In addition to plasma, albumin for the treatment of shock and trauma and Factor VIII for treatment of hemophilia are important products of this industry. A major reason for the continued involvement of the United States in for-profit plasma production is the role that the country plays in the supply of plasma to world markets; in recent years, the United States has produced approximately one-third of the world supply of albumin and one-half the Factor VIII (U.S. Congress, Office of Technology Assessment, 1985). In contrast, many western European countries collect more blood than they require for whole-blood transfusions through purely voluntary donations, and use the overage to produce sufficient plasma. This overbleeding to produce a sufficient supply of plasma results in an oversupply of red blood cells, some of which are exported to the United States. Overbleeding in western Europe introduces commercialism into what is commonly thought of as a purely voluntary system and raises a set of issues for treatment of donors.

AIDS and the blood supply

Current estimates of the safety of the blood supply vary widely, but recent studies suggest that the overall risk of HIV infection through transfusion is 1 in 225,000 per unit, while the risk of transfusion-transmitted infection with hepatitis B is estimated to be about 1 in 50,000 per unit, and the risk of hepatitis C through transfusion is estimated to be less than 1 in 3,300 per unit (Winslow, 1992).

Concerns about the safety of the blood supply took on new significance in 1982 when the possibility of contracting AIDS from blood transfusion became clear. Although the actual risk of contracting AIDS through transfusion is less than the risk of contracting hepatitis B or C, AIDS, unlike other diseases transmitted through the blood, is inevitably fatal. Thus it has radically altered the relationship between donors and recipients of blood. AIDS has raised profound questions about the potential conflict between protection of the rights of donors and the right of society to a safe blood supply. AIDS is also an example of a situation where public perception, rather than actual data based on relative risks, guides what we tell a patient. Physicians tend to have patients sign special consents for transfusion that clarify the AIDS-related risks but do not always include information about other risks. Provision of more complete information might, however, result in too much complexity for the patient to deal with.

Not until 1985 was a test for the presence of antibodies to the AIDS virus introduced. This test, however, allows some blood with the AIDS virus to remain undetected because there is a forty-five-day window of vulnerability (Dodd, 1992), in which an infected individual may not have developed sufficient antibodies to be detected. Only the development of a test for the virus itself will further reduce the danger of contracting AIDS through use of blood or blood products.

Prior to the introduction of the test, donor deferral guidelines were the basis for protecting the safety of the blood supply. Self-deferral involves asking individuals who are members of high-risk groups, such as homosexual men and intravenous drug users of both sexes, not to donate blood (U.S. Congress, Office of Technology Assessment, 1985). Adoption of such guidelines, however, was resisted at first by many of the involved groups. The homosexual community, particularly in San Francisco, was concerned about the consequences of self-deferral to the progress they were making through the increasingly successful homosexual rights movement. In addition there were some general concerns about the violation of the civil rights of individuals excluded from donating through self-deferral. The fact that the groups first seen as potential carriers of AIDS were drug abusers and male homosexuals led some to suggest that, because these groups were personally responsible for having contracted the disease, they had forfeited their civil rights and should be banned from giving blood.

Gradually, however, a sophisticated system for self-deferral was developed. The health history now taken when an individual comes to give blood contains questions about high-risk behaviors including homosexual or bisexual behavior, intravenous drug use, and travel to sub-Sahara Africa. Potential donors may choose to defer after reading the reasons why they should not donate. Testing and self-deferral have substantially reduced the risk factor of contracting AIDS.

The group approach to a safer blood supply involves exclusion of certain categories of individuals from the donor population because they are deemed high-risk groups. Selection of groups to be excluded may reflect societal prejudices rather than scientific judgment. For example, Haitians were first an excluded group, but the exclusion has since been removed as a result of political pressure by Haitians in the United States and of evidence that their infection rate, though higher than the general rate in the United States, is considerably lower than that of persons from countries in sub-Sahara Africa. With the exception of homosexual men, those excluded in the United States are predominantly racial minorities.

Exclusion of high-risk groups raises substantial problems of confidentiality and informed consent. The names of individuals who test positive for HIV antibodies or hepatitis B or C, or who carry other viral agents, are placed on registries maintained by agencies within the blood supply system (e.g., the American Red Cross, the American Association of Blood Banks). Individuals are not always informed, in advance of volunteering, of the possibility of being listed on a registry.

In addition, individuals placed on a registry in one system may or may not be identified as at risk in another, which has led to recent efforts to try to coordinate this information. Since all blood is tested and registries are not checked until after the blood is taken, it is not clear that registries significantly increase safety. Moreover, some tests, including the test for hepatitis C, have produced high false-positive rates. The test for hepatitis C is so new that many who have given blood for decades suddenly find themselves deferred from future donations, resulting in their alienation from the system of collection. In this case, weighing the consequences of this alienation of individuals who have been long-term donors against the potential for life-threatening disease for the recipient has led to a decision to protect the recipient.

Problems of confidentiality also arise because potential donors are asked intimate questions about their sexual life and drug usage. While asking these questions may be justified on public-health grounds, past cases in which government agencies have obtained confidential information raise justifiable belief that the information should not be recorded. There is no federal statute that prohibits disclosure of the information except to blood banks, and there is no assurance under most state law that a court might not order disclosure in unexpected circumstances. In fact, some lawsuits resulting from transfusion-related AIDS have led to court decisions to permit identification of donors (Willett, 1986). Although the issues are similar in some respects to those arising in current debates regarding the testing of alleged rapists to determine HIV status, in the latter case the courts have taken the position that the primary concern is protecting the rights of the accused.

Alternatives to the system of transfusion

Although the gift relationship is founded on altruistic motivation, anthropologists have long recognized that giving gifts creates bonding and an expectation of receipt of gifts (Titmuss, 1971). In the context of the blood supply, voluntary donors expect the availability of blood when they need it and that the blood will be safe. Because of the fatal nature of AIDS, many have begun to fear that the exchange feature of donating has been taken away and have sought alternative ways to assure themselves of a safe, adequate blood supply. These techniques wholly or partially sever the broad community relationship.

For example, autologous transfusion, in which individuals store their own blood for future use, has increased substantially and is safe. A technique has also been developed to recycle the patient's own blood during surgery (interoperative blood salvage). Another alternative is directed donation, in which the patient receives blood from family and friends who are asked to donate. While directed donation may seem a safe alternative to patients, there is no evidence that the blood of directed donors is safer than that of the general donor pool; and if directed donors are unwilling to identify high-risk behavior, the risk may actually be greater because many directed donors are first-time donors. To reduce this risk, donors are given an opportunity to have their blood taken but to indicate through a choice of bar codes that their blood should not be used for transfusion (Shulman, 1991).

Considerable work is being done on the development of artificial blood substitutes. Research has continued for more than twenty-five years on the development of red-cell substitutes but has not yet resulted in an alternative approved for human use (Winslow, 1992). Applied researchers are also at work on the manufacture of biological proteins that plasma now supplies, and a biosynthetic version of one such protein, clotting Factor VIII, has been in clinical trials for several years. Success in the development of artificial blood substitutes would increase the safety of the blood supply and resolve a number of the issues discussed here.

The right to refuse transfusion

Both the right to receive transfusions and the right to refuse them have become increasingly significant issues. In the years since the development of transfusions as a treatment technique, the supply of blood has been increased, and today an inadequate supply is not a barrier to treatment. Therefore, as is the case with other issues in medical decision making, the physician determines the need for transfusion without regard to the economic status of the patient. In U.S. society, however, there are many ways in which the economic status of the patient affects the type of treatment he or she receives, and these factors also affect decisions about transfusions.

General questions of the right to refuse treatment have been raised in recent years, particularly with regard to the terminally ill. Related issues apply, specifically in connection with transfusion, because of the view of Jehovah's Witnesses that the transfusion of whole blood and most of its components is prohibited. This refusal raises dilemmas including the right to informed consent, the ability to help versus the respect for autonomy, and the potential liability for treating versus the potential liability for failing to treat. In the case of adults, court decisions have generally upheld the right to informed consent. Where a child's life is in danger, however, the decisions have favored the transfusion of blood (Lentz, 1990).

The operation of the blood-supply system demonstrates how what initially appears to be a technical or scientific advance frequently gives rise to fundamental ethical and political issues. As explained above, transfusion involves a technology that enables blood to be taken from one individual and given to another, frequently to sustain the life of the recipient. This technical definition, however, is too simplistic. In the collection and distribution of blood, we encounter significant issues of community, social justice, privacy, and the equitable distribution of the gift of life that extend far beyond the promise of the technology.

LOUANNE KENNEDY

Directly related to this entry are the entries AIDS, *article on* PUBLIC-HEALTH ISSUES; ECONOMIC CONCEPTS IN HEALTH CARE; HEALTH-CARE RESOURCES, ALLOCATION OF; ORGAN AND TISSUE PROCUREMENT, *article on* ETHICAL AND LEGAL ISSUES REGARDING LIVING DONORS; *and* PUBLIC HEALTH. *For a further discussion of topics mentioned in this entry, see the entries* BENEFICENCE; CONFIDENTIALITY; ETHICS, *article on* RELIGION AND MORALITY; INFORMED CONSENT; JUSTICE; PRIVACY; *and* TECHNOLOGY, *article on* PHILOSOPHY OF TECHNOLOGY. *Other relevant material may be found in the entry* METAPHOR AND ANALOGY.

Bibliography

DODD, ROGER Y. 1992. "The Risk of Transfusion-Transmitted Infection." *New England Journal of Medicine* 327, no. 6:419–421.

DRAKE, ALVIN W.; FINKELSTEIN, STAN N.; and SAPOLSKY, HARVEY M. 1982. *The American Blood Supply.* Cambridge, Mass.: MIT Press.

LENTZ, SUSAN. 1990. "The Right to Refuse Treatment." In *Transfusion Medicine in the 1990s.* Edited by Sandra T. Nance and Sherrill Slichtes. Arlington, Va.: American Association of Blood Banks.

MURRAY, THOMAS H. 1991. "The Poisoned Gift: AIDS and Blood." In *A Disease of Society: Cultural and Institutional Responses to AIDS,* pp. 216–240. Edited by Dorothy Nelkin, David P. Willis, and Scott V. Parris. New York: Cambridge University Press.

SHULMAN, IRA A. 1991. "A Review of Transfusion Medicine, 1980–1990." *American Journal of Clinical Pathology* 96, no. 4 (supp. 1):S25–S31.

TITMUSS, RICHARD M. 1971. *The Gift Relationship: From Human Blood to Social Policy.* New York: Pantheon.

U.S. CONGRESS. OFFICE OF TECHNOLOGY ASSESSMENT. 1985. *Blood Policy and Technology.* Washington, D.C.: U.S. Government Printing Office.

WILLETT, DAVID E. 1986. "Transfusion-Transmitted Diseases: Legal Aspects." In *Legal Issues in Transfusion Medicine.* Edited by Gilbert M. Clark. Arlington, Va.: American Association of Blood Banks.

WINSLOW, ROBERT M. 1992. "Red Cell Substitutes: Current Status, 1992." In *Blood Safety: Current Challenges.* Edited by Sandra T. Nance. Bethesda, Md.: American Association of Blood Banks.

BODY

I. Embodiment: The Phenomenological Tradition
    Richard M. Zaner
II. Social Theories
    M. Therese Lysaught
III. Cultural and Religious Perspectives
    Thomas J. Csordas

I. EMBODIMENT: THE PHENOMENOLOGICAL TRADITION

Philosophical and ethical issues are closely connected with medical and health professional self-understanding, knowledge, research, and practice. The human body occupies a central place in those contexts, but especially within medicine—certainly one of the sources for understanding the human body. In this article, after a brief review of ideas about the body in the history of medicine, its place in philosophical thought since René Descartes is addressed. This history plays an important role in more recent philosophical reflections on human life, especially in writings directed to the experience of embodiment. After reviewing that history and the understanding of embodiment, some suggestions are made about the relationship between embodiment and the variety of ethical issues presented by medicine, biomedical research, and clinical practice. This discussion is un-

avoidably difficult, because both that history and the issues raised by efforts to explicate and understand embodiment are complex. Addressing those complexities, however briefly, will be helpful in delineating the specific concepts, terms, and methods used in the phenomenological tradition regarding embodiment.

From the earliest stirrings of human fetal life through old age, individuals are embodied. Whether their bodies are more or less healthy, or are sick, injured, compromised by congenital or genetic defects, or are such that they arouse social prejudice, individuals experience the surrounding world by means of a particular body. Being embodied, furthermore, means having a certain sexuality and thus experiencing the milieu in ways that both structure and are socially structured by that sexuality. Even slight reflection also shows that the human body has aesthetic, economic, political, and other dimensions specific to every cultural time: the body figures prominently in clothing styles, pornography, labor, torture, and the like. The experience of the body by oneself and others plays other important roles in broader terms: in the "body politic," for instance, or in the manufacture of automobiles, or in contexts such as physical examinations in the military.

Underlying all of these, however, is a striking phenomenon: regardless of the state of health, skin coloration, sexuality, or sociopolitical usages, one body is uniquely singled out for a person's experience as "mine," as that sole body through which anything else is experienced. While any full explication of embodiment must address each of these fascinating dimensions, the first question concerns that core sense of "mineness": How are we to understand that? It is to this that the present essay is devoted. First, however, an equally brief word is needed about the place of the body in medicine.

The body in medicine

Historically, physicians have sought to understand the body's structures (anatomy), functions (physiology), cellular makeup (biology, biochemistry), activating and regulatory mechanisms (neurology, immunology), the several organ systems and their connections (cardiac, pulmonary, renal, hepatic, etc.), and the variety of diseases, injuries, noxious environmental influences, and genetic and congenital conditions that govern the body's development and underlie personal life.

Even with this focus, however, historical medical views of the body have varied over time (Edelstein, 1967). For example, the "dogmatic" or "rational" view understood the human body as fundamentally causal in nature—events inside the body were thought to cause outer symptoms (a pathological understanding of the body and disease). By contrast, according to the "empiricist" and "skeptical" traditions, the body and the embodied person form an experiential, temporally developing "whole" in continuous and multiple interactions with the surrounding world (a holistic view). Physicians in later historical times who were convinced of the dogmatic, rational view literally looked inside the body—by dissection and vivisection—and understood its structures and functions. Those who held the empiricist view turned instead to history (the patient's history and the collective histories of other physicians) in treating diseases. These two basic, conflicting models have continued to have an important place in medical understanding (Leder, 1990; Zaner, 1988).

Although these views continue to be present in current medicine, the rationalist tradition (emphasizing the body as a material, causally determined organic system) has been clearly dominant in more recent times. The first major steps in the historical development of a rationalist view of the human body were taken in the early fourteenth century by Mondino de' Luzzi and his student Guido da Vigevano (Singer, 1925). By far the most significant steps are found in the seminal work on anatomy by Andreas Vesalius (1514–1564) and later in the important discoveries in physiology by William Harvey (1578–1657), strongly endorsed by René Descartes and continued in the work of seventeenth- and eighteenth-century post-Cartesian physicians, such as Robert Boyle (1627–1691) and Friedrich Hoffmann (1660–1742) (King, 1978) and Jerome Gaub (1705–1780) (Rather, 1965).

In modern times, the body was first proposed as a fundamentally causally determined organic system by Giovanni Battista Morgagni (1682–1771) and Xavier Bichat (1771–1802). Before this time, even though abundant autopsy reports had been published, such recorded data had not offered any correlation between clinical and anatomical findings (King, 1978). With Morgagni and Bichat, however, this changed profoundly. The introduction of the "clinicopathological correlation" radically altered medical understanding. For the first time, what was found at autopsy was taken as "explaining" clinical symptoms observed while the patient was alive. Now disease took on a highly specific form—the "organic lesion" found inside the body—and was no longer associated with a more or less loosely collected set of clinically observed symptoms or patient reports (King, 1978; Zaner, 1988). Because this "correlation" fundamentally changed the way physicians understood disease, it has been called a "revolution" (Laín Entralgo, 1969) comparable to what Copernicus effected in astronomy when he proposed that instead of thinking that the sun moves around the earth, we should perceive it to be the other way around.

The marriage of clinical medicine to biological science, definitively begun in the nineteenth century, was consummated through the work of neurologists such as

John Hughlings Jackson (1834–1911) and clinicians such as William Osler (1849–1919), and the educational reforms recommended by Abraham Flexner (1866–1959) in the early twentieth century. Medical thinking then incorporated the idea that the body is a complex system of physiologically interacting structures and mechanisms governed by multiply interrelated controls seated in the neurological system. Some physicians, appreciating that this complex organism (or set of organ systems) serves as the embodied person's means of expression and action, advocated a type of "medical dualism" or "epiphenomenalism"—there must be a place for the "person," whether thought of as a distinct entity or as a causal consequence of the body complex's functional stability across time.

The body in philosophy

While the history of philosophical and moral deliberations about human life is quite as sophisticated and colorful as medical history, the bulk of reflections have focused on "mind" ("person," "self," "subjectivity," and related notions) (Zaner, 1980). With some notable exceptions, however, there has not been nearly as much reflection about "body" per se. In large part, a basically traditional view of these matters was assumed: that body and soul are distinct (or even separate) realities, and that what is essential in human life is to be found in the soul, not the body. The soul (mind, reason) is the pure and unchanging essence of the human; the body, on the other hand, is a baser sort of affair, belonging to the changeable, the temporal, and the corrupt. The soul, imprisoned within the corporeal, is subject to the body's peculiar "nature," its appetites and inclinations, but has its true destiny and nature elsewhere—a destiny it must pursue by becoming freed from its worldly, bodily prison.

There have been exceptions to this view of the human body. René Descartes (1596–1650), for example, argued that mind (res cogitans) and body (res extensa) are to be understood as "substances": mutually exclusive, self-subsistent, and ontologically distinct entities, neither of which requires the other to be or to be known. This familiar bifurcation of reality (dualism), often said to be at the basis of modern medicine and modern thought more generally (Cassell, 1991; Eccles, 1979), led Descartes to the view that mind and body "interact" in some manner, although specifying that the form of this interaction proved to be inordinately difficult and highly problematic (Leder, 1990).

Hardly satisfied with that, and challenged by Princess Elizabeth (daughter of the exiled king of Bohemia, living at the time in Holland), Descartes's reflections on the body show a surprising turn—one that has not been well appreciated. The mind, he thought, is not "in" the body in the way a boatman is "in" a boat—contingently or accidentally. Rather, the mind is "intimately" connected to the body, an "intimate union" that led him to the view that the human body is intrinsically complex and not at all the simple "extended substance" posited in his metaphysics (Zaner, 1988). As Descartes remarked to Princess Elizabeth, neither mathematics nor metaphysics is capable of apprehending this union. It can by known only in "daily conversation" and in clinical encounters—one might say that the union is essentially a matter of concrete experience (Descartes, 1967; Descartes, 1973; Lindeboom, 1978).

To be sure, from his early work in anatomy, Descartes had learned that the cadaver does indeed seem to be little more than such "extension." But from his earnest attempts to provide medical diagnosis, he knew full well that while it is alive, the body is far more than merely a material entity extended in space. For example, writing of the "dropsical patient" in his *Meditations* (Descartes, 1955), he took pains to point out that there are in fact *two* "natures": the one subject to the laws of nature, the other with its own specific characteristics that must be understood in quite different ways than the other (Kennington, 1978). Indeed, Neils Stenos (1638–1686), a younger physician contemporary of Descartes's who specialized in the brain, contended that nature in the first sense was merely heuristic, a "manner of speaking" (*une pure dénomination* is Descartes's phrase), and should not be taken literally (Lindeboom, 1978). This intrinsic complexity of the body—as cadaver and as embodying the mind—did not attract the attention of many philosophers (or, for that matter, physicians) (Zaner, 1988).

Addressing the Cartesian idea of the "intimate union" of soul and body, Blaise Pascal (1623–1662) argued that one must be able to account for this intimacy. He noted with marked irony that if, like Descartes, one "composes all things of mind and body," surely that mixture would be intelligible—especially to one who so composes all things. Yet not only do we not understand the body, and even less the mind; least of all do we know "how a body could be united to a mind. This is the consummation of [our] difficulties, and yet it is [our] very being" (Pascal, 1941, pp. 27–28).

Benedict de Spinoza (1632–1677) thought that Descartes's bifurcation created insuperable difficulties for understanding how the mind could possibly be connected to the body, much less "intimately" connected. Like others at the time, Spinoza's argument is couched in metaphysical terms: he argued that what Descartes termed "substance" (mind and body) could only be "attributes" of the one and only substance, reality itself. Mind and body are essential to one another; the way in which they are "united," he concluded, then becomes comprehensible. The body is a mirror of the soul; mind, the idea of the body (Spinoza, 1951).

Understanding the body continued to preoccupy physicians but did not become a focal issue for philosophers until the early writings of Henri Bergson (1859–1941). Although he did not fully probe the matter, Bergson argued that the human body should be seen as the person's placement or locus in the world. What makes the body, a sui generis phenomenon, unlike any other worldly object is, he believed, that it is experienced as "mine," as "my center" of action and experience. While it is physical, it is not simply that; it is the "center" of experience, and thus the field of physical objects is spatially organized around it. In addition, the human body and its perceptual capacities are in the service of action. The body is fundamentally an actional center. It is that by means of which the embodied person is able to engage in actions in and on the field of objects. Spatial location and the familiar sensory qualities are thus always experienced within specific contexts of action: for the perceiver, "things" are "menacing," "helpful," "handy," "obstacles," and so on (Bergson, 1970). Correlated to the body as the center of action, physical things are organized as "poles of action" appearing only within specific activities directed toward them, as Jean Piaget (1896–1980) later emphasized (Piaget, 1952). Because of these characteristics, the human body is a critical factor in the development of language and culture.

In the early days of the twentieth century, Max Scheler (1874–1928) devoted serious reflection to the "lived body" (*Leib*), in particular as regards the performance of "deeds" in moral conduct. Scheler's analysis suggests that both "ego" and the ego's "acts" are distinct from what he terms "lived bodiliness" (*Leiblichkeit*). At the same, lived bodiliness must be sharply distinguished from the "thing body" (*Körper*). Although Scheler does not mention it, this idea is a clear echo of the earlier Cartesian insight. The body that embodies the person ("my body") is uniquely singled out for, and experienced by, the person as "mine" (and in this sense is "intimately connected"). As the person's experiential "center," it is that by means of which the person is, as it were, worlded: in the midst of objects, people, language, culture, and so on (Scheler, 1973). These points, which had also impressed Bergson, came to be regarded as fundamental to embodiment, and are crucial for understanding subsequent discussions.

Edmund Husserl (1859–1938) grappled with this phenomenon throughout his career. Its primary feature, he contended, is the experiential relationship of consciousness to its own embodying organism (Husserl, 1952). Granted that this organism (*Leibkörper*) is uniquely singled out (Husserl, 1956–1959), the problem of embodiment is to determine in what sense and in what ways it is actually experienced by the person as his or hers, since it is solely by means of that experience that it is at all possible for the person to experience worldly things (physical, biological, cultural).

What had so impressed and troubled Descartes—the "intimate union"—Husserl calls the experiential relationship to the "body-as-mine"; however, he did not appreciate Descartes's insight any more than had Bergson or Scheler. Descartes seems clearly to have recognized that while a person is alive, there is an "intimate union" between body and soul; yet how are we to understand this "union"—a connection that is all the more peculiar when death occurs and this "alive" body becomes a cadaver that seems no different in kind from any other material thing? Although apparently appreciating this puzzle, Descartes nevertheless obscured matters (as did many others after him) by trying to resolve the very different metaphysical question of the "mind–body" relation.

It is to the embodiment phenomenon that Gabriel Marcel's analysis of the fundamental opacity (the elemental "feeling" or, as he termed it, *Urgefühl*) at the heart of personal life—my body qua mine—is addressed (Marcel, 1940). It is here, too, that Maurice Merleau-Ponty locates the essential ambiguity intrinsic to the body itself (Merleau-Ponty, 1945). So "intimate" is this "union," both Marcel and Merleau-Ponty point out, that one is tempted to say, with Jean-Paul Sartre, "I *am* my body" (Sartre, 1953). "My body qua mine" is thus the paradigm of "belonging" or "having": the sense in which things belong to a person is ultimately derived from the ways in which the "own" body is experienced as belonging to the person. The latter is the condition for the former (Marcel, 1935). This existential source of "belonging" becomes apparent especially in instances where mental disturbances occur and the sense of "mineness" becomes severely compromised or remains seriously undeveloped (Bosch, 1970). A central issue then emerges: By virtue of what is this one animate organism uniquely singled out to exist in my experience as that whereby everything else in the world is experienced? Which specific processes are there without which this organism would cease to be experienced by me as mine, or which give it its sense as mine (Straus, 1958)?

The problem is exceedingly complex and subtle, and is by no means settled (Zaner, 1971; Zaner, 1980). It is one of those regions where philosophy and medicine can productively learn from one another. Within philosophy, however, there seems at least some agreement that the animate organism becomes and remains an embodying organism solely to the extent that (1) it is not just a physical body but a genuinely animate organism, the sole "object" within which the person's own fields of sensation (that whereon sensations occur) belong; (2) it is the only object "in" which the person immediately "rules and governs," within and from each of its "organs" and the total organism itself; (3) it is that whereby the

person's "I can" (walk, perceive, move, grasp, and the like) is most immediately realized and enacted; (4) it is that "by means of which" the person perceives and otherwise experiences the field of worldly objects (things, people, language, etc.) and thus is the person's access to the world and the focus of the world's (objects, people) actions on the person; and (5) it is not only that whereby the person experiences other things, but it is itself experienced by the person (in health and sickness, and these in specific individual ways)—that is, the person's embodying organism is reflexively related to itself (Husserl, 1956, 1959).

The body in medicine and philosophy

It should of course be recognized that, given the uniqueness of each embodiment, individuals experience their bodies (and, correlatively, the surrounding world) in different ways, depending on initial biological endowments, native and cultivated abilities, activities that are available and/or encouraged, and others. Thus, a boy who from birth has been unable to walk experiences "I can" in quite different ways from a boy who has that ability. If the latter has an accident that renders him unable to walk, moreover, his inability is experienced quite differently from that of the former—indeed, while the one undergoes a "loss," the other may not, except perhaps in the indirect way of realizing that while others can walk, he has never been able to. One who is born blind experiences the surrounding world quite differently from one who goes blind due to an accident—while neither experiences a "visual world," the one has "to get used" to the absence of visual space while the other has never experienced anything else. Even in cases where an individual may from birth lack several bodily capabilities (such as Helen Keller), or loses them through illness or injury, the features suggested above still hold: the embodying organism is that whereby one experiences sensations, which most immediately embody wishes and movements, by means of which one perceives (in whatever ways), and through which other things are experienced. Moreover, there are many other meanings the human body acquires—social, political, economic, and others—that a more complete explication of embodiment must address—bodily abilities, stances, comportments, and movements (Buytendijk, 1957) that have their sense and place within the spheres of nature, culture, and history.

Embodiment is thus fundamentally connected with various levels and modalities of bodily actions, attitudes, stances, and movements (Buytendijk, 1957), personal striving or willing, and perceptual awareness of things (including the body itself). Wishing, desiring, noticing, attending, and the like are or can be actualized (embodied, enacted) by means of corporeal movements (kinesthetic flow patterns correlated with muscle activations) that are functionally correlated with the several perceptual fields and what appears in them (turning one's head and looking at . . .). Only to that extent can one sensibly say that this organism is "uniquely singled out" from the field of worldly objects as "mine." Involved in embodiment are processes of sensory "feeling"—coenesthetic (of inner body, e.g., of hunger), kinesthetic (of body motion), proprioceptive (of body stance or posture)—and elementary strivings (reaching, squinting, locomotion, etc.). Together, these contribute not only to the sensing of "this" organism as "belonging to me" but also to the forming of the surrounding field of objects as correlated to bodily feelings and movements, positions, and actions.

But it needs to be emphasized that there is quite another dimension to embodiment. Although surprisingly little attention has been devoted to it, it turns out to be quite essential. However tempting it is to say "I am my body" (when, for example, someone strikes me in the face, I say "Don't hit me!"), many cases in psychopathology literature (Binswanger, 1958), and situations in daily life, suggest that matters are more complicated. The relation between self and its embodying organism seems as much a matter of "otherness" as of "mineness." However intimate and profound the relation between the person and the person's body, it is equally true that a person experiences his or her body as strange and alien, in ways that can be understood (Leder, 1990).

I am my body; but in another sense I am *not* my body, or not simply that. This otherness is so profound that we inevitably feel forced to qualify the "am": it is not identity, equality, or inclusion. It is "mine," but this means that the person is in a way distanced from it, for otherwise there would be no sense to "belonging"; it would not be characterizable in any sense as "mine." So close is the union that a person's experience of his or her "own" body can be psychologically unnerving (its happy obedience that the person notices for the first time, or its hateful refusal to obey his or her wish to do something) (Binswanger, 1958). So intimate is it that the person has moments of genuinely feeling "at home" with it. Yet so other is it that there are times when the person treats the body as a mere thing that is other, obsessively stuffing it with food or otherwise mistreating it; or when it is encountered as "having a life of its own" to which the person must willy-nilly attend: like it or not, "my" hair grows and must be trimmed for certain purposes, "my" hands cleaned, "my" bowels moved, "my" cold cured, and so on (Zaner, 1980; Leder, 1990).

The person finds himself or herself embodied by an animate organism whose peculiar connections to the person (and the person to it) give embodiment its uniquely uncanny character. Nothing is so much "me-

myself," yet nothing seems so strange; so deeply familiar (Who else could "I" be?) yet so oddly alien (Who, indeed, am "I"?). This experience is not indicative of an inability to make up one's mind but, rather, suggests the peculiarity of embodiment. What seems distinctive is this "mineness/otherness" (the most familiar yet the most alien) dialectic that is the core of human body-as-experienced (Engelhardt, 1973; Zaner, 1980).

In these terms, to speak of embodiment is to speak of something that "I" am and not something that can be placed over against me (*ob-jectum*) as an object. As embodied, "I" am in a clear sense a fundamental puzzle to myself—precisely what Pascal had appreciated with remarkable insight. What is expressed by "the problem of the body" is precisely the person's "being as embodied," that is, the fundamental sense of being human in the first place. The "self–body" (or "mind–body") problem is, therefore, a matter of experience: It is enacted at every moment in the ongoing life of the person.

These considerations make it easier to appreciate that the human body is essentially expressive. It is that by means of which the person enacts and expresses feelings, desires, strivings, and so on (albeit in culturally and historically different manners) (Merleau-Ponty, 1945). This expressiveness signifies that embodiment is valorized, that is, deeply textured with a sense of worth (whether positive or negative, as the case may be). After all, what happens to it happens to me: the person, as that which "rules and governs," is at the same time subject to its conditions. What happens to the person's body, in still different terms, matters to the person whose body it is: The embodying organism lies at the root of the moral sense of inviolability of personhood—of the "privacy," "integrity," "consent," "respect," and "confidentiality" that play such profound roles in research ethics, bioethics, and clinical ethics. Nor does the fact that people can and do dissemble and deceive themselves and others—as in cases of factitious illness when a person is thought to "fake" symptoms (Ford, 1983)—belie the body's expressivity. Indeed, these are themselves expressive phenomena, however difficult it may be to discover and to interpret them (Hauerwas and Burrell, 1974).

This value character of the embodying organism also helps elucidate more fully why the continuing discussions of many bioethical issues—pregnancy, prenatal diagnosis, abortion, psychosurgery, withdrawal of life support, euthanasia—are so highly charged and deeply personal. On the other hand, the profound moral feelings evoked by certain medical practices (surgery, chemotherapy) and much biomedical experimentation (in particular the Human Genome Project) are understandable, as they are in effect ways of intervening or intruding into that most intimate and integral of spheres: the embodied person. The person is embodied, enacts himself or herself through that specific animate organism that is his or her own, and is thus expressive of that very person. Bodily schemata, attitudes, movements, actions, and perceptual abilities are all value modalities by which one enacts and expresses one's character, personality, habits, goals, moral beliefs—in short, by which the person is alive as such.

To view medical practice and biomedical research from the perspective of embodiment is to appreciate them as planned or potential interventions into the sphere of personal intimacy, whether this sphere be initial (as in infancy) or more developed. Whether or not such interventions are mainly directed to the body (medicine, surgery) or to the person's mental life or status (psychiatry, psychotherapy), they all unavoidably affect the individual. The person's life as a whole is necessarily affected by surgery no less than by psychotropic medication. Psyche and soma are inextricably bound together as constituents of an integral, contextual whole (Zaner, 1980). The expressive and valuative character of this whole, the embodied person, helps to explain why every medical intervention falls within the moral order. Recognizing this, of course, does not of itself settle any of the ethical issues present in research or clinical situations: when it is morally permissible to withdraw life support, for instance, or whether it is right to restrict a retarded person's ability to procreate. However any such issues may eventually be settled, the point here is that medicine is an inherently moral enterprise, in no small way due to the nature of embodiment and the interventional character of medicine (Cassell, 1973, 1991).

Clearly, the effort to settle the specific ethical issues associated with medical practice and biomedical research requires that the fundamentally ethical nature of any intervention be explicitly recognized and appreciated (Zaner, 1988). It can also be appreciated that the ethical issues associated with the medical profession (medical ethics) can be distinguished from those that arise in research (biomedical ethics) as well as from those that occur in clinical settings (clinical ethics). Each set of issues poses important and distinctive problems.

While embodiment has a place in each of these disciplines, perhaps it is more important in clinical ethics deliberations. Because embodiment is essentially individual, the tasks of identifying, discussing, and (one hopes) settling moral issues that arise in clinical situations require that the specific circumstances of each individual situation be determined. Personal integrity and respect for the unique person are not concerns somehow imported into clinical situations from the outside; they are, on the contrary, intrinsic to the very nature of biomedical research and clinical practice. It might be added that in problematic cases (interventions for an

unconscious or incompetent patient, for instance), the decision to intervene in ways that do not or cannot include the patient's own perspective nevertheless requires other ethical grounds, and thus must be subject to critical ethical assessment. Other problematic situations—involving mental retardation, disabled infants, and so on—do not escape the necessity to respect the patient, though they do require special ways of taking it into account (e.g., consulting family or surrogate) along with the ethical issues involved in decision making (identifying and respecting the moral frameworks of each decision maker).

Medical and other health issues are not only inherently within the moral order but also context-specific. No bioethical or clinical ethics issue can be settled in the abstract. Every medical practice, no matter how apparently trivial, is value-laden to begin with, which means that it either explicitly or (most often) implicitly expresses some vision of what is, or is thought to be, morally good. The primary issue for ethics in clinical situations is to help primary decision makers make explicit what each believes to be most worthwhile, of greatest value, as this is found in ongoing clinical or research situations. Only subsequently does it become possible to make informed judgments about the particular context-specific practices and issues facing people in clinical or research contexts (Zaner, 1988).

How one can come to such truly informed judgments is an obvious problem, but it is not within the scope of this article. It is, one hopes, enough to have delineated the philosophical and ethical dimensions of the human body—in particular, the phenomenon of embodiment, its expressive and value character, and consequently the ethical nature of medicine and biomedical research. What remains to be done is also clear: not only to find appropriate ways to incorporate these philosophical and ethical considerations into the teaching and practices of the health professions and the research community, but also to study the important aesthetic, political, sexual, and other dimensions of the body in social life more broadly.

RICHARD M. ZANER

Directly related to this article are the other articles in this entry: SOCIAL THEORIES, *and* CULTURAL AND RELIGIOUS PERSPECTIVES. *Also directly related are the entries* ACTION; GENDER IDENTITY AND GENDER-IDENTITY DISORDERS; HEALTH AND DISEASE, *article on* THE EXPERIENCE OF HEALTH AND ILLNESS; PERSON; SEXUAL DEVELOPMENT; *and* SEXUAL IDENTITY. *For a discussion of phenomenology and continental philosophy, see the entries* CARE, *article on* HISTORY OF THE NOTION OF CARE; INTERPRETATION; LITERATURE; METAPHOR AND ANALOGY; *and* NARRA-

TIVE. *Other relevant material may be found under the entries* FEMINISM; LIFE; *and* PSYCHOANALYSIS AND DYNAMIC THEORIES.

Bibliography

BERGSON, HENRI. 1953. *Matière et mémoire.* 54th ed. Paris: Presses Universitaires de France. Translated by Nancy Margaret Paul and W. Scott Palmer under the title *Matter and Memory.* London: Allen & Unwin, 1970.

BINSWANGER, LUDWIG. 1958. "The Case of Ellen West." Translated by Werner M. Mendel and Joseph Lyons. In *Existence: A New Dimension in Psychiatry and Psychology,* pp. 237–364. Edited by Rollo May, Ernest Angel, and Henri F. Ellenberger. New York: Basic Books.

BOSCH, GERHARD. 1970. *Infantile Autism: A Clinical and Phenomenological-Anthropological Investigation Taking Language as the Guide.* Translated by Derek Jordan and Inge Jordan. New York: Springer Verlag.

BUYTENDIJK, FREDERIK J. J. 1957. *Attitudes et mouvements: Étude fonctionelle du mouvement humain.* Paris: Desclée de Brouwer.

CASSELL, ERIC. 1973. "Making and Escaping Moral Decisions." *Hastings Center Studies,* no. 2:53–62.

———. 1991. *The Nature of Suffering and the Goals of Medicine.* New York: Oxford University Press.

DESCARTES, RENÉ. 1955. *Philosophical Writings.* Translated by Elizabeth S. Haldane and George R. T. Ross. 2 vols. New York: Dover.

———. 1963–1973. *Oeuvres philosophiques.* Edited by Ferdinand Alquié. 3 vols. Paris: Garner Frères.

ECCLES, SIR JOHN. 1979. *The Human Mystery.* New York: Springer International.

EDELSTEIN, LUDWIG. 1967. *Ancient Medicine: Selected Papers of Ludwig Edelstein.* Edited by Owsei Temkin and C. Lillian Temkin. Baltimore: Johns Hopkins University Press.

ENGELHARDT, H. TRISTRAM, JR. 1973. *Mind-Body: A Categorial Relation.* The Hague: Martinus Nijhoff.

FORD, CHARLES V. 1983. *The Somatizing Disorders: Illness as a Way of Life.* New York: Elsevier Biomedical.

GURWITSCH, ARON. 1964. *Field of Consciousness.* Pittsburgh: Duquesne University Press.

HAUERWAS, STANLEY, and BURRELL, DAVID. 1974. "Self-Deception and Autobiography: Theological and Ethical Reflections on Speer's *Inside the Third Reich.*" *Journal of Religious Ethics.* 2:99–118.

HUSSERL, EDMUND. 1952a. *Allgemeine Einführung in die reine Phänomenologie.* Vol. 1 of *Ideen zu einer reinen Phänomenologie und phänomenologischen Philosophie.* Vol. 3 of *Husserliana: Gesammelte Werke.* The Hague: Martinus Nijhoff. Translated by Fred Kersten under the title *Ideas Pertaining to a Pure Phenomenology and to a Phenomenological Philosophy: First Book: General Introduction to a Pure Phenomenology.* The Hague: Martinus Nijhoff, 1982.

———. 1952b. *Phänomenologische Untersuchen zur Konstitution.* Vol 2 of *Ideen zu einer reinen Phänomenologie und phänomenologischen Philosophie.* Vol. 4 of *Husserliana: Gesammelte Werke.* The Hague. Martinus Nijhoff.

———. 1956–1959. *Erste Philosophie (1923–1924).* Vols. 7 and 8 of *Husserliana: Gesammelte Werke.* The Hague: Martinus Nijhoff.

KENNINGTON, RICHARD. 1978. "Descartes and Mastery of Nature." In *Organism, Medicine, and Metaphysics: Essays in Honor of Hans Jonas on his 75th Birthday, May 10, 1978,* pp. 201–223. Edited by Stuart F. Spicker. Dordrecht, Netherlands: D. Reidel.

KING, LESTER. 1978. *The Philosophy of Medicine: The Early Eighteenth Century.* Cambridge, Mass.: Harvard University Press.

LAÍN ENTRALGO, PEDRO. 1969. *Doctor and Patient.* New York: McGraw-Hill.

LEDER, DREW. 1990. *The Absent Body.* Chicago: University of Chicago Press.

LINDEBOOM, GERRIT A. 1978. *Descartes and Medicine.* Amsterdam: Rodopi.

MARCEL, GABRIEL. 1935. *Être et avoir.* Paris: F. Aubier.

———. 1940. *Du refus à l'invocation.* Paris: Gallimard.

MERLEAU-PONTY, MAURICE. 1945. *Phénoménologie de la perception.* Paris: Gallimard. Translated by Colin Smith under the title *Phenomenology of Perception.* London: Routledge & Kegan Paul, 1962.

PASCAL, BLAISE. 1941. *Pensées: The Provincial Letters.* Translated by William F. Trotter and Thomas McCrie. New York: Modern Library.

PIAGET, JEAN. 1952. *The Origins of Intelligence in Children.* Translated by Margaret Cook. New York: International Universities Press.

RATHER, L. J. 1965. *Mind and Body in Eighteenth Century Medicine: A Study Based on Jerome Gaub's De regimine mentis.* Berkeley: University of California Press.

SARTRE, JEAN-PAUL. 1943. *L'être et le néant.* Paris: Gallimard. Translated by Hazel E. Barnes under the title *Being and Nothingness.* New York: Washington Square Press, 1953.

SCHELER, MAX. 1973. *Formalism in Ethics and Non-Formal Ethics of Values: A New Attempt Toward the Foundation of an Ethical Personalism.* 5th rev. ed. Translated by Manfred S. Frings and Roger L. Funk. Evanston, Ill.: Northwestern University Press.

SINGER, CHARLES J. 1925. *Evolution of Anatomy: A Short History of Anatomical and Physiological Discovery to Harvey.* New York: Alfred Knopf.

SPINOZA, BENEDICT DE. 1951. "Ethics." In vol. 2 of *Chief Works.* Translated by Robert Harvey Monro Elwes. New York: Dover.

STRAUS, ERWIN. W. 1958. "Aesthesiology and Hallucinations." Translated by Erwin W. Straus and Biyard Morgan. In *Existence: A New Dimension in Psychiatry and Psychology,* pp. 139–169. Edited by Rollo May, Ernest Angel, and Henri F. Ellenberger. New York: Basic Books.

———. 1966. *Phenomenological Psychology: The Selected Papers of Erwin Straus.* New York: Basic Books.

ZANER, RICHARD. 1971. *The Problem of Embodiment.* 2d ed. Phaenomenologica, no. 17. The Hague: Martinus Nijhoff.

———. 1980. *The Context of Self: A Phenomenological Inquiry Using Medicine as a Clue.* Athens: Ohio University Press.

———. 1988. *Ethics and the Clinical Encounter.* Englewood Cliffs, N.J.: Prentice-Hall.

II. SOCIAL THEORIES

Everywhere one looks in medicine, one finds bodies. Not only are bodies ubiquitous, they are essential to the practice of medicine. Whenever something seems to go awry with our bodies, we seek the services of medicine and become "patients." Medical personnel often reduce patients' bodies to the particular problems they present, for example, "the coronary bypass in room 14B" or the "end-stage renal disease case." Bodies are the material upon or through which medicine is practiced: clinicians touch, scan, listen to, cut into, comfort, rehabilitate, alter, and monitor the bodies of patients. Likewise, practitioners bring their bodies with them when they enter the clinic. Clinicians not only interact with patients and families through their bodies (e.g., shaking hands, touching, probing, lifting, bathing patients), they also bring to the clinical setting their own unique embodied experience—gendered, professional, perhaps overtired, young or old, ill or healthy, angry or compassionate, prejudiced, and so on. Thus, the body is an indispensable component of those persons experiencing illness and those giving care, as well as to the dynamics of illness and healing. Without a body, there is no person, no identity, no relationship, no health, no illness, no healing.

Yet despite the fact that bodies are so central to medicine, "the body" is rarely mentioned in the literature of bioethics. Discussions in bioethics generally center on concepts of personhood (Is the patient a person? Is the person competent?), issues related to personhood (such as autonomy, informed consent, rights, confidentiality, choice), and questions of cost/benefit analysis (Do the benefits outweigh the risks? How can we achieve the greatest good for the greatest number at the lowest cost?). A patient's "personhood" is generally understood in terms of rationality or mental capacity (rather than, for example, a beating heart, membership in the species *homo sapiens,* or one's ability to form emotional bonds to others), personal values and preferences (rather than, for example, obligations based on relationships or social roles), and ability to function autonomously rather than, alternatively, one's ability to recognize and to function within our essential interdependence and interrelatedness).

Moreover, because "personhood" has been so narrowly defined, and because bioethics has made personhood its central category, many of the significant problems in bioethics center on bodies whose status as "persons" is unclear, bodies that lack or have lost rationality, for example: "defective" neonates, anencephalic newborns, brain-dead potential organ donors, patients in persistent vegetative state, fetuses to be aborted or experimented on, mentally handicapped and incarcerated individuals to be used as research subjects, or elderly individuals suffering from dementia or Alzheimer's disease. When these patients have not left rational and autonomous specifications of what their preferences would be (e.g., living wills, organ donor cards), other individuals possessing rationality, preference, and autonomy (either patient surrogates or the courts) decide what to do with their bodies.

There is a growing consensus that this notion of personhood is too narrow, and that by excluding attention to the body, bioethics does not fully take into account all the morally significant dimensions of the practice of medicine. If we cannot be a self or act in the world without our body, then that body must be included into the description of the moral situation. At the same time, there is a concern that, in spite of the rhetoric of freedom, personal fulfillment, and rights, by overlooking the body, medicine and bioethics can become (some would say "have become") avenues through which society restricts the freedom of its members through repression and control.

The body in medicine and bioethics: Empiricist materialism

The fact that the body is overlooked is due in large part to the ways in which the body is understood by medicine, bioethics, and contemporary Western culture. Richard Zaner has provided a helpful outline of the development of the view of the body that dominates contemporary medicine and is shared by bioethics (Zaner, 1994). This view is called "empiricist materialism" and is chiefly the legacy of, among others, Francis Bacon (1561–1626) and René Descartes (1596–1650). A third philosopher who has also been influential in shaping how bioethics approaches the body is John Locke (1632–1704).

Francis Bacon is credited with the development of the modern scientific experimental method. The development of this method required a new understanding of the meaning of "nature." Bacon demythologized nature, declaring it to be little more than brute, inert, morally neutral, raw material, available to be dissected and manipulated through empirical investigation in order to gain knowledge of its universal laws and regularities. Such knowledge is power, Bacon proposed, for in spite of its status as totally object, nature was also understood as containing within it great power, chaotic power that threatened to undo the orderliness of civilization (take, e.g., the destructive power of tornadoes, earthquakes, and illness). As the human mind gained knowledge of nature, through rational empirical investigation and quantification, this power could be channeled and controlled, thus giving humanity power over nature and making it fulfill human needs.

One aspect of nature affected by this change in understanding was the human body. The body, understood as inert, morally neutral raw material, became likewise amenable to scientific investigation and control. This reconceptualization of the body was accelerated by the work of Descartes. Descartes asserted that the mind (or soul) is both entirely distinct from and morally superior to the body (Descartes, 1968). This view is called "mind/body dualism" and exerted a strong influence on the development of Western philosophy. Allied to this mind/body dualism was Descartes's view of the body as a machine (Descartes, 1968).

This Cartesian metaphor of the body as a machine, in conjunction with Baconian empiricism, has been greatly influential in medical research and contemporary medicine. Medicine has made significant progress by understanding the body as being comprised of separable and identifiable mechanisms. Because the body has been understood as natural and universal, medical science has been able to conduct empirical investigation of the body, yielding statistical standards defining the "normal" human body and methods by which medicine can manipulate and control bodies that diverge from those norms. In fact, some have deemed the body most "human" when it is most completely manipulated, controlled, transformed, or created by human agency (Fletcher, 1971). While medicine has adopted the legacies of empiricism and mechanism, it has been the Cartesian view of mind/body dualism that has most strongly influenced contemporary bioethics, allowing it to focus almost exclusively on the "mind," "self," or "person" when it defines and describes the issues and moral parameters of medicine.

A third influence on contemporary bioethics with respect to the body has been John Locke. In his *Second Treatise on Government*, Locke sought a framework for understanding political society. Locke posited that individuals initially exist in a "state of nature," that is, individual and unconstrained, until they consent to join an ordered society. While Locke's discussion of consent, rights, duties, and so forth are too complex to summarize here (see Copleston, 1964a), these concepts and particularly his notion of private property have notably influenced the worldview of contemporary bioethics. This is especially evident in the way bioethics has become increasingly intertwined with the U.S. legal system and involved in the formation of public policy. While Locke did not discuss the body as such, his views on private property and ownership have been incorporated into the subsequent labor theory of value and applied to contemporary understandings of the body. For Locke, in the state of nature, insofar as an individual invests labor in raw material to produce a product, that individual receives ownership and utilization rights over that product. Correlatively, insofar as the body is a natural resource, a raw material, and insofar as one's body and the bodies of one's offspring are the products of one's labor, the body in bioethics is often treated under the paradigm of property rights (Campbell, 1992; Englehardt, 1985).

A contemporary critique: Social theories of the body

If a primary purpose of bioethics is to reflect on the moral and ethical dimensions of practices and to resolve issues that arise in medicine and scientific research, one must take into account all relevant factors. How one perceives the issues and problems depends largely on how one describes the situation.

Dissatisfaction with a bioethics that employs a philosophical framework rendering the body superfluous to ethical and moral reflection has resulted in the recent emergence of a number of alternative approaches that seek fuller descriptions of the moral situation. These approaches employ philosophical frameworks that envision relationships—between self and body, between persons and their experiences, and between persons—differently than the framework that draws on Descartes, Locke, and other forebears of liberal political philosophy. These approaches (specifically phenomenology, feminism, an ethics of care, virtue, narrative, and hermeneutics) are critical of a medicine that treats merely "the body" and not "the whole person." They are also critical of a bioethics that reduces persons to their rationality and choice, severing the connections between persons and their bodies. (See for example, Zaner, 1988, and Leder, 1990, who take a phenomenological approach; and Sherwin, 1992, who takes a feminist approach. For fuller discussions of virtue ethics, narrative ethics, phenomenology, and hermeneutics, see DuBose et al., 1994.)

An additional alternative framework for describing "what is going on" in medicine and understanding the function of bioethics is an analytical approach called "social theories of the body." Social theories of the body examine the interrelationships between social orders and the bodies within their jurisdiction. To understand their approach to the body, we must first discuss their broader framework. Every society, they suggest, has an "order," that is, integrated structures of power, institutions, codes of behavior, practices, and beliefs. The "order" of a society is also referred to as the "politics" of the society, that is, the formal and informal relations of power and control that govern a society.

One objective of every social order is to perpetuate (or reproduce) itself. Social orders perpetuate themselves by incorporating new members who assume the roles, espouse the beliefs, support the institutions, and participate in the practices of the society. The primary way in which social orders incorporate new members is through the social institutions and practices with which they intersect, touch, or agree not to touch human bodies. Social practices comprise a broad range of activities through which a culture regulates the private actions and public interactions of its members: eating customs (e.g., fasting or *kashrut* [kosher laws]), sexual practices (e.g., monogamy or polygamy, prostitution, adultery, homosexuality), economic structures (e.g., capitalism, communism, barter), practices of dress (e.g., Amish "plain and simple," clerical robes), judicial and penal structures (e.g., public hangings, incarceration, excommunication), religious practices (e.g., confession, pilgrimage, ancestor worship), and so on. Clearly, such practices vary significantly both among and within cultures ("subcultures" are groups which adopt unconventional practices—practices that are often meant to counter the dominant culture).

Through these practices, those bodies within the jurisdiction of a particular social order internalize the order's beliefs and become constructed in conformity with the order's structures. In every culture, certain practices are considered the norm or the ideal, although deviations from the norm are generally tolerated as most cultures hold to beliefs that are often contradictory (for example, a culture that idealizes monogamous marriage may also sanction a thriving prosititution industry). By participating in these practices, individuals learn and internalize the beliefs and norms (as well as the contradictions) of the culture. The more a practice impinges upon one's body, especially the bodies of infants and children, the more deeply the norms are internalized or "embodied," the more unconsciously and effortlessly the "politics" of the culture is learned. (For a display of the dynamic between practices, bodies, and social orders, see Douglas, 1966.)

The interaction between social institutions and human bodies may be potential (government), indirect (media, advertisement), direct but intermittent (medicine, religion), or direct and constant (prisons, asylums). Through these institutions, cultures seek to normalize, discipline, and regulate both the bodies of individuals (in Michel Foucault's term, "anatomo-politics") and the bodies of its total population or subgroups ("biopolitics" or "biopower").

In addition, social theories of the body hold not only that through practices individuals embody the beliefs of their cultures. At the same time, they suggest, cultures require different "kinds" of bodies to maintain their power structures or they find themselves faced with different kinds of bodies that need to be located in the social order, and they subsequently "construct" them to fit the needs of the social order. For example, the economic and social order of antebellum Georgia depended upon the institution of slavery. To maintain this order, a set of practices designed to construct the bodies of blacks as slaves was required to internalize the cultural view that understood them as slaves. These practices included kidnapping and incarceration, physical punishment, rape, total economic dependence upon owners, selling individual family members, marginalized and impoverished dwellings, and so on.

In addition, for whites to participate in these practices in good conscience and for blacks to submit, the practices required conceptual rationalizations that constructed an understanding of blacks as inferior to whites. For example, religious discourse construed blacks as inferior either due to their "heathen" status or due to their descent from Ham, a less privileged son of Noah. Medical discourse, drawing on Darwinian concepts, asserted that blacks were not as advanced as whites on the evolutionary spectrum, or drew normative conclusions from real physiological differences. In short, the order of a given culture requires this interdependence between practices, discourses, and institutions. As will be discussed below, this interdependence is also the location for resistance and change.

While this is a graphic and coercive example of the ways in which the bodies of particular individuals and a particular group were constructed, social theories of the body would maintain that all people's bodies are constructed. Feminist theory has been a major proponent of this view (see Walker, 1991). But because people internalize and generally accept the norms of their culture, they do not generally understand their bodies as constructed. Because of the objective reality of institutions, the official status of discourses, and the embodied dimension of practices, they see the abilities, constraints, limits, perceptions, and experiences of their bodies as "natural," "given," "the way things are," "right," or "true."

The primary analytical and ethical category for social theories of the body is power. Social theories of the body understand bodies as the medium through which social institutions derive power, authority, reality, and meaning as the site upon which power and social control are maintained. Bodies, as Elaine Scarry suggests, are material and real, while political and social configurations are abstractions, precisely lacking material reality. Through the ways in which they intersect human bodies, social orders appropriate the materiality of human bodies and gain the appearance of reality (Scarry, 1985). The most significant analyst of the relationships between power, knowledge, and the body, and therefore the most central figure in the development of social theories of the body, has been Michel Foucault (1973, 1979, 1980).

While not denying that power can and often is exercised in ways that are negative, coercive, or repressive, social theories of the body instead see power as a pervasive and necessary part of every social order. They focus on four other characteristics of power, specifically that it is "productive," "local," "continuous," and "capillary." Power is "productive" insofar as it is that quality that enables individuals and groups to act (generally toward their own advantage) and to effect desired ends and goals. Power is "local" because it is exercised at the level of individual bodies through techniques and technologies of surveillance (quantification, examination, classification, statistical ranking) and discipline. Power operates "continuously" because individuals, by willingly participating in official practices of surveillance, classification, and self-discipline, become self-surveying, internalizing the normative intent of the practices. And finally, power is "capillary" (drawing on the metaphor of arterial and venous capillaries that are the smallest conduits of blood flow, feeding the furthest reaches of the body); power operates through the most common and least formal channels of the social body in everyday practices, such as eating, medicine, and sexuality.

An essential element in establishing systems of power are discourses, as illustrated above by the roles medical and religious discourses played in the institution of slavery. Discourses are verbal and literary constructs through which systems of knowledge are established. Discourses generally belong exclusively to a professional group and are the means by which that profession defines and advances norms for human subjectivity, actions, and bodies. Bioethics would be an example of such a discourse. Bioethics belongs to the professional group of philosophers, theologians, and clinicians who have learned the language. Through this discourse, bioethicists have defined the normative essence of human personhood as rationality, and they have advanced a system of ethical evaluation based on rational autonomous action, and so forth.

When discourses and practices become the exclusive domain of a select group of professionals, domination by that group is almost unavoidable, yet almost imperceivable. Joanne Finkelstein (1990) describes how technology, especially medical technology, is crucial to this dynamic. Through discourse, practices, and technologies, professions cultivate consumer desires and offer the means to satisfy those desires. Yet by exclusively possessing a desired commodity, those providing the service (e.g., in vitro fertilization [IVF]) control access to it. At the same time, since consumers have been cultivated to desire the service (through what Lisa Sowle Cahill has called the "rhetoric of desperation"), they do not perceive the monopoly as dominating or exploitative, even though they (1) are increasing the scope of medical dominance; (2) may bear great burdens and costs in the process (especially women); and (3) may end up with no outcome (for example, there is only a 20 percent success rate with IVF), while the professionals are guaranteed

benefits, such as income, professional status, or social power. When power becomes accumulated in an institution or professional group in such a way that the group can define another's interests, influence individuals to act contrary to their own interests, or influence those individuals to act in ways that simply further the power of the professional group, power becomes domination. (For further discussion of the new reproductive technologies from the perspective of social theories of the body, see Corea et al., 1987.)

Application: Social theories of the body and bioethics

With regard to bioethics, social theories of the body will prove more critical than constructive. In the above discussion of IVF, we have already begun to show how bioethics looks different when approached from a social-theories perspective. Rather than asking the standard questions of bioethics (Is the patient competent? Who decides? Did the patient give an informed consent? Do the benefits outweigh the costs?), it will ask questions of power (Who benefits most from a particular practice or discourse? Is this a practice of surveillance, and if so, for what end? Who has power in this particular situation?). It will describe how power functions within medical institutions; for instance, power rests mainly with physicians or hospital administrators rather than nurses who provide the hands-on, bodily care (see feminist bioethics, especially Sherwin, 1992; Holmes and Purdy, 1992). It will analyze the dynamics of "choice," suggesting what social factors constrain choices (e.g., in the case of IVF described above), and how individual choices are circumscribed so as to further the interests of institutions and professional groups (Corea et al., 1987). It will illuminate how bioethics, with medicine, functions as an agent of social regulation (e.g., bioethics' emphasis on crafting national policies).

For social theories of the body, medicine has emerged as one of the principal agents of social regulation, the crucial actor in contemporary biopower. In his work *The Birth of the Clinic* (1973), Michel Foucault examines the relationships between medical technologies, practices of surveillance, specialization of knowledge, and consolidation of professional power (see also Turner, 1987). Increasingly, medicine offers treatments for aspects of embodied human life—fertility, height, baldness, death (e.g., euthanasia)—thereby defining an expanding number of human conditions as pathological and amenable to treatment and expanding its own influence. Even when treatments are not available, through seemingly benign techniques of surveillance (especially, for example, genetic testing), medicine seeks to bring all individuals, and increasingly all parts of individuals' lives, into its purview in order to "normalize" individuals and populations. The Human Genome Project, the massive research initiative founded by the National Institutes of Health to map "the" human genome, which will be employed as a standard of normality, is just one example. In addition, medicine serves to marginalize and control those who are not considered normal. Through the judgment and practice of medicine, the sick and disabled are removed from the center of public space to the margins—to the home, to the hospital, to the nursing-care facility. Moreover, a movement (advocating euthanasia, assisted suicide, and/or advanced directives) encourages that those "disordered" bodies (bodies that do not fit with the order of the culture) be moved beyond the boundaries of the human community, beyond the boundary of life and death.

It can be likewise argued that this function of medicine as an agent of social regulation is bolstered by bioethics. Generally, bioethics seeks to create arguments and algorithms that justify, rather than challenge or critique, medical "advances." The discourse of bioethics often provides an additional lens by which individuals or groups are rendered more or less "normal," often offering medicine and society moral justifications for practices that further marginalize those deemed nonnormative. Bioethicists increasingly seek to create a professional space for themselves, an area of expertise, from which they can exercise benign dominance in the moral evaluation of medical and biomedical practices; this role is increasingly attested to by the frequency of "bioethicists" in news sound bites.

Bioethics from the perspective of a social theory of the body, however, challenges this trend. How might social theories of the body illuminate the analysis of a typical bioethical issue? Joanne Finkelstein offers a cogent example in her analysis of genetics. She notes how genetic science promises to improve the lives of individuals and populations by monitoring and altering human bodies at the subcellular level through high technology medicine. However, these technologies—for all their apparent neutrality—carry with them significant normative power, that is, "the power of determining which human lives are more valuable, or in utilitarian terms, which individuals are potential welfare burdens to the community in the long term" (Finkelstein, 1990, p. 13). Genetic screening is a technique of surveillance, the penultimate extension of Foucault's "medical gaze." Through a combination of screening, intervention to abort defective fetuses, and interventions to alter human characteristics, genetic technologies undergird cultural efforts to define and institutionalize "normalcy." Genetic science has been granted the ability to define which human characteristics are to be defined as pathological or unacceptable, which are open to genetic remediation, and "which populations will become the experimental subjects used in the future development of the field" (Finkelstein, 1990, p. 14).

One might comment at this point that it seems that even in this approach, one does not hear much about "the body." This illustrates how difficult it is to keep the focus on the body. However, what distinguishes social theories of the body from other approaches is that they consistently begin with bodies—with techniques that are practiced on bodies (e.g., genetic screening), with definitions of bodies or different types of embodiment (e.g., definition of death), with the ways in which the bodies of different groups are treated (e.g., access to health care for the underserved), with the ways in which "political" structures position, appeal to, or ignore the bodies within them (e.g., issues of women's health). For this approach, the point of intersection between institutions, practices, discourses, and human bodies serves as the window through which to analyze political and social structures, relationships of power and dominance, and their moral and ethical effects.

While generally critical and analytical, social theories of the body may also serve a constructive function in the practice of bioethics. For example, analysts may use social theories of the body to identify ideological, oppressive, or coercive power relationships within the practice of medicine; they may then offer alternative "politics" that better embody a preferred set of values. By doing so, they illustrate how bodies, in conjunction with alternative practices, discourses, and institutions, also serve as the context for resistance to domination. Bodies, as the locus for power, are equally the site for control and the site for freedom. However, by illustrating the complexity of embodied social orders, these theories also indicate how difficult resistance can be and how resistance requires community. Those who resist often find themselves de facto members of a subculture. Feminist approaches to bioethics are particularly illustrative in this regard (Corea et al., 1987; Sherwin, 1992; Holmes and Purdy, 1992).

M. Therese Lysaught

Directly related to this article are the other articles in this entry: EMBODIMENT: THE PHENOMENOLOGICAL TRADITION, *and* CULTURAL AND RELIGIOUS PERSPECTIVES. *Also directly related is the entry* HEALTH AND DISEASE, *articles on* HISTORY OF THE CONCEPTS, *and* THE EXPERIENCE OF HEALTH AND ILLNESS. *For a further discussion of topics mentioned in this article, see the entries* AUTHORITY; BEHAVIOR CONTROL; FEMINISM; FREEDOM AND COERCION; GENETICS AND HUMAN SELF-UNDERSTANDING; LIFE; NARRATIVE; *and* NATURAL LAW. *For a discussion of related ideas, see the entries* DEATH; *and* EUGENICS, *article on* ETHICAL ISSUES. *Other relevant material may be*

found in the entries BIOLOGY, PHILOSOPHY OF; META-
PHOR AND ANALOGY; RACE AND RACISM; SEXUAL IDEN-
TITY; *and* SUICIDE.

Bibliography

BYNUM, CAROLINE WALKER. 1991. *Fragmentation and Redemption: Essays on Gender and the Human Body in Medieval
Religion.* New York: Zone.

CAMPBELL, COURTNEY S. 1992. "Body, Self, and the Property
Paradigm." *Hastings Center Report* 22, no. 5:34–42.

COPLESTON, FREDERICK C. 1964a. "Locke." In *Modern Philosophy.* Vol. 5, pt. 1 of his *A History of Philosophy.* Garden
City, N.Y.: Image.

———. 1964b. "Francis Bacon." In *Late Medieval and Renaissance Philosophy.* Vol. 3, pt. 2 of his *A History of Philosophy.* Garden City: N.Y.: Image.

COREA, GENA; DUELLI KLEIN, RENATE; HANMER, JALNA;
HOLMES, HELEN B.; HOSKINS, BETTY B.; KISHWAR,
MADHU; RAYMOND, JANICE; ROWLAND, ROBYN; and
STEINBACHER, ROBERTA. 1987. *Man-Made Women: How
New Reproductive Technologies Affect Women.* Blooming-
ton: Indiana University Press.

DESCARTES, RENÉ. 1968. *Discourse on Method. The Meditations.*
Translated by F. E. Sutcliffe. New York: Penguin.

DOUGLAS, MARY. 1966. *Purity and Danger: An Analysis of the
Concept of Pollution and Taboo.* London: Routledge & Kegan Paul.

DUBOSE, EDWIN R.; HAMEL, RON P.; and O'CONNELL, LAUR-
ENCE J., eds. 1994. *A Matter of Principles? Ferment in U.S.
Bioethics.* Valley Forge, Pa.: Trinity Press International.

ENGELHARDT, H. TRISTRAM, JR. 1985. *The Foundations of
Bioethics.* New York: Oxford University Press.

FINKELSTEIN, JOANNE L. 1990. "Biomedicine and Technocratic
Power." *Hastings Center Report* 20, no. 4:13–16.

FLETCHER, JOSEPH. 1971. "Ethical Aspects of Genetic Controls: Designed Genetic Changes in Man." *New England
Journal of Medicine* 285, no. 14:776–783.

FOUCAULT, MICHEL. 1973. *The Birth of the Clinic: An Archeol-
ogy of Medical Perception.* Translated by Alan M. Sheridan-
Smith. New York: Vintage.

———. 1979. *Discipline and Punish: The Birth of the Prison.*
Translated by Alan M. Sheridan. New York: Vintage.

———. 1980. *Power/Knowledge: Selected Interviews and Other
Writings, 1972–1977.* Translated and edited by Colin Gordon. Sussex, U.K.: Harvester.

FRANK, ARTHUR W. 1991. "For a Sociology of the Body: An
Analytical Review." In *The Body: Social Process and Cul-
tural Theory,* pp. 36–102. Edited by Mike Featherstone,
Mike Hepworth, and Bryan S. Turner. Newbury Park,
Calif.: Sage.

HOLMES, HELEN BEQUAERT, and PURDY, LAURA M., eds.
1992. *Feminist Perspectives in Medical Ethics.* Bloomington: Indiana University Press.

LEDER, DREW. 1990. *The Absent Body.* Chicago: University of
Chicago Press.

LOCKE, JOHN. 1976. *The Second Treatise on Government.* 3d ed.
Edited by John W. Gough. Oxford: Basil Blackwell.

O'NEILL, JOHN. 1985. *Five Bodies: The Human Shape of Modern
Society.* Ithaca, N.Y.: Cornell University Press.

SCARRY, ELAINE. 1985. *The Body in Pain: The Making and
Unmaking of the World.* New York: Oxford University
Press.

SHERWIN, SUSAN. 1992. *No Longer Patient: Feminist Ethics and
Health Care.* Philadelphia: Temple University Press.

TURNER, BRYAN S. 1984. *The Body and Society: Explorations in
Social Theory.* New York: Basil Blackwell.

———. 1987. *Medical Power and Social Knowledge.* London:
Sage.

ZANER, RICHARD M. 1988. *Ethics and the Clinical Encounter.*
Englewood Cliffs, N.J.: Prentice-Hall.

III. CULTURAL AND RELIGIOUS PERSPECTIVES

Scholarly and popular thought alike have typically assumed that the human body is a fixed, material entity
subject to the empirical rules of biological science. Such
a body exists prior to the mutability and flux of cultural
change and diversity, and is characterized by unchangeable inner necessities. Beginning with the historical
work of Michel Foucault and Norbert Elias, the anthropology of Pierre Bourdieu, and phenomenological philosophers such as Maurice Merleau-Ponty, Hans Jonas,
Max Scheler, and Gabriel Marcel, however, scholarship
in the social sciences and humanities has begun to challenge this notion. Late twentieth-century commentators
argue that the body can no longer be considered as a fact
of nature, but is instead "an entirely problematic notion"
(Vernant, 1989, p. 20); that "the body has a history"
insofar as it behaves in new ways at particular historical
moments (Bynum, 1989, p. 171); that the body should
be understood not as a constant amidst flux but as an
epitome of that flux (Frank, 1991); and that "the uni-
versalized natural body is the gold standard of hege-
monic social discourse" (Haraway, 1990, p. 146).

This scholarly perspective—that the body has a
history, and is not only a biological entity but also a
cultural phenomenon—goes hand in hand with the increasing number and complexity of bioethical issues in
contemporary society, many of which have strong religious overtones. Some decades ago the only such issue
arose in cases where religious and biomedical priorities
conflicted in the treatment of illness. Within the majority population, various groups such as Christian Scientists, some Pentecostal Christians, and members of small
fundamentalist sects occasionally have created controversy by refusing medical treatment on the grounds that
faith in medicine undermined faith in God, in other
words, that since healing should occur only at the will
and discretion of the deity, human medicine was pre-
sumptuous upon divine prerogative. This was especially

problematic when young children suffered and were kept from medical treatment by their parents. In Native American communities it has been, and occasionally remains, the practice for ill people to seek biomedical treatment only after having exhausted the resources of their spiritually based traditional medical systems. This occasionally results in the discovery of serious illness such as cancer or tuberculosis at a very advanced stage, and creates a dilemma for health-care personnel who are supportive of indigenous traditions yet concerned that their patients also receive timely biomedical treatment.

More recently, the number of bioethical issues with religious overtones has multiplied. The legality of and right of access by women to abortion have been defined not only as issues of civil rights and feminist politics, but also as religious and moral issues. Surrogate motherhood and donorship of sperm and eggs raise ethical dilemmas regarding the biological, legal, and spiritual connections between parent and child. There is also concern about the apparently godlike ability of biotechnology to determine the genetic makeup of the human species; some see this approaching with the increasing sophistication of genetic engineering and the massive Human Genome Project, which will catalogue all possible human genetic characteristics. At the other end of the life course, the problems of euthanasia, technological prolongation of vital functions by means of life-support machines, and physician-assisted death raise moral and spiritual questions about the prerogative to end the life of oneself or of another. Legal and ethical acceptance of the definition of death as "brain death" has particular significance in that the brain dead individual's other organs are still viable for transplantation to other persons. In the United States the bioethical dilemma is whether the brain-dead person can morally be considered dead until all other vital functions have ceased, or whether removing those organs constitutes killing the patient. In Japan an added dilemma is that a person's spiritual destiny as a deceased ancestor depends in part on maintaining an intact physical body.

Each of these issues has to do with religion, not only because religions often define them as within their moral purview, but also because at a more profound level, each taps a concern that is at the very core of religious thought and practice: the problem of what it means to be human. More precisely, the problem is the nature of human persons, of what it means to have and be a body, of life and death, and of the spiritual destiny of humankind. In the succeeding sections of this article these issues are placed in the context of recent thought about the cultural and historical nature of the human body, about religious conceptualizations of the body, and about religious practices that focus on the body.

The body as a cultural phenomenon

It has been suggested that in contemporary civilization the human body can no longer be considered a bounded entity, in part because of the destabilizing impact of "consumer culture" and its accompanying barrage of images. These images stimulate needs and desires, as well as the corresponding changes in the way the social space we inhabit is arranged with respect to physical objects and other people (Featherstone et al., 1991). In this process, fixed "life-cycle" categories have become blurred into a more fluid "life course" in which one's look and feel may conflict with one's biological and chronological age; some people may even experience conflict between age-appropriate behavior and subjective experience. In addition, the goals of bodily self-care have changed from spiritual salvation, to enhanced health, and finally to a marketable self (Featherstone et al., 1991; cf. Foucault, 1986; and Bordo, 1990). As Susan Bordo has observed, techniques of body care are not directed primarily toward weight loss, but toward formation of body boundaries to protect against the eruption of the "bulge," and serve the purposes of social mobility more than the affirmation of social position (Bordo, 1990). Bodily discipline is no longer incompatible with hedonism but has become a means toward it, so that one not only exercises to look good, but also wants to look good while exercising (Bordo, 1990). This stands in sharp contrast not only to early historical periods but to other societies such as that of Fiji where the cultivation of bodies is not regarded as an enhancement of a performing self but as a responsibility toward the community (Becker, 1994).

This transformation in the body as a cultural phenomenon has been related by Emily Martin (1992) to a global change in social organization. In her view the "Fordist body" structured by principles of centralized control and factory-based production is on the decline. It is being replaced by a body characteristic of late capitalism, a socioeconomic regime characterized by technological innovation, specificity, and rapid, flexible change. She sees these changes particularly vividly in the domains of reproductive biology, immunology, and sexuality, all of which are increasingly intense loci of bioethical debate.

With respect to immunology in particular, Donna Haraway (1991) understands the concept of the "immune system" as an icon of symbolic and material systematic "difference" in late capitalism. The concept of the immune system was developed in its present form as recently as the 1970s, and was made possible by a profound theoretical shift from focus on individual organisms to focus on cybernetic systems. The result has been the transformation of the body into a cybernetic body, one that for Haraway requires a "cyborg ethics and politics" that recognizes radical pluralism, the inevitability of multiple meanings and imperfect communication, and physical groundedness in a particular location.

This groundedness thus extends to biology itself. In addition to immunology, this is evident in recent feminist theory that eliminates "passitivity" as an intrinsic characteristic of the female body and reworks the distinctions between sex and gender, female sexual pleasure, and the act of conception (Jacobus et al., 1990; Bordo, 1990; Haraway, 1990). With biology no longer a monolithic objectivity, the body is transformed from object to agent (Haraway, 1991). The bioethical implications of the body as experiencing agent are evident in recent social science work on the experience of illness (Kleinman, 1988; Murphy, 1987), pain (Good et al., 1992), and religious healing (Csordas, 1990, 1994). New disciplinary syntheses grounded in a paradigm of embodiment are emerging in disciplines such as anthropology (Csordas, 1990, 1994), sociology (Turner, 1986), and history (Berman, 1989).

Many of these new syntheses are predicated on a critique of tenacious conceptual dualities such as those between mind and body, subject and object, and sex and gender (Haraway, 1991; Frank, 1991; Ots, 1991; Csordas, 1990; Leder, 1990). Drew Leder (1990), for example, begins his critique of Cartesian mind–body dualism with the observation that in everyday life our experience is characterized by the disappearance of our body from awareness. He contrasts this with a description of *dysappearance*, the vivid but unwanted consciousness of one's body in disease, distress, or dysfunction. He then argues that it is the very sense of disappearance, itself an essential characteristic of our bodily existence, that leads to the body's self-concealment, and thus to a mistaken notion of the immateriality of mind and thought. That such a notion is cultural is evident in the technological domain if one compares Western navigational techniques, which are based on intellectualist mathematical instruments and calculations, with traditional Polynesian navigation, which in contrast relied on concrete sensory information regarding clouds and light, wave patterns, star movement, and the behavior of birds (Leder, 1990). Leder further suggests that the Western tradition compounds the error by construing the body as a source of epistemological error, moral error, and mortality. In contrast, based on a phenomenological appreciation of unitary embodiment, he suggests the possibility of a new ethics of compassion, absorption, and communion.

The contemporary cultural transformation of the body can be conceived not only in terms of revising biological essentialism and collapsing conceptual dualities, but also in discerning an ambiguity in the boundaries of corporeality itself. Haraway points to the boundaries between animal and human, between animal/human and machine, and between the physical and nonphysical (Haraway, 1991). Michel Feher construes the boundary between human and animal or automaton (machine) at one end of a continuum whose opposite pole is defined by the boundary between human and deity (Feher, 1989). Cultural definitions of the boundary between human and divine can be significant given the circumstances of corporeal flux and bodily transformation sketched above. This is especially the case when the question goes beyond the distinction between natural and supernatural bodies, or between natural corporeality and divine incorporeality, to the question posed by Feher of the kind of body with which members of a culture endow themselves in order to come into relation with the kind of deity they posit to themselves (Feher, 1989). Thus, if the body is a cultural phenomenon in a way that makes its understanding essential to questions of bioethics, religion is an important domain of culture to address in understanding the body.

Religious conceptualizations of the body

Perhaps the most vivid example from the domain of religion that the body is a cultural phenomenon subject to cultural transformations is given in the classic work on New Caledonia by Maurice Leenhardt, the anthropologist and missionary. Leenhardt recounts his discovery of the impact of Christianity on the cosmocentric world of the New Caledonian Canaques via a conversation with an aged indigenous philosopher. Leenhardt suggested that the Europeans had introduced the notion of "spirit" to the indigenous way of thinking. His interlocutor contradicted him, pointed out that his people had "always acted in accord with the spirit. What you've brought us is the body" (Leenhardt, 1979, p. 164). In brief, the indigenous worldview held that the person was not individuated but was diffused with other persons and things in a unitary sociomythic domain:

> [The body] had no existence of its own, nor specific name to distinguish it. It was only a support. But henceforth the circumscription of the physical being is completed, making possible its objectification. The idea of a human body becomes explicit. This discovery leads forthwith to a discrimination between the body and the mythic world. (Leenhardt, 1979, p. 164)

There could be no more powerful evidence that the body is a cultural and historical phenomenon. Insofar as the objectification of the body has the consequences of individuation of the psychological self and the instantiation of dualism in the conceptualization of human being, it has implications for defining a very different regime of ethical relationships and responsibilities. This is not only a relative difference, but—as is clear in the missionary example of Leenhardt—one that has consequences for relations between different cultures.

Ancient Greek conceptualizations. There is much more to the cultural and historical variability of the human body, however. For the ancient Greeks, as described by Jean-Pierre Vernant (1989), the distinction between the bodies of humans and the bodies of deities was not predicated on that between corporeality and incorporeality, but on the notion that the divine bodies were complete and human bodies incomplete. Furthermore, this distinction emphasized not bodily features or morphology, but the being's place on a continuum of value and foulness. Bodies were understood as mutable along these dimensions without losing their identity, and thus deities could be simultaneously very heavy and very light, moving over the earth without quite touching it while leaving exceedingly deep footprints (Vernant, 1989). The deities thus had bodies that were not bodies, but they had characteristics that never ruptured their continuity with human bodies, and which therefore defined human bodies by their very otherness. The existence of the deities guaranteed that in Greek culture qualities such as royalty and beauty were not abstract concepts or categories, since they were concretely embodied in beings like Zeus and Aphrodite (Vernant, 1989).

Hindu conceptualizations. In the Hindu worldview *atman*, "self," is understood not as soul in distinction to body, but as the center in relation to an existential periphery, or as whole in relation to parts (Malamud, 1989). The ritual act of sacrifice is personified and has a body, or in other words the body is both the model for and origin of sacrifice (Malamud, 1989). The individual bodies are inherently sexual and are portrayed as couples, or *mithuna*. The masculine is invariably singular and the feminine plural, as in the sun of day in relation to the multiple stars of night, or the singularity of act/mind/silence in relation to the multiplicity of speech. In contrast to the mutable but distinctly individual body of the Greek deities, Hindu ritual portrays a rich "combinatory of the sexes" that constitutes a way of mythically thinking with the body. The *mithunas* achieve cosmic engenderment (begetting) through diverse body operations including dismemberment, multiplication of body parts, replication of bodies, birth, coupling/copulation, merging/incorporation, transformation and transgendering, and the emission of body products/fluids (Malamud, 1989).

Jewish and Christian conceptualizations. If, in Hinduism, engenderment is timeless and instantiated in the cosmos by the sacrificial act, in Judaism it is linear and instantiated in history by the act of procreation. Creation and engenderment are two moments of the

same process, a "hiero-history" in which human generation does not imitate a divine process, but *is* that process (Mopsik, 1989). Whereas in the Christian perspective the biblical injunction for man and woman to "become one flesh" is understood to refer to the indissolubility of marriage, in the Jewish perspective it is understood as the production of a child, and the birth of Christ outside the historical chain of engenderments is the basis for the Pauline splitting of the spiritual and carnal individual (Mopsik, 1989). This view is elaborated further in the Jewish kabbalistic tradition's notion of the *sefirot,* the ten-gendered emanations of the Infinite that are represented as combining to form a body (Mopsik, 1989).

In sharp contrast to the Jewish kabbalistic elaboration of engenderment as life, the Christian gnostic tradition elaborates it as death (Mopsik, 1989). Gnosticism sees the corporeal form as the creation of monstrous demiurges or archons, foremost among whom is Ialdabaoth, the equivalent of Jehovah. The human condition is symbolized in the gnostic tale of the archons' rape of Eve, who escapes with her psychic body while her "shadow" or material body is defiled (Williams, 1989). The latter is a prison or garment, beastly because humans are created by beasts. Sexuality is an aspect of this beastliness, and hence cannot be part of an embodied sacred process, while the upright posture that distinguishes us from animals is attributed to a separate spark from the authentically spiritual Human (Williams, 1989).

From a more mainstream Christian perspective, the profound cultural implications of Feher's question of the kind of body people endow themselves with in order to come into relation with the sacred (Feher, 1989) can be seen by considering the Eucharist. That the consumption of bread and wine transubstantiated into the body and blood of Christ is essentially a form of ritual cannibalism is emphasized by the story of a miracle in which a priest who doubted the divine reality of the Eucharist was forced to experience the bloody flesh, so that he could come to appreciate God's graciousness in presenting it in the tamer appearance of bread and wine (Camporesi, 1989; see also Bynum, 1989). In earlier periods of Christianity the spiritual power of the Eucharist extended to the nourishment of the body, and this, not through ingestion but by means of its aroma (Camporesi, 1989). Unlike ordinary food, however, it does not become us, but we become it through its sanctifying power (Camporesi, 1989). Great anxiety was created among priests with regard to the immense responsibility of transforming something dead into something alive by the utterance of a few words, and among communicants because of the inclusion of such a sacred substance in such a profane terrain as the digestive tract—hence the importance of a fast before communion (Camporesi,

1989). Yet because the Eucharist was thought to release its grace only in the stomach, sick people who could not eat were excluded (Camporesi, 1989). When later the substantial bread was replaced by thin wafers, it became common to let the wafer melt in one's mouth. Well into the twentieth century, Catholics were taught that biting or chewing the Eucharist was an insult and injury to the deity that could result in divine retribution.

Medieval conceptualizations.   Recent work on medieval Christian spirituality relates to the notion of the body as a cultural phenomenon. Caroline Walker Bynum (1989) has documented the prominence during the years 1200–1500 of a "somatic spirituality" that stands in contrast to gnostic rejection of the body, and that reflects a less dualist mentality than has heretofore been attributed to the thought of this period. In general, a great deal of concern with embodiment was evidenced in speculation about whether the final "resurrection of the body" might be a natural consequence of human nature rather than a discrete divine act to occur at the Last Judgment, and whether we will taste and smell heaven as well as see it (Bynum, 1989).

The medieval body was defined less by its sexuality than by notions of fertility and decay, but the contrast between male and female was as important as that between body and soul (Bynum, 1989). Somatic spirituality was especially evident among female mystics, who—in contrast to their more cerebral male counterparts' experience of stillness and silence—tended to blur the boundaries among the spiritual, psychological, bodily, and sexual by cultivating a sensualized relationship of human body with divine body (Bynum, 1989). Bynum draws on the cultural–historical context to understand why the male-dominated ecclesiastical hierarchy allowed this female spirituality to flourish: evidence was needed against the contemporary dualist heresy of the Cathars; because they were denied education in Latin, they wrote in the less linear and more oral style of the vernacular; they were encouraged to act out maternal roles vis-à-vis Christ (Bynum, 1989).

In this context the relation between the genders took on remarkable properties. Although ideally a woman would die to defend her holy chastity, it was as likely for a holy man to be resurrected in order to complete a virtuous task (Bynum, 1989). In other ways the genders were blurred, since it was thought that all had both genders within, and that men and women had identical organs with only their internal and external arrangements being different (Bynum, 1989). Because of the powerful symbolic association of the female and the fleshly, while holy women sometimes experienced being the mother or lover of Christ, their nature often allowed them to mystically *become* the flesh of Christ (Bynum, 1989). By the same reasoning, since body is equivalent to female, the incarnate Christ had a female nature, and the image of Christ as mother became a feature of medieval iconography (Bynum, 1989).

Religious practices and the body

Fasting.   The cultural-historical transformation of the body is highlighted by comparison of fasting as a technique of the body in the medieval somatic spirituality with the phenomenon of anorexia nervosa in the late twentieth century. In a study of 261 holy women in Italy since the year 1200, Rudolf Bell (1985) distinguishes between contemporary anorexia nervosa and what he calls "holy anorexia." While the former is regarded as a syndrome of clinical pathology, in the latter, "the suppression of physical urges and basic feelings—fatigue, sexual drive, hunger, pain—frees the body to achieve heroic feats and the soul to commune with God" (Bell, 1985, p. 13). There are parallels between the two conditions and historical epochs. Bell suggests that the observation that the internal locus of evil as a corrupting force for women in the Middle Ages, in distinction to the external locus of sin as a response to external stimulus for men, corresponds to the Freudian model of anorexia nervosa as a food/sex oral fixation (Bell, 1985). In addition, in both, "the main theme is a struggle for control, for a sense of identity, competence, and effectiveness" (Hilde Bruch, quoted in Bell, 1985, p. 17). However, there is a critical difference, and "whether anorexia is holy or nervous depends on the culture in which a young woman strives to gain control of her life" (Bell, 1985, p. 20).

Bynum (1987) warns against the assumption that these are precisely the same phenomenon, given theological meaning in one epoch and psychiatric meaning in another. She points out that even medieval writers had more than one paradigm for explaining fasting—that it could be supernaturally caused, naturally caused, or feigned—and that there was a clear distinction between choosing to renounce food and the inability to eat (Bynum, 1987). In both historical cases, the behavior "is learned from a culture that has complex and long-standing traditions about women, about bodies, and about food," including what kind of behaviors are in need of cure (Bynum, 1987, p. 198). It is a profoundly cultural fact that in the patristic era miraculous fasting was attributed largely to men, while in the medieval period it was characteristic of women; likewise it is cultural that in the medieval period the illnesses of men were more likely thought of as needing to be cured, while those of women were to be endured (Bynum, 1987). Furthermore, in the later Middle Ages fasting was associated with a wider array of miracles and practices of somatic spirituality, including subsistence on the Eucharist, stigmata, espousal rings, sweet-smelling bodies, bodily elongation, and incorruptibility (Bynum, 1987).

Some of the behavior of these women fits the pattern of nineteenth-century "hysteria," some is clearly the result of other illnesses, and some follows the thematic of control, altered body concept/perceptions, and euphoria. Yet one cannot be sure whether symptoms are associated with an inability to eat or are the result of freely chosen ascetic fasting. Finally, insofar as psychodynamic explanation can explain only individual cases, Bynum concludes that it is less helpful to know that contemporary labels can in some cases be applied to the medieval phenomenon than to account for cultural symbols that give meaning to the phenomenon, such as body, food, blood, suffering, generativity, or hunger (Bynum, 1987).

Faith healing. Other contemporary religious practices equally require an appreciation of the body as a cultural phenomenon. How, for example, can we understand the imputed efficacy of "faith healing" among contemporary Christians? An understanding of the body as a cultural phenomenon suggests that ritual healing operates on a margin of disability that is present in many conditions. It is well known, for example, that some people who become "legally blind" are able to engage in a wide range of activities, while others retreat to a posture of near total disability and inactivity. Likewise, persons with chronic pain in a limb may be physically able to move that limb, but refrain from doing so for lack of sufficient motivation to make the risk of pain worthwhile. Disability is thus constituted as a habitual mode of engaging the world. The process of healing is an existential process of exploring this margin of disability, motivated by the conviction of divine power and the committed participant's desire to demonstrate it in himself or herself, as well as by the support of the other assembled devotees and their acclamation for a supplicant's testimony of healing. To be convinced of this interpretation one need only consider the hesitant, faltering steps of the supplicant who, at the healer's request, rises from a wheelchair and shuffles slowly up and down a church aisle; or the slowly unclenching fist of the sufferer of chronic arthritis whose hand is curled by affliction into a permanent fist. Ritual healing allows this by challenging the sensory commitment to a habitual posture, by removing inhibitions on the motor tendency toward static postural tone, and by modulating the somatic mode of attention, that is, a person's attention to his or her own bodily processes in relation to others.

Consider also the practice of "resting in the Spirit" or being "slain in the Spirit" among Charismatic and Pentecostal Christians as evidence for the kind of body with which people endow themselves in order to come into relation with the sacred. In this practice, which occurs primarily in healing services, a person is overcome with divine power, and falls into a semi-swoon characterized by tranquility and motor dissociation. Despite its popularity, or perhaps because of it, resting in the Spirit is a controversial phenomenon for Charismatics, and the heart of the issue is its authenticity. More specifically, critics challenge its authenticity while apologists argue for its beneficial effects in terms of healing and spiritual development. Both sides invoke the same biblical scenarios, such as Saul on the road to Damascus and the apostles confronted by the transfiguration of Jesus, and the same religious writers, including the ecstatic mystics Theresa of Avila and John of the Cross, and both sides draw opposing conclusions about whether these constitute examples of resting in the Spirit. They likewise draw opposing conclusions about the historical prototypes of healers known for similar practices, extending backward in time from Kathryn Kuhlman to Charles Finney, George Jeffreys, George Fox, John Wesley, and the fourteenth-century Dominican preacher John Tauler. To be sure, such analogies and precedents suggest that it would be possible to examine the varying meanings of religious falling or swooning across historical and cultural contexts. In the contemporary context, however, the ideological/theological/pastoral debate about authenticity is predicated on the recurrent, constitutive North American psychocultural themes of spontaneity and control, and on the Charismatic cultural definition of the tripartite person as a composite of body, mind, and spirit.

Spirit possession. The sacred swoon leads also to the complex issue of dissociation, common to discussions of "spirit possession." Spirits who inhabit people may be regarded either as malevolent, in which case they must be expelled or exorcised, or as benevolent, in which case becoming possessed is an act of worship and devotion. Possession of both types is widely reported in ethnological literature (Bourguignon, 1976), and is increasingly common in contemporary Western society. Not only is the negative, or demonic, variant reported among some varieties of Christian religions, but the positive variant of possession by deities is characteristic of rapidly growing African religions. These include religions based on the Yoruba tradition of Nigeria, such as *santeria, candomble,* and the related *vodun.* The Yoruba religion, in which the possessing deities are called *orixas,* is rapidly aspiring to membership in that select group of "world religions" that once included only so-called "civilized" faiths such as Christianity, Judaism, Islam, Hinduism, Buddhism, Taoism, and Confucianism. This cultural development requires a more sophisticated understanding of the possession phenomenon not as mental or cognitive dissociation but as physical and existential incarnation; not as a pathological hysterical amnesia to which the devotee becomes abandoned, but as a form of habitual body memory in which the deity's characteristics are enacted in a contemporary form of somatic spirituality.

Abortion healing rituals. A final example of the interplay of religion and bioethics with respect to bodily practices pertains to the contemporary cultural debate over abortion. Among participants in the North American Christian religious movement known as the Charismatic Renewal, and in Japan as a facet of what are called the New Religions, healing rituals are conducted both for the removal of guilt presumed to be experienced by the woman, and for the fetus in order to establish its spiritual status. The American practice is largely a private one that takes place within the membership of a discrete religious movement within Christianity, and is a specific instance of the healing system elaborated within that movement. The Japanese practice has a relatively public profile not limited to a particular social group, and is an instance of a type of ritual common to a variety of forms of Buddhism.

In both societies the affective issue addressed by the ritual is guilt, but whereas in American culture this is guilt occurring as a function of sin, in Japan it is guilt as a function of necessity. For the Americans abortion is an un-Christian act, and both perpetrator and victim must be brought back ritually into the Christian moral and emotional universe; for the Japanese both the acceptance of abortion as necessary and the acknowledgment of guilt are circumscribed within the Buddhist moral and emotional universe. Both rites are intended to heal the distress experienced by the woman, but the etiology of the illness is somewhat differently construed in the two cases. For Charismatics any symptoms displayed by the woman are the result of the abortion as psychological trauma compounded by guilt, along with the more or less indirect effects of the restive fetal spirit "crying out" for love and comfort. In Japan such symptoms are attributed to vengeance and resentment on the part of the aborted fetal spirit that is the pained victim of an unnatural, albeit necessary, act. Finally, not only the etiology but the emotional work accomplished by the two rituals is construed differently. For the Charismatics this is a work of forgiveness and of emotional "letting go." For the Japanese, in whose cultural context gratitude and guilt are not sharply differentiated, it is a work of thanks and apology to the fetus. Thus, "[t]here is no great need to determine precisely whether one is addressing a guilt-pre-supposing 'apology' to a fetus or merely expressing 'thanks' to it for having vacated its place in the body of a woman and having moved on, leaving her—and her family—relatively free of its physical presence" (LaFleur, 1992, p. 147).

Conclusion

The contemporary transformation of the human body and scholarly formulations of it, placed alongside the transformative power of religion in its task of defining what it means to be human, offers an important perspective on issues relevant to bioethics. These range from abortion to brain death, from fasting to resting in the Spirit, from consumer culture to dissociation, and bear on the relation between genders, between cultures, and between the poles of dualities such as mind and body. Such phenomena, and new ways of understanding them, will increasingly come to light with continuing elaboration of the body/culture/religion nexus.

THOMAS J. CSORDAS

Directly related to this article are the other articles in this entry: EMBODIMENT: THE PHENOMENOLOGICAL TRADITION, *and* SOCIAL THEORIES. *Also directly related are the entries* GENDER IDENTITY AND GENDER-IDENTITY DISORDERS; HEALTH AND DISEASE; INTERPRETATION; PERSON; SEXUAL IDENTITY; *and* WOMEN, *article on* HISTORICAL AND CROSS-CULTURAL PERSPECTIVES. *For a further discussion of topics mentioned in this article, see the entries* ABORTION; CIRCUMCISION; DISABILITY, *articles on* ATTITUDES AND SOCIOLOGICAL PERSPECTIVES, *and* PHILOSOPHICAL AND THEOLOGICAL PERSPECTIVES; FERTILITY CONTROL; GENETIC ENGINEERING, *article on* HUMAN GENETIC ENGINEERING; *and* SEXUALITY IN SOCIETY, *article on* SOCIAL CONTROL OF SEXUAL BEHAVIOR. *Other relevant material may be found under the entries* ETHICS, *article on* RELIGION AND MORALITY; FEMINISM; HINDUISM; JUDAISM; LIFE; NATURE; ORGAN AND TISSUE TRANSPLANTS, *article on* SOCIOCULTURAL ASPECTS; PROSTITUTION; PROTESTANTISM; *and* ROMAN CATHOLICISM.

Bibliography

BECKER, ANNE. 1994. "Nurturing and Negligence: Working on Others' Bodies in Fiji." In *Embodiment and Experience: The Existential Ground of Culture and Self.* Edited by Thomas J. Csordas. Cambridge: At the University Press.

BELL, RUDOLPH M. 1985. *Holy Anorexia.* Chicago: University of Chicago Press.

BERMAN, MORRIS. 1989. *Coming to Our Senses: Body and Spirit in the Hidden History of the West.* New York: Simon & Schuster.

BORDO, SUSAN. 1990. "Reading the Slender Body." In *Body/Politics: Women and the Discourses of Science,* pp. 83–112. Edited by Mary Jacobus, Evelyn Fox Keller, and Sally Shuttleworth. New York: Routledge.

BOURGUIGNON, ERIKA. 1976. *Possession.* San Francisco: Chandler and Sharp.

BYNUM, CAROLINE WALKER. 1987. *Holy Feast and Holy Fast: The Religious Significance of Food to Medieval Women.* Berkeley: University of California Press.

———. 1989. "The Female Body and Religious Practice in the Later Middle Ages." In pt. 1 of *Fragments for a History of the Human Body,* pp. 160–219. Edited by Michel Feher. New York: Zone.

CAMPORESI, PIERO. 1989. "The Consecrated Host: A Wondrous Excess." In *Fragments for a History of the Human Body*, Part 1, pp. 220–269. Edited by Michel Feher. New York: Zone.

CSORDAS, THOMAS J. 1990. "Embodiment as a Paradigm for Anthropology." *Ethos* 18, no. 1:5–47.

———, ed. 1994. *Embodiment and Experience: The Existential Ground of Culture and Self.* Cambridge: At the University Press.

FEATHERSTONE, MIKE; HEPWORTH, MIKE; and TURNER, BRYAN S., eds. 1991. *The Body: Social Process and Cultural Theory.* London: Sage.

FEHER, MICHEL. 1989. Introduction. In pt. 1 of *Fragments for a History of the Human Body*, pp. 10–17. Edited by Michel Feher. New York: Zone.

FOUCAULT, MICHEL. 1986. *The Care of the Self.* Vol. 3 of *The History of Sexuality.* Translated by Robert Hurley. New York: Pantheon.

GOOD, MARY-JO DELVECCHIO; BRODWIN, PAUL E.; GOOD, BYRON J.; and KLEINMAN, ARTHUR, eds. 1992. *Pain as Human Experience: An Anthropological Perspective.* Berkeley: University of California Press.

HARAWAY, DONNA J. 1990. "Investment Strategies for the Evolving Portfolio of Primate Females." In *Body/Politics: Women and the Discourses of Science*, pp. 139–162. Edited by Mary Jacobus, Evelyn Fox Keller, and Sally Shuttleworth. New York: Routledge.

———. 1991. *Simians, Cyborgs, and Women: The Reinvention of Nature.* New York: Routledge.

JACOBUS, MARY; KELLER, EVELYN FOX; and SHUTTLEWORTH, SALLY, eds. 1990. *Body/Politics: Women and the Discourses of Science.* New York: Routledge.

KLEINMAN, ARTHUR. 1988. *The Illness Narratives: Suffering, Healing, and the Human Condition.* New York: Basic Books.

LEDER, DREW. 1990. *The Absent Body.* Chicago: University of Chicago Press.

LEENHARDT, MAURICE. 1979. *Do Kamo: Person and Myth in the Melanesian World.* Chicago: University of Chicago Press.

MALAMUD, CHARLES. 1989. "Indian Speculations about the Sex of the Sacrifice." In pt. 1 of *Fragments for a History of the Human Body*, pp. 48–73. Edited by Michel Feher. New York: Zone.

MARTIN, EMILY. 1992. "The End of the Body?" *American Ethnologist* 19, no. 1:121–140.

MOPSIK, CHARLES. 1989. "The Body of Engenderment in the Hebrew Bible, the Rabbinic Tradition, and the Kabbalah." In pt. 1 of *Fragments for a History of the Human Body*, pp. 48–73. Edited by Michel Feher. New York: Zone.

MURPHY, ROBERT F. 1987. *The Body Silent.* New York: Henry Holt.

OTS, THOMAS. 1991. "Phenomenology of the Body: The Subject-Object Problem in Psychosomatic Medicine and Role of Traditional Medical Systems Herein." In *Anthropologies of Medicine: A Colloquium on West European and North American Perspectives*, pp. 43–58. Edited by Beatrix Pfleiderer and Gilles Bibeau. Brunswick, Germany: Vieweg.

TURNER, BRYAN. 1986. *The Body and Society: Explorations in Social Theory.* New York: Basil Blackwell.

VERNANT, JEAN-PIERRE. 1989. "Dim Body, Dazzling Body." In pt. 1 of *Fragments for a History of the Human Body*, pp. 18–47. Edited by Michel Feher. New York: Zone.

WILLIAMS, MICHAEL A. 1989. "Divine Image—Prison of Flesh: Perceptions of the Body in Ancient Gnosticism." In pt. 1 of *Fragments for a History of the Human Body*, pp. 128–147. Edited by Michel Feher. New York: Zone.

BOLIVIA

See MEDICAL ETHICS, HISTORY OF, *section on* THE AMERICAS, *article on* LATIN AMERICA.

BRAIN DEATH

See DEATH, DEFINITION AND DETERMINATION OF.

BRAZIL

See MEDICAL ETHICS, HISTORY OF, *section on* THE AMERICAS, *article on* LATIN AMERICA.

BUDDHISM

A description of Buddhist ethics requires an understanding of the spiritual ends that govern the Buddhist life, its ideal personalities, and the practical display of its ideals. This entry therefore begins with a brief history of the origins and development of Buddhism. It turns next to an outline of its major doctrines and practices. Finally, it reflects on Buddhist ethics, particularly as it is applied to medicine and healing.

In this entry "ethics" refers to the Sanskrit term *sila*, or "virtuous conduct." *Sila* embodies the ideals and doctrines that guide the spiritual life of the Buddhist and the practices through which the devotee approximates those ideals. *Sila* is also a set of precepts.

Origin and spread

Scholars are not certain of the exact dates of Śakyamuni Buddha (ca. 563–483 B.C.E. or 466–386 B.C.E.), who was born in northern India. The earliest biographies, written several hundred years after his death, blend fact and legend and portray him as a warm and caring individual. According to Buddhist lore, Siddhartha Gautama, prince of the Śakya clan and the future Buddha, resided in palatial splendor, isolated from the unpleasant realities of human suffering. At the age of twenty-nine, he ventured for the first time beyond the walls of his palace and chanced upon four individuals: an old person, a sick person, a corpse, and a religious mendicant. These encounters greatly troubled the prince. The first three individuals represented the suffering that we, as human beings, experience. In the fourth individual, the prince observed a quiescence that transcended suffering. The mendicant represented the way the prince would come to understand suffering and, through understanding, transcend it. Soon after, Siddhartha abandoned his princely station and pursued the holy life.

For the next six years, the former prince engaged in, and later abandoned, severe asceticism. Through meditation, he mastered powers of mindfulness, ascended to higher and higher stages of mindful awareness until he realized the Dharma, or Truth, and became the Buddha, "The Enlightened One." The Enlightenment is central to Buddhism. The experience is described as "realizing the undying" and "the discovery of the path to freedom." The Dharma that Gautama apprehended is "interdependence" (*pratityasamutpada*), the doctrinal core of Buddhist thought and practice. The realization of the truth of interdependence freed the Buddha from his ignorance of the three basic features of the world of *samsara*, the realm of change and suffering. The first feature is impermanence; all things are in constant flux. The second is nonsubstantiality; nothing has an enduring reality because of constant change. The third is suffering; insecurity and dissatisfaction are endemic to living in a transient world. Śakyamuni found wisdom (*prajna*) and virtuous conduct (*sila*) to be the paths to *nirvana*, an abiding spiritual reality. Śakyamuni did not reject the belief of rebirth, but it is not a necessary tenet in his teaching. The Buddha's life and teachings have sensitized his devotees to the needs of others and have served as models for Buddhist ethics.

Development of Buddhist thought

Buddhist thought in India can be divided into four phases. Early Buddhism included the period during which the Buddha lived and worked, until about 100 years after his death. During this time the community remained a single unit. Buddhism began its second phase when the community split into two groups, the Theravada (tradition of the Elders, also known as the Sthavira in Sanskrit) and the Mahasanghika. This schism occurred over issues concerning the ideal of the *arahat* (or *arhat*), the status of the historical Buddha, and the *Vinaya*, the monastic rules of conduct. The Theravada subordinated the Buddha to a metaphysical principle. Mahasanghikas, however, went further and argued that the real Buddha is supramundane, free from imperfections or impurities, infinite, and eternal. Any temporal and historical characteristics associated with Śakyamuni

are mere manifestations of a transcendental Buddha. Though he may have died, the Buddha will continue to reappear to deliver beings from suffering. The Theravada accepted the notion that the *arahat* (noble one) is a person who has extinguished ignorance, abandoned all defilements, obtained perfect knowledge, and is worthy of receiving offerings. The Mahasanghikas maintained that the *arahat* is not totally free from imperfections. The Theravada insisted that any deviation from the letter of the *Vinaya* would compromise the original intent of the Buddha. The Mahasanghika believed the spirit of the *Vinaya* to be important. The present-day Theravada claims to observe the Buddhism practiced by the early Buddhists.

Between the second and fourth centuries after the Buddha's passing, the Mahasanghika and Theravada communities fractured further. Buddhist documents mention as many as thirty-four monastic sects. These communities, including the original two, are collectively referred to as Nikaya Buddhism or monastic Buddhism. They believed that the Buddha was a teacher of the Dharma and that understanding the Dharma would lead to Enlightenment or *nirvana*. Their clerics renounced the secular life, rigorously observed the *Vinaya*, and engaged in spiritual exercises that would enable them to become *arahat*. The Nikaya practitioner did not strive to attain Buddhahood. Only a rare person like Gautama could attain Buddahood. Nikaya Buddhism existed as a major force for more than 1,000 years.

The appearance of Mahayana Buddhism in the first century B.C.E marks the beginning of the third phase. The origins of Mahayana (Great Vehicle) are not clear. Many scholars believe Mahayana emerged from ideas within the Mahasanghika and other Nikaya sects and as a reaction to monastic aloofness. Akira Hirakawa, a Japanese scholar, proposes that Mahayana began as a lay movement that appeared almost immediately after the death of the Buddha. The Mahayana evolved from those devotees who worshiped at and maintained monuments that housed the relics of the Buddha. In due time, they developed their own community and their own rituals and liturgies that later evolved into sutras, the sacred scriptures of Buddhism (Hirakawa, 1990). Mahayana has an ordained clergy, some of whom observe a strict monastic life. The demarcation between the clergy and the laity is blurred, especially in Japan, where clerics marry, have children, and live their daily lives much as the laity does.

Early Mahayanists emulated the Buddha. They referred to themselves as *bodhisattvas*, "beings who aspire for wisdom," and strove for Buddahood and to save all beings. The *bodhisattva*, an outgrowth of the idealization of the historical Buddha, vows to save all beings before he or she achieves full enlightenment. The Mahayanist claims that a person saves himself or herself by saving others. In an interdependent world all beings share a common destiny. Since the task is endless, the *bodhisattva* will not achieve liberation until all beings have attained spiritual release. The bodhisattva need not be a cleric. Later Mahayana developed into two major schools: Madhyamika and Yogacara. Together they pondered over such questions as the nature of *sunyata*, or "emptiness," mind, Buddha-nature, ignorance, enlightenment, and practice.

The emergence of Vajrayana (diamond vehicle), later called Tantric Buddhism, in the fifth century C.E. marks the beginning of the last phase of Buddhism in India. Vajrayana, an extension of Mahayana, conceived the Buddha as a cosmic body and all things as its substance. Its practice is based on the Madhyamika principle that *nirvana* and *samsara* are identical. Nagarjunu, the founder, wrote in the *Madhyamaka-learika*, the middle stanzas, "The limit of samsara is the limit of nirvana." We suffer because we are enslaved by *samsaric* forces. These forces can be mastered and channeled to achieve liberation. The goal is to become a *siddha*, "an accomplished one." *Siddhas* are depicted as *bodhisattvas* whose primary mission is to work to benefit others. Unlike the *bodhisattva*, who postpones enlightenment until all beings are saved, *siddhas* achieve Buddahood in this very life and body.

Early teachings were orally transmitted until they were written down in about the first century B.C.E. The *Sutta Pitaka* contains the basic teachings of the Buddha. The *Vinaya Pitaka* discusses the precepts and other rules of conduct. The *Abhidhamma Pitaka* consists of commentaries on the basic teachings. Together they constitute the Buddhist canon, the *Tipitika* (*Tripitaka*).

The Buddhist *sangha*, or community, remained insignificant and strictly regional until the reign of Aśoka (268–232 B.C.E), the third king of the Mauryan empire. Aśoka's conversion to Buddhism and his patronage lent the religion great prestige. The monk Moggaliputta Tissa, a contemporary and possibly a friend of Aśoka, sent missions throughout the king's empire and beyond. From Gandhara and Kashmir in the northwest, Indian Buddhism entered Central Asia and found its way to China, Korea, and Japan; from southern India and Sri Lanka, the new religion spread to what is now Burma, Kampuchea, Vietnam, Laos, Indonesia, and Thailand. Buddhism also filtered into Tibet in the seventh century C.E. Buddhist culture entered North and South America with immigrant Chinese, Japanese, and Korean laborers during the late nineteenth and early twentieth centuries. More recently, refugees from Southeast Asia carried their Buddhist faith to the Americas and Europe. Recent converts have enriched the Buddhist mosaic. Wherever it ventured, Buddhism took on the flavor of its host country, but it has always preserved its essential doctrines and practices.

Buddhist doctrine

On the morning of the Enlightenment, Gautama realized the profound reality that all beings and all things are mutually related, mutually dependent, and concomitantly established. He understood that no single cause or event determines how a being or thing is created or destroyed, or how an event arises and transpires. Rather, the reality of what we are, the events we experience, and the acts we undertake are the result of a complex interplay of countless causes and conditions that do not allow for eternal selves or entities.

Buddhists have based their doctrinal speculations and their practices on two fundamental ideas central to the truth of interdependence. First, interdependence is a principle of cause and effect. Second, interdependence describes the relationship—mutuality and dependence—of all phenomena.

Cause and effect. The Buddha's vision of an interdependent world recognizes that the complexity of human experience and the limits of the law of karma determine a person's moral life. As a moral law karma states that the present moral condition of an individual is determined by past conduct. The future is determined by present decisions and acts. Virtuous behavior leads to spiritual growth and evil acts lead to degeneracy. In an interdependent world an individual lives in resonance and in conflict with other karmic forces. No event or act has a single cause. Countless causes and conditions continually intersect the karmic path of an individual. Molded by his or her past and by the immediate context, an individual's actions affect others, and ultimately, the universe. Though personal free will is assumed, one's every intention cannot be realized because no one lives in a vacuum.

The Four Noble Truths, the Buddha's method for achieving spiritual health, relate directly to karma and the doctrine of interdependence. The Four Truths profile the condition of our lives, explain the cause of suffering, and the means by which we, residing in a *samsaric* world, can extract ourselves and realize an abiding spiritual reality. The Four Noble Truths are: (1) the Noble Truth of Suffering, (2) the Noble Truth of the Cause of Suffering, that is, illusion and desire, (3) the Noble Truth of *Nirvana*, a realm free from suffering, and (4) the Truth of the Noble Eightfold Path, the path to *nirvana*. The Eightfold Path means cultivating Right View, Right Thought, Right Speech, Right Action, Right Livelihood, Right Effort, Right Mindfulness, and Right Meditation. "Right" refers to the wisdom to discover the Middle Path between indulging in sensual delights and engaging in painful spiritual exercises. Right View is the understanding of interdependence.

The Four Noble Truths parallel the steps of medical treatment: diagnosis, etiology, recovery, and therapeutics (Buddhaghosa, 1956). In the First Truth, the Buddha acknowledges that spiritual suffering, though the most serious, is just one of many ills. The Second Truth is that the cause of this suffering stems from illusion and desire. Illusion is the belief in a substantial self and an unchanging world; desire refers to wishing for unattainable things. The Fourth Truth is the Eightfold Noble Path, which releases the individual from ignorance. The Eightfold Path is the spiritual therapy that leads to the Third Truth, *nirvana*. The Four Noble Truths are steps that transcend, not escape, suffering.

Mutuality. The second and more fundamental aspect of the doctrine of interdependence describes the cooperative and mutually supportive relationship among all existing entities. All things and beings arise, exist, and disappear in relation to everything else. We do not simply exist in the world, but we each help to create the world through the manner in which we act and live. We shape the world as we are molded by it. The idea of interdependence envisions a totally integrated universe, wherein all things and all beings are mutually responsible for each other's well-being. All men and women have equal access to the spiritual goal and both sexes are expected to assume equal responsibility for the well-being of each other and the world. Alternative expressions for "interdependence" are "selflessness" (*anatta* or *anatman*), "emptiness" (*sunyata*), and "thusness" (*tathata*). In a world of mutuality there are no substantial "selves"; "selflessness" refers to the self, empty of abiding characteristics, and "thusness" is this reality.

Ethical imperatives. Ethics in an interdependent world is grounded on the laws of karma and mutuality. Karma, the principle of cause and effect, ensures that virtuous actions positively affect the moral life of an individual. The goal is Enlightenment or Buddahood. Mutuality links our lives directly with the well-being of humanity and the world with all its creatures. The realization of interdependence quickens a sense of responsibility and gratitude.

Buddhist ethics

The Buddhist community includes the laity and clerics. All devotees place their faith in the Three Treasures and observe the Five Precepts. The Three Treasures refer to the Buddha; the Dharma, or Truth; and the Sangha, or community. The Five Precepts direct all devotees to refrain from killing, stealing, lying, sexual misconduct, and taking intoxicants. The Precepts and the Eightfold Path are the foundations of the Buddhist life.

Soon after the Buddha's death, the clerics assembled in a great council to compile the teachings and moral injunctions of their Teacher from their collective memories. This compilation resulted in a literary genre called the *pratimoksa* (or *patimokkha*). Originally a confession of faith, the *pratimoksa* contained the fundamental injunctions that renewed the devotees' confidence and commitment to the Dharma and their fellowship as a body. The *Pratimoksa* codes defined offenses against the monastic life and became the basis for the *Vinaya*, the monastic rules that govern the community and clergy behavior. The approximately 250 *Vinaya* rules for monks and 350 rules for nuns are divided into eight categories of offenses and are classified according to the degree of gravity. Stricter societal prescriptions on women during that period required nuns to observe more rules. The community expelled clerics who violated any of the four most serious codes (taking life, stealing, lying about spiritual powers, and sexual misconduct). Lesser violations called for confessions in the presence of the community and penance. Some offenses were simply breaches of etiquette.

Theravada ethics. The Pali *Vinaya Pitaka*, the basis for Theravada ethics, offers detailed descriptions of monastic discipline, standards of virtue and conduct, and monastic relations with the laity and with society. Its *Pratimoksa* and *Vinaya* have remained unchanged since their earliest compilation, approximately 100 and 200 years after the Buddha's death, respectively. Theravadins consider the *Visuddhimagga* (Path of Purification), a commentary on the *Vinaya Pitaka* by Buddhaghosa (ca. 430 C.E.) to be most authoritative (Buddhaghosa, 1956). According to the *Visuddhimagga*, the path to purity requires the practice of Precepts (*sila*), mindfulness (*samadhi*), and wisdom (*prajna*). The goal is to cultivate the four *Brahmaviharas* (sublime virtues). The four virtues, "friendliness" (*metta*), "compassion" (*karuna*), "sympathetic joy" (*mudita*), and "equanimity" (*upekkha*) govern the Theravadin's relationship with others. Friendliness disarms hostility. Compassion quickens the need to remove the suffering of others. Sympathetic joy rejoices in the success of others. Equanimity rouses an attitude of even-mindedness with regard to the actions of others.

The *Sigalovada Sutta*, compiled before the third century C.E., is an important document on lay Buddhist and social ethics. It is still revered in the Theravada tradition. The Buddha appeals to common sense in showing the evils of immoral practices, the need for good friends, and the importance of reciprocal moral relationship among different social classes. The good society is grounded on moral principles.

Mahayana ethics. The major difference between the Theravada and Mahayana, at least according to the Mahayanists, lies in the attitude toward the salvation of others. According to the Mahayanists, the Theravada goal of practice is salvation for oneself and to become an *arahat*, and saving others is not a necessary requirement for the completion of practice, or even after enlightenment had been realized. In Mahayana, compassion governs the *bodhisattva's* conduct toward others. Wisdom perceives the needs of others and how best to relieve their suffering. The unity of compassion and wisdom is acted out through the six *Paramitas*, or perfections: generosity, precepts (*sila*), patience, diligence, mindfulness (*samadhi*), and wisdom (*prajna*). "*Paramita*" alludes to the crossing of the sea of *samsara* to the shore of *nirvana*. The six *Paramitas* combine monastic discipline and lay social virtues. The monastics labored to perfect the precepts, mindfulness, and wisdom. Mahayana added the disciplines of generosity, patience, and diligence, the social virtues of a righteous lay devotee (Dayal, 1932). The *Paramitas* are to be perfected simultaneously. The *bodhisattva* who perfects wisdom does not dwell in a rarefied spiritual bliss, but continually returns to the world of *samsara* to exercise compassion; compassion, in turn, deepens wisdom. Wisdom is manifested in practice. In its broadest sense, anyone who vows to become a Buddha by working to relieve others is a *bodhisattva*.

Many early Mahayana documents expound on ethics. A collection of documents known as the *Prajnaparamita Sutras*, compiled during the first century C.E., links the perfection of wisdom with ethical practice. The "Chapter on Pure Practice" in the *Avatamsaka Sutra*, probably compiled by 350 C.E., speaks of the *bodhisattva's* practice. The Bodhisattva Dharmakara in the "Larger" *Sukhavativyuha Sutra*, probably compiled by 150 C.E., serves as a model for the Buddhist life. The *Bodhicaryavatara* by Shantideva (written in the eighth century C.E.) describes the path to enlightenment of the *bodhisattva* (Shantideva, 1979). This text exerted much influence in Tibet.

East Asian Buddhist ethics. The Chinese reconciled Buddhist precepts with Confucian ethics, particularly filial piety. The effort of reconciliation began as soon as Buddhism entered China in the first century C.E. and continued until the fifth century when the spurious sutra, *Fan-wang ching* (Brahma-net Sutra), was written. The Chinese, who strongly believed in the continuation of the family lineage, objected to the Buddhist practice of celibacy. To accommodate Confucianism, Buddhists identified Confucianism's precepts with the five cardinal virtues. Buddhists equated the precept for not taking life with benevolence; not stealing with righteousness; not committing adultery with propriety; not lying with knowledge; not taking intoxicants with trust. The *Fan-wang ching* synthesizes Mahayana Buddhist and Confucian ethics (Dharma Realm Buddhist University, 1981). It had a wide acceptance in China and in East Asia.

Shinran (1173–1262), a Japanese cleric and founder of the Jodoshin sect, proposed an ethic based on gratitude. Shinran equated the realization of *shinjin*, or "true faith," with enlightenment, or "birth in the Pure Land." Being born in the Pure Land quickens understanding, and the devotee is filled with gratitude that ". . . immediately awakens great compassion and reenters birth and death (*samsara*) to teach and guide sentient beings [to the Pure Land]" (Shinran, 1983, vol. 2, p. 224).

Women and Buddhism

The Buddha admitted women into the Buddhist order with some reluctance. His hesitation had nothing to do with women's capacity for enlightenment or their determination to observe the clerical life. Admitting women into a religious order was unprecedented, and the Buddha felt that public opinion would not be able to sustain such a radical shift in the social structure. Families needed women to run the households and the Buddhist community depended on their support. The Buddha initially admitted Mahaprajapati, his stepmother; Yasodhara, his wife; and other noble ladies from the Śakya clan. Subsequently, the Buddha admitted women prostitutes, bonded servants, courtesans, and widows from all classes. Many achieved spiritual heights equal to those attained by men (Ratnapala, 1993). Queen Śrimala expounds on the Buddha-nature in all beings in the *Srimaladevisimhanada Sutra*, a major Mahayana scripture.

Suffering and healing

Buddhist documents frequently refer to the Buddha as the "Great Physician." Just as a medical physician cares for the ills of the body, the Buddha attends to spiritual ills. The Buddha as a physician is idealized in such celestial beings as Bhaiśajyaguru, the Medicine Buddha, and Avalokiteśvara, the Bodhisattva of Compassion. These celestial healers still enjoy great popularity in East Asia. The Buddha believed that a healthy body is advantageous for cultivating the spiritual life.

Buddhists have expended great effort to relieve physical suffering. King Aśoka commissioned hospitals, banned war as a policy of his government, and encouraged vegetarianism. The Chinese Empress Wu (ca. 627–705) attached hospitals to Buddhist temples. She requisitioned lands, appropriately called "fields of compassion," whose income was dedicated to the care of the indigent, the mentally ill, and orphans. The cleric gYuthog Yon-tan mGon-po (786–911) spread medical science throughout Tibet. In Japan the imperial prince Shotoku Taishi (574–622) established Shitennoji, a temple that served as a hospital, a pharmacy, and a clinic to serve the poor. In 1958, A. Y. Ariyatane, a Sri Lankan school teacher and lay Buddhist, formed the Sarvodaya movement, a rural self-help movement to work on civil and public health projects to combat poverty and disease.

Buddhists continue to be concerned with social and political ethics (Hallisey, 1992) and are increasingly reflecting on issues generated by advances in medicine and technology. Some Buddhists feel that the traditional ethical codes are not adequate for dealing with current issues. They are reflecting on such questions as brain death, organ transplant, and euthanasia and are attempting to formulate a decision-making process for such questions as the right to die and the allocation of resources. They base their reflections on the Buddhist vision of the universe and the nature of humanity, and Śakyamuni Buddha's approach to ethical dilemmas.

The question of brain death and the appropriateness of organ transplant has generated great concern. The controversy hinges, in part, on the meaning of life and death. Buddhists have traditionally associated life with sentience and in a broad sense included animals and plants. Sentience includes consciousness and feeling. Since feeling is part of sentience, many Buddhists are hesitant to endorse organ transplants, especially heart transplants. Death of the mind is not death of the person. Based on the doctrine of interdependence, death is understood to be the dissolution of the mind and body. However, the commonly held definition of death is whole-body death. "Death" is caused by "cutting off the breathing of a living-being" (Sanghabhadra, 1970, p. 319).

Buddhists' belief in impermanence also underlies their concerns about organ transplantation. Since life is transient and death inevitable, and since the spiritual task is to transcend this world, there is a common perception that life and death should take their natural course. Moreover, organ transplantation is often possible only at the expense of another's life. Such a procedure violates the precept against taking life and diminishes the value of life. Consequently, some Buddhists advocate the development and use of artificial organs. Rather than extending life through heroic measures, Buddhists would rather expend energy on care of the dying.

Those who favor transplantation argue that the gift of life is the greatest gift an individual can give. The body is, after all, transient and ultimately to be shared (Masaki, 1993). Buddhists in Sri Lanka seem to agree; Hudson Silva has used the legend of Buddha with great success to persuade people to donate their eyes for corneal transplants. The Buddha is said to have given parts of his body to the first one who asked for them (van Andel, 1990).

Buddhists appeal to the notion of interdependence in their approach to ethical dilemmas. The question of physician-assisted suicide and related issues highlight the Buddhist approach to decision making. Rather than succumbing to the principles of autonomy and paternalism, Buddhists try, by taking into account all aspects of suffering, to balance an individual's wish for a gentle death with the physician's duty to do no harm and society's desire to preserve life.

The dilemmas generated by the advances of modern technology have challenged traditional Buddhist precepts. The Buddha was quite aware of the limitations of the *Vinaya* and its ability to respond to unprecedented problems. The Buddha always stressed that he was a guide, not an authority, and outlined a method for determining proper conduct. Should the *Vinaya*, its commentaries, and current interpreters offer no satisfactory course of action, the Buddha asked his disciples to make their own decisions based on wisdom and compassion (Sanghabhadra, 1970). The Buddha's benevolent skepticism encourages moral imagination concerning difficult ethical questions.

RONALD Y. NAKASONE

Directly related to this entry are the entries DEATH, *article on* EASTERN THOUGHT; ETHICS, *article on* RELIGION AND MORALITY; EUGENICS AND RELIGIOUS LAW, *article on* HINDUISM AND BUDDHISM; *and* POPULATION ETHICS, *section on* RELIGIOUS TRADITIONS, *article on* BUDDHIST PERSPECTIVES. *Also directly related is the entry* MEDICAL ETHICS, HISTORY OF, *section on* SOUTH AND EAST ASIA. *For a further discussion of topics mentioned in this entry, see the entries* ARTIFICIAL ORGANS AND LIFE-SUPPORT SYSTEMS; BENEFICENCE; BIOLOGY, PHILOSOPHY OF; BODY, *article on* CULTURAL AND RELIGIOUS PERSPECTIVES; *and* LIFE. *Other relevant material may be found under the entries* DEATH, DEFINITION AND DETERMINATION OF, *article on* PHILOSOPHICAL AND THEOLOGICAL PERSPECTIVES; ENVIRONMENT AND RELIGION; METAPHOR AND ANALOGY; *and* VALUE AND VALUATION.

Bibliography

BIRNBAUM, RAOUL. 1979. *The Healing Buddha.* Boulder, Colo.: Shambala.

BUDDHAGHOŚA. 1956. *The Path of Purification: Visuddhimagga.* Translated by Bikkhu Nanamoli. Colombo, Sri Lanka: R. Semage.

CARMEN, JOHN B., and JUERGENSMEYER, MARK, eds. 1991. *A Bibliographic Guide to the Comparative Study of Ethics.* Cambridge: At the University Press.

CONZE, EDWARD. 1962. *Buddhist Thought in India: Three Phases of Buddhist Philosophy.* London: George Allen & Unwin.

DAYAL, HAR. 1932. *The Bodhisattva Doctrine in Buddhist Sanskrit Literature.* Delhi: Motilal Banarsidass.

DEMIEVILLE, PAUL. 1985. *Buddhism and Healing: Demieville's Article "Byo" from Hobogirin.* Translated by Mark Tatz. Lanham, Md.: University Press of America.

DHARMA REALM BUDDHIST UNIVERSITY. 1981. *The Buddha Speaks the Brahma Net Sutra: The Ten Major and Forty-Eight Minor Bodhisattva Precepts.* Talmadge, Calif: Buddhist Text Translation Society.

DUTT, SUKUMAR. 1962. *Buddhist Monks and Monasteries of India: Their History and Their Contribution to Indian Culture.* London: George Allen & Unwin.

HALLISEY, CHARLES. 1992. "Recent Work on Buddhist Ethics." *Religious Studies Review* 18, no. 4:276–284.

HIRAKAWA, AKIRA. 1990. *A History of Indian Buddhism: From Śakyamuni to Early Mahayana.* Translated by Paul Groner. Honolulu: University of Hawaii Press.

MASAKI, HARUHIKO. 1993. "Toyotetsugaku to seimei rinri." *Seimei rinri* 1:48–52.

NAKAMURA, HAJIME. 1980. *Indian Buddhism: A Survey with Bibliographical Notes.* Delhi: Motilal Banarsidass.

NAKASONE, RONALD Y. 1990. *Ethics of Enlightenment: Essays and Sermons in Search of a Buddhist Ethic.* Fremont, Calif.: Dharma Cloud.

RATNAPALA, NANDASENA. 1993. *Buddhist Sociology.* Delhi: Sri Satguru.

REYNOLDS, FRANK E. 1979. "Buddhist Ethics: A Bibliographical Essay." *Religious Studies Review* 5, no. 1:40–48.

SADDHATISSA, H. 1970. *Buddhist Ethics: Essence of Buddhism.* New York: George Braziller.

SANGHABHADRA. 1970. *Shan-chien-pi-po-sha: A Chinese Version by Sanghabhadra of Samantapasadika, a Commentary on Pali Vinaya.* Translated by Purushottam V. Bapat and Akira Hirakawa. Poona, India: Bhandarkar Oriental Research Institute.

SHANTIDEVA. 1979. *Bodhicaryavatara.* Translated by Stephen Batchelor under the title *A Guide to the Bodhisattva's Way of Life.* Dharamsala, Tibet: Library of Tibetan Works and Archives.

SHINRAN. 1983. *The Kyo huo shin sho: The Teaching, Practice, Faith, and Enlightenment: A Collection of Passages Revealing the True Teaching, Practice, and Enlightenment of Pure Land Buddhism.* 2d ed. Translated by Hisao Inagaki, Kosho Yukawa, and Thomas R. Okano. Kyoto: Ryukoku Translation Center, Ryukoku University.

TACHIBANA, SHUNDO. 1926. *The Ethics of Buddhism.* London: Oxford University Press.

UPATISSA. 1977. *The Path of Freedom.* Translated by N. R. M. Ehara, Soma Thera, and Kheminda Thera. Kandy, Sri Lanka: Buddhist Publication Society.

VAN ANDEL, M. V. 1990. "King Sivi and Doctor Silva." *Documenta Ophthalmologica* 74, no. 2:141–150.

Vinaya-Pitaka. 1969. Translated by Isaline Blew Horner under the title *The Book of the Discipline.* 6 vols. London: Pali Text Society.

ZYSK, KENNETH G. 1991. *Asceticism and Healing in Ancient India: Medicine in the Buddhist Monastery.* New York: Oxford University Press.

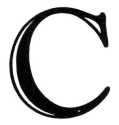

CADAVER DONORS

See ORGAN AND TISSUE PROCUREMENT, *articles on* MEDICAL AND ORGANIZATIONAL ASPECTS, *and* ETHICAL AND LEGAL ISSUES REGARDING CADAVERS.

CANADA

See MEDICAL ETHICS, HISTORY OF, *section on* THE AMERICAS, *article on* CANADA.

CAPITAL PUNISHMENT

See DEATH PENALTY.

CARDIAC-ASSIST DEVICES

See ARTIFICIAL HEARTS AND CARDIAC-ASSIST DEVICES.

CARE

I. HISTORY OF THE NOTION OF CARE

Prior to 1982 scarcely anyone spoke of an "ethic of care." The word "care" had never emerged as a major concept in the history of mainstream Western ethics—as compared, say, with the concepts of freedom, justice, and love. Yet, starting with the 1982 publication of a book by Carol Gilligan that spoke of a care perspective in women's moral development and throughout the 1980s and into the 1990s, an ethic of care emerged very rapidly, questioning earlier assumptions and setting new directions for bioethics. (These contemporary publications and discussions will be reviewed in the third article in this entry.) One characteristic of the literature on an ethic of care is that it has paid virtually no attention to the history of the notion of care prior to 1982. Yet one finds in this history a broad range of meanings and models that both illuminate and challenge the emerging ethic of care.

The "Cura" tradition of care: Ancient Rome

Ancient literary, mythological, and philosophical sources form the roots of the "Cura" tradition of care, named after a mythological figure. The background for this tradition is found in the ambiguity of the term *cura* (care) in the Latin literature of ancient Rome. The term had two fundamental but conflicting meanings. On the one hand, it meant worries, troubles, or anxieties, as when one says that a person is "burdened with cares." On the other hand, care meant providing for the welfare of another; aligned with this latter meaning was the positive connotation of care as attentive conscientiousness or devotion (Burdach, 1923).

319

A literary instance of the first meaning of care—the care that is so burdensome that it drags humans down—is found in the work of the Roman poet Virgil (70–19 B.C.E.), who placed the personified "vengeful Cares" (*ultrices Curae*) before the entrance to the underworld. The philosopher Seneca (4 B.C.E.–65 C.E.), by contrast, saw care not so much as a burdensome force that drags humans down as the power in humans that lifts them up and places them on a level with God. For Seneca, both humans and God have reasoning powers for achieving the good; in God, the good is perfected simply by his nature, but in humans, "the good is perfected by care (*cura*)" (Seneca, 1953, pp. 443–444). In this Stoic view, care was the key to the process of becoming truly human. For Seneca, the word care meant *solicitude*; it also had connotations of attentiveness, conscientiousness, and devotion (Burdach, 1923; Seneca, 1953).

The struggle between the opposing meanings of care—care as burden and care as solicitude—as well as the radical importance of care to being human, were elements in an influential Graeco-Roman myth called "Care," found in a second-century Latin collection of myths edited by Hyginus (Hyginus, 1976; Grant, 1960). More than any other single source, this little-known myth, narrated below, has given shape to the idea of care in literature, philosophy, psychology, and ethics through the intervening centuries.

As Care (Cura) was crossing a river, she thoughtfully picked up some mud and began to fashion a human being. While she was pondering what she had done, Jupiter came along. (*Jupiter was the founder of Olympian society, a society of the major gods and goddesses who inhabited Mount Olympus after most of the gods had already appeared.*) Care asked him to give the spirit of life to the human being, and Jupiter readily granted this. Care wanted to name the human after herself, but Jupiter insisted that his name should be given to the human instead. While Care and Jupiter were arguing, Terra arose and said that the human being should be named after her, since she had given her own body. (*Terra, or Earth, the original life force of the earth, guided Jupiter's rise to power.*) Finally, all three disputants accepted Saturn as judge. (*Known for his devotion to fairness and equality, Saturn was the son of Terra and the father of Jupiter.*) Saturn decided that Jupiter, who gave spirit to the human, would take back its soul after death; and since Terra had offered her body to the human, she should receive it back after death. But, said Saturn, "Since Care first fashioned the human being, let her have and hold it as long as it lives." Finally, Jupiter said, "Let it be called *homo* (Latin for human being), since it seems to be made from *humus* (Latin for earth)" (see Grant, 1960; Shklar, 1972).

The meaning of the word "care" in this myth reflects the Stoic sense of an uplifting, attentive solicitude; it is in light of this positive side of care that we can understand the deeper meaning of the Myth of Care. Yet the word "care" is not without tension: The lifelong care of the human that would be undertaken by Cura entails both an earthly, bodily element that is pulled down to the ground (worry) and a spirit-element that strives upward to the divine (Burdach, 1923; Grant, 1960). The positive side of care dominates in this story, for the primordial role of Care is to hold the human together in wholeness while cherishing it.

It is significant that a myth communicates the meaning of care, for one of the major functions of myths is to offer ancient narratives that make it possible for people to understand the meaning of their experiences regarding the basic characeristics of human life (Doty, 1991; Frye, 1971). The Myth of Care conveys an understanding of how care is central to what it means to be human and to live out a human life. It also provides a genealogy of care in light of which to rethink the value of care in human life.

Myths of origins have often been used to question the established order, both divine and human, and to establish radical moral claims, including claims about power and the social order (Shklar, 1972). Although several prominent political philosophies that have shaped much of modern bioethics are based on myths of origin that emphasize adversarial struggles as the starting point for human societies, the Myth of Care offers a subversively different image of human society, with very different implications for ethics in general and bioethics in particular (Reich, 1993). Indeed, the Myth of Care presents an allegorical image of humankind in which the most notable characteristic of the origins, life, and destiny of humans is that they are cared for (cf. Grant, 1960). At the same time, this gentle myth also speaks about the roots of power. Modern psychology teaches us that those who are cared for from birth (which is the image conveyed in this myth) develop the nurturing power to care for self and others. Furthermore, the fact that the myth's first human being is not named for the most powerful of the gods and goddesses, which would have been a symbol of being dominated by them, suggests that truly solicitous care protects humans from oppressive and manipulative power. The myth also suggests that humankind as a social totality is brought into the world and sustained by care. Since it binds humans together, care is the glue of society.

The care of souls tradition

The moral meaning of care is not only shaped by narratives, it is also historically embedded in practices such as the care of souls (*cura animarum*). The care of souls refers to the care of troubled persons whose difficulties—whether spiritual, mental, or physical—are approached in the context of the pursuit of the religious goals of life or, in nonreligious contexts, the search for ultimate meanings (cf. Clebsch and Jaekle, 1964; Browning, 1983). The care of souls tradition—the explanations offered in its literature and the interpretation of its practices—sheds light on the origins and content of contemporary ideas about care.

The word "care" in the care of souls refers both to the tasks involved in the care of a person or group and to the inner experience of solicitude or carefulness concerning the object of one's care. In the framework of the first meaning of the word, the care of souls consists of helping acts that are directed principally toward "healing" and the means by which healing is brought about, for example, reconciliation (including penitential reconciliation for those who have sinned), sustaining (including compassionate consolation), and guiding (spiritual and moral guidance).

The selection of the term "care of souls" to designate these activities (the word *cura* in the term "care of souls" is frequently translated as "cure" of souls) reflects the historical emphasis on a comprehensive idea of healing in the care of souls tradition (McNeill, 1951; Clebsch and Jaekle, 1964). Socrates regarded himself as the physician or healer of the soul, as did other philosophers (McNeill, 1951); and Gregory of Nazianzus (362 C.E.) said all pastors are physicians of souls, "who must prescribe medicines, or cautery, or the knife" (McNeill, 1951, p. 108).

The word "soul" in the care of souls can have a variety of meanings, depending on the philosophical explanation chosen or the religious tradition in which the term is used. John McNeill calls the soul "the essence of human personality" (McNeill, 1951, p. vii). It is spirit intertwined with the body without being a mere expression of bodily life. The soul is regarded as being susceptible to disorder and anguish, while being endowed with possibilities for well-being and blessedness. The care of *souls*, then, is the healing treatment of persons in those matters that reach beyond the requirements of physical life, in pursuit of the "health of personality" (McNeill, 1951, p. vii). But the welfare of the soul was not isolated: Caring for the healing of the soul, mind, and body have often been integrated (May, 1982). Thus, when we speak today of "the care of the whole person," we are speaking of something comparable to the ancient idea of the care of souls.

The care of souls conveys the primary message that there is invariably a hierarchy of values in what it is that humans choose to care about, and that among those values, care for the spiritual should be preeminent. Socrates exhorted his hearers in Plato's *Apology* "not to care for your bodies or for money above and beyond your souls and their welfare"; and in the *Phaedo* he argued that "the cultivation of the soul is the first concern" (McNeill,

1951, p. 20). Some scholars believe his exhortation greatly influenced the emergence of the idea of the care of the soul in ancient Greece and in Christianity (McNeill, 1951).

Another prominent feature of the care of souls has been the way in which it calls attention to the subjective experience of those who are suffering and their need for relief in the form of personal attention. In the Hebrew scriptures, the Psalmist speaks out of bitter anguish: "I looked . . . and beheld, but . . . no man cared for my soul" (Ps. 142:4–5; McNeill, 1951). The sufferer then appealed to the Lord to be his refuge in the land of the living. In the care of souls tradition, God, self, and other humans care for the troubled soul. The one who gives care must be very attentive to the needs of the individual sufferer. For example, Gregory the Great, renowned for his pastoral leadership in the Western church (590–604), taught that the guide of souls must be a compassionate neighbor to all, a shrewd observer, and watchful and discerning like the physician of the body (McNeill, 1951). But one problem remains constant: whether the sufferer will seek and/or accept care (McNeill, 1951).

The contrast between negative and positive care that one finds in Seneca and the Myth of Care was also presented by Jesus, who contrasted the heavy burdens (the "yoke") that many people bear—the worrisome cares of life—with relief or solicitous care (Matt. 11:28–30). He exhorted his followers not to be anxious about the necessities of life, but instead to trust that they would be cared for by the heavenly Father who knows their needs (Matt. 6:25–34; Davies, 1962).

The care of souls tradition produced three major bodies of literature that are of special historical interest to contemporary bioethics. First, casuistry arose within the context of the *cura animarum*. In contrast to the rigid ethics of the medieval penitential documents, in which priest-confessors were instructed on how to deal with various categories of sinners, casuistry had the objective of bringing the lives of ordinary people under the influence of religious and moral standards by emphasizing practical, case-based moral reasoning that avoided excessive abstractions and complications (McNeill, 1951).

Second, those who cared for souls cared for the sorrows and anxieties of individuals, partly by writing a body of so-called Consolation literature. For example, Seneca and Plutarch in the classical age and Cyprian and Ambrose in the third and fourth centuries C.E. composed Consolation literature, offering sympathy for the ills of life, suffering, and persecution (McNeill, 1951).

Third, in the fourteenth and fifteenth centuries, when the idea of death was so vivid, the care of souls tradition produced a vast *Ars moriendi* literature, commending the art of dying well (willingly and joyfully, rather than in despair) and how to help the dying person (Clebsch and Jaekle, 1964: McNeill, 1951).

Finally, care had the constantly changing function of sustaining souls through the pitfalls of the earthly pilgrimage of each period of history. For example, during the seventeenth and eighteenth centuries, sustaining the troubled soul became the dominant function of the care of souls. Because of the Enlightenment, hopes and human aspirations for this life ran very high, and pastoral sustenance attempted principally to keep believers mindful of their individual destinies beyond this life (Clebsch and Jaekle, 1964). This was precisely the environment in which care (*Sorge*) appeared in Goethe's *Faust*.

Goethe: A romanticist portrayal

The mythic idea of care made a major appearance in German literature in the eighteenth and early nineteenth centuries—a time when the meaning and relevance of myth were being rediscovered as never before—in the work of Johann Wolfgang von Goethe (1749–1832). Taking the Myth of Care from his teacher Johann Gottfried Herder (1744–1803)—specifically from Herder's poem titled "The Child of Care" (Herder, 1990)—Goethe wove the major themes of that myth into his masterpiece, the dramatic poem *Faust* (Grant, 1960; Burdach, 1923).

Dr. Faust, passionately committed to the pursuit of reason and science, also wants to be care-free, that is, free of the disturbing anxieties of care that the pursuit of his goals would entail in working with ordinary human resources. He enters into a pact with Mephistopheles (the devil). In exchange for the knowledge and magical assistance of Mephistopheles, Faust agrees to be his slave; it is agreed at the outset that Faust may lose his soul to the devil in the process (Goethe, 1985).

In the final act of the drama, Faust has become powerful and wealthy, the ruler of a flourishing land that he has reclaimed from the sea. He discovers that the deceitful Mephistopheles, working under orders from Faust, has horribly destroyed by fire the last cottage destined for demolition in the reclamation project; consumed by the flames was a peaceful old couple to whom Faust had promised relocation. Appalled by the horrific consequences of his thoughtless order, Faust breaks with Mephistopheles and his magic. He wants to stand before Nature as the "mere" human being he had been before his pact with the devil. This internal change sets the stage for the struggle over Faust's character, and for the appearance of Care (Goethe, 1959; Burdach, 1923).

Care (*Sorge*), a gray hag calling herself the "eternally anxious companion" ("*Ewig ängstlicher Geselle*"), chides Faust for never having known her: "Have you never known Care?" ("*Hast du die Sorge nie gekannt?*").

She denounces the darkness and ambiguity of Faust's soul—and blinds him because he refuses to acknowledge her fully. The terrible power of the burdens of Sorge's care almost overwhelms Faust but fails to conquer his soul. Linked with Faust's profound horror over his own crime, Sorge's denunciation has the effect of bringing about Faust's turn from burdensome care to the uplifting solicitude of positive care. His "striving," which led him to ruthless acquisition, the oppressive manipulation of masses of people, and the destruction of the old couple, is transformed during his blindness into a genuine solicitude for his people (Jaeger, 1968, pp. 41–43). Faust's experience of a new and very satisfying solicitude (the greatest moment of his life) is represented by his vision of millions of free people living in comfort and freedom on an earth that has been reconciled with itself through human effort.

Goethe's Faustian narrative demonstrates that striving for one's own life goals while shutting out a sometimes worrisome and painful concern for people and institutions results in terrible external and internal harm. In the pursuit of one's destiny, a human cannot avoid care. One must first deal with the heavy side of care, rejecting its power to engulf and destroy, and then convert this care, which is the root of all human striving, into a positive, solicitous concern for people and institutions. For Goethe, care becomes conscientiousness and devotedness (Burdach, 1923). At the same time, care relates in a fundamental way to the human condition, for it may be the key to one's moral "salvation," as it was for Faust. In contrast to today's tendency to associate care exclusively with interpersonal devotion, Goethe works out the meaning of care in a political setting; the problem for Faust is whether he will show solicitous care as a ruler. As a result, Goethe's portrayal of care has important implications for political philosophy.

Kierkegaard and Heidegger: Existentialist and phenomenological approaches

Kierkegaard. Søren Kierkegaard (1813–1855), the Danish philosopher and religious thinker, was the first major philosopher to make significant use of the notion of care or concern, albeit in embryonic fashion. Intimately familiar with the *Sorge* of Goethe's *Faust* (Collins, 1953), Kierkegaard offered creative philosophical explanations of themes that had appeared both in the Myth of Care and in Goethe: that care is central to understanding human life and is the key to human authenticity. The extensive influence of Kierkegaard's idea of care or concern on subsequent thought can be seen in the context of his role as father of existentialism: It was Kierkegaard's idea of the "concerned thinker," pivotal for his own philosophy, that became the central theme of existentialist philosophy and theology (Bochenski, 1968).

Concern and care in Kierkegaard's philosophy. Kierkegaard introduced notions of concern, interest, and care to counteract what he considered the excessive objectivity of philosophy and theology as they were formulated in the early nineteenth century. To recover the sense and significance of individual human existence that he believed modern philosophy's abstract and universal categories had obliterated, Kierkegaard called attention to what he saw as the missing element of concern or care in the kind of philosophical reflection that those systems utilized (Copleston, 1966).

Kierkegaard distinguished between disinterested reflection, on the one hand, and consciousness, which entails interest or concern, on the other. Reflection, he argued, focuses on the objective or hypothetical; it is a merely disinterested process of classifying things in opposition to each other (e.g., the ideal and the real, soul and body); it has "no concern with, or interest in, the knower" (Kierkegaard, 1958, p. 150), or with what happens to the individual person as a result of this kind of knowing (Kierkegaard, 1958).

Consciousness is inherently concerned both with the knower and with the collision of opposites that come to be known through reflection. Indeed, consciousness brings the merely objective elements of reflection into a real relationship with the knowing subject through care or concern (Kierkegaard, 1958). A personal (i.e., a concerned) relationship to truth is the basis of Kierkegaard's whole theory of knowledge (Croxall, 1958). For Kierkegaard the issue of concerned knowledge is a moral issue. To adopt the stance of the impersonally knowing subject rather than that of the concerned human being "as a refuge from the chaos and pain of life," he believes, "is cowardice and escapism" (Rudd, 1993, p. 28).

Kierkegaard also uses the notion of concern to express the nature of the human being and its moral choices. Humans are beings whose greatest interest or concern is in existing; concern or care is subjectively chosen as an intimate part of the individual's being (Kierkegaard, 1958; Stack, 1969). The individual gives form and direction to his or her life, and expresses his or her true self, not by being caught up in a large social system, but by exercising free choice and commitment (Kierkegaard, 1940; Copleston, 1966).

The fundamental question of ethics is: How shall I live? Objective reasoning plays a part in answering this question; but an ethical argument is valid only insofar as it articulates a concerned individual's search for meaning (Rudd, 1993). Thus, ethics starts with the individual. "As soon as I have to act, interest or concern is laid upon me, because I take responsibility on myself . . ." (Kierkegaard, 1958, pp. 116–117, 152–153). Without care or concern, action would not be possible:

Concern is the impetus for the resolute moral action of the self-reflecting individual who acts with purpose (Stack, 1969). Always in the process of becoming, lacking the security of knowledge and facing contradiction, the human is constrained to mold his or her integrity through decision and action. One cannot do this without an "unrelieved and unceasing concern" for the passion and possibility of becoming oneself (Mackey, 1972, p. 71; Hannay, 1982).

Being burdened with cares; being cared for. Kierkegaard offers profound insights into the experience of being laden with cares and being cared for in writings that fall into the category of care of souls literature. He takes the traditional struggle between negative and positive care, previously discussed in the Myth of Care and in Goethe, in a new direction, by turning the subjective experience of worrisome care into reasons for caring for one's self and seeking the care of others.

In his writings on a biblical exhortation regarding human solicitude for material versus spiritual things (Matt. 6:19–34), Kierkegaard remarks that by contemplating the lilies of the field and the birds of heaven, who are not neglected, humans realize that even when they themselves are "outside all human care," neither are they neglected: They are still cared for by a caring God (Kierkegaard, 1940, p. 16). Humans must work to fill their needs; but the human capacity to be weighted down by material care is a mark of perfection, for it also signals the human capacity to cast one's care from oneself, find consolers, accept their sympathy, and choose a caring God (Kierkegaard, 1940). On the other hand, humans can trap themselves into a care-ridden state of mind by worrying about future needs, being convinced they need total security against their anxieties, feeling an exaggerated sense of self-sufficiency, and comparing themselves unfavorably to others (Kierkegaard, 1940).

For Kierkegaard, a special kind of anxious care is created when, in the course of an illness, the question arises whether the sick person is confronting life renewing itself or the looming decay of death. The pathos of this question, which is more moving than the prospect of a terrifying death, can move the sick person to reduce his or her resistance to accepting consolation from others (Kierkegaard, 1940). Finally, Kierkegaard remarks that caring for someone is not always a gentle art. When, for example, there is much that the sick person can do to improve his or her health, stern demands made by the authoritative doctor—sometimes even at the request of the patient—are the expression of concern for the anxious sick person.

Heidegger. For Martin Heidegger (1889–1976), one of the most original and influential philosophers of the twentieth century, care was not just one concept among many; it was at the very center of his philosophical system of thought. Conceptually, Heidegger was strongly influenced by Kierkegaard's teachings on concern and care; yet there is a notable difference. Whereas Kierkegaard saw care or concern always in an individualized, subjective, and psychological fashion, Heidegger used the word at an abstract, ontological level to describe the basic structure of the human self. Although Heidegger insisted that he was not speaking of concrete and practical aspects of care, such as worry or nurturing, it can also be argued that his writings on care do have existential moral significance. He certainly developed some ideas that provide useful insights for a practical ethic of care (Stack, 1969).

Heidegger's starting point and lifelong interest was the philosophical question of being—in particular, the question of the meaning of being. He used the term *Dasein*, or "being-there," to represent the human experience of being in the world through participation and involvement (Heidegger, 1973, 1985). Heidegger's interest was to show how care is the central idea for understanding the meaning of the human self, which is another word for *Dasein*. His philosophy explains how, at a deeper level than the psychological experience of care, care is what accounts for the unity, authenticity, and totality of the self, that is, of *Dasein*. Briefly, Heidegger claims that we are care, and care is what we call the human being (Gelven, 1989).

Heidegger explains the radical role of care by pointing to the tendency of the human self to turn away from its own authentic being to seek security in the crowd. It accommodates itself to what "they" think and forms its conduct in accordance with the expectations of public opinion. Care (*Sorge*) summons the self (*Dasein*) back from the feeling of insignificance and anxiety found in this flight from the self, and instead enables one to be one's own self, that is, to be authentic (Flynn, 1980; Martinez, 1989).

Heidegger also explains care in the context of openness to future possibilities. We are not simply "spectators for whom in principle, nothing would 'matter'" (Olafson, 1987, p. 104). To say that the self (*Dasein*) is care means that we understand and care about ourselves-in-the-world in terms of being connected with what we can and cannot do. Because of the connectedness brought about by care, it *matters* that we can act, and we must act to choose among our own possibilities (Olafson, 1987). In so doing, *Dasein* chooses itself; and the meaning of its existence unfolds in every resolute act. This is all implicit in care (Martinez, 1989).

For Heidegger, care has the double meaning of anxiety and solicitude—the same duality we found among the Romans—and these two meanings of care represent two conflicting, fundamental possibilities (Heidegger, 1973). Anxious, worrisome care (*Sorge*) represents our struggle for survival and for favorable standing among our fellow human beings. It continually drives us to

avoid the significance of our finitude, by immersing ourselves in conventionality and triviality, so as to "conceal from ourselves the question of the meaning of being, and in the process truncate our humanity as well" (Ogletree, 1985, p. 23). Yet care also bears the meaning of solicitude or "caring for" (*Fürsorge*): tending to, nurturing, caring for the Earth and for our fellow human beings as opposed to merely "taking care of" them. However, anxious care never totally dissolves: In the everyday world we cannot avoid the dual sense of care-as-anxiety and care-as-solicitude. Accepting the kinds of beings we are entails embracing a deep ambiguity in which we know that worrisome cares may drive us to escape and that solicitous care can open up all our possibilities for us (Ogletree, 1985).

Heidegger also contrasts *Besorgen* (taking care of, in the sense of supplying the needs of others) with *Fürsorge* (solicitous care). The human self (*Dasein*), which is essentially related to others, enters the world of others by way of care in two ways. On the one hand, we can take care of the "what" that needs to be done for the other, in a rather functional way. This sort of minimal taking care (*Besorgen*) requires few qualities—principally circumspection, so that the service is done correctly. Yet other humans are never merely things like equipment that need to be taken care of in this way; for they, too, are selves oriented to others. Hence they are not simply objects of service but of solicitude (*Fürsorge*). Solicitous care is guided by the subsidiary qualities of considerateness and forbearance. But Heidegger insists that when someone nurses the sick body as a mere social arrangement, that is, without considerateness, the nursing care should still be regarded as solicitude, albeit a deficient solicitude, and never as (mere) service-care (Heidegger, 1973).

Heidegger also speaks of two extreme forms of solicitous care. Intending to show solicitous care, one can "jump in" and take over for the other, who then is dominated and dependent in the caring relationship. Doing what the other can do for himself or herself, the "solicitous" person is actually taking "care" away from the other. In contrast, Heidegger continues, there is a solicitous care that "jumps ahead" of the other, anticipating his or her potentiality—not in order to take away his or her "care" but to give it back. This kind of solicitude is authentic care, for it helps the other to know himself or herself in care, and to become free for care (Heidegger, 1973; Bishop and Scudder, 1991).

Heidegger's substantive development of the notion of care drew from and contributed to the "Cura" tradition of care. At the "highpoint" of his inquiry (Heidegger, 1973), Heidegger directly cited the Myth of Care as a primordial justification of his central claim that the human self (*Dasein*) has the stamp of care (Klonoski, 1984, p. 65). In spite of Heidegger's complexities, some writers are attempting to develop elements of an ethic of care from his insights; and some scholars, such as Anne Bishop and John Scudder, are utilizing Heidegger's ideas in their arguments regarding the moral practice of health care (Bishop and Scudder, 1991).

Rollo May and Erik Erikson: Psychological developments

Rollo May.   Rollo May (1909–1994), a pioneer of the humanistic school of psychology, introduced to U.S. psychology the views of European existentialists. He made Heidegger's views on care more accessible to the average reader by pointing to their psychological and moral implications.

May's 1969 book *Love and Will* was written in a historical period in which, he argued, humans were experiencing a general malaise and depersonalization resulting in cynicism and apathy, which he regarded as "the psychological illnesses of our day" (May, 1969, p. 306). What the youth of the 1960s were fighting in their protests, May claimed, was the "creeping conviction that nothing matters . . . , that one can't do anything." The threat was apathy. Care "is a necessary antidote" to apathy, for care "is a state in which something does matter; care is the opposite of apathy." It is "the refusal to accept emptiness . . . , the stubborn assertion of the self to give content to our activities, routine as these activities may be" (May, 1969, p. 292). Care, regarded as the capacity to feel that something matters, is born in the same act as the infant: If the child is not cared for by its mother, it withers away both biologically and psychologically (May, 1969).

May was concerned that the idea of care would not be taken seriously if it were regarded as mere subjective sentiment. To counteract this attitude, he argued that care is objective. With care, "we are caught up in our experience of the objective thing or event we care about" and about which we must do something (May, 1969, p. 291). Following Heidegger and citing the text of the Myth of Care, May holds that care constitutes the human as human: Care is "the basic constitutive phenomenon of human existence" (May, 1969, p. 290). Drawing from these sources the idea that the human being is constituted in its human attitudes by care, May claimed: "When we do not care, we lose our being; and care is the way back to being." This has moral implications: "If I care about being, I will shepherd it with some attention paid to its welfare . . ." (May, 1969, p. 290).

We could not will or wish if we did not care to begin with; and if we do authentically care, we cannot help wishing or willing. Care makes possible the exercise of will and love; and it is also the source of conscience: "Conscience is the call of Care" (May, 1969, p. 290, quoting Heidegger). Care is a state composed of the rec-

ognition of a fellow human being, of the identification of one's self with the pain or joy of the other . . . and of "the awareness that we all stand on the base of a common humanity from which we all stem." Care of self psychologically precedes care of the other, for care gains its power from the sense of pain; but pain begins with one's own experience of it. "If we do not care for ourselves, we are hurt, burned, injured." And this is the source of identification with the pain of the other (May, 1969, p. 289).

According to May, care must be at the root of ethics, for the good life comes from what we care about. Ethics has its psychological base "in the capacities of the human being to transcend the concrete situation of the immediate self-oriented desire," and to live and make decisions "in terms of the welfare of the persons and groups upon whom his own fulfillment intimately depends" (May, 1969, p. 268).

Erik Erikson.   Partly under the influence of Heidegger's philosophy, Erik Erikson (1902–1994) constructed a richly humanistic theory of psychosocial development in which care played a major role. Like May, Erikson made the idea of care more accessible to the average person; but he went far beyond all his predecessors by developing a fairly comprehensive psychological account of care that is relevant to many of the interests of contemporary ethics.

Based on his study of case histories and of life histories, Erikson developed a theory of psychosocial development in which the human life cycle has eight stages, each of them characterized by a developmental crisis or turning point. From the resolution of that crisis a "specific psychosocial strength" or a "basic virtue" emerges.

In the seventh stage, "adulthood," the developmental crisis is generativity versus self-absorption and stagnation. Generativity—"the concern with establishing and guiding the next generation" (Erikson, 1987, p. 607)—encompasses procreativity, productivity, and creativity. It entails the generation not only of new human beings but also of new products and new ideas, as well as a self-generation concerned with further personal development. Generativity struggles with a sense of self-absorption or stagnation, "the potential core pathology of this stage" that might manifest itself through regression to an obsessive need for pseudo-intimacy (Erikson, 1982, pp. 67–68; 1963, pp. 266–268). The virtue or "basic strength" that emerges from this crisis is care.

Adult caring is "the generational task of cultivating strength in the next generation" (Erikson, 1982, pp. 55, 67–68; 1963, p. 274; 1978, p. 22); that task may be parental, didactic, productive, or curative (Erikson, 1982). For Erikson, care is "the concrete concern for what has been generated by love, necessity, or accident"; it is "a widening commitment to *take care of* the persons, the products, and the ideas one has learned *to care for*" (Erikson, 1978, pp. 27–28.)

The impetus to care has instinctual roots in the "impulse to 'cherish' and to 'caress' that which in its helplessness emits signals of despair" (Erikson, 1982, pp. 59–60). The infant's demeanor awakens in adults a strength that they need to have confirmed in the experience of care; conversely, maternal care enables the infant to trust rather than mistrust and to develop hope rather than a sense of abandonment (Erikson, 1987, p. 600).

The tasks of taking care of new generations must be given continuity by institutions such as extended households and divided labor (Erikson, 1987). "[A] man and a woman must [define] for themselves what and whom they have come to care for, what they care to do well, and how they plan to take care of what they have started and created" (Erikson, 1969, p. 395). Even if individuals choose not to have children, they have a relationship to "care for the creatures of this world" through participation in those institutions that safeguard and reinforce generative succession (Erikson, 1963, pp. 267–268). Some, like Gandhi, choose, as an expression of their care, to become "father and mother, brother and sister, son and daughter, to all creation . . ." (Erikson, 1969, 399). The task of taking care of the new generation also falls to organized human communities (Erikson, 1987); social and political leadership often entails giving direction to people's capacity to care (Erikson, 1969).

The framework for Erikson's ethic of care is one of dialectic dynamics, that is, it depends on a process of development and change through the conflict of two opposing forces; the moral task is to see to it that a new strength emerges. The negative aspect of adulthood (self-absorption) continues to interact dynamically with the positive aspects (generativity) throughout life (Erikson, 1963). Personal growth and the strength of care emerge from this conflict through an active adaptation that requires that one change the environment, including social mores and institutions, while making selective use of its opportunities (Erikson, 1978).

For Erikson, part of the ethics of care involves the struggle between the willingness to embrace persons or groups in one's generative concerns (a *sympathic* strength, which is the virtue of care) and the unwillingness to include specified persons or groups in one's generative concern (an *antipathic* inclination, which Erikson calls rejectivity). With rejectivity, "one does not care to care for" certain individuals or groups, or may even express hostility toward them (Erikson, 1982, p. 68). Because care must be selective, some rejectivity is unavoidable. "Ethics, law, and insight" must define the allowable extent of rejectivity in any given group. With the purpose of reducing rejectivity among humans, "religious and ideological belief systems must continue to advocate a more universal principle of care for specified

wider units of communities" (Erikson, 1982, p. 69). Consequently, for Erikson, the ethics of care expresses itself in both "small but significant gestures" (Erikson, 1978, p. 15) and in global struggles against uncaring attitudes that contribute to the destruction of public and private morals.

Milton Mayeroff: A personalist vision

The 1971 book *On Caring* by American philosopher Milton Mayeroff (1925–1979) provides a detailed description and explanation of the experiences of caring and being cared for. Although he drew on several major themes from the history of the notion of care, he took the idea of care in new, personalist directions. Mayeroff's book is a philosophical essay that at the same time shares some of the characteristics of the care of souls tradition, inasmuch as Mayeroff's purpose was to show how care could help us understand and integrate our lives more effectively.

To care for another, according to Mayeroff, is to help the other grow, whether the other is a person, an idea, an ideal, a work of art, or a community; for example, the basic caring stance of a parent is to respect the child as striving to grow in his or her own right. Helping other persons to grow also entails encouraging and assisting them to care for something or someone other than themselves, as well as for themselves (Mayeroff, 1971).

The caring relationship is mutual: The parent feels needed by the child and helps him or her grow by responding to the child's need to grow; at the same time, the parent feels the child's growth as bound up with his or her own sense of well-being. Caring, Mayeroff says, is primarily a process, not a series of goal-oriented services. For example, if the psychotherapist regards treatment as a mere means to a future product (the cure), and the present process of therapeutic interaction is not taken seriously for its own sake, caring becomes impossible (Mayeroff, 1971).

According to Mayeroff, caring entails devotion, trust, patience, humility, honesty, knowing the other, respecting the primacy of the process, hope, and courage. Knowledge, for example, means being able to sense "from inside" what the other person or the self experiences and requires to grow. Devotion, which gives substance and a particular character to caring for a particular person, involves being "there" for the other courageously and with consistency. But caring does not entail "being with" the other constantly: That is a phase within the rhythm of caring, followed by a phase of relative detachment (Mayeroff, 1971).

Caring involves trusting the other to grow in his or her own time and way. There is a lack of trust when guarantees are required regarding the outcome of our caring, or when one cares "too much." One who "cares" too much is not showing excessive care for the other so much as deficient trust in the other's process of growing (Mayeroff, 1971).

In Mayeroff's vision, moral values are inherent in the process of caring and growth. When cared for, one grows by becoming more self-determining and by choosing one's own values and ideals grounded in one's own experience, instead of simply conforming to prevailing values. Mayeroff's moral approach to care is that of an ethic of response: He emphasizes the values and goods that are discovered in caring, and the fitting sort of human responsiveness to self and other that these engender. Care-related responsibilities and obligations—such as those that derive from devotion to one's children—arise more from internal sources related to character and relational commitments than from external rules (Mayeroff, 1971). When caring engages one's powers sufficiently, it has a way of ordering the other values and activities of life around itself, resulting in an integration of the self with the surrounding world.

The conviction that life has meaning corresponds with the feeling of being uniquely needed by something or someone and of being understood and cared for. Mayeroff concludes that the more deeply we understand the central role of caring in our own life, the more we realize it is central to the human condition (Mayeroff, 1971). Mayeroff's idea that care is central to the human condition reaches back through several philosophers to the Myth of Care, while his rich descriptions of the nature and effects of care set the stage for an ethic of care in the contemporary health-care setting.

Parallel concepts

Sympathy. The history of the ethics of sympathy provides useful insights for the developing notion and ethics of care. A number of philosophers writing between the end of the seventeenth century and the beginning of the twentieth—principally Joseph Butler (1692–1752), David Hume (1711–1776), Adam Smith (1723–1790), Arthur Schopenhauer (1788–1860), and Max Scheler (1874–1928)—developed an ethic of sympathy. Taken from the Greek word *sympatheia*, meaning "feeling with," sympathy referred to a "felt concern for other people's welfare" (Solomon, 1985, p. 552).

There are several reasons for considering some highlights of an ethic of sympathy in the context of this article. First, there are some links between care and sympathy: Some of the authors who have developed the notion of care include sympathy, empathy, or compassion as elements of care, for example, Rollo May and Milton Mayeroff; yet sympathy differs from care, for care has a deeper role in human life, is broader than sympathy in its tasks, and entails a more committed role with

other people and projects. Second, the ethics of sympathy offers sustained philosophical examination of issues that are of interest to the ethics of care, which has been subjected to relatively little systematic philosophical inquiry. In particular, an ethics of care has much to learn from an ethics of sympathy regarding its most distinctive formal feature: It is based on a fundamental human emotion that is viewed as the central feature of the moral life and the basis of an ethic—a fundamental characteristic that it shares with the ethics of sympathy.

Accordingly, there are questions significant for an ethic of care that could be examined in the context of the ethics of sympathy. For example, there is the question regarding justification for the use of a passion or emotion such as care as the starting point or central point in ethics. Joseph Butler, writing in the sympathy tradition, argued against the view of psychological egoism, which asserted that we cannot be motivated simply by a concern for others, for human psychology is such that we cannot help but act in our own interests when we act on emotion. Against this, Butler argued that passions and affections, which are "instances of our Maker's care and love," contribute to public as well as private good and naturally lead us to regulate our behavior. Benevolence for others and the self-love that prompts care of the self are distinct; they are not in conflict; and they are both governed by moral reflection or conscience. David Hume went much further: Passions, or moral emotions, are primary, for they alone move humans to action; reason must serve the passions by providing the means for achieving the ends that sentiment selects. Consequently, moral judgments, which are the motives moving us to action, must be based primarily on moral sentiments or feelings, not on reason (Hume, 1983; Raphael, 1973).

Another question is whether an altruistic virtue traditionally regarded as soft could have much effect on the ethics of the practice of medicine, which emphasizes principles and objectivity. A comparable issue arose particularly in the writings of John Gregory (1724–1773), a prominent Scottish physician-philosopher, who applied the ethics of "sympathy" and "humanity" (the paired terms were taken from David Hume) to the medical care of the sick. Gregory held that the chief moral quality "peculiarly required in the character of a physician" is humanity, namely "that sensibility of heart which makes us feel for the distresses of our fellow creatures, and which, of consequence, incites us in the most powerful manner to relieve them" (Gregory, 1817, p. 22). The moral quality paired with humanity is sympathy, which "produces an anxious attention to a thousand little circumstances that may tend to relieve the patient" and "naturally engages the affection and confidence of a patient, which, in many cases, is of the utmost consequence to his recovery" (Gregory, 1817, p. 22).

Gregory speaks of the development of a balanced skill of medical compassion in the clinician: Physicians who are truly compassionate, "by being daily conversant with scenes of distress, acquire in process of time that composure and firmness of mind so necessary in the practice of physic. They can feel whatever is amiable in pity, without suffering it to enervate or unman them" (Gregory, 1817, p. 23). In this way, Gregory closely tied the virtue of sympathy to the art of medicine and to medical benefit, while answering the objection that sympathy causes an emotional imbalance in the practitioner.

Not only does Gregory defend the role of the "soft" altruistic virtue in medicine; he pointedly identifies the core of the objection against them. Rejecting as "malignant and false" the view that compassion is associated with weakness, Gregory argues that rough manners are "frequently affected by men void of magnanimity and personal courage" in order to conceal their defects (Gregory, 1817, pp. 22–24). Men can gain from women both "humanity" and "sentiment," qualities that are at the very core of the moral life (Gregory, 1765).

Attention.   Attention (or heed or regard) has, for centuries, been one of the meanings of care; it remains an element of care today. To care for someone is to pay solicitous attention to him or her and to have a disposition of attentiveness. To take good (conscientious) care of a patient means to be attentive both to the needs of the patient and to the duties of proper care. The "attending physician" is one who has primary responsibility for the care of, and is ready for service to, the patient. Thus, the notion of attention is not only a concept parallel to care; it is an ingredient in care. The philosopher Gilbert Ryle says, "To care is to pay attention to something . . ." (Ryle, 1949, p. 135).

The most significant and stimulating thinker on the topic of attention was Simone Weil (1909–1943), a French philosopher and mystic who makes attention the central image for ethics. Attention, she explains, is a negative effort consisting of suspending one's thought, leaving it detached, empty, and ready to receive the being one is looking at, "just as he is, in all his truth" (Weil, 1977, p. 51).

Weil says that solving a philosophical problem (including one dealing with morality) requires a kind of caring contemplation: "clearly conceiving the insoluble problems in all their insolubility, . . . simply contemplating them, fixedly and tirelessly, . . . patiently waiting" (Weil, 1970, p. 335). Being attentive is being open to illumination (Weil, 1978, p. 92); we should look at these problems "until the light suddenly dawns" (Weil, 1952, p. 174). What we sometimes fail to see is what Weil perceives: that solving moral problems sometimes entails facing mystery. Thus, to discover what is causing a person's suffering and how to respond to it, the caring

nurse may need to employ Weil's contemplative attention to all details; and even that exercise of attention is itself a caring act.

Attention offers a powerful approach to ethics. For example, Simone Weil thinks of equality and justice not as abstract concepts or principles that serve the well-ordered society; she conceives of them as virtues that can only be illuminated and developed through attentive knowledge. Thus, for Weil, equality is a certain kind of attention, "a way of looking at ourselves and others" (Teuber, 1982, p. 223). Respect for another person is not respect insofar as the other has a rational nature or is a person: Weil states bluntly that she could put out a man's eyes without touching his person or personality. Rather, we show respect for individuals in their concrete specificity: "There is something sacred in every man, but it is not his person [nor] the human personality. It is this man. . . . The whole of him. The arms, the eyes, the thoughts, everything . . ." (Weil, 1981, p. 13). Respect for others is based more in compassion than in awe for personhood, and compassion does not depend on familiarity: We can and should foster compassion for individuals who are very different from ourselves (Teuber, p. 225).

Attention is also a key part of the practice of compassion. Weil explained that those who are suffering "have no need for anything in this world but people capable of giving them their attention." She contended that the capacity to give one's attention to a sufferer is a very rare and difficult thing; "it is almost a miracle; it *is* a miracle . . ." (Weil, 1977, p. 51).

Attention and the equality it discovers do not suffice for all problems in ethics: They do not in themselves define any principles for adjudicating conflicts; but they can and do convey certain attitudes and forms of conduct without which we would lose sight of the meaning and substance of our obligations and rights (Teuber, p. 228). In addition, Weil's sort of attention can show us duties we did not see before (Nelson, 1992, p. 13) and can instruct us in the skills required for caring.

Conclusion

In a variety of settings—mythological, religious, philosophical, psychological, theological, moral, and practical—the notion of care has developed throughout history, influencing moral orientations and behaviors. The tasks for the future will be to more fully understand the richness and complexity of the history of the idea of care, do justice to the texts that have imaginatively portrayed it and the thinkers who have made this idea central to their work, and enter into dialogue with them.

This history reveals, not a unified idea of care, but a family of notions of care. Yet it is a fairly closely related family, for the ideas of care are united by a few basic sentiments, some formative narratives whose influence stretches over time, and several recurring themes. Furthermore, in the history of the English word "care," this single word serves a range of meanings but with a subtle coherence.

The meanings of the word "care" fall into four clusters. The basic meaning is associated with the origins of the word, which are found in the Middle High German word *kar* and more remotely in the Common Teutonic word *caru*, meaning "trouble" or "grief" (Simpson and Weiner, 1989, pp. 893–894). Correspondingly, the primary meaning of the word "care" is anxiety, anguish, or mental suffering. A second meaning of "care" is a basic concern for people, ideas, institutions, and the like—the idea that something matters to the one who is concerned. Two other meanings of care, sometimes in conflict, are found at a more practical level. One is a solicitous, responsible attention to tasks—taking care of the needs of people and one's own responsibilities; and the other is caring about, having a regard for, or showing attentive care for a person, for his or her growth, and so forth. In a sense, all the meanings of "care" share to some extent a basic element: One can scarcely be said to care about someone or something if one is not at least prepared to worry about him, her, or it. The truly caring health professional is one who worries about—is concerned about—his or her patients, especially the patients who cannot take care of themselves.

Several distinctive features stand out in this history of care. The metaphysical and religious dimensions of care appear forcefully and repeatedly in history, emphasizing that care is essential to understanding humans and the human condition. The history of care shows that, at one level, care is a precondition for the whole moral life. It also manifests various frameworks for an ethic of care, including evolutionary ethics, virtue ethics, an ethic of growth, an ethic of response, and duty ethics, yet one does not find a formal and systematic ethics of care in the sources examined.

Repeatedly in this history one encounters a dialectical element in which pairs of ideas of care struggle against each other: care as worry or anxiety versus care as solicitude; the care that enables growth versus the effort to care that robs a person of self-care; or taking technical care of the other versus caring about the other. There is much to learn from history about the dark side of care and how humans might deal with it.

A key historical puzzle is why the notion of care has not become better known and has not exerted more influence in ethics, in view of its highly significant, if somewhat limited, history. The answer lies, in part, in the fact that care has always been a minority tradition of thought and practice. As this survey exemplifies, care is a deeply engaging emotion/idea that has confronted and challenged rationalist, abstract, and impersonal systems of thought, with far-reaching social, political, ethical, and religious implications. In this sense, care has had a countercultural role.

More recently, care may be acquiring a "mainstream" importance, especially in the area of the ethics of health care. The following two articles will show how some elements in the history of the idea of care have become ingredients in an emerging ethic of care in the context of health care, while other historical elements have been overlooked.

All ethics assumes a vision of the human condition. The ethics of care rests on a vision of the capacity to care or be concerned about things, persons, a whole life-course, a society, one's self. The history certainly is not compatible with reducing care to caregiving. The Myth of Care suggestively offers a care-based genealogy of morals that is deeply ingrained in human psychology, anthropology, religion, and altruistic service. The philosophical and psychological developments in the idea of care have built on this basic vision of being well cared for. That the history of the idea of care also suggests many practical ideas—for example, the call and the limits of taking care of others; dealing with the negative side of care; and the intergenerational function of care—makes it all the more useful for a contemporary ethic of care.

WARREN THOMAS REICH

Directly related to this article are the companion articles in this entry: HISTORICAL DIMENSIONS OF AN ETHIC OF CARE IN HEALTH CARE, *and* CONTEMPORARY ETHICS OF CARE. *Also directly related are the entries* COMPASSION; EMOTIONS; HEALING; INTERPRETATION; METAPHOR AND ANALOGY; NARRATIVE; *and* VIRTUE AND CHARACTER. *For a further discussion of topics mentioned in this article, see the entries* DEATH: ART OF DYING, *article on* ARS MORIENDI; HARM; PAIN AND SUFFERING; PSYCHOANALYSIS AND DYNAMIC THERAPIES; TRAGEDY; TRUST; *and* VALUE AND VALUATION. *For a discussion of related ideas, see the entries* BENEFICENCE; BODY, *article on* EMBODIMENT: THE PHENOMENOLOGICAL TRADITION; CONSCIENCE; *and* FEMINISM. *Other relevant material may be found under the entries* CLINICAL ETHICS, *article on* ELEMENTS AND METHODOLOGIES; FIDELITY AND LOYALTY; HUMAN NATURE; *and* MATERNAL–FETAL RELATIONSHIP.

Bibliography

BAIER, ANNETTE C. 1980. "Master Passions." In *Explaining Emotions*, pp. 403–423. Edited by Amélie Oksenberg Rorty. Berkeley: University of California Press.
———. 1987. "Hume, the Women's Moral Theorist?" In

Women and Moral Theory, pp. 35–55. Edited by Eva Feder Kittay and Diana T. Meyers. Totowa, N.J.: Rowman & Littlefield.

BISHOP, ANNE H., and SCUDDER, JOHN R., JR. 1991. "Nursing as Caring." In their *Nursing: The Practice of Caring*, pp. 53–76. New York: National League for Nursing Press.

BLUM, LARRY; HOMIAK, MARCIA; HOUSMAN, JUDY; and SCHEMAN, NAOMI. 1973. "Altruism and Women's Oppression." *Philosophical Forum* 5:222–247.

BOCHENSKI, JOSEPH M. 1968. *The Methods of Contemporary Thought*. New York: Harper & Row.

BROWNING, DON S. 1983. *Religious Ethics and Pastoral Care*. Philadelphia: Fortress.

BRYANT, S. 1961. "Sympathy." In *Encyclopaedia of Religion and Ethics*, vol. 12, pp. 152–155. Edited by James Hastings. New York: Charles Scribner's Sons.

BURDACH, KONRAD. 1923. "Faust und die Sorge." *Deutsche Vierteljahrsschrift für Literaturwissenschaft und Geistesgeschichte* 1:1–60.

BUTLER, BISHOP JOSEPH. 1950. [1726]. *Five Sermons Preached at the Rolls Chapel; and, A Dissertation upon the Nature of Virtue*. New York: Bobbs-Merrill.

CLEBSCH, WILLIAM A., and JAEKLE, CHARLES R. 1964. *Pastoral Care in Historical Perspective: An Essay with Exhibits*. New York: Harper & Row.

COLLINS, JAMES D. 1953. *The Mind of Kierkegaard*. Chicago: Henry Regnery.

COPLESTON, FREDERICK. 1966. *Contemporary Philosophy: Studies of Logical Positivism and Existentialism*. Westminster, Md.: Newman.

CROXALL, THOMAS HENRY. 1958. "Assessment." In *Johannes Climacus; or, De Omnibus Dubitandum Est; and A Sermon*. By Søren Kierkegaard. Translated by Thomas Henry Croxall. Stanford, Calif.: Stanford University Press.

DAVIES, PAUL E. 1962. "Care, Carefulness." In vol. 1 of *The Interpreter's Dictionary of the Bible*, p. 537. Edited by George Arthur Buttrick. New York: Abingdon.

DOTY, WILLIAM G. 1991. "Myth, the Archetype of All Other Fable: A Review of Recent Literature." *Soundings: An Interdisciplinary Journal* 71, nos. 1 and 2:243–274.

ERIKSON, ERIK H. 1963. *Childhood and Society*. 2d ed., rev. New York: W. W. Norton.

———. 1964. *Insight and Responsibility: Lectures on the Ethical Implications of Psychoanalytic Insight*. New York: W. W. Norton.

———. 1969. *Ghandi's Truth: On the Origins of Militant Nonviolence*. New York: W. W. Norton.

———. 1974. *Dimensions of a New Identity*. New York: W. W. Norton.

———. 1978. "Reflections on Dr. Borg's Life Cycle." In *Adulthood: Essays*, pp. 1–31. Edited by Erik H. Erikson. New York: W. W. Norton.

———. 1980a. *Identity and the Life Cycle: Selected Papers*. New York: W. W. Norton.

———. 1980b. "On the Generation Cycle: An Address." *International Journal of Psycho-Analysis* 61, pt. 2:213–223.

———. 1982. *The Life Cycle Completed: A Review*. New York: W. W. Norton.

———. 1987. *A Way of Looking at Things: Selected Papers from 1930 to 1980*. Edited by Stephen Schlein. New York: W. W. Norton.

FLYNN, THOMAS R. 1980. "*Angst* and Care in the Early Heidegger: The Ontic/Ontologic Aporia." *International Studies in Philosophy* 12 (Spring):61–76.

FRYE, NORTHROP. 1971. *The Critical Path: An Essay on the Social Context of Literary Criticism*. Bloomington and London: Indiana University Press.

GELVEN, MICHAEL. 1989. *A Commentary on Heidegger's Being and Time*. Rev. ed. De Kalb: Northern Illinois University Press.

GILLIGAN, CAROL. 1982. *In a Different Voice: Psychological Theory and Women's Development*. Cambridge, Mass.: Harvard University Press.

GOETHE, JOHANN WOLFGANG VON. 1959. *Faust*. Part 2. Translated by Philip Wayne. London: Penguin.

———. 1985. *Faust*, Part 1. German/English rev. ed. Translated by Peter Salm. New York: Bantam.

———. 1989. *Faust: Der Tragödie erster und zweiter Teil; Urfaust*. Edited with commentary by Erich Trunz. Munich: C. H. Beck.

GRANT, MARY A., trans. and ed. 1960. *The Myths of Hyginus*. Lawrence: University of Kansas.

GREGORY, JOHN. 1765. *A Comparative View of the State and Faculties of Man with Those of the Animal World*. London: J. Dodsley.

———. 1817. *Lectures and Duties on the Qualifications of a Physician*. Philadelphia: M. Carey & Son.

HANNAY, ALASTAIR. 1982. *Kierkegaard*. London: Routledge & Kegan Paul.

HEIDEGGER, MARTIN. 1973. *Being and Time*. Translated by John Macquarrie and Edward Robinson. New ed. Oxford: Basil Blackwell.

———. 1985. *History of the Concept of Time: Prolegomena*. Translated by Theodore Kisiel. Bloomington: Indiana University Press.

HERDER, JOHANN GOTTFRIED. 1990. "Das Kind der Sorge." In *Volkslieder, Übertragungen, Dichtungen*, pp. 743–744. Edited by Ulrich Gaier. Vol. 3 of *Herder's Werke*. Edited by Martin Bollacher, Jürgen Brummack, Ulrich Garer, Gunter E. Grimm, Hans Dietrich Irmscher, Rudolf Smend, and Johannes Wallmann. Frankfurt am Main: Deutscher Klassiker Verlag.

HUME, DAVID. 1983. *An Enquiry Concerning the Principles of Morals*. Indianapolis, Ind.: Hackett.

———. 1992.*A Treatise of Human Nature*. Buffalo, N.Y.: Prometheus.

HYGINUS. 1976. [1535]. *Fabularum Liber*. New York: Garland.

JAEGER, HANS. 1968. "The Problem of Faust's Salvation." In his *Essays on German Literature, 1935–1962*, pp. 41–98. Bloomington: Department of Germanic Languages, Indiana University.

KAELIN, EUGENE FRANCIS. 1988. *Heidegger's "Being and Time": A Reading for Readers*. Tallahassee: Florida State University Press.

KIERKEGAARD, SØREN. 1940. *Consider the Lilies: Being the Second Part of "Edifying Discourses in a Different Vein."* Translated by Amelia Stewart Ferrie Aldworth and William Stewart Ferrie. London: C. W. Daniel.

————. 1958. *Johannes Climacus; or, De Omnibus Dubitandum Est; and A Sermon.* Translated by Thomas Henry Croxall. Stanford, Calif.: Stanford University Press.

————. 1960. *Kierkegaard's Concluding Unscientific Postscript.* Translated by David F. Swenson and Walter Lowrie. Princeton, N.J.: Princeton University Press.

————. 1967. *Stages on Life's Way.* Translated by Walter Lowrie. New York: Schocken.

————. 1971. *Christian Discourses; and The Lilies of the Field and the Birds of the Air; and Three Discourses at the Communion on Fridays.* Translated by Walter Lowrie. Princeton, N.J.: Princeton University Press.

KLONOSKI, RICHARD J. 1984. "*Being and Time* Said All at Once: An Analysis of Section 42." *Tulane Studies in Philosophy* 32:62–68.

KNOWLES, RICHARD T. 1986. *Human Development and Human Possibility: Erikson in the Light of Heidegger.* Lanham, Md.: University Press of America.

MACKEY, LOUIS. 1972. "The Poetry of Inwardness." In *Kierkegaard: A Collection of Critical Essays*, pp. 1–102. Edited by Josiah Thompson. New York: Anchor.

MARTINEZ, ROY. 1989. "An 'Authentic' Problem in Heidegger's *Being and Time.*" *Auslegung* 15, no. 1:1–20.

MAY, GERALD G. 1982. *Care of Mind, Care of Spirit: Psychiatric Dimensions of Spiritual Direction.* San Francisco: Harper & Row.

MAY, ROLLO. 1969. *Love and Will.* New York: W. W. Norton.

MAYEROFF, MILTON. 1965. "On Caring." *International Philosophical Quarterly* 5, no. 3:462–474.

————. 1971. *On Caring.* New York: Harper & Row.

McNEILL, JOHN T. 1951. *A History of the Cure of Souls.* New York: Harper & Brothers.

MERCER, PHILIP. 1972. *Sympathy and Ethics: A Study of the Relationship Between Sympathy and Morality with Special Reference to Hume's Treatise.* Oxford: Oxford University Press.

MOONEY, EDWARD F. 1992. "Sympathy." In vol. 2 of *Encyclopedia of Ethics*, pp. 1222–1225. Edited by Lawrence C. Becker and Charlotte B. Becker. New York: Garland.

NELSON, HILDE. 1992. "Against Caring." *Journal of Clinical Ethics* 3, no. 1:11–15.

OGLETREE, THOMAS W. 1985. *Hospitality to the Stranger: Dimensions of Moral Understanding.* Philadelphia: Fortress.

OLAFSON, FREDERICK A. 1987. *Heidegger and the Philosophy of Mind.* New Haven, Conn.: Yale University Press.

RAPHAEL, DAVID D. 1973. "Moral Sense." In vol. 3 of *Dictionary of the History of Ideas.* Edited by Philip P. Wiener. New York: Charles Scribner's Sons.

REICH, WARREN THOMAS. 1993. "Alle origini dell'etica medica: Mito del contratto o mito di Cura?" In *Modelli di Medicina: Crisi e Attualità dell'Idea di Professione.* Edited by Paolo Cattorini and Roberto Mordacci. Milan: Europa Scienze Umane Editrice.

RUDD, ANTHONY. 1993. *Kierkegaard and the Limits of the Ethical.* Oxford: At the Clarendon Press.

RYLE, GILBERT. 1949. *The Concept of Mind.* London: Hutchinson.

SCHELER, MAX. 1954. *The Nature of Sympathy.* Translated by Peter L. Heath. London: Routledge & Kegan Paul.

SCHOPENHAUER, ARTHUR. 1965. *On the Basis of Morality.* Indianapolis, Ind.: Bobbs-Merrill.

SENECA. 1953. *Seneca ad Lucilium Epistulae.* Vol. 3 of *Epistulae Morales.* Translated by Richard M. Gummere. Cambridge, Mass.: Harvard University Press.

SHKLAR, JUDITH N. 1972. "Subversive Genealogies." *Daedalus* 101, no. 1:129–154.

SIMPSON, J. A., and WEINER, S. C., eds. 1989. *The Oxford English Dictionary.* 2d ed., vol. 2. Oxford: Oxford University Press.

SOLOMON, ROBERT C. 1985. *Introducing Philosophy: A Text with Readings.* 3d ed. San Diego, Calif.: Harcourt Brace Jovanovich.

STACK, GEORGE J. 1969. "Concern in Kierkegaard and Heidegger." *Philosophy Today* 13 (Spring):26–35.

TEUBER, ANDREAS. 1982. "Simone Weil: Equality as Compassion." *Philosophy and Phenomenological Research* 43, no. 2:221–237.

WEIL, SIMONE. 1952. *Gravity and Grace.* New York: G. P. Putnam's Sons.

————. 1970. *First and Last Notebooks.* London: Oxford University Press.

————. 1977. *The Simone Weil Reader.* Edited by George A. Panichas. New York: David McKay.

————. 1978. *Lectures on Philosophy.* Cambridge: At the University Press.

————. 1981. *Draft for a Statement for Human Obligations.* Lebanon, Penn.: Sowers.

II. HISTORICAL DIMENSIONS OF AN ETHIC OF CARE IN HEALTH CARE

In the context of health care, the idea of care has two principal meanings: (1) taking care of the sick person, which emphasizes the delivery of technical care; and (2) caring for or caring about the sick person, which suggests a virtue of devotion or concern for the other as a person. At times these two aspects of care have been united; at other times they are in conflict.

Taking care of: Competent, technical care

When speaking of the medical aspects of "taking care of" the patient, one often uses the language of taking good care, or receiving appropriate care. This practical vision of care can be viewed historically from the perspectives of medical competence and technical excellence. The Greek demigod Asklepios, because of his reputation for competence, became the "patron of human healers" (Jonsen, 1990). The virtue that motivated the physician of classical Greece was *philotechnia*, or love of the art (May, 1983; Laín Entralgo, 1969). In the Greek tradition, "the love of technical skill included not only an appreciation of the good which the application of that skill might achieve but also a kind of natural piety that recognized the limits of the art" (May, 1983, pp. 92–93). The ethic of competent care can also be called a Hippocratic ethic, after Hippocrates (ca. 460–378 B.C.E.), the "father of medicine." One phrase in the Hippocratic oath—"I will act for the benefit of my patient according to my ability and judgment"—implies the imperative of the competent practice of the art of medicine (Jonsen, 1990). Under these historical influences, competence, "in the sense of a disciplined understanding of the science and skilled manipulation of the art [of medicine]," was regarded as the first virtue of medical care at least through the seventeenth century (Jonsen, 1990, p. 22).

In modern times, competence has become the essential and comprehensive virtue of medicine; medical practice and education came to emphasize ever-more-complete scientific knowledge and ever-more-competent clinical performance. This demanding standard of competence in turn fueled a drive toward biomedical excellence and deepened the sense of meaning and pleasure gained from practicing the art of medicine (May, 1983; Jonsen, 1990).

At the turn of the twentieth century, as medical competence focused more and more intently on the principles of pathophysiology and factual diagnostics, medical "care" came to be defined by objective data. Clinical and laboratory efforts to comprehend, apply, and evaluate medical data led physicians increasingly to divorce the disease from the patient, thus marginalizing personal care. The desire for liberation from the sometimes oppressive consequences of emotional involvement in "caring for" the person who is in critical condition may have contributed to this trend. As increased technical expertise raised expectations of what "taking care" should mean, legal and ethical requirements of "due care" spelled out the criteria for medical care, prompting clinicians to focus even more on the technical ideal of competence in "taking care of the sick" (Annas, 1990).

By the 1920s, competent care was becoming *the* moral meaning of "taking care of" the patient. Richard C. Cabot (1868–1939), a renowned professor at Harvard Medical School, articulated and championed this new ethic of competence. The humanistic virtue of "caring for" the patient was quickly pushed to the periphery of medicine, for that sort of care was viewed as bearing no apparent relation to the highly esteemed "hard data." This narrowing of the notion of care placed medical ethics in crisis (Jonsen, 1990).

Caring for the sick person

While "taking care of the patient" in competence had been pushing "caring for" the patient to the periphery of medical concerns, "caring for" the patient received a

major impetus at Harvard during the 1920s. This section will consider what altruistic terms and virtues "caring for" replaced, why they had lost their meaning, an account of the onset of the term "caring for," and its meaning in health care prior to 1982.

The moral term "caring for" was turned to at a time when the altruistic virtues that had shaped the care of the sick for centuries had lost much of their luster, particularly terms like hospitality, philanthropy, charity, love, and sympathy.

For example, hospitality, which meant the friendly and cordial taking in of strangers or travelers, had enormous influence as an altruistic virtue for health care; it was a model in rabbinic Judaism, early Christianity, and Islam (Exod. 23:9). Christianity had transformed hospitality from a private into a public virtue of mercy and beneficence that was often directed to the sick stranger (Bonet-Maury, 1961). Hospitality prompted establishment of travelers' inns, which evolved into hospices where health care was sometimes provided, and eventually to hospitals, especially in the Byzantine East but also eventually in the Latin West (Miller, 1985). But by the 1920s this religious term had lost its force; even Christians no longer spoke of hospitality as a major public virtue motivating health care.

Philanthropy had, for centuries, been a dominant altruistic motive for "caring for" the sick in most religious traditions, but it has virtually disappeared from the moral sphere of health care. The ideal of philanthropy (from the Greek *philanthropos,* meaning humane or benevolent) encouraged a love of humankind that expressed itself in concrete deeds of service to others. Philanthropy, associated with the Christian ideal of charity, made it possible for the sick person to assume a preferential position in society (Sigerist, 1943) and motivated the establishment of hospitals starting in the fourth century in the East, until modern times in the West. The ideal of philanthropy also appeared strongly in the first code of medical ethics, adopted by the American Medical Association in 1847. But by the 1920s, professional philanthropy, from which modern professionals had derived much of their authority and prestige, had lost much of its respect, and the significance of the word philanthropy had been reduced to its meaning of private (and to some extent, public) support of the arts, education, and research (May, 1983, 1986).

Sympathy and compassion have exerted a strong public influence on caring for the sick in times past, in particular by motivating the sensitivities of individual medical practitioners. Codes and oaths have exhorted health practitioners throughout the ages to care for the sick out of motives of compassion and sympathy. John Gregory (1724–1773) spoke of the sensibility of heart that makes us feel for the sick and arouses in us the desire to relieve their distresses. Use of the word sympathy to motivate personalized medical care appeared commonly right up to the 1920s and beyond. But the word sympathy lost its effectiveness as it often came to be regarded as the condescending manifestation of pity; the word compassion was looked on with some disfavor as it came to suggest too much identification with the suffering person.

In addition, there is an overarching reason why the previous caring virtues were discounted, leaving room for the new, secular term of care. In criticizing ecclesiastical institutions in the eighteenth century, Enlightenment thinkers denounced charity for the sick and philanthropic hospitals because these activities were tainted by the essentially self-centered gifts and legacies of pious people who sought to atone for their sins by acts of charity in support of the hospitals. Eighteenth-century rationalists emphasized that the poorly organized philanthropic hospitals of Christian Europe did little to help the sick get well; and some Enlightenment thinkers blamed the very concept of Christian charity for these abuses. Furthermore, Christian charity was regarded as too closely linked to dead traditions and blind superstitions to have a close relationship with science (Locke, 1993). The attempt by some philosophers in the eighteenth, nineteenth, and twentieth centuries to base an altruistic care of the sick on a secular notion of sympathy was, in part, a result of these developments.

By the 1920s, the secular term "care" had begun to replace the earlier altruistic terminology. By this time, the history of the idea of care had progressed to the point that the term was coming to be known for its moral implications. In addition, "care" had special appeal as a virtue for health care because the same word had—for centuries and in a variety of languages—been the descriptive term for "taking care of" sick people. It should be no surprise, then, that for a number of decades prior to 1982—when the idea of care began capturing widespread contemporary attention—there appeared a small body of literature in the clinical ethics of physicians and nurses as well as in religious medical ethics that focused attention on the moral meaning and practice of care, as well as on an ethic of care.

"Caring for" in clinical medical ethics, 1920–1982

In championing the fast-developing technical art of medicine, Richard C. Cabot acknowledged and seemed to acquiesce in the fact that doctors and nurses were not caring for the whole patient: Their attention was "too strongly concentrated" on the difficult tasks of diagnosis and treatment, and "there is not enough attention left to go round" (Cabot, 1926, p. 16). He was certainly in favor of manifesting courtesy and patience with sick people; but under some conditions, he said, it is not advisable for the physician to care for anything but the patient's body; and when care for the whole person is desirable, others—medical students, social workers, and even ministerial students—can suitably offer that kind of care (Cabot, 1926). To carry out his purpose of designating surrogates who would "care for" the patient, Cabot was instrumental in establishing the professions of medical social work and clinical pastoral care.

The following year, Francis Peabody, a physician-professor colleague of Cabot at Harvard, offered the opposite point of view. "Caring for" the patient is essential to the practice of medicine, he argued; physicians must engage in this sort of care in order to achieve the goals inherent in medicine. His 1927 essay "The Care of the Patient" is one of the foundation stones of an ethic of care in twentieth-century medicine in the United States (Peabody, 1987).

Peabody acknowledged that the "enormous mass of scientific material" to which a young doctor must be exposed, the depersonalized aspects of modern hospital practice, and physicians' bias toward organic disease could jeopardize the personal aspects of the art of medicine. To remedy these problems, he urged the physician to form and be attentive to a personal relationship with the patient and with the patient's "environmental background." The treatment of a disease, which may be impersonal, "takes its proper place in the larger problem of the care of the patient" (Peabody, 1987, p. 396), which "must be completely personal" (Peabody, 1987, p. 389). His oft-quoted principle was: "One of the essential qualities of the clinician is interest in humanity, for the secret of the care of the patient is in caring for the patient" (Peabody, 1987, p. 401).

The physician must be attentive to particular circumstances of the patient, "not from the abstract point of view of the treatment of the disease, but from the concrete point of view of the care of the individual" (Peabody, 1987, p. 398). Peabody was clearly attempting to exonerate the usefulness—indeed, the necessity—of care in the practice of good clinical medicine when he argued that neglect of careful attention to the true situation of the whole patient, including functional disorder, jeopardizes diagnosis, treatment, and effectiveness of care. Furthermore, the mere caring effort in the relationship with the patient, aside from drugs or other treatments, can help patients get well. This sort of care requires attentiveness and alertness to what kind of a person the patient is; sympathy for the patient's total situation; friendliness that elicits trust; and a consideration expressed in "little incidental" actions that assure the patient's comfort—which may require that the physician learn much from the nurse regarding practical care and comfort of the patient (Peabody, 1987).

Following Peabody's clarion call for care in 1927, several physicians, writing in the 1960s and 1970s, advocated a caring perspective in professional attitudes, practices, and moral analysis in medicine. The starting point that convinced these writers of the need for "caring for" was the depersonalization of medical care in hospitals. Clinical care oriented to the disease in the body leads caretakers to allow technical considerations to dominate, avoid death at any cost, and ignore patients' preferences; this produces indignities for patients and suffering for caregivers (Benfield, 1979).

The concept of caring is defined in the literature of the 1960s and 1970s as implying a broader concern for the whole patient, or for the quality of the patient's life, rather than just for the patient's disease (Menninger, 1975; Benfield, 1979). Caring involves sympathy with the patient, which entails entering into or sharing the feelings of the patient. To prevent loss of objectivity and perspective, "compassionate detachment" (Blumgart, 1964, p. 451) is recommended, which is "to sense the patient's experience empathically without becoming so involved sympathetically that the physician's rational and effective clinical judgment is impaired by emotional involvement" (Menninger, 1975, p. 837).

Caring for the patient embraces both the science and art of medicine; both are oriented to the patient, and both should meet in the individual physician (Blumgart, 1964). A caring solicitude for the individual patient is integral and essential in the practice of clinical medicine (Tisdale, 1979); failure to practice caring medicine leads to incomplete or inaccurate diagnosis and ineffective treatment (Blumgart, 1964). On the other hand, patients manifest care-seeking behavior (Tisdale, 1979). Receiving the sought-for care can be crucial for the patient's "adaptation to various maladjustments, including illness" (Menninger, 1975, p. 836). The role of the physician and other health-care providers in our society is one of a surrogate caregiver, who has the power to give attention to the ill and excuse them from the performance of everyday duties (Menninger, 1975).

There are several obstacles to caring in medicine. The demands of the scientific and technological aspects of medicine, combined with physicians' fascination with disease, achieve great progress for humankind but tend to block out compassionate attention to suffering and the particular needs of the ill individual who has the disease. In addition, patients and families are reluctant to communicate their feelings with health professionals, who are too busy monitoring the patient's physical condition to listen. Other factors that obstruct person-oriented caring are (1) lack of teamwork among health-care providers, coupled with overemphasis on the physician's hierarchical authority; (2) caregivers' feelings of inadequacy due to lack of training in caring for critically ill or dying patients and their families; and (3) time pressures on health professionals (Blumgart, 1964; Benfield, 1979).

Acts of caring, some of which counteract the obstacles to caring, include: listening to patients with personal attentiveness, particularly as a history-taking technique that enables patients to relate their experiences in terms of their own values and concerns (Tisdale, 1979; Blumgart, 1964); being attentive to both the physical and the emotional components of illness (even though medical education and practice tend to focus on the physical—in fact, all medicine is psychosomatic, since the emotional and bodily factors always interact in every disease) (Blumgart, 1964; Menninger, 1975); and offering maximum understanding, freedom, and support to the individual patient (Tisdale, 1979).

Caring is also expressed through acting as companion to a bereaved family; solicitous communication regarding the nature of the illness and its expected course; sharing the patient's and family's responsibility and agony of deciding whether to continue care; relieving the patient of suffering from pointless dehumanizing treatment, and caring for caretakers who suffer the stress of the combined roles of technical caregiver and concerned caregiver (Benfield, 1979).

William Tisdale, writing in 1979, contended that modern medical ethics, with its concern for "the neon problems" of high controversy, is ill-adapted to account for an ethic of care. Because clinical caring pertains to the usual and the commonplace in medicine, it is more difficult to isolate and analyze. William Tisdale appealed for an inquiry into the unresolved and even the unrecognized problems inherent in basic clinical care and the problems inherent in care that are more demanding from an ethical perspective than the usual moral quandaries in medicine. In formal ethical terms, Tisdale saw clinical caring as characterized by the ideals of love and charity that also being a form of duty beneficence, a duty to benefit others apart from special relationships and responsibilities (Tisdale, 1979). Making certain that expected benefits of a particular procedure outweigh the definite risks is a characteristic of caring for one's patients.

In the highly influential book published in 1970, *Patient as Person*, Paul Ramsey linked care with "covenant fidelity," which he saw as the appropriate norm for the relationship between physician and patient. Covenant fidelity always requires care, which is directed to the person of the patient. But at the end of life, when attempts to cure are no longer appropriate, one must always care even if one only cares—through keeping company and offering comfort—while permissibly withdrawing medical care (Ramsey, 1970).

Caring for the sick, the wounded, and the troubled has been characterized through the centuries by altruistic motives and virtues. By the 1920s an interest had arisen in the virtue of care as the basic moral orientation to health care, based in feelings for the other. Practitioners felt that care could provide the grounding for the moral practice of health care and for mitigating some of the excesses of medical technique. Still, very little by way of a formal ethic had arisen.

Caring in nursing theory, philosophy, and ethics

It required the intellectual and moral energy of feminist perspectives on care in the 1980s to establish a noteworthy movement promoting an ethic of care that reached deep into the field of bioethics.

Nursing theorists, educators, and philosophers explored and applied a more extensive theory and ethic of care prior to 1982 than any other single group had. Their contributions differed considerably from those of physician-writers: The nursing theorists paid much more attention to the meaning and theories of nursing, examined the structures and functions of care, turned occasionally to philosophers who had explained the meaning of care (such as Martin Heidegger and Milton Mayeroff), developed the implications of care for nursing practices and skills, considered the status of caregivers, showed an interest in the historical links between nursing and maternal care, and proposed educational improvements to foster professional care.

The strongest impetus for an examination of the role of caring in nursing came from Madeleine Leininger, who has organized national conferences on caring and published on the topic (Leininger, 1981). Leininger was one of the pioneers who fostered the idea that caring is the essence of nursing and the unique focus of the profession. Leah Curtin went a step further when she claimed that the distinctiveness of nursing cannot be located in functions, but in "the moral art of nursing," in its primary moral conviction, by virtue of which nurses "are committed to care for, as well as to the care of, other human beings" (Curtin, 1979, p. 26).

Nursing theorists offer a variety of definitions of care: for example, the explanation that caring in nursing is a process in which one shows "compassionate concern for the individual" (Gaut, in Leininger, 1981, p. 18). Leininger suggests this definition of professional nursing care: "those cognitively learned humanistic and scientific modes of helping or enabling an individual, family, or community to receive personalized services through specific culturally defined or ascribed modes of caring processes, techniques, and patterns to improve or maintain a favorably healthy condition for life or death" (Leininger, 1981, p. 9). This definition includes concepts of compassion, concern, nurturance, stress alleviation, comfort, and protection.

The precise historical origins of a concern for caring in nursing are unclear, but a number of authors trace them to the writings of Florence Nightingale. However, nurse theorists have relied not so much on a history of care in nursing as on the writings of social scientists and existentialists such as Buber, Erikson, and Rogers (Gaut, in Leininger, 1981).

Why did nursing theorists turn so strongly to the idea of care in the 1970s? Marilyn Ray explains that as nursing became increasingly technological, bureaucratic, managerial, and supervisory, nurses began experiencing a struggle relative to their central focus as a "direct caring profession" (Ray, in Leininger, 1981, p. 28). Barbara Carper (1979) answers the question by mentioning two factors that have had the effect of eroding care in health generally, not just in the experience of nurses: depersonalization of health care due to the fragmentation of specialized treatment, the subdivision of tasks, and highly institutionalized bureaucracy; and technological progress and technical expertise, which she saw as having the potential of overshadowing individuals, "reducing them to objects or abstractions" (p. 13). Within such a system, even when competent, scientifically based care is delivered, it "is often perceived by the client as lacking the 'personally experienced feeling of being cared for'" (p. 13, quoting Menninger, 1975, p. 837). This depersonalization of the individual entails the devaluing and loss of identity of the individual. She sees a compelling metaphor for the relationship of technology to care in the novel in which Dr. Frankenstein created a monster. Frankenstein's tragedy was not due to his scientific triumph over nature, but "his *failure to care* for what he had created. He was unable to recognize or experience the humanness of another's self" (Carper, 1979, p. 13).

Finally, even prior to the emergence of an ethic of care in other disciplines, nurses were already applying the idea of care both to nursing practice and to nursing ethics. For example, Carper argued that caring is the most essential ingredient in the curative process, because caring acts and decisions "make the crucial difference in effective curing consequences" (Carper, 1979, p. 14, quoting Leininger, 1977, p. 2). Anne J. Davis stimulated reflection on the relationship between caring and ethical principles in the context of taking care of the dying. She contrasted the compassionate meaning of care (to undergo with, to share solidarity with) with the technical terms "nursing care" or "medical care." She argued that situations of serious illness and dying call for putting aside the instrumental meaning of caring and instead manifesting "the most demanding and deeply human aspect of caring: the expressive art of being fully present to another person" (Davis, 1981, p. 1). A caring attitude would incline the nurse not to turn away from the stranger's world of suffering, but to appreciate the other person's independent existence and enter into and share his or her pain as much as possible. Caring for the sufferer is an ethical obligation inherent in the health professional's role. But caring transcends role obligations: It acknowledges the vulnerable humanness of the other and reinforces the caring of the one who cares. Ethical principles are not at variance with care: They provide specific judgments in the context of caring for another person. A caring disposition inclines caregivers to respect the patient as an autonomous agent and to recognize the patient's considered value judgments, even if they go contrary to what the clinician expects.

The foregoing presents a few indications of the pioneering work in nursing care theory and ethics in the 1970s. As the following article indicates, the ethics of nursing care expanded considerably after the notion of care came to be more widely acknowledged through the writings of women social scientists.

WARREN THOMAS REICH

Directly related to this article are the companion articles in this entry: HISTORY OF THE NOTION OF CARE, *and* CONTEMPORARY ETHICS OF CARE. *Also directly related are the entries* COMPASSION; EMOTIONS; HEALING; MEDICINE, ART OF; NARRATIVE; NURSING ETHICS; TRUST; *and* VIRTUE AND CHARACTER. *For a further discussion of topics mentioned in this article, see the entries* BENEFICENCE; BIOETHICS; CASUISTRY; COMPETENCE; FEMINISM; FIDELITY AND LOYALTY; HARM; PAIN AND SUFFERING; VALUE AND VALUATION; *and* WOMEN, *section on* WOMEN AS HEALTH PROFESSIONALS. *Other relevant material may be found under the entries* CLINICAL ETHICS, *article on* ELEMENTS AND METHODOLOGIES; CONSCIENCE; ETHICS, *article on* NORMATIVE ETHICAL THEORIES; INTERPRETATION; MEDICAL CODES AND OATHS; MEDICAL ETHICS, HISTORY OF, *section on* THE AMERICAS, *article on* UNITED STATES IN THE TWENTIETH CENTURY; METAPHOR AND ANALOGY; *and* NURSING, THEORIES AND PHILOSOPHY OF.

Bibliography

ANNAS, GEORGE J. 1990. *American Health Law.* Boston: Little, Brown.

BENFIELD, D. GARY. 1979. "Two Philosophies of Caring." *Ohio State Medical Journal* 75, no. 8:508–511.

BLUMGART, HERMANN L. 1964. "Caring for the Patient." *New England Journal of Medicine* 270, no. 9:449–456.

BONET-MAURY, G. n.d. "Hospitality (Christian)." In vol. 6 of *Encyclopaedia of Religion and Ethics,* pp. 804–808. Edited by James Hastings. New York: Charles Scribner's Sons.

CABOT, RICHARD C. 1926. *Adventures on the Borderlands of Ethics.* New York: Harper & Brothers.

CARPER, BARBARA A. 1979. "The Ethics of Caring." *Advances in Nursing Science* 1, no. 3:11–19.

CURTIN, LEAH. 1980. "Ethical Issues in Nursing Practice and Education." In *Ethical Issues in Nursing and Nursing Education,* pp. 25–26. New York: National League for Nursing.

DAVIS, ANNE J. 1981. "Compassion, Suffering, Morality: Ethical Dilemmas in Caring," *Nursing Law & Ethics* 2, no. 5:1–2,6,8.

GRUBB, EDWARD. n.d. "Philanthropy." In vol. 9 of *Encyclopaedia of Religion and Ethics,* pp. 837–840. Edited by James Hastings. New York: Charles Scribner's Sons.

JONSEN, ALBERT R. 1990. *The New Medicine and the Old Ethics.* Cambridge, Mass.: Harvard University Press.

LAÍN ENTRALGO, PEDRO. 1969. *Doctor and Patient.* Translated by Frances Partridge. New York: McGraw-Hill.

LEININGER, MADELEINE. 1977. "Caring: The Essence and Central Focus of Nursing." In *The Phenomenon of Caring: Part V.* Washington, D.C.: American Nurses Foundation, Nursing Research Report 12, no. 1:2–14.

———. 1981. *Caring: An Essential Human Need: Proceedings of Three National Caring Conferences.* Thorofare, N.J.: Charles B. Slack.

LOCKE, JOHN. 1993. [1690]. *An Essay Concerning Human Understanding.* Edited by John W. Yolton. 3d ed., rev. London: Dent.

MAY, WILLIAM F. 1983. *The Physician's Covenant: Images of the Healer in Medical Ethics.* Philadelphia: Westminster Press.

———. 1986. "Philanthropy." In *The Westminster Dictionary of Christian Ethics,* pp. 474–475. Edited by James F. Childress and John Macquarrie. Philadelphia: Westminster Press.

MENNINGER, W. WALTER. 1975. "'Caring' as Part of Health Care Quality." *Journal of the American Medical Association* 234, no. 8:836–837.

MILLER, TIMOTHY S. 1985. *The Birth of the Hospital in the Byzantine Empire.* Baltimore: Johns Hopkins University Press.

NUMBERS, RONALD L., and AMUNDSEN, DARREL W. 1986. *Caring and Curing: Health and Medicine in the Western Religious Traditions.* New York: Macmillan.

PEABODY, FRANCIS W. 1987. [1927]. "The Care of the Patient." In *Encounters Between Patients and Doctors: An Anthology,* pp. 387–401. Edited by John Stoeckle. Cambridge, Mass.: MIT Press.

RAMSEY, PAUL. 1970. *The Patient as Person: Explorations in Medical Ethics.* New Haven, Conn.: Yale University Press.

SIGERIST, HENRY ERNEST. 1943. *Civilization and Disease.* Ithaca, N.Y.: Cornell University Press.

TISDALE, WILLIAM A. 1979. "On Clinical Caring." *Pharos* 42, no. 4:23–26.

III. CONTEMPORARY ETHICS OF CARE

A major contemporary impetus to scholarly discussions of caring occurred with the 1982 publication of Carol Gilligan's *In a Different Voice: Psychological Theory and Women's Development* (Gilligan, 1982). Nursing theorists—and, to a lesser extent, physicians—were exploring moral dimensions of caring prior to the publication of Gilligan's work; but her book led, for the first time in the history of the idea of care, to widespread efforts to develop a systematic philosophical ethic of care beyond the world of health-care practitioners.

Contemporary elements of an ethic of care

In a Different Voice begins by contrasting the primary moral orientation of boys and men with the primary orientation of girls and women. Gilligan proposes that females and males tend to employ different reasoning strategies and apply different moral themes and concepts when formulating and resolving moral problems. According to Gilligan's analysis, females are more likely than males to perceive moral dilemmas primarily in terms of personal attachment versus detachment. From this perspective, which she dubs the "care" perspective, central concerns are to avoid deserting, hurting, alienating, isolating, or abandoning persons and to act in a manner that strengthens and protects attachments between persons. In this analysis, the moral universe of girls and women tends to be primarily "a world of relationships and psychological truths where an awareness of the connection between people gives rise to a recognition of responsibility for one another, a perception of the need for response" (Gilligan, 1982, p. 30). For example, Amy, an eleven-year-old girl whom Gilligan interviews in her book, describes herself in terms of her connection with other people: "I think that the world has a lot of problems, and I think that everybody should try to help somebody else in some way . . ." (Gilligan, 1982, p. 34).

By contrast, Gilligan argues that the primary moral orientation of men and boys tends to focus on moral concerns related to inequality versus equality of individuals. Rather than emphasizing the importance of sustaining personal relationships, this approach emphasizes abstract ideals of fairness and rights, and requires abiding by impartial principles of justice, autonomy, reciprocity, and respect for persons. Viewed from this perspective, which Gilligan refers to as the "justice" perspective, moral dilemmas are defined by hierarchical values and impersonal conflicts of claims. The moral agent, like the judge, is called upon to "abstract the moral debate from the interpersonal situation, finding in the logic of fairness an objective way to decide who will win the dispute" (Gilligan, 1982, p. 32). To illustrate justice reasoning, Gilligan describes the moral reasoning of Jake, an eleven-year-old boy interviewed for her book. Asked how he would resolve a conflict between responsibility to himself and other people Jake answers, "You go about one-fourth to the others and three-fourths to yourself," and adds that "the most important thing in your decision should be yourself, don't let yourself be guided totally by other people . . ." (Gilligan, 1982, pp. 35–36). Gilligan concludes that Jake understands this moral dilemma as an abstract mathematical equation and perceives his responsibility for others as potentially interfering with his personal autonomy.

Gilligan refers to the moral orientation that she finds most prevalent among girls and women as an ethic of "care," and she calls the moral orientation that is most common among boys and men an ethic of "justice." Gilligan, a developmental psychologist, argues that an ethic of care has been generally ignored in the past because girls and women have been excluded as subjects in the study of moral development. For example, accounts of moral maturation described by Lawrence Kohlberg (1981, 1984) and Jean Piaget (1965) were based entirely on studies and observations of boys and men. These male-based theories of moral psychology, when applied to girls and women, were interpreted as showing girls and women to be deficient in moral development. Gilligan identifies an ethic of care as a distinctive form of moral reasoning.

Implications for ethics of health care

The implications of Gilligan's analysis for contemporary bioethics are the subject of ongoing discussion. First, an ethic of care may lead to positive changes in bioethical education, including placing greater emphasis on health-care providers' communication skills and emotional sensitivity, and on the effects that ethical issues have on relationships (Carse, 1991). To the extent that bioethicists with formal training in ethics are inclined to emphasize justice over care, it may be desirable to broaden their training to include an ethic of care (Self et al., 1993a).

In addition to producing changes in ethics education, a care orientation within bioethics arguably requires placing greater emphasis on beneficence as the health-care provider's primary responsibility to the patient (Sharpe, 1992). Finally, an ethics emphasizing caring for others may produce substantive changes in the way we resolve moral problems. It may encourage resolutions of moral problems that give greater authority to family members in health-care decision making (Hardwig, 1990, 1991; Jecker, 1990), or it may lead to paying greater attention to how various relationships are affected by moral decisions (Jecker, 1991).

One area within bioethics where an ethic of care has been studied in some detail is abortion. Gilligan found that women who face abortion decisions tend to frame moral issues in terms of a responsibility to care for and avoid hurting others (Gilligan, 1982). These women often base decisions about having an abortion on "a growing comprehension of the dynamics of social interaction . . . and a central insight, that self and others are interdependent" (Gilligan, 1982, p. 74). In other words, rather than conceptualizing abortion in terms of abstract values, such as "life," or in terms of competing claims or rights, these women tend to see abortion as a problem of how best to care for and avoid harming the particular people and relationships affected by their choices. Considered in this light, the resolution of abortion requires taking stock of how any decision might affect not only the pregnant woman and fetus, but also the relationship between the pregnant woman and biological father, and relationships and persons within the wider family circle (Jecker, 1993b). Arguably, an ethic of care illuminates the moral issues abortion raises better than an ethic of justice, because only an ethic of care portrays individuals as uniquely constituted by their connections to others (Gatens-Robinson, 1992).

In addition to these proposed changes, introducing a care orientation within bioethics may shed a negative light on more traditional forms of bioethical analysis (Walker, 1989). For example, Virginia Sharpe claims that a justice orientation has dominated bioethics in the past, and this has encouraged ethicists to treat provider–patient relationships as free exchanges between equals (Sharpe, 1992). She argues that this picture of the provider–patient relationship is seriously distorted. Rather than being equals in relationships with health-care providers, patients typically experience diminished power and authority as a result of being physically and emotionally vulnerable and in need of the provider's help (Sharpe, 1992). Others charge that a justice orientation has traditionally prevailed within bioethics, resulting in too much focus on competition for power, status, and authority and too little focus on the human relationships at stake (Warren, 1989, pp. 73–87). For example, the autonomy–paternalism debate within bioethics concentrates on who has the authority to make treatment decisions. Similarly, when bioethicists emphasize impersonal ethical principles, such as autonomy, nonmaleficence, beneficence, and justice, this can have the effect of making the particular persons and relationships involved in ethical dilemmas incidental, rather than essential, to the crafting of moral responses.

Feminist versus feminine ethics

Gilligan's ongoing effort (Gilligan et al., 1988; Gilligan et al., 1989; Brown and Gilligan, 1992) to characterize girls' and women's moral reasoning in terms of care has occurred in tandem with important developments in feminist ethics. It is useful, however, to distinguish between the care ethic that Gilligan describes, which has been called a "feminine ethic," and the development of "feminist ethics." According to Susan Sherwin (1992), the primary concern of feminine ethics is to describe the moral experiences and intuitions of women, pointing out how traditional approaches have neglected to include women's perspectives.

In addition to Carol Gilligan, both Nel Noddings (1984) and Sara Ruddick (1989) have made important contributions to feminine ethics. Whereas Gilligan emphasizes the unique form of moral reasoning that caring engenders, Noddings focuses on caring as a practical activity, stressing the interaction that occurs between persons giving and receiving care. From this perspective, she identifies two distinctive features of caring: engrossment and motivational shift. "Engrossment" refers to a receptive state in which the person caring is "receiving what is there as nearly as possible without assessment or evaluation"; "motivational shift" occurs when "my motive energy flows towards the other and perhaps . . . towards his ends" (Noddings, 1984, pp. 33, 34). Critics of Noddings's approach raise the concern that her interpretation of caring may lead to exploitation (Houston, 1990) or complicity in the pursuit of evil ends (Card, 1990).

Unlike Gilligan and Noddings, Ruddick emphasizes "maternal thinking," which she says develops out of the activity of assuming regular and substantial responsibility for small children. Although Ruddick acknowledges that the work of mothering falls under the more general category of "caring labor," she argues that it cannot simply be combined with other forms of caring because each form of caring involves distinctive kinds of thinking arising from different activities (Ruddick, 1989). Ruddick delineates maternal thinking as a response to the small child's demands for preservation, growth, and acceptability. These demands elicit in the mothering person the responses of "preservative love," "fostering growth," "conscientiousness," and "educative control," which Ruddick identifies as the hallmarks of maternal thinking.

In contrast to feminine ethics, the primary concern of feminist ethics is to reject and end oppression against women. Susan Sherwin defines "feminist ethics" as "the name given to the various theories that help reveal the multiple, gender-specific patterns of harm that constitute women's oppression," together with the "diverse political movement to eliminate all such forms of oppression" (Sherwin, 1992, p. 13). By "oppression," Sherwin means "a pattern of hardship that is based on dominance of one group by members of another. The dominance involved . . . is rooted in features that distinguish one group from another" and requires "exaggerating these features to ensure the dominant group's supremacy" (Sherwin, 1992, p. 24). Feminism aims, in this interpretation, to show that the suffering of individual women is related because it springs from common sources of injustice. According to Rosemarie Tong, feminist ethics is typically far more concerned than feminine ethics with making political changes and eliminating oppressive imbalances of power (Tong, 1993).

In many respects, however, feminine and feminist ethics are interrelated. The careful study of women's lives and moral reasoning that feminine ethics undertakes can contribute substantially to dismantling habits of thought and practice that enable women's oppression to continue. Both feminine and feminist ethics share the goal of adding women's voices and perspectives to various fields of scholarly inquiry. Finally, as Ruddick notes, feminist ethics can lend important support to the ideals that feminine ethics upholds. For example, feminist ethics can help to ensure "women's economic and psychological ability to engage in mothering without undue sacrifice of physical health and nonmaternal projects" (Ruddick, 1989, p. 236).

Objections to an ethic of care

Since the publication of *In a Different Voice,* the proposal to develop a feminine ethic of care has met with a variety of concerns and objections. One set of concerns is that a feminine ethic of care may unwittingly undermine feminism. These concerns stem, in part, from a belief that the qualities in girls and women that feminine ethics esteems have developed within the context of a sexist culture. Thus, some suspect that women's competency at caring for and serving others is an outgrowth of their subordinate status within modern societies (Sherwin, 1992; Moody-Adams, 1991), and worry that emphasizing caring as a virtuous feminine quality may simply serve to keep women on the down side of power relationships (Holmes, 1989). Others urge women to aspire to assertiveness, rather than caring, in order to challenge conventional images of women as concerned with serving and pleasing others (Card, 1991). Feminist critics also warn that caring cannot function as an ethic that is complete unto itself. Observing that caring can "be exploited in the service of immoral ends," Card insists on the need to balance caring with justice and other values (Card, 1990, p. 106). Exclusive attention to caring can also lead to overlooking "the lack of care of women for women" and may preclude "the possibility of our looking at anything but love and friendship in women's emotional responses to one another" (Spellman, 1991, p. 216).

A second family of concerns about a feminine ethic of care relates to the belief that caring for others can lead to neglect of self. The phenomenon of "burnout," for example, refers to the situation of parents, nurses, family caregivers, or other individuals who become utterly exhausted by the physical and emotional demands associated with giving care. Especially when care is conceived to be an ethic that is sufficient unto itself, the tendency may be to continue caring at any cost. Attention to other values, such as the rights and dignity of the one caring, may be necessary in order to place reasonable limits on caring. Arguing along these lines, Judith Jarvis Thomson criticizes those who suppose it possible to exclude the language of rights from morality, replacing this language with moral prescriptions to care for others (Thomson, 1990). She cautions that "what has oppressed women in the past is precisely the socially engendered expectation that they will melt into their

personal relationships; the women's movement succeeded in bringing home to many that women, like men, have inherently individual interests . . ." (Thomson, 1990, p. 288). Others suggest that in order to care for others—which is an inherently limited ability—one must first be cared for by other individuals, by communities, and by oneself (Reich, 1991).

A third group of objections to developing a feminine ethic of care holds that the concept of care is not helpful at the social and institutional level. This group of objections may acknowledge that an ethic of care serves well within the limited sphere of personal ethics, but finds care unhelpful outside of this sphere. One form this objection takes is to argue that an ethic of care cannot be formulated in terms of the general rights and principles that are necessary for designing public policies. Proponents of a care ethic sometimes acknowledge this limitation. Thus, Noddings states, "to care is to act not by fixed rule but by affection and regard" (Noddings, 1984, p. 24). Similarly, Patricia Benner and Judith Wrubel maintain that caring is always specific and relational; hence, there exist no "context-free lists of advice" on how to care (Benner and Wrubel, 1989, p. 3). They reject the idea of formulating ethical theories or rules about caring on the grounds that general guides cannot "capture the embodied, relational, configurational, skillful, meaningful, and contextual human issues" that are central to an ethic of care (Benner and Wrubel, 1989, p. 6). Despite this view, there exist historically important examples of using the vocabulary of general rights and principles to formulate an ethic of care. For example, the *Universal Declaration of Human Rights* identifies "motherhood and childhood" as "entitled to special care and assistance," and the *Declaration of the Rights of the Child* asserts general principles of caring for children, noting that children need "special safeguards and care" on the basis of their "physical and mental immaturity" (U.N. General Assembly, 1948, 1960).

Another reason why care may be assumed unworkable at a social or institutional level is that historically, public and private spheres have been distinguished as separate moral domains (Elshtain, 1981). During the nineteenth century, for example, the doctrine of separate spheres held that the family constituted a private sphere in which a morality of love and self-sacrifice prevailed; this private domain was distinguished from the public life associated with business and politics, where impersonal norms and self-interested relationships reigned (Nicholson, 1986). To the extent that these historical attitudes continue to shape present thinking, they may lead to the mutual exclusivity of care-oriented and justice-oriented approaches. In response to this structural objection, some ethicists have argued that justice and care are compatible forms of moral reasoning (Jecker, 1993a).

A final set of objections to a feminine ethic of care does not deny the importance of care, but rather argues that care is properly interpreted as a broad human ethic, rather than an ethic that expresses an exclusively feminine form of moral reasoning. Defenders of feminine ethics often meet this objection by claiming that their approach has been misunderstood. Thus advocates of feminine ethics may deny that care is an ethic that only women articulate, or an ethic that is valid only within the moral experience of women. According to Noddings, caring is an important ingredient within all human morality, and moral education should teach all people how and why to care. She concludes that "an ethical orientation that arises in female experience need not be confined to women"; to the contrary, "if only women adopt an ethic of caring the present conditions of women's oppression are indeed likely to be maintained" (Noddings, 1990, p. 171). Gilligan and Jane Attanucci also reject the idea that an ethic of care correlates strictly with gender, and instead report that most men and women can reason in accordance with both care and justice (Gilligan and Attanucci, 1988). Gilligan's research supports the more modest claim that care is gender-related. That is, although women and men can reason in terms of both care and justice, women are generally more likely to emphasize care while men generally emphasize justice. Thus she states that the so-called different voice she identifies is characterized "not by gender, but by theme," and cautions that its association with gender "is not absolute" and is not a generalization about either sex (Gilligan, 1982, p. 2).

Caring and contemporary nursing

Within health care, attention to caring is perhaps most evident within nursing. Emphasizing caring as a central value within nursing often provides a basis for arguing that nursing requires its own description, possesses its own phenomena, and retains its own method for clarification of its own concepts and their meanings, relationships, and context (Jameton, 1984; Fry, 1989a, 1989b; Watson, 1988; Gadow, 1987; Swanson, 1990; Reverby, 1987a, 1987b). For example, Jean Watson holds that nurses should reject the impersonal, objective models that she says currently dominate ethics and choose instead an ethic that emphasizes caring.

Those who invoke caring in developing a theory of nursing ethics often assign caring a privileged or foundational role. For example, Sarah Fry posits caring as "a foundational, rather than a derivative, value among persons" (Fry, 1989b, pp. 20–21). She argues that other ethical values, such as personhood and human dignity, are an outgrowth of nurses' caring activity. Similarly, Benner and Wrubel argue for the primacy of caring on the grounds that skillful technique and scientific knowledge do not suffice to establish ethical nursing in the absence of a basic level of caring and attachment (Benner and Wrubel, 1989).

Like Fry, Kristen Swanson regards caring as central to nursing ethics. According to her analysis, caring requires acting in a way that preserves human dignity, restores humanity, and avoids reducing persons to the moral status of objects. Specifically, caring requires

(1) knowing, or striving to understand an event as it has meaning in the life of the other; (2) being with, which means being emotionally present to the other; (3) doing for, defined as doing for the other as he or she would do for himself or herself if that were possible; (4) enabling, or facilitating the other's passage through life transitions and unfamiliar events; and (5) maintaining belief, which refers to sustaining faith in the other's capacity to get through an event or transition and to face a future of fulfillment. (Swanson, 1990)

Susan Reverby finds caring to be a central ethic throughout nursing's history. Tracing the history of nursing to its domestic roots during the colonial era, when nursing took place within the family, Reverby argues that caring for the sick was originally a duty rather than a freely chosen vocation for women. Reverby suggests that nurses today possess "some deep understandings of the limited promise of equality and autonomy in a health care system. In an often implicit way, such nurses recognize that those who claim the autonomy of rights often run the risk of rejecting altruism and caring itself" (Reverby, 1987a).

Some have challenged the proposal to consider care as a concept unique to nursing ethics (Veatch, 1981). Others identify nursing with maternal practice, a specific kind of caring activity (Newton, 1990; O'Brien, 1987). For example, Patricia O'Brien defends the importance of nursing's maternal function by noting that historically the source of nurses' prestige has been the manner in which nurses blend home and hospital. That is, nursing's strength has come from nurses' skill at the traditionally female tasks of feeding, bathing, cleaning, coaching, and cajoling those in one's care. Just as mothers make a home, it is female nurses who have been able to make a home of the hospital, to personalize an increasingly impersonal environment.

Critics of the maternal paradigm for nursing fault this approach as casting women in traditional and stifling roles. Historically, for example, nurses were socialized into the health-care field to know their place and were relegated to the bottom of the pyramid and taught not to ask questions (Murphy, 1984). Casting nursing practice in terms of mothering potentially reverses progress made in the late 1970s when nurses began to see themselves as shared-decision makers rather than handmaidens to physicians (Stein et al., 1990).

A further objection to identifying ethical ideals of nursing with ethical ideals of mothering holds that nurses' proper function is to serve as patients' advocates, rather than as patients' parents. Sally Gadow and Gerald Winslow, for example, argue that advocacy of patients' autonomy, rather than paternalistic promotion of patient benefit, should guide nursing ethics (Gadow, 1980a, 1980b; Winslow, 1984).

Caring and contemporary medicine

Whereas nursing is often associated with a caring function, doctoring has traditionally been associated with a curing function. However, the tendency to associate caring exclusively with nursing is misleading for a variety of reasons (Jecker and Self, 1991). First, both doctors and nurses are engaged in caring for patients. In addition, assigning caring activities to nurses and curing activities to doctors is misleading because certain meanings of "curing" are actually derived from "caring." Thus, the Latin definition of "cure" comes from the word "curare," meaning "care, heed, concern; to do one's busy care, to give one's care or attention to some piece of work; or to apply one's self diligently."

Although there has been less explicit attention to an ethic of care in medicine than in nursing, caring for patients represents a central component of ethics in medicine. Caring is inextricably linked to the physician's obligation to relieve suffering, a goal that stretches back to antiquity (Cassell, 1982)

There are several more specific ways in which an ethic of care becomes manifest in the practice of medicine. First, caring is manifest in the activity of healing the patient. Whereas curing disease typically requires the physician to understand and deal with a physical disease process, healing requires that the physician also respond to the patient's subjective experience of illness (Cassell, 1989). For example, healing a patient who is suffering from a serious infection requires not only administering antibiotics to kill bacteria but also addressing the patient's feelings, questions, and concerns about his or her medical situation. In cases of serious illness where cure is not possible, caring for the patient may become the primary part of healing. For example, when patients are terminally ill and imminently dying, physicians' primary duty may become providing palliative and comfort care. Under these circumstances, healing emphasizes touch and communication, psychological and emotional support, and responding to the patient's specific feelings and concerns, which may include fear, loss of control, dependency, and acceptance or denial of death and final separation from loved ones.

Caring is also evident in what Albert Jonsen calls the "'Samaritan principle': the duty to care for the needy sick, whether friend or enemy, even at cost to oneself"

(Jonsen, 1990, p. 39). The tradition of Samaritanism dates to the early Christian era and the parable of the Good Samaritan described in the Gospel according to Luke; it persists during the modern, secular era as a central ethic for medicine. Jonsen argues that although the original Christian parable of the Samaritan refers to giving aid to a particular individual, the ethical tradition of Samaritanism within medicine bears relevance to entire groups of patients. So understood, Samaritanism underlies the physician's broader social duty to care for indigent persons. In contrast to the past, when physicians provided charity care for indigent persons without financial remuneration, today universal health insurance is the norm in most developed countries. Therefore, in contemporary times physicians are generally compensated for their services through a private or government health insurance mechanism. In the United States, however, large numbers of patients continue to lack health insurance. A principle of Samaritanism continues to be evident in the legal and ethical requirement that U.S. physicians provide emergency treatment to any patient regardless of the patient's ability to pay for care. A stronger Samaritan ethic, mandating access to all forms of basic health care, would require, in the United States, successful implementation of health-care reform.

A third way in which caring is manifest in the ethics of medicine is through the healing relationship of doctor and patient. Edmund Pellegrino and David Thomasma regard this relationship as one of inherent inequality because the patient is vulnerable, ill, and in need of the physician's skill (Pellegrino and Thomasma, 1988). In light of the patient's diminished power, Pellegrino and Thomasma argue that the physician incurs a duty of beneficence, a duty requiring the physician to respond to the patient's needs and promote the patient's good. Other ethical values in medicine can presumably be derived from the physician's primary duty of beneficence. For example, according to Pellegrino and Thomasma, a duty to enhance patients' autonomy is based on the duty to benefit patients.

Some (Sharpe, 1992) have sought to identify the principle of beneficence that Pellegrino and Thomasma delineate with an ethic of care. However, beneficence and care differ in crucial respects. Whereas a principle of beneficence identifies promoting the patient's good as a requirement for right action, an ethic of care is a type of virtue ethic that is basically concerned about the affective orientation and moral commitment—that is, the concern—of the one who cares. For example, a physician may perform actions that promote a patient's good, and thus meet the requirement of beneficence, without caring about or feeling any commitment toward the patient. If this analysis is correct, then actions that fulfill the principle of beneficence do not necessarily fulfill standards associated with an ethic of care. An ethic of care suggests both a feeling response directed to the object of care and a commitment to ensuring that things go well for that person.

Despite the integral role that an ethic of caring plays in medicine, contemporary physicians sometimes neglect to offer adequate palliative and comfort measures to patients (Angell, 1982). This may stem from a failure to teach and nurture empathy in medical education (Spiro et al., 1993), and from financial incentives that discourage spending time at patients' bedsides and getting to know patients as persons. In addition, physicians may overlook caring for patients when conflicts exist about the use of futile treatments (Schneiderman et al., 1994). For example, members of the health-care team may become distracted debating the appropriateness of high-technology interventions and neglect to care for patients' spiritual and emotional needs.

Ethics of care in environmental ethics

Attempts have been made to rethink environmental issues in bioethics—those affecting the health, for example, of nonhuman animals and plant life—on the basis of an ethic of care. Contemporary critics of a rights-based approach to environmental bioethics often criticize it as inadequate to express insights into why we value nonhuman animals and the environment. In an effort to attribute rights to nature, rights-based theorists seek to establish parallels between nature and humans—such as their equality—on the basis of which rights can be granted. But, critics object, it seems that our moral interests may rest on the differences between humans, nonhuman animals, and the environment rather than on their similarities; it seems too that these interests may be better expressed in an ethic of care.

This approach entails reconceiving the grounds on which we understand our relationship to "the world of nature," including a reconsideration of the domination of nonhuman animals according to a patriarchal mindset that has also accounted for the domination of women (Curtin, 1991, p. 60). In addition, the care approach involves a shift from an ethic of rights, rules, and principles to an ethic that "makes a central place for values of care, love, friendship, trust and appropriate reciprocity—values that presuppose that our relationships to others are central to our understanding of who we are" (Curtin, 1991, p. 65). Whether or not animals have rights, we certainly can and do care for them (Curtin, 1991). While a rights-based ethic tries to prevent infringements on individual rights, an ethic of care tries to prevent people from neglecting other people and things. It stresses the importance of recognizing our interconnected web of relationships with elements of the environment, dialoguing with them, and strengthening those bonds. Claims that we ought to protect and respect the environment are made on the grounds that we are in a relationship of interdependence with the environment, a relationship expressed through care. Finally, while animal rights have been argued for on the basis of such criteria as animal sentience, it may be more coherent to argue for the respect and protection of animals on the basis of our caring relationship with them and the responsibilities incurred by that relationship.

Conclusion

Although the development of theories of an ethic of care for health care is new, the idea of care has long presented a moral standard or ideal for health care. Although caring has been an abiding concern within nursing practice, within medicine care has sometimes been overshadowed by other ethical values and goals. The emergence of feminine ethics can play an important role in reemphasizing the value and importance of caring within medicine. However, the close association of care with gender and with the feminine voice may hinder efforts to develop a broader human understanding of care, such as the understanding of care that emerged earlier in human history.

NANCY S. JECKER
WARREN THOMAS REICH

Directly related to this article are the companion articles in this entry: HISTORY OF THE NOTION OF CARE, *and* HISTORICAL DIMENSIONS OF AN ETHIC OF CARE IN HEALTH CARE. *Also directly related are the entries* FEMINISM; NURSING ETHICS; COMPASSION; EMOTIONS; HEALING; NARRATIVE; VIRTUE AND CHARACTER; *and* ENVIRONMENTAL ETHICS, *article on* ECOFEMINISM. *For a further discussion of topics mentioned in this article, see the entries* BENEFICENCE; BIOETHICS; CASUISTRY; HARM; INTERPRETATION; METAPHOR AND ANALOGY; PAIN AND SUFFERING; TRUST; VALUE AND VALUATION; *and* WOMEN, *section on* WOMEN AS HEALTH PROFESSIONALS. *Other relevant material may be found under the entries* CLINICAL ETHICS, *article on* ELEMENTS AND METHODOLOGIES; CONSCIENCE; ETHICS, *articles on* TASKS OF ETHICS, NORMATIVE ETHICAL THEORIES, *and* SOCIAL AND POLITICAL THEORIES; FIDELITY AND LOYALTY; HUMAN NATURE; NURSING, THEORIES AND PHILOSOPHY OF; *and* WOMEN, *article on* HISTORICAL AND CROSS-CULTURAL ISSUES.

Bibliography

ANGELL, MARCIA. 1982. "The Quality of Mercy." *New England Journal of Medicine* 306, no. 2:98–99.
BENNER, PATRICIA, and WRUBEL, JUDITH. 1989. *The Primacy of Caring.* Menlo Park, Calif.: Addison-Wesley.

BROWN, LYN M., and GILLIGAN, CAROL. 1992. *Meeting at the Crossroads: Women's Psychology and Girls' Development.* Cambridge, Mass.: Harvard University Press.

CARD, CLAUDIA. 1990. "Caring and Evil." *Hypatia* 5, no. 1:101–108.

———. 1991. "The Feistiness of Feminism." In *Feminist Ethics,* pp. 3–13. Edited by Claudia Card. Lawrence: University Press of Kansas.

CARSE, ALISA L. 1991. "The 'Voice of Care': Implications for Bioethical Education." *Journal of Medicine and Philosophy* 16, no. 1:5–28.

CASSELL, ERIC J. 1982. "The Nature of Suffering and the Goals of Medicine." *New England Journal of Medicine* 306: 639–645.

———. 1989. *The Healer's Art.* Cambridge, Mass.: MIT Press.

CURTIN, DEANE. 1991. "Toward an Ecological Ethic of Care." *Hypatia* 6, no. 1:60–74.

ELSHTAIN, JEAN BETHKE. 1981. *Public Man, Private Woman: Women in Social and Political Thought.* Princeton, N.J.: Princeton University Press.

FRY, SARAH T. 1989a. "The Role of Caring in a Theory of Nursing Ethics." *Hypatia* 4, no. 2:88–103.

———. 1989b. "Toward a Theory of Nursing Ethics." *Advances in Nursing Science* 11, no. 4:9–22.

GADOW, SALLY. 1980a. "Existential Advocacy: Philosophical Foundations of Nursing." In *Nursing: Images and Ideals, Opening Dialogue with the Humanities,* pp. 79–101. Edited by Stuart F. Spicker and Sally Gadow. New York: Springer Press.

———. 1980b. "A Model for Ethical Decision Making." *Oncology Nursing Forum* 7, no. 4:44–47.

———. 1985. "Nurse and Patient: The Caring Relationship." In *Caring, Curing, Coping: Nurse, Physician, Patient Relationships,* pp. 31–43. Edited by Anne H. Bishop and John R. Scudder, Jr. Birmingham: University of Alabama Press.

GATENS-ROBINSON, EUGENIE. 1992. "A Defense of Women's Choice: Abortion and the Ethics of Care." *Southern Journal of Philosophy* 30, no. 3:39–66.

GILLIGAN, CAROL. 1982. *In a Different Voice: Psychological Theory and Women's Development.* Cambridge, Mass.: Harvard University Press.

GILLIGAN, CAROL, and ATTANUCCI, JANE. 1988. "Two Moral Orientations." In *Mapping the Moral Domain: A Contribution of Women's Thinking to Psychological Theory and Education,* pp. 73–86. Edited by Carol Gilligan, Janie V. Ward, and Jill M. Taylor. Cambridge, Mass.: Harvard University Press.

GILLIGAN, CAROL; LYONS, NONA P.; and HANMER, TRUDY J., eds. 1989. *Making Connections: The Relational Worlds of Adolescent Girls at the Emma Willard School.* Cambridge, Mass.: Harvard University Press.

GILLIGAN, CAROL; WARD, JANIE V.; and TAYLOR, JILL M., eds. 1988. *Mapping the Moral Domain: A Contribution of Women's Thinking to Psychological Theory and Education.* Cambridge, Mass.: Harvard University Press.

HARDWIG, JOHN. 1990. "What About the Family?" *Hastings Center Report* 20, no. 2:5–10.

———. 1991. "Treating the Brain Dead for the Benefit of the Family." *Journal of Clinical Ethics* 2, no. 1:53–56.

HOLMES, HELEN B. 1989. "A Call to Heal Medicine." *Hypatia* 4, no. 2:1–8.

HOUSTON, BARBARA. 1990. "Caring and Exploitation." *Hypatia* 5:115–119.

JAMETON, ANDREW. 1984. *Nursing Practice: The Ethical Issues.* Englewood Cliffs, N.J.: Prentice-Hall.

JECKER, NANCY S. 1990. "The Role of Intimate Others in Medical Decision Making." *Gerontologist* 30, no. 1:65–71.

———. 1991. "Giving Death a Hand: When the Doctor and Patient Stand in a Special Relationship." *Journal of the Geriatrics Society* 39, no. 8:831–835.

———. 1993a. "Impartiality and Special Relations." In *Kindred Matters: Rethinking the Philosophy of the Family,* pp. 41–58. Edited by Diana T. Myers, Kenneth Kepnis, and Cornelius F. Murphy, Jr. Ithaca, N.Y.: Cornell University Press.

———. 1993b. "Abortion." In *Ethics Applied.* Edited by Michael L. Richardson and Karen White. New York: McGraw-Hill.

JECKER, NANCY S., and SELF, DONNIE J. 1991. "Separating Care and Cure: An Analysis of Historical and Contemporary Images of Nursing and Medicine." *Journal of Medicine and Philosophy* 16, no. 3:285–306.

JONSEN, ALBERT R. 1990. "The Good Samaritan as Gatekeeper." In his *The New Medicine and the Old Ethics,* pp. 38–60. Cambridge, Mass.: Harvard University Press.

KING, ROGER J. H. 1991. "Caring About Nature: Feminist Ethics and the Environment." *Hypatia* 6, no. 1:75–84.

KOHLBERG, LAWRENCE. 1981. *The Philosophy of Moral Development: Moral Stages and the Idea of Justice.* San Francisco: Harper & Row.

———. 1984. *The Psychology of Moral Development: The Nature and Validity of Moral Stages.* San Francisco: Harper & Row.

MOODY-ADAMS, MICHELE M. 1991. "Gender and the Complexity of Moral Voices." In *Feminist Ethics,* pp. 195–212. Edited by Claudia Card. Lawrence: University Press of Kansas.

MURPHY, CATHERINE P. 1984. "The Changing Role of Nurses in Making Ethical Decisions." *Law, Medicine, and Health Care* 12, no. 4:173–175, 184.

NEWTON, LISA H. 1990. "In Defense of the Traditional Nurse." In *Ethics in Nursing: An Anthology,* pp. 13–20. Edited by Terry Pence and Janice Cantrall. New York: National League for Nursing.

NICHOLSON, LINDA J. 1986. *Gender and History: The Limits of Social Theory in the Age of the Family.* New York: Columbia University Press.

NODDINGS, NEL. 1984. *Caring: A Feminine Approach to Ethics and Moral Education.* Berkeley: University of California Press.

———. 1990. "Ethics from the Standpoint of Women." In *Theoretical Perspectives on Sexual Difference,* pp. 160–173. Edited by Deborah L. Rohode. New Haven, Conn.: Yale University Press.

O'BRIEN, PATRICIA. 1987. "'All a Woman's Life Can Bring': The Domestic Roots of Nursing in Philadelphia, 1830–1885." *Nursing Research* 36, no. 1:12–17.

PELLEGRINO, EDMUND D.; and THOMASMA, DAVID C. 1988.

For the Patient's Good: The Restoration of Beneficence in Health Care. New York: Oxford University Press.

PIAGET, JEAN. 1965. *The Moral Judgment of the Child.* New York: Free Press.

REICH, WARREN THOMAS. 1991. "The Case: Denny's Story," and "Commentary: Caring as Extraordinary Means." *Second Opinion* 17:43–45.

REVERBY, SUSAN. 1987a. "A Caring Dilemma: Womanhood and Nursing in Historical Perspective." *Nursing Research* 36, no. 1:5–11.

———. 1987b. *Ordered to Care: The Dilemma of American Nursing, 1850–1945.* New York: Cambridge University Press.

RUDDICK, SARA. 1989. *Maternal Thinking: Toward a Politics of Peace.* Boston: Beacon Press.

SCHNEIDERMAN, LAWRENCE J.; FABER-LANGENDOEN, KATHY; and JECKER, NANCY S. 1994. "Beyond Futility to an Ethic of Care." *American Journal of Medicine* 96, no. 2:110–114.

SELF, DONNIE J.; SKEEL, JOY D.; and JECKER, NANCY S. 1993a. "A Comparison of the Moral Reasoning of Physicians and Clinical Ethicists." *Academic Medicine* 68, no. 11: 852–855.

———. 1993b. "The Influence of Philosophical Versus Theological Education on the Moral Development of Clinical Medical Ethicists." *Academic Medicine* 68, no. 11: 848–852.

SHARPE, VIRGINIA A. 1992. "Justice and Care: The Implications of the Kohlberg-Gilligan Debate for Medical Ethics." *Theoretical Medicine* 13, no. 4:295–318.

SHERWIN, SUSAN. 1992. *No Longer Patient: Feminist Ethics and Health Care.* Philadelphia: Temple University Press.

SPELLMAN, ELIZABETH V. 1991. "The Virtue of Feeling and the Feeling of Virtue." In *Feminist Ethics,* pp. 213–232. Edited by Claudia Card. Lawrence: University Press of Kansas.

SPIRO, HOWARD M.; MCCREA, MARY G. M.; PESCHEL, ENID; and ST. JAMES, DEBORAH. 1993. *Empathy and the Practice of Medicine: Beyond Pills and the Scalpel.* New Haven, Conn.: Yale University Press.

STEIN, LEONARD I.; WATTS, DAVID T.; and HOWELL, TIMOTHY. 1990. "The Doctor-Nurse Game Revisited." *New England Journal of Medicine* 322, no. 8:546–549.

SWANSON, KRISTEN M. 1990. "Providing Care in the NICU: Sometimes an Act of Love." *Advances in Nursing Science* 13, no. 1:60–73.

THOMSON, JUDITH JARVIS. 1990. *The Realm of Rights.* Cambridge, Mass.: Harvard University Press.

TONG, ROSEMARIE. 1993. *Feminine and Feminist Ethics.* Belmont, Calif.: Wadsworth.

U.N. GENERAL ASSEMBLY. 1948. *Universal Declaration of Human Rights.* New York: Author.

———. 1960. *Declaration of the Rights of the Child: Adopted by the General Assembly of the United Nations, New York, November 20, 1959.* New York: Author.

VEATCH, ROBERT M. 1981. *A Theory of Medical Ethics.* New York: Basic Books.

WALKER, MARGARET URBAN. 1989. "Moral Understandings: Alternative Epistemology for a Feminist Ethics." *Hypatia* 4, no. 2:15–28.

WARREN, VIRGINIA L. 1989. "Feminist Directions in Medical Ethics." *Hypatia* 4, no. 2:73–87.

WATSON, JEAN. 1988. *Nursing: Human Science and Human Care: A Theory of Nursing.* New York: National League for Nursing.

WINSLOW, GERALD R. 1984. "From Loyalty to Advocacy: A New Metaphor for Nursing." *Hastings Center Report* 14, no. 3:32–40.

CASUISTRY

Casuistry, a term derived from the Latin word meaning "event, occasion, occurrence" and in later Latin, "case," was coined in the seventeenth century to refer pejoratively to the practice described by contemporary Christian theologians as "cases of conscience" (*casus conscientiae*). Today the word might be defined as the method of analyzing and resolving instances of moral perplexity by interpreting general moral rules in light of particular circumstances. This article will relate the origins and development of casuistry in Western culture, its decline, and its current revival as a method of ethical analysis, particularly in bioethics.

Origins of casuistry

The earliest discussions of morality in Western philosophy reveal the tension between general moral norms and particular decisions. The Sophists of fifth-century Greece maintained that since no universal truths could be affirmed in moral matters, right and wrong depended entirely on the circumstances: ethics consisted in the rhetorical ability to persuade persons about "opportune" action. Plato devoted his *Republic* to a vigorous refutation of this thesis, placing moral certitude only in universal moral truths: ethics consisted in transcending particularities and grasping permanent ideals from which right choice could be deduced. Aristotle proposed that in ethical deliberations, which deal with contingent matters, formal demonstration was not possible. Rather, plausible argument would support probable conclusions. Ethics belongs, he maintained, not in the realm of scientific knowledge but in the domain of practical wisdom (*phronesis*). *Phronesis* is a knowledge of particular facts and is the "object of perception rather than science" (*Nicomachean Ethics,* VI. viii. 1142a). Criticism, interpretation, and amplification of these theses constitutes much of the history of moral philosophy. The Aristotelian viewpoint, which places moral certitude in the domain of practical judgments about what ought to be done in the actual circumstances of a situation, is the remote philosophical ancestor of the casuistry that developed in Western culture.

The Roman philosopher and statesman Marcus Tullius Cicero (106–43 B.C.E.) designed an approach to moral problems that would powerfully influence the casuistic authors of the Middle Ages and Renaissance. Cicero, although a philosophical eclectic, inclined to Stoic thought in ethics. Drawing from the Stoics Panaetius and Posidonius and inspired by the Roman passion for practicality, he held that to be a virtuous person one must become "a good calculator of one's duty in the circumstances, so that by adding and subtracting considerations, we may see where our duty lies" (*On Duties*, I, 59). This adding and subtracting was done by offering and evaluating "probable reasons." The primary moral problem was the continual conflict between duty and utility, a conflict resolved only by examining the circumstances of cases. In his *On Duties*, Cicero proposed a number of cases, some drawn from the Stoic philosophers and others from Roman history. Each case, representing an apparently insoluble conflict between duty and utility, was then analyzed to show how, if circumstances were taken into account, one could discern one's moral duty. Cicero also espoused the Stoic doctrine of natural law and often referred to its overarching precepts in his analyses of cases; but the problem, he affirmed, was how these precepts were to be interpreted in context. *On Duties* remained one of the most studied texts of antiquity through the subsequent centuries. By its organization of material and its methods of reasoning, *On Duties* powerfully influenced the way in which morality was conceived and taught in the Western world, and thus sanctioned subsequent casuistry.

While moral discourse always moves between the broad generalizations of principle and the particular decisions made in specific circumstances, religions that are monotheistic and moral in nature face a particular problem in moving from the general to the particular. The three "religions of the Book"—Judaism, Christianity, and Islam—have in common a Scripture in which the word of God is recorded; that is, in which God speaks to believers in concrete and specific language. Also, the divine message contains imperatives that enjoin moral obligations, sometimes stated in broad terms and sometimes referring to specific forms of behavior. It becomes necessary for believers to understand how the broad general imperatives apply to the great variety of daily life, and to learn how specific commands expressed in the language and cultural setting of the past are to be followed in the circumstances of later times. Thus, each religion of the Book developed a moral teaching that begins with affirmations from the divine text, moves through traditional interpretations of that text by the saintly and the scholarly, and comes, finally, to the task of bringing text and interpretation to bear on particular circumstances of time and place. Each of these religions, then, has developed a casuistry or manner of working at the task of concrete application. The particular forms of Jewish and Islamic casuistry are discussed elsewhere; this

entry will relate the development of casuistry in Western Christianity.

Christianity introduced a powerful and original morality into the Graeco-Roman world. The thought of its founder, Jesus, both reflected the dedication of Jewish law to the sovereignty of God and refashioned it to include a demanding commitment to himself as Lord as well as self-sacrifice for one's neighbors, spelled out in strenuous, often paradoxical commands. His early disciples, seeking to follow these commands, preached an ascetic repudiation of "the ways of the world." This meant that the moderate virtues prized by the pagans among whom the early Christians lived were often deprecated and the vices of pagan life, which even pagan authors often criticized, were reviled. The morality of the Hebrew Scriptures and the Christian Gospels, which condemned many attitudes and practices common in pagan culture and demanded adherence to self-discipline and altruism, posed profound difficulties to believers. How were they to live in a world that held different values? How were the "hard commandments" of the Gospels to be carried out in daily life? These problems perplexed Paul of Tarsus, the most influential of Jesus' first followers, whose efforts to answer them, especially in his First Letter to the Corinthians, adumbrated the work of later Christian casuists. In addition, early Christian thinkers were suspicious of the philosophical thought of the Graeco-Roman world. However, by the third century, many Christian scholars had come to accept that Christian belief and "pagan" philosophy were compatible in important respects. The authors of the patristic era (second to sixth centuries) reflected on Christian moral problems with the help of Plato, Aristotle, and Cicero. The framework of virtues, natural law, and practical reasoning elucidated in these and other pagan authors were modified and incorporated by Christian authors and teachers. They sought, as did their pagan mentors, to understand the nature of the moral life but were concerned, above all, with providing practical advice about how the faithful should live a Christian life in a non-Christian world. Many Christian authors used Cicero's *On Duties* as a model for treatises on morality: St. Ambrose of Milan (339–397), friend and teacher of the great St. Augustine, also entitled a book *On Duties* and, closely following Cicero, attempted to refashion the latter's thoughts within the perspective of Christian faith.

Christian teaching does not merely require belief; it strongly stresses the importance of morally correct behavior. While killing, deception, and adultery are condemned as sins, and charity, self-denial, and honesty are commanded, inevitably questions arise about what sorts of behavior belong in these general categories. Early Christians were intensely aware that failure to follow the rigorous commandments of their faith separated them from God and from their fellow believers. The practice of confession of one's sins before the community of believers and the imposition of penance that would once again reconcile the sinner to God and to the community became common in the early centuries. By the eighth century, private confession to a priest, who had the ecclesiastical authority to absolve the repentant sinner from guilt, had been introduced. This practice of sacramental confession and penance enhanced the need for clear descriptions of the moral dimensions of various behaviors and of the ways in which various circumstances excused or aggravated the seriousness of those behaviors. From the eighth to the twelfth centuries, educators of the clergy produced penitential books that presented systematic catalogs of sinful and virtuous actions under various typical circumstances (e.g., the killing of another out of vengeance, in fear, in ignorance, etc.). The motives, the consequences, and the social status of the agent were important considerations in evaluating the responsibility and seriousness of behavior. Appropriate penances were assigned in view of the gravity of the sin.

These penitential volumes, the earliest examples of which came from the Irish and Welsh churches, became widespread throughout Europe. In the course of four centuries, their content became more elaborate and their format more systematic. The first were collections of crudely described cases with simple distinctions, elaborated with biblical or patristic quotations. Later examples incorporated advancing biblical and theological scholarship and, above all, the work of the canon lawyers who, since the rediscovery of Roman law in the eleventh century, had exercised increasing influence over the formulation of church law as it touched the organization and practices of Christian life. The work of Peter the Chanter (d. 1197), Alain of Lille (d. ca. 1203), and Thomas Chobham (c. 1200) were filled with well-described cases of moral perplexity, analyzed with reference to biblical texts, maxims from the fathers of the church, and the growing body of church law. These books were not only for the education of the parish priest but also to guide the ecclesiastical hierarchy in the formulation of policy and the making of judicial decisions. Some of these books were written for the instruction of the laity in making a proper confession and leading a good life.

During the twelfth through fourteenth centuries, great theological scholars such as Abelard, Peter Lombard, Albert the Great, Thomas Aquinas, Duns Scotus, and William of Ockham elaborated systematic treatises or *summas* in which they attempted to present the full range of Christian belief and to support it with rational argument. In doing so, they placed the questions of morality within larger frameworks of interpretation and jus-

tification, drawing heavily on philosophers of antiquity. These treatises did not discuss cases, as did the penitential literature, but created theoretical foundations for the discussion of cases. The relevance of scriptural admonitions, natural law, custom, and civil and canon law to moral decisions was explored in great depth; the relevance of principle, motive, and circumstances was carefully examined. These theologians, while not casuists, greatly influenced the next generations of casuists.

Casuistic writings

Through the fourteenth and fifteenth centuries, many books of cases of conscience were published. The *Summa Angelica* (1480) and the *Summa Sylvestrina* (1516) were the most famous. However, these works were staid, unimaginative, and formalistic; many authors simply plagiarized from more celebrated authors. But casuistry properly speaking came into its own in the mid-sixteenth century. In 1556 a Spanish canonist, Martin Azpilcueta, published *A Handbook for Confessors and Penitents*, which revitalized the literature of cases of conscience. This book abandoned the practice of listing moral problems alphabetically and adopted a less frequently used device of organizing various sins under the Decalogue. This allowed for a more flexible and nuanced treatment and for comparison between various categories of moral behavior. Above all, it introduced the analysis of issues from the more clear and obvious to the more complex, a method that later casuists would exploit and that is described below as reasoning by paradigm and analogy.

Azpilcueta's style was widely copied. The Jesuit order, founded in 1534, was dedicated to the work of moral education and guidance of conscience, especially in sacramental confession. The Jesuits introduced Azpilcueta's approach into their own training of priests as ministers of the sacrament of penance. They published many volumes of cases of conscience. John Azor's *Moral Instruction* (1600) was the preeminent work. Jesuit casuistry was, in general, careful, scholarly, sensible, and practical. It was also comprehensive. While the general rubric of the Decalogue was used to organize materials, the duties of various occupations, the obligations of princes and bishops, and the moral dimensions of diplomacy, Jesuit casuistry also dealt with economics, warfare, and exploration. It has been suggested that the origins of modern economics, sociology, and political science lie in the work of the seventeenth-century casuists. Certainly, their advice was often sought by popes and kings in matters that we would today consider political or economic rather than moral. But in the seventeenth century, the moral questions on a king's or pope's conscience often concerned politics and finance.

The seventeenth-century casuists not only analyzed and resolved complex cases. They also elaborated speculative positions, writing treatises on topics such as justice, usually as prolegomena to their analyses of cases of government or trade. Among the central speculative questions was that of the degree of moral certitude required to act in good conscience, that is, how sure a person must be that a casuistic resolution of a moral problem is the correct one before acting upon it. A vigorous intellectual debate on this question took place in the last half of the seventeenth century between the Jesuits and their theological rivals, the Dominicans, and among the Jesuits themselves. From that debate, the position of the leading Jesuit theologians emerged as dominant. That position, probabilism, maintained that a person was entitled to act in good conscience if there were probable arguments in favor of the choice; probable arguments are those supported by solidly reasoned opinion and defended by respected authors. Probabilism, while defended with elegant argument and sanctioned by ecclesiastical authority, remained a contentious issue and led to the tarnishing of the casuists' reputation in the seventeenth century, since many critics accused them of being able to find any probable argument to justify their preferences.

The Jesuits were by no means the only authors of casuistry; many other Catholic theologians were so engaged. Anglican divines produced clear and sensible books of casuistry; and since most works of classical casuistry have not been translated from their original Latin, Anglican casuistical books offer the best access to casuistry for English readers (see Perkins, 1970). Lutherans were not well disposed toward casuistic analysis: Luther had cast into the flames the *Summa Angelica,* calling it "Summa Diabolica." Still, the Jesuits attained the reputation of being the premier casuists. Since they were deeply involved in the religious and secular politics of the era, they won enemies on every side and their casuistry appeared to many to serve their own interests rather than the good conscience of their penitents. In particular, the genius mathematician Blaise Pascal found distressing the Jesuits' opposition to Jansenism, a particularly rigoristic Catholic theology that he favored; and at the urging of other Jansenists, he set out to destroy the Jesuits' anti-Jansenist arguments.

Pascal's *Provincial Letters* (1656) was a brilliant and wittily written refutation of the Jesuit arguments against Jansenist theology and, in particular, of the casuistry that, he claimed, made a mockery of Christian moral beliefs. He gave numerous examples of Jesuit resolution of cases of conscience and found them tainted by a probabilism that bred moral laxity, intellectual sophistry, and disguised heresy. Despite the fact that Pascal took cases out of context and chose only those that suited his po-

lemical purposes, his diatribe became immensely popular. At best, it can be said that his critique demolished not casuistry itself but the lax casuistry that was counted reprehensible even by the Jesuits whom he accused.

It was not only Pascal's popular book that tarnished casuistry's reputation. Certain casuists, few of them Jesuits, did take the skill at case analysis to an extreme: Almost any argument could be presented plausibly and fine distinctions could be drawn to make, as Plato said of the Sophists, "the worse appear the better." Casuistry and sophistry became invidious synonyms, as did casuistry and Jesuitry. And casuistic argument, once quite liberal, became legalistic in tone and content, promoting a morality of observance rather than of conscience. Finally, casuistry was falling out of step with the prevailing intellectual progress. The interest in intellectual systems, seen in Isaac Newton, Gottfried Wilhelm Leibniz, Baruch Spinoza, and Hugo Grotius, made the casuists' interest in particular cases appear disorderly and without solid foundation. By the end of the seventeenth century, casuistry was discredited in the European intellectual world. The word "casuistry" was invented as a term of abuse (earlier the word *casista* was used merely to describe a scholar who presented cases of conscience). Bayle's *Dictionary* (1697) defined "casuistry" as the "art of quibbling with God." At the close of the eighteenth century, Kant, who was familiar with traditional casuistry as a way of teaching ethics, found the only interesting question to be how to transform the limited and probable maxims of moral discourse into categorical certitude.

Casuistic writing continued through the eighteenth and nineteenth centuries within the Roman Catholic tradition, particularly in the education of the clergy, but it was a desiccated casuistry, wary of innovative solutions and bound by ecclesiastical pronouncements on moral matters. The work of the French Jesuit J. Gury (1862) was representative of the fading tradition; a journal entitled *The Casuist,* published for American Catholic clergy (1906–1917), shows the tradition at its nadir. Still, casuistry continued to serve the practice of sacramental penance for which it had been created. Outside this tradition, remnants of casuistry lingered in the teaching of ethics. The textbooks of the time included fragments of Aristotle and Cicero and many of the classical cases, loosely grouped around virtues and duties. In 1870, revolted by the untidy and incoherent presentations of these texts, Henry Sidgwick, professor of casuistical divinity at Cambridge University (he had his chair renamed "moral philosophy"), undertook to construct a systematic presentation of an ethical theory, utilitarianism, in which tenets were tightly argued, inconsistencies rectified, and opponents refuted. The progress of moral philosophy from Sidgwick's time until recently has been toward greater articulation of theory and away from analysis of cases of conscience.

The practical need for casuistry

Casuistry then almost disappeared from the formal academic disciplines that study moral discourse. However, in the 1960s, a number of important moral questions began to trouble the American conscience, and moral philosophers were spurred to attend to the practical application of their discipline. The war in Vietnam required many to examine their consciences concerning support of and participation in what they felt was an immoral war. At the same time, the civil rights movement stimulated consciences concerning discrimination and racial injustice. The analytic moral philosophy current in academic circles had little advice to offer. Even the widely accepted and elaborate utilitarian theory seemed to lead to no firm conclusions.

The emerging interest in the ethics of medical and health care also opened vistas for a new casuistry. Medical care is about cases: the illness and the treatment of particular persons with particular diseases. Philosophers and theologians who engaged in this work had initially tried to bring the standard ethical theories to the analysis of medical problems, but they found themselves discussing cases, not theories, and felt the need for an approach that would stay closer to the particulars of the case under discussion than did the standard theories. Above all, they realized that cases were being discussed not merely to elucidate the meaning of concepts but also to arrive at a resolution: physicians, nurses, and patients were interested in what moral philosophy had abandoned: answers to practical moral perplexity. By the late 1970s, talk of "case method" had become common in bioethics. At the same time, ethical issues in business, government, and journalism seem to call for study of individual cases rather than flights into ethical theory. Also, influential moral philosophers were beginning to criticize the dominance of moral theory in practical ethics and to call for approaches that were more concrete than speculative.

Albert Jonsen and Stephen Toulmin published *The Abuse of Casuistry* in 1988. Aware that many were interested in inventing a "case method" for ethics, they hoped to show that such a method had been invented long ago and that, although discredited and seemingly outmoded, classical casuistry had much to offer modern ethicists. Case method in ethics might be similar in many respects to the case method in Anglo-American common law, which had developed in parallel with classical casuistry. Both the common law, about which much research has been done, and casuistry, which has been invisible to the scholarly world for several centu-

ries, need to be explored if a case method for ethics, of "morisprudence," is to be re-created. These authors attempted to restore casuistry to intellectual respectability. After a historical survey of the rise and fall of casuistry, they contrast it with current approaches to moral philosophy and define it as follows:

> [T]he analysis of moral issues, using procedures of reasoning based on paradigms and analogies, leading to the formulation of expert opinion about the existence and stringency of particular moral obligations, framed in terms of rules and maxims that are general but not universal or invariable, since they hold good with certainty only in the typical conditions of the agent and circumstances of the case. (Jonsen and Toulmin, 1988, p. 257)

Methodology

The term "methodology" may be too formal a word to describe how casuistry works. The casuists of the past left almost no formal description of their way of working; the casuists of the present, pressed by their critics based in moral philosophy, are still asking themselves questions about methodology. Still, certain characteristics of the casuistic approach can be noted. These characteristics appear to have their origins in the classical discipline of rhetoric rather than in philosophy as such. The historical casuists had, like all educated persons of their time, been educated thoroughly in rhetoric. Aristotle and Cicero, the authors from whom they learned rhetoric, also taught them ethics. Classical rhetoric was defined as having a moral purpose: the persuasion of persons toward right and just action. Indeed, the classical books of rhetoric, because they were so rich in comments about and examples of moral behavior, were often used as texts in ethics. In the centuries during which casuistry flourished, moral philosophy was not a clearly defined discipline. Thus, it is not surprising to find the historical casuists implicitly using the techniques of rhetoric in their analysis of cases of conscience. Both rhetoric and casuistry had morally correct attitudes and action as their ultimate goal.

Two characteristics of rhetorical technique are particularly important for casuistry: topics and the comparison of paradigm and analogy. Rhetoricians taught that discourse in general could be divided into a set of common ideas, such as "causality," "temporal sequence," and so on, which they called "topics." Each of these topics had sets of definitions and forms of argumentation that were invariant. Also, each special realm of discourse, such as discourse about politics, art, or economics, has its own set of "special topics," the features of the field that must be understood and discussed if an adequate argument is to be made about what should be done. A casuistic approach to an ethical problem, then, requires that the field of discourse be analyzed to designate the invariant features. For example, it has been suggested that the topics of clinical ethics are (1) medical indications, (2) patient preferences, (3) quality of life, and (4) contextual features, such as costs of care and allocation of resources (Jonsen et al., 1992). Each of these topics has certain definitions, maxims, and arguments that must be taken into account in discussion of any case. The particular circumstances of time, place, personal characteristics, various behaviors, and so on that are the details of any case are viewed in the light of these topics.

Once the particular case is described by its circumstances and topics, casuistical analysis seeks to place this case into a context of similar cases. The classical casuists were accustomed to line up cases of similar sorts, so that cases describing various sorts of homicide, for example, were aligned in order that the similarities and differences between cases would become clear. This enabled the casuist to see those cases in which the moral principles and maxims appeared to lead to an unambiguous resolution. Thus, the prohibition against killing another human being seemed most obviously to hold if the circumstances described a vicious, unprovoked attack on an unoffending person; the prohibition would allow an exception if the circumstances described a killing that resulted from that unoffending person's self-defense against a lethal attack. This technique of lining up cases, rather than seeing them in isolation, is the essence of casuistical analysis. It is called by some authors the technique of paradigm analogy: The paradigm case is the case in which circumstances allow moral maxims and principles to be seen as unambiguously relevant to the resolution of the case; the analogies are those cases in which particular circumstances justify exceptions and qualifications of the moral principles. A high degree of assurance, or moral certitude, pertains to the resolution of paradigm cases, while varying degrees of moral probability, or probabilism, attach to the resolution of analogous cases.

Finally, the resolution of each case depends on what Aristotle called *phronesis*, or moral wisdom: the perception of an experienced and prudent person that, in these circumstances and in light of these maxims, this is the best possible moral course. As one commentator on modern casuistry has written, "for casuistry, moral truth resides in the details . . . the meaning and scope of moral principles is determined contextually through the interpretation of factual situations in relation to paradigm cases" (Arras, 1991, p. 37).

Bioethics is the most prominent field in which casuistry is beginning to be reintroduced as a method for ethical analysis. This is not surprising, since a strong interest of bioethics is the clinical care of patients, and many cases that came to the early attention of bioethicists involved life-and-death decisions arising from the use of new medical technologies. Cases about whether life-supporting technologies should or should not be continued for particular patients lend themselves to casuistic analysis. The differing circumstances of individual patients, the topics (the significant categories into which a medical-ethical decision can be factored), and the maxims (such as "do no harm" or "respect the patient's informed choices") are each in their own way crucial to the resolution of any case. The placing of the case in a lineup of paradigm and analogy, from the most obvious—in which the patient is brain-dead, or continued care is manifestly futile—to the problematic, in which diminished quality of life or unclear preferences are at issue, allows for discretionary judgment between cases (Jonsen, 1991). This sort of casuistry can also be applied to questions of health-care policy, such as those surrounding the various programs proposed for allocation of resources, although relatively little of such analysis has been done.

Casuistry, then, keeps moral reflection close to cases. Neither classical nor modern casuistry repudiates principles: Casuistry is not merely another name for situationism or contextualism. Rather, principles are seen to be relevant to cases in varying degrees: In some cases, principles will rule unequivocally; in others, exceptions and qualifiers will be appropriate. Modern casuists dislike the description of casuistry as "applied ethics," since they explicitly repudiate the notion that an ethical theory must be elaborated and then "applied to" the circumstances of the case. Still, the relationship between cases and ethical theory is unclear and poses the principal speculative problem that casuists and moral philosophers must ponder, just as the historical casuists pondered the problem of the certitude of practical judgment. On the one hand, casuistry is not simply applied ethical theory; on the other, it is not simply immersion in the factual circumstances of cases, which would reduce it to situationism. Casuistry is not tied to any single theory of ethics but can be comfortable with selected elements of multiple theories. For example, a casuistic argument might draw on utilitarian, deontological, and contractual justifications in a single case. Also, the designation of topics and the selection of paradigms have theoretical presuppositions. Finally, the normative nature of principles and maxims, which must be clarified in order to specify the obligatory nature of casuistic resolutions, requires reference to theory. Casuistry, then, is not "theory free" but is rather, as one commentator has suggested, "theory modest" (Arras, 1991, p. 41). Theories, for contemporary casuistry, are not mutually exclusive, a priori foundations for practical ethical discourse but limited and complementary perspectives that illuminate practical judgment. Much work remains to be done on the relationship between theory and practical judgment. Still, as suits the style of casuistry through its history, it can grapple effectively with difficult cases even though all speculative and theoretical questions about its methods and presuppositions have not yet been answered.

ALBERT R. JONSEN

For a further discussion of topics mentioned in this article, see the entries CONSCIENCE; ETHICS, *especially the article on* RELIGION AND MORALITY; ISLAM; JUDAISM; METAPHOR AND ANALOGY; NARRATIVE; NATURAL LAW; *and* ROMAN CATHOLICISM. *This article will find application in the entries* BIOETHICS; CLINICAL ETHICS, *article on* ELEMENTS AND METHODOLOGIES; LAW AND MORALITY; *and* NURSING ETHICS. *Other relevant material may be found under the entries* INTERPRETATION; *and* MEDICAL ETHICS, HISTORY OF, *section on* EUROPE.

Bibliography

ARRAS, JOHN D. 1991. "Getting Down to Cases: The Revival of Casuistry in Bioethics." *Journal of Medicine and Philosophy* 16:29–51.

CARSON, RONALD A. 1986. "Case Method." *Journal of Medical Ethics* 12, no. 1:36–39.

GURY, J. 1862. *Casus conscientiae in Praecipuas Quaestiones, Theologiae Moralis.* 1st ed. Lepuy: Marchesson.

JONSEN, ALBERT R. 1991. "Casuistry as Methodology in Clinical Ethics." *Theoretical Medicine* 12, no. 4:295–307.

JONSEN, ALBERT R.; SIEGLER, MARK; and WINSLADE, WILLIAM. 1992. *Clinical Ethics: A Practical Approach to Ethical Decisions in Clinical Medicine.* 3d ed. New York: Macmillan.

JONSEN, ALBERT R., and TOULMIN, STEPHEN E. 1988. *The Abuse of Casuistry: A History of Moral Reasoning.* Berkeley and Los Angeles: University of California Press.

JUENGST, ERIC. 1989. "Casuistry and the Locus of Certainty in Ethics." *Medical Humanities Review* 3, no. 1:19–28.

KIRK, KENNETH. 1927. *Conscience and Its Problems: An Introduction to Casuistry.* London: Longman's Green.

LEITES, EDMUND, ed. 1988. *Conscience and Casuistry in Early Modern Europe.* Cambridge: At the University Press.

MAHONEY, JOHN. 1987. *The Making of Moral Theology: A Study of the Roman Catholic Tradition.* Oxford: Oxford University Press.

McHUGH, JOHN AMBROSE, ed. 1906. *The Casuist: A Collection of Cases in Moral and Pastoral Theology.* New York: Joseph E. Wagner.

PASCAL, BLAISE. 1967. *The Provincial Letters.* Edited and translated by Alban Krailscheimer. Harmondsworth, U.K.: Penguin.

PERKINS, WILLIAM. 1970. *Works.* Abingdon, U.K.: Sutton Courtenay Press.

CATHOLIC BIOETHICS

See ABORTION, *section on* RELIGIOUS TRADITIONS, *article on* ROMAN CATHOLIC PERSPECTIVES; EUGENICS AND RELIGIOUS LAW, *article on* CHRISTIANITY; POPULATION ETHICS, *section on* RELIGIOUS TRADITIONS, *article on* ROMAN CATHOLIC PERSPECTIVES; *and* ROMAN CATHOLICISM.

CATHOLIC HOSPITALS

See HOSPITAL; *and* ROMAN CATHOLICISM.

CENTRAL AMERICA

See MEDICAL ETHICS, HISTORY OF, *section on* THE AMERICAS, *article on* LATIN AMERICA.

CHAPLAINS

See PASTORAL CARE.

CHEMICAL AND BIOLOGICAL WARFARE

See WARFARE, *article on* CHEMICAL AND BIOLOGICAL WARFARE.

CHILD ABUSE

See ABUSE, INTERPERSONAL, *article on* CHILD ABUSE; *and* CHILDREN. *See also* INFANTS.

CHILDBEARING AND CHILDBIRTH

See MATERNAL–FETAL RELATIONSHIP; *and* WOMEN, *article on* HEALTH-CARE ISSUES.

CHILDREN

I. History of Childhood
    Joseph M. Hawes
    N. Ray Hiner
II. Rights of Children
    Francis Schrag
III. Health-Care and Research Issues
    Loretta M. Kopelman

I. HISTORY OF CHILDHOOD

Childhood is a culturally determined social construct that might be thought of as a set of expectations for children. The principal dynamic in the history of childhood involves changes in these expectations. The history of childhood can be organized around three fundamental concepts: socialization, maturation, and modernization. Socialization is the process whereby a child incorporates the principal elements of the culture into which she or he is born. Maturation is the biological process of growing up. Modernization is the large-scale transformation of economies and societies—of European countries first, and then others. This process includes industrialization, urbanization, and the expansion of capitalistic systems of economic organization. The most dramatic changes in socialization and maturation of children come from the impact of modernization.

In traditional societies, socialization usually took place within families at a gradual pace and in informal ways. Sons learned the skills and practices of adult males by working alongside their fathers. Similarly, daughters worked and learned in close contact with their mothers. In the modern world new agencies such as schools appeared and became part of the socialization process; and the process of maturation, formerly a natural process marked, perhaps, by rites of passage from youth to adulthood, now became the focus of serious social thought and practice. Put another way, maturation has been redefined in the modern age as a time of "identity crisis" for youth. In the modern age youths have a greater range of choices for adult roles than did their ancestors.

The pioneering work in the history of childhood is *L'Enfant et la vie familiale sous l'ancien régime*, published by Philippe Ariès in 1960 (and translated into English as *Centuries of Childhood: A Social History of Family Life* [1962]). Ariès not only wrote one of the first modern scholarly treatments of the history of childhood, he also made the central point that childhood is socially constructed; that is, that ideas about and expectations for children are determined by social leaders and experts (advice-givers). Another early writer on the history of childhood, Lloyd deMause, in a work titled *The History of Childhood*, argued that "The further back in history one goes, the lower the level of child care and the more likely children are to be killed, abandoned, beaten, terrorized, and sexually abused" (deMause, 1974, p. 1). Professional historians have modified the views of Aries and deMause as they have developed deeper knowledge of the ways earlier societies regarded and treated children. The lasting importance of both scholars is that they founded the field of history of childhood and stimulated others to further investigations and revisions.

Childhood in the ancient Western world

We know that childhood, a period of relative freedom from work, existed in the ancient world because children's play was depicted on Greek vases and Roman sarcophagi. There were several ancient treatises on the diseases of children and a recognition that children were to be treated differently from adults. Thus there was a tradition of childhood in the ancient world that saw children as passing through stages of growth, as being malleable, as being fragile, playful, and sometimes headstrong. This tradition saw children as individually different and in need of protection from abuse by adults. Ancient philosophers, particularly Plato and Aristotle, wrote about child-rearing practices and regarded children as a link to the future. Some children's toys have survived—dolls, small versions of weapons, and the like—and they point to adult agendas for future citizens. Epitaphs remind us that ancient parents mourned the death of their children.

The Greeks and Romans devoted special attention to children and child-rearing practices. Women were the child rearers, and a number of other adults worked with children: midwives, teachers, tutors, and physicians. Both Plato and Aristotle recognized five stages of childhood (expressed in modern terms):

1. Babyhood, from birth to about two years—that is, until the child is weaned and can talk
2. The early preschool age, from two to three years or later—when the child is separating emotionally from the mother, becomes more active physically, and begins to play games alone
3. Later preschool age, from ages three to seven—a stage when children become more active and more involved in social groups
4. School-age children (up to puberty)—a time of intense competition, especially among boys
5. The stage between puberty and adulthood—which continues into the late teens or early twenties.

The last stage may have been brief or nonexistent for girls, who married at a relatively early age. In their broad outline, however, these stages closely resemble modern child-development theory.

Threats to children in the ancient world

Childhood in the ancient world had a darker side: some people practiced infanticide as a means of birth control or eugenics (French, 1991); some children were sold into slavery; and some of the little slaves were maimed so that they could be more pitiable beggars. Additionally, the use of wet nurses for the newborn was common and undoubtedly led to higher infant mortality rates. Wet nursing led to higher infant mortality because there was a greater possibility of disease, the wet nurse had less concern for the child than the mother did, and the amount of nourishment from the wet nurse might have been less. Infanticide was common, and such evidence as there is suggests that it was more common for female children than for male children to be killed by being abandoned and left to starve. A Roman law, for instance, said that all boy children and at least one girl born to a family had to be raised. In Sparta (from 700 to about 350 B.C.E.) infanticide was part of a program of eugenics whereby defective children were exposed. Illegitimate children were also disposed of through infanticide. Most children grew up in small nuclear families with one or two siblings. These small families were of concern to the Romans, who sought to increase the birth rate through incentives.

Childhood in medieval and early modern times

Very little is known about child-rearing practices and childhood in the early centuries of the Middle Ages because the historical sources for this period are very scattered and fragmentary. But it is known that children were valued. Among the Visigoths, for example, a male baby had a blood price (wergild) of one-tenth that of an adult male. As the child aged, the wergild increased. Female children had a blood price half that of male children, but adult women's wergild was five-sixths that of an adult male. There was some schooling in this period; scattered references attest to schools in palaces and monasteries, although the practice of taking in small boys as oblates by monastic orders was already declining. For much of the population the process of maturation involved a long apprenticeship with children working alongside adults and thereby learning adult roles and responsibilities.

Literary references suggest that adults treated young children in a kindly fashion but that they had little regard for young people in their teens. Laws set the age of criminal responsibility (when a child could be charged with a crime) at seven and the age of majority (when a person could make a binding contract) at eighteen or older. As in the ancient world, medieval parents clearly mourned the deaths of their children. Medieval commentaries on childhood saw three stages in place of the ancient world's five (again expressed in modern terms):

1. *Infancy*—up to the age of two
2. *The preschool period*—from age two to age seven
3. *Puerility*—from age seven to age fourteen.

There were texts that stressed the importance of breast-feeding (and by inference pointed to the dangers of wet nurses), but the use of wet nurses was common among the upper classes. An English bishop wrote of the importance of cradles (which would prevent infant deaths resulting from suffocation in the parental bed). Some children's toys—miniature figurines, for example—have survived from the period.

Infanticide was still common for female babies, but illegitimate children were sometimes added to the father's household. To counter the pattern of infant exposure and abandonment, orphanages appeared, the first being established in 787 at Milan. By the early fourteenth century, there were two hospitals in Florence that accepted foundlings, and in 1445 a separate foundling hospital, the Innocenti, was established. Other foundling hospitals appeared in Rome, Bologna, Pavia, and Paris by the end of the fifteenth century.

During the course of the Middle Ages, opportunities for schooling expanded from the limited possibilities offered by palaces, monasteries, or nunneries. Schools began to appear in the major cities of Europe; many of them, such as the grammar school at St. Paul's Cathedral in London, which was revived by John Colet early in the sixteenth century, were founded for the express purpose of training boys in business.

Most medieval children left home fairly early. Girls entered the work force at around age eight as servants, and boys typically were apprenticed to learn a trade. In effect these children traded their labor for their upkeep in their new households.

The death rate for children in the medieval world was extremely high—from 30 to 50 percent of children did not live to maturity. Besides disease, infanticide, and wet nursing, accidents claimed a great many children. There was little supervision of young children. Newborn children were swaddled (tightly wrapped with strips of cloth so that they could not move about or even move their limbs). Older siblings might provide some care, but most children were left alone; many of them suffered accidents, such as falling into an open fire, as a result.

European living patterns in the medieval and early modern period are comparable in some ways with traditional Japanese households. In traditional Japan the household was a residence as well as a legal, economic, affective, and ritual unit. In it children were regarded as treasures, although only one child would remain in the household as heir (the heir could be either male or female). The other children became apprentices or spouses or servants or remained in the household as dependents. The successor inherited all the assets of the household and was responsible for the continuity of the household and its reputation. The household was child-centered and stressed socialization into traditional roles.

In recent times, as a result of the modernization of Japanese society, the process of socialization has changed. Japanese children do not remain in the traditional households, and younger families move to cities, where schools and other institutions have replaced the household as the primary agent of socialization because new occupations require different forms of preparation.

A similar transformation occurred in the Muslim Middle East. Ironically, it began with a reemphasis on the traditional household, which had been devalued by Westerners since the modern colonial period began in 1798. The family became a point for resistance to colonialism and strengthened paternal authority at a time when Western families were becoming more democratic. As the nations of the Middle East gained independence in the last half of the twentieth century, these traditional households began to give way before the process of modernization. And, as was the case in Japan and early modern Europe, schools and other institutions supplemented the family as agents of socialization.

Childhood in the modern Western world

As modernization transformed western Europe and North America in the eighteenth and nineteenth centuries, a new and distinctive pattern of childhood emerged that was the result of a number of influences—economic changes such as the intensification of a market economy, a decline in family size, the rise of rationalism in public discourse, to name a few. In addition, several important European thinkers were midwives to this new form of childhood. John Locke helped to undermine the dominant Puritan conception of children as innately evil, that is, born in sin, when he published his *Essay Concerning Human Understanding* in 1690. In it he argued that ideas could come from experience and thus were not innate. In 1693 he issued *Some Thoughts Concerning Education,* in which he attacked the doctrine of infant depravity. Locke did not regard children as innately good; rather, he argued that they were morally neutral—blank tablets.

Another central figure was the French philosopher Jean-Jacques Rousseau, whose *Émile* (1762) was the story of a boy and his tutor. Rousseau argued that children should be reared more naturally, making use of their innate curiosity to motivate their learning. For Rousseau both nature and the child were innately good. Evil arose from the corruptions of civilization. One of Rousseau's followers who put his ideas into practice was Johann Heinrich Pestalozzi, who founded a school in Switzerland in 1799.

Yet another important figure in the emergence of the modern concept of childhood was the English novelist Charles Dickens, whose well-known child characters Oliver Twist, Charley Bates, Jack Dawkins, and the Artful Dodger personalized some of the tragic effects of the industrial revolution in England. Dickens vividly described the desperation of the urban working classes and the processes whereby homeless children had to fend for themselves. His writings, supported by the findings of royal commissions and by the work of social reformers, helped transform the social attitudes of the Western world. In 1848 the English established "Ragged Schools" for the children of the urban working classes. Later they created a system of universal public education with the Forster Education Act of 1870.

In the United States in the nineteenth century, Charles Loring Brace, a New York clergyman and reformer, founded the Children's Aid Society in 1853 to ship "surplus" urban children—whether orphaned or not—to rural areas. The Children's Aid Society also founded lodging houses for homeless newsboys and industrial schools for homeless girls of the streets. (It was hoped that by teaching the latter unfortunates a trade such as sewing, they might be rescued from prostitution.) Later in the nineteenth century another New York reformer, Elbridge Thomas Gerry, founded the Society for the Prevention of Cruelty to Children in 1875. Popularly known as "the Cruelty," the organization sought to reduce or eliminate the worst instances of child abuse and neglect.

While these reforms and the expansion of public schools sought to provide opportunities for the child victims of modern society, the problem of child labor proved more difficult to solve. In part this was because few people—and certainly not most parents or employers—regarded child labor as a problem. For one thing, children had always worked before the modern era. Only the sons and daughters of the privileged elite escaped labor during their childhood. In the preindustrial world most families, whether urban or rural, relied on the labor of their children. Children in that world were regarded as a renewable labor supply. They began doing simple chores as early as possible, and they continued to work throughout adulthood and into old age, as long as they were able. Children also functioned as safety nets for parents. As parents became too infirm to work, they relied on their offspring for food and shelter. This family labor system moved with families to industrial cities. Thus, in nineteenth- and twentieth-century factories children joined their parents on the shop floor, first as helpers and later as hands. Industries welcomed child labor because it guaranteed a steady supply of trained workers, and families depended on the income the children produced.

But modern society demanded more skills from its work force than the family labor system was able to deliver. As a result, families had to forgo the income from some of their children so that they could learn the skills necessary to obtain employment. At the same time, reformers began to define child labor as a social problem and to expand the availability of schools. By the 1920s, child labor was on the decline in the Western world as schools, child labor laws, and technological innovation finally reduced the supply of child laborers and the demand for them.

In the process of expanding schools and trying to reduce child abuse and to regulate child labor, Western society was redefining childhood. Childhood now became a special, protected status, a time during which biological maturation could run its course, and children could come to know the complexities of the modern world and find their places in it. Two other social developments were significant in this process of redefinition: the creation of the federal Children's Bureau and a federally funded program to reduce infant mortality in the United States. The Children's Bureau, established in 1912, was an outgrowth of the First White House Conference on Children, convened by President Theodore Roosevelt in 1909. At first it concentrated on the reduction of infant mortality, which led in 1921 to the passage of the Sheppard-Towner Act, a program of matching grants for states. The grants helped states set up programs of education and prenatal clinics. This program of prevention and education had the desired effect, but was killed by lobbying from the American Medical Association in 1929.

Other social advances in the nineteenth and twentieth centuries included the rise of pediatrics as a medical specialty and the rise of child psychologists, psychiatrists, and social workers. By the late twentieth century virtually all advanced industrial countries, including many outside the West, had made significant strides in reducing some of the threats to children's health and well-being.

Conclusion

The experiences of children in the recent past cannot be reduced to simple generalizations; there are too many variables. But it is obvious that region, economic health, and aspects such as race, class, and gender all have a major impact on children and childhood. Having noted these difficulties, some observations are possible. Abortion is more common in the industrialized world, whereas infant mortality is much lower. Children are less likely to become orphans in industrialized countries, to experience the death of a sibling, or to die before reaching adulthood. Children in industrialized countries will probably know their grandparents, and their parents may well have been divorced; many of them live in single-parent households, a sharp contrast to the extended households of traditional cultures.

Children in industrialized countries will spend more time in schools than children did in the medieval world, or than they do now where traditional cultures prevail. They will spend more time in groups with children of the same age. Their parents will have relied more heavily on experts, and they will probably have only a few siblings and perhaps a room of their own. They will have money of their own, and parts of the media will cater especially to them. They will also have a legal status that is clearly spelled out, although their status will vary from country to country. Of course even in industrialized countries poorer children will enjoy fewer privileges than the children of middle-class or elite parents.

In the twentieth century the improvements in children's lives in industrialized countries have been dramatic. In the United States, for example, in 1900 infant mortality was estimated to be more than 160 per 1,000 live births; by 1990 this rate had dropped to around 10 per 1,000. In Japan the rate was 5 per 1,000. Similar improvements occurred in access to schooling and literacy. In 1900 high school graduates in the United States constituted less than 4 percent of the seventeen-year-old population. By 1990 they represented approximately 75 percent. Similar evidence of significant improvement in children's health and education can be cited for most, if not all, industrialized nations.

In the modern world childhood has been extended, redefined, and supported by an array of experts and social institutions. Maturity, once a biological matter worth little notice, has become a complex process perhaps more social and psychological than physical in nature. Similarly, the process of socialization is now much more complex, reflecting, as always, the society into which children are to be socialized. In complex modern societies, the preparation necessary to become a productive adult is much longer and more intensive than formerly. In recognition of this, students now extend their schooling well into their twenties and even beyond. Maturation, modernization, and socialization as they have interacted have created an entirely new world of childhood.

JOSEPH M. HAWES
N. RAY HINER

Directly related to this article are the other articles in this entry: RIGHTS OF CHILDREN, HEALTH-CARE AND RESEARCH ISSUES, MENTAL-HEALTH ISSUES, *and* CHILD CUSTODY. *For a further discussion of topics mentioned in this article, see the entries* ABORTION; ABUSE, INTERPERSONAL, *article on* CHILD ABUSE; ADOLESCENTS; ADOPTION; DEATH; EUGENICS; EUGENICS AND RELIGIOUS LAW; FAMILY; HOSPITAL; INFANTS; LIFE; *and* MARRIAGE AND OTHER DOMESTIC PARTNERSHIPS. *For a further discussion of related ideas, see the entries* FEMINISM; HUman Nature; Literature; Prostitution; Public Health, *article on* determinants of public health; Race and Racism; Sexism; Sexual Development; Sexual Identity; *and* Women, *article on* historical and cross-cultural perspectives. *Other relevant material may be found under the entries* Circumcision; Fetus; Maternal–Fetal Relationship; Medical Ethics, History of, *section on* europe; Person; *and* Reproductive Technologies.

Bibliography

Ariès, Philippe. 1962. [1960]. *Centuries of Childhood: A Social History of Family Life.* Translated by Robert Baldick. New York: Random House.

deMause, Lloyd, ed. 1974. *The History of Childhood.* New York: Psychohistory Press.

Fingerhut, Lois A., and Kleinman, Joel C. 1989. *Trends and Current Status in Childhood Mortality, United States, 1900–1985.* Washington, D.C.: U.S. Government Printing Office.

French, Valerie. 1991. "Children in Antiquity." In *Children in Historical and Comparative Perspective: An International Handbook and Research Guide,* pp. 3–29. Edited by Joseph M. Hawes and N. Ray Hiner. Westport, Conn.: Greenwood.

Gillis, John R. 1974. *Youth and History: Tradition and Change in European Age Relations, 1770–Present.* New York: Academic Press.

Golden, Mark. 1990. *Children and Childhood in Classical Athens.* Baltimore: Johns Hopkins University Press.

Greenleaf, Barbara Kaye. 1978. *Children Through the Ages: A History of Childhood.* New York: McGraw-Hill.

Hanawalt, Barbara A. 1986. *The Ties That Bound: Peasant Families in Medieval England.* Oxford: Oxford University Press.

Hawes, Joseph M. 1971. *Children in Urban Society: Juvenile Delinquency in Nineteenth-Century America.* New York: Oxford University Press.

———. 1991. *The Children's Rights Movement: A History of Advocacy and Protection.* Boston: Twayne.

Hawes, Joseph M., and Hiner, N. Ray, eds. 1985. *American Childhood: A Research Guide and Historical Handbook.* Westport, Conn.: Greenwood.

———. 1991. *Children in Historical and Comparative Perspective: An International Handbook and Research Guide.* Westport, Conn.: Greenwood.

Hiner, N. Ray, and Hawes, Joseph M., eds. 1985. *Growing Up in America: Children in Historical Perspective.* Urbana: University of Illinois Press.

Hunt, David. 1970. *Parents and Children in History: The Psychology of Family Life in Early Modern France.* New York: Basic Books.

Jordan, Thomas E. 1987. *Victorian Childhood: Themes and Variations.* Albany: State University of New York Press.

King, Charles R. 1993. *Children's Health in America: A History.* New York: Twayne.

Korbin, Jill E., ed. 1981. *Child Abuse and Neglect: Cross-Cultural Perspectives.* Berkeley: University of California Press.

Maynes, Mary Jo. 1985. *Schooling in Western Europe: A Social History.* Albany: State University of New York Press.

Pollock, Linda A. 1983. *Forgotten Children: Parent–Child Relations from 1500 to 1900.* Cambridge: At the University Press.

Sommerville, C. John. 1990. *The Rise and Fall of Childhood.* Rev. ed. New York: Vintage.

II. RIGHTS OF CHILDREN

Since about 1970, philosophical interest in the rights of children has grown substantially. This growth owes much to the social upheavals of the 1960s and 1970s, especially the civil rights and women's movements, both of which employed the rhetoric of rights. When the plights of children, homosexuals, and the disabled began to be highlighted, it was natural that advocates for these groups also used the rhetoric of rights.

The invocation of rights in connection with children, however, predated the 1960s. In 1959 the United Nations General Assembly (1960) adopted a ten-principle Declaration of the Rights of the Child, itself a descendant of one adopted by the League of Nations in 1924.

Why rights?

Why do activists concerned with the lives of children attempt to protect children's interests by invoking the notion of rights? The key features of the rhetoric of basic rights are (1) that rights are entitlements, and (2) that they impose duties on others. To claim something as a fundamental right is to make the strongest kind of claim one can make; it is to claim that something is an entitlement, not a privilege—something it would be not merely inadvisable or regrettable, but wrong and unjust, to withhold. And, typically, if one person is the bearer of rights, some or all others are the bearers of obligations. In the case of basic rights, the responsibilities fall either on all others as individuals or on the government, which in the case of democracies means on individuals acting as representatives of the citizenry. This is easily seen in the cases of the rights of adults to free speech and to health care.

The rights to free speech and health care illustrate two broad classes of rights given a variety of names by theorists. These may be designated "option" rights and "welfare" rights respectively (Golding, 1968). The idea behind option rights is that there is a sphere of sovereignty within which the individual cannot be intruded upon by government, even for the greater good. This idea is at the heart of classical liberal theory. Option rights are rights to choose. For instance, although persons have the right to speak, they may remain silent if they wish. Welfare rights, on the other hand, are rights to direct provision of services, such as medical care, that meet a basic need.

Do both categories apply to children? The notion of option rights motivated children's rights activists who saw children as oppressed by adults. Psychologist Richard Farson stated, "Children, like adults, should have the right to decide the matters which affect them most directly. The issue of self-determination is at the heart of children's liberation" (Farson, 1974, p. 27). The authors of the United Nations Declaration, on the other hand, focused almost exclusively on welfare rights. For example:

> The child, for the full and harmonious development of his [sic] personality, needs love and understanding. He shall, wherever possible, grow up in the care and under the responsibility of his parents, and in any case in an atmosphere of affection and of moral and material security; a child of tender years shall not, save in exceptional circumstances, be separated from his mother. (United Nations, 1960, p. 113)

Although some children's advocates urge recognition of both option and welfare rights, the underlying rationales are quite different. While the rationale for according children option rights conceives of minor status *itself* as a disabling condition that ought to be removed, the rationale for welfare rights urges that various goods and services be provided to minors *as minors*.

Most sensible people would look askance at putting children, especially young children, on a par with adults, insofar as freedom to live as they wish is concerned. The notion of a protected sphere of autonomous decision making is closely linked to the presence of developed capacities for rational choice, capacities that usually are only potential in young children. It may well be that the development of autonomy is impeded when children are not permitted to exercise choices in their lives, but advocating that children be given some options is a far cry from asserting that children have the same rights as adults to live their lives as they please. Paternalism, the coercion of individuals for their own good, is odious only when those coerced are capable of exercising rational choice.

Why not rights?

Rights discourse does have some limitations in the context of advocacy for children. An initial difficulty lies in identifying universal rights while taking account of the limited resources and diverse values of particular societies. It may not be possible in some countries to fulfill the universal right to grow up in an atmosphere of material security, due to lack of resources. A second difficulty is that alleged welfare rights may be in tension with each other—for example, the right of a child to grow up

in material security and the right to love and understanding.

A danger of rights discourse derives from the fact that, taken literally, respect of children's rights may permit substantial intrusion into parents' lives. For example, should government agents monitor parents to make sure they provide their children with the love and understanding they need? A less obvious danger derives from the fact that some of a child's most important needs, such as the need for love, cannot be coerced. If love fails, must the child be taken from the parent and given to another who is known to love the child? It is apparent that the struggle for children's rights may have the potential of making parents and children into adversaries.

Alternatives to rights

Given children's vulnerability to abuse and neglect by immediate caregivers and by society at large, what ethical bases other than rights might serve to enhance children's welfare? Philosopher Onora O'Neill (1989) suggests that Immanuel Kant's notion of imperfect duty provides such a basis. An "imperfect" duty—the duty to contribute to charity is an illustration—differs from a "perfect" duty in the latitude allowed for fulfillment; toward whom and how much the duty requires is not specified. Thus, although we all have an obligation to help the next generation not only to survive but also to develop its capacities, we may meet this obligation in different ways—some as parents, some as professional caregivers, some as taxpaying citizens. The idea is attractive philosophically, but it admittedly lacks the precision, and hence the force, of the language of rights. Since the precise nature of the duty cannot be specified, it will be difficult to determine when people have or have not done enough to help needy children.

Another stream of ethical reasoning centers on character and virtue. So-called virtue ethics takes the focus away from whether particular acts are obligatory, permitted, or forbidden, and explores the notion of a good or virtuous person, a notion it alleges is fundamental. Proponents of virtue ethics would say, for example, that the idea of a virtuous or good mother cannot be reduced to that of a mother who performs or refrains from performing specific actions viewed as duties. A decided advantage of virtue ethics is that it encourages us to ask a key question: What legal and economic structures are conducive to "good parenting"? Virtuous parents, for example, take time to be with their children, especially when they are ill, but such virtuous actions will be more likely if employed parents enjoy legal protection against punitive actions by employers for their taking family leave.

Unlike the children's rights approach, which may pit parents against children, this approach does not put parents on the defensive. But virtue ethics also has theoretical difficulties, chief of which is defining character traits in ways that do justice to the diverse cultural ideals present in a heterogeneous population like that of the United States. Everyone will agree that virtuous parents, for example, need to teach their children to distinguish right from wrong, but may they use corporal punishment in the process? Here, consensus will break down. Another limitation of the approach is that virtue ethics has little to say about what precisely is owed to, or what ought to be done for, children whose primary caregivers have *already* failed them.

Care ethics, a variant of virtue ethics, is utterly antithetical to the Kantian emphasis on general principles and the development of rational agency. Deriving primarily from the work of feminist psychologists and philosophers, this approach takes close personal relationships, such as that between mother and child, as a model for all moral relations. Emphasis is placed on the need for compassion and empathy in the context of relationships to particular others in concrete settings, rather than on allegiance to abstract principles. Parents, for example, often succeed in meeting the needs of their children because they can empathize with them in particular situations; no abstract duty to care for one's children needs to be evoked. The ethic of care counters a philosophical focus on rationality as the defining essence of humanity.

Is care ethics sufficient to meet the needs of *all* children? For example, should affluent citizens provide funds for intensive professional care of babies born with drug addictions, babies they never will meet? If the answer to such a question is yes, then the notion of duty may provide a more secure basis for persuading people that such contributions are obligatory, since emotional identification with those one does not know is likely to be weak.

If both justice and care are regarded as virtues, then virtue ethics may have the potential to offer moral grounds for the protection and care of all children. Whether such a reconciliation of alternative approaches is possible remains an open question. If it is not possible, then philosophical ethics offers a number of lenses through which to view the status of children. As in the case of actual lenses, however, there may be no single lens that fits all purposes.

FRANCIS SCHRAG

Directly related to this article are the other articles in this entry: HISTORY OF CHILDHOOD, HEALTH-CARE AND RESEARCH ISSUES, MENTAL-HEALTH ISSUES, *and* CHILD CUSTODY. *For a further discussion of topics mentioned in this article, see the entries* ABUSE, INTERPERSONAL, *article on* CHILD ABUSE; AUTONOMY; CARE; FAMILY; PATER-

NALISM; RIGHTS; *and* VIRTUE AND CHARACTER. *Other relevant material may be found under the entries* ADOLESCENTS; FEMINISM; FUTURE GENERATIONS, OBLIGATIONS TO; INFANTS; LOVE; OBLIGATION AND SUPEREROGATION; *and* PATIENTS' RIGHTS.

Bibliography

AIKEN, WILLIAM, and LAFOLLETTE, HUGH, eds. 1980. *Whose Child? Children's Rights, Parental Authority, and State Power.* Totowa, N.J.: Littlefield, Adams.

FARSON, RICHARD E. 1974. *Birthrights.* New York: Macmillan.

FREEDEN, MICHAEL. 1991. *Rights.* Minneapolis: University of Minnesota Press.

GOLDING, MARTIN P. 1968. "Towards a Theory of Human Rights." *Monist* 52, no. 4:521–549.

HOULGATE, LAURENCE D. 1980. *The Child and the State: A Normative Theory of Juvenile Rights.* Baltimore: Johns Hopkins University Press.

KRUSCHWITZ, ROBERT B., and ROBERTS, ROBERT C., eds. 1987. *The Virtues: Contemporary Essays on Moral Character.* Belmont, Calif.: Wadsworth.

NODDINGS, NEL. 1984. *Caring: A Feminine Approach to Ethics and Moral Education.* Berkeley: University of California Press.

O'NEILL, ONORA. 1989. "Children's Rights and Children's Lives." In her *Constructions of Reason: Explorations of Kant's Practical Philosophy,* pp. 187–205. Cambridge: At the University Press.

O'NEILL, ONORA, and RUDDICK, WILLIAM, eds. 1979. *Having Children: Philosophical and Legal Reflections on Parenthood.* New York: Oxford University Press.

UNITED NATIONS. GENERAL ASSEMBLY. 1960. *Declaration of the Rights of the Child: Adopted by the General Assembly of the United Nations, New York, November 20, 1959.* London: H.M.S.O.

III. HEALTH-CARE AND RESEARCH ISSUES

Access to good parenting, food, housing, and sanitation remain the primary aids to enhancing children's well-being and opportunities. The consensus that children should also have basic health-care and social services grew over the twentieth century. Initially, advocates for better health and social care for the many impoverished, neglected, abused, and exploited children included those active in the women's rights movement, the newly recognized specialty of pediatrics, and the visiting home-health nursing programs. As the century progressed, lawyers and social scientists joined the reform movement. They attacked the long-dominant views that children were the property of their parents or guardians and that the state had no authority to intervene even if the children were abused or neglected. Children gained rights to certain medical services and to be protected from abuse, poverty, neglect, or exploitation; adolescents gained liberties such as the right to consent to some kinds of treatments or services without parental approval or notification (Holder, 1985, 1989). Scientists further helped transform children's programs through study of children's growth, development, needs, experiences, illnesses, and perspectives, showing the importance of candor and respect for children's views. A distinctive feature of advocacy for improved health and social care for children remains: Others make most decisions for minors, both in terms of their personal care and in allocation of funds for their programs.

Moral disputes about children's health care generally fall into four areas: First, who should make decisions for children? Second, how should decisions be made? Third, when should children be enrolled as research subjects? Fourth, how much of society's health-care funds should be allocated to children's programs?

Basic moral values

Different solutions to these questions will be evaluated in terms of basic moral values: Solutions are judged superior when they fairly promote children's well-being and opportunities to flourish and help children become empowered, self-fulfilled persons who can develop their potential. The U.N. *Declaration of the Rights of the Child* (U.N. General Assembly, 1960) endorsed these basic values, underscoring their wide acceptance. These values received international support because most adults want to help children and recognize some responsibilities to help them. These values also promote stability by helping to address inequalities of the "natural lottery" (the inequalities caused by nature, such as health status) and of the "social lottery" (inequalities caused by social factors, such as wealth, schooling, or family). Children are not responsible for such inequalities, yet they affect whether children will thrive and flourish. Adequate health-care and social services enhance children's well-being and opportunities by treating diseases, in some cases returning children from the brink of death or permanent disability to full and healthy lives. These services also restore or maintain compromised function, avert or ameliorate suffering, and prevent disease or disabilities through interventions or counseling. Basic prevention, diagnosis, treatment, rehabilitation, and social services not only make children's lives better, they profit society with healthier and more productive citizens. The focus of this article is primarily on preadolescent children, who are clearly not responsible for their quality of life or its inequities and who need help making prudent decisions for themselves.

Who has authority to decide for children?

Adults are presumed competent and minors incompetent to consent to medical treatment or participation in research. Minors generally lack the capacity, maturity, foresight, and experience to make important choices for themselves, and cannot determine what choices promote their well-being or opportunities. In general, the younger and less experienced the child, the greater the presumption that he or she cannot competently participate in health-care decisions. Some children, especially older adolescents, may overturn this presumption.

Shared decision making.   Ideally, important health-care choices should represent a consensus among parents, doctors, nurses, and the child, if he or she is mature enough and willing to participate. Together they find the option best suited to the child and family (U.S. President's Commission, 1982). In the final analysis, however, parents or guardians generally have legal and moral authority to make medical decisions for minor children.

Parent's or guardian's authority.   Parents and guardians have the authority to make decisions for many of the same reasons they have authority to select their children's religion and schooling. Philosophers Allen Buchanan and Dan Brock (1989) discuss several reasons for this policy. First, parents and guardians are generally most knowledgeable and interested in their children, and so are most likely to do the best job for them. Second, the family usually bears the consequences of the choices that are made for the child. Some choices and their resulting consequences suit certain families better than others. Third, children learn values and standards within their families, and different values and standards may lead to different health-care choices. Within limits, it is important to honor the standards and values of families, because it is within the family structure more than anywhere else that people in society learn values. Fourth, families need intimacy with minimal state intrusion. Thus, unless the child is placed at risk, there is reason to tolerate choices that families make for their children and give families wide discretion in selecting health care for their children.

Parents or guardians maintain this authority as long as they promote the well-being and opportunities of those under their care, and prevent, remove, or minimize harms to their minor children. Their authority can be contested, however (Rodham, 1973; Holder, 1985). Moral disputes over when to challenge parental authority to make health-care decisions often center on practical and theoretical issues about when harms or dangers to children warrant interfering with parental authority, and what restrictions on the parental choice are needed to secure the child's well-being.

Parents who abuse, neglect, or exploit their children may lose custody of them temporarily or permanently. Physical, sexual, or emotional abuse inflicted on their children constitutes grounds for loss of parental authority. In addition, parents who make imprudent or neglectful decisions may lose custody temporarily or permanently. For example, parents might temporarily lose custody if they endanger a child by declining standard antibiotic care to treat their child's bacterial meningitis, preferring the use of herbal teas for treatment. Parents might also lose custody temporarily if they endanger a child by acting upon certain beliefs. For example, Christian Scientists object to surgery and Jehovah's Witnesses object to blood transfusions, yet courts can order either intervention if the child is endangered (Holder, 1985; Rodham, 1973). Because children cannot protect themselves, health-care professionals, teachers, neighbors, or other members of the community have a duty to report suspected child abuse, neglect, or exploitation to state agencies for investigation. When parental acts or omissions pose an imminent danger to children, then doctors, nurses, hospital administrators, or social workers have a moral and legal duty to seek a court order for proper care (Holder, 1985).

Children's assent and competence. Decisions about when to consult or inform children about their health-care options usually become important for children with serious illnesses where distinct choices result in different outcomes. Some, but not all, children want to understand the decisions about their health care. Older children will often have an opinion about their care (Brock, 1989; Holmes, 1989; Matthews, 1989). Moreover, adolescents do not always need parental consent to gain certain services such as treatment for substance abuse, abortion, or contraception (Holder, 1985, 1989).

This trend to inform or consult children stems from several sources. First, it results from research about what children of different ages and stages of development can understand. Social-science research has found that many children understand a great deal about their diseases and even their imminent death (Bluebond-Langner, 1978). They sense when people are not truthful, and this can cause them to suffer by feeling isolated from discussions, decisions, and support (Bluebond-Langner, 1978; Matthews, 1989). When children are competent and prepared appropriately, truthfulness generally has good consequences by promoting cooperation and enhancing trust in the credibility of their caretakers. Truthfulness can also foster decision-making abilities and maturity. When children have life-threatening or chronic illnesses, it may be especially important to them to gain some control in their lives and some respect for their views. For those facing death, opportunities to become self-fulfilled and self-determining persons may be restricted to choices about how they will live their last months.

Second, this trend stems from understanding that competency is task related. In assessing competency, the question needs to be asked: Competence for what? People are competent to do some things and not others, and so may be competent to make some health-care decisions but not others (Brock, 1989; Faden et al., 1986; Matthews, 1989; U.S. President's Commission, 1982). An eleven-year-old child with cancer may understand a great deal about the illness, because he or she has had experiences beyond those of most eleven-year-old children. Consequently, the child may be better able than most children of the same age to understand or participate in health-care decisions.

Children are increasingly competent to participate in health-care decisions as they become better able to understand and reason about their options and life plans. While young children cannot do this, some adolescents may be as competent as most adults in these respects (Holmes, 1989).

How should decisions be guided?

There are four important standards for health-care decision making.

1. The first standard, self-determination, applies primarily to competent and informed adults, who should be generally free to make their own choices about their well-being and opportunities as long as they do not harm or violate the rights of others. As minors become more mature and competent, they are accorded more self-determination, but their preferences need not be honored as those of adults (Holder, 1985, 1989). An adolescent with cancer insisting that he or she would rather die than lose a leg needs help in order to understand this reaction. The degree of irreversibility and severity of the consequences often determines whether the minor's preferences should be honored. Minors' choices generally become more morally binding upon adults when minors show that they understand and appreciate the nature of the situation in relation to life goals. Adult guidance is needed when minors cannot demonstrate that their choices enhance their own well-being and opportunities.

2. Second, adults and some older children may prepare advance directives about their health-care choices should they become incompetent. While a minor's choice need not be honored as an adult's decision, it may be an important consideration or even seem morally binding under some circumstances. Dying children may, for example, indicate that they wish to donate organs or plan their funerals. Parents may want to follow such instructions carefully.

3. A third standard, that of substituted judgment, applies to someone who was once competent enough to express preferences. Using this standard, people select the option they believe the person would have chosen were he or she able. Families often know their relatives well enough to make choices their relatives would have made. Children, especially those with serious or chronic illnesses, may also express general preferences that guide parental choices. One child who was very sick insisted

that he did not want to be maintained in a persistent vegetative state (PVS), "like a zombie."

4. The best-interest standard applies to those who do not have the ability or authority to make decisions for themselves. This standard maintains that decision makers should try to identify the person's immediate and long-term interests and then determine whether the benefits of an intervention or procedure outweigh the burdens. It does not mean they seek what is absolutely best, since that may be impossible (the best doctor cannot treat everyone), but the best among the available options. The best-interest standard permits complex judgments about what, on balance, is likely to be best for that individual given the available options (Buchanan and Brock, 1989; Kopelman, 1993). For example, the benefit of obtaining a long and healthy life would outweigh the burden of enduring intense pain for a short time. The best-interest standard, however, might be used by parents, doctors, and nurses to consider withholding or withdrawing maximal life-support treatment from children whose lives are filled with intense and chronic pain, with no prospects of improvement or foreseeable pleasures, understanding, or capacities for interaction.

In some cases, objective or intersubjectively confirmable estimates about pain and a well-understood prognosis force parents and doctors to choose between preserving biological life and providing comfort. Some children live in considerable discomfort from the very technologies that keep them alive, such as a gastrostomy (a tube through which food goes directly into the stomach, and which is irritating), intravenous lines, ventilators (breathing machines), long stays in intensive-care units (which can be extremely disorienting), or a tracheotomy (a hole in the throat that aids breathing but often clogs with saliva).

One goal of medicine, to be balanced against others, is to preserve and prolong biological life when possible. Since ancient times, this ideal has been understood to mean that one ought to prevent untimely death. However, a question remains regarding the best interests of a person whose life is continued by means of maximal treatment that is a burden to that person (U.S. President's Commission, 1983; Buchanan and Brock, 1989; Kopelman, 1993; Clouser, 1973). In cases where doctors and others disagree about what is best, it is hard to apply the best-interest standard. In such situations, and for the general reasons given above that allow parents wide discretion when doctors disagree about what is best, an established legal and moral consensus using the best-interest standard allows parents to choose from options advanced as best (Buchanan and Brock, 1989; Holder, 1985, 1989; U.S. President's Commission, 1982, 1983).

The best-interest standard was challenged by President Ronald Reagan (1986) and Surgeon General C. Everett Koop (1989), who rejected this standard, believing that quality-of-life considerations were likely to be abused. Under their influence, the federal government in 1984 amended its child-abuse laws and adopted the so-called Baby Doe guidelines ("Child Abuse and Neglect," 1985). These rules forbid withholding or withdrawing lifesaving care from a sick infant unless the child is dying or in an irreversible coma or when treatment is both virtually futile in terms of survival and inhumane. To forgo lifesaving treatments, it is not sufficient that the treatment is inhumane or gravely burdensome, as it would be in Roman Catholic tradition. If the care cannot honestly be deemed virtually futile, then according to these rules, it must be given even if it is inhumane and not very likely to succeed. Suffering cannot be taken into account except where the child cannot survive even with maximal treatment (Kopelman, 1989a, 1993). The Baby Doe rules are controversial because they radically restrict parental discretion and standard medical practice. In a 1988 survey, U.S. neonatologists indicated that the use of this policy for judging when to withdraw or withhold care for infants would result in overtreatment, poor use of resources, and insufficient attention to suffering (Kopelman et al., 1988).

Many commentators disagree with claims that the best-interest standard is open to abuse or that it is excessively vague (Rodham, 1973). For example, the U.S. President's Commission states, "This is a very strict standard in that it excludes considerations of the negative effects of an impaired child's life on other persons, including parents, siblings and society" (U.S. President's Commission, 1983, p. 219). Allen Buchanan and Dan Brock argue that quality-of-life assessments are not especially open to abuse if carefully limited to judgments about what is best for the individual patient. The courts and others who reject quality-of-life judgments made on behalf of incompetent people, they argue, fail to distinguish two kinds of quality-of-life judgments. Quality-of-life judgments based on considerations of social worth try to decide the interests or value of a person's life in relation to the interests or value of other people's lives; they are comparative. In contrast, noncomparative quality-of-life judgments try to consider the value of the life to the person, comparing the value of living the individual's life to having no life at all. While this comparison is difficult to make, it can be guided by choices made by competent adults who decide that there are worse things than death, including certain treatments keeping them alive. Buchanan and Brock hold that in using the best-interest standard, we should use noncomparative estimates, contemplating only the quality of the person's life for that individual; a person's social value should not be a part of this assessment. These noncomparative quality-of-life judgments, then, should be very carefully and strictly circumscribed. We can reflect, for example, upon whether most people would want to live such a life (Buchanan and Brock, 1989).

The debate between those who want to consider the person's quality of life and those who reject such considerations continues. The solution depends, in part, on whether one believes that, in the end, quality-of-life decisions can be avoided. For example, the Baby Doe regulations state that one need not provide maximal treatment to those who are permanently comatose, and this is a quality-of-life judgment. The solution also depends upon whether one believes laws should permit parents, nurses, and doctors to have some discretion in selecting what is the best available option.

Children as research subjects

Children who become sick are not responsible for their illnesses. The natural and social lotteries leave some children with a diminished quality of life due to illness. Good health and social services may be essential to give these children a chance to flourish and develop their potential as self-fulfilled and self-determining persons empowered to develop their talents. In addition, good health care helps children by preventing many illnesses and allows for early diagnosis and treatment. Good health care, however, is the product of study and research, and the problem is how research should be conducted to help children.

The ethical basis for research policy with children concerns promoting the same primary values that shape treatment decisions, namely, fairly enhancing well-being and opportunities. Since children, like adults severely impaired with mental illness or retardation, lack the capacity to give informed consent, they are regarded as vulnerable research subjects. Like policy regarding treatment, research policy with children is also shaped by different authority principles (stating who decides) and guidance principles (substantive directions about how decisions should be made). Four important policy options for vulnerable subjects balance these primary values differently.

1. The "surrogate" or "libertarian" solution allows the same sort of research with children as with other subjects, if parents give consent. This solution may not offer adequate protection to children because it permits parents to enroll them in potentially harmful research. Parents' legal and moral authority presupposes the promotion of children's opportunities and well-being, and prevention, removal, or minimization of harms to them. Parents have no authority to enroll their children in potentially harmful research. Volunteering to put another in harm's way is not admirable, and may violate the guardian's protective role.

2. The "no consent–no research" or "Nuremberg" solution excludes children because children are not considered competent to give informed consent to being en-

rolled as research subjects. This view, expressed in the Nuremberg Code (Germany [Territory Under . . .], 1947), seems too restrictive. It prohibits enrolling a child in a study even if the project could directly benefit the child. Moreover, to test the efficacy of treatments for distinctive groups, some members of the groups must be subjects. Competent, normal adults cannot serve as subjects in projects that test for children's growth or maturity, drugs for premature infants, or treatments for children's life-threatening asthma.

3. The "no consent–only therapy" or "Helsinki" solution holds that persons who lack the capacity to give informed consent may be enrolled only in therapeutic studies. This view, found in the World Medical Association's (1991) Declaration of Helsinki, is controversial because, first, classifying studies as either therapeutic or nontherapeutic may be misleading and arbitrary. Therapeutic studies may have burdensome, nontherapeutic features such as additional tests, hospitalizations, or visits to the doctor. Second, important medical research may hold out benefits other than therapy to subjects, such as gaining special care. Third, nontherapeutic studies that involve little or no risk to children (e.g., identifying at what age children are mature enough to name animals) may be important sources of information about children.

4. The "risk–benefit" or "U.S. federal regulation" solution allows research with children if it holds out direct benefit to them or does not place them at unwarranted risk of harm, discomfort, or inconvenience. To try to balance the social utility of research with respect for and protection of children, this option stipulates that the greater the risk, the more rigorous and elaborate the procedural protection and consent requirements. Many countries, such as the United States, Canada, the United Kingdom, and Norway, and international organizations, such as the Council for the International Organizations of Medical Science, favor this solution. Research needs approval by local boards known as institutional review boards (IRBs) or research ethics committees (RECs), and in some cases, by federal boards as well. Approval is based on findings that subjects have been selected fairly and that the risks to subjects are minimized and reasonable in relation to anticipated benefits of the study ("Protection of Human Subjects," 1993). Adequate provisions must also be made for the safety and confidentiality of subjects. Investigators must seek parents' informed consent. When possible, they must also obtain the child's assent, where assent means a positive agreement, not merely a failure to refuse. Children's refusals are not binding where their parents and doctors judge it is in the interests of the children to participate, as in studies where children may obtain a scarce resource to treat their deadly disease. This risk–benefit solution tries to determine whether the risks are proportional to the benefits for each individual, and uses

risk assessment to try to balance the social utility of encouraging studies that maintain respect for and protection of children's rights and welfare.

Using a likely harms-to-benefit calculation, U.S. regulations ("Protection of Human Subjects," 1993), outlined below, specify four categories of research with children. As risks increase, the regulations require increasingly more rigorous documentation of appropriate parental consent, children's assent, direct benefits to each child, and benefits to other children with similar conditions. Local IRBs can approve studies only in the first three categories.

The first category of research permits research with no greater than a minimal risk, provided it makes adequate provisions for parental consent and children's assent. Many important studies are safe, like asking children to perform simple and pleasant tasks. Using this category, investigators might gain approval to study at what ages preschool children can name colors, identify animals, and perform simple tasks like stacking blocks upon request.

The second category of research permits approval of studies with greater than a minimal risk if (1) the risk is justified by the anticipated benefit to each subject; (2) the risks in relation to these benefits are at least as favorable to each subject as available alternatives; and (3) provisions are made for parental consent and the child's assent. This category permits a child to get an investigational drug that is available only in a research study. Moreover, because children have unique diseases and reactions, to study the safety and efficacy of many conventional, innovative, or investigational treatments for children, some children will have to serve as subjects in controlled testing.

The third category of research permits research (1) with a minor increase over minimal risk that holds out no prospect of direct benefit to the individual subject; (2) where the study is like the child's actual or expected medical, dental, psychological, or educational situation; (3) where the study is likely to result in very important information about the child's disorder or condition; and (4) when provisions are made for parental consent and the child's assent. Investigators using this category have been permitted to conduct, for example, additional lumbar punctures on children with leukemia, who get them anyway, to help study leukemia.

Research that cannot be approved under the first three categories might be approved if (1) it presents a reasonable opportunity to understand, prevent, or alleviate a serious problem affecting the health or welfare of children; and (2) the study is approved by the secretary of the Department of Health and Human Services (DHHS) after consulting with a panel of experts about the value and ethics of the study and determining that adequate provisions have been made for the parental consent and the child's assent. Using this category, investigators might gain approval to conduct studies to prevent or treat epidemics affecting children, such as the acquired immunodeficiency syndrome (AIDS) epidemic, or a new infectious disease like the killers of the past (pneumonia, scarlet fever, diphtheria, or polio).

Difficulties. Unfortunately, the risk–benefit solution leaves key terms vaguely defined, allowing different interpretations about when risks of harm are warranted and what constitutes a benefit (Freedman et al., 1993; Kopelman, 1989b). In particular, the pivotal concepts of a "minimal risk" and a "minor increase over minimal risk" are problematic (Kopelman, 1989b). The federal rules state: "*Minimal risk* means that the probability and magnitude of harm or discomfort anticipated in the research are not greater in and of themselves than those ordinarily encountered in daily life or during the performance of routine physical and psychological examinations or tests" ("Protection of Human Subjects," 1993, sec. 102i). The Council for International Organizations of Medical Science (CIOMS) has a similar definition (CIOMS, 1993).

One difficulty with this definition of minimal risk is that it is vague. People's daily risks include dangers such as car accidents or getting mugged. Do we know the nature, probability, and magnitude of these everyday hazards well enough that they could serve as a baseline to estimate research risks for children? It seems easier to determine that a study asking children to stack blocks and name colors is a minimal-risk study than to estimate the nature, probability, and magnitude of whatever risks of harm people normally encounter.

A second problem with the definition of minimal risk is that it offers little guidance about how to assess psychosocial risks, such as breach of confidentiality, stigmatization, labeling, and invasion of privacy. Risks are allegedly minimal if they are either ordinarily encountered in daily life or during routine examinations. Doctors, nurses and psychologists, however, "ordinarily encounter" many psychosocially sensitive discussions in routine examinations and testing, including those about family abuse, substance abuse, sexual preference, and diagnoses, any of which could affect how people are viewed or whether they will be able to gain jobs or buy insurance. Moreover, psychosocial-risk assessment is an increasingly difficult problem. Some genetic and other testing has low physical risks—like taking a drop of blood—but high psychosocial risks. For example, Huntington disease is a genetic condition causing progressive dementia and loss of motor function when the person becomes an adult. A person known to have this condition could be denied a job or insurance or become stigmatized in the community. Thinking of risks of harm as merely physical ignores such profound psychosocial risks.

Third, there is no definition of "a minor increase over minimal risk," the crucial upper limit of what local boards can approve, and it is even unclear what constitutes a minimal risk. The second part of the definition seems to set an upper limit for physical interventions that have a minimal risk: Arterial puncture and gastric and intestinal intubation are not part of routine examinations; they exceed a minimal risk. The difficulty, however, is that there are considerable differences among pediatric experts, in both treatment and research settings, about how to assess the risk of such procedures as venipuncture, arterial puncture, and gastric and intestinal intubation (Janofsky and Starfield, 1981). Investigators and others concluded that better standards of risk assessment in children's research need to be formulated (Janofsky and Starfield, 1981; Lascari, 1981).

Even when it is agreed that the ethical basis for research policies with children is to promote their opportunities, well-being, fair treatment, and self-determination, it is difficult to determine when research involving children can be permitted. On the one hand, if research is not conducted with children as subjects, children may be denied the benefits of advances stemming from research and good information about what procedures or interventions effectively promote health and prevent, treat, or diagnose disease. On the other hand, if children are enrolled as research subjects, then vulnerable individuals who cannot give informed consent are being used.

Resource allocation

Many children throughout the world do not receive basic health-care or social services. In some cases, countries that can afford to do so provide insufficient funds for this purpose. For example, the main health problems of children in the United States arise from a failure to provide such basic care for children's allergies, asthma, dental pathology, hearing loss, vision impairments, and many chronic disorders (Starfield, 1991). Basic health-care and social services promote children's well-being, enhancing their opportunities in fundamental ways and correcting some inequities due to the natural and social lotteries. Children who are sick cannot compete as equals and thus are denied equality of opportunity with other children. The more these conditions are easily correctable, as many of them are, the more unjust it is to leave the children sick or disabled. Failing to provide children with basic health-care and social services, when a society has the means, is unjust based upon any one of four important theories of justice: utilitarianism, egalitarianism, libertarianism, and contractarianism. This point of agreement among widely divergent positions serves as a powerful indictment and proof that as a matter of justice we should redistribute goods, services, and benefits more fairly to children in order to provide them with basic health-care and social services.

Four theories of justice offer different guidance about how to allocate goods, services, and benefits. Proponents have used them to determine children's fair share of health-care funding in relation to adults (intergenerational allocation) and how to set priorities for funding within children's health-care programs (intragenerational allocation). Each theory addresses problems about what kinds of goods and services should be provided to people as a matter of justice and how to choose from among programs when not all can be funded. Although there are many variations of these positions, each seeks a defensible standard to help make choices fairly.

Utilitarianism. Utilitarianism offers one solution to the problem of how to allocate health care justly between generations and among children's programs. In one well-known version, philosopher John Stuart Mill (1863) argued that a just allocation provides the greatest good to the greatest number of people; the utility of following principles of justice was so great, he held, that these were among the most fundamental moral principles. We should not just consider the utility of isolated acts, he maintained, but the rules of conduct that, if adopted and adhered to, maximize utility. Actions are right insofar as they fall under such a rule.

In their efforts to maximize utility for the greatest number in accordance with just rules, utilitarians seek to prevent or cure the most common illnesses, adopt programs that help many rather than few persons, and generally use funds where they will have the greatest impact for most people. For example, utilitarians would resist funding expensive organ transplantations that help relatively few persons for a short time if such transplantations sidetrack programs that could help many people.

Some of the least expensive and most beneficial interventions are education about the benefits of exercise, a good diet, prevention of teenage pregnancy, and avoidance of alcohol, tobacco, and harmful drugs (U.S. DHHS, 1992). Relatively inexpensive interventions can aid in the treatment of many problems common in childhood, including vision impairments, hearing loss, dental pathology, allergies, and asthma as well as the variety of chronic disorders that come in the aggregate and cause considerable functional impairment (Starfield, 1991). Utilitarians favor providing such health care for children because it greatly increases their well-being and opportunities. It is socially useful and cost-effective since it can prevent later costly illnesses and benefit the current generation of adults who, when aged, will need to be supported by a healthy, stable, and productive work force.

Utilitarians might even favor preferential consideration of children. Interventions that benefit both children and adults generally offer children the most years of benefit. These added years of benefit increase the net good and, thus, could justify some preference toward children. For example, in some countries children receive dental care unavailable to adults because it has lifelong benefits and avoids later costly problems. Daniel Callahan (1987, 1990) believes that the young have a stronger claim to health care than the old and that the young should be given priority; the health-care system should see as its first task helping young people become old people, and then helping older people become still older only if money is available. He argues, moreover, that medicine should give its highest priority to the relief of suffering rather than the conquest of death.

In choosing from among children's programs for funding, defenders of utilitarianism assess net benefit for the community of children. A utilitarian would favor funding routine care, mass screening, and prevention programs that help many children rather than the development of costly therapies that help few children. Consequently, utilitarians would probably resist using state funds to give otherwise normal short children growth hormone for many years, at a cost of many thousands of dollars a year, to add several centimeters or inches to their adult height. Utilitarians, however, might permit private insurance or payment (in a multi-tiered health-care system) for these and other services if it increased or did not diminish the net good.

Defenders of utilitarianism presuppose that we can calculate what is best for the greatest number, and critics question this presumption (Brock, 1982). Moreover, the critics continue, whole groups could be excluded from beneficial health care for the sake of the common good; people with expensive or rare conditions, and those with illnesses that are stigmatizing, might be excluded from care. Utilitarians might respond that we would suffer from such exclusions, thus showing that this is not a good option even using utilitarian calculations. This presupposes, however, that enough people would know about the exclusions and be distressed enough to alter the calculation. Sympathy for utilitarianism may depend upon beliefs about whether we can make utility calculations, and whether a theory is acceptable if it permits us to exclude some groups for the common good regardless of the results of the utility calculation (see Brock, 1982). Defenders of rule utilitarianism, a version of utilitarianism clarifying the role of rules in assessing utility, respond that, properly understood, utility prohibits such unfair exclusions of individuals or groups; we adopt rights and justice principles because they are useful, and unjust exclusions undercut the utility of these rights and principles for all (Buchanan, 1991; Mill, 1863). Even if it might be cost-effective or politically expedient to exclude a particular person or group, such an exclusion undercuts something more important: fair rules.

Utilitarians favor basic health-care and social services for all children because of the utility to the children and to society. For example, suppose we could save a great deal of money by excluding certain children from health-care services. Although this might save some money in the short run, defenders of rule utilitarianism might argue that it is unjust because adapting and adhering to the rule that all should receive basic services is more useful in the long run than excluding a few to save money. Accordingly, the rule that all children should receive basic care is vindicated because the rule is useful and making exceptions is less useful.

Egalitarianism. Egalitarianism is a theory of justice whose defenders attempt to solve allocation issues and intergenerational disputes by holding that access to the same benefits, goods, and services should be provided to everyone on the same basis. It is a principle of justice that requires us to try to make all people's objective net well-being as equal as possible. Most of us do not want dialysis treatment since we do not have kidney disease, but we want access to it if we should need it. Egalitarians, then, do not want exactly the same treatment for everyone as a condition of justice, but for everyone to have access to the same goods, services, and benefits on the same footing. Egalitarians look at outcomes of distribution schemes to determine whether distributions are fair. Accordingly, defenders of egalitarianism judge it to be unfair, for example, that adults over sixty-five could get their diabetes and asthma treated free of charge in the United States but children could not. Age might be a determinant in deciding who gets benefits, goods, and services, but only as one among other prognosticators of success. For example, people over eighty or under two years of age might be excluded from consideration for a certain type of surgery because they are unlikely to survive the procedure.

Defenders of egalitarianism hold that what is provided to one person should be available to all who are similarly situated. The advantages of good health care are such that, in fairness, they should be distributed on as equal a basis as possible. There should not be a multitiered system with one level of goods and services for the rich and another for the poor. If we are going to allow some normal short children to have growth hormone for many years at a cost of thousands of dollars a year, then all who are similarly situated should have access to similar services. For expensive or scarce resources, many egalitarians favor lotteries so all those similarly situated have an equal opportunity and are recognized as having equal worth (Childress, 1970; Veatch, 1986). Consequently, if organs for transplantation can only be provided to some children, there should be a lottery among those who meet whatever standards are set. In this way, we acknowledge the value of each person and the importance of fair access of each to scarce or costly benefits, goods, or services. One difficulty for egalitarians is that some people's needs are so great they could consume most of the resources of a health-care system. Robert Veatch (1986) tries to defend a commitment to those who are so disadvantaged they could use unlimited resources, while placing limits on their claims upon other members of society.

In defending egalitarianism, it is difficult to clarify what kind of equality is important. On the one hand, if it is access to the same benefits, goods, and services, age bias and discrimination could be introduced through preference for certain benefits, goods, and services. For example, treatment for prostatic hyperplasia and Alzheimer's disease only helps adults; other care helps adults much more than children, such as treatments for heart disease or lung cancer or treatments at the end of life. Some funding choices discriminate by excluding services equally and for all diseases afflicting people with stigmatizing conditions, such as sexually transmitted diseases. This parallels a problem of utilitarianism, where whole groups could be excluded if society decides, to save money, that none will have treatments for certain conditions.

On the other hand, if equality is understood in terms of outcomes, age bias and discrimination can also be introduced just by the method of collecting and presenting data (Starfield, 1991). In the United States, for example, data collection to determine the health of different populations focuses upon life-threatening illnesses and death. Relatively few children have such morbidity or mortality in comparison to adults, giving the impression that children are generally healthy. This impression, however, is a consequence of how the data are collected. Most children's needs stem from problems that are not life-threatening illnesses, but that have a profound effect on health, such as dental problems, vision impairments, allergies, and asthma. Moreover, although the death rate of children in the United States is low when compared with that of adults, it is the highest in the world when compared with equally affluent countries (Starfield, 1991). Looking at certain outcomes, then, promotes an unfair view of childhood health and morbidity. Programs based upon such data can create unjust age bias against children. Thus, treating everyone as equals is problematic if the measures favor certain groups.

People's willingness to defend egalitarianism depends, in part, on whether they believe it is fair to restrict choices by insisting that no one can have health care that cannot be provided to all on the same basis. If people can squander their assets on frivolous entertainment and flashy clothes, it seems unfair to insist that they cannot spend it on marginally beneficial, exotic, or expensive health care for their families. Some defenders respond that rich people dread single-tiered systems, be-cause it means that they cannot have their usual advantages through money and forces them to live by the same rules as others. They argue that allocation of health care (especially in life and death situations) is too important to be left to unregulated personal choice and market forces. Some defenders of egalitarianism modify their view to permit people to use their discretionary resources as they wish.

Libertarianism. Libertarians generally agree that competent adults should not be forced to do anything by the state unless it prevents harm to third parties. Their coercion is permissible to prevent theft, murder, physical abuse, and fraud, to enforce contracts, or to punish competent people for harming others (Buchanan, 1981). The best-known defender of this view, Robert Nozick (1974), follows the eighteenth-century philosopher John Locke in maintaining that people's right to their fairly obtained property is fundamental and also determines the proper functions of the state and the moral interactions among individuals. People are entitled to their holdings and may dispose of them as they wish, according to this view. States should not redistribute people's wealth in accordance with some pattern of distribution that examines outcomes (such as utilitarianism or egalitarianism) or that uses coercive measures to take people's holdings; and adults should be free to fashion social arrangements out of their ideas of compassion, justice, and solidarity (Engelhardt, 1992). People do not have a responsiblity to be charitable, say libertarians, but acts of charity are praiseworthy and should be encouraged.

Libertarians hold that children's health care is the responsibility of their guardians, not the state. Market forces of supply and demand, and choices about how to use their own money, should shape the kind of health care people select for themselves and their children. If parents want to pay for special services, such as growth hormones or repeated organ transplants, they should be permitted to do so. H. Tristram Engelhardt, Jr., argues that societies can decide morally who is entitled to health care of a certain kind, within certain limitations. But a society does not, for example, have "the moral authority to forbid consensual acts among agreeing adults, such as agreement to sell an organ" (Engelhardt, 1992, p. 10).

Sympathy for libertarianism depends upon whether it is believed to offer enough protection for people, especially for children and impoverished or incompetent adults. This view arguably benefits the wealthy and powerful; since most children are neither, it might create an age bias against children. Libertarians argue that competent adults should pay their own way, but when do people really pay their own way? Typically, people's health-care insurance has gained them access to institutions heavily subsidized by public money. People who "pay their own way" may pay just a bit more for a great deal more in the way of services. Those who cannot pay more are unfairly excluded. Libertarians might agree that separate institutions should be set up where people truly pay their full share, even if that would mean few could afford such added care.

Libertarians usually favor special state protection for children, allowing the state to interfere with parents who endanger, neglect, or harm children. This has included providing children with a "safety net" of basic health-care and social services. A system favoring special benefits based upon redistribution of wealth for competent adults, however, is judged unjust. Hence, a system like that in the United States that provides many social and health benefits to competent—even wealthy—adults but not to children, such as in the allocation of health-care benefits, goods, and services, would be viewed by libertarians as unjust.

Contractarianism.   Contractarians hold that distributions of social goods are fair when impartial people agree upon the procedures used for distribution. The best-known defender of this position is John Rawls, who in A Theory of Justice (1971) and Political Liberalism (1993) contends that the way in which we form stable and just societies is through building consensus that merits endorsement by rational and informed people of good will. This entails commitment to three principles of justice. First, "each person is to have an equal right to the most extensive system of equal basic liberties compatible with a similar system compatible for all." Second, "offices and positions are to be open to all under conditions of equality of fair opportunity—persons with similar abilities and skills are to have equal access to offices and positions." Finally, "social and economic institutions are to be arranged so as to benefit maximally the worst off" (Rawls, 1971, p. 60). These principles are ordered lexically such that the first, or greatest equal-liberty principle, takes precedence over the others when they conflict; and the second, the principle of fair equality of opportunity, takes precedence over the third, the difference principle. Nowhere is health care as a right specifically mentioned in Rawls's attempt to frame the basic structure of a just society. This is understandable, in part, because a society might not have any decent health-care goods, services, or benefits to distribute. In a society that does have such goods, services, and benefits, however, their fair distribution seems central to promoting fair equality of opportunity and benefits to the worst off.

Norman Daniels (1985), building on Rawls's work, argues that we should provide basic care to all, but redistribute health-care goods and services more favorably to children. The moral justification for giving children access to basic health care, argues Daniels, rests on social commitments to what he and Rawls call "fair equality of opportunity" (or affirmative action). Health-care

needs are basic insofar as they promote fair equality of opportunity. Health care for children is especially important in relation to other social goods, because diseases and disabilities inhibit children's capacity to use and develop their talents, thereby curtailing their opportunities. For example, children cannot compete as equals among their peers if they are sick or cannot see or hear the teacher. Thus, a society committed to a fair equality of opportunity for children should provide adequate health care. Daniels holds that in order to assess whose needs are greatest, we have to use objective ways of characterizing medical and social needs; the ranking of needs helps determine what is basic and who profits most from certain services. Using the difference principle, free, additional service might be provided to the poorest children so they could compete more effectively with those from more affluent homes. Unlike utilitarians, who would be guided by where money would have the greatest overall impact on the health of the greatest number of children, contractarians try to bring all children of similar talents to the same level of functioning so they can compete as equals.

Contractarianism has its difficulties. Some regard it as a method for arriving at ethical principles, not as an alternative to views like utilitarianism, egalitarianism, or libertarianism (Veatch, 1986). Accordingly, those who think it generates a unique theory need to clarify how it has a distinct content. In addition, it is hard to specify what is meant by people's normal opportunity ranges or how to apply fair equality of opportunity. It seems to suggest (arguably similar to egalitarianism) the unsatisfactory consequence that we should fund treatments, however exotic and costly, offering a chance for the most disadvantaged to improve their normal opportunity range irrespective of the needs of the many; gifted children could be denied opportunities to excel, as a matter of justice, so others can enhance their normal opportunity range or be brought to roughly the same level of well-being and opportunities of average children. Another problem is that contractarianism presupposes, like utilitarianism, that we have a fair and objective system for ranking which medical and social needs are greatest and who benefits most from given services (Brock, 1982). It is unclear if such a comprehensive and objective ranking is possible. Such "objective" choices about appropriate or useful programs might be heavily mixed with social and personal biases about what promotes a fair equality of opportunity for people with similar talents. These problems, however, do not undermine the contractarians' commitment to the justice of equal opportunity for children, including the fairness of providing basic health and social care for children.

A proposed consensus.   Each of these four theories of justice supports the claim that children are entitled to basic health-care and social services to correct inequalities and promote their flourishing as free and self-determining people who can develop their potential. That defenders of such divergent approaches agree on this entitlement reflects a remarkable consensus that children's distress ought to be relieved whether it is related to inadequate health care, poverty, abuse, neglect, malnutrition, or exploitation. A primary duty of a just society is to promote fairly its children's well-being and opportunities to become self-fulfilled persons through access to basic health-care and social services and to address the inequities resulting from life's natural and social lotteries. Children living in low-income homes in the United States, the richest country in the world, are two to three times as likely as children in high-income homes to be of low birth weight, to get asthma and bacterial meningitis, to have delayed immunizations, and to suffer from lead poisoning. Poor children are also three to four times as likely as rich children to become seriously ill and get multiple illnesses when they get sick (Starfield, 1991). The gap between the rich and the poor is increasing and the rise of poverty is most rapid among children in the world. Health-care costs, driven higher by an aging population and increased demands for expensive technologies, will make it harder for societies to allocate costs justly. Consequently, disputes involving intergenerational and intragenerational allocation are likely to continue as programs compete for funding. Since children depend upon others to advocate on their behalf, adults should continue to set aside their individual interests and consider children's well-being, needs, and opportunities as a matter of justice.

LORETTA M. KOPELMAN

Directly related to this article are the other articles in this entry: HISTORY OF CHILDHOOD, RIGHTS OF CHILDREN, MENTAL-HEALTH ISSUES, *and* CHILD CUSTODY. *For a further discussion of topics mentioned in this article, see the entries* ABUSE, INTERPERSONAL, *article on* CHILD ABUSE; ADOLESCENTS; COMPETENCY; DEATH AND DYING: EUTHANASIA AND SUSTAINING LIFE, *article on* ADVANCE DIRECTIVES; FAMILY; HEALTH-CARE RESOURCES, ALLOCATION OF, *article on* MACROALLOCATION; INFANTS; LIFE, QUALITY OF, *article on* QUALITY OF LIFE IN CLINICAL DECISIONS; *and* RESEARCH POLICY, *especially the article* RISK AND VULNERABLE GROUPS. *For further discussion of surrogate decision making, see* DEATH AND DYING: EUTHANASIA AND SUSTAINING LIFE, *article on* ETHICAL ISSUES. *For a discussion of related ideas, see the entries on* INFORMATION DISCLOSURE; JUSTICE; PATERNALISM; TRUST; UTILITY; *and* VALUE AND VALUATION. *Other relevant material may be found under the entries* CIRCUMCISION; ECONOMIC CONCEPTS IN HEALTH CARE; ETHICS, *article on* TASK OF ETHICS; FUTURE GENERATIONS, OBLIGATIONS TO; *and* MENTALLY DISABLED AND MENTALLY ILL PERSONS.

Bibliography

BLUEBOND-LANGNER, MYRA. 1978. *The Private Worlds of Dying Children.* Princeton, N.J.: Princeton University Press.

BROCK, DAN W. 1982. "Utilitarianism." In *And Justice for All: New Introductory Essays in Ethics and Public Policy,* pp. 217–240. Edited by Tom Regan and Donald VanDeVeer. Totowa, N.J.: Rowman and Allanheld.

———. 1989. "Children's Competence for Health Care Decisionmaking." In *Children and Health Care: Moral and Social Issues,* pp. 181–212. Edited by Loretta M. Kopelman and John C. Moskop. Dordrecht, Netherlands: Kluwer.

BUCHANAN, ALLEN E. 1981. "Justice: A Philosophical Review." In *Justice and Health Care,* pp. 3–21. Edited by Earl E. Shelp. Dordrecht, Netherlands: D. Reidel.

BUCHANAN, ALLEN E., and BROCK, DAN W. 1989. *Deciding for Others: The Ethics of Surrogate Decisionmaking.* New York: Cambridge University Press.

CALLAHAN, DANIEL. 1987. "Terminating Treatment: Age as a Standard." *Hastings Center Report* 17, no. 5:21–25.

———. 1990. *What Kind of Life: The Limits of Medical Progress.* New York: Simon & Schuster.

"Child Abuse and Neglect Prevention and Treatment Program." 1985. *Federal Register* 50, no. 72 (April 15): 14878–14892.

CHILDRESS, JAMES F. 1970. "Who Shall Live When Not All Can Live?" *Soundings* 53 (Winter):339–354.

CLOUSER, K. DANNER. 1973. "'The Sanctity of Life': An Analysis of a Concept." *Annals of Internal Medicine* 78, no. 1:119–125.

COUNCIL FOR INTERNATIONAL ORGANIZATIONS OF MEDICAL SCIENCE (CIOMS). 1993. *International Ethical Guidelines for Biomedical Research Involving Human Subjects.* Geneva: Author.

DANIELS, NORMAN. 1985. *Just Health Care.* Cambridge: At the University Press.

ENGELHARDT, H. TRISTRAM, JR. 1992. "The Search for a Universal System of Ethics: Post-Modern Disappointments and Contemporary Possibilities." In *Ethical Problems in Dialysis and Transplantation,* pp. 3–19. Edited by Carl M. Kjellstrand and John B. Dossetor. Dordrecht, Netherlands: Kluwer.

FADEN, RUTH R.; BEAUCHAMP, TOM L.; and KING, NANCY M. P. 1986. *History and Theory of Informed Consent.* New York: Oxford University Press.

FREEDMAN, BENJAMIN; FUKS, ABRAHAM; and WEIJER, CHARLES. 1993. "*In Loco Parentis:* Minimal Risk as an Ethical Threshold for Research upon Children." *Hastings Center Report* 23, no. 2:13–19.

GERMANY (TERRITORY UNDER ALLIED OCCUPATION, 1945–1955: U.S. ZONE) MILITARY TRIBUNALS. 1947. "Permissible Medical Experiments." In vol. 2 of *Trials of War Criminals Before the Nuremburg Tribunals Under Control Law No. 10,* pp. 181–184. Washington, D.C.: U.S. Government Printing Office.

HOLDER, ANGELA. 1985. *Legal Issues in Pediatrics and Adolescent Medicine.* 2d ed. New Haven, Conn.: Yale University Press.

———. 1989. "Children and Adolescents: Their Right to Decide About Their Own Health Care." In *Children and Health Care: Moral and Social Issues,* pp. 161–172. Edited by Loretta M. Kopelman and John C. Moskop. Dordrecht, Netherlands: Kluwer.

HOLMES, ROBERT L. 1989. "Consent and Decisional Authority in Children's Health Care Decisionmaking: A Reply to Dan Brock." In *Children and Health Care: Moral and Social Issues*, pp. 213–219. Edited by Loretta M. Kopelman and John C. Moskop. Dordrecht, Netherlands: Kluwer.

JANOFSKY, JEFFREY, and STARFIELD, BARBARA. 1981. "Assessment of Risk in Research on Children." *Journal of Pediatrics* 98, no. 5:842–846.

KOOP, C. EVERETT. 1989. "Mercy, Murder, and Morality: Perspectives on Euthanasia: The Challenge of Definition." *Hastings Center Report* 19, no. 1 (special supplement, January–February):2–3.

KOPELMAN, LORETTA M. 1989a. "Charlotte the Spider, Socrates, and the Problem of Evil." In *Children and Health Care: Moral and Social Issues*, pp. 121–131. Edited by Loretta M. Kopelman and John C. Moskop. Dordrecht, Netherlands: Kluwer.

———. 1989b. "When Is the Risk Minimal Enough for Children to Be Research Subjects?" In *Children and Health Care: Moral and Social Issues*, pp. 89–99. Edited by Loretta M. Kopelman and John C. Moskop. Dordrecht, Netherlands: Kluwer.

———. 1993. "Do the 'Baby Doe' Rules Ignore Suffering?" *Second Opinion* 18, no. 4:101–113.

KOPELMAN, LORETTA M.; IRONS, THOMAS G.; and KOPELMAN, ARTHUR E. 1988. "Neonatologists Judge the 'Baby Doe' Regulations." *New England Journal of Medicine* 318, no. 11:677–683.

LASCARI, ANDRE D. 1981. "Risks of Research in Children." *Journal of Pediatrics* 98, no. 5:759–760.

MATTHEWS, GARETH B. 1989. "Children's Conceptions of Illness and Death." In *Children and Health Care: Moral and Social Issues*, pp. 133–146. Edited by Loretta M. Kopelman and John C. Moskop. Dordrecht, Netherlands: Kluwer.

MILL, JOHN STUART. 1863. *Utilitarianism.* London: Parker, Son and Bourn.

NOZICK, ROBERT. 1974. *Anarchy, State and Utopia.* New York: Basic Books.

"Protection of Human Subjects." 1993. 45 CFR 46.

RAWLS, JOHN. 1971. *A Theory of Justice.* Cambridge, Mass.: Harvard University Press.

———. 1993. *Political Liberalism.* New York: Columbia University Press.

REAGAN, RONALD. 1986. "Abortion and the Conscience of the Nation." In *Abortion, Medicine, and the Law*, 3d ed, pp. 352–358. Edited by J. Douglas Butler and David F. Walbert. New York: Facts on File.

RODHAM, HILLARY. 1973. "Children Under the Law." *Harvard Educational Review* 43, no. 4:487–514.

STARFIELD, BARBARA. 1989. "Child Health and Public Policy." In *Children and Health Care: Moral and Social Issues*, pp. 7–22. Edited by Loretta M. Kopelman and John C. Moskop. Dordrecht, Netherlands: Kluwer.

———. 1991. "Childhood Morbidity: Comparisons, Clusters, and Trends." *Pediatrics* 88, no. 3:519–526.

U.N. GENERAL ASSEMBLY. 1960. *Declaration of the Rights of the Child: Adopted by the General Assembly of the United Nations, New York, November 20, 1959.* New York: Author.

U.S. DEPARTMENT OF HEALTH AND HUMAN SERVICES. 1992. *Healthy People 2000: National Health Promotion and Disease-Prevention Objectives. Full Report with Commentary.* DHHS publication no. (PHS) 91–50212. Washington, D.C.: U.S. Government Printing Office.

U.S. PRESIDENT'S COMMISSION FOR THE STUDY OF ETHICAL PROBLEMS IN MEDICINE AND BIOMEDICAL AND BEHAVIORAL RESEARCH. 1982. *Making Health Care Decisions: A Report on the Ethical and Legal Implications of Informed Consent in the Patient-Practitioner Relationship.* Washington, D.C.: Author.

———. 1983. *Deciding to Forego Life-Sustaining Treatment: A Report on the Ethical, Medical, and Legal Issues in Treatment Decisions.* Washington, D.C.: Author.

VEATCH, ROBERT M. 1986. *The Foundation of Justice: Why the Retarded and the Rest of Us Have Claims to Equity.* New York: Oxford University Press.

WORLD MEDICAL ASSOCIATION. 1991. "Declaration of Helsinki." *Law, Medicine and Health Care* 19, nos. 3–4: 264–265.

IV. MENTAL-HEALTH ISSUES

Conceptualizing a domain of "mental health and children" represents an advance in cultural and societal thinking. The various impediments to this view are well known among students of the history of childhood—at least in Western cultures. These include the concept of children as property, and the broader ignorance and denial of children's affective and cognitive development that has found expression in the concept of children as "unfeeling and unthinking."

More modern concepts of children and childhood provide a foundation for focusing on the mental health of children as a vital concern. One testament to this development is the passage in 1989 of the United Nations Convention on the Rights of the Child. The convention provides a view of children and childhood in which mental-health concerns are central, one that goes beyond the ideas contained in the 1959 Declaration of the Rights of the Child.

The convention makes it clear that mental-health issues (e.g., policies that facilitate prevention, access to services, etc.) are primary implications of children's rights. Children, the convention asserts, are entitled to basic psychological resources. These include mandates to ensure family and social identity, empathic and stable care, protection from exploitation, and rehabilitative treatment when experiencing mental-health problems or being exposed to trauma, such as war and abuse.

This rights-focused orientation to the mental health of children reflects a growing appreciation for the scope, depth, range, and subtlety of children's experience. Indeed, in the field of children's mental health there has been a growing recognition and empirical exploration of the existence and characteristics of child variants of most major adult mental-health problems. Two important examples are depression and post-traumatic stress disorder.

Acknowledging the child's perspective

Until the 1970s, many clinicians and scholars expressed doubt that children experience "genuine" depression. The common view held that children (and, according to some observers, even adolescents) were incapable of experiencing full-blown depression (White and Watt, 1973). It is now clear that children do experience depression, but do so and express it differently from adults (e.g., in offering less verbalization concerning mood and symptoms).

Children often mask their depression by denying symptoms to avoid humiliation and embarrassment, to "protect" vulnerable adults who do not appear to be able to tolerate the child's sadness, or to avoid therapeutic intervention that children perceive adversely (e.g., a child may resist the idea of missing recreational activities to attend therapy or may not acknowledge symptoms of depression to avoid causing parental upset or even conflict).

More generally, one of the important breakthroughs in understanding the mental health of children has been the recognition that "what children can tell us depends upon what adults are prepared to hear" (cf. Garbarino et al., 1989). That is, children reveal their mental-health status in ways that make sense to adults *if* the adults have the technical skill and psychological availability necessary to receive the child's messages. For adults to be responsive to the mental-health issues facing children, they need to understand some basic features of child development, particularly the operation of risk and opportunity.

Children face a variety of opportunities and risks for health and development because of their mental and physical makeup and because of the social environments they inhabit. Moreover, social environment affects mental health through its impact on the physical makeup of the child—a notion expressed by the term "social biology." In contrast to sociobiology, which emphasizes a genetic origin for social behavior, social biology concentrates on the social origins of biological phenomena. An example is the impact of economic conditions and social policy on brain growth and development; for example, environmental lead poisoning of children may lead to mental retardation and/or behavioral problems.

These social biological effects are often negative—for example, the impact of poverty and famine on mental retardation, or the mutagenic influence of industrial carcinogens. But they may also be positive—for example, intrauterine surgery or nutritional therapy for a fetus with a genetic disorder. When these social influences operate in psychological or sociological terms, we refer to them as sociocultural opportunities and risks.

"Opportunities for development," then, mean relationships in which children find material, emotional, and social encouragement compatible with their needs and capacities at a specific point in their developing lives. For each child, the exact combination of factors depends upon temperament, family resources, potential, skill, and the role of culture in defining the meaning and social significance of specific characteristics or behaviors, within some very broad guidelines of basic human needs that are renegotiated as development proceeds and situations change.

The effects of risk factors

This complex and important phenomenon has profound implications for understanding the mental health of children. We can start from recent findings regarding the "accumulation of risk." For example, according to a 1987 investigation, the average IQ scores of four-year-old children are related to the number of psychological and social risk factors present in their lives, which include socioeconomic conditions as well as intrafamilial, psychosocial factors (Sameroff et al., 1987).

But this research reveals that the relationship is not simply additive. Average IQ for children with none, one, or two of the factors is above 115. With the addition of a third and then a fourth risk factor, the average IQ score drops precipitously to nearly 85, with relatively little further decrement as there is further accumulation of five through eight risk factors. This is important because IQ plays an important role in resilience and coping. Thus, low IQ is a risk factor for children's mental health. And, as Carl Dunst and Charles Trivett's work reveals (1992), understanding developmental opportunities helps to explain the differences among children that are unaccounted for in an analysis that includes only "risk."

"Windows of opportunity" (opportunity that arises at particular points in development) for intervention on behalf of the mental health of children appear repeatedly across the life course. What may be a threat at one point may be harmless or even developmentally good for a child at another. Classic analysis of the impact of the Great Depression of the 1930s in the United States reveals that its mental health effects were felt most negatively by young children (Elder, 1974). However, some adolescents, particularly girls, benefited from the fact that paternal unemployment often meant special opportunities for enhanced responsibility and status in the family.

The stress of urban life associated with "family adversity" appears to be most potent for young children and most negative for their mental health, yet it can stimulate some adolescents who have had a positive childhood (Bronfenbrenner, 1986). Research on the mental health of children may contribute a great deal to our understanding of the circumstances and conditions that constitute "growth-inducing" rather than debilitating challenges and adversity.

Risks to the mental health of children can come both from direct threats and from the absence of normal, expectable opportunities. The experience of homelessness is one example of a sociocultural risk factor with profound implications for child mental health.

How children integrate experiences

Children create narrative accounts of their lives, accounts that are represented as a worldview, as "social maps" of the world. The child's social maps are both a product and a cause of behavior and development. These social maps reflect the child's experience and competence, and serve to motivate and guide the child in ways that influence the course of his or her development (Garbarino et al., 1992).

Of special concern is the role of traumatic experiences, such as the loss of parents or home, in shaping the processes of memory and "narrative accounting" that provide the raw materials for the child's social maps. Central to the process of social mapping is locating the concept of "home."

The importance of "home"

"Home" implies permanence, a lack of contingency. You have a home when you have a place to go, no matter what. You have a home when there is a place with which you are connected permanently, a place that endures, a place that represents you. Or, as a young homeless child wrote, "A home is where you can grow flowers if you want" (Daly, 1990, p. 2).

It is only a small step from this concept of "home" to the political concept of "homeland" as a sense that one is part of a nation, that one belongs somewhere in the political sense. Both home and homeland may be important resources in identity formation, and a childhood lack of either or both may lead to mental-health problems associated with alienation, conduct disorder, rootlessness, violence, and depression in adolescence. Shame—individual and collective—can be both a product and a cause of aggression (Gilligan, 1991). Thus, we are driven to seek to improve the mental health of children as both a primary and a secondary issue in the larger issue of violence.

Understanding the child's experience of "home" may help sort out the divergent psychological impacts and characters of experiences that appear similar on the surface, such as being an "immigrant" and a "refugee," or having "moved" and being "displaced." With millions of children worldwide suffering homelessness, this is a crucial issue for further study (cf. Garbarino et al., 1991). Seeing homelessness as traumatic reminds us that trauma is one of the central underlying concepts in understanding the mental health of children.

Childhood experience of trauma

Trauma—the overwhelming arousal and cognitive dislocation that results from experiencing horrible events—is an important field of study for those who seek to understand mental health in childhood. As with depression, it was once thought that children were incapable of experiencing genuine trauma (Van der Kolk, 1987). But research and clinical experience since 1980 have established that trauma and post-traumatic stress disorder play significant roles in the mental health of children.

Children experience trauma in many settings: televised violence, community violence, domestic violence, war, homelessness. All point to the need to develop a better understanding of the impact of trauma on childhood (Garbarino et al., 1992) as part of a larger commitment to understand the mental-health issues facing children.

Children may suffer from post-traumatic stress disorder as a consequence of their experiences at home, in school, or in the community. Its symptoms in children include sleep disturbances, daydreaming, re-creating trauma in play, extreme startle responses, diminished expectations for the future, and even biochemical changes in their brains that impair social and academic behavior. Trauma can produce significant psychological problems that interfere with learning and appropriate social behavior in school and the family, the bedrocks for mental health in childhood.

It is clear that the children least prepared to master trauma outside the home are those who experience psychological, physical, or sexual maltreatment at home. When children are traumatized, they can have memory problems and distort information (Terr, 1990). This increases the importance of improving our ability to help children tell their stories. In seeking information from children, we must be sensitive to their need to construct a narrative account of self and family that meets their emotional needs in a way that is consistent with their cognitive resources (Garbarino et al., 1989).

Hundreds of thousands of children face the mental-health challenge of living with chronic community violence, whether it derives from war or domestic crime. For example, since 1974, the rate of serious assault in Chicago has increased 400 percent; other major metropolitan areas reveal similar patterns. Interviews with families living in public housing projects in Chicago and other urban centers reveal that virtually all the children have had firsthand experiences with shooting by the age of five. Some 30 percent of the children living in high-crime neighborhoods of the city have witnessed a homicide by the time they are fifteen years old, and more than 70 percent have witnessed a serious assault (Garbarino et al., 1992). In Brazil, death squads terrorize and assassinate impoverished "street children." In refugee camps around the world, children witness and are subject to violence and exploitation.

The experience of community violence takes place within a larger context of risk for these children. They are often poor; often live in families where the father is absent; often contend with their parents' depression or substance abuse; often are raised by parents with little education or few employment prospects; and often are exposed to domestic violence. This constellation of risk by itself creates enormous mental-health challenges for young children. For them, the trauma of community violence is often literally the straw that breaks the camel's back.

Conclusion

The task of dealing with the effects of this environmental conspiracy falls to the people who care for these children—their parents and other relatives, teachers, and counselors. But these adults who take on this task face enormous challenges of their own. Human-service professionals and educators working in the high-violence areas of our communities are themselves traumatized by their exposure to violence, and mental-health agencies often "evacuate" from these areas, thus exacerbating the mental-health issues facing the children who remain. Finding the will and resources to address this "ecological conspiracy" against children is one of the major ethical issues faced by professionals, policymakers, and citizens everywhere.

JAMES GARBARINO

Directly related to this article are the other articles in this entry: HISTORY OF CHILDHOOD, RIGHTS OF CHILDREN, HEALTH-CARE AND RESEARCH ISSUES, *and* CHILD CUSTODY. *Also directly related to this article are the entries* MENTAL HEALTH; *and* MENTAL ILLNESS. *For a further discussion of topics mentioned in this article, see the entries* ABUSE, INTERPERSONAL, *article on* CHILD ABUSE; ADOLESCENTS; CARE; ENVIRONMENTAL HEALTH; FAMILY; FETUS; HOMICIDE; NARRATIVE; PUBLIC HEALTH, *articles on* DETERMINANTS OF PUBLIC HEALTH, *and* HISTORY OF PUBLIC HEALTH; RIGHTS; SUBSTANCE ABUSE; TRAGEDY; *and* WARFARE. *For a further discussion of related ideas, see the entries* POPULATION POLICIES, *section on* DONOR AGENCIES, *article on* MIGRATION AND REFUGEES; RISK; SEXUAL DEVELOPMENT; SEXUAL ETHICS; SEXUAL IDENTITY; SUICIDE; *and* VALUE AND VALUATION. *Other relevant material may be found under the entries* ADVERTISING; AIDS; CIRCUMCISION; COMMITMENT TO MENTAL INSTITUTIONS; DEATH; DEATH, ATTITUDES TOWARD; DEATH EDUCATION; FOOD POLICY; HAZARDOUS WASTES AND TOXIC SUBSTANCES; *and* PAIN AND SUFFERING.

Bibliography

BRONFENBRENNER, URIE. 1986. "Ecology of the Family as a Context for Human Development: Research Perspectives." *Developmental Psychology* 22, no. 6:723–742.

DALY, MARTIN. 1990. "The True Meaning of 'Home.'" In *The Better Homes Foundation 1989 Annual Report.* Boston: Better Homes Foundation.

DUNST, CARL, and TRIVETT, CHARLES. 1992. "Risk and Opportunity Factors Influencing Parent and Child Functioning." Paper presented at the Ninth Annual Smoky Mountain Winter Institute, Asheville, N.C., March.

ELDER, GLEN H. 1974. *Children of the Great Depression: Social Change in Life Experience.* Chicago: University of Chicago Press.

GARBARINO, JAMES. 1992. *Children and Families in the Social Environment.* 2d ed. Hawthorne, N.Y.: Aldine de Gruyter.

GARBARINO, JAMES; DUBROW, NANCY; KOSTELNY, KATHLEEN; and PARDO, CAROLE, eds. 1992. *Children in Danger: Coping with the Consequences of Community Violence.* San Francisco: Jossey-Bass.

GARBARINO, JAMES; KOSTELNY, KATHLEEN; and DUBROW, NANCY. 1991. *No Place to Be a Child: Growing up in a War Zone.* Lexington, Mass.: Lexington Books.

GARBARINO, JAMES; STOTT, FRANCES M.; and THE FACULTY OF THE ERIKSON INSTITUTE. 1989. *What Children Can Tell Us: Eliciting, Interpreting, and Evaluating Critical Information from Children.* San Francisco: Jossey-Bass.

GILLIGAN, JAMES. 1991. "Shame and Humiliation: The Emotions of Individual and Collective Violence." Paper presented at the 1991 Erikson Lectures, Carpenter Center, Harvard University, May 23.

SAMEROFF, ARNOLD J.; SEIFER, ROBERT; BAROCAS, ROGER; ZAX, MARTIN; and GREENSPAN, STANLEY. 1987. "Intelligence Quotient Scores of 4-Year-Old Children: Social–Environmental Risk Factors." *Pediatrics* 79, no. 3: 343–350.

TERR, LENORE. 1990. *Too Scared to Cry: Psychic Trauma in Childhood.* New York: Harper & Row.

VAN DER KOLK, BESSEL A., ed. 1987. *Psychological Trauma.* Washington, D.C.: American Psychiatric Press.

WHITE, ROBERT W., and WATT, NORMAN F. 1973. *The Abnormal Personality.* 4th ed. New York: Ronald Press.

V. CHILD CUSTODY

Child custody disputes arise in various ways, but by far the most common need for resolution occurs when the child's parents separate or divorce. When the previously intact family splits into two new households and the parents cannot agree on the child's future care, some external authority like a court or arbitrator must determine arrangements. Even after a custody order is imposed as part of the divorce judgment, parents quite often return to court seeking to enforce the terms of the decree or to modify them in light of the inevitable adaptations that accompany the upheaval of divorce.

Divorce and child custody

Divorce in the United States now occurs every thirteen seconds, and estimates are that by the year 2000, one out of every two marriages will end in divorce. As the concept of marriage evolves away from a status controlled by the state and toward a privately negotiated agreement fixing spousal rights and obligations, the legal action for divorce has also changed. Modern divorce now rather closely resembles ancient divorce recognized by Talmudic and Roman law, when marriages were privately arranged and quite routinely dissolved upon petition of one or both spouses. This has not been always so.

With the rise of Christianity in the fourth century, marriage was reconceptualized as a sacramental and civilly binding relationship, dissoluble only by death or annulment. In the Anglo-American legal system, divorce was not authorized until the mid-nineteenth century, and even then could be granted only upon proof that one spouse had committed a specific marital fault, such as desertion, adultery, or cruel treatment. Furthermore, if both spouses were guilty of fault, the divorce would be denied because this equitable remedy was available only to the "faultless." Occasionally, doctors and other health professionals would be summoned as witnesses in divorce proceedings—for example, to prove that one of the spouses had sought treatment for emotional or physical abuse inflicted by the other, or to support a charge that one was a chronic alcoholic or mentally ill (in states that recognized those additional grounds for divorce).

The fault system created a constellation of ethical issues for the spouses, for their lawyers, for health-care professionals, and for society as a whole. Some spouses agreed to perjury or the suppression of evidence in order to end what they deemed an intolerable union. Other desperate spouses simply abandoned their families and began new relationships with others, creating for their legal spouse, new mate, and children legal entanglements that were often not unraveled until their deaths. Perhaps most important, forcing husband and wife to publicly accuse each other of serious marital misconduct destroyed whatever goodwill might have existed between them and imperiled their willingness to work cooperatively in providing care and support for any children of the marriage.

With the 1966 publication in England of *Putting Asunder,* an influential study of the fault system of divorce initiated by the Archbishop of Canterbury, and with the 1971 promulgation of the Uniform Marriage

and Divorce Act in the United States, divorce became more easily and inexpensively available. Now all states have modified their laws to authorize the granting of a divorce on "no-fault" grounds, that is, upon the assertion by one spouse that the marriage is irretrievably broken or by proof of the spouses' voluntary separation for some stated period. As a matter of public policy, all states now acknowledge that marital misconduct cannot be neatly circumscribed in any enumeration of spousal faults, that the law cannot force intimacy or even goodwill, and that requiring proof of fault engenders more social harm than good.

Although many mischiefs of the divorce fault system have been eliminated, there remain personal, moral, and economic costs for many divorcing spouses and their children. Members suffer not only emotionally but also economically when their family falls apart (Weitzman, 1985; Wallerstein and Kelly, 1980; Wallerstein and Blakeslee, 1989). As Margaret Mead observed:

> Each American child learns, early and in terror, that his whole security depends on that single set of parents who, more often than not, are arguing in the next room over some detail in their lives. A desperate demand upon the permanence and all-satisfyingness of monogamous marriage is set up in the cradle. What will happen to me if anything goes wrong? If Mommy dies, if Daddy dies, if Daddy leaves Mommy, or Mommy leaves Daddy? are the questions no American child can escape. (1970)

Children's well-being can become further compromised when the parents engage in a legal battle over their custody.

No one knows precisely how many custody disputes are litigated each year, but some national assessments indicate that 35,000 (10 percent of all divorces) involve custody trials (Crippen, 1990). When the numbers of postdivorce disputes and challenges to a parent's custody by nonparents are added, it is obvious that child custody determinations consume significant social and legal resources.

Custody disputes between parents

Legal doctrine governing child-custody determinations has swung like a pendulum in its preferences for fathers vis-à-vis mothers. As a result of Roman law's doctrine of *patriae potestas* (paternal authority), the father possessed full authority over his child, originally including the power of life or death. This patriarchal legal system denied a child's mother the right to challenge her husband's decision making as long as he was alive and competent. Even if the child's mother and father lived apart, the mother had no cause of action for custody because her natural rights to the child were held to be subordinate to the father's. However, in the 1840s, with the beginning of the women's rights movement, equal custody and guardianship rights were among the reformers' primary objectives.

By the end of the nineteenth century, the "tender years" doctrine was entrenched and the mother replaced the father as the preferred parent in child-custody disputes. The definition of a child of tender years varied from state to state, ranging from preschoolers to any dependent child. Some scholars attribute this doctrinal shift to the influence of Sigmund Freud's work on the importance of the mother–child relationship in early childhood. Others credit the shift in custodial preference to an amalgam of social developments: the change from an agrarian, home-centered economy to an industrial economy; the greater earning power of men in the labor force; and the efficiencies of role diversification in parenting and family life.

Until the middle of the twentieth century, marital fault as grounds for divorce also affected the award of child custody. Proof of a mother's marital misconduct was commonly used to overcome the "tender years" preference that would otherwise favor her. Proof of any ground for divorce tended to disqualify a parent, and custody was bluntly granted as a bonus to whichever spouse prevailed in the divorce action. When hearing evidence of adultery or fault causing or justifying the end of the spouses' adult relationship, courts rarely sought to determine whether the parent's conduct affected his or her capability of being a conscientious and loving caretaker of the child.

It was not until the 1960s that U.S. legal doctrine settled into what is now the nearly universal standard of awarding custody in parent–parent disputes: "best interests of the child." Theoretically the "best interests of the child" rule avoids a presumption or preference based purely upon the gender of the parent. This standard encourages a court to focus upon the unique needs of the particular child and his or her parents' comparative capabilities for meeting those needs. Advocates of the "best interests of the child" rule also point out that acceptance of this rule is evidence that the law has moved away from considering the child purely as property, having no needs or rights of his or her own.

Custody disputes between parents and nonparents

Child-custody disputes can also arise in actions unrelated to the parents' divorce. Typically, such conflicts stem from formal or informal arrangements made with relatives or friends by parents seeking temporary care for their children. When the terms of these arrangements are not clearly articulated as to the duration of care or other conditions, disputes can occur, usually when a parent seeks the return of the child. Litigation can also arise when a relative or family friend asserts that the parent-caretaker is providing inadequate care for the child or is abusing the child.

Until the mid-eighteenth century, no one had a legal claim to contest a child's care and control except the child's biological parents. Although in time the legal authority of the child's father became extended to the mother, the "parental rights" doctrine stopped there, foreclosing any challenge about the quality of parental care from concerned outsiders. Finally, the Chancery courts of England began accepting petitions addressed to the king as *parens patriae* (the father of the country), asking that he exercise his authority "for the benefit of such who are incapable to protect themselves" from mistreatment by living parents (*Butler v. Freeman*, 1756, p. 302). As a result, courts' doors were opened to charges that a child's parent or parents had failed in the performance of their parental duties. Today the *parens patriae* doctrine is the justification underlying the assertion of U.S. courts' jurisdiction over abuse, neglect, and delinquency cases as well as over child-custody disputes pitting parents against relatives, foster parents, and other would-be caretakers.

Some U.S. courts still adhere to the parental-rights doctrine in parent–third party custody disputes, requiring a demonstration that the biological parent is unfit or has relinquished his or her rights to custody before custody will be awarded to a nonparent claimant. "Unfitness" is usually quite narrowly defined to include only certain types of extreme parental misconduct—such as cruel treatment of the child, failure to provide necessities, and abandonment—as well as mental illness, drug or alcohol addiction, and other types of incapacity. According to the parental-rights doctrine, biological connection between parent and child is superior to any other adult's claim of concern for or actual caretaking of the child. The needs or preferences of the child are ignored as irrelevant.

In the 1970s, the force of this ancient doctrine began to dissipate with the publication of psychological evidence challenging the law's nearly impregnable presumption that custody should be awarded on the basis of the existence of blood ties between the claimants and the child (Goldstein et al., 1973, 1979). Child psychologists and psychiatrists urged that in custody disputes, the child's interests and needs should be paramount and that courts should discount parents' claims to proprietary "rights." They urged the universal adoption of the "best interests of the child" standard to resolve all custody disputes, noting that the most important determinants of healthy child development are stability and continuity of caregiving that permit the child to form strong emotional attachments. Thus, logically, whoever has served as a child's "psychological parent" should be preferred over an adult who, though related by blood, has not been involved in nurturing the child. As a result of the influence of this social-science research, the majority of U.S. courts have now adopted the "best interests of the child" rule in deciding custody disputes between parents and other claimants. Consequently, some unrelated but longtime caretakers of a child can now prevail in a dispute with the child's biological parents even if the parents are fit, able, and willing to provide for the child's needs.

Determining the "best interests of the child"

Critics of the "best interests" rule have scoffed that it is a nonrule, so broad as to be meaningless as a control on a court's discretion. What information is relevant to an assessment of a specific child's interests or needs and of the comparative capabilities of the mother or father or other caregiver to meet these needs? The question may be better formulated as, What is *irrelevant* to such a determination? since over the years, scholars have identified hundreds of factors cited by various courts as criteria for a "best interests" evaluation. Expert witnesses such as psychiatrists, psychologists, social workers, or other mental health professionals can assist the court in properly weighting the most important of these usually conflicting criteria. For example, in a change-of-custody dispute, a psychologist might testify that stability and continuity of care are more important to the child's healthy development than the challenging parent's greater affluence, better health, or superior moral character.

The role of witness. Health-care professionals are often summoned to present their assessments of both the child's needs and the strengths and weaknesses of the parents. According to the rules of evidence of every state, expert testimony is admissible to assist a court in making a just decision. In custody disputes, a litigant is permitted to hire an expert, such as a child psychiatrist or child psychologist, to evaluate parents and child, and to offer an assessment and advisory recommendation as to which parent should be named the child's primary custodian. Such expertise certainly provides information relevant to custody determinations, and the training and skills of such clinicians seem superior, in this regard, to the exclusively legal training received by most judges.

Many ethical issues confront medical professionals who agree to serve as expert witnesses. First, any evaluation or description of treatment may be privileged. When a patient subpoenas his or her own physician or therapist to testify, the privilege is waived. The privilege becomes a bar to testimony only when the nonpatient party attempts to force such disclosures. Even so, the patient may be caught in a dilemma: He or she may be more damaged by the inference that there is an attempt to hide relevant but damaging information. Even if not legally privileged, information related by a patient to the professional may be confidential. Ethical conflicts can occur when the physician or therapist is forced by candor to supply information that will jeopardize any future therapeutic relationship.

Second, when asked to evaluate a person's fitness for custody, and having no treatment relationship with that person, the health-care professional may find that he or she lacks sufficient case history or contact time with all family members to make an adequate assessment of children's special needs, and other critical aspects of family dynamics. Some lawyers, misperceiving their profession's ethical restraints upon zealous advocacy, may search for an expert willing to ratify their client's objectives by writing an evaluation biased in the client's favor. In every city there are "guns for hire," health-care professionals who are willing to shape an evaluation or testimony to support the claims of the employing attorney. Yet there are other professionals who, refusing to compromise their objectivity and integrity, prepare candid evaluations that may damage the prospects of the referring lawyer's client.

There is nothing in the Model Rules of Professional Conduct that requires an attorney to offer in evidence an unfavorable evaluation of the client in a custody dispute. Although the trial court has inherent authority to appoint its own expert witness or to summon an evaluator as the court's witness, this power is rarely exercised. Furthermore, under the child-abuse reporting laws of most states, a mental-health professional is required only to report the physical, psychological, or sexual abuse of a child. However, short of reasonable grounds to suspect such extreme harm to the child, the professional need not report lesser concerns to the child-welfare authorities. Of course, the lawyer–client and health-care professional–patient privilege also prevents the revelation of some damning disclosures made in the context of consultation. Consequently, both lawyers and health-care professionals experience significant ethical problems when a custody-seeking parent is perceived as being seriously flawed but yet not abusive. In this instance, the legal system depends on the adversarial system, including pretrial discovery and trial cross-examination, to bring out such damaging evidence for the court's consideration.

These intractable ethical issues have prompted some critics to propose that expert evaluations and testimony should not be permitted in most child-custody disputes. Many social scientists have argued that health-care professionals ordinarily are concerned with therapeutic issues that may be irrelevant to a custody decision, and consequently, health-care professionals are ill-equipped to answer the sorts of questions that the legal system poses.

Only the grossest sorts of projections can be made regarding the future behavior of any individual on the basis of past reports or current observations. Anna Freud called such predictions "difficult and hazardous" (1958). The expert's task is further complicated by the fact that the relationships, responsibilities, and adaptations forged in the triad of the former intact family will radically change upon divorce. Furthermore, children are always "moving targets" of concern: As the child matures, his or her needs will change (Coons et al., 1991).

Even if the medical expert were able to avoid or minimize these conflicts in a particular case, many social critics have expressed concern about converting child-custody determinations into a battle of medical experts. The embattled parents may have unequal ability to retain expert witnesses; hired experts may be tempted to tailor their recommendations to the cut of their employer; and judges may lack the ability to make a proper evaluation of the expertise of the evaluator. To mitigate these problems, some courts contract with independent clinicians who can provide neutral assessments at state expense for parents who cannot afford the fees.

"Best-interests" theory. More fundamental societal issues inhere in the "best interests of the child" decision-making formulation. While there may be collective agreement about what constitutes extremely harmful or grossly inadequate parenting behaviors or "parental unfitness," "good" or "better" parenting is more likely to be determined on the basis of individualized values (Mnookin, 1975). Between two parents who are eager and able to meet the ordinary needs of their child, is the warmth and nurturing of one to be preferred over the other's high expectations or consistent discipline? Any custody decision maker or adviser brings to an evaluation his or her own hierarchy of desirable parental qualities, and reasonable persons can differ about the weight to be accorded to a parent's sense of humor, flexibility, sensitivity, punctuality, moral rectitude, and countless other aspects of personality and character. Similarly, reasonable persons can differ about the needs and flexibility of a child. Is cultural mainstreaming of a child with an urban parent better for the child than preservation of the child's ethnic heritage with a parent who lives in a tribal community? Is a child "harmed" by living with a parent who has remarried a person of a different race or who has established a new intimate relationship with someone of the same gender?

As a result of the ambiguities of the "best interests" rule, scholars, legislatures, and courts continue to search for ways to refine the substantive standard for child-custody decision making. Some states direct the trial court to award custody to the "primary caretaker" when considering the child's best interests, unless there is evidence of the caretaker's unfitness to continue in that role. Accentuating the child's need for stability and continuity of care and seeking to minimize child-custody litigation, the "primary caretaker" standard functions to confirm as custodian whichever parent had been the child's primary caregiver before the family's breakup. Of course, the difficulty of this standard is that in families that share child care, it may not always be possible to determine which parent has assumed the lead; thus the rule may lead to unjust results by focusing upon the quantification of caregiving. The "primary caretaker" standard also reinforces role attributions previously assumed for reasons other than the mother's or father's talent or desire to be the primary parent, such as the greater earning ability in the labor market of the "secondary" caretaker. (For other criticisms, see the summary in Crippen, 1990.)

Many U.S. jurisdictions modify the "best interests" rule when the custody of an adolescent is at stake. At some point, typically around age twelve, a child is thought to have matured to the extent that his or her own perceptions of needs and of the parents' comparative capabilities ought to be taken in account. Although no state law forces an unwilling child to state a preference, courts in most states are instructed to consider the opinions of older children. Aside from considerations of maturity, such rules tacitly acknowledge that a custody order forcing an adolescent to remain where he or she does not want to be is unlikely to be enforceable. Such rules have been justified not only on notions of maturity but also on adolescents' capability of frustrating any order in opposition to their desires by running away to the preferred custodian or otherwise expressing antipathy to the appointed one. While such a rule permits an older child to voice personal needs free from the potential distortions of interpreters or representatives, critics point out that such rules can subject children to intolerable pressure from competing parents and can create estrangement between the child and the rejected parent.

Finally, there is now a clear trend toward "joint custody" judgments. Traditionally a judgment in a disputed custody case resulted in one parent's being named the child's legal custodian, with residual rights, including visitation, granted to the other parent. The sole legal custodian had full authority to make major and minor decisions affecting the child's care and development, thus effectively barring the other parent from the decision-making process. Reformers urged that custody judgments should mirror as closely as possible the coparenting model of the intact family and should maintain the authority and involvement of both parents in the child's life. Most U.S. jurisdictions now encourage judgments of joint custody. Although typically one parent will become the child's primary physical custodian, usually for the school year, joint custody requires at least the consultation of both parents, if not their agreement, before important decisions affecting the child are made.

The major stumbling block to a joint-custody judgment is that it is unlikely to reduce future acrimony and relitigation unless the parents can learn mutual accommodation skills that they may have lacked when living together.

The process for determining custody

Although since the 1890s both law and the social sciences have concentrated upon the development of the substantive standard that ought to govern custody determinations, many critics now believe that the more fruitful reform lies in redesigning the process for making such judgments.

The traditional process of adjudicating custody rights in U.S. courtrooms exacts heavy costs. Each adult contestant is represented by his or her attorney, and the trial is conducted as an adversarial proceeding. Contested child-custody matters can cost thousands of dollars in pretrial preparation, and the trials can last for many days. Each of the adult parties presents lay and expert witnesses who relate their supportive and highly subjective observations about the adult's parenting capabilities. Each party has the right to cross-examine the other's witnesses. From this welter of conflicting evidence and often acrimonious battle, what Andrew Watson (1969) has called a modern Armageddon, the court is asked to determine who should be named a child's legal custodian.

Most custody disputes, like other controversies, are resolved by a negotiated settlement between counsel for the parents, and the proposed judgment is submitted to the court for its review and approval. Yet the "shadow" of litigation and its combative tactics infects these more informal negotiations. The parent less able to bear the costs of litigation and more fearful of losing custody may feel pressure to settle for less property or support in exchange for some secure custody rights. In negotiated settlements, the discretion inherent in the "best interests of the child" rule may simply be transferred from the court to the parents' lawyers, causing the agreement to reflect their personal values (Mnookin and Kornhauser, 1979).

One of the earliest suggested reforms of the U.S. adversarial system was motivated by concerns about the unrepresented child caught in the middle of a custody dispute. Certainly the lawyers retained by the parents often experience substantial conflicts of interest. If the client insists on purely vindictive strategies or is known to be abusive toward the child, the attorney should withdraw as counsel. Otherwise, the *Standards of Conduct* of the American Academy of Matrimonial Lawyers (1991) and the "Model Rules of Professional Conduct" of the American Bar Association (1992) provide little guidance to an attorney whose client's expressed wish or exhibited conduct is contrary to the attorney's assessment of the child's needs and best interests. Reformers have urged that independent counsel be appointed for the child during custody litigation. In most states, by express statutory authorization or by what is perceived as the court's inherent power, a lawyer or specially trained person can be appointed by the court to serve as a court-appointed special advocate or guardian *ad litem.* A guardian *ad litem* is a person appointed to represent a child for the duration of particular litigation, such as the custody dispute. Such appointments are quite common in Canada and Great Britain but are rare in most U.S. jurisdictions. Many critics question whether adding yet another lawyer to the fray is worth the added expense, delay, and potentially heightened adversarial character of the proceedings. Others point out that the guardian's role is unclear: Is the guardian bound by the child's wishes and perception of interests, or should the guardian exercise his or her personal judgment about how the child's needs would be best served? Is the guardian an advocate or a judge?

Since the 1970s, some critics have sought more radical changes in the way custody disputes are resolved, arguing that both litigation and lawyer-dominated negotiation provide a forum for continuing hostility. Externally imposed, authoritarian judgments are unworkable and unwise modes of conflict resolution within the context of ongoing relationships. Instead, reformers have asserted that parents should be encouraged to use mediation as a means of working out coparenting plans for their child's future care. Most states now broadly define by statute the professional groups that can be approved or licensed as mediators. Typically, lawyers, psychiatrists, psychologists, and professionals with graduate degrees in counseling, social work, psychology, or marriage and family counseling are authorized to serve as mediators. Some advocates of mediation have proposed that custody disputes should be removed from courts and replaced by mediation. If they cannot be resolved by mediation, then binding arbitration should be employed.

Longitudinal studies of children's adjustment after their parents' divorce indicate that the greatest risk of emotional and mental illness stems from the parents' continuing hostility and the child's loss of meaningful contact with both parents (Wallerstein and Kelly, 1980). As a modest beginning, many U.S. courts now offer programs conducted by mental-health professionals to educate divorcing parents about the fears and needs of their child after the divorce, if reconciliation and reconstitution of the family are impossible. Furthermore, in some states, parents are required to attempt to mediate and custom-tailor the terms and conditions of their personalized custody and visitation arrangements. Under the tutelage of a skilled mediator, parents can learn conflict management and accommodation of mutual needs, skills crucial to the peaceful resolution of future disagreements.

Skeptics of mediation document the recent trend toward joint custody and mediation as a professional power shift from lawyers and the legal system to the "helping professions" and a therapeutic model of decision making. They point out that the justice of any resolution depends upon the reflection of widely held values and the accuracy of fact-finding, essentials best preserved by laws and the legal process (Fineman, 1988). Feminists have expressed alarm that mediation cannot correct persistent power imbalances that disadvantage mothers in private ordering of custody arrangements. However, while mediation is not a panacea for dispute resolution, it offers bright hope for many parents and seems preferable to the fang and claw of litigation.

Conclusion

Twentieth-century family law has completed two revolutions: the conversion to "no-fault" divorce and the adoption of the "best interests of the child" standard in custody disputes. The third reform wave, recognition of alternatives like mediation for the resolution of custody disputes, is still in progress.

Child-custody law has been enormously influenced by the disciplines of psychology and psychiatry. As a result, statutory law and court decisions now demonstrate a greater sensitivity to the needs of all family members, and the children have been repositioned at the center of the process of resolution. The search for the perfect standard for resolving child-custody disputes will continue, but the brightest prospects for minimizing trauma for both children and parents now seem to lie in refashioning the process of deciding custody. Predictably, the future role of health professionals will shift from giving expert testimony at trials to serving as dispute mediators or providing counseling to adults and children who are adjusting to new family life patterns. Health professionals will also bear a continuing responsibility to ensure that the law and legal processes reflect the findings of social science.

Courts may continue to play an authoritative role when parents are unable to mediate their differences or when they are abusive or otherwise unfit, but resort to judges is now being seen as the last resort in resolving custody disputes. As a reflection of the need to reduce present and future discord over the parenting of a child, alternatives to adversarial litigation are now being implemented that empower the best decision makers, the child's parents or caretakers, to work cooperatively for the best interests of the child.

LUCY S. McGOUGH

Directly related to this article are the other articles in this entry: HISTORY OF CHILDHOOD, RIGHTS OF CHILDREN, HEALTH-CARE AND RESEARCH ISSUES, *and* MENTAL-HEALTH ISSUES. *For a further discussion of topics mentioned in this article, see the entries* ABUSE, INTERPERSONAL, *especially the article on* CHILD ABUSE; ADOLESCENTS; CONFIDENTIALITY; EXPERT TESTIMONY; FAMILY; MARRIAGE AND OTHER DOMESTIC PARTNERSHIPS; PRIVACY IN HEALTH CARE; PROTESTANTISM; *and* ROMAN CATHOLICISM. *For a discussion of related ideas, see the entries* LOVE; PATERNALISM; *and* VALUE AND VALUATION. *Other relevant material may be found under the entries* ADOPTION; FEMINISM; PROFESSIONAL–PATIENT RELATIONSHIP; SOCIAL WORK IN HEALTH CARE; *and* WOMEN, *article on* HISTORICAL AND CROSS-CULTURAL PERSPECTIVES.

Bibliography

AMERICAN ACADEMY OF MATRIMONIAL LAWYERS. 1991. *Bounds of Advocacy: American Academy of Matrimonial Lawyers Standards of Conduct.* Chicago: Author.

AMERICAN BAR ASSOCIATION. 1992. "Model Rules of Professional Conduct." In *Selected Statutes, Rules and Standards on the Legal Profession.* Edited by John S. Dzienkowski. St. Paul, Minn.: West.

ARCHBISHOP OF CANTERBURY'S GROUP ON THE DIVORCE LAW. 1966. *Putting Asunder: A Divorce Law for Contemporary Society.* London: SPCK.

Butler v. Freeman. 1756. Amb. 301, 302, 27 Eng. Rep. 204.

CHAMBERS, DAVID L. 1984. "Rethinking the Substantive Rules for Custody Disputes in Divorce." *Michigan Law Review* 83, no. 3:477–569.

CLARK, HOMER H. 1988. *The Law of Domestic Relations in the United States.* 2d ed. St. Paul, Minn.: West.

COONS, JOHN E.; MNOOKIN, ROBERT H.; and SUGARMAN, STEPHEN D. 1991. "Puzzling over Children's Rights." *Brigham Young University Law Review* 1991:307–350.

CRIPPEN, GARY. 1990. "Stumbling Beyond Best Interests of the Child: Reexamining Child Custody Standard-Setting in the Wake of Minnesota's Four-Year Experiment with the Primary Caretaker Preference." *Minnesota Law Review* 75, no. 2:427–503.

ELLSWORTH, PHOEBE C., and LEVY, ROBERT J. 1969. "Legislative Reform of Child Custody Adjudication: An Effort to Rely on Social Science Data in Formulating Legal Policies." *Law and Society Review* 4, no. 2:167–233.

FINEMAN, MARTHA. 1988. "Dominant Discourse, Professional Language, and Legal Change in Child Custody Decision-making." *Harvard Law Review* 101, no. 4:727–774.

FREUD, ANNA. 1958. "Child Observation and Prediction of Development: A Memorial Lecture in Honor of Ernst Kris." *Psychoanalytic Study of the Child* 13:92–116.

GLENDON, MARY ANN. 1986. "Fixed Rules and Discretion in Contemporary Family Law and Succession Law." *Tulane Law Review* 60, no. 6:1165–1197.

GOLDSTEIN, JOSEPH; FREUD, ANNA; and SOLNIT, ALBERT J.

1973. *Beyond the Best Interests of the Child*. New York: Free Press.

———. 1979. *Before the Best Interests of the Child*. New York: Free Press.

"Lawyering for the Child: Principles of Representation in Custody and Visitation Disputes Arising from Divorce." 1978. *Yale Law Journal* 87, no. 6:1126–1190.

MARLOW, LENARD, and SAUBER, S. RICHARD. 1990. "In Whose Best Interests?" In their *The Handbook of Divorce Mediation*, pp. 73–87. New York: Plenum Press.

MCGOUGH, LUCY S., and SHINDELL, LAWRENCE M. 1978. "Coming of Age: The Best Interests of the Child Standard in Parent–Third Party Custody Disputes." *Emory Law Journal* 27:209–245.

MNOOKIN, ROBERT H. 1975. "Child-Custody Adjudication: Judicial Functions in the Face of Indeterminancy." *Law and Contemporary Problems* 39, no. 3:226–293.

MNOOKIN, ROBERT H., and KORNHAUSER, LEWIS. 1979. "Bargaining in the Shadow of the Law: The Case for Divorce." *Yale Law Review* 88, no. 5:950–997.

NEELY, RICHARD. 1984. "The Primary Caretaker Parent Rule: Child Custody and the Dynamics of Greed." *Yale Law Policy Review* 3, no. 1:168–186.

POUND, ROSCOE. 1960. "Discretion, Dispensation, and Mitigation: The Problem of the Individual Special Case." *New York University Law Review* 35:925–937.

REPPUCCI, N. DICKON. 1984. "The Wisdom of Solomon: Issues in Child Custody Determination." In *Children, Mental Health, and the Law*, pp. 59–78. Edited by N. Dickon Reppucci, Lois A. Weithorn, Edward P. Mulvey, and John Monahan. Beverly Hills, Calif.: Sage.

SCOTT, ELIZABETH, and DERDEYN, ANDRE. 1984. "Rethinking Joint Custody." *Ohio State Law Journal* 45, no. 2: 455–498.

STEINMAN, SUSAN. 1983. "Joint Custody: What We Know, What We Have Yet to Learn, and the Judicial and Legislative Implications." *University of California at Davis Law Review* 16:739–762.

UVILLER, RENA K. 1978. "Fathers' Rights and Feminism: The Maternal Presumption Revisited." *Harvard Women's Law Journal* 1:107–130.

WALLERSTEIN, JUDITH S., and BLAKESLEE, SANDRA. 1989. *Second Chances: Men, Women, and Children a Decade After Divorce*. New York: Ticknor & Fields.

WALLERSTEIN, JUDITH S., and KELLY, JOAN B. 1980. *Surviving the Breakup: How Children and Parents Cope with Divorce*. New York: Basic Books.

WATSON, ANDREW S. 1969. "The Children of Armageddon: Problems of Custody Following Divorce." *Syracuse Law Review* 21:55–86.

WEITZMAN, LENORE J. 1985. *The Divorce Revolution: The Unexpected Social and Economic Consequences for Women and Children in America*. New York: Free Press.

CHILE

See MEDICAL ETHICS, HISTORY OF, *section on* THE AMERICAS, *article on* LATIN AMERICA.

CHINA

See MEDICAL ETHICS, HISTORY OF, *section on* SOUTH AND EAST ASIA, *subsection on* CHINA.

CHIROPRACTIC

See ALTERNATIVE THERAPIES; *and* UNORTHODOXY IN MEDICINE. *See also the* APPENDIX (CODES, OATHS, AND DIRECTIVES RELATED TO BIOETHICS), SECTION III: ETHICAL DIRECTIVES FOR OTHER HEALTH-CARE PROFESSIONS, CODE OF ETHICS *of the* AMERICAN CHIROPRACTIC ASSOCIATION.

CHRISTIAN SCIENCE

See ALTERNATIVE THERAPIES.

CHRONIC CARE

The term "chronic condition" encompasses a great variety of long-term health problems that cause symptoms and disability over months and years for individuals. They include pathologies, injuries with lasting effects, and enduring structural or sensory/communication abnormalities. The conditions can be of a physical or mental, including cognitive and emotional, nature. Their time of onset ranges from before birth to late life.

The defining aspect is duration: A chronic condition is one that has lasted or can be expected to last for a "long" time, defined variously in health statistics as three months, six months, or twelve months. After crossing some symptomatic or clinical threshold, chronic conditions become permanent features of individuals' lives. It is rare for them to disappear, to be cured. More typically, they are static or progressive (increasing in severity over time). The time course often has uneven and unpredictable features, as interventions in the disease process and its functional consequences succeed or fail.

This combination of fundamental permanence together with dynamic course and consequences affects people's happiness, future outlook, use of time, residence, and financial planning. Health statistics never reflect the lengthy burden that chronic conditions pose for quality of life among affected persons.

Comorbidity

Older persons are likely to have multiple chronic conditions, called comorbidity. There are many ways this occurs: First, an initial condition can cause additional problems that are directly related (e.g., eye disease related to diabetes) or indirectly related (e.g., arthritis can reduce mobility, thereby causing circulatory problems). These secondary conditions are of special medical concern in two situations: youths with severe conditions who may live many more years and frail older persons with progressive conditions. Second, diseases with the same risk factor are more likely to occur simultaneously in a person; for example, obesity can cause both diabetes and arthritis. Third, aging increases a person's chances of acquiring new chronic conditions that may have little or no causal relationships to each other. Having multiple chronic conditions increases an individual's chances of disability, institutionalization, and death.

Epidemiology of chronic conditions

Scientific efforts are being made to identify the risk factors that influence the onset and progression of specific conditions. In contrast to many acute conditions, chronic ones tend to have multiple and delayed causes. Genetic, hormonal, metabolic, and wear-and-tear factors are all implicated in osteoarthritis; rheumatologists describe the disease as a "final common pathway" of numerous causes. To identify causes, researchers must look not only at contemporary and recent features of a person but also at behaviors across his or her whole lifetime.

Nonfatal and fatal conditions

Chronic conditions can be divided into two main types: fatal and nonfatal. Fatal conditions swiftly or eventually lead to death (unless another disease accomplishes that first); examples are malignant neoplasms, ischemic heart disease, and cerebrovascular disease. Nonfatal conditions are much more common than fatal conditions; examples are visual impairment, arthritis, and chronic low back pain. Though often progressive, they do not prompt death directly even at severe stages.

Arthritis is the leading chronic condition for middle-aged (forty-five to sixty-four years) and older (sixty-five and over) persons, ranking first for women and first or second for men (Verbrugge, 1991). Besides arthritis, the ten most prevalent conditions among adults (ages eighteen to forty-four, forty-five to sixty-four, and sixty-five and over) include many nonfatal conditions such as hearing impairment, visual impairment, cataracts, deformity of a lower extremity, deformity of the back, varicose veins, hemorrhoids, migraine headache, dermatitis, chronic sinusitis, high blood pressure, and hay fever without asthma. With increasing age, fatal conditions such as heart disease and cancer rise in rank and are more likely to be among the top ten conditions in an age group. Nevertheless, nonfatal conditions remain preeminent even at older ages.

Prevalence rates indicate the proportion of the population with a certain condition at a particular time. The rates reflect both incidence (the time of onset) and duration (how long the condition lasts). Prevalence statistics are available for many conditions from population-based studies with medical evaluations or health interviews, but it is difficult to find information about incidence and duration. Why? First, incidence statistics are not common. They exist for a few major fatal conditions through government-sponsored surveillance programs and surveys. But incidence rates are rare for nonfatal conditions that have very gradual onset or highly uneven course, conditions such as osteoarthritis, urinary incontinence, tinnitus, and low back pain. Second, for accurate information about duration, one must follow up affected people from diagnosis to death. The case-survival rates sometimes reported for fatal conditions come from such follow-ups; they state the average number of years after diagnosis that people live. There may also be some relationship between nonfatal conditions and mortality; for example, arthritis could weaken stamina and resistance to fatal conditions, resulting in higher mortality among persons with arthritis than those without arthritis.

Disability

Interest in disability has burgeoned in clinical, scientific, and public-health domains. Disability refers to the impacts that chronic conditions have on the functioning of specific body systems and on people's ability to act in necessary, expected, and personally desired ways in their society. Usually, disease causes dysfunctions (called impairments) in specific body systems. These impairments, in turn, prompt restrictions in basic actions of body and mind (called functional limitations), leading to restrictions in roles and activities (called disability). For example, arthritis induces pain and restricts joint flexibility, causing trouble walking and running and, eventually, difficulties doing errands and favorite sports. The term "handicap" indicates social disadvantages that people with disabilities experience, namely, restrictions on doing what they can and wish to do because of social conventions, ranging from attitudes to laws, or because of environmental barriers. Epidemiologists are studying pathways of disease consequences on physical, mental, and social function over time for individuals and the whole population. They also want to know the factors that speed up or slow down the pace of those consequences.

About 14 percent of the noninstitutionalized population of the United States has activity limitations due to chronic conditions. The figure rises steeply with age, from 6 percent for males under age eighteen to 35 percent for those aged seventy and over and from 4 percent to 40 percent for females (Adams and Benson, 1991). Limitations can occur in a person's major activity (i.e., principal role, whether school, job, or keeping house) or secondary ones (e.g., doing errands, attending religious services, going to movies). Nine percent of the population is limited in major activity. The percentage rises from 4 percent to 14 percent for males across the ages noted before, and from 3 percent to 22 percent for females.

What conditions are most often cited by people as causing activity limitations? In young adulthood (ages eighteen to forty-four), nonfatal conditions are the leading limiters, especially musculoskeletal disorders (deformities of back, lower extremity, and upper extremity and intervertebral disc disorders) (Verbrugge, 1991). At older ages (seventy and over), the top ten limiters are an even mixture of nonfatal and fatal conditions. Standing out most of all is arthritis, the foremost cause of activity limitation for middle-aged and older persons of both genders.

In political settings, many chronic conditions have strong advocacy. Some get their power from the sheer number of affected people, and some from their devastating (though rare) impact. This difference in emphasis is matched by a difference in age groups affected: High prevalence usually occurs among older persons, whereas dire and lasting consequences often result from chronic conditions in children and youths. Late-life and lifelong disability experiences do differ, making it difficult for advocacy groups to perceive similar goals for older and younger persons with disabilities.

Persons disabled in late life have experienced the accretion and expression of personal skills, and they have enjoyed life's variety and change. By contrast, persons disabled in childhood or youth are blunted from that process. Older persons with chronic conditions strive to regain lost abilities. Young persons, often facing nonmodifiable limitations, turn instead to technological and social adaptations. Despite profound differences in causes, trajectories, and interventions, all age groups have the same underlying goal—the desire to maintain function in spite of chronic health problems, to enjoy social opportunities for productive and pleasurable activities, and to have long life. In coming decades, advocacy groups will perceive this similarity and combine the voices of younger and older persons for medical, technological, and societal changes to reduce disability.

Future health of the population

What are the health prospects for the U.S. population and those of other developed countries?

The twentieth century produced a striking epidemiologic transition from a population whose morbidity (illness), disability, and death profile was characterized by acute conditions to a profile dominated by chronic conditions. It is uncertain whether the degenerative diseases that are now killers (ischemic heart disease, cere-

brovascular disease, malignant neoplasms) are new pathologies distinctive to the twentieth century or old pathologies uncovered in the century by different diagnostic procedures, changes in disease names, and population aging. Immense scientific energy has gone toward locating personal and environmental factors that cause these diseases, and the knowledge has penetrated medical care and personal lifestyles in a widespread way. Population aging occurred throughout the century, fueled first by fertility declines and in the last quarter of the century by mortality declines concentrated at the oldest ages. Although mortality trends are well documented, long series of data with age-specific rates of chronic conditions and disability do not exist, so we cannot know their course over the whole century. Data series collected since the 1950s often, but not always, show rises in age-specific prevalence of chronic conditions and disability in recent decades.

Population health depends on the population's age structure and age-specific rates of acute conditions, chronic conditions, and disability. The pace of population aging is slowing, but it will continue to push upward both the numbers of people with chronic morbidity and disability and the prevalence rates for the total population. Because age distribution can be projected quite well (specific projections vary depending on assumptions about mortality, fertility, and migration), its implications for societal health burden can be readily calculated. Most reports about how future population health will affect medicine, long-term care, and health insurance are based solely on changes in age distribution. What will happen to age-specific illness and disability rates is less certain. Yet the rates will be influential in determining population health status. Will age-specific prevalence rates of illness and disability rise, fall, or stay essentially constant?

A frequently discussed scenario is the "compression of morbidity." It proposes that incidence of illness and disability can be markedly delayed for fatal and nonfatal conditions so that the fraction of life spent ill and disabled declines from one generation (cohort) to the next. Stated another way, improvements in morbidity and disability will outpace mortality reductions. Incidence and prevalence rates fall for morbidity/disability. For this scenario to result, great strides in primary prevention—helping people to avoid disease for most or all of their lifetimes—must occur for numerous diseases. This is unlikely in the near future.

Instead, the recent situation of falling age-specific mortality rates with possibly rising age-specific morbidity and disability rates suggests a scenario of "longer life but worsening health," also called "expansion of morbidity." This strikes many as contradictory. Instead, it should be viewed as an expected stage in the ongoing epidemiologic transition: Since midcentury, medicine's forte has become secondary prevention, the early diagnosis and management of chronic conditions, especially key killers. With treatment, people live longer than before, often with less severe illness and symptoms. Efficacious therapies cause a shift toward symptom mitigation in the whole distribution of persons with a condition. People live longer; the number of ill/disabled persons in an age group increases, propelling age-specific rates upward. Although some people may move back to wellness, the typical situation is continued presence of disease/disability of less severity during the extra years of life. Assuming that medicine remains oriented toward diagnosis and management for some decades, the situation of longer life with worsening health is likely to continue and ultimately find solid empirical verification. Furthermore, assuming that biomedical research remains oriented toward fatal diseases, with research results being gradually translated into medical care and lifestyles, the significance of nonfatal conditions will increase in individuals' health profiles and medical complaints. Societal investments in research have concentrated on "saving lives" and thus invested most resources in research on fatal diseases. Some ethicists argue that more money should be invested in research on chronic disabling diseases that affect the quality, not the quantity, of life.

Without rich historical data about trends in morbidity and disability, discussions of the future are based largely on reasoned speculation and formal statistical modeling of disease-disability-death relationships. Both of these can be excellent bases for thinking and planning when they include well-stated assumptions about incidence, duration, and prevalence of chronic conditions, incidence and duration of disability, and mortality (all age-specific). Population health tends to change slowly; so a future scenario that has continuity with the past is more likely to be right than one premised on a vastly different milieu of medicine and lifestyles than now exists. This is already a chronic disease society and probably will become more so in decades ahead.

Prevention

Physicians and public-health experts use a typology of prevention strategies to indicate where professional efforts are aimed. Primary prevention strives to avert the onset of illness or injury. Secondary prevention is early detection and management of illness/injury. Tertiary prevention is intervention to reduce the impacts of disease; it includes efforts to avoid onset of secondary conditions, to maintain and restore function, and to sustain life (heroic care). The broad sweep of tertiary care reflects the relative disinterest in disease consequences that characterized medicine earlier in this century, when the words were coined. Some scientists and clinicians now think that "tertiary prevention" should be used just for medical efforts directed against secondary conditions and death, preferring the term "quaternary prevention" for function-related efforts.

There is a fine match between the four types of prevention and the pathology-to-disability pathway. Primary prevention acts ahead of pathology, secondary acts between pathology and impairment, tertiary blunts feedback effects to new pathology and impairment from any point on the pathway, and quaternary reduces consequences of impairment for function/disability.

The twentieth century excelled first in primary prevention of acute conditions and next in secondary prevention of chronic ones. To achieve high quality of life for the growing number of persons with chronic morbidity and activity limitations, dedicated attention must go to tertiary prevention (avoiding the pernicious cycles of deconditioning in older persons that prompt frailty) and especially to quaternary prevention (helping older persons keep and regain function so that they are independent, active, and productive). Changes in medical practice to emerging health needs are fostering the development of geriatrics, rehabilitation medicine, and specialties in musculoskeletal, sensory, and mental domains; focusing closely on function and its trajectory over time; developing genuine interest in protracted symptoms and dysfunctions whose toll lies in duration rather than severity; and attending to the whole person instead of just his or her ailing portions. Broad social changes are also needed, such as better insurance coverage for home-based and equipment services, deeper sensitivity to both visible and invisible disabilities, technological development and wide marketing of assistive equipment, environmental accommodations in buildings and public spaces, and expanded opportunities for work and pleasure for disabled persons.

Chronic conditions and the care they necessitate can occur at any age, but they are disproportionately the experience of older persons. And because that age group is predominantly female, chronic care is mainly (but not stereotypically) a concern of older women. In efforts to achieve comfort and good function, chronic care can become a time-consuming activity. Chronic care occurs mostly on one's own or with the aid of relatives and friends. The more swiftly medical research and practice shift toward nonfatal conditions and toward disability, the sooner older persons will have professional helpers in the long process of chronic care.

Lois M. Verbrugge

For a further discussion of topics mentioned in this entry, see the entries Aging and the Aged; Disability; Health and Disease; *and* Public Health. *Other relevant material may be found under the entries* Hos-

PICE AND END OF LIFE CARE; LIFESTYLES AND PUBLIC HEALTH; *and* LONG-TERM CARE.

Bibliography

ADAMS, PATRICIA F., and BENSON, VERONICA. 1991. "Current Estimates from the National Health Interview Survey, 1990." *Vital and Health Statistics, Series 10: Data from the National Health Survey.* No. 181. DHHS Publication no. (PHS) 92–1509. Hyattsville, Md.: National Center for Health Statistics.

CORBIN, JULIET M., and STRAUSS, ANSELM L. 1988. *Unending Work and Care: Managing Chronic Illness at Home.* San Francisco: Jossey-Bass.

CRIMMINS, EILEEN M.; SAITO, YASUHIKO; and INGEGNERI, DOMINIQUE. 1989. "Changes in Life Expectancy and Disability-Free Life Expectancy in the United States." *Population and Development Review* 15, no. 2:235–267.

FRIES, JAMES F. 1989. "The Compression of Morbidity: Near or Far?" *Milbank Quarterly* 67, no. 2:208–232.

HAAN, MARY N.; RICE, DOROTHY P.; SATARIANO, WILLIAM A.; and SELBY, JOE V., eds. 1991. "Living Longer and Doing Worse? Present and Future Trends in the Health of the Elderly." *Journal of Aging and Health* 3, no. 2. Special issue.

INSTITUTE OF MEDICINE (U.S.). COMMITTEE ON A NATIONAL AGENDA FOR THE PREVENTION OF DISABILITIES. 1991. *Disability in America: Toward a National Agenda for Prevention.* Edited by Andrew M. Pope and Alvin R. Tarlov. Washington, D.C.: National Academy Press.

KATZ, SIDNEY, ed. 1987. "The Portugal Conference: Measuring Quality of Life and Functional Status in Clinical and Epidemiological Research." *Journal of Chronic Diseases* 40, no. 6. Special issue.

LAPLANTE, MITCHELL P. 1991. "Disability Risks of Chronic Illnesses and Impairments." *Disability Statistics Report,* no. 2. Washington, D.C.: National Institute on Disability and Rehabilitation Research, U.S. Department of Education.

LAST, JOHN M. 1988. *A Dictionary of Epidemiology.* 2d ed. New York: Oxford University Press.

MANTON, KENNETH G. 1982. "Changing Concepts of Morbidity and Mortality in the Elderly Population." *Milbank Memorial Fund Quarterly/Health and Society* 60, no. 2: 183–244.

———. 1988. "A Longitudinal Study of Functional Change and Mortality in the United States." *Journal of Gerontology* 43, no. 5:S153–S161.

MCKINLAY, JOHN B.; MCKINLAY, SONJA M.; and BEAGLEHOLE, ROBERT. 1989. "A Review of the Evidence Concerning the Impact of Medical Measures on Recent Mortality and Morbidity in the United States." *International Journal of Health Services* 19, no. 2:181–208.

OLSHANSKY, S. JAY, and AULT, A. BRIAN. 1986. "The Fourth Stage of the Epidemiologic Transition: The Age of Delayed Degenerative Diseases." *Milbank Quarterly* 64, no. 3:355–391.

OMRAN, ABDEL R. 1971. "The Epidemiologic Transition: A Theory of the Epidemiology of Population Change." *Milbank Memorial Fund Quarterly* 49, no. 4, pt. 1:509–538.

ROTHENBERG, RICHARD B., and KOPLAN, JEFFREY P. 1990. "Chronic Disease in the 1990s." *Annual Review of Public Health* 11:267–296.

STAHL, SIDNEY M., ed. 1990. *The Legacy of Longevity: Health and Health Care in Later Life.* Newbury Park, Calif.: Sage.

VERBRUGGE, LOIS M. 1984. "Longer Life but Worsening Health? Trends in Health and Mortality of Middle-Aged and Older Persons." *Milbank Memorial Fund Quarterly/Health and Society* 62, no. 3:475–519.

———. 1989. "Recent, Present, and Future Health of American Adults." *Annual Review of Public Health* 10:333–361.

———. 1991. "Physical and Social Disability in Adults." In *Primary Care Research: Theory and Methods: Conference Proceedings,* pp. 31–57. Edited by Heddy Hibbard, Paul A. Nutting, and Mary L. Grady. AHCPR publication no. 91–0011. Rockville, Md.: U.S. Department of Health and Human Services, Agency for Health Care Policy and Research.

VERBRUGGE,, LOIS M., and JETTE, ALAN M. 1994. "The Disablement Process." *Social Science and Medicine* 38, no. 1:1–14.

VERBRUGGE, LOIS M.; LEPKOWSKI, JAMES M.; and IMANAKA, YUICHI. 1989. "Comorbidity and Its Impact on Disability." *Milbank Quarterly* 67, nos. 3–4:450–484.

CIRCUMCISION

I. Female Circumcision
   Olayinka A. Koso-Thomas
II. Male Circumcision
   Jeffrey R. Botkin

I. FEMALE CIRCUMCISION

"Female circumcision" is the term used to identify the practice of removing healthy normal female genitalia by surgical operation. Because of the severity of the operation and its known harmful effects, the term "female genital mutilation" is now generally used. There are three increasingly severe types of this operation, and each makes orgasm impossible. Clitoridectomy, or sunna (Type 1), is the removal of the prepuce of the clitoris and the clitoris itself (Figure 1-1). When excited, the clitoris swells and becomes erect, and it is this excitement that causes female orgasms. Excision, or reduction (Type 2), is the removal of the prepuce, the clitoris, and the labia minora, leaving the majora intact. The labia minora produce secretions that lubricate the inner folds of the lips and prevent soreness when these lips rub against each other (Figure 1-2). Infibulation, or pharaonic circumcision (Type 3), is the removal of the prepuce, the clitoris,

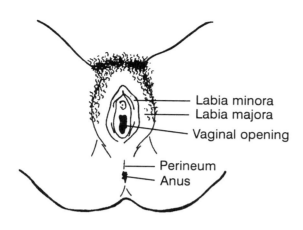

1-1 Vulva after clitoridectomy.

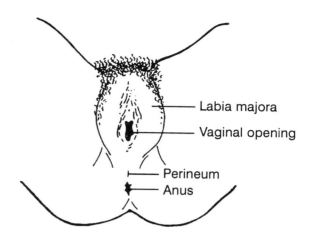

1-2 Vulva after excision.

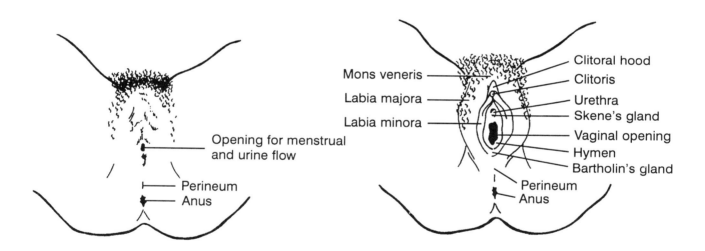

1-3 Vulva after infibulation.

1-4 Normal vulva before circumcision.

FIGURE 1 The vulva.

the labia minora and majora, and the suturing of the two sides of the vulva, leaving a very small opening for the passage of urine and menstrual blood (Figure 1-3). This type of circumcision is referred to as pharaonic probably because it is identified with circumcision methods of ancient Egypt under the pharaohs.

In a study of the various types of circumcision undergone by women in Sierra Leone (Koso-Thomas, 1987), it was found that 39.03 percent of the women had undergone Type 1, 59.85 percent, Type 2, and 1.12 percent, Type 3. In Somalia, 80 percent of the opera-

tions are Type 3 (El Dareer, 1982). The prevalence of circumcision in Africa ranges from 10 percent in Tanzania to 98 percent in Djibouti (Toubia, 1993).

The most common and basic procedure followed during circumcision is the traditional method. In this method, usually employed by circumcisers who have no medical training, the female is firmly held down on dry ground with her legs wide apart to expose the genitalia and the parts to be removed. In some cases, the genital part to be excised is held with a special hemostatic leaf before excision, or the candidates are made to lie near a cold flowing stream so the excised area can be bathed in chilled water to numb the pain. The implements used are often unsterilized razor blades, knives, scissors, broken bottles, or any other sharp implement. Some form of herbal dressing is applied to the raw wound after the operation. The same implement is used for successive operations without sterilization. When the operation is carried out in modern clinics, standard modern surgical practice is followed.

Origin of the practice

We do not know with any precision when, why, and how female circumcision began. There is evidence that female circumcision and female genital surgery have been done in many parts of the world, although currently it is mainly done in different communities in parts of Africa, Asia, the Far East, Europe, and South America.

The early Romans, concerned about the consequences of sexual activity among female slaves, adopted the technique of slipping rings through their labia majora (Figure 1-4) to block access to the vagina. In the twelfth century c.e., Crusaders introduced the chastity belt in Europe for the same purpose; the belt prevented girls and women from engaging in unlawful or unsanctioned sex. This method caused little permanent physical damage to the individual. Genital surgery was permitted in North America and Europe in the late nineteenth century with the intention of curing nymphomania, masturbation, hysteria, depression, epilepsy, and insanity. There is no evidence that such surgery was associated with any ritualistic activity. Elsewhere, the surgery has historical links with either religious or ethnic rituals. It is believed that the ancient Egyptians and ancient Arabs practiced this form of surgery. Genital mutilation seems to have been transplanted to Latin America from Africa during the slave trade and may have taken root first in the central part of Brazil, where groups of West Africans were resettled after the abolition of the slave trade in the middle of the nineteenth century, and to eastern Mexico and Peru through migration. In Asia genital mutilation is found among Islamic religious groups in the Philippines, Malaysia, Pakistan, and Indonesia. Where the mutilation exists in the Middle East and Asia, it is strongly associated with Islam. Female genital mutilation is not practiced in all Islamic countries. Those societies known to practice it, namely, the United Arab Emirates, South Yemen, Oman, and Bahrain in the Middle East, and northern Egypt, Mauritania, Sudan, Somalia, Mali, and Nigeria in Africa, probably inherited it from pre-Islamic cultures.

Alleged benefits of female circumcision

The modern defense of female circumcision allows us to reconstruct the ancient rules that governed moral action or behavior in polygamous communities. The defense enumerates a wide range of health-related and social benefits alleged to result from the practice:

1. maintenance of cleanliness
2. maintenance of good health
3. preservation of virginity
4. enhancement of fertility
5. prevention of stillbirths in women pregnant for the first time
6. prevention of promiscuity
7. increase of matrimonial opportunities
8. pursuance of aesthetics
9. improvement of male sexual performance and pleasure
10. promotion of social and political cohesion

Cleanliness is regarded as a great virtue by women in countries where the practice is common. In some cultures, particularly in Africa, women are required to cleanse their genitalia with soap and water after urinating. Those who justify removing parts of the genitalia that produce secretions cite this preoccupation with the cleanliness of the genital organs. Some traditional circumcision societies claim that circumcised women are generally healthy and that the operation cures women suffering from problems resembling those identified in nontraditional societies as depression, melancholia, nymphomania, hysteria, insanity, epilepsy, and the social disorder of kleptomania. In situations where proof of virginity is essential for concluding a marriage transaction, circumcision is believed to be the guarantee against premarital sex. This guarantee benefits parents who are able to demand a high bridal price for their daughters. Marriage immediately after the transaction ceremony is common, and such marriages, involving pubertal girls, are usually followed by pregnancy within a very short time. Circumcised girls and women are regarded as having an advantage over the uncircumcised in marrying. Where female genital mutilation is an established custom, tradition forbids men to marry uncircumcised girls; hence, circumcision of girls ensures they will be marriageable. Certain traditional communities, such as the Mossi of Burkina Faso and the Ibos of Nigeria, believe that a firstborn child or even subsequent babies will die if their heads touch a mother's clitoris during the birth process. The clitoris is therefore removed at the time of delivery if this has not already been done. Since female genital mutilation reduces or even eliminates sexual pleasure, the practice presumably eliminates the risk of female promiscuity. The justification of the practice to preserve chastity, eliminate promiscuity, foster or improve sexual relations with men, generate greater matrimonial opportunities, protect virginity, and increase fertility reflects the existence in traditional societies of strict controls on social behavior.

The belief that circumcision enhances beauty stems from the claim that the male prepuce or foreskin is removed mainly for aesthetic reasons, and that the clitoris, the female counterpart to the penis, should be removed for the same reason. If left intact, the clitoris is believed likely to grow to an embarrassing and uncomfortable size. In some patriarchal societies, female genital mutilation is also said to benefit the male by prolonging his sexual pleasure, since the clitoris is thought to increase male excitement during sexual intercourse with a female partner and may rush a man's orgasm. Of great importance to women in such cultures is the status circumcision bestows on the circumcised. It entitles them to positions of religious, political, and social leadership and responsibility.

The argument in favor of circumcision serves narrow social interests and does not achieve the goods desired or guaranteed. Failure to achieve these goods, moreover, is often blamed on the woman rather than the ritual. For example, maintaining cleanliness becomes an agonizing task. The hardened scar and stump that result from circumcision are unsightly, and they halt the flow of urine and menstrual blood through the normal channels. This obstruction causes unnecessary fluid retention and results in odors more disagreeable than those from the natural hormonal secretions that tradition teaches are degrading. Associating the death of babies at childbirth with clitoral contact is clearly refuted by the evidence that millions of healthy babies are born to uncircumcised mothers.

While the desire of organized society to maintain control over people's actions may be understandable, not all such control promotes their well-being or self-determination. Such rituals also cause harm to society by increasing morbidity and mortality levels. In addition, although these rites may promote social and political cohesion, they thwart the individual's freedom to determine what is right and in her best interests. Even women who learn that circumcision is an unsafe and harmful practice may feel pressure from society to agree to it for themselves or their children in order to marry or remain members of the group.

Harmful effects of female circumcision or female genital mutilation

The medical consequences of female genital mutilation are quite grave (El Dareer, 1982; Koso-Thomas, 1987). In Africa an estimated ninety million females are affected (Hosken, 1982). Three levels of health problems are associated with the practice. Immediate problems include pain, shock, hemorrhage, acute urinary retention, urinary infection, septicemia, blood poisoning, fever, tetanus, and death. Occasionally, force is applied to position candidates for the operation, and as a result, fractures of the clavicle, humerus, or femur have occurred.

Intermediate complications include pelvic infection, painful menstrual periods, painful and difficult sexual intercourse, formation of cysts and abscesses, excessive growth of scar tissue, and the development of prolapse and fistulae. A fistula is an abnormal passage: a hole (opening) between the posterior urinary bladder wall and the vagina or a hole between the anterior rectal wall and the vagina. Late complications include accumulation of menstrual blood of many months or even years, primary infertility, painful clitoral tumors, recurrent urinary tract infections, and kidney or bladder stone formation. Obstetric complications such as third-degree perineal tear, resulting in anal incontinence and fissure formation, and prolonged and obstructed labor are also known to occur. Psychological problems of anxiety, frigidity, and depression, as a result of the physical inability to have a clitoral orgasm, may also develop.

Women who undergo circumcision suffer various degrees of emotional and mental distress depending on the nature of complications following their operation. Records show that 83 percent of all females undergoing circumcision are likely to be affected by some condition related to that surgical procedure requiring medical attention at some time during their lives. This level of health risk should be of concern to nations with a large proportion of circumcised women, because such women may never make the progress toward the economic and social development required of them.

Application of modern medical practice to female genital mutilation

Modern medicine has made impressive strides in investigating, preventing, and treating a wide range of ailments. Through its investigative approaches it has judged that unwarranted surgery is wrong. In the case of female genital mutilation, studies have found that certain of the resulting medical conditions are serious and can lead to complications and permanent health damage requiring both medical treatment and counseling (Koso-Thomas, 1987). Awareness of female genital mutilation's harmful effects has encouraged changes in how the operation is performed, changes that may include sterilization of equipment and dressings and administration of local anesthetic, antibiotics, and antitetanus injections prior to circumcision.

Ethical aspects

Since some followers of Islam in Africa, the Far East, and the Middle East endorse circumcision, it has been widely identified as an Islamic rite. However, female genital mutilation is not practiced in Saudi Arabia, Algeria, Iran, Iraq, Libya, Morocco, or Tunisia. Many Islamic and Christian religious leaders have categorically denied that female circumcision or female genital mutilation is an injunction in the Qur'an or a "commandment" in the Bible. Since the foundations of the practice lie outside Islamic or Christian religious law, the origins of circumcision and its justification must lie in the moral, social, and religious structure and operation of societies practicing it. Individuals practicing it act within a system of rules that strictly regulate sexual behavior in society. Female genital mutilation generally thrives in communities with strictly enforced conventions and social rules. With the knowledge of its harmful effects now common, no social system endorsing this kind of mutilation can be said to promote a favorable climate for a fulfilling life.

The attitudes of women toward circumcision depend on their experiences and level of education. Most women affected by the practice are unaware that circumcision is the cause of their health difficulties (Koso-Thomas, 1987). Once aware of this relationship, however, many women who have some education and training and who are exposed to a modern environment are better able to assess what is involved in circumcision actions and, on that basis, to make a reasoned judgment of its rightness or wrongness. Many such women have come to believe that the practice is unacceptable and have refused to allow their female children to go through the same traumatic experience. Many feminists and health professionals have openly displayed a higher regard for women's health than for tradition.

It has been shown, however, that some women who admit to suffering under the unexpected effects of the operation still feel obliged to support the practice. A study carried out to obtain opinions on circumcision involving 135 men and 120 women showed that 25 percent were shocked at what happened to them on their circumcision day, as it was not what they had expected (Koso-Thomas, 1987). The majority of them, either semi- or nonliterate, believed that they had done the right thing and planned to have their daughters circumcised. Those women who were not shocked by their experiences were also mainly illiterate and did not see why their daughters should not undergo circumcision. The attitude of men in the sample also varied according to their level of education. Illiterate men insisted that all women should be circumcised to keep them in their place, while the literate men argued that women should be given a choice as to whether or not to be circumcised. They felt that to deny women this choice was a violation of their human rights. It has also been found that circumcision is supported in most women's organizations, particularly political and social groups, since these groups reflect the feelings of the majority in the community.

Usually the decision to have a girl circumcised is made by the female elder members of the family/clan who insist on carrying out the procedure. An aura of secrecy, celebration, and pride surrounds the circumci-

sion and encourages voluntarism on the part of recruits by making membership in the group seem more attractive. A few educated women, however, who have had access to modern medical assessment of their health as well as information on the dangers of the practice also support circumcision but advocate changes to reduce its health hazards. A few health-care personnel have felt that medical intervention at the early stages of the operation might prevent the more serious health consequences of circumcision. Since circumcision cannot take place without health consequences, the position of these women and health practitioners is untenable.

Women who live in a traditional environment tend to judge their actions on the basis of traditional rules and principles of their society. There may be some misogynistic attitudes among such women, but the dominant force directing their actions comes from the society that demands, among other things, that this ritual be performed in order for them to qualify for marriage and social acceptance.

There are also attitudes inherent in African sexuality that not only permit circumcision but foster it. In most African cultures, sexuality is regarded as a gift to be used for the procreation of the human species, and any public or even private display of sex-related feeling or enjoyment is seen as debasing this gift. In some communities, only a token expression of the sexual self is permitted. The issue of sexual fulfillment is unimportant. Thus, controls over the sexual behavior of women are designed to curb female sexual desire and response and to encourage disregard for the sexual aspects of their lives. The removal of the organ or organs responsible for sexual stimulation is therefore taken as necessary for the fixation of certain values within the community and for ensuring the acceptance of rigid standards of sexual conduct. Thus, the underlying concern of those who defend the institution of female circumcision is that women's sexuality will be corrupted if women are allowed the freedom to control it or indeed to pursue the personal satisfaction of their sexual desire. Implicit in this argument is the major premise that it is immoral for a woman to act on her sexual desire. Women who still support the practice continue to promote injury with confirmed medical consequences. In this respect the role of the health-care practitioner in the society is crucial and may lead to personal dilemmas that have to be resolved. Many feel anger against the executors and supporters of the ritual and sadness at the futility of the exercise and at the intransigence of traditional circumcising communities. Health-care professionals presented with the choice of treating or not treating women who have chosen to be circumcised are often determined to rescue a life they see as poised on the brink of destruction. On the other hand, traditional circumcisers have no moral dilemmas about the practice. They believe that they have no choice in a matter which concerns the preservation of their cultural heritage. That heritage dictates how women must live, and to them, life should be one of happiness in subservience to the will of the people and in obedience to customary and religious laws.

OLAYINKA A. KOSO-THOMAS

Directly related to this article is the companion article in this entry: MALE CIRCUMCISION. *Also directly related are the entries* SEXISM; SEXUALITY IN SOCIETY; *and* WOMEN, *articles on* HISTORICAL AND CROSS-CULTURAL PERSPECTIVES, *and* HEALTH-CARE ISSUES. *For a further discussion of topics mentioned in this article, see the entries* AFRICAN RELIGIONS; FEMINISM; FREEDOM AND COERCION; ISLAM; JUSTICE; *and* VALUE AND VALUATION. *Other relevant material may be found under the entries* AUTONOMY; *and* BODY, *articles on* SOCIAL THEORIES, *and* CULTURAL AND RELIGIOUS PERSPECTIVES.

Bibliography

AUNE, BRUCE. 1979. *Kant's Theory of Morals.* Princeton, N.J.: Princeton University Press.

EL DAREER, ASMA. 1982. *Woman, Why Do You Weep? Circumcision and Its Consequences.* London: Zed.

FRANCOEUR, ROBERT T. 1983. *Biomedical Ethics: A Guide to Decision Making.* New York: Wiley.

HOSKEN, FRAN P. 1982. *The Hosken Report on Genital and Sexual Mutilation of Females.* 3d rev. ed. Lexington, Mass.: Women's International Network News.

KOSO-THOMAS, OLAYINKA. 1987. *The Circumcision of Women: A Strategy for Eradication.* London: Zed.

MACINTYRE, ALASDAIR C. 1967. *A Short History of Ethics.* London: Routledge & Kegan Paul.

"Report of the Workshop on African Women Speak." 1984. Khartoum: Scientific Association for Women's Studies.

SCHWEITZER, ALBERT. 1947. *Civilization and Ethics.* 3d rev. ed. London: A. and C. Black.

THIAM, AWA. 1986. *Speak Out, Black Sisters: Feminism and Oppression in Black Africa.* London: Pluto.

TOUBIA, NAHID. 1993. *Female Genital Mutilation: A Call for Global Action.* New York: New York Women.

WALKER, ALICE. 1990. *Possessing the Secret of Joy.* New York: Harcourt Brace Jovanovich.

WALKER, ALICE, and PARMAR, PRATIBHA. 1993. *Warrior Marks: Female Genital Mutilation and the Sexual Blinding of Women.* New York: Harcourt Brace.

II. MALE CIRCUMCISION

Male circumcision entails the surgical removal of the foreskin that covers the glans of the penis. The relative simplicity of the surgical procedure itself belies the complexity of the conflicting values surrounding male circumcision. The primary ethical issue can be simply stated: Are the pain, risks, and costs of routine neonatal circumcision justified by the potential benefits to those who undergo this procedure? Given the strong opposing opinions surrounding circumcision, it is questioned whether children should undergo the procedure prior to an age when they can provide informed consent on their own behalf. Circumcision in adults is less common and will not be the focus of discussion here.

The prevalence of male circumcision

Circumcision is the most common procedure performed on males in the United States; an estimated one million procedures are performed per year. Only about 20 percent of the procedures are performed for religious reasons; the majority are performed in newborns for medical, cultural, or aesthetic reasons (Wallerstein, 1985). Estimates suggest that circumcision is performed on 60 percent to 90 percent of boys in the United States. Although observers have noted some variations by region and by cultural group in the use of this procedure, accurate rates for circumcision have not been obtained (Wallerstein, 1985). The best documented rates of newborn circumcision in the United States come from a study of infants delivered in U.S. military hospitals (Wiswell, 1992). The rate of circumcision in 1971 was estimated to be 89 percent, falling to 70 percent in 1984, with a subsequent rise to 80 percent in 1990. These differences show that parents' decisions about circumcision were influenced by debate over the procedure.

The high rate of nonritual circumcision places the United States in a unique position in the world. In regions where the majority of the world's population lives, including western Europe, the former Soviet Union, China, and Japan, male circumcision is not performed. Edward Wallerstein provides the following estimates of circumcision rates: In Great Britain an estimated 1 percent of the male population is circumcised; for New Zealand the figure is about 10 percent; for Australia, 35–40 percent; and for Canada, 35–40 percent (Wallerstein 1985). Circumcision is performed commonly as a religious ritual by Jews, Muslims, many black Africans, and nonwhite Australians.

The history of circumcision

The walls of Egyptian tombs depict male circumcision, so the practice is known to be at least 5,000 years old. The Jewish and Muslim traditions of circumcision have their origin in the Old Testament. Jews accept the practice as a sign of the covenant between God and Abraham. In Gen. 17:12, God instructs Abraham: "He that is eight days old shall be circumcised among you, every male throughout your generations" (Robson and Leung, 1992). As a Jew, Jesus was circumcised, and the early Christian church debated the need for circumcision as a criterion for joining the Christian fellowship; it decided that circumcision was not necessary for salvation. According to the apostle Paul, "For in Jesus Christ neither circumcision availeth nor uncircumcision; but faith which worketh by love" (Gal. 5:6). These religious traditions remain strong, although the health debate has led to a questioning of the religious practice by a few members of the Jewish community (Milos and Macris, 1992).

The practice of routine neonatal circumcision has been controversial within the U.S. medical profession for over a century. Circumcision was initially advocated in the Victorian era as a measure to reduce masturbation. Medical benefits from the procedure were first widely proposed in 1891 by P. C. Remondino, who claimed that circumcision prevented or cured a host of diseases, including alcoholism, epilepsy, asthma, and renal disease (Wallerstein, 1985). More scientific studies of the potential medical benefits of circumcision began to appear in the professional literature in the 1930s. Urologists observed an association between penile cancer and an intact foreskin (Schoen, 1992). During World War II, American troops stationed in the Pacific and in desert climates had problems with irritation and infection of the penis because of sand and the inability to maintain adequate hygiene. The military response was to circumcise many of the affected soldiers. However, the Japanese did not use circumcision despite their war experience in the same environments (Wallerstein, 1985).

Circumcision became popular, indeed almost universal, after the war. Rates remained high until the 1970s, when both the medical profession and the general public began to question the widespread use of the procedure for newborns. The American Academy of Pediatrics issued two separate statements in 1971 and 1975 declaring there were no valid medical indications for neonatal circumcision (Committee on Fetus and Newborn, 1975). Specific concerns were raised over the pain of the procedure and over potential complications in the face of questionable medical benefits. In 1985, the first in a series of papers was published that documented an increased risk of urinary tract infections in uncircumcised neonates (Wiswell et al., 1985). These reports came in association with an apparent increased risk of sexually transmitted disease, specifically the human immunodeficiency virus (HIV), in uncircumcised males (Schoen, 1993). In 1989 the American Academy of Pediatrics issued a revised statement that concluded that there were both medical advantages and medical disadvantages to the procedure and that full information and informed consent were important for parents who were making this decision (American Academy of Pediatrics, 1989).

Medical and ethical issues

The basic ethical question involved is whether it is justified to perform a surgical procedure on a healthy, unconsenting child to prevent the possibility of future disease. The primary ethical task is to balance the pain and potential complications with the potential benefits. Although the full details of the risks and benefits are beyond the scope of this discussion, key issues will be outlined.

Proponents of circumcision claim several advantages for the procedure: decreased incidence of urinary tract infections in infancy, decreased risk of penile cancer in adults, and decreased risk of sexually transmitted diseases (Wiswell, 1992; Wiswell et al., 1985). In addition, routine circumcision prevents occasional penile problems such as phimosis (a narrowing of the foreskin that prevents its retraction), balanitis (an infection of the head of the penis), and posthitis (an infection of the foreskin). Significant complications of the procedure are quite rare, occurring in less than 1 percent of circumcised neonates (Kaplan, 1983). Until the mid-1980s, circumcision was performed commonly without anesthesia. With the introduction of a variety of simple techniques (Kirya and Werthmann, 1978; Stang et al., 1988), it is claimed that the pain of the procedure can be minimized. In contrast to female circumcision, the procedure has no significant effect on sexual function or pleasure.

Social issues are raised in the debate. Many parents would like their sons to look like the majority of their peers in the locker room, and many parents would like their sons to look like their fathers, the majority of whom are circumcised. Finally, parents who have grown up in a society of circumcised men may find a circumcised penis to be more aesthetically pleasing.

Those who question the value of the procedure counter that the case for reductions in urinary tract infections, cancer rates, and sexually transmitted diseases is not convincing, or that many of the same benefits may be achieved through better personal hygiene (Poland, 1990; Milos and Macris, 1992). While the prodecure is generally safe, there are risks of excessive bleeding, infection, removal of too much tissue, tissue damage and scarring, reactions to anesthetic agents, and retention of urine (Kaplan, 1983). It is argued that the penile problems that may arise in uncircumcised males, such as balanitis, can be treated like any other local skin problems or infections. Further, it is noted that pain-control measures are often ineffective, carry their own risks (Snellman and Stang, 1992), and are associated with some pain as well. It is claimed that the foreskin provides a protective covering for the glans, making the uncircumcised penis more sensitive during sexual activity (Milos and Macris, 1992). Since the 1960s, a cultural shift has placed a higher value on preserving the natural look. Uncircumcised males are now common enough, the argument goes, that the appearance of an uncircumcised penis in the locker room will not be cause for embarrassment. Finally, it is claimed that a simple explanation from father to son will prevent a son's confusion about a different look to his penis.

Of all of the potential medical advantages of circumcision, the reduced risk of urinary tract infection in the infant is the best documented, and this is the benefit most likely to be experienced by the child (Wiswell, 1992; Schoen, 1993). Urinary tract infections in neonates are potentially serious infections that may be life-threatening and may lead to the later development of renal insufficiency and hypertension. However, the risk of urinary tract infection in uncircumcised infants is still relatively small, occurring in approximately 1 to 4 percent of infants (Wiswell, 1992). Of those infected, only a small minority will suffer long-term kidney damage (Chessare, 1992).

Parents are thus left with a difficult decision. Circumcision might be delayed until the child is old enough to make his own choice, but this alternative obviates the primary medical advantage, that is, decreasing the risk of urinary tract infection in infancy. In addition, performing the procedure beyond the newborn period may be associated with greater risks (Wiswell et al., 1993). Therefore, reliance on surrogate decision making by the parents for the newborn boy remains an ethically appropriate approach. With all of the current data in hand, many physicians and parents find themselves falling between the polar positions in this debate. As the 1989 American Academy of Pediatrics statement concluded, there is no clear answer to the question of whether the benefits of circumcision outweigh the risks. For many parents, the final decision will be made primarily on cultural and social grounds, with less weight placed on the potential health benefits or risks. Fortunately, there is some evidence that most adult men like the way they are, whether circumcised or not (Lee, 1990).

Unless additional medical research documents significantly greater benefits or harms of male circumcision, the social debate over the procedure in the United States is likely to continue. In this context, the responsibilities of both the physician and the parents are to make sure that all are fully informed about the benefits and risks of this procedure, and that the procedure, if elected, is performed in a competent and humane manner.

JEFFREY R. BOTKIN

Directly related to this article is the companion article in this entry: FEMALE CIRCUMCISION. *For a further discussion of the topics mentioned in this article, see the entries* INFANTS;

INFORMED CONSENT; JUDAISM; *and* ROMAN CATHOLICISM. *For a discussion of related ideas, see the entries* COMPASSION; PAIN AND SUFFERING; *and* VALUE AND VALUATION. *Other relevant material may be found under the entries* CHILDREN, *articles on* RIGHTS OF CHILDREN, *and* HEALTH-CARE AND RESEARCH ISSUES; LIFESTYLES AND PUBLIC HEALTH; *and* SEXUAL IDENTITY.

Bibliography

AMERICAN ACADEMY OF PEDIATRICS. TASK FORCE ON CIRCUMCISION. 1989. "Report of the Task Force on Circumcision." *Pediatrics* 84, no. 2:388–391.

CHESSARE, JOHN B. 1992. "Circumcision: Is the Risk of Urinary Tract Infection Really the Pivotal Issue?" *Clinical Pediatrics* 31, no. 2:100–104.

COMMITTEE ON FETUS AND NEWBORN. 1975. "Report of the Ad Hoc Task Force on Circumcision." *Pediatrics* 56, no. 4:610–611.

KAPLAN, GEORGE W. 1983. "Complications of Circumcision." *Urologic Clinics of North America* 10, no. 3:543–549.

KIRYA, CHRISTOPHER, and WERTHMANN, MILTON W. 1978. "Neonatal Circumcision and Penile Dorsal Nerve Block—A Painless Procedure." *Journal of Pediatrics* 92, no. 6:998–1000.

LEE, PETER A. 1990. "Neonatal Circumcision." *New England Journal of Medicine* 323, no. 17:1204–1205.

MILOS, MARILYN F. and MACRIS, DONNA. 1992. "Circumcision: A Medical or a Human Rights Issue?" *Journal of Nurse-Midwifery* 37, no. 2 (suppl):87s–96s.

POLAND, RONALD L. 1990. "The Question of Routine Neonatal Circumcision." *New England Journal of Medicine* 322, no. 18:1312–1315.

ROBSON, WILLIAM LANE, and LEUNG, ALEXANDER K. 1992. "The Circumcision Question." *Postgraduate Medicine* 96, no. 6:237–242, 244.

SCHOEN, EDGAR J. 1992. "Urologists and Circumcision of Newborns." *Urology* 40, no. 2:99–101.

———. 1993. "Circumcision Updated—Indicated?" *Pediatrics* 92, no. 6:860–861.

SNELLMAN, LEONARD W., and STANG, HOWARD J. 1992. "Prospective Evaluation of Complications of Local Anesthesia for Neonatal Circumcision." *American Journal of Diseases of Children* 146, no. 4:482. Abstract of a paper presented at the Annual Meeting of the Ambulatory Pediatric Association, May 5.

STANG, HOWARD J.; GUNNAR, MEGAN R.; SNELLMAN, LEONARD; CONDON, LAWRENCE M.; and KESTENBAUM, ROBERTA. 1988. "Local Anesthesia for Neonatal Circumcision: Effects on Distress and Cortisol Response." *Journal of the American Medical Association* 259, no. 10:1507–1511.

WALLERSTEIN, EDWARD. 1985. "Circumcision: The Uniquely American Enigma." *Urologic Clinics of North America* 12, no. 1:123–132.

WISWELL, THOMAS E. 1992. "Circumcision—An Update." *Current Problems in Pediatrics* 22, no. 10:424–431.

WISWELL, THOMAS E.; SMITH, FRANKLIN R.; and BASS, JAMES W. 1985. "Decreased Incidence of Urinary Tract Infection in Circumcised Male Infants." *Pediatrics* 75, no. 5: 901–903.

WISWELL, THOMAS E.; TENCER, HEATHER I.; WELCH, CATHERINE A.; and CHAMBERLAIN, JOHN L. 1993. "Circumcision in Children Beyond the Neonatal Period." *Pediatrics* 92, no. 6:791–793.

CIVIL COMMITMENT

See COMMITMENT TO MENTAL INSTITUTIONS.

CIVIL DISOBEDIENCE AND HEALTH CARE

Organized civil disobedience as a political act designed to challenge and change unjust laws has a long history in working-class protest, alongside strikes and riots, as well as in nonviolent resistance to oppression by religious pacifists. Carried out in a setting that involves the delivery of health services or the protest of health-care policy and law, civil disobedience in the United States occurred at least as early as 1916. In that year Margaret Sanger and other women in New York City sought to disseminate birth control information, knowingly violating the law. In the 1980s, People for the Ethical Treatment of Animals (PETA) and other animal-rights groups used direct action (trespass, breaking and entering) to prevent animal experimentation for human benefit by releasing the animals from the laboratories where they were confined. In the 1990s, members of the AIDS Coalition to Unleash Power (ACT-UP) staged sit-ins at the offices of major drug companies in an effort to force the companies to reduce the cost of drugs used to treat HIV and AIDS. As the end of the century approached, the most frequent, widely publicized, and controversial protests have been carried out by Operation Rescue. Founded by Randall E. Terry in 1987 in Binghamton, New York, Operation Rescue has organized blockades of more than 400 abortion clinics around the nation in the effort to "rescue" the unborn by preventing abortions and abortion counseling. Some 25,000 Operation Rescue protesters were arrested between 1988 and 1990 for trespass and related offenses.

Definition

The variety of goals and methods of civil disobedience makes it difficult to generalize about its nature and justification. Central to its definition are the illegality and nonviolence of the conduct, the purpose of the protest, and the nature of the justification. What is distinctive about civil disobedience in the setting of health care is thus neither the definition of the concept nor the justification of the act. It is, rather, the application of the concept and the justification of acts so described in this particular context.

If the term is used strictly, civil disobedience must be contrasted with forms of protest that are permitted by law. Boycotts, poster parades, and heckling are not civil disobedience, so long as no laws are broken by the protesters. But trespass and blockades that prevent public access are unlawful (criminal misdemeanors), and such tactics are typically incorporated in strategies of civil disobedience. On the other hand, a doctor who refuses to sign a contract to provide health care for a certain class of patients because the reimbursement for the services is judged to be woefully inadequate is not committing civil disobedience—not even if the refusal is public, conscientious, and designed to change the reimbursement practices—since no law requires the doctor to sign such a contract in the first place.

Yet in the United States, with its complex federal system (local and state vs. national jurisdictions) and constitutional provisions for reviewing statutory law, it is often difficult to determine what is and what is not unlawful. The distribution of contraceptive devices by William Baird in the 1960s in New Jersey and elsewhere, which violated criminal statutes in those states and led to his arrest, is plausibly viewed as civil disobedience: Baird knew he was violating state statutes. A subsequent decision by the U.S. Supreme Court, however, vindicated his actions by holding the state statutes unconstitutional (*Eisenstadt v. Baird*, 405 U.S. 438 [1972]). Some would say this showed his civil disobedience was justified; but others might argue that this showed his acts were not civil disobedience at all, because they were not ultimately illegal. But allowing forty-three infants to die in a special-care nursery in Connecticut between 1970 and 1972, on the ground that their "prognosis for meaningful life was extremely poor or hopeless," was probably illegal—though the doctors who permitted these deaths may have thought otherwise and their conduct was not prosecuted. Whether permitting these deaths would qualify as civil disobedience depends not only on their legality but also on their purpose or aim.

Civil disobedience (as in Baird's case) is distinctive in that it uses unlawful conduct, in an open and public manner, in an effort to try to change the law by raising the consciousness of the majority to the (alleged) injustice being protested. This purpose contrasts sharply with other forms of conscientious illegal conduct, such as principled refusal to obey the law and evasive violation of the law (as perhaps was true of the special-care physicians). A doctor opposed to capital punishment who refuses (as recommended by the American Psychiatric Association) to participate in a court-ordered execution by lethal injection of a condemned prisoner does not commit civil disobedience, even if he loses his job as a public employee. No law requires any doctor to perform this service. Neither is there a law that requires a nurse to obey a "Do Not Resuscitate" (DNR) order for a dying patient. However strong and well-founded her convictions to save human life may be, her violating the DNR order is conscientious refusal, not civil disobedience.

Capt. Yolanda Huet-Vaughn, M.D., however, who refused to join her Army Reserve unit for service in the Persian Gulf War in 1990, is a more interesting borderline case. She publicly argued that "the Department of Defense was interfering with the doctor–patient relationship" on the ground that military policy required doctors to give soldiers headed for the Persian Gulf anthrax toxin and botulin toxin without their informed consent. She sought, unsuccessfully, status as a conscientious objector. Early in 1991, after a month-long tour of talk shows on radio and television, she was arrested and charged with desertion; she served eight months of a thirty-month prison sentence. In its illegality, publicity, and nonviolence, her conduct is typical of civil disobedience. But it is also typical of personal conscientious refusal to participate in what the individual believes is immoral conduct required by law, regardless of its effects on the law or policy being protested.

Covert law violation and evasion, as found in the Stamp Act protests (against taxation in the form of stamps on documents, newspapers, and other items) the American colonists of the 1760s and as practiced by the abolitionists who operated the Underground Railroad (to assist fugitive slaves) prior to the U.S. Civil War, may effectively defeat an unjust law. But they do not do so by appealing openly to principles of justice shared by the common conscience of the majority. Such an appeal was essential to the civil disobedience preached and practiced by Henry David Thoreau in the 1840s in Massachusetts, by Mohandas Gandhi in South Africa and India from 1907 until his death in 1948, and by Martin Luther King, Jr., in Georgia and Alabama during the civil rights movement of the 1960s. In this respect, evasion of a law and a conscientious refusal are alike: Their primary purpose is not to mount an openly political effort to change the law but to avoid participation in it and, to that extent, to nullify it. Therefore, unlike civil disobedience, refusal and evasion need not be conducted in the glare of publicity.

Many, like Gandhi and King, argue that civil disobedience must be nonviolent, at least in intention, so far as persons (if not also property) are concerned; and that nonviolence includes passive obedience, the willingness to suffer the lawful punishment for breaking the law (even though the law is believed to be unjust). Others argue that civil disobedience may be either violent or nonviolent; some, like Thoreau, are essentially silent on the point. In any case, few would deny that, other things being equal, nonviolent illegal acts are much more likely to be justified than is violence to persons or property. The antiabortion protests conducted by the group known as the Lambs of Christ, founded in 1989 by Father Norman Weslin, is a militant but nonviolent group that practices passive obedience and silent protest as it blockades abortion clinics. But the better-known Operation Rescue, although claiming to be "nonviolent in word and deed," has often used tactics that damage or deface property as well as violate the legal rights of pregnant women seeking abortion or abortion counseling. (It should be noted that Operation Rescue does not characterize its protests as civil disobedience, on the ground that civil disobedience is necessarily "political," whereas fetal rescues are not.)

Finally, civil disobedience may be either direct or indirect. It is direct whenever the law being violated is the law believed to be unjust (as when birth control advocates, like Sanger and Baird, distribute contraceptives in direct violation of a law prohibiting such distribution). It is indirect whenever the law violated is itself not under protest—perhaps the injustice being protested is inaccessible to direct violation (as when pro-choice protesters commit trespass and theft to protest substandard medical care available to patients seeking abortions). In the nature of the case, it is almost always possible for citizens to protest any government law or regulation indirectly, by refusing to pay their taxes. However, indirect civil disobedience often becomes largely symbolic because it lacks sufficient causal proximity to the moral wrong that inspires it. Nevertheless, the symbolism itself may be important both as an expression of deep moral conviction by the protesters (especially if it leads to their arrest and punishment) and as an effective tactic in drawing public attention to the issue.

Some have argued that indirect civil disobedience in a constitutional democracy can never be justified. But that is a minority view. From the time of Thoreau, who withheld his taxes to protest the Mexican War, the Fugitive Slave Law, and mistreatment of American Indians, to Martin Luther King, Jr., who in 1963 refused to obey a court injunction forbidding him to march in the streets of Birmingham, Alabama, in protest of racial segregation, indirect civil disobedience has been widely practiced in the United States.

Justification

Quite apart from differences in how best to characterize civil disobedience, theorists also differ over the grounds required to justify an act of civil disobedience. Given American history and traditions, few argue that civil disobedience (whether direct or indirect, violent or nonviolent) is never justified. Equally few would argue the extreme reverse, that all acts of civil disobedience are justified. At most, some would insist that any conscientious act, including even illegal and violent acts, can be justified simply by virtue of its conscientiousness. This is particularly true of those who see in human conscience "the voice of God within us."

Traditionally, justifications of conscientious disobedience of the law have been based on more objective grounds and sophisticated reasoning. Christian thinkers have for centuries appealed to "higher law" doctrines, according to which human laws that do not conform to divine "natural" law establish no obligation to be obeyed. This view is succinctly expressed in the epigram of Saint Augustine (endorsed by Saint Thomas Aquinas and invoked by Martin Luther King, Jr.) that "an unjust law is no law at all." Secular thinkers have often favored a utilitarian criterion of justified disobedience. On this view, an act of civil disobedience is justified whenever more overall good than harm results. Both these approaches tend to obscure the fact that any prospect of success for mass illegal protest or even individual conscientious refusal depends upon a certain degree of constitutional protection of the rights of dissenters, protections not found under every government.

In recent decades both higher law and utilitarian justifications have been displaced by theories designed to understand civil disobedience from within the framework of the rule of law, constitutional democracy, and respect for minority rights. On such views (developed in the 1970s by the philosopher John Rawls), an act of civil disobedience is justified if and only if four criteria are satisfied.

First, the dissenters must have made some good-faith effort to use normal political means to achieve the change in the law that they desire. It is difficult to defend breaking the law, even in a good cause, if the law-breaking is unnecessary (lawful means of change would have sufficed) or premature (lawful means of change were not even tried). Second, the protester must accord the right to others also to use illegal tactics to try to overturn laws these others regard as unjust. No cause is unique, and no protesters on behalf of any cause are uniquely privileged. Third, the law or policy that is the target of protest must involve some fundamental injustice, or violation of individual rights. It is not enough that the law being protested merely departs from good judgment or ideal policy on matters that raise no fundamental question of injustice. Of course, protesters and their critics may well disagree in any given case whether the law under protest is unjust. Resolving such a dispute rationally can be done only if both sides can agree on some fundamental theory of social justice that provides the relevant criteria to distinguish just from unjust laws. Finally, if civil disobedience (rather than conscientious refusal) is in question, there must be some reasonable prospect of success that does not jeopardize the framework of the society itself. Civil disobedience normally respects the rule of law even though it involves unlawful conduct. It is a rare cause that will justify unlawful disobedience at the cost of social disorder and political chaos.

Even with such criteria, it may be difficult to decide in any given case whether the act of civil disobedience is justified. Much turns on the moral convictions relevant to the third criterion above. For example, if one believes that abortion is murder, then one may well believe that preventing murder by fetal rescue cannot be wrong. (Ethicists, of course, will counsel that, here as elsewhere, not every means is permissible to achieve a just end.) However, insofar as the belief that abortion is murder rests on a conception of the human person that depends on sectarian religious convictions, using illegal direct action to force the conduct of nonbelievers into compliance with this conception is not legitimate. For it rests on a ground that is not available and acceptable—even in principle—to all as a product of sound reason and shared experience. Where the relevant facts and moral principles held by the protesting minority are not shared by the majority, acts of civil disobedience are not likely to succeed, and—more important—neither will their justification.

Hugo Adam Bedau

For a further discussion of topics mentioned in this entry, see the entries Medical Codes and Oaths; Natural Law; Rights, *article on* rights in bioethics; *and* Strikes by Health Professionals. *This entry will find application in the entries* Nursing Ethics; Profession and Professional Ethics; *and* Whistleblowing. *For a discussion of related ideas, see the entries on* Law and Bioethics; Obligation and Supererogation; Utility; *and* Virtue and Character.

Bibliography

American Psychiatric Association. 1980. "Position Statement on Medical Participation in Capital Punishment." *American Journal of Psychiatry* 137, no. 11:1487.

Bedau, Hugo A., ed. 1969. *Civil Disobedience: Theory and Practice.* New York: Pegasus. Reprints twenty articles and essays.

———, ed. 1991. *Civil Disobedience in Focus.* New York and London: Routledge. Reprints twelve essays, four classics and eight by contemporary philosophers.

Bernal, Ellen W.; Hoover, Patricia S.; and Aroskar, Mila Ann. 1987. "Commentary: The Nurse's Appeal to Conscience." *Hastings Center Report* 17, no. 2:25–26.

Bonnie, Richard J. 1990. "Healing-Killing Conflicts: Medical Ethics and the Death Penalty." *Hastings Center Report* 20, no. 3:12–18.

CARTER, GEORGE M. 1992. *ACT UP, the AIDS War and Activism.* Westfield, N.J.: Open Media.

CHILDRESS, JAMES F. 1971. *Civil Disobedience and Political Obligation: A Study in Christian Social Ethics.* New Haven, Conn.: Yale University Press.

COHEN, CARL. 1989. "Militant Morality: Civil Disobedience and Bioethics." *Hastings Center Report* 19, no. 6:23–25. This essay is followed by a symposium to which nine authors contributed brief essays.

DUFF, RAYMOND, and CAMPBELL, A. G. M. 1973. "Moral and Ethical Dilemmas in the Special-Care Nursery." *New England Journal of Medicine* 289, no. 2:890–894.

FAGLIONI, KELLY L. 1991. "Balancing First Amendment Rights of Abortion Protesters with the Rights of Their 'Victims.'" *Washington and Lee Law Review* 48:347–380.

GANDHI, MOHANDAS K. 1942–1949. *Non-Violence in Peace & War.* 2 vols. Ahmedabad, India: Navajivan.

HARRIS, PAUL, ed. 1989. *Civil Disobedience.* Lanham, Md.: University Press of America. A selection of recent articles by philosophers; valuable introduction and extensive bibliography.

KING, MARTIN LUTHER, JR. 1963. "Letter from Birmingham City Jail." Reprinted in *Civil Disobedience in Focus,* pp. 68–84. Edited by Hugo A. Bedau. New York and London: Routledge.

MADDEN, EDWARD H., and HARE, PETER H. 1978. "Civil Disobedience in Health Services." In *Encyclopedia of Bioethics,* vol. 1, pp. 159–162. Edited by Warren T. Reich. New York: Free Press.

RAWLS, JOHN. 1971. *A Theory of Justice.* Cambridge, Mass.: Harvard University Press. Civil disobedience and conscientious objection are discussed on pp. 363–391.

TERRY, RANDALL E. 1988. *Operation Rescue.* Springdale, Pa.: Whitaker House.

THOREAU, HENRY DAVID. 1849. "Civil Disobedience." Reprinted in *Civil Disobedience in Focus,* pp. 28–48. Edited by Hugo A. Bedau. New York and London: Routledge.

WHITEHEAD, JOHN W. 1991. "Civil Disobedience and Operation Rescue: A Historical and Theoretical Analysis." *Washington and Lee Law Review* 48:77–122. One of nine articles in the Winter issue devoted to abortion protest.

YODER, JOHN H.; ZINN, HOWARD; CHRISTIANSEN, DREW; LIPPMAN, MATTHEW; CAVANAUGH-O'KEEFE, JOHN; McEWEN, STEPHEN J., JR.; DAVIS, PAUL R.; DAVIS, WILLIAM C.; DOHERTY, MAURA C.; and LOESCH, MARTIN C. 1991. "Symposium on Civil Disobedience." *Notre Dame Journal of Law, Ethics, & Public Policy* 5, no. 4:889–1119. Contains eight articles focused on abortion protests.

CLIMATIC CHANGE

In recent years many environmental problems have come to public consciousness. Of all of these problems, global climate change could prove to be the most dramatic and least reversible. It could have profound implications for the health of humans and other beings.

A climate change is quite different from a change in the weather. While weather constantly changes, climate is relatively stable. We can discuss the North American climate during the last ice age, but when we talk about the cold and snow in Boulder, Colorado, yesterday, we are talking about the weather. Weather systems last from a few hours to a few weeks and range from about 10 to 10,000 horizontal kilometers in size. A climate regime may persist for millennia, with variability in temperature and precipitation being part of a stable climate system. The climate system involves complex interactions between the atmosphere, oceans, land surface, snow and ice cover, and the biosphere. We are learning that human activity is also a part of the dynamic that affects climate.

The discovery of anthropogenic climate change

On June 23, 1988, a sweltering day in Washington, D.C., in the middle of a severe drought in the United States, James Hansen of the National Aeronautics and Space Administration testified before the U.S. Senate Committee on Energy and Natural Resources. It was 99 percent probable, Hansen contended, that global warming had begun. His testimony, which was covered by media all over the world, appeared to many people to come from nowhere. But like most "overnight" sensations, speculation about climate change has a history.

In the eighteenth century, Benjamin Franklin surmised that the hard winter of 1783–1784 was due to excessive dust in the air, either from the destruction of meteorites or from volcanic eruptions. Early in the nineteenth century, the French mathematician Jean Baptiste Fourier (1768–1830) speculated that the atmosphere might function like the glass in a greenhouse, warming Earth's surface by preventing heat from escaping. In 1861 John Tyndall showed that slight changes in the composition of the atmosphere could significantly raise Earth's temperature. The Swedish Nobel Prize winner Svante Arrhenius theorized in 1896 that the use of fossil fuels would increase atmospheric carbon dioxide, thereby changing climate and affecting biological processes. He calculated that a doubling of atmospheric carbon dioxide would lead to an increase of four to six degrees centigrade in Earth's mean surface temperature. In the 1930s the British engineer George Callendar revived Arrhenius's ideas and asserted that global warming had already begun. Working in the United States, Gilbert Plass, Roger Revelle, and Hans Suess brought these ideas into the scientific mainstream in the 1950s. A very influential article by Revelle and Suess in 1957 asserted that because of the exponentially increasing use of fossil fuels, an experiment was in progress that could not have happened in the past and that could not be reproduced in the future. Their work led to the establishment of the Mauna Loa Observatory in Hawaii, which has been measuring carbon dioxide concentrations in the atmosphere since 1958.

The climate anomalies of 1972 and the global food shortages of 1972–1973 brought the possibility of climate change to the attention of a broader audience. Droughts in the Sahel region of Africa in the late 1960s and early 1970s had reminded people how dependent on climate humans remain. When drought also occurred in the Soviet Union in 1972, world grain prices doubled; global food shortages followed. During the same year, frost destroyed coffee plantations in Brazil, and changes in seawater temperatures (related to a climate anomaly called "El Niño") had a severe impact on Peru's anchovy fisheries. U.S. Secretary of State Henry Kissinger raised the possibility of climate change in a 1974 speech to the United Nations.

The climate change scare of the early 1970s was a fear of cooling. From the 1940s through the 1960s, Earth's mean surface temperature had declined; there was concern that another ice age was beginning. The Central Intelligence Agency undertook a study of how such a cooling might affect agricultural production in the Soviet Union; and the same Senate committee that fifteen years later would hold hearings on global warming held hearings on global cooling.

Whether the fear was of a cooling or a warming, climate increasingly came to be viewed as a dynamic system that is vulnerable to human action. By the mid-1970s the possibility of climate change had been discovered.

The current scientific view

Throughout the late 1970s and 1980s, conferences and studies were instituted by a wide range of national and international organizations. The culmination of this activity was the 1990 report of the Intergovernmental Panel on Climate Change (IPCC). The process that led to the development of this report (published in 1991) involved 170 scientists from 25 countries; 200 other scientists reviewed the results. The goal of the IPCC process was to determine the international scientific consensus about climate change. The conclusion was that if emissions of "greenhouse gases" (primarily carbon dioxide, methane, chlorofluorocarbons, and nitrous oxide) continue as usual, Earth's mean surface temperature could rise 0.2 to 0.5 degree centigrade per decade, with a likely warming of 1 degree centigrade by 2025, and 3 degrees centigrade by the end of the twenty-first century. This would be the greatest temperature change to have occurred on Earth for at least 10,000 years.

In a 1992 update the IPCC noted new research developments, but stood by its 1990 projections with only minor revisions. A 1992 assessment by leading climatologists Tom M. L. Wigley and Sarah C. B. Raper reduced the IPCC estimates of expected temperature increases on what they called a "business as usual" scenario; but they concluded that even on the revised projections, temperature increases are likely to occur that are four to five times more dramatic than any change that has occurred since the 1890s.

Some scientists remain skeptical: Some believe that there will be no climate change; others believe that there will be a cooling. At this point there is too much uncertainty to rule the skeptics out of court. One thing certain is that there is a "greenhouse effect." According to climatologist Stephen Schneider, it is "one of the best, most well-established scientific theories in the atmospheric sciences" (Boyle and Ardill, 1989, p. 12). Were it not for the greenhouse effect, all of the planets of the solar system would be cold and lifeless. But as we have learned in other areas, such as medicine, too much of a good thing can be a bad thing.

The greenhouse effect occurs when a planetary atmosphere, due to its physical/chemical composition, permits solar radiation to heat the surface of the planet but traps some of the heat that would otherwise radiate back into space. The greenhouse effect explains, at least partially, the differences between conditions on the surfaces of Venus, Mars, and Earth. Venus has an extremely dense, carbon dioxide–rich atmosphere that traps so much heat that life is not possible on the surface of the planet. Mars has a very thin, carbon dioxide–poor atmosphere, and mid-latitude surface temperatures on Mars are about the same as those of Earth's polar winters. Earth is just right for evolving and sustaining life—at least for the moment.

Another fact about which we are certain is that human activity is affecting the chemical composition of Earth's atmosphere. From 1800 to 1990 there has been an increase of about 26 percent in atmospheric carbon dioxide, nearly half of that occurring since the 1960s. Other greenhouse gases have increased by even greater percentages during the same period. Concentrations of these gases have risen as a result of activities that are essential to economic growth and development, at least as they are presently conceived: fossil fuel combustion, deforestation, food-animal production, rice-paddy agriculture, and fertilizer use.

What is certain, then, is that the greenhouse effect exists, and that concentrations of greenhouse gases in the atmosphere are increasing. However, not all scientists agree about what the effects of these increasing concentrations are likely to be. There are extremely complicated and ill-understood feedbacks in the climate system. The effects of these feedbacks could be to stabilize climate even in the face of changes in the atmosphere, or to exaggerate the effects of climate change. Since these feedbacks could be positive or negative and are not well understood, the scientific community's prediction of a significant greenhouse warming is a cautious one.

The effects of climate change

The image that many people have of a global warming is that all regions of Earth would be warmed equally, as if one turned up the thermostat in the global house. This image is quite misleading. The impacts of global warming would be very diverse. Some regions would warm while others would cool. Precipitation patterns would change, and extreme events (e.g., droughts and hurricanes) would become more frequent. While this much is clear, it is extremely difficult to say how particular regions would be affected. The predictions generally agree about the global effects of climate change but disagree to a great extent about its regional effects.

Impacts of climate change fall into three categories. First-order impacts involve physical changes such as rises in sea level, effects on biological systems and circulation of water and so on. A large number of species will become extinct and many ecosystems will fracture and disintegrate. Some of the most dramatic first-order effects of a global warming could be the inundation of island nations, such as the Maldives, Kiribati (Gilbert Islands), and the Marshall Islands. Egypt could lose 1 percent of its land due to flooding. Second-order impacts involve the direct social, economic, and health effects of first-order impacts. An example would be the economic, social, and cultural consequences of Egypt's loss of 1 percent of its land. The part of Egypt that would be threatened by a sea-level rise is the Nile delta, home to 48 million people and contributor of 15 percent of Egypt's GNP. Third-order impacts of climate change involve the indirect social and political responses to the first- and second-order effects. Third-order impacts might include massive emigration from affected regions such as the Nile delta, and international conflicts resulting from economic dislocations and changing patterns of resource use.

In the late 1980s, when climate change was born as an important contemporary issue, it was commonly said that all people would suffer from climate change. However it has become increasingly clear that climate change will involve winners and losers, and most experts believe that the rich countries will do better than the poor ones. Rich countries can build seawalls and dikes to protect coastal areas against rising sea levels. They can even gain economically by developing and exporting technologies that will help in adapting to climate change. Rich countries can pay more for food if climate change adversely affects agriculture. In general, their control of capital can be used to shield them from many effects of a changing climate. Poor countries do not have resources to protect themselves in these ways. Moreover, some poor countries (e.g., Bangladesh) already suffer enormously from extreme climatic events.

But even though it may generally be true that the rich would do better than the poor in adapting to climate change, there are still reasons for the rich to be concerned. Rich people are often more averse to risk than poor people, for they have more to lose. Moreover, if climate change occurs, there will be differential effects across both rich and poor countries. For example, according to some scenarios, agriculture in the U.S. Great Plains might dry up and blow away, while in some arid regions of Africa precipitation might increase.

Although the regional effects of global climate change are very uncertain, it is clear that there will be winners and losers. When human action has consequences that benefit some and burden others, it becomes a matter for moral evaluation.

Risk and insurance

Some commentators have tried to transform the ethical problems implicit in the possibility of climate change into problems of rational choice. One approach has been to think of the possibility of climate change as a risk, and the costs of emission reduction, mitigation, and adaptation as the premium paid for insurance against this risk. However tempting this approach may be, the insurance metaphor is misleading. An insurance company is able to set rational premiums because of actuarial tables that are based on the frequency with which compensable losses occur. But however strong our theoretical reasons are for thinking that climate change will occur, we have nothing like actuarial tables that tell us about the frequency of climate change when the atmosphere is loaded with greenhouse gases. Moreover, the idea that we are in a position to reasonably assess the potential damages of climate change is quite absurd. No one knows what all the economic and health effects of a greenhouse warming would be, much less how to attach meaningful economic values to the loss of many wild species and the destruction of societies and cultures. Although economists such as William Nordhaus (1992) have estimated the costs of various emissions-reduction scenarios, neither he nor his colleagues have tried to estimate the damages that such reductions might help us to avoid. While it is easy to talk about the importance of taking out insurance against the possibility of a greenhouse warming, there is no way to determine what it would be rational to pay for such insurance.

Finally, the insurance metaphor defers rather than evades the ethical questions. Even if we were able to determine a rational premium, the question of how the costs should be distributed would remain. Talk of purchasing insurance against the risk of a greenhouse warming does not free us from the hard ethical discussions.

Moral and political issues

Philosophers often distinguish duties of justice from other sorts of duties. For present purposes, however, we can think of climate change as posing questions of justice with respect to our human contemporaries (intragenerational justice), our descendants (intergenerational justice), and possibly nonhuman nature. Because climate change is by its very nature global in scope, the questions of justice that it provokes are international.

The rich countries of the world have loaded the atmosphere with the greenhouse gases that may already be changing climate. They have benefited from their actions by developing economically. While rich countries have gained the benefits, the deleterious effects of their emissions will be felt by everyone. If climate change-induced floods occur in Bangladesh, it will not be due to the actions of the Bangladeshis. They will not have caused the floods, nor will they have benefited from the past emissions of greenhouse gases that caused them.

In addition to these historical inequities in emissions, there are important differences in present emissions. A handful of industrial countries emit between one-half and three-quarters of all greenhouse gases. Yet at the United Nations–sponsored Conference on Environment and Development, held in Rio de Janeiro in June 1992, the rich countries were unwilling to agree to timetables and targets even for stabilizing their emissions, much less reducing them, mainly due to the intransigence of the United States.

Rich countries became rich in part by taking actions that may be changing the global climate. This climate change may have devastating impacts on poor countries. What do the rich owe the poor as a consequence of their actions? This question arises against the background of an international system characterized by radical and increasing inequality. According to Sir Crispin Tickell (1992), in 1880 the ratio of real per capita income between Europe, on the one hand, and India and China, on the other, was two to one; in 1965 it was forty to one; and in the 1990s it is seventy to one. According to the World Bank (1992), poverty is increasing: 1.1 billion people are living in poverty, more than 20 percent of the world's population. Yet because of the burden of international debt and the trade relations between rich and poor nations, resources are being sent from poor countries to rich ones. According to Susan George (1992), between 1982 and 1990 rich countries transferred about 900 billion dollars in loans, credits, and grants to poor countries. Over the same period poor countries transferred more than 1.3 trillion dollars to rich countries in interest and principal payments on loans.

Underlying these problems of inequality and poverty are an exploding population in some parts of the developing world and increasing overconsumption in the developed world. The United States, with 5 percent of the world's population, annually consumes 25 percent of the world's fossil fuels, 33 percent of its paper, 24 percent of its aluminum, and 13 percent of its fertilizer. A child born in 1994 in the United States will in his or her lifetime drive 700,000 miles, using 28,000 gallons of gasoline; produce 110,250 pounds of trash; eat 8,486 pounds of red meat; and consume enough electricity to burn 16,610 pounds of coal. Earth simply cannot support many Americans. The world population is now more than 5 billion, and is increasing by 300 million per year. An "optimistic" scenario calls for world population to stabilize at 9 billion in the twenty-first century. Many observers expect population to grow far beyond that.

One way of trying to understand the joint impact of overconsumption and exploding population is to consider the following facts. Sweden is a country that enjoys one of the highest standards of living in the world, yet its per capita carbon dioxide emissions are only 40 percent of those of the United States. If Sweden's level of per capita emissions were to be established as an international ceiling, the United States would have to reduce its emissions by two or three times what most environmentalists are now calling for. Yet even given such painful reductions on the part of some countries, according to this scenario world emissions would nearly triple, reflecting the large populations of some less developed countries, despite their current very low consumption of energy. A tripling of emissions is far beyond any of the IPCC scenarios, and its effects on the climate system could well be catastrophic.

Philosophical theorizing about international justice is underdeveloped, and very little work has been done on international environmental justice. The most influential philosophical theories of justice were formulated with an eye to what constitutes a just national distribution of private goods. Pattern theories such as that of John Rawls (1993), and entitlement theories such as that of Robert Nozick (1974), have received the most attention. Although we can speculate about what these theories might imply with respect to climate change, neither philosopher has had much to say about global justice, much less global environmental justice.

Rawls's principle of distributive justice is the "Difference Principle": Social and economic inequalities are to be attached to positions and offices that are open to all under conditions of fair equality of opportunity, and they are to be to the greatest benefit of the least advantaged members of society. Whether we take the subjects to be individuals or societies, it seems quite obvious that the global distribution of social and economic benefits is unjust according to this principle. Moreover, if we were to use the Difference Principle as a test for who should benefit from further releases of greenhouse gases and who should bear the costs of reduction, it seems equally clear that current policies would not satisfy this principle.

Nozick argues that the moral acceptability of a distribution depends entirely on how it came about. If the present distribution resulted from a just initial distribution through voluntary exchanges, then it is just, regardless of how unequal it may be. But given the global history of domination, imperialism, and exploitation, it seems clear that the present global distribution is unjust on Nozick's grounds. According to Nozick, any complete theory of justice must include a principle specifying how past injustices are to be rectified, but he has little to say about what such a principle may require.

Although it appears that both Rawls and Nozick are committed to the view that the current international order is unjust, neither deals specifically with this question or with the distribution of environmental benefits and burdens. Moreover, there are reasons for supposing that many environmental goods resist treatment as distributable benefits and burdens. The bad effects of climate change would include spillover effects suffered by some parties who had virtually no role in bringing them about. On reasonable human time scales, a stable climate is irreplaceable and irreversible. Furthermore, modeling aspects of the environment as distributable goods may be misleading and inappropriate. Such an approach neglects the fact that we humans are situated in an environment that conditions and affects everything we do, and in part constitutes our identities.

While there is good reason for supposing that both historical and current patterns of greenhouse gas emissions are part of an unjust system of intragenerational relationships, philosophical theories of justice have not yet given us the conceptual resources to address these issues in a detailed and meaningful way. More work needs to be done.

In addition to questions about intragenerational justice, global climate change poses moral questions about intergenerational justice. Those who come after us will live in a very different world than the one we inhabit, due in part to actions that we are now taking. Some who are influenced by utilitarian philosophers such as Henry Sidgwick (1874) may think that we owe just as much to future people as to present ones, since once they come to exist, they will be just as real as present people and will have the same moral status. On this view, the claims of future people should not be treated less seriously than those of present people simply because they

are remote from us in time. But barring a complete collapse of Earth's human population, over the course of millennia there will be vastly more people in the future than exist now. If we take each future person as seriously as each present person, it would appear that the interests of the present would be swamped by virtue of the size of our future human population.

Other thinkers, impressed by an argument of Derek Parfit's (1984), may conclude that we have no obligations to future people (although this is not Parfit's conclusion). On this view, future people who feel disadvantaged would have no cause for complaint against us because their very existence would be contingent on actions that we have taken. If our present actions were other than they are, then different people would come to exist in the future. Thus, no future person can say that he or she would have been better off had we made different choices; for if we had made different choices, then that person would not have existed at all.

Many economists would grant that we have obligations to those who will follow us, but they would argue that these obligations are easily fulfilled. Suppose that, because we are now acting in such a way as to change the climate, our descendants living in 2094 will incur damages valued at N dollars. In order for our climate change activities to be justified, we must profit enough from them to provide our descendants with N dollars when they come into existence. Because of the power of compound interest, small present benefits justify large future damages. If N dollars come due in a century and we can obtain a 5 percent return on our investments, our present benefit from climate-changing activities would have to be only .0068N dollars (compounded monthly) in order for them to be justified. In other words, a present benefit of $100,000 would justify inflicting a compensation of $14.68 billion on those living a century hence.

There are many problems with such an approach. Even if we were able to compensate future people adequately in this way, they will have been deprived of the ability to make some significant choices. For example, they will not have been able to choose to preserve a stable climate regime, even if that implies a lower standard of living.

This approach also involves the ludicrous idea that we can attach meaningful economic values to the loss of many wild species, the destruction of societies and cultures, and the unknown health effects of significant climate change. There simply are no credible attempts to carry out a benefit–cost analysis of the warming of Earth's median surface temperature by three degrees centigrade. This is hardly surprising, since there is often a great deal of disagreement about such relatively simple questions as the short-term effects of a change in the marginal tax rate of a single country.

Peter Brown (1992) and Edith Brown Weiss (1988) have argued that we have a fiduciary trust to preserve Earth's natural and human heritage at a level at least as good as that we received. On this basis, Weiss argues that we should reduce greenhouse gas emissions, take steps to minimize the damage that results from climate change, and develop strategies to assist future generations in adapting to climate change. This is a sensible approach that has the virtue of squaring with many people's moral intuitions. It suggests that we have significant obligations to future people, but that they do not entirely swamp the interests of the present.

Unfortunately, the fiduciary view verges on the platitudinous. Among those who believe that the buildup of greenhouse gases poses a threat, not many would deny that we need to reduce emissions, minimize harms, and develop adaptation strategies. What people disagree about is how aggressively we should pursue these policies, what the proper mix of them is, and who should bear the burdens. The fiduciary approach stops short of trying to answer these hard questions.

Furthermore, if we take seriously the idea that each generation has an obligation to preserve Earth's natural and human heritage at a level at least as good as what was received, then we are immediately plunged into questions about how to evaluate the goodness of our own heritage and various changes that we might make with respect to it. These are the sorts of questions that economists try to answer, using various techniques of benefit–cost analysis, such as interviewing people about their willingness to pay (or accept compensation) for environmental good, that ethicists typically find unsatisfactory.

In addition to the problems of human health and welfare that are likely to be caused by climate change, nonhuman nature will also be affected. Climate change is likely to be much too rapid for most plants and animals to adapt to or migrate from. Even when migration would in principle be possible, no migration routes will be available for most plants and animals in a densely populated and developed world.

In recent years a powerful literature has developed that argues humans have obligations to nonhuman nature. Some philosophers, such as Peter Singer (1990), argue that our direct obligations end at the border of sentience; others, such as Holmes Rolston III (1988), argue that we have obligations to virtually every element of the natural order. Whatever we may think about this dispute, only someone who believes that our obligations are exhausted by our duties to humanity can remain unmoved in the face of this anticipated destruction of nonhuman nature.

Indeed, even someone who believes that our obligations are only to humans may feel that massive destruction of nonhuman nature is morally appalling. Humans have preferences about what happens to nature, and insofar as nature's destruction is contrary to human preferences, this destruction can be morally condemned. Moreover, anyone can be morally appalled by the character of a culture that would so willingly destroy nature in order to preserve a way of life that is rooted in overconsumption. Think of nature as being like a work of art. We may not think that works of art are the direct objects of moral concern, yet we may morally condemn those who would vandalize them—say by burning the contents of the Louvre in order to warm their houses by one or two extra degrees for a year or so.

Climate change poses serious threats to human health and welfare and raises questions about our global duties and perhaps our duties to nonhuman nature. As the concentration of greenhouse gases in the atmosphere continues to increase, the moral issue of climate change will grow in importance.

DALE JAMIESON

For a further discussion of topics mentioned in this entry, see the entries AGRICULTURE; ANIMAL WELFARE AND RIGHTS, *articles on* ETHICAL PERSPECTIVES ON THE TREATMENT AND STATUS OF ANIMALS, *and* WILDLIFE CONSERVATION AND MANAGEMENT; ENDANGERED SPECIES AND BIODIVERSITY; ENVIRONMENTAL ETHICS; ENVIRONMENTAL HEALTH; FUTURE GENERATIONS, OBLIGATIONS TO; HARM; HAZARDOUS WASTES AND TOXIC SUBSTANCES; JUSTICE; POPULATION ETHICS, *especially the article* IS THERE A POPULATION PROBLEM?; RISK; UTILITY; *and* VIRTUE AND CHARACTER. *For a discussion of related ideas, see the entries* CONFLICT OF INTEREST; ENVIRONMENT AND RELIGION; FREEDOM AND COERCION; LIFE; POPULATION POLICIES, *article on* MIGRATION AND REFUGEES; *and* SUSTAINABLE DEVELOPMENT.

Bibliography

ABRAHAMSON, DEAN E., ed. 1989. *The Challenge of Global Warming.* Washington, D.C.: Island Press.

AGARWAL, ANIL, and NURAIN, SUNITA. 1991. *Global Warming in an Unequal World: A Case of Environmental Colonialism.* New Delhi: Centre for Science and the Environment.

BOYLE, STEWART, and ARDILL, JOHN. 1989. *The Greenhouse Effect.* London: New English Library.

BROWN, PETER G. 1992. "Climate Change and the Planetary Trust." *Energy Policy* 20, no. 3:208–222.

GEORGE, SUSAN. 1992. *The Debt Boomerang: How Third World Debt Harms Us All.* Boulder, Colo.: Westview.

GLANTZ, MICHAEL, ed. 1988. *Societal Responses to Regional Climatic Change: Forecasting by Analogy.* Boulder, Colo.: Westview.

HOUGHTON, JOHN T.; JENKINS, GEOFFREY J.; and EPHRAUMS, J. J., eds. 1990. *Climate Change: The IPCC Scientific Assessment.* Cambridge: At the University Press.

INTERGOVERNMENTAL PANEL ON CLIMATIC CHANGE (IPCC). 1991. *Climate Change: The IPCC Response Strategies.* Washington, D.C.: Island Press.

JAMIESON, DALE. 1992. "Ethics, Public Policy, and Global Warming." *Science, Technology, and Human Values* 17, no. 2:139–153.

———. 1994. "Global Environmental Justice." In *Philosophy and the Natural Environment.* Edited by Robin Attfield and Andrew Belsey. Cambridge: At the University Press.

NORDHAUS, WILLIAM D. 1992. "An Optimal Path for Controlling Greenhouse Gases." *Science* 258, no. 5086:1315–1319.

NOZICK, ROBERT. 1974. *Anarchy, State, and Utopia.* New York: Basic Books.

PARFIT, DEREK. 1984. *Reasons and Persons.* Oxford: Oxford University Press.

RAWLS, JOHN. 1993. *Political Liberalism.* New York: Columbia University Press.

REVELLE, ROGER, and SUESS, HANS E. 1957. "Carbon Dioxide Exchange Between Atmosphere and Ocean and the Question of an Increase of Atmospheric CO_2 During the Past Decades." *Tellus* 6, no. 1:18–27.

ROLSTON, HOLMES, III. 1988. *Environmental Ethics: Duties to and Values in the Natural World.* Philadelphia: Temple University Press.

SIDGWICK, HENRY. 1874. *Methods of Ethics.* London: Macmillan.

SINGER, PETER. 1990. *Animal Liberation.* 2d ed. New York: New York Review of Books.

STREETS, DAVID. 1991. "Equity and Equality in the Greenhouse." In *Report of a Workshop on Assessing Winners and Losers in the Context of Global Warming, St. Julians, Malta, 18–21 June 1990.* Edited by Michael H. Glantz, Martha F. Price, and Maria E. Krenz. Boulder, Colo.: Environmental and Societal Impacts Group, National Center for Atmospheric Research.

TEGART, W. J. McGREGOR; SHELDON, GORDON; and GRIFFITHS, D. COLIN, eds. 1990. *Climate Change: The IPCC Impacts Assessments.* Canberra: Australian Government Publishing Service.

TICKELL, SIR CRISPIN. 1992. "The Quality of Life: What Quality? Whose Life?" *Interdisciplinary Science Reviews* 17, no. 1:19–25.

WEISS, EDITH BROWN. 1988. *In Fairness to Future Generations: International Law, Common Patrimony, and Intergenerational Equity.* Dobbs Ferry, N.Y.: Transnational Publishers.

WIGLEY, TOM M. L., and RAPER, SARAH C. B. 1992. "Implications for Climate and Sea Level of Revised IPCC Emissions Scenarios." *Nature* 357, no. 6376:293–300.

WORLD BANK. 1992. *World Development Report 1992: Development and Environment.* New York: Oxford University Press.

CLINICAL ETHICS

I. Elements and Methodologies
   John C. Fletcher
   Howard Brody

II. Clinical Ethics Consultation
   George A. Kanoti
   Stuart Youngner
III. Institutional Ethics Committees
   Charles J. Dougherty

I. ELEMENTS AND METHODOLOGIES

Clinical ethics is concerned with the ethics of clinical practice and with ethical problems that arise in the care of patients. Those who write about clinical ethics and shape its practices do so from within the larger interdisciplinary domain of bioethics and draw upon disciplines that inform and shape bioethics. However, due to its emphasis on clinical practice, clinical ethics relies strongly on narrative accounts of clinicians and patients in struggles with disease and illness. The primary characteristics of clinical ethics are its focus on ethical problems in patient care, its discomfort with a theoretical model of ethical inquiry, and its emphasis on an equal role for service activities in balance with teaching and research.

The emergence and activities of clinical ethics

During the 1980s, several postgraduate training programs, some textbooks (e.g., Jonsen et al., 1992), and one journal declared that they addressed "clinical ethics," a term that had not been used in the earlier bioethics movement. Although clinicians themselves probably coined the term "clinical ethics" during the mid-1970s when discussing various approaches to cases, Joseph Fletcher may have been the first to refer formally to "clinical ethics" in a 1976 commencement address at the University of Minnesota School of Medicine. He said that physicians often responded to his arguments for "situation ethics" in contrast to "rule ethics" by identifying his approach as "clinical ethics" or "deciding what to do case by case, using guidelines to be sure, but deciding what to do by the actual case or situation of the patient." Whether the term clinical ethics accurately describes a new discipline or subdiscipline has been debated; however, there can be little disagreement that the term correctly denotes an important activity characterized by unique features that emerged in the 1980s and early 1990s.

In the United States and Canada, clinical ethicists are associated primarily with service activities, that is, clinical care, but they also perform important teaching and research functions. The typical clinical ethicist works within a program in a health-care institution such as a large hospital, and provides services that include staff and community education, policy critique and formulation, retrospective and prospective case review, and case consultation. Some institutions with programs in clinical ethics offer advanced education and training in fellowship or degree programs. They may also have outreach efforts to assist in the formation of clinical ethics programs and the training of leaders for these programs.

A distinctive feature of inquiry in clinical ethics is that it tends to start from the reality of the clinician–patient encounter and to end in a practical case judgment that impacts upon an identifiable patient. Earlier bioethical inquiry, when case-oriented, had often begun from a less than full factual description of the case that then proceeded to address those problematic "facts" from an ethical viewpoint. Such cases and inquiries were widely criticized, especially by experienced clinicians (Sider and Clements, 1985), as impoverished and distant from the realities of practice. The clinical ethicist, by contrast, is actively engaged in accumulating and developing as rich a set of facts as possible as well as interpreting them (Siegler et al., 1990).

Clinical ethicists may be involved in teaching at all levels of health-professional education (preclinical, clinical, graduate, postgraduate, and continuing education). In these academic settings the teaching activity most associated with the term "clinical ethics" is the postgraduate fellowship or master's program of one or two years' duration. By 1992, there were at least nine such programs in the United States. The number of these programs will undoubtedly grow with the demand for clinical ethicists in hospitals, long-term care facilities, home health agencies, and hospices. Candidates in these programs are usually clinicians (M.D.s and R.N.s) who are fully qualified within a practice specialty and other professionals who work in health-care settings (e.g., attorneys, clergy, social workers, administrators). They share the desire for advanced education in clinical ethics and allied subjects, but without completing a more traditional graduate degree program in philosophical or theological ethics. Many clinical ethicists employed by predominantly nonacademic health-care institutions have no teaching responsibilities besides staff education.

Some clinical ethicists, especially those employed by academic centers and those who have graduated from fellowship programs, are actively engaged in research. This may be empirical research to measure the frequency of various ethical problems or the practical impact of various ethical policies; or it may be analytic research to describe and refine the methods and approaches of ethical inquiry most suitable for clinical application (Singer et al., 1990).

According to one important review of the field (Siegler et al., 1990), two developments led to the inception of clinical ethics as a distinct field of activity: first, the need for bedside teaching of ethics (Siegler, 1978) in the tradition of William Osler (1849–1919), a professor of medicine renowned for his bedside teaching and power of observation; and second, the elaboration of a method of inquiry especially suitable to individual cases in clinical settings (Siegler, 1982; Jonsen et al., 1992). Implicit within both developments was the assertion that ethics, properly understood, was intrinsic to the practice of good clinical medicine. This assertion and its view of medicine and ethics were not new. First, Ludwig Edelstein (1967), and later Richard Zaner (1988), discerned an intrinsic view of ethics in the Hippocratic tradition. On the other hand, Galen, a distinguished physician of antiquity, held that ethics was external to medicine, an influence on the individual physician but not essential to characteristics of practice.

When nonclinicians spoke of the "intrinsic" nature of ethics within medicine, the message was often heard with skepticism as self-serving. So long as only those with Ph.D.s taught and wrote about the field, skeptical physicians and nurses could conclude that ethics was a sort of artificial graft that was not woven into the fabric of medicine or nursing in any essential way. But when fully qualified physicians and nurses achieved competence in ethical vocabulary and methodology to make the case for ethics as intrinsic to clinical practice, these same skeptics probably found it much harder to dismiss the message.

Clinical ethics is now pursued by clinicians—physicians, nurses, social workers, and other health professionals—as well as by lawyers and those with graduate training in philosophical or theological ethics who choose to focus their attention upon, and develop the necessary medical knowledge and interpersonal skills to function well within, the clinical setting. The knowledge base for clinical ethics also includes legal and public policy trends that affect the clinical setting. It also appears that the emergence of "clinical ethics" as an activity seeking distinctiveness within the larger enterprise of bioethics began in the early 1980s, largely in the United States and Canada, where the value of patient-centered "shared decision making" in health care is strongly supported (U.S. President's Commission, 1983, p. 4). As a phenomenon in these cultures, clinical ethics is an organized effort to make shared decision making a reality. The emergence of clinical ethics as a special set of concerns, as well as the tasks of clinical ethicists, can also be explained in terms of deficits within the earlier expressions of bioethics in these two nations.

Concerns and elements of clinical ethics

Renée Fox (1976) and David Rothman (1991) argue that bioethics began in the 1960s as a social and intellectual movement. The earliest concerns of bioethics were focused on acute ethical problems in research settings. Influenced by the U.S. civil rights movement, bioethical inquiry also exposed weaknesses in institutional arrangements that no longer adequately protected research subjects or patients (Fletcher, 1991). From its origins to the present, the bioethics movement has had two arms: (1) an interdisciplinary dialogue, known as bioethics, that became a new academic subdiscipline in the larger field of ethics; and (2) an agenda for institutional and social change to prevent abuses and enhance the values that guide decision making with research subjects and patients. Social changes in research settings to protect human subjects preceded such changes in patient-care settings by almost a decade.

In the 1970s, scholars in bioethics increasingly taught new courses as faculty members of medical, nursing, and other professional schools. Bioethics scholars also served the growing number of "medical humanities" programs. Some of these scholars were among the first nonclinicians to provide ethics consultation in cases involving patients (Jonsen, 1980). A practice of ethics consultation began to be defined in the early to mid-1980s (Fletcher et al., 1989), and ethics committees multiplied in clinical settings to protect shared decision making with patients and family members.

Did the bioethics movement and other currents of change in the larger society influence clinicians and their practices? It is remarkably apparent that they did, but it was not without criticisms. The responses and criticisms of clinicians required changes and adaptation by bioethicists who desired to teach, do research, and serve in clinical settings. These criticisms resulted in two goals for conceptual and practical change.

The first goal was to develop modes of ethical inquiry in clinical care and with ill and suffering patients. The prevailing approach to bioethical inquiry (Beauchamp and Childress, 1989) used systematic reflection on moral principles and their relevance for resolving ethical problems in biomedicine by weighing and balancing the claims of competing principles. Although this mainstream approach achieved valuable work, criticisms pointed to three ways that it required strengthening: (1) to give more attention to the nature of diseases and the clinical contexts in which clinicians and patients face ethical problems (Sider and Clements, 1985); (2) to meet criticism that "principlism" appeared to promote a hierarchical form of reasoning that deduced ethical resolutions for complex clinical problems from fixed moral principles and rules (Jonsen and Toulmin, 1988); and (3) that more conceptual and methodological resources for ethical inquiry needed development, in addition to moral principles; because principlism appeared too vague and flexible to yield well-reasoned conclusions (Clouser and Gert, 1990).

In response to these perceived inadequacies in the forms of ethical inquiry, Glenn Graber and David Thomasma (1989) attempted to recast the theory and practice of medical ethics in terms of a "unitary ethical theory" founded in clinical medicine itself. Their con-

tribution, with strengths and weaknesses, was expertly reviewed by Zaner (1990), a philosopher with significant clinical experience who enriched the literature with narratives of illness and ethical conflicts over uses of high technology that are frequent in tertiary-care centers. Other contributors to the clinical ethics literature responded by drawing on writings of feminist (Gilligan, 1982; Noddings, 1984) and theological (Hauerwas, 1986) writers who criticized bioethics for neglecting the ethical significance of specific clinical virtues, such as caring for persons in concrete human relationships.

Additional methodological resources for ethical inquiry appeared in the renewal of interest in casuistry, the art of ethical analysis that compares and contrasts relevantly similar cases (Jonsen and Toulmin, 1988; Brody, 1988; Arras, 1991). Clinical decision making is case-specific: it is directed at the care of a particular patient faced with a particular illness or injury. Each case has a history preceding the problems that need medical attention, what needs to be done, and what was done to address the problems presented by the patient. Since it focuses on the ethics of clinical practice, clinical ethics strives for the richest possible descriptions of cases and their interpersonal dynamics and power differentials. In this vein, several anthologies of cases have appeared with well-informed clinical discussions (Pence, 1990; Veatch and Fry, 1987; Levine, 1989), including one with cases in ethics consultation (Culver, 1990). Like the practice of clinical medicine, casuistry builds on the accumulated experience, both individual and of the professions, of dealing with a variety of cases. Comparison and contrast of related cases can reveal important ethical considerations that may not be apparent in isolated focus on a particular case.

Yet another response to critiques of earlier bioethics was to deepen and enrich the study of larger issues and themes in clinical practice, both by using cases and by drawing on knowledge available only through the intimacies of the clinician–patient encounter. Authors of such studies tend to be clinician–ethicists or ethicists who have adapted to the clinical setting sufficiently to share in such intimacies. Four examples among many are discussions of informed consent (Katz, 1984), life-and-death decision making (Brody, 1988), pain and suffering (Cassell, 1991), and the uses of power by clinicians (Brody, 1992). These studies draw on a variety of disciplines and experiential data obtained in clinical settings. As such, they encourage ethical scrutiny and reform of understandings and practices in the clinical encounters between patients and clinicians (Zaner, 1988). In this way, clinical ethics strengthens the conceptual underpinnings of bioethics with experiential data and helps motivate clinicians to reform their practices.

A second goal for clinical ethicists was to develop a set of practical services to clinicians and their patients, in addition to their activities in teaching and research. Clinical ethicists today serve in several ways: (1) technical assistance to a variety of ethics groups in health-care organizations (research involving human subjects, patient care, research involving animals, scientific integrity, etc.), (2) outreach efforts to health-care institutions for assistance in starting or strengthening an ethics program and training resource persons, and (3) providing ethics consultation. Rules of the Joint Commission for the Accreditation of Healthcare Organizations (1993) state that member institutions must have a "mechanism" for "the consideration of ethical issues arising in the care of patients and to provide education to caregivers and patients on ethical issues in health care" (R.1.1.6.1, p. 9). These rules intensified the need for competence and leadership in clinical ethics. In practice, these and other rules bearing upon patient rights are being met through the activities of multidisciplinary ethics programs. These programs need nurturance by well-informed leaders. Such assistance can be provided by persons trained in clinical ethics fellowships and master's programs who continue to serve patients and the institution in their primary disciplines.

Scholarly assessment of clinical ethics

Clinical ethics has provided a valuable impetus to scholarly investigation and reassessment of bioethics generally, as evidenced by important conferences and collections of papers (e.g., Ackerman et al., 1987; Hoffmaster et al., 1989).

A major and recurring debate, as noted above, deals with the importance of general ethical principles in clinical-ethical inquiry. On one side, it is claimed that ethical knowledge and insights emerge from a careful study of concrete cases, and general or abstract principles play only a small role (Jonsen and Toulmin, 1988). On the other side, some claim that the study of a set of principles and ethical theory constitutes useful ethical knowledge to be applied to specific cases (Veatch, 1987). Not surprisingly, several proposals for clinical-ethical inquiry fall in between these positions. Proponents of "middle ground" approaches have to explain how to bridge the gaps between abstract general principles and specific concrete cases, and also how one can extract defensible judgments from particular cases in a rigorous and methodical fashion without appealing solely to general principles and theories (Brody, 1988; Brody, 1992).

Another area of debate focuses on the proper role assumed by the consulting clinical ethicist and the moral warrant underlying that role. Again, a spectrum may be described. At one end, patient autonomy is viewed as the overriding moral consideration in any clinical decision, and so it follows that the clinical ethicist has a legitimate role only if called in by the patient as an adviser to the patient on value issues in clinical care (Veatch, 1987). At the other end, the clinical ethicist is seen as analogous to the hospital pharmacist; the attending physician might ask the pharmacist a question about drug dosages or interactions, simply presuming that by consenting to hospitalization, the patient implicitly agreed to any and all ancillary consultations of this sort that might improve the quality of care. Again, more proposals lie somewhere between these views and must address questions of appropriate patient consent for ethics consultation or review (Agich and Youngner, 1991; Wolf, 1991) and appropriate involvement of patients and/or family members in the consultation process. When consultation occurs within a committee setting, one may ask whether the ability of such a committee to reach a consensus provides any additional moral warrant for the recommendation (Caws, 1991).

Another role-related question is the analysis of activities the clinical ethicist might be asked or tempted to assume but that lie outside the proper roles. Terrence Ackerman (1987) suggests four such illegitimate roles: moral policeman, modified social worker, secular clergy, and patient advocate. To some extent the clinical ethicist might occasionally perform within one of these roles, but should do so as part of more general responsibilities as a member of the institutional staff and not because of any special role responsibilities as ethicist. For example, if blatantly unethical behavior occurs within the institution, all employees, not only or especially the ethicist, have a duty to try to stop it. Others would argue that the lines of distinction between these "illegitimate" roles and the proper role of the clinical ethicist are much more blurred. Giles Scofield (1993) warns of a trend toward professionalization among clinical ethicists and is skeptical about their qualifications as ethics consultants and advisers. He emphasizes the role of clinical ethicists as educators. Benjamin Freedman (1989) has stated that clinical ethicists need a professional code of ethics.

Such debates are, in themselves, a sign that clinical ethics has become a social reality in many settings in the United States and Canada. It remains to be seen whether the bioethics movement in other nations will evolve in a similar way in patient-care settings. We predict that in nations where shared decision making in patient care is a value to be prized or where significant numbers of clinicians become involved in bioethics, clinical ethics will develop a clearer identity.

JOHN C. FLETCHER
HOWARD BRODY

Directly related to this article are the other articles in this entry: CLINICAL ETHICS CONSULTATION, *and* INSTITUTIONAL ETHICS COMMITTEES. *For a further discussion of methodologies in bioethics, see the entries* AUTONOMY; BE-NEFICENCE; BIOETHICS; CASUISTRY; ETHICS, *article on* NORMATIVE ETHICAL THEORIES; FEMINISM; JUSTICE; NARRATIVE; UTILITY; *and* VIRTUE AND CHARACTER. *For a discussion of related ideas, see the entries* BIOETHICS EDUCATION, *especially articles on* NURSING, OTHER HEALTH PROFESSIONS, *and* SECONDARY AND POSTSECONDARY EDUCATION; INFORMED CONSENT, *article on* CLINICAL ASPECTS OF CONSENT IN HEALTH CARE; *and* PROFESSIONAL–PATIENT RELATIONSHIP.

Bibliography

ACKERMAN, TERRENCE F. 1987. "Medical Ethics in the Clinical Setting: A Critical Review of Its Consultative, Pedagogical, and Investigative Methods." In *Clinical Medical Ethics: Exploration and Assessment,* pp. 145–173. Edited by Terrence F. Ackerman, Glenn C. Graber, Charles H. Reynolds, and David C. Thomasma. Lanham, Md.: University Press of America.

ACKERMAN, TERRENCE F.; GRABER, GLENN C.; REYNOLDS, CHARLES H.; and THOMASMA, DAVID C., eds. 1987. *Clinical Medical Ethics: Exploration and Assessment.* Lanham, Md.: University Press of America.

AGICH, GEORGE J., and YOUNGNER, STUART J. 1991. "For Experts Only? Access to Hospital Ethics Committees." *Hastings Center Report* 21, no. 5:18–21.

ARRAS, JOHN D. 1991. "Getting Down to Cases: The Revival of Casuistry in Bioethics." *Journal of Medicine and Philosophy* 16, no. 11:29–52.

BEAUCHAMP, TOM L., and CHILDRESS, JAMES F. 1989. *Principles of Biomedical Ethics.* 3d ed. New York: Oxford University Press.

BRODY, BARUCH A. 1988. *Life and Death Decision Making.* New York: Oxford University Press.

BRODY, HOWARD. 1992. *The Healer's Power.* New Haven, Conn.: Yale University Press.

CASSELL, ERIC J. 1991. *The Nature of Suffering and the Goals of Medicine.* New York: Oxford University Press.

CAWS, PETER. 1991. "Committees and Consensus: How Many Heads Are Better Than One?" *Journal of Medicine and Philosophy* 16, no. 4:375–391.

CLOUSER, K. DANIEL, and GERT, BERNARD. 1990. "A Critique of Principlism." *Journal of Medicine and Philosophy* 15, no. 2:219–236.

CULVER, CHARLES M., ed. 1990. *Ethics at the Bedside.* Hanover, N.H.: University Press of New England.

EDELSTEIN, LUDWIG. 1967. *Ancient Medicine: Selected Papers of Ludwig Edelstein.* Baltimore: Johns Hopkins University Press.

FLETCHER, JOHN C. 1991. "The Bioethics Movement and Hospital Ethics Committees." *Maryland Law Review* 50, no. 3:859–894.

FLETCHER, JOHN C.; QUIST, NORMAN A.; and JONSEN, ALBERT R. eds. 1989. *Ethics Consultation in Health Care.* Ann Arbor, Mich.: Health Administration Press.

FOX, RENÉE C. 1976. "Advanced Medical Technology: Social and Ethical Implications." *Annual Review of Sociology* 2:231–268.

FREEDMAN, BENJAMIN. 1989. "Bringing Codes to Newcastle: Ethics for Clinical Ethicists." In *Clinical Ethics: Theory and Practice,* pp. 125–139. Edited by Barry Hoffmaster, Benjamin Freedman, and Gwen Fraser. Clifton, N.J.: Humana.

GILLIGAN, CAROL. 1982. *In a Different Voice: Psychological Theory and Women's Development.* Cambridge, Mass.: Harvard University Press.

GRABER, GLENN C., and THOMASMA, DAVID C. 1989. *Theory and Practice in Medical Ethics.* New York: Continuum.

HAUERWAS, STANLEY. 1986. *Suffering Presence: Theological Reflections on Medicine, the Mentally Handicapped, and the Church.* South Bend, Ind.: Notre Dame University Press.

HOFFMASTER, C. BARRY; FREEDMAN, BENJAMIN; and FRASER, GWEN, eds. 1989. *Clinical Ethics: Theory and Practice.* Clifton, N.J.: Humana.

JOINT COMMISSION FOR ACCREDITATION OF HEALTHCARE ORGANIZATIONS. 1993. "Patient Rights." In *1992 Accreditation Manual for Hospitals,* pp. 1–16. Chicago: Author.

JONSEN, ALBERT R. 1980. "Can an Ethicist Be a Consultant?" In *Frontiers in Medical Ethics: Applications in a Medical Setting,* pp. 157–171. Edited by Virginia Abernathy and Harry S. Abram. Cambridge, Mass.: Ballinger.

JONSEN, ALBERT R.; SIEGLER, MARK; and WINSLADE, WILLIAM J. 1992. *Clinical Ethics: A Practical Approach to Ethical Decisions in Clinical Medicine.* 3d ed. New York: McGraw-Hill.

JONSEN, ALBERT R., and TOULMIN, STEPHEN E. 1988. *The Abuse of Casuistry: A History of Moral Reasoning.* Berkeley: University of California Press.

KATZ, JAY. 1984. *The Silent World of Doctor and Patient.* New York: Free Press.

LEVINE, CAROLE, ed. 1989. *Cases in Bioethics: Selections from the Hastings Center Report.* New York: St. Martin's Press.

NODDINGS, NEL. 1984. *Caring, a Feminine Approach to Ethics and Moral Education.* Berkeley: University of California Press.

PELLEGRINO, EDMUND D.; SIEGLER, MARK; and SINGER, PETER A. 1990. "Teaching Clinical Ethics." *Journal of Clinical Ethics* 1, no. 3:175–180.

PENCE, GREGORY E. 1990. *Classic Cases in Medical Ethics.* New York: McGraw-Hill.

ROTHMAN, DAVID J. 1991. *Strangers at the Bedside: A History of How Law and Bioethics Transformed Medical Decision Making.* New York: Basic Books.

SCOFIELD, GILES R. 1993. "Ethics Consultation: The Least Dangerous Profession?" *Cambridge Quarterly of Healthcare Ethics* 2, no. 4:417–426.

SIDER, ROGER C., and CLEMENTS, COLLEEN D. 1985. "The New Medical Ethics: A Second Opinion." *Archives of Internal Medicine* 145, no. 12:2169–2173.

SIEGLER, MARK. 1978. "A Legacy of Osler: Teaching Clinical Ethics at the Bedside." *Journal of the American Medical Association* 239, no. 10:951–956.

———. 1982. "Decision-Making Strategy for Clinical–Ethical Problems in Medicine." *Archives of Internal Medicine* 142, no. 12:2178–2179.

SIEGLER, MARK; PELLEGRINO, EDMUND D.; and SINGER, PETER A. 1990. "Clinical Medical Ethics." *Journal of Clinical Ethics* 1, no. 1:5–9.

SINGER, PETER A.; PELLEGRINO, EDMUND D.; and SIEGLER, MARK. 1990. "Ethics Committees and Consultants." *Journal of Clinical Ethics* 1, no. 4:263–267.

SINGER, PETER A.; SIEGLER, MARK; and PELLEGRINO, EDMUND D. 1990. "Research in Clinical Ethics." *Journal of Clinical Ethics* 1, no. 2:95–99.

U.S. PRESIDENT'S COMMISSION FOR THE STUDY OF ETHICAL PROBLEMS IN MEDICINE AND BIOMEDICAL AND BEHAVIORAL RESEARCH. 1983. *Making Health Care Decisions: A Report on the Ethical and Legal Implications of Informed Consent in the Patient-Practitioner Relationship.* Washington, D.C.: U.S. Government Printing Office.

VEATCH, ROBERT. 1987. "The Medical Ethicist as Agent for the Patient." In *Clinical Medical Ethics: Exploration and Assessment*, pp. 59–67. Edited by Terrence F. Ackerman, Glenn C. Graber, Charles H. Reynolds, and David C. Thomasma. Lanham, Md.: University Press of America.

VEATCH, ROBERT M., and FRY, SARA T. 1987. *Case Studies in Nursing Ethics.* Philadelphia: J. B. Lippincott.

WOLF, SUSAN M. 1991. "Ethics Committees and Due Process: Nesting Rights in a Community of Caring." *Maryland Law Review* 50, no. 3:798–858.

ZANER, RICHARD M. 1988. *Ethics and the Clinical Encounter.* Englewood Cliffs, N.J.: Prentice-Hall.

———. 1990. "The Discipline of Clinical Ethics." *Bioethics Books* 2:21–24.

II. CLINICAL ETHICS CONSULTATION

The dictionary defines consulting as "providing professional or expert advice." A clinical ethics consultant is defined here as a person who upon request provides expert advice to identify, analyze, and help resolve ethical questions or dilemmas that arise in the care of patients. Although the ethics consultant also may provide ethics education and help formulate policy, the bedside role is central to the definition of an ethics consultant (Jonsen, 1980).

In the United States, clinical ethics consultation began in some academic medical centers in the late 1960s and early 1970s (La Puma and Schiedermayer, 1991), and was given great impetus by the development of hospital ethics committees in the late 1970s and 1980s. During this period the rapid growth of medical technology confronted critically ill patients, their families, and health professionals with difficult ethical choices. At the same time, the traditional authority of the physician was challenged not only by the patient-rights and consumer-rights movements, but also by changes in the way medical care was delivered in tertiary-care hospitals, where patients were often treated by teams consisting of physicians, nurses, social workers, medical technicians, and others. Decisions about for-going life-sustaining treatment for incompetent adults or premature infants were being made in a legal vacuum often filled by the fears of civil and even criminal litigation. In this atmosphere there was considerable uncertainty about the optimum process for resolving difficult ethical decisions without resorting to the public arena of the courts.

In its 1976 Quinlan decision, the New Jersey Supreme Court tentatively suggested the use of ethics committees to assist persons who faced difficult end-of-life decisions. In the early 1980s, the federal "Baby Doe" regulations spurred hospitals to develop internal mechanisms for dealing with decision making for severely handicapped infants. In 1983 the U.S. President's Commission for the Study of Ethical Problems in Medicine and Biomedical and Behavioral Research endorsed the notion of shared decision making between patients and physicians. It suggested consultation with an ethics committee as a possible means for resolving disputes that arose in the clinical setting, but noted that the efficacy of such consultation had not been demonstrated (U.S. President's Commission, 1983).

In 1985 the National Institutes of Health and the University of California at San Francisco cosponsored a conference in Bethesda, Maryland, for persons designated by their institutions as ethics consultants. The conference was attended by fifty-three invitees, and fifty additional persons expressed interest in attending a future meeting of this group (Fletcher, 1986). By 1987 the Society for Bioethics Consultation was formed for the support and continuing education of clinical ethics consultants. In 1992 the Joint Commission for the Accreditation of Health Care Organizations (JCAHO) published a requirement for health-care institution accreditation that all health-care institutions must have in place a mechanism for resolving disputes concerning end-of-life decisions.

Structures of clinical ethics consultation

Clinical ethics case consultation is provided in several ways: by an ethics consultative group as a whole (such as an ethics committee), by a subgroup of the consultative group, or by individual consultants. Clinical ethics case consultation by a large group has the potential for having diffused accountability and being depersonalized, bureaucratic, insensitive, closed-ended, and removed from the clinical setting. But it has the advantage of providing multiple perspectives and opportunities for queries from persons of diverse backgrounds, and for correcting the potential for narrow or idiosyncratic views of an individual consultant.

In contrast, clinical ethics case consultation by an individual consultant is an open-ended process that can extend over a period of time, and permit ongoing discussion and pursuit of issues that require clarification. The individual consultant can decide what information is necessary and obtain it firsthand. Interviews with patients, families, and health professionals can be scheduled flexibly and conducted in private settings more conducive to diminishing apprehension, establishing trust, sharing information, and allowing the kind of give-and-take that is so important to exploring emotionally powerful and intensely personal issues. Furthermore, an individual ethics consultant is more visible and accountable than a committee (Agich and Youngner, 1991). For these reasons, many ethics consultative groups and health-care professionals have found the individual clinical ethics consultant more effective than the committee. Many ethics consultative groups have created a middle ground that involves small teams who serve as an extension of the ethics consultation group or ethics committee.

Some see an advantage to a relationship between the ethics consultant and an ethics consultative group or committee because the large group regularly can review the individual consultant's activities. This arrangement provides peer review and quality assurance for the consultant as well as education for the larger group or committee. The ethics consultant or consultation team can ask the entire group to become involved in particularly controversial or complex cases.

The role of the clinical ethics consultant

Despite the growing interest in and practice of clinical ethics consultation, important questions remain about its purpose, requisite skills, methods, specific responsibilities, evaluation, and effect. Unlike traditional medical consultants, clinical ethics consultants are not subject to widely accepted standards and procedures for training, credentialing, maintaining accountability, charging fees, obtaining informed consent, or providing liability coverage (Purtilo, 1984; Agich, 1990).

While the role of the ethics consultant generally has been pragmatic, that is, to provide practical assistance with actual patient-care decisions (Cranford, 1989; Glover et al., 1986; Siegler and Singer, 1988; Fletcher, 1986), there has been little consensus about how this role should be implemented. For example, although some see the ethics consultant, like the traditional medical consultant, as an expert who uses specific skills and knowledge to help "answer" ethical questions, exactly what constitutes the appropriate skills and knowledge base is a matter of debate. Does the expertise come from the wisdom of practical clinical experience (La Puma et al., 1988), or is it derived from a knowledge of moral theory and ethical principles?

Others see the clinical ethics consultant's role not so much as an expert but as someone who facilitates de-

cisions in a "community of reflective persons" (Glover et al., 1986, p. 24). This approach stresses the importance of involving all persons connected with the case—the patient, family members, physicians, nurses, medical students and residents, social workers, friends, and clergy. In this view, a shared decision-making process should extend beyond the physician–patient dyad so that a greater range of personal values and interests can be considered. This view is less compatible with the traditional model of medical consultation, which focuses more narrowly on the physician as decision maker.

Some commentators have worried that the individual ethics consultant, the ethics consultative group, or the ethics committee will act as moral "police" or "God Squad" (Siegler and Singer, 1988, p. 759), and erode the decision-making authority of the physician. Troyen Brennan has voiced a more subtle concern: that by turning increasingly to ethics consultants and ethics committees, we "run the risk of forcing the ethics of the caring relationship to the periphery of clinical practice as something that is best left to experts" (Brennan, 1992, p. 4). Furthermore, the role of the ethics consultant may be confused with other institutional roles, such as risk management, peer review, quality assurance, or resource allocation. Taking on these roles could create a conflict of interest for the ethics consultant.

Reasons for ethics consultation

Ethics consultations are requested for a variety of reasons that include prevention of litigation; mediation of disputes and resolution of conflicts between or among the patient, health-care professional, and family; confirmation of or challenges to decisions already made; emotional support for difficult decisions; and identification of morally acceptable alternatives. For example, ethics consultation may be requested because physicians and family members disagree about how aggressively to treat a dying, incompetent cancer patient, or because there is difficulty interpreting a patient's living will. Ethics consultants may be called because there is disagreement about the acceptability of a family request to stop tube feeding for an Alzheimer patient who refuses to eat. Requests for ethics consultation may come because nurses or house officers are concerned that competent patients are being left out of the decision-making process.

Goals of ethics consultation

There is disagreement about the appropriate goals of ethics consultation. John La Puma and E. Rush Priest have suggested that ethics consultation's primary goal should be "to effect ethical outcomes in particular cases and to teach physicians to construct their own frameworks for ethical decisions making" (La Puma and Priest, 1992,

p. 17). Patient-rights advocates disagree. They argue that the primary goal of ethics consultation is the promotion of patient autonomy by encouraging shared decision making (Tulsky and Lo, 1992). John Fletcher takes a broader view. He identifies four goals of ethics consultation: (1) to protect and enhance shared decision making in the resolution of ethical problems; (2) to prevent poor outcomes; (3) to increase knowledge of clinical ethics; and (4) to increase knowledge of self and others through participation in resolving conflicts (Fletcher, 1992).

Contributions to the practice of ethics consultation

While the general purpose of clinical ethics consultation is to help resolve ethical questions or dilemmas in patient care, persons who perform ethics consultation come from diverse professional backgrounds and do not share the same problem-solving methods or theoretical assumptions. This diversity has left its stamp on the way clinical ethics consultation is performed, and has profound implications not only for the practice of clinical ethics consultation but also for the training of its practitioners.

Despite this diversity, a common ground can be seen in the shared goal of identifying an ethically supportable solution to a clinical ethical question or dilemma, and in a recognition that the process of arriving at a solution requires knowledge of law, ethics, medicine, psychosocial issues, and at times, religion.

The legal tradition has influenced clinical ethics consultation by placing emphasis on rights and on formal mechanisms of decision making and arbitration, such as due process. The protection and nurturing of individual rights are central to this style (Wolf, 1991). Strict adherence to this style, however, may encourage adversarial rather than collaborative or nurturing relationships between patients and health-care professionals (Agich and Youngner, 1991).

The medical tradition has contributed methods, assumptions, and traditions of clinical practice: a combination of technical knowledge and clinical experience (La Puma and Toulmin, 1989). Some argue that physicians are best suited to provide clinical ethics consultation because (1) their advice will be easily accepted by their medical colleagues, since they have clinical experience and speak the same language; and (2) only physicians can understand the ethos of physician-patient relationships. Critics caution that because they are "insiders," physicians may promote the values of medicine rather than those of their patients or the larger community. They argue that the ethics consultant should serve as a bridge between medical and other values, and

cannot function properly from a position entirely within medicine (Glover et al., 1986; Churchill, 1978).

Moral philosophy has offered three major approaches to clinical ethics consultation. The first is principle-based ethics, which argues that the answer to a given ethical question or dilemma may be discovered by applying the correct ethical theory (e.g., utilitarianism) or principle (e.g., autonomy) to the case. The second is virtue ethics, which emphasizes that the possession of certain virtues (e.g., honesty, loyalty, compassion) is essential to sound ethical decision making. The third is a case-based or casuistic ethic, which holds that by examining the particulars of a given case and comparing them with similar cases, a moral maxim that applies to the case can be discovered. An advantage of casuistry is that it sues a decision-making method already employed by clinicians (Jonsen and Toulmin, 1988). Casuistry relies upon teachable medical moral maxims that build upon experience. Because casuistry is not principle-based, it has been criticized as "situational," that is, pragmatically driven to solve individual problems without reference to a broader moral framework.

While principle-based clinical ethics reasoning has the advantage of providing a consistent moral reference point, its principles are necessarily abstract, often conflict with each other, and may create a rigid paradigm that is insensitive to differences in specific cases.

Theology and religion contribute to clinical ethics consultation by recognizing that specific religious positions may either facilitate the resolution of an ethical question or contribute to its intensity. For example, the Jehovah's Witness position on blood transfusions can create serious ethical dilemmas in the case of a Jehovah's Witness patient who is in urgent need of extensive, life-saving surgery but refuses blood. One of the disadvantages of this perspective is that many physicians are suspicious of or even hostile to religious or theological interpretations of medical problems. However, insight into the religious morality of patients, family members, and health-care professionals is useful in establishing communication and reaching understanding among physicians, patients, and family members.

Consultation liaison psychiatry and clinical psychology have influenced clinical ethics consultation by addressing dynamic and interpersonal elements of clinical ethics cases. This style involves using insight into the motivations and values of those involved in the ethics case to resolve conflicts among decision makers. The goal is to produce a consensus or compromise solution rather than to evoke rights language, ethical principles, or religious codes. A disadvantage of this approach is that a compromise solution is not always a just one. Its strength is that it skillfully manages confrontation and addresses the emotional needs of the participants.

Knowledge and skills needed for ethics consultation

While there is not unanimity about how rigorously schooled in specific academic disciplines or how proficient in specific skills the consultant should be, there is general agreement about the kind of skills, knowledge, and personal qualities ethics consultants require. These include knowledge of ethical language and ethical theory; skills of ethical analysis and reflective moral judgment; knowledge of clinical medicine (e.g., medical terminology, the natural history of disease and its treatment); knowledge of and familiarity with hospital structure, sociology, and politics; knowledge of and familiarity with the professional ethos of physicians and nurses; knowledge of the law and legal reasoning; knowledge of psychological and social theories of behavior; communication and teaching skills; personal qualities such as the ability to establish rapport, empathy, and compassion; and professional attributes such as dedication, ability to maintain confidentiality, and comfort with cultural and ethical diversity.

Access to ethics consultation

Who should be able to request an ethics consultation? The answer to this question has political as well as moral implications. On the one hand, if only physicians have access to ethics consultation, many important ethical issues may never be examined (Tulsky and Lo, 1992). On the other hand, permitting patients, families, and other health professionals to request ethics consultation, especially without the physician's concurrence, might discourage more direct communication, disrupt physician–patient relationships, or undermine physician authority. The last possibility would be most threatening to authoritarian-minded physicians and very likely would challenge the traditional power structure of many hospitals. This may explain the gap between the argument in the literature for the ideal—that patients, families, and nurses should be able to request an ethics consultation—and the impression that many institutions do not permit, and almost none actively encourage, patient, family, or other health professional requests for ethics consultation.

The ability to ask for consultation is only one question concerning patient and family access to and control over the consultation process. Other questions include whether the patient or family should have authority to (1) call a consultation when the physician refuses to do so; (2) be informed routinely when consultations are requested by physicians; (3) veto physician-initiated consultation requests; (4) participate in all ethics consultations if they wish; and (5) receive verbal or written information about the consultant's findings and recommendations. Some argue that an insistence on a rights-based approach to these questions would doom ethics consultation services to failure in modern hospitals because of political considerations (Agich and Youngner, 1991).

Standards and evaluation

The fact that standards and methods for evaluating clinical ethics consultation are not established comes as no surprise. The infancy of clinical ethics consultation and the disagreement about its goals, as well as the diverse academic and professional backgrounds of its practitioners, account for this lack. Most studies to date have employed physician satisfaction and usage as outcome measures. By this standard, ethics consultations have been judged to be helpful. Critics have pointed out, however, that by not including patient and surrogate satisfaction and reactions of house staff and nurses, an incomplete and perhaps inaccurate picture of ethics consultation is painted (Tulsky and Lo, 1992). For example, "it would be hard to argue that it is desirable for an ethics consultant to reject the choices of a competent and informed patient, even if the attending physician expresses satisfaction with such a consultation" (Tulsky and Lo, 1992, p. 591). More objective measures like changes in physician behavior, reduction in use of limited resources (Kanoti et al., 1992), and decreased litigation are attractive, but could confuse matters if these goals were achieved at the expense of more traditional values, such as patient autonomy and well-being.

Credentialing and accreditation

As ethics consultation becomes more widespread and perceived as part of the standard of medical care, society will hold accountable its practitioners and the institutions that employ them. Individual institutions and national accrediting bodies, such as the Joint Commission for the Accreditation of Health Care Organizations, will undoubtedly become more concerned with setting standards for clinical ethics consultation: consultation through traditional professional methods, such as standardized education and training, accreditation of training programs, and credentialing of ethics consultants. This process will be a major challenge to an interdisciplinary field that has yet to agree on its goals and how to evaluate them.

Fees

By and large, ethics consultants have not charged patients or third-party payers for their services. This may be explained by at least two factors. First, the efficacy of ethics consultations has not been clearly demonstrated; and second, ethics consultations are called as frequently to assist health professionals as they are to help patients. Generally, ethics consultants have been paid by the institutions where they practice, either directly for their consultations or indirectly, as part of their overall responsibility in directing ethics programs or committees.

As our health-care system becomes increasingly constrained by economic factors, health-care institutions may find it more difficult to support clinical ethics consultation. This will put pressure on ethics consultants to charge patients or third-party payers or to demonstrate that their activities save money by decreasing litigation or reducing resource consumption.

Conclusion

Clinical ethics consultation arose in the United States in the latter half of the twentieth century amid the moral and legal uncertainty spawned by the rapid expansion of choices produced by medical advances, the emergence of the tertiary-care medical center, and the individual-rights movement that challenged traditional authority structures. Although it holds great promise, clinical ethics consultation remains a nascent profession. Many of the theoretical and practical questions about its goals, training, evaluation, accountability, and support remain unanswered. Nonetheless, clinical ethics consultation is growing and even flourishing. As the U.S. health system evolves over the coming years, the role and place of clinical ethics consultation in the health-care system certainly will be addressed.

GEORGE A. KANOTI
STUART YOUNGNER

Directly related to this article are the other articles in this entry: ELEMENTS AND METHODOLOGIES, *and* INSTITUTIONAL ETHICS COMMITTEES. *Also directly related to this article are the entries* BIOETHICS; BIOETHICS EDUCATION, *the* INTRODUCTION; *and* CONFLICT OF INTEREST. *For a discussion of related topics, see the entries* COMMUNICATION, BIOMEDICAL, *article on* MEDIA AND BIOETHICS; EXPERT TESTIMONY; HEALTH-CARE DELIVERY, *article on* HEALTH-CARE INSTITUTIONS; HOSPITAL, *article on* CONTEMPORARY ETHICAL PROBLEMS; LICENSING, DISCIPLINE, AND REGULATION IN THE HEALTH PROFESSIONS; PROFESSION AND PROFESSIONAL ETHICS; PUBLIC POLICY AND BIOETHICS; TEAMS, HEALTH-CARE; *and* WHISTLEBLOWING. *For a discussion of issues encountered in clinical ethics consultation, see the entries* CONFIDENTIALITY; DEATH AND DYING; EUTHANASIA AND SUSTAINING LIFE; GENETIC COUNSELING; INFORMATION DISCLOSURE; *and* INFORMED CONSENT, *article on* CLINICAL ASPECTS OF CONSENT IN HEALTH CARE.

Bibliography

AGICH, GEORGE J. 1990. "Clinical Ethics: A Role Theoretic Look." *Social Science Medicine* 30, no. 4:389–399.

AGICH, GEORGE J., and YOUNGNER, STUART J. 1991. "For Experts Only? Access to Hospital Ethics Committees." *Hastings Center Report* 21, no. 5:17–31.

BRENNAN, TROYEN A. 1992. "Quality of Clinical Ethics Consultation." *QRB: Quality Review Bulletin* 18, no. 1:4–5.

CHURCHILL, LARRY R. 1978. "The Role of the Stranger." *Ethicists in Professional Education: Hastings Center Report* 8, no. 6:13–15.

CRANFORD, RONALD E. 1989. "The Neurologist as Ethics Consultant and a Member of the Institutional Ethics Committee: The Neuroethicist." *Neurologic Clinics* 7, no. 4:697–713.

FLETCHER, JOHN C. 1986. "Goals and Process of Ethics Consultation in Health Care." *Biolaw* 2, no. 2:37–47.

———. 1992. "Needed: A Broader View of Ethics Consultation." *QRB: Quality Review Bulletin* 18, no. 1:12–14.

GLOVER, JACQUELINE J.; OZAR, DAVID T.; and THOMASMA, DAVID C. 1986. "Teaching Ethics on Rounds: The Ethicist as Teacher, Consultant, and Decision-Maker." *Theoretical Medicine* 7, no. 1:13–32.

JONSEN, ALBERT R. 1980. "Can an Ethicist Be a Consultant?" In *Frontiers in Medical Ethics: Applications in a Medical Setting,* pp. 157–171. Edited by Virginia Abernathy and Harry S. Abram. Cambridge, Mass.: Ballinger.

JONSEN, ALBERT R., and TOULMIN, STEPHEN E. 1988. *The Abuse of Casuistry: A History of Moral Reasoning.* Berkeley: University of California Press.

KANOTI, GEORGE A.; GOMBESKI, WILLIAM; GULLEDGE, A. DALE; KNORADS, DALE; COLLINS, ROBERT; and MEDENDORP, SHARON. 1992. "Impact of Do-Not-Resuscitate Policies on Length of Stay." *Cleveland Clinic Journal of Medicine* 59, no. 6:591–594.

LA PUMA, JOHN, and PRIEST, E. RUSH. 1992. "Medical Staff Privileges for Ethics Consultants: An Institutional Model." *QRB: Quality Review Bulletin* 18, no. 1:17–20.

LA PUMA, JOHN, and SCHIEDERMAYER, DAVID L. 1991. "Ethics Consultation: Skills, Roles and Training." *Annals of Internal Medicine* 114:155–160.

LA PUMA, JOHN; STOCKING, CAROL B.; SILVERSTEIN, MARC D.; DiMARTINI, ANDREA; and SIEGLER, MARK. 1988. "An Ethics Consultation Service in a Teaching Hospital: Utilization and Evaluation." *Journal of the American Medical Association* 260, no. 6:808–811.

LA PUMA, JOHN, and TOULMIN, STEVEN E. 1989. "Ethics Consultants and Ethics Committees." *Archives of Internal Medicine* 149, no. 5:1109–1112.

PERKINS, HENRY S., and SAATHOFF, BONNIE S. 1988. "Impact of Medical Ethics Consultation on Physicians: An Exploratory Study." *American Journal of Medicine* 85, no. 6:761–765.

PURTILO, RUTH B. 1984. "Ethics Consultations in the Hospital." *New England Journal of Medicine* 311, no. 15: 983–986.

SIEGLER, MARK, and SINGER, PETER A. 1988. "Clinical Ethics

Consultation: Godsend or God Squad." *American Journal of Medicine* 85, no. 6:759–760.

TULSKY, JAMES A., and LO, BERNARD. 1992. "Ethics Consultation: Time to Focus on Patients." *American Journal of Medicine* 92, no. 4: 343–345.

U.S. PRESIDENT'S COMMISSION FOR THE STUDY OF ETHICAL PROBLEMS IN MEDICINE AND BIOMEDICAL AND BEHAVIORAL RESEARCH. 1983. *Deciding to Forego Life-Sustaining Treatment: A Report on the Ethical, Medical, and Legal Issues in Treatment Decisions.* Washington, D.C.: Superintendent of Documents.

WOLF, SUSAN M. 1991. "Ethics Committees and Due Process: Nesting Rights in a Community of Caring." *Maryland Law Review* 50:798–858.

III. INSTITUTIONAL ETHICS COMMITTEES

Ethics committees have played clinically relevant roles in U.S. health-care contexts since the 1960s. At that time, some hospitals established committees to approve requests for abortion and sterilization and to allocate scarce dialysis machines. Universities and hospitals created human subjects committees to scrutinize research protocols and consent forms; in the 1970s, these committees became federally mandated institutional review boards (IRBs).

In the 1976 *Quinlan* case, in which parents won the authority to remove a ventilator from an incompetent adult child, the New Jersey Supreme Court recommended that hospitals establish ethics committees to confirm prognoses in cases involving withdrawal of life support. The 1982 "Baby Doe" ruling that allowed parents to withhold a life-saving operation from an infant with Down syndrome led to the establishment of infant-care review committees in cases of withholding or withdrawing life support from disabled newborns. In 1983, a report from the U.S. President's Commission for the Study of Ethical Problems in Medicine and Biomedical and Behavioral Research encouraged the formation of hospital ethics committees to review cases that raised ethical dilemmas and to resolve ethical conflict.

By the mid-1980s, a movement had begun to establish institutional ethics committees in health-care facilities, especially in hospitals. In 1982, only 1 percent of all U.S. hospitals had ethics committees; by 1987, over 60 percent did (Fleetwood et al., 1989). Ethics committees were endorsed in this period by leading professional groups, including the American Medical Association, the American Hospital Association, the American Academy of Pediatrics, and the American Academy of Neurologists. Growth in the number of institutional ethics committees continued into the 1990s and spread to nursing homes and hospices (Glaser, 1989). It is likely that the number and influence of these committees will grow as the length of stay in hospitals continues

to decline and more patient days are spent outside hospitals. Moreover, with the shift of many kinds of care to alternative sites, it is likely that other institutional ethics committees will develop and spread—in home-health-care agencies and managed-care networks, for example. Hospital ethics committees remain, however, the most common institutional ethics committees and the most closely analyzed in bioethics literature.

There is a paucity of empirical studies of hospital ethics committees. Committees have a "grass-roots" character, reflecting a variety of local circumstances and personalities. These factors make it hard to generalize. Nevertheless, some typical features have emerged. One of these features is interdisciplinary composition. Generally, committees are composed of doctors, nurses, social workers, pastoral-care professionals, and philosophers or theologians trained in ethics. Committee members can also include administrators, hospital attorneys, and consumer or community representatives. Committees are sometimes authorized by the medical staff; sometimes by the hospital governing board; sometimes by the administration.

Functions of ethics committees

Committee functions vary but generally include one, two, or all three of the following. First, institutional ethics committees create a vehicle for education on ethical dimensions of patient care. Committees typically have dual efforts in this respect: education of the committee itself, through discussion of current bioethics literature, for example; and education of the medical staff and hospital employees, by organizing periodic lectures, panel discussions, and "ethics grand rounds."

Second, committees draft institutional policies on ethical questions. This may arise through committee initiative. For example, a hospital panel discussion may reveal the need for a new policy on withholding resuscitation from dying patients, and the ethics committee takes the lead by preparing a first draft. New policies or review of existing policies may also be requested from the ethics committee by the hospital administration, or other hospital committees may route drafts of proposed policies and revisions of existing policies to the committee for review and comment.

Third, many institutional ethics committees offer ethics consultations, prospectively or retrospectively, on difficult clinical cases, often those involving the withholding or withdrawal of life-support measures. This last function—ethics consultation, especially for ongoing cases—has been the main focus of discussion in the bioethics literature. Seven issues have dominated these discussions: questions of competence and authority; impact on the doctor–patient relationship; access to consultation; recordkeeping and charting; problems of evaluation; unsettled legal questions; and questions about the purpose or purposes of consultations.

Competence and authority.   Some committees that offer consultation services, generally smaller committees, consult as a committee of the whole. Larger committees typically have a subcommittee that consults prospectively and reports to the committee as a whole for retrospective review of its work. Some committees offer consultation through a single ethics consultant who may be on the committee or have a formal relationship with it. Some critics have expressed concern that when committees consult, difficult ethical choices will be affected by compromise, hospital politics, professional rivalries, and conformism (Wikler, 1989). Concerns about competence have been raised when individuals provide consultations. Clinicians typically have few of the skills of trained ethicists and vice versa.

Continued spread of ethics committee consultation to more hospitals and nonhospital settings is indirect evidence that the challenges to competence and authority are being met successfully. Furthermore, most published concerns about the competence of committees or individuals are from the 1970s "first wave" of writing about institutional ethics committees, at a time when the idea of ethics consultation was new and controversial. The literature of the 1980s and 1990s displays a growing confidence about the concept of ethics consultation and more attention to resolving specific problems. Apparently, committees had learned to negotiate without conformism or loss of principle. Individuals have been acquiring the proper expertise: clinicians gaining the analytic techniques of ethicists, and ethicists learning to apply their analyses in clinically relevant ways.

Gender-related questions have not been raised directly in the bioethics literature on ethics committees. However, they are raised indirectly when the focus is on the role of nurses, given the fact that most nurses are women. Nurses have been excluded from some committees, could not access them for consultation, or have found their special ethical concerns omitted from consideration. In addition to the gender issue, this situation raises questions of professional status in relation to other health-care providers. In some hospitals, these problems have been addressed by the formation of nursing ethics committees (Edwards and Haddad, 1988).

There has also been a suggestion in the literature that ethics committees, especially those that are or function as infant-care review committees, should include persons with disabilities on the committee (Mahowald, 1988). This step could help ensure that the quality of life of persons with disabilities is not undervalued in deliberations about treatment decisions.

Doctor–patient relationship.   Trust in the doctor–patient relationship is grounded in the doctor's professional obligation to the patient. Some have expressed concern that ethics consultations will undermine that obligation and trust by limiting doctors' authority to act for their patients or by encouraging abdication of the responsibility (Siegler, 1986). These concerns are addressed or attenuated by the fact that use of a committee's consulting service is generally optional and its findings are advisory (Fost and Cranford, 1985). It should be admitted, however, that when an ethics consultation is sought and its findings are received, a de facto "burden of proof" may be imposed on those doctors who choose to reject or ignore the ethics committee's advice. They will probably need to muster strong reasons for doing so.

Access to consultation.   Who should have the authority to request an ethics consultation? Some committees use a medical model whereby only the attending physician can initiate a consultation; he or she alone joins in the deliberations and receives the advice. But many committees allow other physicians, nurses, other professionals, and the patient and family to initiate consultations.

There are two main reasons why ethics committees reject the medical model. First, ethical dilemmas in patient care, especially those surrounding withholding or withdrawing life support, are felt acutely by all professionals involved. Second, if the consulting process helps to delimit or set priorities for a patient's options, the patient's right of informed consent may require that he or she, or a surrogate, be able to participate in the consultation. There is no clear pattern for such participation in the literature. Some consulting teams interview competent patients; others do not. Some encourage the presence of patients or surrogates at consultations; others do not. While most committees that reject the medical model respond to patient requests for consultation, it is not clear generally whether objection by a patient or surrogate can prevent an ethics consultation or stop one that has been initiated by others.

Recordkeeping and charting.   Some committees and consultants keep no records in order to ensure patient confidentiality and to prevent the use of committee deliberations in legal proceedings. Plainly, all institutional ethics committees must carefully adhere to the norms of medical confidentiality, but the prevailing wisdom is that ethics committees should keep good records and should enter their advice and reasons for it into the patient's active chart (Cranford et al., 1985). Such procedures build trust in the committee, educate the medical and nursing staffs on ethical issues, and provide accountability for committee advice in what are often literally life-and-death decisions.

Evaluation.   The brief history of most ethics committees, the confidential status of what they do, and the ambiguity many of them experience about their roles, especially in consultation, have made it difficult to conduct comprehensive evaluation of their effectiveness. Moreover, there is no independent standard of right and wrong against which the advice of these committees can be measured. However, committees can be evaluated by reference to their own mission statements, by written assessments of those who request consultations, and by the informal measures of success as an interdisciplinary forum: enhanced institutional sensitivity to ethical issues and increased requests for consultation (Van Allen et al., 1989).

Some ethics committees use very explicit regulations or ethical guidelines for consulting. These documents could provide norms for more focused evaluation of consultation. Hospitals in the Veterans Administration system, for example, employ detailed national protocols on withholding and withdrawing life support. Catholic hospitals make explicit use of ethical guidelines contained in the Ethical and Religious Directives for Catholic Health Facilities (Craig et al., 1986).

Unsettled legal questions. A number of legal questions about ethics committees remain unsettled for want of legislation and court decisions. Can an ethics committee and/or its members be sued and held accountable in civil or criminal actions? Are the records of an ethics committee discoverable? If used in court, what weight should they be given (Wolf, 1986)? There is also a widely held, but undocumented, view that the availability of an ethics committee can lessen the likelihood of litigation because it provides a forum for resolving conflict and because it allows for thorough examination of ethical issues that frequently have significant legal components.

The purpose or purposes of consultations. Several authors have argued that protection of patients' interests should be the single purpose of an institutional ethics committee's consultation (Hoffmann, 1993). But it is also clear that consultations often serve other purposes: to assist caregivers, to support patients' families, to negotiate compromise when disputes arise, to protect the hospital, to offer the correct or best moral advice. Sometimes these other purposes can conflict with the purpose of protecting the patients' best interests. Moreover, in some cases a patient's apparent best interest is incompatible with what the patient demands. Clear strategies for dealing with such conflicts have not yet emerged in the bioethics literature, but they are plainly needed.

Conclusion

Much remains to be done to sharpen the focus of the work of institutional ethics committees and to evaluate the strengths and weaknesses of various committee and consultation models. This area is one of social experi-

mentation and will remain so into the foreseeable future. Nevertheless, in a very short time, ethics committees have contributed greatly to the general bioethics agenda of creating dialogue on ethics issues in health care. Most acute-care hospitals in the United States, and many other settings where chronically ill and dying patients receive care, have an established institutional vehicle for explicit, interdisciplinary discussion of difficult ethical issues.

CHARLES J. DOUGHERTY

Directly related to this article are the other articles in this entry: ELEMENTS AND METHODOLOGIES, *and* CLINICAL ETHICS CONSULTATION. *For a further discussion of the topics mentioned in this article, see the entries* COMPETENCE; CONFIDENTIALITY; INFORMED CONSENT; PROFESSIONAL–PATIENT RELATIONSHIP; *and* TRUST. *Also directly related are the entries* RESEARCH ETHICS COMMITTEES; *and* TEAMS, HEALTH-CARE. *For a discussion of related ideas, see the entries* CONFLICT OF INTEREST; HOSPITAL; KIDNEY DIALYSIS; VALUE AND VALUATION; *and* WOMEN, *section on* WOMEN AS HEALTH PROFESSIONALS. *See also the entries* ALLIED HEALTH PROFESSIONS; BIOETHICS EDUCATION, *article on* SECONDARY AND POSTSECONDARY EDUCATION; PASTORAL CARE; *and* SOCIAL WORK IN HEALTH CARE.

Bibliography

CRAIG, ROBERT P.; MIDDLETON, CARL L.; and O'CONNELL, LAURENCE J. 1986. *Ethics Committees: A Practical Approach.* St. Louis, Mo.: Catholic Health Association.

CRANFORD, RONALD E.; HESTER, F. ALLEN; and ASHLEY, BARBARA ZIEGLER. 1985. "Institutional Ethics Committees: Issues of Confidentiality and Immunity." *Law, Medicine, and Health Care* 15, no. 2:52–60.

EDWARDS, BARBA J., and HADDAD, AMY M. 1988. "Establishing a Nursing Bioethics Committee." *Journal of Nursing Administration* 18, no. 3:30–33.

FLEETWOOD, JANET E.; ARNOLD, ROBERT M.; and BARON, RICHARD J. 1989. "Giving Answers or Raising Questions?: The Problematic Role of Institutional Ethics Committees." *Journal of Medical Ethics* 15, no. 3:137–142.

FOST, NORMAN, and CRANFORD, RONALD. 1985. "Hospital Ethics Committees: Administrative Aspects." *Journal of the American Medical Association* 253, no. 18:2687–2692.

GLASER, JOHN W. 1989. "Hospital Ethics Committees: One of Many Centers of Responsibility." *Theoretical Medicine* 10, no 4:275–288.

HOFFMANN, DIANE E. 1993. "Evaluating Ethics Committees: A View from the Outside." *Milbank Quarterly* 71, no. 4:677–701.

MAHOWALD, MARY B. 1988. "Baby Doe Committees: A Critical Evaluation." *Clinics in Perinatology* 15, no. 4: 789–800.

Quinlan, in re. 1976. 355 A.2d 647 (N.J.).

SIEGLER, MARK. 1986. "Ethics Committees: Decisions by Bureaucracy." *Hastings Center Report* 16, no. 3:22–24.

U.S. PRESIDENT'S COMMISSION FOR THE STUDY OF ETHICAL PROBLEMS IN MEDICINE AND BIOMEDICAL AND BEHAVIORAL RESEARCH. 1983. *Deciding to Forgo Life-Sustaining Treatment: A Report on the Ethical, Medical, and Legal Issues in Treatment Decisions.* Washington, D.C.: Author.

VAN ALLEN, E.; MOLDOW, D. G.; and CRANFORD, RONALD. 1989. "Evaluating Ethics Committees." *Hastings Center Report* 19, no. 5:23–24.

WIKLER, DANIEL. 1989. "Institutional Agendas and Ethics Committees." *Hastings Center Report* 19, no. 5:21–23.

WOLF, SUSAN M. 1986. "Ethics Committees in the Courts." *Hastings Center Report* 16, no. 3:12–15.

CLINICAL RESEARCH

See RESEARCH BIAS; RESEARCH ETHICS COMMITTEES; RESEARCH METHODOLOGY; *and* RESEARCH POLICY. *See also* RESEARCH, HUMAN: HISTORICAL ASPECTS; *and* RESEARCH, UNETHICAL.

CLINICAL TRIALS

See RESEARCH METHODOLOGY, *article on* CONTROLLED CLINICAL TRIALS.

CODES OF ETHICS

See MEDICAL CODES AND OATHS; *and the* APPENDIX (CODES, OATHS, AND DIRECTIVES RELATED TO BIOETHICS), *the introductory article on* THE NATURE AND ROLE OF CODES AND OATHS, *and* SECTIONS I–VI.

COERCION

See FREEDOM AND COERCION; *and* POPULATION POLICIES, *section on* STRATEGIES OF FERTILITY CONTROL, *articles on* COMPULSION *and* STRONG PERSUASION. *See also* BEHAVIOR CONTROL; COMMITMENT TO MENTAL INSTITUTIONS; INFORMED CONSENT; *and* PATIENTS' RIGHTS.

COLOMBIA

See MEDICAL ETHICS, HISTORY OF, *section on* THE AMERICAS, *article on* LATIN AMERICA.

COMA, IRREVERSIBLE

See DEATH, DEFINITION AND DETERMINATION OF. *See also* DEATH AND DYING: EUTHANASIA AND SUSTAINING LIFE.

COMFORT CARE

See HOSPICE AND END OF LIFE CARE; *and* DEATH AND DYING: EUTHANASIA AND SUSTAINING LIFE. *See also* CARE.

COMMERCIALISM AND PROFIT IN HEALTH CARE

See HEALTH-CARE FINANCING, *article on* PROFIT AND COMMERCIALISM.

COMMERCIALISM IN SCIENTIFIC RESEARCH

Scientific research has never been entirely insulated from the incentives provided by the profit motive and the need to secure financial support. Scientists have always required funding, whether it be from personal funds, patrons, universities, or industry. Similarly, opportunities for scientific entrepreneurship have always existed. In the past two hundred years, however, scientific research has both required increasing amounts of capital investment and promised progressively greater financial returns. Consequently, scientists have been forced to rely on a broader range of funding sources and have become more willing to involve themselves in the financial implications of their work. This incremental "commercialization" of science poses interrelated challenges for both society and the research community.

Although there were notable exceptions, well into the early nineteenth century scientists were frequently indifferent to the commercial potential of their work and typically did not pursue large-scale or external financial support. This posture arose both because research did not require huge capital expenditures and because many researchers held the belief that scientific research was the work of disinterested amateurs—a calling devoted to the pursuit of truth. Few scientists took advantage of financial opportunities even where they existed. In the mid- to late nineteenth century the development of the large-scale laboratory in Europe and ultimately in the United States increased the costs associated with research and foreshadowed the decline of the solitary, amateur researcher. At the same time, a variety of connections between industry and science developed. Many businesses employed their own scientists, but an increasing number established relationships with universities and employed academic scientists as consultants and researchers. While this trend continued in the early twentieth century, industry-sponsored research typically focused on applied-science projects. Basic research areas had yet to be viewed as fruitful areas of investment (Etzkowitz, 1983).

In the last half of the twentieth century, several developments have enhanced the commercial aspects of science. The cost of basic science research has continued to soar as it requires sophisticated equipment and resources, larger laboratories, and more staff. Basic research therefore has become increasingly dependent on financial support, provided by both the government and the private sector. Scientific research, especially in the biomedical fields, promises to generate tremendous profits for those who control new discoveries. Moreover, the gap between basic and applied science has narrowed, so that discoveries can be translated into usable and profitable products with less energy and time (Etzkowitz, 1983). These changes have accelerated the commercialization of basic as well as applied science.

Commercialization, the ideals of science, and the public good

Despite the clear need for broad-based and generous funding and the right of scientists to reap rewards for their efforts and ingenuity, financial incentives may create conflicts of interest that can undermine and corrupt the ideal of disinterested scientific inquiry. While the phrase "conflict of interest" is frequently employed to suggest that an ethical violation has already occurred, it is more accurate and useful to view conflict of interest as a set of conditions under which an ethical violation is more likely to occur. More specifically, a conflict of interest exists when any professional judgment or activity relating to a primary interest (e.g., intellectual honesty, validity, openness, or objectivity), equivalent to the scientific norms articulated by Robert K. Merton and others, may be influenced by secondary interests (e.g., financial gain, profit, position, or fame). Primary interests or scientific norms are typically considered superior to secondary interests, and their subversion must be avoided by prophylactic measures, or in extreme cases the secondary interests must be removed from the relationship so as to end the conflict and danger (Thompson, 1993; Merton, 1942; Cournand, 1977).

Even when no conflict of interest is created, financial incentives may also induce researchers and institutions to behave in ways that may be detrimental to society; for example, a scientist may forgo research on an important project in favor of another that is more profitable. Personal, institutional, and societal responses to the two challenges necessarily differ. In conflicts of interest, the primary values of the institution or profession should ordinarily prevail. In situations where commercial incentives appear to work against the public good without creating conflicts of interest, the financial arrangements and the research choices they encourage should be judged by their fairness and social utility.

Industry investment in academic research

Private investment in university research may take a number of forms. Companies may offer universities large grants in exchange for patent rights to anticipated discoveries or establish lucrative consulting arrangements with faculty members who provide sponsoring corporations with priority access to valuable research. Faculty members sometimes own equity interests in biotechnology firms related to their work, or they may found their own corporations. And in what is so far a rare agreement, a corporation may provide an academic research institute generous payments in exchange for the right to market all the institution's discoveries. These secondary, financial interests threaten to undermine the university's primary interests of advancing basic knowledge, promoting the open exchange of ideas, providing a source of expertise for society, and training future scientists (Etzkowitz, 1983; Ashford, 1983).

Some scientists admit that financial arrangements have led them to delay publication of research results or communication of findings to others in the field in order to protect potential trade secrets. Researchers, of course, may have other reasons (professional rivalry, jealousy, etc.) for withholding research findings from their colleagues and others in the scientific community. But the increasing financial value associated with biotechnological research may greatly magnify these existing tendencies. David Blumenthal and his colleagues report that biotechnology academics with industrial connections were four times as likely as other biotechnology academics to report that their research had produced information that was kept secret to protect its proprietary value, but larger empirical studies of the impact of commercialism on intellectual openness and data sharing within the scientific community are sorely lacking (Blumenthal et al., 1986). If free exchange through traditional scholarly mediums of conferences and publications is blunted, scientists working in the same and affiliated fields will be unable to examine and replicate experiments, promising advances may be slowed, and scientific progress may be endangered. Some contractual agreements with industries specifically require scientists to withhold submission to professional journals until the corporation has determined if the information warrants patent protection. After patent protection is secured, obviously, the findings can be released to the general scientific community. The propriety of these arrangements depends in part on the length and impact of the delay of release of scientifically important information and varies from contract to contract. It is possible that much of the research that is withheld from the scientific community as trade secrets has little intrinsic scientific value or applicability and is limited to information such as scientifically unimportant formulas for products, scientific instrument calibrations, or engineering tolerances (Snapper, 1992). Without a clearer view of what information is withheld and for how long, it is impossible to evaluate definitively the dangers posed by these trends. But while empirical evidence of commercialism's impact on the free flow of scientific information is incomplete, current industry–scientist relationships pose a clear potential threat to the traditional scientific norms of openness.

Commercial considerations can distort academic life in other respects. Researchers may be tempted to devote time earmarked for the university to their commercial projects and to use university resources, including graduate assistants and laboratory staff, for their own financial benefit. Graduate students are particularly vulnerable to the availability of funds; the entire course of their careers may be guided by the source of their mentors' grants (Porter, 1992a; Blumenthal, 1992). The prospect of large infusions of money into a cash-starved university might make an institution less scrupulous when evaluating potential research projects. For example, an institutional review board might be less likely to point out minor, yet problematic, aspects of an experimental study at the institution if they believe that the corporate sponsor will withdraw its funds and go elsewhere with the proposal. An existing or potential grant might influence a university's decision on the composition of its faculty, the structure of a department, and the granting of tenure (Nelkin and Nelson, 1987). Financial incentives have encouraged some university researchers to redirect their work toward projects that are more likely to yield financial rewards. Such a redirection of research might encourage researchers to value applied projects with clear commercial ends and patentable uses over basic science projects whose practical applications are uncertain. While society benefits from applied research, fundamental breakthroughs and scientific progress are predicated on a strong commitment to basic research.

Despite these caveats, private funding of university research serves as an effective and essential supplement to government funding. Some reports demonstrate that industry-funded scientists tend to publish more, produce more patentable discoveries, and yet teach as much and serve as many administrative roles as colleagues without corporate financial support (Blumenthal, 1992). Industrial subsidies allow universities to support a more talented and larger faculty and to improve their facilities. Therefore, some authors argue that the danger of increased commercial presence in universities must be weighed against the positive contributions made by industry funding (Blake, 1992).

Conflicts and scientists' social duties

Professional researchers are the public's and policymakers' most important source of scientific expertise. Gov-

ernment agencies that evaluate biomedical proposals and projects must rely on scientists to analyze the safety and efficacy of research and products. Active scientists also serve as reviewers for governmental grant applications and as authors, editors, and referees for professional publications. Conflicts of interest arise when industry, regulatory agencies, government committees, and editors all seek out the same individuals—a likely prospect when many of the most talented researchers have already established commercial interests (Culliton, 1982).

Few scientists will purposely present biased conclusions, but researchers' commercial interests may influence their professional life in other respects. Scientists might be hesitant to participate in the evaluation of an industry with which they maintain a financial connection. Following a large oil spill on the California coast in the late 1960s, for example, government investigators found it difficult to recruit scientists willing to testify against the oil companies. Most qualified scientists had commercial ties to the industry (Kenney, 1986). Corporations frequently employ researchers as consultants to determine if their facilities meet governmental health standards or if their new product induces disease. A researcher's desire to please the employer and to preserve the potential of future affiliations may influence the study design and methodology selected for the investigation. A study that monitors employee health for only a short time, for example, would be less likely to uncover an occupation-related disease with a long latency period. Different methods of statistical analysis and characterization can yield conclusions that either highlight or minimize potential health risks. A corporation facing liability for a suspect drug would prefer its researchers to find that the product presented no danger and was not responsible for the maladies suffered by current users (Ashford, 1983; Porter, 1992a, 1992b).

Similarly, reviewers of grant applications may have commercial interests that unconsciously lead them to undervalue a potential competitor's proposal. Journal referees may denigrate articles or reports that threaten their commercial interests or their industry employer. A researcher with a consulting arrangement or an equity interest in a new development might tend toward findings that would laud the benefits of the innovation. In one egregious case, a researcher who owned over 500,000 shares of biomedical stock altered a study design to delay the release of negative findings until he could sell his holdings for a tremendous profit (Council on Scientific Affairs, 1990). In each of these cases, the secondary interest of financial gain created by the industry–scientist relationship endangered the primary scientific interest of a disinterested quest for truth.

Physician-researchers with commercial interests in innovative treatments or research protocols bear additional responsibilities. A central tenet of medical professionalism holds that the welfare of the patient be placed before the benefit to the physician. If a physician-researcher is testing an experimental therapy, the treatment must be in the best interests of the patient and considered at least as effective as the standard therapy. In extreme cases, physician-researchers with financial interests in their protocol might tend to recruit subjects aggressively, downplaying the risks and exaggerating the benefits associated with the research.

In addition, some scientists participate in innovative "fee-for-service research" in which seriously ill patients finance the development of new treatments. Supporters of patient-financed research argue that individuals should have the freedom to purchase the type of care they desire and that such projects will benefit society by either highlighting the availability of a new treatment or demonstrating its ineffectiveness. This knowledge, they reason, would not otherwise be available. Critics claim that the practice will place the primary interests of both the medical profession and the scientific community (e.g., patient benefit, objectivity, and validity) in direct conflict with the secondary interests created by the profit motive. For example, a paying research subject's unwillingness to participate in double-blind studies in which the subject may receive a placebo could jeopardize the reliability of the study results. Researchers might undermine the scientific reliability of studies further by accepting subjects who do not meet inclusion criteria but who are willing to support the project with financial contributions. Researchers may also be hesitant to report negative results if they have a financial interest in the continuation of the research. Moreover, patient investors are particularly vulnerable and may be unable to fully judge the merits, potential, and risks of the research project in which they are being asked to participate. These problems are exacerbated in that much of this research may be beyond the supervisory powers of government agencies and institutional review boards (Lind, 1986).

Remedies and safeguards

The integrity of individual researchers is clearly the most important guard against the malevolent potential of conflicts of interest. But honesty alone may sometimes be insufficient, as damage can occur from unconscious bias and error as well as from conscious falsification. While all conflicts of interest have the potential to undermine a scientist's or institution's primary goals of truth, objectivity, and openness, all conflicts do not pose the same degree of danger or require the same response. The danger of a particular conflict of interest depends both on how likely the arrangement is to corrupt the scientist's professional duty and on how much damage that corruption is likely to cause. Larger financial payments, and longer and closer relationships between researchers and business, will typically pose greater dangers than small financial incentives and one-time contacts with corporations (Thompson, 1993). While supervisory and regulatory measures can usually be tailored to the degree of the risk, there may be some situations in which the danger of harm to scientific integrity and society is so high that no protective measure can remedy it.

Universities might limit the amount of support they accept from industry, limit the amount of time that faculty may devote to outside endeavors, or prohibit particularly suspicious arrangements. In addition, research institutes can require the disclosure of all commercial links and interests and institute prospective administrative review of all proposals for outside funding (Varrin and Kukich, 1985; Association of American Medical Colleges, 1990). Disclosure rules not only assist university officials and peers in policing conflicts of interest but may also make researchers more scrupulous in evaluating the potential bias in their own work. Researchers sometimes end or eschew questionable relationships rather than disclose them to the academic community. Universities have employed a wide range of these safeguards. For example, Stanford University's policy relies greatly on the integrity of the individual researcher, explicitly barring no commercial relationship but demanding comprehensive disclosure to department and university officials of any potential financial conflict. Johns Hopkins University demands reporting of financial ties and allows its faculty to accept paid consultancies but forbids researchers from holding equity interests in the company that supports their research (Blumenthal, 1992). The most effective and defensible policies impose greater safeguards for arrangements that create the greatest danger of abuse.

Government agencies and professional publications also institute policies to guard against conflicts of interest. The U.S. Food and Drug Administration and the National Institutes of Health require extensive disclosure of all advisers' commercial interests. Some professional journals demand that authors and reviewers disclose any commercial relationships that might be construed as creating conflicts of interest. According to this view, conflicts of interest should not automatically disqualify a reviewer or author, but the revelation will allow readers, editors, and administrators to scrutinize conclusions more carefully (Koshland, 1992). Other publications have adopted somewhat more stringent guidelines. The *New England Journal of Medicine,* for example, requires that authors disclose their financial conflicts, that its editors have no financial interest in any business related to clinical medicine, and that authors of review articles and editorials have no financial connection to their topics (Relman, 1990). Physician-researchers who hold financial interests in their research projects carry an additional responsibility. They have a duty to ensure that the commercial potential of a re-search therapy does not undermine their ethical duty to act in the best interest of the patient. Some observers argue that the physician-researcher's commercial ties should be revealed to the patient-subject through the mechanism of informed consent and to the investiga-tor's institution through a formal reporting mechanism. Finally, institutional review boards can scrutinize pro-tocols that promise great financial rewards for physician-investigators.

Patents and the public interest

Patenting is another commercially motivated practice that may create conflicts between the primary interests of good science and the secondary interests created by the profit motive. Patenting is based on the theory that innovators will be more likely to share their knowledge because they know that they will receive remuneration and credit and that entrepreneurs will be more willing to invest in the development of discoveries because they know that they have exclusive or protected access and will recoup their expenditures in profits. Patenting's skeptics, however, argue that the very nature of patent-ing undermines the traditional scientific norm of open-ness. Researchers may be tempted to withhold socially valuable information until they are certain that their pe-cuniary interests are protected by a patent (Kass, 1981; Wiener, 1987). Especially in the biomedical fields, a de-lay in the release of information can lead to postponed development and dissemination and the loss of lives. Others speculate that potentially patentable, lucrative discoveries will lead researchers away from less profitable yet socially important projects. Finally, some critics claim that entrepreneurs who purchase rights to a basic discovery often do not use or develop it in a socially responsible way. And, their monopoly advantage makes it impossible for the market to force them to distribute the breakthrough in an equitable and useful manner (Goldman, 1987).

The government can also provide patentlike incen-tives to encourage the development of products with marginal profitability that are intended to treat a small patient population or that are ineligible for normal pat-ent protection—so-called orphan drugs. Orphan-drug programs might include research grants, investment tax credits, expedited approval processes, and exclusive li-censes to produce and distribute the drug. Critics of or-phan-drug programs argue that the policy excessively favors drug manufacturers, inflates the costs of lifesaving medications, and delays the development of lower-cost alternatives. Private corporations sometimes reap profits far in excess of their expectations and effort while ef-fectively denying life-sustaining remedies to patients through monopoly pricing practices (Ackiron, 1991). Incentives are sometimes overgenerous, and corpora-tions are able to enrich themselves on drugs that serve only a small number of patients and occasionally pro-duce limited benefits (Wagner, 1992). It is important to scrutinize the incentive structure of the orphan-drug policy in an attempt to eliminate unnecessary windfall profits for drug manufacturers. Policymakers must bal-ance the cost of the incentives, including monopoly pricing practices and tax abatements, against the bene-fits provided by the new drug (i.e., the number of people served and the efficacy of the remedy).

Marketable products from human sources

Another challenging problem arises when an individu-al's body parts or cells are transformed into valuable commodities. In one such case, a patient's removed spleen contained unique cells that a physician-re-searcher cultured into a patented cell line. Should the patient have been apprised, as part of the informed-con-sent procedure, that the cells had potential commercial value? Fully informed consent would have allowed the patient to evaluate the physician's potential conflict of interests and choice of treatments more effectively. Be-cause society and the law have typically been hesitant to "commodify" the body and do not allow the sale of organs, it might seem inappropriate to grant the patient a share of the profits based on the theory that the tissue is his or her "property." On the other hand, the present system appears to allow the biomedical entrepreneur to benefit from the sale of body parts. Developers of such innovative products might argue that the resulting cell line is not a body part but rather the result of their labor and ingenuity and that these efforts deserve to be re-warded and encouraged by traditional patents. Even granting this argument, it may be unjust to allow others to benefit from an innovation while the person upon whose existence the development rests receives nothing. Consequently, it seems fair and equitable that an indi-vidual receive some benefit from his or her unique phys-ical characteristics that have been used to create great profits. The amount of remuneration could depend upon the nature of the informed-consent agreement, the de-gree to which the body tissue contribution was changed by the researcher before it was offered as a product, and the uniqueness of the physical material utilized (Murray, 1985).

Crisis or witchhunt?

Some observers have suggested that the fears associated with the commercialization of scientific research have been overstated. While the profit motive can subvert the integrity of the research enterprise in a variety of ways, it must also be acknowledged that the scientific ideal of free and open exchange of information has never been fully realized. Conflicts of interest are not new. Re-searchers have always competed for fame, if not for profit, and this competition has sometimes bred secrecy and encouraged the withholding of useful information. Society and the scientific community have relied on peer review and professional integrity to limit these sorts of conflicts and will continue to do so as financial conflicts arise. Some writers have even argued that the selfish race for profit and fame may enhance scientific productivity. They agree that researchers may be drawn toward the most profitable projects, but argue that in many cases profitability is a plausible and accurate gauge of the value society places on a particular line of research (Lomasky, 1987). Careful investors will not reward incompetent and unimaginative researchers who have little chance of developing genuine or useful discoveries. And scientists, anxious for a marketable discovery, will be more likely to pursue innovative projects than to focus their work on more conventional research (Kitcher, 1993).

A few observers warn that excessive concern over conflicts of interest and current safeguards may hinder scientific progress and undermine the scientific objectivity that they are designed to preserve. These writers claim that focusing reviewers' and readers' attention on potential outside influences instead of the content of the data, findings, and ideas generates a subjective skepticism unrelated to the objective merit of the work (Rothman, 1993). These sometimes cogent criticisms of orthodox views of conflicts of interest neither suggest solutions to the insidious problem of unconscious bias nor appear to recognize that commercial affiliations frequently remain hidden and are therefore difficult to assess. And while fame and prestige may also create conflicts and endanger scientific ideals, these motives are well known, unavoidable, and shared by all scientists.

Conclusion

It would be unrealistic to expect modern capital-intensive scientific research to thrive entirely without the support and influence of commercial interests and incentives. Similarly, it would be unwise and impractical to suggest that scientists who maintain commercial connections, and therefore conflict of interests, should disqualify themselves from all advisory duties. Instead, researchers need to be personally sensitive to the variety of insidious pitfalls of their multifaceted role. For their part, government agencies, universities, and editors can employ safeguards to eliminate the worst and most obvious abuses and can establish education and training programs to highlight and mitigate the more subtle and ambiguous conflicts engendered by commercial research opportunities.

KENNETH ALLEN DE VILLE

For a further discussion of topics mentioned in this entry, see the entries COMMUNICATION, BIOMEDICAL, *article*

on SCIENTIFIC PUBLISHING; CONFLICT OF INTEREST; PATENTING ORGANISMS; RESEARCH, UNETHICAL; RESEARCH BIAS; RESEARCH ETHICS COMMITTEES; RESEARCH METHODOLOGY; *and* RESEARCH POLICY. *Other relevant material may be found under the entries* AIDS, *article on* HEALTH-CARE AND RESEARCH ISSUES; ANIMAL RESEARCH; BIOMEDICAL ENGINEERING; BIOTECHNOLOGY; FETUS, *article on* FETAL RESEARCH; GENETICS AND HUMAN BEHAVIOR, *article on* SCIENTIFIC AND RESEARCH ISSUES; MULTINATIONAL RESEARCH; PRIVACY AND CONFIDENTIALITY IN RESEARCH; *and* RESEARCH, HUMAN: HISTORICAL ASPECTS. *See also the* APPENDIX (CODES, OATHS, AND DIRECTIVES RELATED TO BIOETHICS), SECTION IV: ETHICAL DIRECTIVES FOR HUMAN RESEARCH, *and* SECTION V: ETHICAL DIRECTIVES PERTAINING TO THE WELFARE AND USE OF ANIMALS.

Bibliography

ACKIRON, EVAN. 1991. "Patents for Critical Pharmaceuticals: The AZT Case." *American Journal of Law and Medicine* 17, nos. 1–2:145–180.

ASHFORD, NICHOLAS A. 1983. "A Framework for Examining the Effects of Industrial Funding on Academic Freedom and the Integrity of the University." *Science, Technology, and Human Values* 8, issue 2:16–23.

ASSOCIATION OF AMERICAN MEDICAL COLLEGES. AD HOC COMMITTEE ON MISCONDUCT AND CONFLICT OF INTEREST IN RESEARCH. 1990. *Guidelines for Dealing with Faculty Conflicts of Commitment and Conflicts of Interest in Research.* Washington, D.C.: Author.

BLAKE, DAVID A. 1992. "The Opportunities and Problems of Commercial Ventures: The University View." In *Biomedical Research: Collaboration and Conflict of Interest*, pp. 87–92. Edited by Roger J. Porter, Thomas E. Malone, and Christopher C. Vaughn. Baltimore: Johns Hopkins University Press.

BLUMENTHAL, DAVID. 1992. "Academic-Industry Relationships in the Life Sciences: Extent, Consequences, and Management." *Journal of the American Medical Association* 268, no. 23:3344–3349.

BLUMENTHAL, DAVID; GLUCK, MICHAEL; LOUIS, KAREN SEASHORE; STOTO, MICHAEL A.; WISE, DAVID. 1986. "University-Industry Research Relationships in Biotechnology: Implications for the University." *Science* 232: 1361–1366.

COUNCIL ON SCIENTIFIC AFFAIRS and COUNCIL ON ETHICAL AND JUDICIAL AFFAIRS. AMERICAN MEDICAL ASSOCIATION. 1990. "Conflicts of Interest in Medical Center/Industry Research Relationships." *Journal of the American Medical Association* 263, no. 20:2790–2793.

COURNAND, ANDRÉ. 1977. "The Code of the Scientist and Its Relationship to Ethics." *Science* 198, no. 4318:699–705.

CULLITON, BARBARA J. 1982. "The Academic-Industrial Complex." *Science* 216, no. 4549:960–962.

ETZKOWITZ, HENRY. 1983. "Entrepreneurial Scientists and Entrepreneurial Universities in American Academic Science." *Minerva* 21, nos. 2–3:198–233.

FINKEL, MARION J. 1991. "Should Informed Consent Include Information on How Research Is Funded?" *IRB*: 13, no. 5:1–3.

GOLDMAN, ALAN H. 1987. "Ethical Issues in Proprietary Restrictions on Research Results." *Science, Technology, and Human Values* 12, issue 1:22–30.

KASS, LEON R. 1981. "Patenting Life." *Commentary* 72, no. 6:45–57.

KENNEY, MARTIN. 1986. *Biotechnology: The University-Industrial Complex.* New Haven, Conn.: Yale University Press.

KITCHER, PHILIP. 1993. *The Advancement of Science: Science Without Legend, Objectivity Without Illusions.* New York: Oxford University Press.

KOSHLAND, DANIEL E., JR. 1992. "Conflict of Interest Policy." *Science* 257, no. 5070:595.

LIND, STUART E. 1986. "Fee-for-Service Research." *New England Journal of Medicine* 314, no. 5:312–315.

LOMASKY, LOREN E. 1987. "Who Should Profit from the Business of Science? Public Money, Private Gain, Profit for All." *Hastings Center Report* 17, no. 3:5–7.

MERTON, ROBERT K. 1942. "Science and Technology in a Democratic Order." *Journal of Legal and Political Sociology* 1:115–126.

MURRAY, THOMAS H. 1985. "Ethical Issues in Genetic Engineering." *Social Research* 52, no. 3:471–489.

NELKIN, DOROTHY, and NELSON, RICHARD. 1987. "Commentary: University-Industry Alliances." *Science, Technology, and Human Values* 12, issue 1:65–74.

PORTER, ROGER J. 1992a. "Conflicts of Interest in Research: Investigator Bias—The Instrument of Conflict." In *Biomedical Research: Collaboration and Conflict of Interest,* pp. 151–162. Edited by Roger J. Porter, Thomas E. Malone, and Christopher C. Vaughn. Baltimore: Johns Hopkins University Press.

———. 1992b. "Conflicts of Interest in Research: Personal Gain—The Seeds of Conflict." In *Biomedical Research: Collaboration and Conflict of Interest,* pp. 135–150. Edited by Roger J. Porter, Thomas E. Malone, and Christopher C. Vaughn. Baltimore: Johns Hopkins University Press.

RELMAN, ARNOLD S. 1990. "New 'Information for Authors'— and Readers." *New England Journal of Medicine* 323, no. 1:56.

ROTHMAN, KENNETH J. 1993. "Conflict of Interest: The New McCarthyism in Science." *Journal of the American Medical Association* 269, no. 21:2782–2784.

SHIPP, ALLAN C. 1992. "How to Control Conflict of Interest." In *Biomedical Research: Collaboration and Conflict of Interest,* pp. 163–184. Edited by Roger J. Porter, Thomas E. Malone, and Christopher C. Vaughn. Baltimore: Johns Hopkins University Press.

SNAPPER, JOHN W. 1992. "Doing Science While Keeping Trade Secrets." *Phi Kappa Phi Journal,* winter, pp. 22–25.

THOMPSON, DENNIS F. 1993. "Understanding Financial Conflicts of Interest." *New England Journal of Medicine* 329, no. 8:573–576.

VARRIN, ROBERT D., and KUKICH, DIANE S. 1985. "Guidelines for Industry-Sponsored Research at Universities." *Science* 227, no. 4685:385–388.

WAGNER, JUDITH L. 1992. "Orphan Technologies: Defining the Issues." *International Journal of Technology Assessment in Health Care* 8, no. 4:561–565.

WIENER, CHARLES. 1987. "Patenting and Academic Research: Historical Case Studies." *Science, Technology, and Human Values* 12, issue 1:50–62.

COMMISSION AND OMISSION

See ACTION; *and* DEATH AND DYING: EUTHANASIA AND SUSTAINING LIFE, *article on* ETHICAL ISSUES.

COMMITMENT TO MENTAL INSTITUTIONS

Throughout the world, there are legal mechanisms whereby mentally ill persons can be sent to psychiatric hospitals even when they do not wish to go. In the United States this is sometimes done through the criminal justice system: A person may be judged incompetent to stand trial for a crime because of mental illness, or may be tried for a crime and found not guilty by reason of insanity, and subsequently be committed to an institution for mentally ill criminal offenders. The more common type of commitment is civil, and usually no criminal offense is involved: A person is judged to require hospitalization because of his or her mental condition but does not consent to it; nevertheless, if certain specified legal criteria are fulfilled, the person may be hospitalized against his or her will. Commitment is a legal process and can be discussed mainly in terms of its case and statutory legal history (Wexler, 1981). This article, however, emphasizes important ethical issues underlying the process of civil commitment.

Commitment raises serious ethical concerns. It involves depriving persons of their freedom for days, weeks, or longer, usually by incarcerating them in a locked psychiatric facility. In most states, this violation of a person's civil liberties can be carried out initially on an "emergency" basis, on the strength of one physician's signature on an appropriate form. Most agree that it is preferable that a psychiatrist be the initial committing physician, but psychiatrists are too few in many rural areas to allow this usually to be mandated by law.

After the emergency commitment form is signed, the person is taken to the nearest locked psychiatric facility authorized to receive committed persons. Medical personnel there usually have the authority to question the appropriateness of the commitment and even to refuse to detain the person. In most states, under modern law, a probable-cause judicial hearing is held within two to three working days, in an appropriate local court, to determine the justifiability of continued detainment.

The vast majority of admissions to psychiatric hospitals, however, are voluntary and do not involve the commitment process. A small minority of these voluntary admissions, however, result from persons being told that they will be committed if they do not enter the hospital "voluntarily." There seems nothing inherently unethical about giving a person, who would otherwise be committed, the opportunity to avoid the commitment process in this way, assuming that the planned commitment itself is ethically justified. It seems clear, however, that these persons have not entered the hospital entirely voluntarily. It would, in addition, be prima facie unethical for a physician to use this process deceptively: to manipulate a person into entering a hospital by deceptively threatening a commitment that in fact would not be carried out.

Legal criteria for commitment

Both within and outside of psychiatry, there is dispute about what commitment criteria should be written into state statutes. Statutory language varies from state to state (Arthur et al., 1988). All U.S. state statutes stipulate that, to be committed, the person must be mentally ill, though this concept is variously defined. The existing continuum of positions is based upon how wide or narrow the additional statutory commitment criteria are.

The broadest criteria are advocated by those who think physicians should be able to commit anyone they sincerely believe would profit from commitment. At one time many states had statutes of this breadth. Arizona law, for example, as recently as 1981 allowed persons to be detained if they were "mentally ill and in need of supervision, care or treatment" (Wexler, 1981, p. 74). Criteria of this breadth seem unsupportable to most commentators. For example, many persons with a moderate degree of depression are mentally ill, in that they satisfy the criteria in *DSM-III-R* (American Psychiatric Association, 1987) of having a psychiatric disorder, and treatment almost certainly would make them feel better. No one, however, would think that in most cases they should be forced into a psychiatric hospital if they do not wish to go.

A narrower position is taken by many psychiatrists (see Chodoff, 1976, for a good description of this position; and Buchanan and Brock, 1989, for clear arguments supporting it). In addition to requiring that the person be mentally ill, supporters advocate a criterion stipulating that the person be "gravely disabled" or manifest a "serious disruption of functioning" due to the mental illness. Being physically dangerous to oneself (suicidal) or to others (homicidal or physically threatening) is one kind of serious disruption of functioning but not the only one. The kind of behavioral and social dis-

organization shown by many manic persons, for example, while often not immediately physically threatening to themselves or to others, may in the long run cause the persons serious social and financial harm. Under a "serious disruption" criterion, many such persons could be committed.

A narrower position still is that advocated by many civil libertarians and by some psychiatrists as well (see American Bar Association, 1977, for a well-documented and well-argued presentation of this position). A diagnosis of mental illness is required, and there must be a high probability that, because of this mental illness, the person is a serious physical threat to himself or herself or to others. A minority within this group would restrict the criterion still further and require that there be good evidence of recent *behavior* toward self or others that was in fact physically harmful, but most believe that evidence of strong *threats* of physical harm is sufficient. Most also believe that dangerousness toward self can be evidenced not only by threats of suicide but also by extreme self-neglect, so that, for example, starvation or untreated serious disease can constitute an immediate threat. However, without the threat of imminent dangerousness of some kind, commitment would not be allowed.

The final point on the continuum is taken by those who believe that psychiatric commitment is never ethically justified and, thus, that there should be no commitment criteria at all. Thomas Szasz (1970), a psychiatrist, has been the foremost spokesperson for this position. Szasz believes that the concept of mental illness is mythical, and argues that those who manifest what others regard as the symptoms of mental illness should be judged only by the standards of criminal law: If they have broken a law, they may be arrested or otherwise constrained; if they have not, their freedom should be preserved. Szasz believes that commitment is based on a false theory that "medicalizes" deviant behavior into illness, and that psychiatrists who commit persons thereby become unwitting arms of the criminal justice system.

For several reasons, Szasz's position has not been persuasive to many inside or outside of psychiatry, including most civil libertarians. First, most scholars do feel that some psychological conditions satisfy the criteria of a definition of "illness" (Culver and Gert, 1982; Margolis, 1976), and that Szasz's position has serious theoretical problems (Moore, 1975) he has never addressed. Second, and more important, most believe that paternalistic interventions of the kind that commitment usually represents are at least sometimes ethically justified.

The principal and enduring tension is between those holding the two middle positions described above. Some states have commitment statutes closer to one, some closer to the other. Those who advocate a broader criterion believe that dangerousness to self and others is only one of many manifestations of severe mental illness, and that it is cruel and theoretically incorrect to ignore the needs of disordered or disabled persons, often homeless and wandering the streets, who would clearly benefit from treatment (Treffert, 1985). References are made to people "dying with their rights on," or to Janis Joplin's song line, "Freedom's just another word for nothin' left to lose."

Those who advocate the narrower grounds fear that relaxing the criterion in the direction of "disruption of functioning" leaves the door open too wide to psychiatric paternalism and represents a threat to the civil liberties of everyone. Images of forced psychiatric internment of political dissidents in the Soviet Union may be invoked as a frightening example of giving psychiatrists the power to confine those who are not physically dangerous but only "disrupted" in their functioning. One of the necessary and willing prices we pay in a free society, they argue, is that people are free to make self-defeating choices and, sometimes irrationally, to reject opportunities for help.

There is a cohort of persons who are commitable under a broader but not under a narrower set of criteria. One example is a person with a history of bipolar disorder who has become increasingly hypomanic and is now squandering his carefully accumulated savings in what are almost certainly hopeless financial schemes. He refuses all treatment. Everyone who knows him believes that his spending spree is due to his hypomania and that if his behavior were curtailed, he would later almost certainly be grateful. Although his current behavior is harmful to his long-term interests, he is not "dangerous to himself or others" as that criterion is explicated in many states.

Many persons, like this man, whose behavior meets broader but not narrower commitment criteria, suffer from cyclical disorders: Their aberrant behavior occurs only episodically. Some authors have suggested that such persons might be offered, during nonsymptomatic times, the opportunity to create a contract stating that if their future behavior deviates from their usual behavior in certain specified ways, they would sanction the use of appropriate interventions (confiscation of funds or forced hospitalization, "voluntary commitments") that might not otherwise be legally permissible (Howell et al., 1982; Culver and Gert, 1982).

Conceptual issues underlying commitment

Ethical justification. In discussing the ethical justification of commitment, a distinction must be made between whether the commitment is intended primarily to help the person committed or to help others whom the person may be putting at risk (Culver and Gert,

1982; Buchanan and Brock, 1989). This distinction is sometimes not clear-cut, because it is usually to the advantage of mentally ill persons to be prevented from harming others. The harm they might cause would usually be serious and thus constitute a crime. Committing the crime would often be clearly a result of the mental illness—for example, obeying a voice commanding that someone be killed—and it usually is highly likely that the mentally ill offender would be apprehended, incarcerated, and then punished, or at least hospitalized for a long time. Nonetheless, there is a distinction to be made between paternalistic and nonpaternalistic commitments, and there is no doubt that the protection of others is the predominant reason for some commitments.

Paternalistic commitment. To the extent that commitment is intended to help the person committed, it essentially always qualifies as a paternalistic action. That is, the commitment is intended to benefit the person; it violates at least one moral rule (deprivation of freedom) and usually several; it is done without the consent of the person; and the person is at least minimally competent to give consent (Culver and Gert, 1982).

Whether paternalistic commitment is ethically justified, then, depends upon whether a particular commitment meets whatever theoretical criteria for justified paternalism are thought to be adequate. Various sets of criteria, partly overlapping, have been proposed by Tom Beauchamp and James Childress (1989), Allen Buchanan and Dan Brock (1989), Childress (1982), and Charles Culver and Bernard Gert (1982). The criteria depend upon theoretical concepts like the degree of irrationality and voluntariness of the person's behavior. None of these authors seems to believe that, as a species of paternalism, there is anything qualitatively unique about committing the mentally ill. Thus, particular acts of commitment are measured directly against the theoretical criteria of the particular justification procedure proposed.

However, the presence of mental illness does, in the judgment of many authors (Culver and Gert, 1982; Buchanan and Brock, 1989), play an indirect role in the justification of paternalistic commitment by sometimes affecting concepts that these authors believe are centrally important in the justification process. Thus, some suicidal desires may be regarded as not truly expressing an individual's autonomous wishes (Beauchamp and Childress, 1989), or some conditions of mental illness may be thought to affect a person's competence to make decisions (Buchanan and Brock, 1989).

Nonpaternalistic commitment. When commitment is not paternalistic, it must be ethically justified on other grounds. To commit persons to try to prevent their harming others represents a kind of preventive detention, which ordinarily is not legally permitted in the

United States. In the presence of some kinds of mental illness, however, it is argued that nonpaternalistic commitment may be ethically justified. Consider the following example. Two men are separately brought to the emergency room by the police. In each instance the police have been called because the man has just threatened to kill his wife. Each man admits to the emergency room psychiatrist that this is true. The first man has a history of paranoid psychotic episodes and in recent days has heard voices instructing him to kill his wife. The second man has no symptoms nor history of any major mental illness, though he and his wife have a history of chronic marital discord. In both cases the psychiatrist feels there is a reasonably high probability of the man's harming his wife if he returns home.

Based on the fact that in some kinds of mental illness, persons are not held responsible for their actions, it may be argued that it is ethically justified to commit the first man but not the second. The second man, for example, presumably has the volitional ability to will or to refrain from willing to harm his wife, while the first man may not have the volitional ability to will not to harm her (Culver and Gert, 1982). Dangerous, mentally ill persons are sometimes not considered capable of guiding their behavior by promulgated social rules (Brock, 1980).

Predicting possible future harm. Civil commitment always involves a doctor's appraising a person's physical and mental status and deciding whether commitment seems warranted. Sometimes persons may be committed because they are currently in such a disabled condition that even more serious future harm seems all but inevitable. A man may, for example, be continuously hallucinating, unresponsive to the questions or actions of others, and significantly malnourished because of a lack of interest in food. Much more often, however, serious future harm is only a possibility: For example, the person has threatened suicide or is hearing voices urging her to harm someone, and the physician must try to predict how likely it is that the harm will occur.

The process of predicting possible future harm in the commitment setting has the following components (Grisso, 1991): The *criterion* is what is being predicted (for example, the person's suicide); the *cues* are discrete pieces of available information about a particular case (for example, the person's age, sex, state of intoxication, and history of impulsivity); and the *judgment* is the physician's conclusion after assessing the case (for example, to commit or not to commit). These are three separate elements. Empirical research can be and has been done that separately focuses on the correlations among them. The *judgment–criterion* correlation shows how well physicians do in predicting that particular persons will kill themselves. The *cues–criterion* correlation shows the extent to which persons' suicides can be pre-

dicted from whatever facts about cases can be isolated and measured independently of physicians' judgments. Finally, the *cues–judgment* correlation shows which data about cases do in fact lead physicians to make one judgment or another.

One critically important issue, with respect to prediction, is the extent to which commitment does in fact prevent future serious harm. There are few data addressing this issue. If we knew, for example, that 90 percent of the persons committed would have seriously harmed themselves or others had they not been committed, most people would probably feel that commitment was ethically justified. Committing one hundred persons would avoid ninety instances of serious harm, albeit at the "cost" of committing ten persons who would not have caused harm if not committed. By contrast, if only one in one hundred persons would have harmed themselves or others, few would feel commitment justified that ninety-nine persons should suffer the evils of detainment in order to prevent one bad future outcome.

This kind of utilitarian calculus seems central to most writers who discuss the ethical justifiability of commitment. Commitment always inflicts significant harms, but only sometimes does it prevent significant harms. Almost everyone acknowledges that even among those at relatively high risk of causing harm—for example, suicidal persons brought to an emergency room—only a small minority would, if left alone, subsequently harm themselves. The emergency room physician thus faces a difficult task. To commit every person would be to commit too many, but which persons should be committed? Certain characteristics of persons (cues) are known to increase the likelihood of future harmful acts (for example, a history of impulsive or suicidal behavior, being inebriated, having access to lethal weapons, being male), but the physician must make a binary, yes–no decision about commitment, not a probability estimate.

Research (Monahan, 1984) suggests that physicians are poor predictors of whether later harmful behavior will occur (that is, *judgment–criterion* correlations). There is reason to believe that basing predictions on discrete, measurable pieces of information about a case (*cues–criterion* correlations) might yield greater accuracy (Monahan, 1984). There is, however, probably an upper limit to predictive accuracy: Whether a person commits a harmful act in the hours or days after a physician's assessment may depend at least as much on later fortuitous situational factors (for example, whether a friend returns a telephone call) as on factors that can be measured during the assessment.

An important statistical feature of prediction plays a key role in understanding the commitment process. When predicting relatively rare events (for example, the occurrence of a future suicide) with the use of predictive signs of relatively low accuracy (for example, a physician's judgment, or whether a person has access to a lethal weapon), one will inevitably make a high proportion of false positive predictions; that is, one will frequently predict future harm when in fact none will occur. This actuarial problem, described by Paul Meehl and Albert Rosen (1955), was later applied to the issue of commitment by Joseph Livermore, Carl Malmquist, and Paul Meehl (1968).

Suppose that 10 percent of suicidal persons who are brought to an emergency room, but are unwilling to be hospitalized, would kill or seriously harm themselves if not committed. Suppose further that by collecting all available information, physicians can make predictions that are 70 percent accurate; that is, of those persons who would truly kill themselves unless committed, 70 percent are correctly identified and 30 percent are missed, and of those who would not kill themselves, 70 percent are correctly labeled and 30 percent are missed. Therefore, the physician will commit and thus "save" seven of the ten persons destined for suicide, but also commit twenty-seven persons (30 percent of ninety) who would not have killed themselves. These latter are "false positives."

The ratio between the number of "true positives" (seven) and "false positives" (twenty-seven) shows that nearly four persons would be needlessly committed in order to save one. (These are hypothetical figures. Many would argue that subsequent suicide is rarer than 10 percent in this population and that 70 percent is too high an estimate of predictive accuracy, and thus that the proportion of false positives would be much higher.) Note that the physician would be correct a higher percentage of the time (90 percent) if he or she simply predicted no one would commit suicide, but then none of the ten persons would be saved.

Is it ethically justified to commit four unwilling persons needlessly to save one life? Suppose empirical data existed (they do not) that enabled the construction of actuarial tables correlating the signs and symptoms shown by mentally ill persons in emergency rooms with their subsequent likelihood of harming themselves or others if not committed (cue–criterion correlations). Each person could thus be assigned to a cohort: Some would have a one in five chance of harming themselves or others, others a one in ten chance, one in twenty, one in forty, and so forth. Where should the line be drawn? What is the appropriate trade-off between saving one life and needlessly depriving many persons of their freedom? Reasonable persons might disagree about where the line should be drawn, but this is a matter that could be open to public debate. Psychiatrists probably have no special expertise in deciding where the threshold for commitment should be placed.

Some persons, confronted with the inevitable large numbers of false positive commitments, recall the injunction often cited in connection with the U.S. criminal justice system, "Better that ten guilty persons go free than one innocent person suffer," and conclude that civil commitment is ethically unjustified (Sartorius, 1980). Others, however, while concerned about the "false positive" problem, believe there are sufficient differences between the underlying conceptual justifications of the criminal justice system and the civil commitment system that some number of false positives can be tolerated in the latter (Brock, 1980).

Conclusion

Although debates about involuntary hospitalization are sometimes framed in legal rather than ethical terms, it is important to be clear about the underlying ethical issues. Civil commitment involves incarcerating an unwilling person, who has committed no crime, for days, weeks, or longer. Such a prima facie unethical action requires clear justification in terms of some general moral theory. Current theoretical discussions of commitment emphasize concepts like the degree of irrationality and extent of voluntariness of the person's behavior. In applying theoretical concepts to the process of commitment, it is critical to describe the components of the process clearly and to take into account certain statistical features that are inherent in making predictions about a person's future behavior.

CHARLES M. CULVER

Directly related to this entry are the entries INSTITUTIONALIZATION AND DEINSTITUTIONALIZATION; *and* PATIENTS' RIGHTS, *article on* MENTAL PATIENTS' RIGHTS. *For a further discussion of topics mentioned in this entry, see the entries* COMPETENCE; INFORMED CONSENT, *article on* ISSUES OF CONSENT IN MENTAL-HEALTH CARE; PATERNALISM; *and* SUICIDE. *This entry will find application in the entry* PSYCHIATRY, ABUSES OF. *For a discussion of related ideas, see the entries on* AUTONOMY; FREEDOM AND COERCION; HARM; *and* TRUST. *Other relevant material may be found under the entries* BEHAVIOR CONTROL; MENTAL HEALTH; MENTAL-HEALTH SERVICES; MENTAL-HEALTH THERAPIES; MENTAL ILLNESS; *and* MENTALLY DISABLED AND MENTALLY ILL PERSONS.

Bibliography

AMERICAN BAR ASSOCIATION. 1977. "Legal Issues in State Mental Health Care: Proposals for Change." *Mental Disability Law Reporter* 2, no. 1:57–159.

AMERICAN PSYCHIATRIC ASSOCIATION. 1987. *Diagnostic and Statistical Manual of Mental Disorders: DSM-III-R.* 3d ed., rev. Washington, D.C.: Author.

ARTHUR, LINDSAY G.; HAIMOVITZ, STEPHAN; LOCKWOOD, ROBERT W.; DOOLEY, JEANNE A., and PARRY, JOHN W., eds. 1988. *Involuntary Civil Commitment: A Manual for*

Lawyers and Judges. Washington, D.C.: American Bar Association.

BEAUCHAMP, TOM L., and CHILDRESS, JAMES F. 1989. *Principles of Biomedical Ethics.* 3d ed. New York: Oxford University Press.

BROCK, DAN W. 1980. "Involuntary Civil Commitment: The Moral Issues." In *Mental Illness: Law and Public Policy,* pp. 147–173. Edited by Baruch A. Brody and H. Tristram Engelhardt, Jr. Boston: D. Reidel.

BUCHANAN, ALLEN E., and BROCK, DAN W. 1989. *Deciding for Others: The Ethics of Surrogate Decision Making.* New York: Cambridge University Press.

CHILDRESS, JAMES F. 1982. *Who Should Decide? Paternalism in Health Care.* New York: Oxford University Press.

CHODOFF, PAUL. 1976. "The Case for Involuntary Hospitalization of the Mentally Ill." *American Journal of Psychiatry* 133, no. 5:496–501.

CULVER, CHARLES M. 1991. "Health Care Ethics and Mental Health Law." In *Law and Mental Health: Major Developments and Research Needs,* pp. 25–47. Edited by Saleem A. Shah and Bruce D. Sales. Rockville, Md.: U.S. Department of Health and Human Services.

CULVER, CHARLES M., and GERT, BERNARD. 1982. *Philosophy in Medicine: Conceptual and Ethical Issues in Medicine and Psychiatry.* New York: Oxford University Press.

GRISSO, THOMAS. 1991. "Clinical Assessments for Legal Decision Making: Research Recommendations." In *Law and Mental Health: Major Developments and Research Needs,* pp. 49–80. Edited by Saleem A. Shah and Bruce D. Sales. Rockville, Md.: U.S. Department of Health and Human Services.

HOWELL, TIMOTHY; DIAMOND, RONALD J.; and WIKLER, DANIEL. 1982. "Is There a Case for Voluntary Commitment?" In *Contemporary Issues in Bioethics,* 2d ed., pp. 163–167. Edited by Tom L. Beauchamp and LeRoy Walters. Belmont, Calif.: Wadsworth.

LIVERMORE, JOSEPH M.; MALMQUIST, CARL P.; and MEEHL, PAUL E. 1968. "On the Justifications for Civil Commitment." *University of Pennsylvania Law Review* 117, no. 1:75–96.

MARGOLIS, JOSEPH. 1976. "The Concept of Disease." *Journal of Medicine and Philosophy* 1, no. 3:238–255.

MEEHL, PAUL E., and ROSEN, ALBERT. 1955. "Antecedent Probability and the Efficiency of Psychometric Signs, Patterns, and Cutting Scores." *Psychological Bulletin* 52, no. 3:194–216.

MONAHAN, JOHN. 1984. "The Prediction of Violent Behavior: Toward a Second Generation of Theory and Policy." *American Journal of Psychiatry* 141, no. 1:10–15.

MOORE, MICHAEL S. 1975. "Some Myths About 'Mental Illness.'" *Archives of General Psychiatry* 32, no. 12:1483–1497.

SARTORIUS, ROLF E. 1980. "Paternalistic Grounds for Involuntary Civil Commitment: A Utilitarian Perspective." In *Mental Illness: Law and Public Policy,* pp. 137–145. Edited by Baruch A. Brody and H. Tristram Engelhardt, Jr. Boston: D. Reidel.

SZASZ, THOMAS S. 1970. *Ideology and Insanity: Essays on the Psychiatric Dehumanization of Man.* Garden City, N.Y.: Anchor.

TREFFERT, DAROLD A. 1985. "The Obviously Ill Patient in Need of Treatment: A Fourth Standard for Civil Commitment." *Hospital and Community Psychiatry* 36, no. 3:259–264.

WEXLER, DAVID B. 1978. "Institutionalization." In vol. 2 of *Encyclopedia of Bioethics,* pp. 779–784. Edited by Warren T. Reich. New York: Macmillan.

———. 1981. *Mental Health Law: Major Issues.* New York: Plenum.

COMMUNICATION, BIOMEDICAL

I. Media and Medicine
   Deni Elliott
II. Scientific Publishing
   Richard M. Glass
   Annette Flanagin
III. Media and Bioethics
   Bette-Jane Crigger

I. MEDIA AND MEDICINE

Mass-market media are vital in communicating important medical information to consumers. What the general public understands about medical breakthroughs is attributable to the stories that appear in the lay press. While media and medical practitioners share a common goal of informing the public, there is often serious disagreement between the professions over the quality and focus of the information provided. What follows is a description of the unique role of the media in terms of disseminating medical information and a description of complexities that affect the quality of that dissemination.

Journalists and social function

Media professionals have a distinct function in society: to tell citizens what they need to know so that they can participate as informed members of a self-governing society. The function of advertisers and public relations practitioners is to promote their clients' products or messages, a far different social function that will not be discussed here. The media–medicine relationship described here, instead, rises from the nonadvocate position of the mainstream, mass-market, professional news media.

Unlike the sets of governmental and professional controls to which health-care practitioners must subscribe, there is no regulation of function and little social accountability for newsmedia. News media comprise the only industry in the United States that has constitutional protection. The First Amendment of the U.S.

Constitution guarantees a free and independent press, providing a check on the power of government. Over the years, news media have broadened their watchdog role to include checks on other social institutions, including the health-care industry.

News organizations produce reports that reflect the editors' and reporters' professional judgment of what should be covered and how thoroughly. Social accountability comes into play only at the level of minimalist legal standards. News organizations can be held legally accountable for their actions, but only after the fact, in the narrowly prescribed areas of libel, invasion of privacy, and obscenity. News organizations cannot be held legally accountable for failure to provide information.

Despite the unequaled freedom that news organizations have in determining what they will cover and how they will cover it, they have social responsibilities. Role-related responsibilities for journalists, like other social roles, derive from societal needs, not from rules and regulations. Even in the most primitive cultures, communities need people to care for the health and well-being of individuals, and need information to facilitate the provision of health care. News media are organizations that voluntarily take on the responsibility of providing needed information to the community. Because the United States has a political system that depends on citizen participation, the primary social function of the U.S. news media is to provide citizens with the information that they need for self-governance.

The fact that news media have a social role does not deny that privately owned news organizations operate out of a set of economic motivations. Print news organizations need to sell papers; electronic news media must bring in advertising revenue. However, the economic realities do not negate ethical responsibilities. News media have a moral obligation to meet their role-related responsibilities despite the economic pressures, just as for-profit hospitals have a moral obligation to provide a minimal level of care. News media also play other, less vital roles in the community. There is nothing wrong with news organizations providing advice columns and human interest stories as long as they are also fulfilling their primary function.

The social function of journalism provides a basis for news judgment—the process by which the media choose news stories and create emphases within them—and a criterion for judging the adequacy of medical reporting. News media and medical professionals have a shared goal of getting information to consumers so that they can make informed decisions about their medical care. But conflicts can hinder journalists in their efforts to do their job. Some of these pressures and how they function in the definition and reporting of medical news are detailed in this article.

Generalist and specialty reporters

Traditionally, journalists have been expected to cover important events and issues with the curious, but ignorant, perspective of a representative of the lay audience. A lack of specialized training was considered an advantage in that the reporter could be more sensitive to the needs of the audience. It meant that the journalist would provide information that was accessible to someone who lacked formal training or sophisticated understanding of the field.

More recently, while journalism school is not legally required for someone who wants to become a journalist, the trend is increasingly in that direction. News organizations report that an increasing number of those they hire have formal journalism education. A prominent media analyst has predicted that by the year 2000, virtually all journalists will be the products of formalized journalism education (Merrill, 1974). By the early 1980s, the majority of working journalists in the United States had at least a bachelor's degree. About half of these degrees were degrees in journalism (Weaver and Wilhoit, 1986).

Journalism students leave this formal education with a set of investigative, writing, and editing skills; an understanding of news judgment; and a liberal arts education with a strong humanities component. No particular specialization, such as medicine or science or economics, is required or even encouraged. There are no necessary qualifications by which journalists become medical reporters. The reporter investigating a medical story may lack background, experience, or even interest in the field.

Most journalists are generalists and, representative of their audiences, may be just as dependent upon expert interpretation as the most naive reader. Although scientists and health-care practitioners have at times been frustrated by the banality of generalist reporter questions, they have also commanded instant (and sometimes undeserved) respect and trust from these reporters. As a result, journalists may not recognize the pressures and interests that can drive medical sources to be self-serving. Lack of a science background may cause a journalist's reporting to be biased rather than balanced. The primary medical and science sources continue to be the American Medical Association and the American Association of the Advancement of Science, both of which exist to promote the interests of their memberships.

Both the growing complexity of some reporting areas such as medicine, economics, and the environment as well as the fear of manipulation by self-interested sources have resulted in the appearance of specialized journalists. Instead of reader representatives, these journalists are teachers, interpreters, and experts who use their knowledge of the field to create meaning for the lay audience. In the early 1990s as many as 26 percent of the 3,800 members of the American Medical Writers Association had some specialized training in medicine or in medical research at the doctoral level (personal communication, AMWA, Dec. 1992). Through conferences, publications, and networking, professional organizations like this one reflect the increasing sophistication of specialty writers.

Specialty reporters face a danger, however, of becoming advocates for the specialties that they cover, thereby losing objectivity. Medical research reporters believe in the promise of medical breakthroughs; science and technology reporters sometimes start with the assumptions that technology is progress and that announced findings equal new knowledge. Specialty reporters are also more likely to become aligned with mainstream rather than alternative medicine. The audience can thus suffer by receiving noncritical presentations of medical care and research.

Despite these problems, the increasing complexity of medical stories has also made a positive change in traditional journalistic methods. For example, journalists have traditionally shunned the notion of "readbacks," the practice of reading back to a source information as it is planned to appear in the story. The reporter's concern that a source would take back a quote has given way, among reporters who specialize in complex fields, to a commitment to making sure that complicated or technical material is accurate.

Specialist reporting, however, is a luxury that few news organizations can afford. Specialty reporters are generally found at the networks, large market broadcast stations, and newspapers with large circulation. Editors of smaller news organizations turn to national wire services to fulfill their reporting needs in these areas. With little local specialty coverage, readers or viewers get little medical news tailored toward their specific community.

Formula stories

Journalists as well as their audiences rely on certain formulas in news stories. Readers or viewers find it easier to follow a news article or to take in information from a ninety-second broadcast news story if they know what to expect from its structure. Within seconds, the audience can recognize a conflict story, a portrait of a famous person, hero, or villain, or a story explaining an important issue. Structure helps readers and viewers put the story into context that, in turn, helps them create meaning. A similar perception pattern is followed by journalists confronting information to present as news.

Sometimes, however, journalists formulize a story without realizing that the larger point has been lost.

Stories focusing on the drama of human illness or on the thrill of technological discovery are cases in point. Many newsrooms run stories about patients—often children—who need treatment such as transplant or gene therapy, stories likely to be interesting to the general population. The audience can then participate in the life-and-death drama as the search for the needed donor or funds races against the patient's deteriorating medical condition.

These dramas rarely provide space and time for careful interviews in which policymakers can explain how funding for only a small number of bone marrow transplants may deplete resources that would provide years of childhood care for several hundred others, or why Medicaid or insurance funds are chronically limited. Instead, the audience is usually offered tearful interviews with parents, who thank the community for pitching in to help.

Because the story fits into a predictable journalistic formula—person in need is rescued (or dies)—the journalist may simply miss the policy aspects of the story. However, it is in telling these policy aspects that citizens become informed members of a self-governing society. What citizens need to know about transplantation is not the private story of the one photogenic person with an interesting disease who was lucky enough to get news coverage on a "slow" news day. To make informed decisions about health care, citizens need to know how transplantation works, about the likelihood of various procedures becoming standards of care, about the accessibility of the procedure, about the funding of the procedure, and about participating in decisions on how public-health dollars are spent.

Another formula story is the "wonders of technology" story of discovery. Such stories begin with the assumptions that new knowledge is good knowledge and that new knowledge carries a moral requirement to act. There are two recognizable elements of this story: wonderful new knowledge and how people should change to accommodate it. For example, the "wonders of technology" story presents prenatal screening and diagnostic testing as a way to ensure perfect babies. News stories that concentrate on the glorification of new knowledge rarely mention the uncertainty of the information provided or the fact that the most certain types of information arise in the context of many other unknowable fetal traits. The new technology stories relating to genetic testing, for instance, rarely note that the only cure for genetic anomaly is termination of a pregnancy. Reporters sometimes miss the moral dilemmas that prospective parents face in confronting prenatal information. The cost of prenatal screening and the resultant cost of making fetal diagnosis is another topic not usually discussed when genetic testing is the subject of a technology story.

Only with some stories about xenografting—the practice of grafting tissue from a donor of one species to a recipient of a different species—do reporters routinely ask if this practice is really a good idea. Even here, reporters rarely provide full context for the discussion, responding usually only to an assumption that some part of the lay audience would question using primate organs to save dying humans. Such stories rarely remind readers that porcine heart valves and other xenografts are commonly used in human patients.

The number of Americans who lack medical insurance has not changed substantially between the mid-1980s and the mid-1990s. Nor have the problems caused to individuals or the community changed. But the problem of under- or uninsured Americans did not become "a story" for many news organizations until it was made an issue by candidates in political campaigns of the early 1990s. The story of how industry supports and shapes scientific and medical research is still not a story that often hits the news columns nor is the connection between scientific progress and financial gain for the medical researcher who owns a biotechnology firm or for one who secures a patent. Journalists blame their lack of financial resources to pursue such complicated multifaceted stories, but business backgrounds are as rare for journalists as are science backgrounds. In addition, these are not the stories that are volunteered by traditional medical sources.

Language and presentation

News media help shape consumers' opinions about medical care and medical research with their choice of language and their style of presentation. If the media are confused or inaccurate, the public will magnify that confusion and inaccuracy in their own misunderstandings or prejudices. The coverage of the acquired immunodeficiency syndrome (AIDS), which matured through the 1980s, provides a good example. Early media coverage included references to "high-risk groups" (rather than high-risk behavior). Journalists talked about "bodily fluids" without clarifying that this meant blood but not sweat, semen but not saliva. Media helped perpetuate an "us/them" atmosphere by dividing people with AIDS into the victims (who had done something wrong in the process of contracting the disease) and the redundant "innocent victims" (who had not).

Media participated in the isolation of people living with AIDS by identifying those who were known to be HIV-positive with the justification of "protecting the community." For example, editors justified the identification of a pediatrician who was found to be HIV-posi-

tive with the argument that referring only to a "local pediatrician," without identifying the individual, would put other physicians under suspicion. During the 1980s, newsmedia also participated in giving citizens a false sense of security by implying that someone who was HIV-positive but not symptomatic was also not infectious.

Another example of problematic media presentation and language involves the presentation of people with disabilities, which continues to reflect a medical model of disability as malady at a time when people with disabilities are making claims for their normalcy and rights to equal access in society. News stories that celebrate the accomplishments of normal tasks by people with disabilities work from the medical description of disability as individual deficiency rather than disability as social construct that classifies only those without a handicap as normal.

Issues of confidentiality and privacy

Medical and media professionals have differing concepts of confidentiality and privacy. Despite the intrusion of insurance companies, managed-care systems, and easily accessible data bases, medical professionals assume the confidential nature of any physician–patient relationship. Journalists, however, believe that the circle of valid privacy claims shrinks in direct proportion to the importance or popularity of the individual.

The health problems of public officials and celebrities are considered fair game for news stories. Reporting the health problems of public officials is connected to the role-related responsibilities of newsmedia on the basis that citizens have a legitimate interest in knowing anything that might affect the performance of an elected official or one who makes decisions of importance in a democratic society. Reporting the health problems of celebrities rarely has such connection.

But, medical personnel are at least partly responsible for creating an atmosphere in which journalists think they have a right to private medical details. Medical personnel generate news stories. Research centers benefit by attracting funds and patients when experimental patients are willing to give testimonials to their treatment. Transplant center financial service representatives and information service officers coach patients and their families on how to attract media coverage so that they can solicit community help when transplant candidates lack necessary funds.

Journalists are not likely to share the medical perspective that sometimes it is acceptable to tell patients' stories and sometimes it is not. Journalists see themselves as separate from the interests of the medical community and even from the patients. No matter how good the cause the medical community hopes to promote, once the story is in the hands of the journalists, they, not the medical personnel or patient, have control over how information is used. Once a patient consents to giving up confidentiality and privacy for the purposes of public disclosure, it is difficult to get it back.

Medicine sells itself

Journalists are producing news stories in a context in which some medical researchers and medical journals are working hard at self-promotion. This is complicated because journalists, particularly generalist reporters, may come to medical reporting with the assumption that anyone in a white coat is an "expert" and that medical researchers are releasing information only with the interest of providing needed medical information to consumers. But medical researchers, health-care practitioners, and even medical journals sometimes have other agendas.

The *Journal of the American Medical Association* (JAMA), for example, changed its publication date so that, as of 1990, it was published a day before its competitor, the *New England Journal of Medicine*, rather than trailing it by a day. JAMA's editor explained that it was "nicer to be first" (Scott, 1990).

The time lag between important clinical discovery and actual publication creates pressure for researchers to enlist the lay press. The peer-review system provides an important check on the accuracy of scientific claims, but patients can die waiting for such information to filter through the screens and into the hands of general practitioners. In addition, funds for research result from the researcher's good work and from the researcher's willingness to talk about the importance of the research to the medical concerns of the public (Nelkin, 1987; Martin, 1990; Cohen and Peter, 1988). These pressures on the medical community can lead to hyped stories in the media. Sophisticated medical reporters are needed to understand the complex field that they attempt to explain to the public.

DENI ELLIOTT

Directly related to this article are the other articles in this entry: SCIENTIFIC PUBLISHING, *and* MEDIA AND BIOETHICS. *For a further discussion of topics mentioned in this article, see the entries* ADVERTISING; CONFIDENTIALITY; NARRATIVE; *and* PRIVACY IN HEALTH CARE. *For a discussion of related ideas, see the entries* INTERPRETATION; *and* VALUE AND VALUATION. *Other relevant material may be found under the entries* HEALTH OFFICIALS AND THEIR RESPONSIBILITIES; HEALTH POLICY; *and* HEALTH PROMOTION AND HEALTH EDUCATION.

Bibliography

BURNHAM, JOHN C. 1987. *How Superstition Won and Science Lost: Popularizing Science and Health in the United States.* New Brunswick, N.J.: Rutgers University Press.

COHEN, LYNNE, and MORGAN, PETER P. 1988. "Medical Dramas and the Press: Who Benefits from the Coverage?" *Canadian Medical Association Journal* 139, no. 7:657–661.

COHN, VICTOR. 1989. *News and Numbers: A Guide to Reporting Statistical Claims and Controversies in Health and Other Fields.* Ames: Iowa State University Press.

———. 1992. "Science and Medicine: Corrective Surgery." *Quill* 80, no. 9:17–18.

CONQUEST, WENDY; DRAKE, BOB; and ELLIOTT, DENI. 1993. *The Burden of Knowledge: Moral Dilemmas in Prenatal Testing.* Videodocumentary. Hanover, N.H.: Duma Productions.

CREWSDON, JOHN. 1993. "Perky Cheerleaders: By Accepting Research Reports Without Adequate Checking Science Writers Do a Disservice to the Public." *Nieman Reports* 47, no. 4:11–16.

ELLIOTT, DENI. 1989. "Media and Persons with Disabilities: Ethical Considerations." In *Reporting on Disability: Approaches and Issues: A Sourcebook.* Edited by Mary Johnson and Susan Elkins. Louisville, Ky.: Avocado Press.

———. 1991. "A Case of Need: Media Coverage of Organ Transplants." In *Risky Business: Communicating Issues of Science, Risk and Public Policy,* pp. 151–158. Edited by Lee Wilkins and Philip Patterson. New York: Greenwood.

ELLIOTT, DENI; CONQUEST, WENDY; and DRAKE, BOB. 1991. *Buying Time: The Media Role in Healthcare.* Videodocumentary. Hanover, N.H.: Duma.

HEUSSNER, RALPH, and SALMON, MARLA E. 1988. *Warning: The Media May Be Harmful to Your Health! A Consumer's Guide to Medical News and Advertising.* Kansas City, Mo.: Andrews and McMeel.

KEMP, SID. 1993. "The Case for Reporting on Medical Alternatives." *Nieman Reports* 47, no. 4:40–43.

KINSELLA, JAMES. 1989. *Covering the Plague: AIDS and the American Media.* New Brunswick, N.J.: Rutgers University Press.

KLAIDMAN, STEPHEN. 1991. *Health in the Headlines: The Stories Behind the Stories.* New York: Oxford University Press.

MARTIN, ROBERT G. 1990. "Scientific Hype." *New Biologist* 2, no. 9:747–749.

MERRILL, JOHN. 1974. *The Imperative of Freedom: A Philosophy of Journalistic Autonomy.* New York: Hastings House.

MEYERS, BOB. 1993. "Tsunami, Wavelets and Medical News: Journalists and Experts, Riding in Different Boats, Fail to Communicate with Each Other." *Nieman Reports* 47, no. 4:8–10.

MOORE, MICHAEL, ed. 1989. *Health Risks and the Press: Perspectives on Media Coverage of Risk Assessment and Health.* Washington, D.C.: Media Institute.

NELKIN, DOROTHY. 1987. *Selling Science: How the Press Covers Science and Technology.* New York: W. H. Freeman.

SCOTT, JANNY. 1990. "Medical Journals: Eye on the Scoop." *Los Angeles Times,* February 26, p. A24.

SIGNORIELLI, NANCY. 1993. *Mass Media Images and Impact on Health: A Sourcebook.* Westport, Conn.: Greenwood.

Steinbrook, Robert, and Lo, Bernard. 1990. "Informing Physicians About Promising New Treatments for Severe Illnesses." *Journal of the American Medical Association* 263, no. 15:2078–2082.

Weaver, David H. and Wilhoit, G. Cleveland. 1986. *The American Journalist: A Portrait of U.S. News People and Their Work:* Bloomington: Indiana University Press.

II. SCIENTIFIC PUBLISHING

During the late 1970s and the 1980s, an ethics of scientific publication began to evolve. Competition among scientists for academic rewards and research funds, the continued fragmentation and commercialization of science, and reports of scientific misconduct, as well as increasing governmental and legal interference with the inner workings of the scientific community led many within that community to perceive a need for reforms to guide both the conduct of science and the dissemination of scientific information. Journal editors, universities, professional associations, funding agencies, and governments have taken active roles in debating and setting ethical standards and editorial policies for the dissemination of scientific information. In 1978, a self-appointed group of editors, the International Committee of Medical Journal Editors (ICMJE), representing leading general medical journals, met in Vancouver, British Columbia, to set technical guidelines for the submission of manuscripts. These guidelines, the Uniform Requirements for the Submission of Manuscripts to Biomedical Journals, have evolved to include statements for the ethical conduct of authors, editors, and peer reviewers. While the ICMJE statements set international standards for biomedical publishing, the number of journals that adhere to them is unknown (ICMJE, 1991, 1993b). This article presents an overview of the major ethical issues in biomedical and scientific publishing.

Editorial and peer review

The prestige and influence of biomedical journal publication are closely related to the quality control and selection process that precedes publication. Thus, the essential tasks of medical editing are the selection and improvement of articles submitted for publication. These tasks are generally accomplished through processes of editorial review (evaluation by the journal's editorial staff) and peer review (evaluation by experts in a given field who are considered the authors' "peers"). These two processes may overlap, particularly when an editor is also an expert in a manuscript's topic, but editorial review usually focuses on the appropriateness, clarity, and priority of articles for the journal's readership. Peer reviewers are selected by the editor to assess the quality of an article's scientific and technical content and to offer advice about publication. Since decisions regarding rejection, revision, or acceptance are made solely by the editor, the term "referee" exaggerates a reviewer's advisory role and should be avoided.

Peer review was first used for biomedical publications by the Royal Societies of London and Edinburgh in the eighteenth century, but evolved haphazardly; it was not employed regularly until after World War II (Lock, 1986). Two striking aspects of peer review are that it is based almost entirely on uncompensated, voluntary labor and that the peer review system itself has only recently come under scientific scrutiny (Lock, 1986; "Guarding the Guardians," 1990; Rennie and Flanagin, 1994b).

Journals follow differing policies about revealing reviewers' identities to authors and authors' identities to reviewers (Lock, 1986; "Guarding the Guardians," 1990; Rennie and Flanagin, 1994b). Some editors believe that disclosure of reviewer identities to authors decreases the potential for bias, while others believe such disclosure leads to less critical reviews. Many biomedical journals do not attempt to remove the identities of authors or their institutions from submitted manuscripts; studies have shown that author identities may be discerned by reviewers from the paper's content or from bibliographic citations, especially in narrow subspecialties (Lock, 1986). On the other hand, these same journals do not reveal the identities of peer reviewers to authors. While most editors are impressed by the care and objectivity usually reflected in reviewer comments and recommendations, the anonymous review of papers whose authors are known obviously involves potential for abuse. To maintain integrity in the peer review process, reviewers are expected to disclose any conflicts of interest involved in their review, and editors are expected to be alert to any signs of bias that may interfere with an objective evaluation of the merits of the paper.

Maintaining the confidentiality of an author's work before publication is an important ethical principle in scientific publishing. Most journals inform peer reviewers that the information in unpublished manuscripts is privileged and should be kept confidential, and also require manuscripts to be either returned to the editorial office or destroyed after review. However, maintaining confidentiality depends on an honesty among editors, authors, and reviewers that is nearly impossible to guarantee. Conscious or unconscious intellectual theft by peer reviewers may occur but cannot be measured. Journal editors have a particular responsibility to maintain strict confidentiality about the peer review process, editorial decisions, and all manuscript submissions.

How well do the processes of editorial and peer review work? Many persons involved in publishing recognize the improved quality of articles that have been revised after review, and this has been clearly demonstrated with regard to improvements of study designs and statistical methods ("Guarding the Guardians," 1990; Rennie and Flanagin, 1994b). Nevertheless, both editorial and peer review are based on human judgments that carry the potential for bias and error.

One form of publication bias is the tendency for papers with statistically significant "positive" results (for example, those showing that a new treatment works better) to be published in favor of papers with statistically nonsignificant "negative" results (for example, those showing that a new treatment does not have any effect or does not work any better than other treatments). Studies have shown that such publication bias exists, but its extent is unknown and controversial ("Guarding the Guardians," 1990; Rennie and Flanagin, 1992, 1994b). Prepublication bias (the tendency of authors not to submit negative results for publication because the findings are incomplete or nonsignificant or because funding runs out) and postpublication bias (bias in the reception and interpretation of published research data by researchers, funding agencies, editors, and the media) may be more substantial problems. All of these forms of bias can lead to inappropriate medical policies and treatment decisions, especially with new or controversial therapies. Hence, the evaluation of scientific results should be based on their quality and importance, not on their direction.

Authorship

Despite the fact that university promotion committees evince some shift in the emphasis from the quantity to the quality of publication, academic pressures to publish remain. In many academic circles, achievement is still measured by the length of an individual's bibliography. As a result, authorship of an article published in a peer-reviewed scientific journal carries considerable merit, and consequently, considerable responsibility (Rennie and Flanagin, 1994a).

During the past several decades, the meaning of authorship has become diluted as the number of names appearing in scientific article bylines has grown. Authors have justified lengthy bylines by the increasing specialization of science and the need for collaboration among many subspecialists. But the once-accepted practices of adding the names of a department chair or laboratory chief to the end of bylines (guest authorship), and hiring someone to write up a paper without credit (ghost authorship), have caused many editors to adopt formal policies to curtail inflated bylines (Huth, 1986a, 1986b; Lundberg and Flanagin, 1989; Rennie and Flanagin, 1994a) and limit the number of names that can appear in a byline without formal justification.

In 1985, the ICMJE recommended that only those persons who have participated sufficiently to take public responsibility for the work should be authors and that "authorship credit should be based solely on substantial contributions to (a) conception and design, or analysis and interpretation of data; (b) drafting the article or revising it critically for important intellectual content; and (c) final approval of the version to be published" (ICMJE, 1991). Each of these criteria must be met by each person listed in the byline, and the authors must state that they meet these criteria in the cover letter accompanying each submitted manuscript. In the latter half of the 1980s, a number of medical journals, including the *Annals of Internal Medicine* and the *Journal of the American Medical Association* (JAMA), began requiring authors to sign authorship statements based on the ICMJE criteria. Anyone who does not meet these conditions but has contributed or assisted significantly can be recognized in an acknowledgment within the article, if he or she has given written permission to be so named (ICMJE, 1993b).

Group authorship results when investigators from many different institutions or participants in study groups, consensus conferences, or working groups prepare reports of their works. Frequently these groups comprise hundreds of investigators, technicians, and specialists. While it is conceivable that each of these individuals contributed critical time and information to the overall work, it is unlikely that each meets the ICMJE authorship criteria. In these cases, those participants who do meet the authorship criteria can be listed with the name of the study group in the byline. Those participants who do not qualify for authorship are then listed in a group box or in an acknowledgment. If all of the participants do meet the criteria for authorship, then the group name can be listed as the sole byline, with the individuals composing the group named in a separate box or the acknowledgment.

Unlike the definition of authorship, there are no established standards for order of authorship, although a number have been proposed, ranging from alphabetical listings to mathematical formulas for determining individual contribution levels and ranking. Many editors agree that authors should be listed according to how much they contributed, with the author who contributed the most listed first and the author who contributed least listed last (Huth, 1986a, 1986b; Riesenberg and Lundberg, 1990). In addition, a number of publications and indexes limit the number of names to be published in a reference list to three, six, or ten. But there is still no consensus on the order of authorship, mostly because there are no widely accepted objective measures of individual coauthors' contribution levels. Editors recommend that authors determine the order of authorship before writing their papers, or before beginning their study, with an agreement to reevaluate the order later if necessary. Editors also recommend that authors solve disagreements over order among themselves, since the authors are in the best position to determine levels of contribution (Riesenberg and Lundberg, 1990; ICMJE, 1991).

Duplicate publication

Another result of the pressures to publish and a driving force behind the need for ethical standards in scientific publication is the practice of duplicate publication. Also known as multiple, dual, or redundant publication, duplicate publication is the simultaneous or subsequent publication of the same article or major parts of an article—methods, results and data, discussion, conclusions, and graphic or illustrative material—in two or more journals or other media, including electronic journals and databases, without notifying the editors (Huth, 1986a, 1986b; ICMJE, 1993b; Iverson et al., 1989). The types of duplicate publication range from self-plagiarism (publishing two or more identical articles or large parts of an article in different journals without citing each article in the texts and references lists) to "salami slicing" (dividing up different parts of the same study for publication in different journals) to sequential publication (reporting follow-up of the same study with additional subjects but without new results). Word-for-word duplication is uncommon, as duplicators usually attempt to alter or disguise the similarities.

Duplicate publication should be distinguished from secondary publication, in which an article or abbreviated version is subsequently republished, in the same or another language, with the consent of both editors. The secondary article should include a footnote on the title page, informing all readers that the information was published previously, and a complete citation to the primary article. Duplicate publication may violate copyright law, and it is unethical for an author to submit duplicate papers to different journals without notifying the editors. By doing so, authors clutter the literature with redundant information; waste the valuable time and resources of editors, reviewers, and readers; and prevent other authors from publishing their work because of limited journal space. To discourage such practices, many scientific journals state in their instructions for authors that they will only consider papers that have not been previously published or submitted to other journals, and some journals will publish notices of duplicate publication, publicly admonishing those authors who publish duplicate articles in violation of the journal's written policies (Iverson et al., 1989).

Conflicts of interest

Reflecting the increasing commercialization of science and the public doubts about researchers' once hallowed and rarely questioned integrity, financial conflicts of interest are now recognized as another ethical problem for authors and editors. During the 1980s, the public's trust of the scientific community diminished as a result of a number of public scandals and government investigations of biomedical researchers' ties to drugs with potential public health benefits and high financial rewards for stockholders and manufacturers (Relman, 1984; Lundberg and Flanagin, 1989; U.S. Congress, 1990). These cases have generally involved researchers being biased by their direct but undisclosed financial interests, such as stock ownership and paid consultancies. However, there are several other potential sources of author bias: funds from granting agencies, any research or material support, employment, money paid for expert testimony, and honoraria paid for public speaking.

Recognizing that not all financial interests will bias an author, editors disagree over how to handle these financial interests. Most journals publish an author's source of funding or material support, but that is usually because the funding institution requires that it be published. Some journals require authors to disclose all financial interests relevant to the work reported in their submitted manuscripts. If a manuscript is subsequently accepted for publication, the editors of these journals will determine whether it is necessary to publish such financial interests. In this manner, readers can judge for themselves the author's potential for bias from a financial interest just as they can judge an author's potential for intellectual bias based on his or her previously published works or specialty status (Rennie et al., 1991). In 1990, the *New England Journal of Medicine* instituted a stringent policy prohibiting anyone with relevant financial interests from publishing editorials or review articles in that journal. Critics have argued that such prohibition is scientific censorship.

In 1989, the American Federation for Clinical Research and the Association of American Medical Colleges recommended full disclosure of all relevant financial interests and the possible divestiture of any stock or equity in a company that makes a product the researcher is studying (U.S. Congress, 1990). The Editorial Policy Committee of the Council of Biology Editors (CBE) recommends that authors disclose all relevant financial interests to the editors at the time of manuscript submission, and that editors disclose authors' financial interests to reviewers and readers when appropriate (CBE, 1990). There is no consensus among editors for the need and extent of such disclosure. In 1993, however, the ICMJE approved a statement that all participants in the peer review and publication process disclose any conflicting interests (ICMJE, 1993a). Some journals with disclosure policies have applied the basic principles of disclosure to everyone in the editorial process, including editors, editorial board members, and in some cases, reviewers (Relman, 1984; Rennie et al., 1991).

Fraudulent publication resulting from scientific misconduct

The publication of a fraudulent article remains the most serious transgression of the ethics of scientific publication. The once generally accepted view that scientific misconduct was rare and committed by a few deviants has been replaced by a view, unsubstantiated, that it is more common and can involve respected scientists from leading institutions. Scientific misconduct has been defined as plagiarism (presenting another's ideas without attribution), fabrication (presenting data or facts that do not exist), falsification (changing or selecting certain data to obtain a desired result, misrepresenting evidence or facts, or misrepresenting authorship), or other serious deviations from accepted practice in the proposing, conducting, or reporting of research (U.S. Department of Health and Human Services, 1990). Policy makers have disagreed over the merits of including the phrase "deviations from accepted practice" in the definition. Some argue that the phrase is too vague and thus open to misinterpretation and overuse (Committee on Science, 1992–); others argue that it must be included to address misconduct that would not technically be considered plagiarism, fabrication, or falsification. Examples of such deviations include misuse or theft of privileged information by a reviewer or editor, submitting a paper listing several coauthors who are unaware that they are named as coauthors, misrepresenting publication status of articles in a bibliography, or failing to perform funded research while filing reports stating that such work has been done (U.S. Department of Health and Human Services, 1991).

Variations in the definition of fraud have caused some confusion, but most editors acknowledge a major difference between fraud and unintentional errors. Although unprofessional and in some cases unethical, the following usually are not considered fraudulent: errors in study design or application of methods, inappropriate use or interpretation of statistics, faulty interpretation or overgeneralization of study results, failure to cite relevant literature or studies, duplicate publication or fragmentary reporting of results, prepublication release of information, publication bias, failure to disclose intellectual or financial conflicts of interests, or violations of experimentation rules protecting humans or animals.

Plagiarism is probably more commonly acknowledged, since it is easier to detect and prove. Detecting and proving falsification or fabrication of data in a published article is not so easy, and it carries grave ethical and legal consequences for editors, authors, institutions, and funding agencies. While an editor has a duty to see that questions of fraud are appropriately and confidentially pursued, the Association of American Medical Colleges, the National Academy of Sciences, and the

ICMJE recommend that primary responsibility for investigating cases of suspected fraud rests with the author's institution or funding agency (Association of American Medical Colleges, 1992; Committee on Science, 1992–; ICMJE, 1991). If it is determined that a fraudulent paper has been published, the journal should print—in a timely manner—a retraction, written by the author(s) or an appropriate representative of the institution. Since the validity of any previous work by the author of a fraudulent paper cannot be assumed, the editor must ask the institution to verify the validity of any of the author's articles previously published in the journal or to retract them (ICMJE, 1991).

Protecting patient rights

The two major issues regarding patient rights in medical publishing are requirements for the ethical conduct of published research and the protection of patient confidentiality. A now well-established principle followed by all credible medical journals is that reports of experimental investigations of human or animal subjects must include a statement that the research project has been approved by an appropriate institutional review board (IRB). For investigators not covered by a formal ethics review board, the report should state that the researchers have followed the principles of the Declaration of Helsinki (World Medical Association, 1990), which includes requirements for freely given informed consent and for the review of the research protocol by a committee independent of the investigator and the sponsor. Many journals also require an additional statement of the manner in which informed consent was obtained from human subjects, since informed consent is a central tenet for ethical research.

Many editors now agree that journal publication should protect patient confidentiality. For example, placing a black bar over the eyes in a facial photograph does not effectively disguise identity. Patients may also be identified from detailed case descriptions. In 1991, the ICMJE published expanded guidelines for the protection of patients' right to anonymity (ICMJE, 1991). These guidelines state that identifying information should be avoided unless it is essential for scientific purposes; informed consent should be obtained for the publication of identifying descriptions or photographs; changing patient data should not be used as a way of securing anonymity; and journals should publish editorial policies to preserve patient confidentiality (ICMJE, 1991).

One problematic area regarding patient anonymity is the publication of pedigrees from genetics research, since the family as a whole or individual family members can sometimes be identified from pedigree information. Following the ICMJE guidelines, identifying information should be deleted if possible, but pedigree data should not be altered. Pedigree publication is complicated by the fact that a large number of family members may be involved, not all of whom may have given consent for, or even be aware of, the collection of family data. A requirement for informed consent for publication from each individual member of a large pedigree may be impossible to meet, particularly if family members disagree about publication. Whether some kind of group consent would be ethically permissible, or whether identifiable pedigrees should not be published without the consent of each individual family member, remains an unsettled issue.

Release of information

Scientific journals play a major role in informing the public, as well as health professionals, about biomedical developments. This function involves a balance between the timely release of information and the adequate evaluation of the quality of the information. Conflicts sometimes occur between scientists, who want rapid dissemination of new or controversial research findings; editors, who as gatekeepers want to make sure that only accurate and valid scientific information is released; and the news media, which compete with each other to be the first to publicize new scientific information. The process of scientific publication after peer review takes time. Some investigators have chosen to short-circuit this traditional process by announcing results at a news conference rather than waiting for a paper to be evaluated by a scientific journal. Advocates for a particular disease (acquired immunodeficiency syndrome [AIDS], for example) have also pressed for faster release of research results. Even if well-intended, such attempts to bypass careful evaluation and publication may result in the dissemination of misinformation (Angell and Kassirer, 1991).

In 1969, Franz Ingelfinger, then editor of the *New England Journal of Medicine*, promulgated a policy (subsequently known as the "Ingelfinger rule") that manuscripts would be considered for publication only if their substance had not been submitted or reported elsewhere. Other journals adopted similar policies to discourage both duplicate publication and the public dissemination of results before peer review and publication. Such policies have been criticized as self-serving on the part of journals, but they usually exempt presentations at scientific meetings (including published abstracts and media coverage from such meetings) and the rare situations when an appropriate public health authority determines that there is an immediate need for dissemination. Some medical journals also ask news media to observe a press embargo for a brief period to allow physician subscribers to read and evaluate information before their patients begin seeing it in the media.

Copyright

Copyright protection covers text and illustrative material—whether in print or electronic (digital) format. U.S. copyright law provides that the creator of a written work, the author, owns all legal rights to that work for his or her life span plus fifty years, unless the author transfers those rights to another party. Two exceptions to individual copyright ownership are works prepared by employees of the U.S. government and works made for hire, in which an individual, either by an employment mandate or by contract, agrees in writing that all work prepared within the scope of employment or contract is the property of the employer or contractor (*Copyright Law of the United States of America*, 1993). Different countries have different copyright laws, but the Universal Copyright and Berne Conventions protect works published and distributed in other countries.

Most journals require authors to transfer copyright to their publishers before publication, giving the publisher exclusive rights to the work after publication. Therefore, anyone who wishes to reprint or adapt from an article (in part or whole) must receive written permission to do so from the publisher. However, certain uses of a published work without permission from the owner—such as photocopying for teaching, scholarship, or research purposes—may not be an infringement of copyright under the provisions of "fair use." Fair use can be difficult to justify in court and must take into account the following factors: (1) the purpose of the use, including whether it is educational or commercial; (2) the nature of the copyrighted work; (3) the amount of the copyrighted work to be used; and (4) the effect of use on the potential marketability or value of the copyrighted work (*Copyright Law of the United States of America*, 1993).

Rights to unpublished data

Unlike rights to copyrighted work, rights to unpublished data are difficult to define, and most ethical dilemmas concern access to rather than ownership of such information. Unpublished scientific data include written and electronic laboratory notes, experimental materials, project records and observations, databases, descriptions of methods and processes, analyses, and illustrative material. Traditionally, unpublished scientific data have been owned by their creators—the scientific investigators—and most scientists believe they have a duty to share data with their peers and, when appropriate, with the public. Any data reported in a published article become the property of the publisher, but rights to relevant, supportive data not reported in a published article (sometimes called raw data) are not transferred to the publisher. Problems arise when investigators, institutions, the government, and the public compete for control of and access to the same data. For example, who should have first rights to publication of research data: the principal investigator, the coinvestigators, or the institution that funded the research?

Legally, the investigator controls access to unpublished data, except under the following circumstances: (1) the investigator is an employee of an organization that claims rights to any work conducted by its employees; (2) the investigator is under federal contract or has received a federal grant to perform the work; or (3) a court decides that public interest in the data outweighs the interest of the owner (CBE, 1990). Government or industrial sponsorship of research may impose specific restrictions on data control and sharing, particularly when such data are proprietary or commercial. This area of law will continue to evolve as electronic technology makes data ownership and access more difficult to define and control by narrow standards and laws.

While it is generally agreed that data must be kept in an accessible format for a reasonable period of time, no standard has been universally accepted, because different types of data from different specialties require various modes and spaces for storage, which can be prohibitively expensive. Some institutions have recommended three or five years, and longer periods for data that support publications (Committee on Science, 1992–). The National Research Council Committee on National Statistics recommends and many journals require that editors have access to data during the peer review process, which means that the data must be maintained until publication (CBE, 1990). Some journals require authors to provide data to editors for their evaluation if requested, but this requirement does not have a time limit. Some journals require authors to send their data to national or international storage centers at the time of publication.

Disputes over who has rights to use scientific data have caused ethical dilemmas for editors. For example, what should an editor do with a manuscript from an author that reports an analysis of unpublished data originally collected and analyzed by another author? The ICMJE and the Committee on National Statistics recommend that editors consider such secondary analyses on their scientific merit as long as full credit and appropriate citations are given to the original data collections (ICMJE, 1991; CBE, 1990).

Other open questions concern the nature of sharing data, which is a vital part of the scientific enterprise. Should there be restrictions on the access, use, and citation of unpublished works by other authors and investigators? Most scientists and editors would argue that such restrictions would stifle scientific exchange. But what about access to unpublished data by those outside the scientific community, such as representatives of the media, the courts, and people with commercial interests? Many of these questions are currently under de-

bate, and whether or not access will be widened or restricted is difficult to predict.

Advertising

Advertisements for pharmaceutical products and medical/laboratory devices provide major financial support for biomedical publications. Advertising income is essential for many large biomedical publications since their costs would not be met by subscription revenue. Whether this situation represents one aspect of the success of the free enterprise system or a major ethical problem for editors is a matter of controversy.

To protect a journal's integrity and credibility, complete separation between advertising and editorial decisions is essential, and advertisers should have no influence on editorial content. Advertisements, including advertorials, should have a distinct appearance or labeling so that readers can readily distinguish them from editorial content, and ads for a product should not be placed adjacent to editorial material dealing with the product or disorders for which it might be used (Rennie, 1991). Publication of industry-sponsored journal supplements is problematic, since the supplement's editorial content may be selected or influenced by the sponsor to favor their products, and the review process may not be as rigorous or as independent as it is for the journal's regularly published issues.

The accuracy of advertisements in medical publications is more controversial. The purpose of advertisements is promotional, and studies have shown that the prescribing behavior of physicians is indeed influenced by advertisements. Because of their effect on the health of the public, advertisements for drugs and medical devices are regulated by a government health agency in many countries. In the United States, this responsibility lies with the Food and Drug Administration (FDA), which reviews and approves marketing and "labeling" (the package insert that describes the indications and side effects of a drug) but does not routinely review or approve advertisements prior to their dissemination. However, the FDA does review advertisements after publication and can require companies to withdraw or publicly correct ads that it determines to be inaccurate or misleading.

The standards by which print advertisements should be judged and the method of enforcing standards remain unsettled. Some have recommended the development of multidisciplinary review boards, such as the Canadian Pharmaceutical Advertising Advisory Board, to review and approve medical advertisements before their dissemination.

Enforcement of ethical standards

The enforcement of ethical standards in scientific publishing is a responsibility shared among authors, institutions, funding organizations, peer reviewers, and editors. Authors are primarily responsible for upholding the scientific commitment to a search for truth, accepting responsibility and credit for the work that bears their names, and fully disclosing any conflicts of interest. Institutions where research is performed and organizations that fund research share the main responsibility for ensuring that studies are designed and conducted ethically, and also for investigating and sanctioning allegations of misconduct. Peer reviewers are charged with performing objective and timely appraisals of papers submitted for publication, while maintaining strict confidentiality and disclosing their own conflicts of interest. Editors should exercise sound judgment and objectivity in selecting papers for publication, maintaining vigilance for any ethical problems, and ensuring that authors, reviewers, and institutions fulfill their responsibilities.

Clear ethical standards and implementation policies are certainly desirable, and editors have taken the lead in setting standards and policies (U.S. Congress, 1990). Yet the ethics of scientific publication is based on trust, and obsessive "policing" of the research community and the publication enterprise could be counterproductive. Persistent emphasis on the importance of maintaining ethical standards in the entire research process, from initial research ideas to their eventual publication, should be an expectation shared by all involved in that process. However, defining and enforcing such standards will be an even greater challenge as the electronic revolution extends the traditional boundaries of authorship and scientific publication.

RICHARD M. GLASS
ANNETTE FLANAGIN

Directly related to this article are the other articles in this entry: MEDIA AND MEDICINE, *and* MEDIA AND BIOETHICS. *For a further discussion of topics mentioned in this article, see the entries* ADVERTISING; COMMERCIALISM IN SCIENTIFIC RESEARCH; FRAUD, THEFT, AND PLAGIARISM; *and* RESEARCH, UNETHICAL. *For a discussion of related ideas, see the entries on* CONFLICT OF INTEREST; INFORMATION DISCLOSURE; *and* PRIVACY AND CONFIDENTIALITY IN RESEARCH. *See also the* APPENDIX (CODES, OATHS, AND DIRECTIVES RELATED TO BIOETHICS), SECTION IV: ETHICAL DIRECTIVES FOR HUMAN RESEARCH, *and* SECTION V: ETHICAL DIRECTIVES PERTAINING TO THE WELFARE AND USE OF ANIMALS.

Bibliography

ANGELL, MARCIA, and KASSIRER, JEROME P. 1991. "The Ingelfinger Rule Revisited." *New England Journal of Medicine* 325, no. 19:1371–1373.

ASSOCIATION OF AMERICAN MEDICAL COLLEGES. AD HOC COMMITTEE ON MISCONDUCT AND CONFLICT OF INTEREST IN RESEARCH. 1992. *Beyond the "Framework": Institutional Considerations in Managing Allegations of Misconduct in Research.* Washington, D.C.: Author.

COMMITTEE ON SCIENCE, ENGINEERING, AND PUBLIC POLICY. PANEL ON SCIENTIFIC RESPONSIBILITY AND THE CONDUCT OF RESEARCH. 1992–. *Responsible Science: Ensuring the Integrity of the Research Process.* Vol. I. Washington, D.C.: National Academy Press.

Copyright Law of the United States of America, as Contained in Title 17 of the United States Codes. 1993. Washington, D.C.: U.S. Government Printing Office.

COUNCIL OF BIOLOGY EDITORS (CBE) EDITORIAL POLICY COMMITTEE. 1990. *Ethics and Policy in Scientific Publication.* Bethesda, Md.: Author.

"Guarding the Guardians: Research on Editorial Peer Review: Selected Proceedings from the First International Congress on Peer Review in Biomedical Publication." 1990. *Journal of the American Medical Association* 263, no. 10:1317–1441.

HUTH, EDWARD J. 1986a. "Guidelines on Authorship of Medical Papers." *Annals of Internal Medicine* 104, no. 2: 269–274.

———. 1986b. "Irresponsible Authorship and Wasteful Publication." *Annals of Internal Medicine* 104, no. 2:257–259.

INTERNATIONAL COMMITTEE OF MEDICAL JOURNAL EDITORS (ICMJE). 1991. "Statements from the International Committee of Medical Journal Editors." *Journal of the American Medical Association* 265, no. 20:2697–2698.

———. 1993a. "Conflicts of Interest." *Annals of Internal Medicine* 118, no. 8:646–647.

———. 1993b. "Uniform Requirements for Manuscripts Submitted to Biomedical Journals." *Journal of the American Medical Association* 269, no. 17:2282–2286.

INTERNATIONAL CONGRESS ON PEER REVIEW IN BIOMEDICAL PUBLICATION. 1991. *Peer Review in Scientific Publishing.* Chicago: Council of Biology Editors.

IVERSON, CHERYL; DAN, BRUCE B.; GLITMAN, PAULA; KING, LESTER S.; KNOLL, ELIZABETH; MEYER, HARRIET S.; RAITHEL, KATHRYN SIMMONS; RIESENBERG, DON; and YOUNG, ROXANNE K. 1989. *American Medical Association Manual of Style.* 8th ed. Baltimore, Md: Williams & Wilkins.

LOCK, STEPHEN. 1986. *A Difficult Balance: Editorial Peer Review in Medicine.* Philadelphia: ISI Press.

LUNDBERG, GEORGE D., and FLANAGIN, ANNETTE. 1989. "New Requirements for Authors: Signed Statements of Authorship Responsibility and Financial Disclosure." *Journal of the American Medical Association* 262, no. 14:2003–2004.

RELMAN, ARNOLD S. 1984. "Dealing with Conflicts of Interest." *New England Journal of Medicine* 310, no. 18:1182–1183.

RENNIE, DRUMMOND. 1991. "Editors and Advertisements: What Responsibility Do Editors Have for the Advertisements in Their Journals?" *Journal of the American Medical Association* 265, no. 18:2394–2396.

RENNIE, DRUMMOND, and FLANAGIN, ANNETTE. 1992. "Publication Bias: The Triumph of Hope Over Experience."

Journal of the American Medical Association 267, no. 3:411–412.

———. 1994a. "Authorship! Authorship! Guests, Ghosts, Grafters, and the Two-Sided Coin." *Journal of the American Medical Association* 271, no. 6:469–471.

———. 1994b. "Selected Proceedings from the Second Internatinal Congress on Peer Review in Biomedical Publication." *Journal of the American Medical Association* 272, no. 2:91–173.

RENNIE, DRUMMOND; FLANAGIN, ANNETTE; and GLASS, RICHARD M. 1991. "Conflicts of Interest in the Publication of Science." *Journal of the American Medical Association* 266, no. 2:266–267.

RIESENBERG, DON, and LUNDBERG, GEORGE D. 1990. "The Order of Authorship: Who's on First?" *Journal of the American Medical Association* 264, no. 14:1857.

U.S. CONGRESS. HOUSE COMMITTEE ON GOVERNMENT OPERATIONS. 1990. *Are Scientific Misconduct and Conflicts of Interest Hazardous to Our Health?* Washington, D.C.: U.S. Government Printing Office.

U.S. DEPARTMENT OF HEALTH AND HUMAN SERVICES. OFFICE OF THE ASSISTANT SECRETARY FOR HEALTH. 1991. *First Annual Report: Scientific Misconduct Investigations: Reviewed by the Office of Scientific Integrity Review, March 1989–December 1990.* Washington, D.C.: Author.

WORLD MEDICAL ASSOCIATION. 1990. "Declaration of Helsinki." *Bulletin of the Pan American Health Organization* 24, no. 4:606–609.

III. MEDIA AND BIOETHICS

Common sense, physician Victor Sidel has said, suggests that the relationship between the media and bioethics should be a symbiotic one. To the extent that both journalists and bioethicists take their job to be informing public debate about important issues, they ought to complement one another. In practice, however, their relationship is often stressed and hostile (American Public Health Association, 1992).

The antagonism is no doubt partly a function of the relative youth of their professional association; bioethics itself is a young discipline, and the media have attended to the issues of bioethics more or less explicitly only since the mid- to late 1970s. More important, there are very real tensions between the practices of the media and bioethics that frustrate both parties. Reporters may argue that bioethicists simply do not understand the purposes and needs of print or broadcast journalism; bioethicists may contend that the media skimp coverage of important issues, reduce complex considerations to simple black-and-white questions, or inappropriately favor the ethically bizarre in choosing which stories to pursue. Each party still has much to learn about the other; and both have yet to attend critically to the matter of how they might collaborate most effectively.

Medicine makes the evening news

Arthur Caplan has noted that the advent of truly efficacious medicine after World War II was clearly reflected in increased media coverage of medical matters (Caplan, 1985). Combined with this in recent years has been a growing interest in ethics—or the lack thereof—in public life (see, e.g., Callahan, 1980; for a more biting perspective, see Baker, 1990; Bennett, 1980; McEnroe, 1990). Journalists have responded by giving the public what they seem to want: stories about medical miracles and the ethical dilemmas they raise. Both hard news and feature stories on new developments in medicine and the life sciences now often incorporate reflection on ethical issues.

Identifying the "first" bioethics story to make headlines is, of course, somewhat arbitrary. One possibility might be the "Life or Death Committee" at the Swedish Hospital's kidney dialysis program, a group of seven community members in Seattle, Washington, charged with determining which of many medically eligible patients would win one of the limited places in the new program to treat end-stage renal disease. Shana Alexander's story in the November 9, 1962, issue of *Life* magazine described how the committee evaluated dialysis candidates and also described the uncertainties the committee weighed in deciding who would receive treatment (Alexander, 1962).

Another leading candidate is certainly the Tuskegee syphilis study. Jean Heller's article in the *New York Times* on July 27, 1972, broke the story of how over 400 poor black men in rural Alabama were deliberately denied penicillin in a longitudinal study of the effects of untreated syphilis. The bulk of the article discussed details of the study itself and who might have been responsible for allowing it to go forward. Ethical commentary consisted of a single quotation from Senator William Proxmire, who labeled the research "a moral and ethical nightmare" (Heller, 1972, p. A1).

In 1975–1976, the New Jersey Supreme Court considered the Karen Ann Quinlan case, which quickly became a primary point of reference in arguments about the right to die. At the time, media coverage focused at least as heavily on questions of Quinlan's clinical condition and prognosis and on the legal argument as on moral questions of how treatment decisions are to be made for incompetent patients. Stories in the *New York Times*, for example, sought commentary from "religious spokesmen" largely as a preliminary to discussion of physicians' role in making such decisions (see Altman, 1976; Goldstein, 1976; Sullivan, 1976a, 1976b).

By the time Louise Brown, the first "test-tube baby," was born in Great Britain in July 1978, however, the media had clearly discovered bioethics. Front-page stories in the *New York Times* announced her birth, described the scientific history of her conception by in vitro fertilization (IVF), and noted that one British parliamentarian had expressed concerns about the implications of the technique for genetically engineering a "master race" (Reed, 1978). One companion article described the IVF procedure in detail, noted ethical concerns about the destruction of unused embryos, and quoted Robert Edwards, one of the physicians involved in the experiment, on questions of when human life begins (Sullivan, 1978). Another article canvassed theologians and religious leaders, citing a common fear that IVF techniques would lead to what is now called gestational surrogacy, that is, a woman bearing a child conceived by IVF to whom she is genetically unrelated (Vecsey, 1978).

In 1983, with *Newsday's* coverage of the Long Island case of Baby Jane Doe, bioethics became the stuff of Pulitzer Prize–winning journalism. In a series of articles over several weeks, *Newsday* reporters explored the story of an infant born with spina bifida and other serious birth defects and her parents' decision not to authorize surgery that would prolong her life. The lead article in the series highlighted ethical concerns as a topic and solicited comments from religious, legal, and philosophical experts, giving each several paragraphs to identify and discuss issues they found germane to the case—parental autonomy, state obligations to protect life, the legal rights of the handicapped, and questions centering on quality of life (Kerr, 1983; see also Colen, 1983a, 1983b, 1983c).

Bioethics still has not acquired the status of a formal "beat" comparable to medical or science reporting. Stories may be covered by medical or science writers, sometimes by religion reporters, but more often than not, for most publications or programs, by general-assignment reporters who have no special background in covering medical or ethical issues (Klaidman and Beauchamp, 1986; American Public Health Association, 1992). Nonetheless, bioethics has become reasonably well established as a feature of the journalistic landscape, both print and broadcast. In part this is because bioethics emerged as part of a larger movement toward civil rights and empowerment, as Daniel Callahan has noted (1980, 1993). But at least arguably as important is the fact that bioethics can be used to tell a news story as a modern-day morality tale. It can be used, that is, to bring the language of right and wrong, good and evil into the "factual" realm of science reporting.

Bioethics thus has come to be part of the way reporters "frame" stories, as well as a way to present an important dimension of a story. An emerging, if perhaps still tacit, professional standard seems in fact to require that a journalist discuss his or her story with an ethicist, either for background or, ideally, for a pithy quotation or two, when the topic falls within the purview of bioethics (see, e.g., Rachels, 1991; Murray, 1988).

For the media, one definition of what constitutes a "bioethics" story would be those medical or quasi-medical matters that reach the courts—virtually all of the foregoing cases, for example, or *Baby M*, the New Jersey surrogate motherhood case (1987); *Davis v. Davis*, the Tennessee frozen embryo case (1989); *Cruzan v. Director, Missouri Department of Health*, the Missouri "right to die" case that reached the U.S. Supreme Court (1992); or efforts in the early 1990s to indict Michigan pathologist Jack Kevorkian on charges of murder for assisting patients to take their own lives with his "suicide machine."

As a result, the media and the general public tend to define bioethics more narrowly than bioethicists themselves. While abortion, termination of treatment, euthanasia and assisted suicide, organ transplantation, and assisted reproduction (and all its variations) are frequently covered as "bioethics," other questions—of priority setting, access to health care, and the broader interplay of health care with other social goods like education or housing—tend to be covered by the media as political issues. This, presumably, is because such issues often achieve public prominence when they are linked to election campaigns and so tend to be treated as "political" matters and are less often recognized as having particularly "ethical" implications. Moreover, for journalists, bioethics stories tend to hinge on particular cases, whose identifiable participants and gripping dilemmas capture public attention in ways that the media can accommodate—and exploit. Thus, as Caplan has noted, coverage of bioethics still often has a sensational quality to it; stories focus on new technologies or wonder drugs, or on "science fiction" topics like the cloning of human embryos (for further comment, see Caplan, 1985; Schwitzer, 1992).

Journalism as a practice imposes some very real constraints on the way issues and topics, bioethical or otherwise, can be handled. Hard-news stories, with their focus on getting information out as succinctly as possible, impose stringent limitations on what can be offered in the way of ethical commentary and leave little opportunity to plumb the moral depths of stories. The broader scope and greater length of feature articles more readily accommodate thoughtful reflection on issues (e.g., Carson, 1991).

In broadcast journalism, the format of the half-hour news show is not conducive to sustained ethical reflection but rather reduces discussion to a series of "ethical sound bites," short, provocative quotations couched in highly polarized, and thus memorable, terms (see Nelson, 1991; Rachels, 1991; Murray, 1988). Stephen Klaidman and Tom Beauchamp wonder whether television can do a good job of covering ethically complex stories at all, particularly when one person in the story may be much more appealing to viewers than others, quite independently of his or her role or moral position (Klaidman and Beauchamp, 1986). Yet while many, with some justification, decry this kind of "soundbite" commentary and those who offer it, there may be valid reasons for bioethicists to participate. As Caplan suggests, working with the media—even when it cannot accommodate sustained reflection—helps assure that bioethics is heard as a real and important voice on significant public issues (Caplan, 1982).

The opportunities to explore complex issues are greater, clearly, in the context of television news magazines such as "Nightline" or "Sixty Minutes"; documentaries and other special programs, of course, may focus particularly on ethical concerns in a biomedical context (e.g., public television's "Hard Choices" or the 1993 "Frontline" exploration of euthanasia, "Choosing Death," etc.). All of these considerations shape the way bioethics can be and is covered by print and broadcast journalism.

But if bioethics has come to be recognized as somehow a distinctive domain of stories, what of the experts who offer commentary on those stories? Who qualifies as a "bioethicist"? Since there is no universally recognized curriculum for training bioethicists, no fixed criteria by which expertise may be tested, nor any credentialling body or procedure, just who can legitimately call him- or herself a bioethicist remains one of the more contentious questions in the field. In many ways, not all of them desirable, media recognition itself—both of bioethics as a distinct discipline and of those willing to offer comment as practitioners—is becoming a form of credentialling every bit as compelling, for the public at any rate, as a doctorate in philosophy or a degree in medicine (for discussion, see Caplan, 1992).

Conflicting professional goals

To say that journalists cover stories—with or without bioethical content—because they are newsworthy is a truism. Yet defining just what "news" is, or what makes a given story "newsworthy," is hardly a straightforward task. Joshua Halberstam has suggested that we tend to feel stories are newsworthy if the information is of a kind that interests (or should interest) us and is likely to make a difference in our lives (Halberstam, 1992).

The criteria of interest and importance help to explain two different and potentially conflicting goals of journalism: entertainment and education. News stories may be intended to do little more than play on our curiosity; as Philip Hilt, a science reporter for the *New York Times,* has put it, reporting is essentially gossip carried

out under rules. We are mistaken if we think of journalism as a profession rather than a trade, or expect journalists to do more than simply relate interesting news. When the media do educate or influence the public, that is an epiphenomenon. So too, according to Hilt and colleague Malcolm Gladwell of the *Washington Post,* stories are covered as much by serendipity—who happens to call a reporter with information on a potential story, what the journalist's current interests are personally, whether someone is available to work on the story just then, who does or does not return a reporter's phone calls, what other stories are competing for space or air time, and so forth—as by design or a clear sense of broader professional goals (see American Public Health Association, 1992; Klaidman and Beauchamp, 1986).

The more common perspective on journalism, however, sees the media's role as fundamentally educational, rooted in a professional obligation to benefit the public. As Klaidman and Beauchamp note, arguments supporting the institution and privileges of a free press in the United States have rested on the premise that the press promotes the commonweal "as monitor of the public's business and as an educator" (Klaidman and Beauchamp, 1987, p. 128).

As part of the perceived professional obligation to inform and educate, the media have adopted what Michael O'Neill has criticized as a "reactive, adversarial, action-oriented" posture (Klaidman and Beauchamp, 1987, p. 151). The contemporary popular paradigm of investigative reporting is inherently critical, of course, requiring that the reporter uncover information and/or practices in the interest of bringing public scrutiny to bear on events or situations. And to the extent that contemporary journalistic practice maintains a skeptical stance toward the subject matter of its stories, it welcomes the kind of critical commentary bioethics tends to offer. Indeed, it may not only welcome it but insist on it. As James Rachels notes, journalists are rarely "eager to hear reassurances that the alarming events really aren't alarming. That doesn't make good copy. What makes good copy is the idea that the events being reported are morally troubling, or worse" (Rachels, 1991, p. 67). As Rachels goes on to argue, bioethicists reinforce this trend when their comments hinge on "slippery slope" arguments about the evils to which a new development might ultimately lead (p. 70). The more slippery the slope and the morally nastier its endpoint, the better the copy. And all too often, it seems, bioethicists are prepared to envision some very nasty slides indeed.

There is a range of professional goals within bioethics as well, spanning reflection on the foundations of ethical theory, to examination of how developments in medicine and the life sciences challenge deeply held values, to consultation at the bedside regarding treatment decisions for individual patients. Among the tasks of the bioethicist are identifying which problems raise moral issues, providing systematic means of thinking about those issues, and helping physicians and others make right decisions in particular cases (Callahan, 1973; Bouton, 1990; Callahan, 1980; Caplan, 1982, 1992).

Journalists and bioethicists may thus envision their respective professional goals as benefiting the public and serving the political, social, and moral needs of a democratic society—especially by bringing to light and clarifying hitherto unappreciated dilemmas and problematic practices. They may employ similar methods, moreover, since as critical practices both journalism and bioethics take as their points of departure specific, concrete moments in the flow of daily life.

Stories such as those of Louise Brown, Karen Quinlan, and Baby M capture the attention of journalists and ethicists not simply because of their individual drama but also because they "resonate with meanings and dilemmas larger than [themselves]" (Morrow, 1991; see also Altman, 1984). They raise issues of concern to all of us. And in reporting and discussing these stories, the professional goals of journalists and bioethicists may converge in a common enterprise of—as the code of ethics of the American Society of Newspaper Editors phrases it—"informing the people and enabling them to make judgments on the important issues of the times" (Klaidman and Beauchamp, 1987, p. 130).

Sharing a broadly defined goal is not in and of itself sufficient to ensure that the collaboration between journalism and bioethics will be smooth or successful, however. Bioethicists may not be aware of their own agendas in agreeing to be interviewed, and so, as pediatrician-ethicist Alan Fleischman has argued, move in and out of their potential roles as educators, advocates, or agents of social change (American Public Health Association, 1992). Or they may fail to recognize or take seriously enough the constraints under which journalists must routinely work—among others, the need to meet deadlines on important breaking stories, the limited air time or column space allocated to the story by producers or editors, and the commercial need to reach as broad an audience with as lively and compelling a story as possible.

For their part, journalists who do not adequately appreciate the nature of bioethics as a discipline may approach the encounter seeking clear, straightforward answers that bioethics cannot provide. Thus reporters may chafe at the ("sterile," "academic") qualifying, the attention to nuance, the attempt to offer a scrupulously thorough analysis that bioethicists take (or at least profess) as their ultimate professional obligation. The experience can leave both parties distrustful of further collaboration.

Even under the best conditions there are special risks for bioethicists in their relationships with the media. In important ways, bioethics as a discipline is known to the general public as it is presented in media accounts of dilemmas in medicine and the life sciences. What the public generally take to be the subject matter and methods of bioethics are shaped in no small measure by the glimpses afforded on television and in the daily papers. And that does risk conveying a skewed image of the bioethicist as either a prophet of moral doom or an effete, hypercritical "talking head," waiting to offer uniquely erudite commentary.

Recourse to experts, Cheryl Noble has argued, reinforces the notion that problems, including ethical ones, are best solved by turning them over "to the correct set of problem solvers" (Noble, 1982, p. 7). Moreover, she observes, applied ethics' habit of privileging techniques of moral reasoning tends to undervalue not only possession of substantive moral wisdom, but also the social and political dimensions of moral problems, and so to set morality apart from social life. The emphasis on expert commentary also risks playing into what Daniel Callahan has identified as the problem of "disciplinary reductionism," the tendency to reduce complex moral dilemmas to a single "transcendent issue" (Callahan, 1973, p. 69).

Caplan analyzes these problems somewhat differently as shortcomings of what he calls the "engineering model" that prevails in contemporary applied ethics. This model takes the business of applied ethics to be a neutral, value-free process of "mechanically deducing conclusions" from the normative ethical theories that comprise the discipline's distinctive, self-defining body of knowledge. In Caplan's view, the engineering model is simply wrong—it is unable to explain which theories count as part of the canon and offers no insight into how properly to weight different theories when, inevitably, they conflict in individual cases (Caplan, 1982).

Such a model of expertise, coupled with the fact that ethicists are most often asked to comment on events that are in progress or have already taken place, means that bioethicists are effectively called upon to act as if moral inquiry were little more than a matter of offering post hoc moral judgment. This reduces bioethics to simply a practice of critical-case commentary, obscuring the larger normative and theoretical questions with which the field is equally concerned. Yet it is, of course, precisely this illusory clarity about cases that best suits the media's approach to bioethics stories, and that reporters seek in interviewing bioethicists.

In combination with broader societal trends toward specialization within disciplines, journalism's invocation of bioethical expertise further risks driving that expertise to coalesce around particular sets of issues. There is an increasing tendency to identify individual ethicists as particularly knowledgeable about, for example, organ transplantation, assisted reproduction, national health, or other single issues. Commenting for the press may reinforce tendencies to identify particular ethicists with particular substantive positions as well, creating cadres of "pro-choice," "anti-euthanasia," or "pro-national-health" specialists, and so on, available to trot out their analyses on cue. This is not to deny that some individuals have thought through certain issues more thoroughly than others and so are better situated to comment on them, or to deny that individual ethicists do or should come to substantive conclusions on given moral issues. Rather, it is to point out that the press may exploit these disciplinary realities in ways that, while they may make for good copy, can be problematic for bioethics—and the public.

Working with journalists to cover stories of significant moral interest may frustrate the goals and ethos of bioethics, but this should not serve as an excuse for bioethicists to avoid the media. Bioethicists may well have a professional obligation to collaborate with the press in bringing important issues before the public to insure that debate is as informed and as sensitive to ethical complexity as possible. In contemporary American culture, media recognition is also a powerful way to ensure participation in important social decisions. If bioethics is actively to join debates on health care and other issues, it must gain the kind of recognition accorded economics, law, and public policymaking. Yet with their journalist colleagues, bioethicists also have an obligation to recognize when not to comment: because they do not have enough information, because a story does not actually raise significant issues, because they themselves have not thought through the issues carefully, or because they feel compassion for the principals (see, e.g., Crigger, 1990; Murray, 1988).

It may be that contemporary journalistic practice can generally support little more than impoverished exploration of ethical issues. That is no argument for journalists not to cover bioethics stories (as ethical stories), however, nor for ethicists to decline to shed what light they can on pressing moral questions. It is, rather, an argument for both journalists and bioethicists to work creatively within the inevitable constraints on their joint undertaking. Understanding those limitations can help to assure that "ethical soundbites," instead of being the last word on moral problems, serve as the first impulse toward sustained ethical reflection.

BETTE-JANE CRIGGER

Directly related to this article are the other articles in this entry: MEDIA AND MEDICINE, *and* SCIENTIFIC PUBLISH-ING. *For a discussion of related ideas, see the entries* INTERPRETATION; *and* VALUE AND VALUATION. *Other relevant material may be found under the entries* HEALTH OFFICIALS AND THEIR RESPONSIBILITIES; HEALTH POLICY; *and* HEALTH PROMOTION AND HEALTH EDUCATION.

Bibliography

ALEXANDER, SHANA. 1962. "They Decide Who Lives, Who Dies: Medical Miracle Puts a Moral Burden on a Small Committee." *Life*, November 9, pp. 102–117.

ALTMAN, LAWRENCE K. 1976. "New Questions in Quinlan Case." *New York Times*, May 27, p. A22.

———. 1984. "After Barney Clark: Reflections of a Reporter on Unresolved Issues." In *After Barney Clark: Reflections on the Utah Artificial Heart Program*, pp. 113–128. Edited by Margery W. Shaw. Austin: University of Texas Press.

AMERICAN PUBLIC HEALTH ASSOCIATION. 1992. "The Media and the Message: News Coverage of Bioethical Issues." Panel Presentation, November 11. Washington, D.C.

Baby M, in re. 1987. 109 N.J. 396, 537 A.2d 1227.

BAKER, RUSSELL. 1990. "Ethicizationism." *New York Times*, October 27, p. A23.

BENNETT, WILLIAM J. 1980. "Getting Ethics." *Commentary*, December, pp. 62–65.

BLAKESLEE, SANDRA, ed. 1986. *Human Heart Replacement: A New Challenge for Physicians and Reporters*. Los Angeles: Foundation for American Communications and the Gannett Foundation.

BOUTON, KATHERINE. 1990. "Painful Decisions: The Role of the Medical Ethicist." *New York Times Magazine*, August 5.

CALLAHAN, DANIEL. 1973. "Bioethics as a Discipline." *Hastings Center Studies* 1, no. 1:66–73.

———. 1980. "Shattuck Lecture—Contemporary Biomedical Ethics." *New England Journal of Medicine* 302, no. 22:1228–1233.

———. 1993. "Why America Accepted Bioethics." Special Supplement, *Hastings Center Report* 23, no. 6:58–59.

CAPLAN, ARTHUR L. 1982. "Mechanics on Duty: The Limitations of a Technical Definition of Moral Expertise for Work in Applied Ethics." *Canadian Journal of Philosophy*, supplementary volume 8, pp. 1–17.

———. 1985. "Press Has Much to Learn about Medical Courage." *Times Union* (Albany, N.Y.), April 28.

———. 1991. "Bioethics on Trial." *Hastings Center Report* 21, no. 3:19–20.

———. 1992. "Moral Experts and Moral Expertise: Does Either Exist?" In his *If I Were a Rich Man, Could I Buy a Pancreas?* Bloomington: Indiana University Press.

CARSON, ROB. 1991. "Initiative 119: The Right to Die." *Tacoma Morning News Tribune*, October 6–9.

———. 1993. "What Bioethics Brought to the Public." Special Supplement, *Hastings Center Report* 23, no. 6: S14–S15.

COLEN, B. D. 1983a. "A Life of Love—and Endless Pain." *Newsday*, October 26.

———. 1983b. "Open Question of Life or Death." *Newsday*, November 13.

———. 1983c. "Prognosis of One Doctor for a Spina Bifida Baby." *Newsday*, November 9.

CRIGGER, BETTE-JANE. 1990. "Private Lives, Public Scrutiny." *Hastings Center Report* 20, no. 5:2–3.

Cruzan v. Director, Missouri Department of Health. 1992. 497. U.S. 261.

Davis v. Davis. 1992. 8425.W.2d 588 (Tennessee).

FRIEDMAN, SHARON M.; DUNWOODY, SHARON; and ROGERS, CAROL L. 1986. *Scientists and Journalists: Reporting Science as News*. New York: Free Press.

GOLDSTEIN, TOM. 1976. "Life, Death and the Law." *New York Times*, April 2, p. A38.

HALBERSTAM, JOSHUA. 1992. "A Prolegomenon for a Theory of News." In *Philosophical Issues in Journalism*, pp. 11–21. Edited by Elliot D. Cohen. New York: Oxford University Press.

HELLER, JEAN. 1972. "Syphilis Victims in U.S. Study Went Untreated for 40 Years." *New York Times*, July 27, pp. 47–48.

KERR, KATHLEEN. 1983. "An Issue of Law and Ethics." *Newsday*, October 26.

———. 1984. "Reporting the Case of Baby Jane Doe." *Hastings Center Report* 14, no. 4:7–9.

KLAIDMAN, STEPHEN, and BEAUCHAMP, TOM L. 1986. "Baby Jane Doe in the Media." *Journal of Health Politics, Policy and Law* 11, no. 2:271–284.

———. 1987. *The Virtuous Journalist*. New York: Oxford University Press.

MCENROE, COLIN. 1990. "Was It Ethical for You Too?" *Mirabella*, November, pp. 130, 133.

MORROW, LANCE. 1991. "When One Body Can Save Another." *Time*, June 17, pp. 54–58.

MURRAY, THOMAS H. 1988. "Mediagenic Ethics." *Hastings Center Report* 18, no. 6:3–4.

NELSON, JAMES LINDEMANN. 1991. "Not Quite Live from Briarcliff Manor: Bioethics on Television." *CenterPiece*, December, p. 1.

NOBLE, CHERYL N. 1992. "Ethics and Experts." *Hastings Center Report* 12, no. 3:7–9.

RACHELS, JAMES. 1991. "When Philosophers Shoot from the Hip." *Bioethics* 5, no. 1:67–71.

REED, ROY. 1978. "Early Insertion of Embryo into Womb Is Linked to Successful Gestation." *New York Times*, July 27, pp. A1, A16.

SCHWITZER, GARY J. 1992. "Doctoring the News: Miracle Cures, Video Press Releases, and TV Medical Reporting." *Quill* 80, no. 9:19–21.

SULLIVAN, JOSEPH F. 1976a. "Court Rules Karen Quinlan's Father Can Let Her Die by Disconnecting Respirator If Doctors See No Hope." *New York Times*, April 1, pp. A1, A23.

———. 1976b. "Court's Ruling to Let Miss Quinlan Die Stirs Much Praise and Condemnation." *New York Times*, April 2, p. A38.

SULLIVAN, WALTER. 1978. "Doctors' Success in Conception in the Laboratory Intensifies the Debate over Reproductive Control." *New York Times*, July 27, pp. A1, A16.

VECSEY, GEORGE. 1978. "Religious Leaders Differ on Implant." *New York Times*, July 27, p. A16.

ZUCKER, ARTHUR. 1992. "Baby Marrow: Ethicists and Privacy." *Journal of Medical Ethics* 18, no. 3:125–127, 141.

COMPANION ANIMALS AND PETS

See ANIMAL WELFARE AND RIGHTS, *article on* PET AND COMPANION ANIMALS.

COMPASSION

The word "compassion" comes from the Latin *compati*, which means "to suffer with" or "to experience with." Compassion, with its cognate notions of pity, mercy, sympathy, empathy, fellow feeling, benevolence, care, and love, is variously described as a visceral passion, as a kind of emotion or emotional attitude, as an intuitive identification with the pain and suffering of another, or as a duty enjoined upon the moral agent to respond actively to another's plight. Those different descriptions, subjects of controversy in their own right, may also carry different prescriptive implications.

Compassion can be distinguished from its cognates, despite their affinities in common usage. Pity, while similar to compassion as a feeling in response to the plight of another, may also connote passivity toward the one who suffers as a mere "object" of feeling. Compassion, in contrast, connotes both a sense of "shared humanity" and an "active regard for the [other's] good" (Blum, 1980, p. 509), even if one is not able to respond with direct action. Mercy, with deep roots in religious worldviews, is closely associated with compassion as an active response to suffering. Mercy, however, may suggest a difference in status between the agent and the object of mercy; in the societal context of class differences, for example, acts of mercy may be associated with attitudes of condescension. Sympathy refers to a shared sense of the other's suffering through some power or mechanism of transference or to an imaginative identification with the other's plight. Empathy refers to a capacity to participate in the state of another's feelings but, unlike sympathy, without the same possibility of being overwhelmed in the process. Benevolence, care, and love, while often motivated by compassion as an emotion or an attitude, are richer notions, ordinarily connoting a fuller sense of what active concern for the other implies, beyond or in addition to the motivation that compassion may provide.

Philosophical perspectives on compassion

The Greek Stoic tradition enjoins *apatheia* ("without feeling") as the appropriate attitude of the moral person and assesses compassion as a "sickness of the soul." While the Stoic sage is not hard-hearted or indifferent to the plight of others, a rational and impartial concern, rather than compassion, is praised as the proper motive for ethical action.

Plato's work contains only two specific references to compassion or its cognates. In the *Menexenus*, Socrates notes the "deserved accusation" that could be made against Athens for being too compassionate toward its vanquished enemy (Plato, 1969, 244e). In the *Protagoras*, pity is commended as an appropriate reaction to those faults in others due to "nature or chance," whereas indignation or admonition are appropriate responses to flaws of character that can be reformed through training (Plato, 1969, 323e).

Aristotle provides extended discussion of pity as a passion, in light of his understanding of what constitutes excellence. According to Aristotle, pity is elicited by unpleasant, painful, and/or destructive things (death, bodily injuries and afflictions, old age, diseases, lack of food), serious evils resulting from chance (friendlessness, scarcity of friends, deformity, weakness, mutilation), and evil coming from a source that should have effected good (Aristotle, 1984, 1386a). Pity is also limited by several factors: (1) We pity persons we know who are "not very closely related to us," since in the latter case, we respond not with pity but "as if we were in danger ourselves" (Aristotle, 1984, 1386a); (2) we pity those who suffer unmerited misfortune (Aristotle, 1984, 1385b); and (3) we pity "those who are like us in age, character, disposition, social standing, or birth, since in such cases we are more likely to view the same misfortune as possible for us" (Aristotle, 1984, 1386a). Aristotle's general principle here is that "what we fear for ourselves excites our pity when it happens to others" (Aristotle, 1985, 1386a). Nonetheless, as a passion pity is not in itself virtuous or vicious, for "we are not called good or bad on the ground of our passions, but are so called on the ground of our excellences and our vices, which depend upon us feeling in a certain mode or manner" (Aristotle, 1984, 1105b).

In the modern period, the cognate notion of sympathy is a central constituent of the moral theory of David Hume (1711–1776), Adam Smith (1723–1790), and Arthur Schopenhauer (1788–1860). According to the Earl of Shaftesbury (1671–1713) and Francis Hutcheson (1694–1746), morality requires a separate "moral sense" by which primary sentiments such as pity are made reflective objects of approval or disapproval. By contrast, Hume denies that an additional "moral sense" is required. Instead, he affirms the presence of universally shared moral sentiments that function according to the same laws that operate in our nonmoral thinking. While Hume and Smith both view sympathy as the primary principle at work in moral attitudes and actions, they conceive of sympathy in different ways. In contrast to Aristotle on pity, Hume understands sympathy not merely as a passion, but as an automatic "propensity to receive by communication the sentiments and inclinations of others" (Brown, 1992, p. 865). Sympathy generates in us approval of virtuous behavior in others, joy in their happiness, and the urge to respond to their suffering. The ability to feel sympathy toward the other varies according to circumstances: We sympathize more readily with those who resemble us, who are contiguous, or who are related to us. Hume concludes, however, that moral judgments based upon sympathy, rather than being variable or arbitrary, can be made uniform as we learn to regulate sympathy according to a general point of view (Hume, 1948). In contrast to some religiously inspired interpretations of sympathy that may link fellow-feeling to excessive self-denial, Hume finds in sympathy the basis of our self-esteem; without a mutuality of persons in sympathetic relatedness, we cannot maintain our own steadfastness as moral agents.

According to Smith, sympathy is not a shared feeling, in the sense of direct participation in what another experiences, but an identification with the sentiments one imagines one would feel in the other's situation (Smith, 1990). As a parallel to Hume's general point of view, Smith develops the regulative role of the well-informed, impartial spectator in order to constrain variations in sympathetic projection.

Arthur Schopenhauer makes compassion the only legitimate motive of moral attitudes and behavior. His argument proceeds in three steps: (1) "The moral significance of an action can lie only in its reference to others" (Schopenhauer, 1965, p. 142). (2) Since "what moves the will is simply weal and woe," the other's "weal and woe must be directly my motive, just as my weal and woe are so in the case of all other actions" (Schopenhauer, 1965, p. 143). (3) But the motive for sympathetic identification "is not one that is imagined or invented; . . . it is the everyday phenomenon of compassion, of the immediate participation, independent of all ulterior considerations, primarily in the suffering of another, and thus in the prevention or elimination of it" (Schopenhauer, 1965, pp. 143–144). In effect, Schopenhauer incorporates central features of Hume's account of sympathy, even as he undergirds the notion by identifying compassion as its motive.

All moral theories that emphasize notions of sympathy stand in marked contrast to the understanding of morality offered by Immanuel Kant (1724–1804). According to Kant, morality requires that one form one's will according to a sense of duty. The moral law is the principle of both moral obligation and autonomy. All feelings, including compassion and sympathy, are items of human experience that reveal nothing about the nature of things in themselves and thus cannot ground moral principles. Kant's theory is an attempt to define morality in transcendental rather than contingent, categorical rather than hypothetical, terms (Kant, 1964). Alternatively, moral theories that emphasize sympathy and compassion can be viewed as experience-based alternatives to the formalism of the Kantian project. Uncertainties persist, at both metaethical and normative levels, about the possibilities of developing a moral theory that can adequately combine the sense of binding obligation characteristic of Kantian approaches and concern for the good central to experiential accounts (the metaethical level concerns itself with the meanings of ethical terms, the nature of ethical judgments, and the types of ethical arguments).

Religious perspectives on compassion

In religious traditions, compassion and mercy are moral attitudes, enjoined as moral requirements, praiseworthy virtues, or superfluous ideals. Compassion refers to the emotional attitude or perspective that should shape and inform the appropriate response of religious believers to the suffering of others. Differences in religious discussions are to be found less at the level of moral attitude and response than in the ground or warrant that justifies compassion.

Buddhism espouses compassion as central to the moral vision set forth in the Fourfold Holy Truths and the Noble Eightfold Path. The Holy Truths describe all existence as suffering, all suffering as caused by attachment and craving, and all craving as capable of being overcome by heeding the tenets of the Eightfold Path. Although the goal of Buddhist practice is ultimately transcendental enlightenment, the fourth tenet of the Eightfold Path stresses the importance of "right acts" (samma-kammanta). Especially in the Mahayana school, right action requires compassion as the central motive for perfection to be attained in thought and behavior. Buddhist priestly practice, from the time of its introduction into China in the first century c.e., has emphasized succor of the poor, including their medical care.

In Judaism, raham (from the Hebrew for "bowels") refers to the seat of compassion. Compassion, a "feeling with and for others," is described, in literally visceral terms, as an attribute of God and as the source of the ethical obligation to respond to the neighbor in need. In the Hebrew scriptures, mercy is an essential attribute of God himself (Ps. 116:5; Prov. 12:10), and Yahweh's constant and certain mercy is inextricably linked to his

covenantal love (hesed). The ethical imperative follows from this understanding of God's merciful love: As God has been merciful in establishing his covenantal concern, so God's people are to show mercy to one another. Although the basis for compassionate love is clear, the nature and scope of the injunction to "love your neighbor as yourself" (Lev. 19:18) remains the subject of rabbinical controversy.

In the Christian scriptures, as in Judaism, compassion is described in literally visceral terms (from the Greek splangchnizomai, "being moved to the bowels"). Jesus' deeply felt reaction to human suffering is an essential attribute of his person and ministry. In direct response to the merciful love of God in the saving action of Jesus Christ, Christians are likewise to be compassionate to all. The universalizing impulse in the scope of Christian compassion is emphasized in the literature of the early Church, and provides the ethos for the formation of hospitals as early as the fourth century. Yet, as in Judaism, the Christian tradition has understood the nature and scope of compassion-inspired love (agape) in a number of ways: as equal regard, as self-sacrifice, as mutuality, or as active concern with the neighbor's welfare (Outka, 1972).

Islam stresses universal mercy as an attribute of Allah and as an ethical obligation. Compassion and mercy are central aspects of one's dealings with fellow Muslims, as well as with "people of the Book" (Jews and Christians). Islam also emphasizes justice and fairness as moral requirements in dealing with non-Muslims who are not hostile to Allah's cause. A number of texts emphasize the duty of kindness and generosity to both Muslim and non-Muslims, using the same term (birr) to describe both this duty and the Muslim's obligation to his or her parents.

An attitude of compassion toward all sentient beings follows from certain key tenets of the Hindu worldview. Because atman (one's inmost self) is brahman (impersonal world spirit) and essentially immutable, and because rebirth (samsara) depends upon one's present action (karma), certain attitudes and behaviors are required to progress toward release (mokśa) from the cycle of birth and death. Hinduism stresses an attitude of nonviolence or noninjury (ahimsa) toward all sentient beings, especially toward particularly vulnerable forms of life. Ahimsa also carries the positive implication of working to benefit others (Coward et al., 1989).

Compassion and the practice of medicine

Links between compassion and the practice of medicine can be drawn at several levels. First, as a matter of medical history and professional self-understanding, numerous oaths and codes proclaim compassionate care for patients as an ideal. Second, commentators underscore the need for a technologically sophisticated medicine to respond to the patient's suffering, rather than merely to treat the physical symptoms of disease. Third, in contrast to the recent stress upon midlevel principles in bioethical method, an emphasis on compassion and care has been proposed as a preferable alternative.

Compassion in the history of medicine.   In classical treatises of medicine, one finds a fusion of *techne* (skill in healing) and *philanthropia* (love of humankind). For example, the Hippocratic precepts recommend that physicians sometimes offer their services without fees and that they provide aid to all needy strangers, "for where there is love of man, there is also love of the art" (Reiser et al., 1977, p. 5). A close reading of these Greek texts, however, suggests that "love of humankind" is espoused as an ideal rather than as a regulative virtue for all physicians. Moreover, no univocal basis for medical ethics derives from a shared vision of general humanistic duties; rather, "medical ethics remains relative to the respective philosophies" of practitioners (Reiser et al., 1977, p. 44).

The history of a professionally based medical ethics can be read as an increasingly self-conscious attempt of the medical guild to define the nature of its own commitments, to both patients and society at large. Written codes, from the Hippocratic oath through the various codes of the American Medical Association, profess philanthropy as an ideal, even as the less formal codes that guide clinical apprenticeship increasingly focus on technical proficiency (see Appendix, vol. 5). The informal codification of medical ethics, by characterizing medicine primarily in terms of technique, tends to discourage compassionate involvement with the patient as a requirement of professional practice. Formal codes of medical ethics, even when they emphasize compassion as a virtue necessary to patient care (along with self-effacement, tenderness, and gentleness), remain conspicuously silent on how these qualities of character are to be nurtured and sustained in a clinical climate often dominated by high-technology interventions and increasing regulation and regimentation.

Compassion and the art of medicine.   Any account of compassion proposed either as a general duty or as a professional ideal confronts two serious obstacles. Unlike the philosophical and/or metaphysical commitments that served as background assumptions to classic treatises on physicians' responsibilities, today's professional standards do not articulate and cannot presume such shared premises. But in the absence of shared religious or philosophical convictions, compassion—whether discussed as virtue, duty, or ideal—remains inadequately explicated and justified. Even if a common set of assumptions were available to ground compassion as a binding obligation for health-care professionals,

fundamental differences in expectation, experience, and language between the perspectives of professionals and patients would continue to pose significant challenges to a comprehensive account of compassion as the basis of medical practice.

Warren T. Reich argues that an adequate account of compassion must derive from the internal dynamic of suffering rather than from external sources (Reich, 1989). As a first step in internal definition, compassion requires that a distinction be drawn between "suffering" and "pain." Suffering, unlike pain, is experienced by persons, not merely by bodies. Although suffering often occurs along with pain, suffering transcends the physical: "Most generally, suffering can be defined as the state of severe distress associated with events that threaten the intactness of the person" (Cassell, 1991, p. 33). Moreover, suffering is not experienced only with regard to the restoration of bodily integrity, but in relation to various aspects of persons, including their family and social roles and their beliefs in a transcendent source of meaning.

Reich develops a tripartite process of suffering and compassionate response to it that emphasizes the dialectic between the one who suffers and the one who responds. Mute suffering, literal speechlessness in the face of distress, takes as its fitting response a silent compassion: One is quiet in the presence of the suffering other, but respectfully so, in a space potentially open to genuine, albeit unvoiced, meaning. Next, in the phase of expressive suffering, the sufferer gives voice to experience, often with cries of lament, by placing suffering within a larger narrative context. Corresponding to this second phase of suffering is the response of expressive compassion, whereby the caregiver works with the sufferer to help "find a voice for the voiceless," by sharing thoughts and feelings with the sufferer in an attempt to connect the patient to "a wider spectrum of meaning and value" (Reich, 1989, p. 94). In a third phase, the sufferer, by finding a voice, discovers a "new identity in suffering." Correlatively, the compassionate caregiver, in the process of expressing compassion, comes to a new awareness of the self as compassionate, thereby strengthening the very dispositions necessary to overcome the tendencies toward objectivity and depersonalization so prevalent in clinical medicine.

Nonetheless, the desiderata of expressive suffering and compassion are often thwarted by the vocabulary of physicians. The language of "disease" is the argot of the health-care professional, a language of classification based on categories rather than the particular circumstances of the patient. Despite the penchant of physicians for particular case studies as the best entree to clinical education, medical vocabulary, as scientifically based, may remain a language of generalization rather than a description of unique events. Alternatively, medicine might be seen to involve, by its very nature, the personal application of general information. According to this view, while generalizations concerning biology and pathology underlie the epistemology of allopathic medicine, the function of the practitioner is to abstract essential information from these generalizations relevant to individual patients.

Whichever of the above interpretations one adopts, the patient's experience of suffering does not admit either of medical generalizations or of easy abstraction from such generalizations to particular circumstances. The question remains, then, how the health-care professional can bridge the gap between diagnostic generalizations and the patient's unique experience of illness (McCullough, 1989).

A compassion-based medicine must involve the quest for a commonly shared language of suffering through an awareness of the patient as a person rather than the patient as the passive locus of disease (the latter is a view that the metaphors of medicine as warfare serve to reinforce). To view the patient as a person requires a careful entering into the patient's own life-world, attention to the patient's unique efforts to restore integrity and meaning, and the recognition that medicine, by touching upon life-transforming events, often involves the need to encounter the transcendent. The organizational and institutional obstacles to this interpersonal encounter between health-care professionals and their patients remain formidable.

According to Howard Brody, if compassion is to become a standard of excellence for clinical practice, the physician must be willing "to adopt a position of relative powerlessness," to "acknowledge that the patient's suffering has incredible power over him and that he cannot remain unchanged in the face of it" (Brody, 1992, p. 259). Compassion, then, will emerge from a sense of shared vulnerability that can serve as an antidote to potential abuses of power in a structurally unequal relationship. At the same time, compassion has the potential to empower patient and physician to find new identities in their vulnerability to the reality of suffering. Indeed, vulnerability provides an interesting cipher to the mystery of compassion; besides its usual passive sense of "being liable to be wounded," it retains an archaic active sense of "having the power to wound." The art of compassionate medicine, then, will require of the physician an openness to the wounding power of the patient's vulnerability.

Care and compassion as an alternative paradigm for ethics. In recent years, an ethic of care has been proposed as an alternative to the regnant emphasis in ethics on principles and rules. Compassion and care are not identical. Compassion refers primarily to the attitude or disposition to identify with and respond to another's suffering, whereas a substantive notion of care requires one to specify more fully what compassion motivates in particular circumstances. Moreover, care may involve several different underlying attitudes, including impersonal respect, although it is very often associated with the disposition that characterizes compassion. Thus, while care and compassion remain distinct notions, they are sufficiently similar that they can be jointly considered as providing an alternative basis for understanding morality and ethics.

Carol Gilligan argues that the language of "justice and rights" has shaped male norms, values, and virtues, while that of "care and responsiveness" has defined female norms, values, and virtues. Women construe moral problems from the perspective of conflicting responsibilities rather than competing rights; moral resolution requires, therefore, a particularism that stresses the dimensions of interpersonal narrative and embedded context (Gilligan, 1982). Other theorists suggest that a "feminine" ethic of caring is an effect of patriarchal domination, rather than a distinctive expression of gender-based differences (Kymlicka, 1990).

The differences proposed between an ethic of care and an ethic of principles involves three characteristic aspects: Care emphasizes moral dispositions rather than moral principles, is characteristically case-oriented and particularistic rather than universal in scope, and speaks primarily about responsibilities and relationships rather than rights and justice (Kymlicka, 1990).

Reactions to Gilligan's thesis vary. Some see the languages of principles and caring as used more or less equally by both men and women, depending upon the context of ethical reasoning. In interpersonal relations, for example, an ethic of compassion and care may resolve problems in ways that an appeal to impartial principles fails to address. In the case of larger societal and institutional concerns, however, appeals to impartiality, especially when compromise and trade-offs are necessary, may better comport with our considered judgments about justice and public policy. Others argue, moving beyond Gilligan, that dispositions of compassion or care are not merely necessary but also sufficient for morality. Nel Noddings suggests that principles provide us with prima facie duties, but that such duties "yield no real guidance in concrete situations" (Noddings, 1984, p. 85). Only particular caring relations can specify our moral choices and actions. Noddings claims that her position avoids relativism because right and wrong are always specified according to one ideal: "maintenance of the caring relation" (Noddings, 1984, p. 85). Critics of the position Noddings defends suggest that principles, rather than abstractions from particularity, often function as general considerations that help one to determine which features are morally salient (Grimshaw, 1986). Moreover, if compassion is "misguided" or "grounded in superficial understanding of a situation," it can be harmful (Blum, 1980, p. 516). The appeal to principles can often serve to widen the lens of compassion's narrower focus.

Finally, the dichotomy between the languages of responsibility and rights, central to Gilligan's thesis, has drawn sharp criticism from a number of quarters. Distinctions drawn between care and responsibility, on the one side, and rights and impartiality on the other, may be overdrawn. For all but libertarian conceptions of rights, positive rights are meaningful entitlements that require correlative responsibilities from those against whom claims are lodged. A number of feminists also dispute the dichotomy drawn between care and impartiality, suggesting that benevolence as a motive can support principled commitments to justice (Okin, 1989). The discussion of compassion and care as an alternative paradigm to principlism will continue, but more nuanced depictions of both approaches are called for, and some form of "complementarity thesis" seems likely to emerge.

B. ANDREW LUSTIG

For a further discussion of topics mentioned in this entry, see the entries BUDDHISM; CARE; EMOTIONS; FEMINISM; HINDUISM; ISLAM; JAINISM; JUSTICE; LOVE; MEDICAL CODES AND OATHS; MEDICAL ETHICS, HISTORY OF, *section on* EUROPE, *subsection on* ANCIENT AND MEDIEVAL, *article on* GREECE AND ROME, *and subsections on* RENAISSANCE AND ENLIGHTENMENT, *and* NINETEENTH CENTURY; NARRATIVE; OBLIGATION AND SUPEREROGATION; PAIN AND SUFFERING; PROFESSION AND PROFESSIONAL ETHICS; PROTESTANTISM; RIGHTS; ROMAN CATHOLICISM; *and* VIRTUE AND CHARACTER. *For a further discussion of related ideas, see the entries* AUTONOMY; CONFUCIANISM; EASTERN ORTHODOX CHRISTIANITY; MEDICINE, ART OF; NURSING, THEORIES AND PHILOSOPHY OF; PASTORAL CARE; PROFESSIONAL–PATIENT RELATIONSHIP; SIKHISM; TAOISM; *and* WOMEN. *See also the* APPENDIX, (CODES, OATHS, AND DIRECTIVES RELATED TO BIOETHICS), SECTION I: DIRECTIVES ON HEALTH-RELATED RIGHTS AND PATIENT RESPONSIBILITIES; SECTION II: ETHICAL DIRECTIVES FOR THE PRACTICE OF MEDICINE; *and* SECTION III: ETHICAL DIRECTIVES FOR OTHER HEALTH-CARE PROFESSIONS.

Bibliography

ARISTOTLE. 1984. *Complete Works.* Edited by Jonathan Barnes. Princeton, N.J.: Princeton University Press.
BLUM, LAWRENCE. 1980. "Compassion." In *Explaining Emotions,* pp. 507–517. Edited by Amelie Oksenberg Rorty. Berkeley: University of California Press.
BRODY, HOWARD. 1992. *The Healer's Power.* New Haven, Conn.: Yale University Press.
BROWN, CHARLOTTE. 1992. "Moral Sense Theorists." In vol. 2 of *Encyclopedia of Ethics,* pp. 862–868. Edited by Lawrence C. Becker and Charlotte B. Becker. New York: Garland.
CAIRNS, HUNTINGTON, and HAMILTON, EDITH, eds. 1969. *The Collected Dialogues of Plato.* Princeton, N.J.: Princeton University Press.
CASSELL, ERIC J. 1991. *The Nature of Suffering and the Goals of Medicine.* New York: Oxford University Press.
COWARD, HAROLD G.; LIPNER, JULIUS J.; and YOUNG, KATHERINE K. 1989. *Hindu Ethics: Purity, Abortion, and Euthanasia.* Albany: State University of New York Press.
GILLIGAN, CAROL. 1982. *In a Different Voice: Psychological Theory and Women's Development.* Cambridge, Mass.: Harvard University Press.
GRIMSHAW, JEAN. 1986. *Philosophy and Feminist Thinking.* Minneapolis: University of Minnesota Press.
HUME, DAVID. 1948. "A Treatise of Human Nature. Book III: 'Of Morals.'" In *Hume's Moral and Political Philosophy,* pp. 31–169. Edited by Henry D. Aiken. New York: Hafner.
KANT, IMMANUEL. 1964. *Groundwork of the Metaphysic of Morals.* 3d ed. Translated by Herbert James Paton. New York: Harper & Row.
KYMLICKA, WILL. 1990. *Contemporary Political Philosophy: An Introduction.* New York: Oxford University Press.
MCCULLOUGH, LAURENCE B. 1989. "The Abstract Character and Transforming Power of Medical Language." *Soundings* 72:111–125.
NODDINGS, NEL. 1984. *Caring: A Feminine Approach to Ethics and Moral Education.* Berkeley: University of California Press.
OKIN, SUSAN MOLLER. 1989. "Reason and Feeling in Thinking About Justice." *Ethics* 99, no. 2:229–249.
OUTKA, GENE H. 1972. *Agape: An Ethical Analysis.* New Haven, Conn.: Yale University Press.
PLATO. 1969. *The Collected Works of Plato, Including the Letters.* Edited by Edith Hamilton and Huntington Cairns. Princeton, N.J.: Princeton University Press.
REICH, WARREN THOMAS. 1989. "Speaking of Suffering: A Moral Account of Compassion." *Soundings* 72 (Spring): 83–108.
REISER, STANLEY J.; DYCK, ARTHUR J.; and CURRAN, WILLIAM J., eds. 1977. *Ethics in Medicine: Historical Perspectives and Contemporary Concerns.* Cambridge, Mass.: MIT Press.
SCHOPENHAUER, ARTHUR. 1965. *On the Basis of Morality.* Translated by E. F. J. Payne. Indianapolis, Ind.: Bobbs-Merrill.
SMITH, ADAM. 1990. *The Theory of Moral Sentiments.* 6th ed. Charlottesville, Va.: Ibis.

COMPETENCE

Competence is a necessary condition before a physician can accept a patient's treatment consent or refusal. Competence confers decision-making authority on those who are competent, while disenfranchising those who are not (Beauchamp, 1991). A determination of patient competence promotes respect for self-determination as well as patient participation in health-care and other decision making. In most nonemergency situations, those who are legally competent may consent to or refuse health care. A patient maintained for years on outpatient hemodialysis, for example, may be allowed to terminate hemodialysis, resulting in death, if the patient decides that he or she can no longer tolerate the stress of the procedure (Neu and Kjellstrand, 1986). And based upon religious reasons, a Jehovah's Witness may even refuse a blood transfusion that would otherwise save his or her life. In contrast, the consent or refusal of those who are legally incompetent or clinically incapacitated need not be respected. A psychotic woman who refuses to have a cardiac pacemaker inserted because she believes that others could then monitor and control her activities would not be permitted to refuse this life-sustaining surgical procedure. Competence is usually not a relevant issue in health-care emergencies, when treatment delay would be substantially harmful to the patient.

Competence and autonomy are often conflated, although their meanings are quite distinguishable (Beauchamp, 1991). Competence allows a person to exercise his or her autonomy. One must be autonomous to be competent, yet competent persons may act nonautonomously when, for example, compelled to do so by another person. Further, an autonomous person may act incompetently (e.g., a professional negligent at work).

This entry considers some of the issues in defining, determining, and assessing competence, as well as some of the applications of competence to the field of mental-health care.

Definitions

Generically, "competence" means simply the ability to perform a particular task (Beauchamp, 1991), although it has often been used loosely in several senses. In health-care contexts, competence is the capacity to make autonomous health-care decisions (Morreim, 1991). In most accounts of competence, competence is specific to the task or issue, since a person may be able to perform one task but not another. Few people are globally competent or incompetent. Since one's abilities change over time, in either direction, competence is also specific to time. Abilities may also be a function of the conditions or the situation in which they are tested or the person who tests them.

Competencies, of course, relate to all areas of function (Grisso, 1986). While competence to consent to health care or research is of primary concern in the present context, issues are often raised about a person's abil-

ity to work, manage personal finances, make a contract, write a will, live independently, drive a car, marry and divorce, parent a child, or testify in court. In legal contexts, competence questions arise in civil actions as well as in criminal litigation (competence to stand trial, commit a crime, enter a plea, or be sentenced) (Bonnie, 1992). Legal competencies implicate past decision making (e.g., competence to write a will), present decision making (e.g., competence to stand trial), or future decision making (e.g., competence to manage one's financial affairs).

A person's competence may be questioned in more than one area. In the case of a mother with cancer and a psychotic depressive disorder who is separated from her husband, for example, questions may arise about her capacity to parent her children, manage her finances, and consent to medical or psychiatric care. If she were employed, questions may arise about her ability to function at work if she failed to meet deadlines or otherwise fulfill her job duties due to a medical or psychiatric disorder. Her or her husband's attorney may question her ability to consult with her attorney and participate in the divorce litigation.

This contextualized, decision-specific notion of competence may be contrasted with a more generalized conception that reflects the general legal and moral autonomy enjoyed by most adults in contemporary Western cultures (Wear, 1991). Many more adults are considered competent under the general conception than the task-specific one; therefore, establishing that a person is incompetent is more difficult under the former than the latter.

"Incompetence" has come to mean the loss in court of a person's legal right to function in some particular area. Such a narrow legal definition of competence or incompetence contrasts with the more common clinical use of incompetence according to which a person has a legal right to function but is unable to do so. Clinical and legal competence may not correspond. An elderly, demented person, for example, may have the legal right to drive a car or make his or her own health-care decisions but may no longer be substantially able to do so. Similarly, an adolescent may not be legally competent to consent to health care but may be clinically or functionally able to do so.

The increasingly prevalent view is that individuals have various specific abilities or capacities as well as incapacities, each along a continuum. A person is considered incapacitated when the person is no longer able to perform that specific function and incompetent when a court has so ruled. Legally, there is a presumption of competence, which may be overcome when the court is presented with adequate evidence of incapacitation. In the clinical literature, however, competence refers either to an individual's capacities (a descriptive definition) or to whether that individual's particular capacities are sufficient to render legal decision-making authority to him or her (a threshold definition).

Finally, although competence usually refers to a person's abilities, it may also refer to his or her actions or behavior (Beauchamp, 1991). For example, a person of general competence may autonomously choose to act incompetently in a given situation (e.g., intentionally fail an examination).

Managing incompetence

Because functional or decision-making capacities occur on a continuum and because a person's capacities can be expected to fluctuate over time, in most cases a clinician need not be resigned to accept a patient as permanently incapacitated. The clinician frequently has opportunities to enhance the person's functional or decision-making capacity. Hearing aids, eyeglasses, psychotropic medication, counseling and psychotherapy, and specific behavioral training in the area of incapacity are examples of remedial efforts that can be made to improve a person's capacity. When such efforts fail, disposition of those who are incapacitated is a complex matter and varies with the context in question. In a case where life-saving treatment may be needed, the clinician may have to obtain an adjudication of legal incompetence in order to treat an incompetent refusing patient.

Although competence is a necessary precondition to respecting patient choice, incompetence is not a sufficient condition to overriding it, contrary to much clinical and lay understanding. The clinician may wish to, and often should, respect a person's preferences even if the person is legally incompetent or functionally incapacitated. The clinician may ask a young boy with which parent he prefers to live following his parents' divorce; the clinician probably will ask an elderly, demented woman whom she prefers to manage her estate should the appointment of a legal guardian be authorized.

Before intervening over the person's objection, the clinician needs to specifically assess the risks, benefits, and alternatives; this includes an evaluation of the potential harms of a proposed intervention to the person. Overriding treatment refusals, whether by a health-care professional, family member, or court, ethically and legally requires evidence that (1) such treatment would benefit the patient (the "best interests" test); (2) such treatment would have been the decision of the patient had he or she been able to make the decision (the "substituted judgment" test); or (3) the patient had provided some previous direction or instruction about the treatment in question ("expressed interest" test). The test of substitute decision making varies with the decision, the decision maker, and the legal jurisdiction. Use of the substituted-judgment or the expressed interest test, in contrast to the best-interests test, better respects the person's autonomy and self-determination.

Competence criteria

There is no international clinical, legal, philosophical, or ethical consensus about competence criteria or standards, and many are in use. In other words, there is no agreement about the threshold of decision-making or functional capacity necessary to consider a person legally or morally competent. In a given case, there may be wide consensus among clinicians, legal professionals, and ethicists that a particular person is, or is not, competent in some respect; however, disagreement is likely in many cases. In part, this derives from the fact that competence determinations are not essentially factual, objective, or empirical matters but rather are value-laden judgments about the relative importance of autonomy and beneficence to the person, as assessed by the clinician or others. Competence is typically inferred from the person's behavior and thinking rather than observed directly, and evaluators may differ in their judgment of the person's competence. Such differences about the person's competence occur in part due to evaluators' varying perceptions of the person's values or of the person's rationality. Under the most common view, competence is not a fixed property of an individual applicable to all decisions and all potential risks; rather, competence is a context-dependent, decision-specific, interpersonal process (Buchanan and Brock, 1989; Drane, 1985).

Criteria for competence involve whether the person can make a choice, communicate that choice, understand relevant information about the choice and its alternatives, and rationally manipulate information about the choice and its alternatives (Appelbaum and Grisso, 1988). The person must be able to apply the relevant information about a prospective decision to his or her own case rather than in the abstract or as applied to someone else.

The influential U.S. President's Commission for the Study of Ethical Problems in Medicine and Biomedical and Behavioral Research adopted a standard of capacity that requires (1) possession of a set of values and goals; (2) the ability to communicate and to understand information; and (3) the ability to reason and to deliberate about one's choices (U.S. President's Commission, 1982). This standard emphasizes the process of reasoning or decision making rather than the particular outcome of the decision. A competence standard that focuses upon the outcome of the decision can be faulted for granting greater priority to the values of the person assessing the patient's competence than to the values of the patient.

A similar definition of competence is offered by the Canadian province of Ontario: "Mentally competent means having the ability to understand the subject-matter in respect of which consent is requested and able to appreciate the consequences of giving or withholding consent" (Ontario Ministry of Health, 1987). This "appreciation" component, however, involves emotional rather than strictly cognitive considerations, and broadens the competence standard.

As noted by the U.S. President's Commission, assessment of the individual's current and previous personal values is an essential component of evaluating competence. Obtaining a values history for the individual provides critical information about the person's past major life decisions relevant to the present decision making. Judgments about a person's competence must be individualized according to his or her attitudes and values history rather than reflect only the person's knowledge, skills, and cognitive capacities.

It is unrealistic to expect that competence criteria are, or will remain, fixed over time. Competence criteria are likely to evolve as society seeks to resolve the conflict between the competing principles of respect for autonomy and concern for the person's well-being.

Sliding scale of competence criteria.   The predominant approach to selecting competence criteria, at least with regard to competence to consent to health care, depends on the actual decision at issue. In this scheme, named the "sliding scale," the criteria for competence vary with the particular decision and its risks and benefits. As the risks of the proposed health care increase or as the benefits to the proposed health care decrease, more capacity is required for the patient to be considered competent to consent to the health care (Drane, 1985; Roth et al., 1977). For example, it is less difficult to decide to consent to a course of conventional antibiotic medication for a urinary tract infection than a course of experimental chemotherapy for stomach cancer, and less capacity should be required to do so. Likewise, more capacity is required for the patient to be considered competent to refuse health care when its risks decrease or its benefits increase.

Although the sliding-scale approach to competence criteria is commonly used in health-care decision making, some problems accompany its use. Given the strong bias of health-care professionals—and society—in favor of treatment, one concern is that professionals will manipulate or selectively use those competence criteria that result in labeling competent someone who consents to health care, while labeling incompetent someone who refuses care. Another concern of the variable standard approach is that, counterintuitively, a patient could be considered competent to consent to a particular intervention but incompetent to refuse that same intervention (Buchanan and Brock, 1989). This may occur because refusing health care is more complicated than

consenting to it, but here too a protreatment bias is evident.

Competence assessments

Clinicians frequently make informal judgments about a patient's competence in their daily work; but some cases, such as treatment refusals or consents by questionably competent patients, necessitate formal, detailed assessments. Competence assessments should focus on the specific area of function in question. Assessments of global or general competence are unlikely to adequately respond to the presenting question. Among the procedural considerations in conducting competence assessments, the time and place of examination and the need for reexamination are especially important (Weiner and Wettstein, 1993). These assessments sometimes use written structured or formal assessment inventories of functioning, observational functional assessments (e.g., observing a patient grocery shopping and preparing a meal), psychological testing, or formal psychiatric interviews. History taking and collateral reports from third-party informants such as family, friends, and other health-care personnel can be valuable additions to individual contact with the person being assessed. The examiner pays particular attention to eliciting information about the patient's decision-making history and the values he or she has placed on personal autonomy, health care, disability, and death. Consultations with colleagues or second opinions may also be helpful to the examiner in difficult cases. In general medical hospitals, competence assessments are conducted initially by nonpsychiatric physicians; if necessary, psychiatric consultants are called to assist in the evaluation.

Competence assessments raise many problematic clinical issues including denial of illness; subtle forms of incapacity; impact of elevated or depressed mood on decision-making capacity; fluctuating mental status (due to intermittent treatment compliance, the natural course of the disorder, or side effects of treatment); treatment refusals based on religious reasons; lack of information about the patient, including personal values and goals or history of treatment refusals; lack of formal staff training to do competence assessments; and disagreements among staff about the appropriate competence criteria or threshold. Typically, competence is not challenged, investigated, or formally assessed in clinical practice until a patient refuses treatment or is noncompliant with it.

Competence and mental-health care

The presence of a mental disorder does not automatically negate the presumption of a person's competence. Although some severely mental ill persons are indeed incapacitated in many areas of their functioning, most mentally ill persons have only some discrete areas of decision-making incapacity, often confined to episodes of their illness. A paranoid delusional patient who denies that he is mentally ill, for example, may be unable to rationally decide whether or not to consent to antipsychotic medication while he is mentally ill but may have adequate decision-making ability to consent to treatment for diabetes and heart disease. In such a case, the content of the patient's paranoid delusions would be irrelevant to the patient's diabetes and heart disease, and the patient would not deny the fact of his medical illnesses. A patient in a manic episode may be unable to manage his finances because he will rapidly dissipate them, but his decision-making capacity will return as the episode ends. Subtle forms of decision-making incapacity can also arise from mildly altered mood states (depression, hopelessness, anxiety, euphoria), from cognitive dysfunction (impairment in memory or attention from head injury), or from personality traits (guilt, self-punishment, feelings of worthlessness).

Competence to refuse psychotropic medication. In contrast to admission to a medical-surgical hospital, admission to a psychiatric hospital may be accomplished by voluntary or involuntary means. In either facility, however, there may be uncertainty about the patient's ability to consent to voluntary hospitalization. Patients who are demented or seriously depressed or psychotic often have difficulty understanding that they are ill, need treatment, or should be hospitalized. They may have difficulty comprehending the risks and benefits of treatment and hospitalization. Nevertheless, decisions about the person's ability to consent to voluntary hospitalization precede, and differ from, decisions about the person's ability, once hospitalized, to consent to treatment with medication.

Managing a person's refusal of psychotropic medication (e.g., antipsychotic or antidepressant medication), once he or she has been hospitalized, has been one of the most controversial issues in mental-health care in recent years. Before the 1980s, many rejected the notion of a psychiatric patient's right to refuse medication, suggesting that the purpose of psychiatric hospitalization would be defeated if patients were permitted to refuse treatment with medication (Appelbaum, 1988). In part, the controversy about involuntary treatment of psychiatric inpatients with medication arose from the nature and effects of psychotropic medication. Psychotropic medications have been viewed somewhat inaccurately as powerful and dangerous substances whose use is akin to "mind control." Their risks, whether short-term dry mouth and constipation or long-term involuntary movement disorders, relative to their benefits, the treatment of the mental disorder, have been greatly exaggerated, at least by many attorneys and courts (Gutheil and Appelbaum, 1983).

Once patients enter psychiatric hospitals, especially on an involuntary basis by court order, they sometimes refuse recommended treatment with psychotropic medication, particularly antipsychotic medication. Patients refuse treatment based on problems in the physician–patient relationship, such as rebelliousness towards authority figures and reality-based side effects of medication (e.g., dry mouth, constipation, weight gain, restlessness), or most relevant in the present context, symptoms of the patient's illness, such as a delusional belief that the medication is poison. Decisions about hospitalizing a person involuntarily differ from those about medicating that person involuntarily once hospitalized; the former are largely a function of the person's future risk of violence to self or others due to a mental disorder, while the latter usually depend upon the person's ability to make decisions about accepting medication or his or her best interests. An involuntarily hospitalized patient, even one committed by a court, is not necessarily deemed unable to consent to medication. In most cases, a person who has been involuntarily hospitalized does not lose the legal right to object to or to refuse medication.

Voluntarily hospitalized patients who refuse medication for whatever reason may not be medicated involuntarily, except briefly in emergency situations. It is argued that patient autonomy regarding treatment refusal should be respected despite the consequences of continued illness, hospitalization, and incapacity. This legal right to refuse medication is based on the patient's right to free speech and thought, to freedom from bodily intrusion, the right to bodily integrity, a ban on cruel punishment, and the right to autonomy and self-determination.

Nevertheless, involuntarily hospitalized patients who refuse medication may sometimes be medicated involuntarily in nonemergency situations, as well as briefly in emergencies. Many states in the United States use a judicial model for these cases in which forced medication of involuntarily hospitalized patients may be accomplished only after a judicial hearing and court determination that the patient is incompetent to refuse the mediation because of the mental illness (Weiner and Wettstein, 1993). A substitute decision maker is sometimes appointed by the court to determine whether the patient should be compelled to take medication. This is the same procedure that would be followed if the physician sought involuntary surgery (e.g., amputation of a gangrenous extremity) on the patient. In contrast, in some U.S. states and in some Canadian provinces, the attending physician or a medical or administrative review panel decides whether or not to override the patient's refusal; the patient may then appeal the physician or panel's decision to involuntarily medicate to a court (Weiner and Wettstein, 1993; Ontario Ministry of Health, 1987). In England, the Mental Health Act of 1983 permits the treating physician to authorize medication for up to three months to an incompetently refusing, involuntarily hospitalized patient (section 56); after that, a second physician opinion is needed to continue the involuntary treatment (section 58) (Appelbaum, 1985). In this nonjudicial model, the patient's decision-making capacity about medication as assessed by the attending physician may still be the most important factor in the disposition of the case. However, the U.S. Supreme Court has held that decision-making capacity is not relevant to determining whether prisoners should be medicated involuntarily with psychotropic drugs (*Washington v. Harper*, 1990).

According to empirical data about the right to refuse psychotropic medication, the judicial-review model, using a formal incompetence declaration, carries substantial fiscal costs, given the delays inherent in obtaining the required court hearing. It also involves prolonged periods of nontreatment pending the hearing, which often results in injuries to the patient, other patients, and staff (Ciccone et al., 1993; Hoge et al., 1990). Few courts ultimately grant the patient a right to refuse medication.

Competence for execution.   According to U.S. law civil or criminal litigants must be legally competent before they can bring suit or have suit brought against them. In criminal law, defendants must be competent to stand trial, plead guilty, be sentenced, or be executed before those proceedings can occur.

Executing a person who is considered incompetent (i.e., "insane") at the time of execution, as opposed to at the time of the crime, has been ruled unconstitutional by the U.S. Supreme Court (*Ford v. Wainwright*, 1986). Execution in such cases offends humanity, has no deterrent value to others, and offers no retribution to the condemned person. The courts, however, have yet to articulate a competence standard by which to adjudicate a death-row inmate as incompetent (Winick, 1992).

The courts have not yet decided whether, once death-row inmates have been found incompetent, the state may involuntarily medicate them to restore competence and then execute them (*Louisiana v. Perry*, 1990). Such an eventuality places the treating psychiatrist, who ethically must not participate in an execution, in a difficult dilemma: Medicate the inmate to relieve suffering, which leads to the inmate's death, or do not medicate the inmate, which spares the inmate's life but fails to reduce suffering (Heilbrun et al., 1992). Only automatic commutation of an incompetent death-row inmate to life in prison would definitively resolve the matter.

Conclusion

Whether in health-care, financial, legal, or any other area of decision making, the stakes for both persons and professionals in competence definitions are substantial.

Identifying and labeling someone as incompetent can be stigmatizing and deprives the person of self-determination. Legal and health-care delivery systems are then confronted with, and disrupted by, the need for surrogate decision making for the incapacitated or incompetent person. On the other hand, failure to protect the incapacitated person from making erroneous and harmful decisions (e.g., refusing necessary medical care) may not honor the person's best interests. The question then is when and how to respect people's choices and maximize their decision-making autonomy while protecting them from their own harmful choices (Drane, 1985). In most cases in the health-care system, clinicians agree that the person should, or should not, be considered competent, even if there is no universal consensus on how much rationality and understanding are sufficient for the person to be considered legally competent and granted authority to decide for him- or herself. Still, there are other cases in which judgments about the person's decision-making capacity are problematic, and clinicians, administrators, patients, families, and the courts become involved in emotionally charged disputes about how to manage the person's medical care. Such cases are unlikely to abate in the future as long as our society continues to value, and attempts to balance, autonomy and beneficence.

Robert M. Wettstein

Directly related to this entry is the entry Autonomy. *For a further discussion of topics mentioned in this entry, see the entries* Adolescents; Aging and the Aged, *article on* health-care and research issues; Children, *articles on* health-care and research issues, *and* mental-health issues; Death and Dying: Euthanasia and Sustaining Life, *article on* ethical issues; Informed Consent, *article on* legal and ethical issues of consent in health care *(with its* postscript*)*; Law and Bioethics; Mental-Health Services, *article on* ethical issues; Mental Illness; Mentally Disabled and Mentally Ill Persons; Patients' Rights, *article on* mental patients' rights; Prisoners; *and* Psychopharmacology. *For a discussion of related ideas, see the entries on* Beneficence; Paternalism; *and* Value and Valuation. *Other relevant material may be found under the entries* Behavior Control; Commitment to Mental Institutions; *and* Women, *especially the articles on* health-care issues, *and* research issues.

Bibliography

Appelbaum, Paul S. 1985. "England's New Commitment Law." *Hospital and Community Psychiatry* 36, no. 7:705–706, 713.

———. 1988. "The Right to Refuse Treatment with Antipsychotic Medications: Retrospect and Prospect." *American Journal of Psychiatry* 145, no. 4:413–419.

APPELBAUM, PAUL S., and GRISSO, THOMAS. 1988. "Assessing Patients' Capacities to Consent to Treatment." *New England Journal of Medicine* 319, no. 25:1635–1638.

BEAUCHAMP, TOM L. 1991. "Competence." In *Competency: A Study of Informal Competency Determinations in Primary Care*, pp. 49–78. Edited by Mary Ann Gardell Cutter and Earl E. Shelp. Dordrecht, Netherlands: Kluwer.

BONNIE, RICHARD J. 1992. "The Competence of Criminal Defendants: A Theoretical Reformulation." *Behavioral Sciences and the Law* 10, no. 3:291–316.

BUCHANAN, ALLEN E., and BROCK, DAN W. 1989. *Deciding for Others: The Ethics of Surrogate Decision Making.* Cambridge: At the University Press.

CICCONE, J. RICHARD; TOKOLI, JOHN F.; GIFT, THOMAS E.; and CLEMENTS, COLLEEN D. 1993. "Medication Refusal and Judicial Activism: A Reexamination of the Effects of the *Rivers* Decision." *Hospital and Community Psychiatry* 44, no. 4:555–560.

DRANE, JAMES F. 1985. "The Many Faces of Competency." *Hastings Center Report* 15, no. 2:17–21.

Ford v. Wainwright. 1986. 477 U.S. 399.

ONTARIO MINISTRY OF HEALTH. 1987. *Mental Health Act: Revised Statutes of Ontario.* Toronto: Queen's Printer for Ontario.

GRISSO, THOMAS. 1986. *Evaluating Competencies: Forensic Assessments and Instruments.* New York: Plenum.

GUTHEIL, THOMAS G., and APPELBAUM, PAUL S. 1983. "'Mind Control,' 'Synthetic Sanity,' 'Artificial Competence,' and Genuine Confusion: Legally Relevant Effects of Antipsychotic Medication." *Hofstra Law Review* 12:77–120.

GUTHEIL, THOMAS G., and BURSZTAJN, HAROLD. 1986. "Clinicians' Guidelines for Assessing and Presenting Subtle Forms of Patient Incompetence in Legal Settings." *American Journal of Psychiatry* 143, no. 8:1020–1023.

HEILBRUN, KIRK; RADELET, MICHAEL L.; and DVOSKIN, JOEL. 1992. "The Debate on Treating Individuals Incompetent for Execution." *American Journal of Psychiatry* 149, no. 5:596–605.

HOGE, STEVEN K.; APPELBAUM, PAUL S.; LAWLOR, TED; BECK, JAMES C.; LITMAN, ROBERT; GREER, ALEXANDER; GUTHEIL, THOMAS G.; and KAPLAN, ERIC. 1990. "A Prospective, Multicenter Study of Patients' Refusal of Antipsychotic Medication." *Archives of General Psychiatry* 47, no. 10:949–956.

Louisiana v. Perry. 1990. 498 U.S. 38.

MORREIM, E. HAAVI. 1991. "Competence: At the Intersection of Law, Medicine, and Philosophy." In *Competency: A Study of Informal Competency Determinations in Primary Care*, pp. 93–125. Edited by Mary Ann Gardell Cutter and Earl E. Shelp. Dordrecht, Netherlands: Kluwer.

NEU, STEVEN, and KJELLSTRAND, CARL M. 1986. "Stopping Long-Term Dialysis: An Empirical Study of Withdrawal of Life-Supporting Treatment." *New England Journal of Medicine* 314, no. 1:14–20.

ROTH, LOREN H.; MEISEL, ALAN; and LIDZ, CHARLES W. 1977. "Tests of Competency to Consent to Treatment." *American Journal of Psychiatry* 134, no. 3:279–284.

U.S. PRESIDENT'S COMMISSION FOR THE STUDY OF ETHICAL PROBLEMS IN MEDICINE AND BIOMEDICAL AND BEHAVIORAL RESEARCH. 1982. *Making Health Care Decisions: A Report on the Ethical and Legal Implications of Informed Consent in the Patient–Practitioner Relationship.* Washington, D.C.: Author.

Washington v. Harper. 1990. 110 S.Ct. 1028.

WEAR, STEPHEN. 1991. "Patient Freedom and Competence in Health Care." In *Competency: A Study of Informal Competency Determinations in Primary Care*, pp. 227–236. Edited by Mary Ann Gardell Cutter and Earl E. Shelp. Dordrecht, Netherlands: Kluwer.

WEINER, BARBARA A., and WETTSTEIN, ROBERT M. 1993. *Legal Issues in Mental Health Care.* New York: Plenum.

WINICK, BRUCE J. 1992. "Competency to Be Executed: A Therapeutic Jurisprudence Perspective." *Behavioral Sciences and the Law* 10, no. 3:317–337.

CONFIDENTIALITY

Confidentiality has its roots in the human practice of sharing and keeping secrets (Bok, 1984). For children, the desire to keep a secret is a manifestation of an emerging sense of self; the desire to share a secret stems from a need to retain or establish intimate relationships with others (Ekstein and Caruth, 1972). The willingness to share secrets presupposes an implicit trust or an explicit promise that they will be dept. Keeping and sharing secrets is a more complex social practice among adults. Some adults keep secrets simply to preserve their personal privacy; others may have something illegal or immoral to hide. Some persons do not reveal private thoughts, feelings, or behavior for fear of embarrassment, exploitation, stigmatization, or discrimination. Still others feel a need to disclose secrets to others to help resolve emotional conflicts or seek solutions to problems arising out of interpersonal relationships. The sharing and keeping of secrets among friends, for instance, creates a context in which ethical issues concerning promises, trust, loyalty, and interests of others may come into conflict. For example, I may promise a friend to keep a secret that she feels an urgent need to tell me. She trusts me not to tell anyone else about her revelation. Out of loyalty to my friend, I promise in advance to keep her secret. But I am thrown into a moral conflict when she unexpectedly discloses her impulse and plan to kill a family member who she believes is plotting against her. I realize that my obligations to keep my promise and preserve loyalty and trust conflict with a desire, if not a responsibility, to prevent my friend's harm to herself as well as serious harm to another. Do I preserve confidentiality or protect others? Similar ethical conflicts arise for health professionals and their clients or patients.

The following discussion clarifies the concept of confidentiality and the related ideas of privacy and privileged communication in health-care settings. The rights of clients/patients and the responsibilities of health professionals to their clients, their professions, and society bring out key ethical issues. Legal regulations both protect and limit confidentiality, sometimes in ways that create ethical conflicts for clients as well as professionals. In health-care contexts neither absolute protection nor total abandonment of confidentiality is plausible. Yet sometimes it is uncertain where boundaries should be drawn because legitimate interests come into conflict. Personal privacy, professional integrity, effective care, economic considerations, and public health and safety influence both general policies and specific practices concerning confidentiality.

Conceptual analysis

Confidentiality is closely related to the broad concept of privacy and the narrower concept of privileged communications. All three concepts share the idea of limiting access of others in certain respects (Gavin, 1980; Allen, 1988). Privacy refers to limiting access of others to one's body or mind, such as through physical contact or disclosure of thoughts or feelings. The idea of limited access describes privacy in a neutral way. But privacy is closely linked to normative values. Privacy is usually thought to be good; it is something that individuals typically desire to preserve, protect, and control. Thus privacy and a right to privacy are sometimes not clearly distinguished. In law and ethics "privacy" usually refers to privacy rights as well as limited access. Thus, privacy in law is linked to freedom from intrusion by the state or third persons. It may designate a domain of personal decision, usually about important matters such as personal associations, abortion, or bodily integrity.

Confidentiality concerns the communication of private and personal information from one person to another where it is expected that the recipient of the information, such as a health professional, will not ordinarily disclose the confidential information to third persons. In other words, other persons, unless properly authorized, have limited access to confidential information. Confidentiality, like privacy, is valued because it protects individual preferences and rights.

Privileged communications are those confidential communications that the law protects against disclosure in legal settings. Once again, others have limited access to confidential information. A person who has disclosed private information to a spouse or certain professionals (doctor, lawyer, priest, psychotherapist) may restrict his or her testimony in a legal context, subject to certain exceptions (Smith-Bell and Winslade, 1994; Weiner and Wettstein, 1993).

Privacy and confidentiality are alike in that each stands as a polar opposite to the idea of "public": what is private and confidential is not public. Yet privacy and confidentiality are not the same. Privacy can refer to singular features of persons, such as privacy of thoughts, feelings, or fantasies. Confidentiality always refers to relational contexts involving two or more persons. Privacy can also refer to relational contexts, such as privacy of personal associations or private records. Thus, in this respect the concepts overlap. In many relational contexts the terms "privacy" and "confidentiality" are used interchangeably and sometimes loosely. Professional codes of ethics, for example, often use these terms in this way (Winslade and Ross, 1985).

It should be noted, however, that privacy and confidentiality are significantly different in one important respect. Relinquishing personal privacy is a precondition for establishing confidentiality. Confidentiality requires a relationship of at least two persons, one of whom exposes or discloses private data to the other. An expectation of confidentiality arises out of a special relationship between the parties created by their respective roles (doctor–patient, lawyer–client) or by an explicit promise. Confidentiality, as with its linguistic origins (con and fides: with fidelity), assumes a relationship based on trust or fidelity. Between strangers there is no expectation of trust. Privacy is given up because confidentiality is assured; unauthorized persons are excluded.

Yet confidentiality does not flow simply from the fact that personal or private information is divulged to another. If persons choose to announce their sexual preferences in street-corner speeches, in books, or on billboards, this information, though private in its origin, is not confidential. Confidentiality depends not only on the information, but also on the context of the disclosure as well as on the relationship between the discloser and the recipient of the information. Confidentiality applies to personal, sensitive, sometimes potentially harmful or embarrassing private information disclosed within the confines of a special relationship. It should be noted, however, that the disclosure of private information from client to professional is one-way, unlike other interpersonal confidentiality contexts (Winslade and Ross, 1985).

Rights of patients/clients

When clients enter into a health-care relationship, they relinquish some personal privacy in permitting physical examinations, taking tests, or giving social and medical histories. Usually this information is documented in a medical record, often stored electronically and held by the health professional or an institution. In exchange for the loss of privacy, clients expect and are promised some degree of confidentiality. In general, all personal medical information is confidential unless the client requests disclosure to third parties or a specific exception permits or requires disclosure. For example, clients may request disclosure to obtain insurance coverage or permit disclosure to a scientific researcher. The law requires health professionals to report certain infectious diseases to public-health departments or to report suspected child abuse to appropriate agencies. Unilateral disclosure of otherwise confidential information to third parties by health professionals or institutions is unethical unless it is authorized by the client or by law.

In the United States and other Western societies, the values of privacy, confidentiality, and privileged communications are closely tied to the values of personal rights and self-determination. These rights include freedom from the intrusion of others into one's private life, thoughts, conduct, or relationships. Interest in protection of personal rights has grown in response to public and private surveillance of individuals through the use of data bases to collect, store, and transmit information about individuals (Flaherty, 1989). In the United States the ideas of privacy and confidentiality have generated much legal and philosophical scholarship, influenced important judicial decisions, and prompted federal and state legislation (Winslade and Ross, 1985). The legal doctrine and ethical ideal of informed consent in health care reinforces the importance of personal autonomy (Beauchamp and Childress, 1989). The right to informed consent, applied specifically to confidentiality, gives patients/clients the right to control disclosure of confidential information. Other countries with less individualistic traditions do not place such high ethical value on privacy or personal rights. Even persons in cultures where privacy is not a prominent value can be harmed, however, by revelations of personal information (Macklin, 1992).

Traditional ethical theories can be interpreted to provide additional support for the values of privacy and confidentiality. Deontology stresses the rights of persons and the duties of others to respect persons as ends in themselves, to respect especially their personal rights. To the extent that the social practices tied to privacy and confidentiality enhance the welfare of all, utilitarianism may also be invoked on behalf of individuals. Virtue theory advocates personal moral aspiration and achievement. Privacy and confidentiality provide a context and an opportunity for cultivation of virtues without outside interference.

Despite the value of privacy and confidentiality to individuals, however, other values—such as collective need for information or public health and safety—limit individual rights. Confidentiality conflicts often arise about information contained in medical records. Cli-

ents usually want information to remain confidential. Others—such as employers, insurers, family members, researchers, and litigants—exert pressure to limit confidentiality and to gain access to personal information. Health professionals are often pulled in both directions by their professional loyalty to patients/clients and their broader social responsibilities.

Responsibilities of health professionals

The responsibilities of health professionals, as articulated in codes of professional ethics, reinforce the value of confidentiality. For example, the Hippocratic oath states:

> What I may see or hear in the course of the treatment or even outside of the treatment in regard to the life of men, which on no account one must spread abroad, I will keep to myself, holding such things shameful to be spoken about. (see Appendix)

Modern codes of professional ethics, like the Principles of Ethics of the American Medical Association, instruct physicians to "safeguard patient confidences within the constraints of the law" (see Appendix). Similarly, ethics codes for psychotherapists, nurses, and other allied health professionals make general, though not always coherent, reference to protection of professional–client confidentiality (Winslade and Ross, 1985). The American Psychiatric Association, however, has also issued detailed official Guidelines on Confidentiality pertaining to special situations, records, special settings, and the legal process (Committee on Confidentiality, 1987). The American Bar Association has offered a handbook, *AIDS/HIV and Confidentiality Model Policy and Procedures*, that addresses the value of confidentiality, consent to disclosures, third-party access to information, and penalties for unauthorized disclosures (Rennert, 1991). The Council on Ethical and Judicial Affairs of the American Medical Association (1992) outlines the scope and value of confidentiality and addresses in detail confidentiality in the context of computerized medical records. These documents stress individual rights and specify professional responsibilities concerning confidentiality.

Despite the explicit attention given to confidentiality in oaths and codes, practical ethical problems arise, occasionally causing heated controversy. For instance, in 1991 an authorized biography of the deceased poet Anne Sexton relied in part upon audiotapes of psychotherapy sessions. One of Sexton's psychiatrists permitted the biographer to listen to some 300 hours of psychotherapy tapes. Prior to the publication of the biography, a front-page story in the *New York Times* about the disclosure of the tapes to the biographer generated a furious ethical debate. On the one hand, some critics believed that release of the tapes violated the deceased patient's privacy. Others pointed out the harm to surviving family members. Still others stressed the duty of the psychiatrist not to reveal anything about the content of therapy. Unless the therapist was required by law to release the information on the tapes, these critics argued, confidentiality should have been preserved. On the other hand, the psychiatrist claimed that his duty was primarily to protect his patient's interests—including her interest in self-revelation, in being understood, and in helping others. The psychiatrist believed that the patient, when competent, had specifically authorized him to use his own best judgment about what to do with the tapes. He also believed that he should cooperate with the request of the patient's literary executor—her daughter—to help make the biography accurate and complete. None of the relevant ethics codes sufficiently clarified or specifically addressed a case of this kind. Although charges were brought that the psychiatrist violated the code of ethics of the American Psychiatric Association, eventually a decision was reached that no ethics violation occurred. But a still-unsettled controversy swirls around these issues.

Professionals are often more aware of confidentiality issues than patients or clients. Professionals realize that privacy and confidentiality may give way to the institutional, governmental, and other third-party pressures for specific information about patients or clients. Health professionals desire to protect the integrity and special value of the professional–client relationship itself. Confidentiality is one basis of professionals' reciprocity with clients who reveal private information. (Other aspects of reciprocity include the clients' payment for the professionals' services in response to the professionals' expertise to meet the clients' needs.)

It should be emphasized that the primary justification for confidentiality is derived from the individual rights of clients and is supplemented by the responsibilities of professionals and the benefits of the health-care relationship. This is why the client, rather than the health professional, determines what information is to remain confidential. Except where laws or other rules limit clients' rights to confidentiality, the client may not only request but require professionals to disclose otherwise confidential information. It is, after all, the client's private information that has been revealed to the professional.

Some recent critics, including feminist theorists, have questioned the adequacy of rights-based approaches. They argue that an ethics of care or caring must take account of a web of relationships, emotions, and values that include but go beyond individual rights. A care-based ethics stresses the interactive relationships, not only of patients and clinicians, but also families and society. Within the context of caring, humans—especially those who experience special suffering or discrimination—need more than just protection of their legal rights. In the specific context of privacy and confidentiality in medical genetics, for example, an ethics of care rather than rights may better explain the moral reasoning of geneticists (Wertz and Fletcher, 1991). This is discussed further in the later section on genetic and other medical screening.

Other critics think that the preservation of confidentiality should take priority over clients' and professionals' autonomy. This idea is based on the idea that total confidentiality is essential to protect both the integrity and the effectiveness of the professional–client relationship. No third parties should ever be permitted to penetrate the boundaries of a protected professional relationship. Neither the client nor the professional, according to this view, should be required or even permitted to disclose confidential information. Something close to this extreme position was considered but rejected by the California Supreme Court in *Lifshutz* (1970). Neither professional organizations nor their ethics codes endorse this idea, but it does highlight the importance that can be ascribed to confidentiality.

Even if the ideal of complete confidentiality cannot be justified in theory, it can sometimes be achieved in practice. A dyadic, exclusive relationship between client and health professional can sometimes fully preserve confidentiality. For example, a client establishes a relationship with a psychotherapist to explore the meaning of a significant personal loss. The client may not want others to know about the consultation. It is nobody else's business.

The therapist's office may have a separate entrance and exit to decrease the likelihood that clients will encounter each other. The therapist may answer personally all phone calls. The therapist may keep no client-specific records and take no notes. The client may pay cash, not file a claim for insurance coverage, explicitly request that all discussions be kept confidential, and take other precautions to prevent others from learning even that the relationship with the therapist exists at all. The client reveals his or her feelings, fantasies, thoughts, or dreams only to the therapist, who seeks to understand and help interpret their meaning only to the client.

If client confidentiality and professional secrecy were always as unambiguous as the foregoing scenario, there would be little more to say. However, professionals as well as clients have widely divergent attitudes, beliefs, expectations, and values concerning confidentiality (Wettstein, 1994). A few professionals espouse the absolute value of confidentiality in dyadic therapeutic relationships while many others acknowledge only its limited and relative value. Others lament the declining value of confidentiality while accepting the encroachment of legal, economic, public-health and safety, or research interests. A few others view confidentiality as an inflated value that some professionals or clients use as a shield to conceal fraud, malpractice, or even criminal activity.

Rather than a simple dyadic relationship, a more complex, polycentric model is necessary to capture the nuances of confidentiality in health care. Clients, health professionals, and third parties may have varying claims on ethical grounds to protection of or access to confidential information. Clients may waive their rights to confidentiality to obtain other benefits such as insurance coverage or employment. Professionals may discern a conflict between ethical obligations to their clients and legally required reports. Third parties may have a legitimate need to know otherwise confidential information to assess quality of health-care services, uncover fraud, or determine appropriate allocations of health-care resources. Loss of confidentiality may result not only from ethical, legal, or economic factors, but also because of client ignorance or misunderstanding, professional or institutional carelessness, or third-party overreaching. The interplay of those various factors can best be understood by examining in more detail selected problem areas where confidentiality comes into conflict with competing ethical and social interests.

AIDS

The acquired immunodeficiency syndrome (AIDS) epidemic brings with it a full range of confidentiality issues. Patients who think that they might be HIV-positive are reluctant to be tested for fear that disclosure of such sensitive information may cause them to lose employment or insurance coverage or may make them subject to other types of discrimination. Yet if they are not tested, the benefits of clinical care to diminish the damage of the disease are not available. Patients who know that they are HIV-positive may not want others to know of their status to prevent discrimination. But third parties, such as sexual partners, who are at risk of being infected with a lethal virus, have a legitimate interest in access to otherwise confidential information. If the infected person is unwilling to inform others who may be at risk of getting AIDS, health professionals may be permitted or even required to warn persons who have been or may be put at risk of being infected. Family members may want to know why their relative is sick; they may need to know if they become caretakers. But patients may not be willing to disclose their diagnosis. Health-care workers want to know their patients' HIV status just as patients want to know if their caretakers are infected. Both desire to avoid becoming infected themselves. Those

who are at risk of infection may have a justifiable need to know; others may not.

Confidentiality is not the only value at stake, but it does impose substantial burdens on others. For example, in institutional settings, confidentiality of personal information, such as a patient's diagnosis, must be protected by written policies and actual practices. In a recent court case in Maryland, a hospital failed to protect adequately a patient's medical record that included a diagnosis of AIDS. It is not sufficient to state a policy that access to medical records is limited. It is also necessary to have and implement policies that actually restrict physical access to the records (Brannigan, 1992). The hospital was negligent because it did not go far enough to limit physical access of unauthorized persons to the records.

Required reporting

Legal rules that require health professionals to report child or elder abuse, infectious diseases, or gunshot wounds preempt many of the specific ethical conflicts between confidentiality and public health or safety. However, not all ethical issues are resolved by legal rules. For example, some child-abuse–reporting laws are overly broad; health professionals may fail to make mandated reports in part because of the value ascribed to client confidentiality. Other reporting laws are so narrow that protection of threatened victims is undermined by confidentiality rules and practices (Miller and Weinstock, 1987). Some commentators have pointed out, for example, the conflicts created by statutes that require the reporting of not only actual but also suspected child abusers. Some parents alleged to have abused their children have been required to undergo therapy; but to require them to admit abuse before conducting therapy conflicts with the constitutional privilege against self-incrimination.

Professionals, caught between the need for confidentiality in therapy and the legal demand for reporting abuse, sometimes underreport abuse; they protect therapeutic relationships at the risk of legal liability. Other professionals may overreport child abuse because of their concerns about legal liability, strained therapeutic relationships, vulnerability of potential victims, or uncertainty about the value of confidentiality. Some commentators have suggested that child-abuse statutes should be revised to be more specific and limited, requiring professionals to report only when their patients are victims of child abuse, but to give professionals greater discretion about whether to report abusers who are in treatment (Smith-Bell and Winslade, 1994).

Another ethical problem for health professionals that arises in connection with legally required disclosures of otherwise confidential information is what to tell clients prior to or near the outset of therapy. If clients are inadequately apprised about the limits of confidentiality, their trust in health professionals is damaged and their relationship may be ruptured. If clients are fully advised of the legal limits placed on confidentiality, they may withhold essential information, terminate therapy, or not even start it. A further problem is that professionals may not know precisely where legal lines have been drawn. For example, a therapist may know that notification must be made to authorities but may not know how much, if any, of the content of therapy must be disclosed.

Genetic and other medical screening

Genetic and other types of medical screening by epidemiologists, physicians, employers, schools, and other public and private agencies give rise to situations in which confidentiality is threatened by a demand for personal medical information. Individuals who are screened want to control information about themselves to prevent stigma, loss of insurance or employment, or other forms of discrimination. Screeners desire access to such information to promote their interests in knowledge, scientific discovery, publication, or economic considerations as well as therapeutic purposes. Control over the information raises moral issues as well as practical problems. These values must be balanced against individuals' rights to preserve their informational privacy. Blood tests, family medical histories, personal medical histories, DNA assays, and data banking, for instance, all raise questions about confidentiality, access, and control of personal information (De Gorgey, 1990). Lack of consensus about ethical priorities, gaps in legal policies and remedies to individuals, and political uncertainty about jurisdiction and control over medical screening combine to create controversy. Protection of individual rights of privacy and confidentiality requires careful monitoring of the use of data banks to store information obtained by the Human Genome Project (Macklin, 1992).

Health professionals in genetics differ in their beliefs about the value of privacy and confidentiality. Considerable disagreement has been documented, for example, in an international study in nineteen countries of the attitudes of geneticists toward privacy and disclosure. These health professionals were asked to respond to vignettes concerning disclosure of false paternity; of a patient's genetic makeup to a spouse; to relatives at genetic risk; of ambiguous test results; and to institutional third parties, such as employers and insurers (Wertz and Fletcher, 1991). Some consensus as well as numerous differences were discovered among the geneticists' opinions about what disclosures are appropriate.

Dorothy Wertz and James Fletcher also found that geneticists' reasoning was more likely to be based on the complex needs and relationships of the various parties rather than the rights of individuals. A care-based ethics approach poses a theoretical and practical alternative to a rights-based approach.

Legal protections and limitations

Legal protection of confidentiality in the United States has been sporadic and uneven. The 1974 Federal Privacy Act (P.L. 93-579) included some medical information and records; its passage signaled heightened congressional awareness of threats to privacy and confidentiality. The National Privacy Commission's report (U.S. Domestic Council, 1976) seemed to set the stage for further protective federal legislation. Several subsequent attempts to pass comprehensive federal laws to protect medical information failed; a patchwork of state statutes provides only limited protection of patients' confidentiality. The reason is that patients' interests in confidentiality are balanced against powerful interests of third parties, such as health-care payers, governmental agencies, researchers, and law-enforcement agencies, who wish to have access to otherwise confidential medical information (Hendricks et al., 1990).

Courts have been as hesitant as federal and state legislatures to provide stringent protection of patient confidentiality. The U.S. Supreme Court considered but rejected the idea that patients enjoy a constitutional right to "informational privacy" with regard to treatment records (*Whalen v. Roe*, 1977). This decision was rendered when the rhetoric of privacy was prominent in Supreme Court opinions; in the 1980s the right to privacy was restricted, and the rhetoric of privacy diminished. State courts, such as those in Florida and California, whose constitutions make explicit reference to a right to privacy, have been more inclined to protect confidentiality of medical information. But state laws provide infrequently enforced bureaucratic protections or opportunities for recovery of damages only after confidentiality has been violated. Even then, litigation is rare because patients are reluctant to further expose confidential matters, damages are difficult to prove, and awards are often limited by statute (Winslade, 1982).

In some settings, such as substance-abuse treatment programs, the federal government has established special rules to protect confidentiality. To encourage persons in need of treatment to enter substance-abuse programs, records are not disclosed to law-enforcement agencies that might otherwise seek to prosecute substance abusers. In sensitive human subject research, special "privacy certificates" can be obtained by researchers from the federal government to give added protection to confidential information. Similarly, coded and locked files, limited access even to authorized personnel, and other precautionary measures against leakage further enhance confidentiality (McCarthy and Porter, 1991).

Public concern about confidentiality surfaces periodically, especially concerning the potential evils of misuses of patient-identifiable information. For example, implications of the Human Genome Project and health-care reform have most recently evoked anxiety about discrimination, violation of personal rights, and commerce in patient information. The potential for a new health-care information infrastructure that relies heavily on computer technology to facilitate the flow of medical information dramatically increases the threat to confidentiality of medical records (Brannigan, 1992). Recent commentaries remind us that current legal policies are inadequate to protect individuals against unwarranted disclosure, to provide security for complex medical-information systems, and to preserve individuals' rights to consent and control the uses of personal medical information (Alpert, 1993; Gostin et al., 1993).

A specific area of law that directly affects confidentiality concerns the obligations of psychotherapists whose potentially violent patients place other individuals at risk of harm. The California Supreme Court, in the case of Tarasoff v. Regents of the University of California (1974), ruled that psychotherapists of dangerous patients have a duty to use reasonable care to protect threatened victims from harm. To do so may require the disclosure of otherwise confidential patient information. In balancing public safety and confidentiality, the Court observed that "the protective privilege ends where the public peril begins."

In the Tarasoff case, a psychotherapist believed that his patient was potentially dangerous to a young woman who had rejected his interest in her. The patient was obsessed with her at the expense of his studies, his work, and his friends. When the patient talked of revenge and was thought to have a gun, the therapist sought to have his patient evaluated for involuntary hospitalization. But the police declined to bring the patient in for an assessment of his mental status. The patient, angry with his therapist, abruptly terminated treatment. A couple of months later the former patient killed the young woman. Her parents sued the therapists and their employer for failing to warn the victim or her family about the dangerous patient. Although this case was settled out of court without a trial, the reasonable-protection rule was articulated by the court for future cases.

Subsequently, a series of judicial decisions have elaborated the duty of psychotherapists to third parties. Some courts have restricted the duty to situations in which there is an imminent threat of serious violence toward an identifiable victim. Others have focused on the broader duty of health professionals to control the conduct of the dangerous patient. Still others have applied the Tarasoff standard even when the risk to others is neither serious nor specific. And a few courts have protected confidentiality rather than endorse the Tarasoff standard (Felthous, 1989).

The complexity of particular cases and the variability of judicial interpretations of facts and laws inevitably cause some uncertainty. In this context, as in many others, confidentiality is limited by other important values. For example, suppose a voluntary psychotic in-patient with no history of violence leaves the hospital against medical advice. He leaves behind some written notes that include violent fantasies about a family member. His therapist discovers the notes (which were left unsealed). Assume the therapist consults the patient, who demands confidentiality; but the therapist is concerned that the patient may be dangerous. The therapist must assess the probability of harm to the patient or the potential victim, consider alternatives to revealing confidential information, and decide what, if anything, to tell the patient, the threatened victim, or others. This delicate balancing inevitably occurs in contexts where information is incomplete, contextual nuances are elusive, and human behavior is notoriously difficult to predict. Nevertheless, decisions must be made and actions taken that will affect the scope of confidentiality as well as bring about other consequences.

Information about limits of confidentiality

When entering into a professional–client relationship, clients have a right to receive explicit information about the scope and limits of confidentiality. Most nonprofessionals assume that disclosures made in the context of health care are confidential (Weiss, 1982). Most clients are uninformed about the limits of confidentiality and pressures to reveal presumably confidential information to third parties. Some clients realize that there are legal and ethical restrictions on confidentiality in health care, but others learn of them only after an undesired disclosure (Siegler, 1982).

Clients for whom confidentiality is especially important may take steps to preserve it. For example, a medical patient who chooses to file an insurance claim may request the right to review all documents released to the insurance carrier. Or the patient may pay privately rather than file an insurance claim. Other clients may be less concerned with confidentiality. Clients have a responsibility to inform themselves about what expectations about confidentiality are reasonable; then they will not be surprised or dismayed because of false assumptions about confidentiality.

Professionals have a responsibility to inform themselves as well as their clients about legal, ethical, and practical aspects of confidentiality. For example, neither patients nor health professionals usually are familiar with the practices of insurance companies concerning redisclosure of confidential information. Patients often sign a blanket waiver of confidentiality in order to obtain insurance benefits. This information may then be sold by the insurer to the Medical Information Bureau, a clearinghouse to protect against insurance fraud. This goal is laudable, but the data-banking process may include erroneous information that is difficult to detect or correct. In addition, many other interests outside health care—such as employers, government agencies, educational institutions, and the media—may gain access to information contained in these data bases (Linowes, 1989; Alpert, 1993).

At the very least, professionals should ask their clients what they want to know about confidentiality. Some professionals prepare a disclosure statement to give each new client, that is, a document that outlines confidentiality practices the particular professional follows. Policies and procedures concerning written medical records might be given to each new client. Further conversation, including clients' questions and professionals' answers, can clarify details that written statements may not address. Because professionals, like their clients, may differ in their attitudes toward confidentiality, it is important that disclosures about confidentiality be particularized. For example, the values of a psychoanalyst in private practice who never publishes patient case reports significantly differs from those of a research-oriented psychoanalyst who tapes and transcribes every session and publishes detailed case reports. Each should fully inform clients about the nature of his or her practice (Stoller, 1988).

Professionals have an obligation to take precautionary measures to protect confidentiality even if their clients have not requested it. Professionals should assume that all client information (including the very existence of the professional–client relationship as well as personal and private information revealed) is strictly confidential unless the client has requested or waived disclosure or unless the law requires it. Professionals should advise their clients of required disclosures, inform them of waivers, explore with them the consequences of disclosing or not disclosing information, and examine the reasons for and against disclosure. But clients retain the authority to decide what voluntary disclosures are to be made to third parties (Winslade and Ross, 1985).

Professionals also have a special responsibility to protect confidential client information from leakage through lax office procedures, professional or personal gossip, or the inappropriate inquiries of unauthorized persons. This is particularly problematic in institutional settings, where many individuals may have routine access to patient information contained in medical records

(Siegler, 1982). As computerization of medical records expands further and information storage, retrieval, and distribution technologies become more sophisticated, the need for professionals' vigilance increases.

Many third parties—government officials and agencies, insurance interests, employers, family members, researchers, and others—seek specific information about particular patients. Third parties should not assume, however, that mere interest gives them legitimate authority to have access to confidential information. Third parties have a responsibility to justify to patients and professionals their need for access to confidential information. In some instances, this may require only a routine inquiry and documentation, but in other situations, professionals may find it necessary to confirm that their patients have requested, waived, or forfeited their rights to confidentiality. Too often, professionals, especially in an institutional setting, capitulate to pressure to disclose more information than necessary to third parties. At the very least, third parties as well as professionals should notify patients when access is sought, how it will be used, and whether the information will be redisclosed to anyone else. If appropriate disclosures are made to patients before access to confidential information is granted to third parties, not only will confidentiality be better preserved, but patients will also be better served.

WILLIAM J. WINSLADE

Directly related to this entry are the entries PRIVACY IN HEALTH CARE; PRIVACY AND CONFIDENTIALITY IN RESEARCH; PRIVILEGED COMMUNICATIONS; RIGHTS, *article on* RIGHTS IN BIOETHICS; FIDELITY AND LOYALTY; TRUST; *and* PROFESSIONAL–PATIENT RELATIONSHIP, *article on* ETHICAL ISSUES. *For a further discussion of topics mentioned in this entry, see the entries* AIDS; CARE, *article on* CONTEMPORARY ETHICS OF CARE; HEALTH-CARE FINANCING, *article on* HEALTH-CARE INSURANCE; HEALTH OFFICIALS AND THEIR RESPONSIBILITIES; REPRODUCTIVE TECHNOLOGIES, *articles on* ETHICAL ISSUES, *and* LEGAL AND REGULATORY ISSUES; *and* SUBSTANCE ABUSE. *This entry will find application in the entries* ABORTION; FERTILITY CONTROL, *article on* ETHICAL ISSUES; GENETIC COUNSELING; HEALTH SCREENING AND TESTING IN THE PUBLIC-HEALTH CONTEXT; LABORATORY TESTING; LIFESTYLES AND PUBLIC HEALTH; MEDICAL INFORMATION SYSTEMS; *and* MENTAL-HEALTH SERVICES. *Other relevant material may be found under the entries* AUTONOMY; BENEFICENCE; CLINICAL ETHICS, *article on* ELEMENTS AND METHODOLOGIES; ETHICS, *article on* NORMATIVE ETHICAL THEORIES; *and* MEDICAL CODES AND OATHS. *See also the* APPENDIX (CODES, OATHS, AND DIRECTIVES RELATED TO BIOETHICS), SECTION II. ETHICAL DIRECTIVES FOR THE PRACTICE OF MEDICINE, *and* SECTION III. ETHICAL DIRECTIVES FOR OTHER HEALTH-CARE PROFESSIONS.

Bibliography

ALLEN, ANITA L. 1988. *Uneasy Access: Privacy for Women in a Free Society*. Totowa, N.J.: Rowman & Littlefield.

ALPERT, SHERI. 1993. "Smart Cards, Smarter Policy: Medical Records, Privacy and Health Care Reform." *Hastings Center Report* 23, no. 6:13–23.

BEAUCHAMP, TOM L., and CHILDRESS, JAMES F. 1989. *Principles of Biomedical Ethics*. 3d ed. New York: Oxford University Press.

BOK, SISSELA. 1984. *Secrets: On the Ethics of Concealment and Revelation*. New York: Oxford University Press.

BRANNIGAN, VINCENT M. 1992. "Protecting the Privacy of Patient Information in Clinical Networks: Regulatory Effectiveness Analysis." *Annals of the New York Academy of Sciences* 670:190–201.

COMMITTEE ON CONFIDENTIALITY. AMERICAN PSYCHIATRIC ASSOCIATION. 1987. "Guidelines on Confidentiality." *American Journal of Psychiatry* 144, no. 11:1522–1527.

DE GORGEY, ANDREA. 1990. "The Advent of UNA Databanks: Implications for Information Privacy." *American Journal of Law and Medicine* 16, no. 3:381–398.

EKSTEIN, RUDOLF, and CARUTH, ELAINE. 1972. "Keeping Secrets." In *Tactics and Techniques in Psychoanalytic Therapy*, pp. 200–215. Edited by Peter L. Giovacchini. New York: Science House.

FELTHOUS, ALAN R. 1989. *The Psychotherapist's Duty to Warn or Protect*. Springfield, Ill.: Charles C. Thomas.

FLAHERTY, DAVID H. 1989. *Protecting Privacy in Surveillance Societies: The Federal Republic of Germany, Sweden, France, Canada, and the United States*. Chapel Hill: University of North Carolina Press.

GAVISON, RUTH. 1980. "Privacy and the Limits of Law." *Yale Law Journal* 89, no. 3:421–472.

GOSTIN, LAWRENCE O.; TUREK-BREZINA, JOAN; POWERS, MADISON; KOZLOFF, RENE; FADEN, RUTH; and STEINAUER, DENNIS. 1993. "Privacy and Security of Personal Information in a New Health Care System." *Journal of the American Medical Association* 270, no. 20:2487–2493.

HENDRICKS, EVAN; HAYDEN, TRUDY; and NOVIK, JACK. 1990. *Your Right to Privacy: A Basic Guide to Legal Rights in an Information Society*. 2d ed. Carbondale: Southern Illinois University Press.

Lifshutz, In re. 1970. 467 P.2d 557 (Cal.).

LINOWES, DAVID F. 1989. *Privacy in America: Is Your Private Life in the Public Eye?* Urbana: University of Illinois Press.

MACKLIN, RUTH. 1992. "Privacy and Control of Genetic Information." In *Gene Mapping: Using Law and Ethics as Guides*, pp. 157–172. Edited by George J. Annas and Sherman Elias. New York: Oxford University Press.

McCARTHY, CHARLES R., and PORTER, JOAN P. 1991. "Confidentiality: The Protection of Personal Data in Epidemiological and Clinical Research Trials." *Law, Medicine and Health Care* 19, nos. 3–4:238–241.

MILLER, ROBERT D., and WEINSTOCK, ROBERT. 1987. "Conflict of Interest Between Therapist-Patient Confidentiality and the Duty to Report Sexual Abuse of Children." *Behavioral Sciences and the Law* 5, no. 2:161–174.

RENNERT, SHARON. 1991. *AIDS/HIV and Confidentiality: Model Policy and Procedures*. Washington, D.C.: American Bar Association.

SIEGLER, MARK. 1982. "Confidentiality in Medicine—A Decrepit Concept." *New England Journal of Medicine* 307, no. 24:1518–1521.

SMITH-BELL, MICHELE, and WINSLADE, WILLIAM J. 1994. "Privacy, Confidentiality, and Privilege in Psychotherapeutic Relationships." *American Journal of Orthopsychiatry* 64, no. 2:180–193.

STOLLER, ROBERT J. 1988. "Patients' Responses to Their Own Case Reports." *Journal of the American Psychoanalytic Association* 36, no. 2:371–391.

Tarasoff v. Regents of the University of California. 1974. 529 P.2d 553 (Cal.); 551 P.2d 334 (Cal. 1976).

U.S. DOMESTIC COUNCIL. COMMITTEE ON THE RIGHT OF PRIVACY. 1976. *National Information Policy: Report to the President of the United States*. Washington, D.C.: Author.

WEINER, BARBARA A., and WETTSTEIN, ROBERT M. 1993. "Confidentiality." In *Legal Issues in Mental Health Care*. New York: Plenum.

WEISS, BARRY D. 1982. "Confidentiality Expectations of Patients, Physicians, and Medical Students." *Journal of the American Medical Association* 247, no. 19:2695–2697.

WERTZ, DOROTHY C., and FLETCHER, JOHN C. 1991. "Privacy and Disclosure in Medical Genetics Examined in an Ethics of Care." *Bioethics* 5, no. 13:212–232.

WETTSTEIN, ROBERT M. 1994. "Confidentiality." *Review of Psychiatry* 13:343–364.

Whalen v. Roe. 1977. 97 S. Ct. 869.

WINSLADE, WILLIAM J. 1982. "Confidentiality of Medical Records: An Overview of Concepts and Legal Policies." *Journal of Legal Medicine* 3, no. 4:497–533.

WINSLADE, WILLIAM J., and ROSS, JUDITH WILSON. 1985. "Privacy, Confidentiality, and Autonomy in Psychotherapy." *Nebraska Law Review* 64:578–636.

CONFLICT OF INTEREST

In a conflict of interest, one's obligations to a particular person or group conflict with one's self-interest. A physician, for example, is ordinarily obligated to provide his or her patients with only the care that is reasonable and medically necessary, even though the physician may earn more money through unnecessary interventions. Conflicts of interest should be distinguished from conflicts of obligation, in which one's obligations to one person or group conflict with one's obligations to some other person or group. The latter need not per se involve any threat to the agent's own interests. For example, a physician is normally obligated to keep patients' medical problems confidential; however, when a patient poses a danger to others, as by transmitting AIDS to a spouse, the physician may have an obligation to protect that third party by violating the confidentiality that would otherwise be owed to the patient. This essay focuses specifically on conflicts of interest. In the health-care context, conflicts of interest can arise for individual providers such as physicians, dentists, nurses, or physical therapists, or for institutions such as hospitals, health maintenance organizations (HMOs), insurers, or pharmaceutical companies.

Conflicts of interest can be found in any human endeavor; indeed, the clash between self-interest and altruism lies at the heart of morality (Jonsen, 1983). However, conflicts of interest in health care are especially serious because of the patient's vulnerability. Illness can impair a patient physically, emotionally, and rationally. To secure treatment, patients must expose physical and emotional intimacies normally reserved for loved ones, and frequently must face further risks from invasive diagnostic and therapeutic technologies. Patients usually have no choice but to submit to such exposure and risk, because typically they lack the knowledge and skill to identify and treat the illness or, for that matter, to ascertain whether care is being rendered appropriately (Morreim, 1991). This vulnerability creates ample opportunities for providers to exploit patients for personal gain. Physicians or dentists might recommend costly, unnecessary care, or an insurer or HMO might lure subscribers by promising more than it can deliver.

Accordingly, providers are often regarded as fiduciaries, in both a moral and a legal sense. Fiduciaries hold beneficiaries' (here, the patients') interests in trust and are obligated to promote the latter's interests, even above their own. This includes physicians and dentists (*Batty v. Arizona State Dental Board*, 1941; *Berkey v. Anderson*, 1969; *Lockett v. Goodill*, 1967; *Moore v. Regents of the University of California*, 1990), hospitals (*Wohlgemuth v. Meyer*, 1956; *Darling v. Charleston Community Memorial Hospital*, 1965), and insurance companies (*Brown v. Blue Cross & Blue Shield of Alabama*, 1990; Chittenden, 1991). It is a small step from there to regard HMOs similarly (Chittenden, 1991). Nursing and allied health professions are not ordinarily considered fiduciaries in the legal sense but do share a strong ethic of dedication to patients' interests.

For many years a serious commitment to professionalism and an effacement of self-interest seemed a sufficient response to conflicts of interest. The traditional fee-for-service system admittedly encouraged some unnecessary services, but prior to the mid-twentieth century providers had relatively few interventions to offer, beyond their own care and concern. As technologies emerged, a relative shortage of providers meant that each had more than enough to do. Furthermore, in the long-term relationships of mainly rural health care, providers had to live with the consequences of their decisions, right alongside their patients. Exploitive or abusive practices thus carried strong disincentives (Relman, 1983).

Since about the mid-1960s, however, health care has become high cost, and big business. Providers now face a plethora of conflicts of interest, ranging from the traditional but much-exacerbated conflicts implicit in fee-for-service, to powerful pressures to cut the cost of care by doing less for patients. Because physicians play such a central role in the economics of health care, this article initially will focus special attention on their conflicts. These arise in two distinct realms: the clinical setting, where medical care is primarily designed to help the patient; and the research setting, where physicians seek scientific knowledge and only sometimes aim to benefit the patient or research subject. Conflicts faced by other health professionals and by institutions will also be addressed, followed by some remarks concerning the moral management of conflicts of interest.

Physicians: Conflicts of interest in the clinical setting

In the clinical setting, a number of factors can encourage a physician to alter the patient's optimal care to secure a personal gain or to avoid a loss. Conflicts can be posed by third-party payers, institutional health-care providers, private industry, the legal system, and physician investment (Rodwin, 1993).

Third-party payers. Traditional fee-for-service reimbursement encourages physicians to deliver as many services as possible and, in a maneuver called "unbundling," to break down each service into as many separately billable small interventions as possible. Maximizing income may thus mean excessive care that, in turn, threatens needless inconvenience, expense, and iatrogenic injury for patients.

Partly because of this inflationary reimbursement system, health-care costs have grown at an alarming rate, consuming some 12 percent of the gross domestic product by 1990, with projections to reach 15 to 20 percent by the year 2000. In response, those who pay directly for health care—government, businesses, and insurers—have placed powerful pressures on physicians to do less for their patients. Payers have sometimes offered bonuses to physicians to discharge patients earlier, and often have refused to pay for designated tests and surgeries unless they are performed in an outpatient setting. Through extensive utilization review (UR), many payers reimburse only hospitalizations or medical interventions that meet their private criteria of medical necessity. Physicians therefore must spend large amounts of time, usually uncompensated, justifying their plans of care to payers' UR personnel in order to secure reimbursement (Morreim, 1991a).

Capitation systems attempt to save money by paying a single fee for a large unit of care, thereby creating an incentive to avoid rendering care beyond the budgeted fee. Medicare, for example, inaugurated its diagnosis-related-group (DRG) system in the early 1980s, paying hospitals a set amount for a specific episode of illness, based on such factors as the patient's diagnosis, age, and coexisting illnesses. HMOs, in a broader capitation concept, agree to provide all necessary health care for each of their subscribers in exchange for a single annual premium. In order to ensure that their physicians deliver services within the year's budget, virtually all HMOs apply a system of financial incentives. Typically 20 percent or more of the physician's salary or fees is withheld, to be paid (or not) at the end of the year, depending on the HMO's financial health. Many HMOs also set aside a special fund for diagnostic tests, consultants, and hospitalization. Primary-care physicians, acting as gatekeepers whose permission is required for the patient to gain access to these services, share any surplus funds—or debts—that remain at the end of the year (Hillman, 1987). These arrangements can make a substantial difference in the physician's year-end income, thereby providing a powerful incentive for physicians to economize on the level of care they provide or authorize for patients (Berenson, 1987). Some patients have initiated lawsuits alleging that these incentives have caused misdiagnosis or delayed care (Shimm and Spece, 1991).

All payment systems create conflicts of interest. There is incentive to provide more of the services that are best reimbursed and less of those that are not. However, the challenge has been markedly exacerbated through recent expansion of health-care costs. Every medical decision is a spending decision, yet payers ordinarily cannot control their costs by directly dictating what care the physician will and will not provide. To do so would be to practice medicine in the physician's stead. Rather, payers attempt to influence physicians, who control up to 80 percent of health-care costs through their power of prescription and their professional influence over patients. That influence is almost always gained by placing physicians' personal interests in peril as they are rewarded or penalized for fiscally (im)prudent health-care decisions (Morreim, 1991a).

Institutional providers. Institutional health-care providers such as hospitals and clinics often establish incentives that can encourage physicians to do more or to do less, depending on the institution's purpose (proprietary or charitable) and the patient's economic status (well-insured or not). A for-profit walk-in clinic, for instance, makes its money through the tests and treatments its physician-employees order. Hence, high-profit physicians may be praised and invited to share

profits, or even to own a share of the business, while low-profit physicians may receive administrative warnings or lose their jobs if they do not improve (Bock, 1988). A proprietary hospital may induce physicians to join its staff with perquisites such as free office space, bookkeeping services, and malpractice insurance (Institute of Medicine, 1986). Physicians who fail to admit enough well-insured patients, however, may lose such benefits. In other cases, physicians and hospitals may enter into joint ventures to share the profits and risks of running the facility (Institute of Medicine, 1986).

Whether proprietary or charitable, all institutional providers need to contain the costs of the care they provide. Monthly printouts comparing the costs of each physician's care may be publicized at staff meetings to shame the high spenders into delivering more conservative care. And those whose patients consistently leave too many unpaid bills may lose their staff privileges in a strategy called "economic credentialing" (Blum, 1991).

Such incentives systematically place physicians in conflicts of interest. The potential loss of income, peer esteem, staff privileges, or one's job creates powerful pressures to align one's judgment with the institution's best interests, even at some cost to patients' best interests.

Private industry. Many medical drugs and devices are sold only with the prescription of a licensed physician, and are not readily advertised to the general public. Therefore, manufacturers' marketing typically targets physicians. Because physicians tend to be busy people with substantial incomes, advertising can go to great lengths to catch their attention. Promotions have included all-expense-paid trips to exotic locations for physician and spouse, ostensibly to hear a lecture on a new product; payment of cash to the physician who agrees to read literature describing nonapproved uses of a drug; "frequent prescriber" programs awarding frequent flyer points with the physician's preferred airline for every prescription of the company's drug; lavish parties and tickets to entertainment events; costly gifts such as luggage and decorative arts; inexpensive gifts such as pens and notepads; and subsidies for local educational colloquiums and travel to professional meetings (Randall, 1991).

The conflicts of interest are obvious. Physicians are rewarded for prescribing drugs and devices whether or not they are necessary, and whether or not that particular prescription is most appropriate and least costly for the patient. And the acceptance of gifts engenders a sense of personal gratitude and indebtedness that can place corporate loyalty over patients' interests (Chren et al., 1989). Furthermore, patients ultimately bear the costs of the promotional gifts their physicians receive, whether by buying prescription drugs and devices directly, or by paying more for insurance premiums that rise with rising costs, or by forgoing higher salaries or fringe benefits as their employers pay higher insurance premiums.

Legal system.   Parallel to the escalation of health-care costs, the frequency and cost of medical malpractice litigation have increased. Physicians fearful of lawsuits may order extra diagnostic tests and more potent therapies to ensure that no one can accuse them of missing the diagnosis or doing too little for their patients. The cost of such "defensive medicine" has been estimated at about 15 percent of the total cost of physicians' services (Reynolds et al., 1987). When physicians order procedures that are not medically necessary in order to protect their actual or imagined legal interests, they expose patients to extra inconvenience and iatrogenesis—at the patient's expense and usually without the patient's knowledge. It is a clear conflict of interest.

Physician investment.   In some cases physicians create their own conflicts of interest by investing in facilities to which they refer their patients. Examples include freestanding diagnostic imaging centers, home health services, clinical laboratories, and physical therapy services. Although such investments can enhance the availability and quality of health-care facilities in a locale, the physician owners of such facilities nevertheless have an incentive to refer patients there, even when the care is unnecessary, costly, or of poor quality (Morreim, 1989, 1993b).

The conflicts embedded in investments are not limited to freestanding facilities. In one study, physicians who owned radiographic equipment in their own offices tended to use it four times more often, generating costs seven times higher, than physicians who referred patients to independent radiologists for those services (Hillman et al., 1990).

Physicians: Conflicts of interest in the research setting

The research context sometimes involves testing new treatments on ill patients, but it also can involve healthy volunteers as researchers look for toxicities of the very newest drugs. In many instances there is no expectation that participation in research will benefit the patient at all, whether because the subject is a normal control subject or because many people in the study will receive a placebo instead of active medication, or because the patient is too hopelessly ill to benefit from any treatment. Whatever the research protocol, however, the physician must respect the research subject's rights and interests.

Physicians enjoy personal rewards for successful research. Private companies such as drug manufacturers commonly sponsor research, frequently paying the physician investigator a fixed capitation fee up to $5,000 per person enrolled. The sum is intended to cover the costs of each subject's participation in the study, but in fact can result in a considerable surplus of money pocketed by the investigator. The more patients one enters in the study, the higher one's rewards (Shimm and Spece, 1991). An overzealous recruiter may be tempted to understate the inconvenience, discomfort, or risk that research participation may present for the patient, or could even compromise the integrity of the study by signing up patients who are only marginally eligible for the protocol.

Research that is funded by government or other nonprofit sources can avoid some, but not all, of the conflicts of privately sponsored research. Physician researchers still have strong incentives to gain the prestige, larger laboratory, increased technical support, academic promotion, science awards, and institutional power that come with securing grants and producing publishable research. Also, some research projects pay finders' fees to those, particularly young hospital staff physicians, who recruit patients for studies (Lind, 1990). As a result, these investigators have powerful incentives to recruit patients into studies without necessarily taking full account of the patients' best interests.

Physicians can also create their own conflicts of interest. Sometimes physicians invest in corporations sponsoring their research, or serve as their paid spokesmen when research is completed (Kessler, 1991). They may earn money from producing a valuable commodity, such as a cell line, by using tissues that patients either knowingly or unwittingly donate (*Moore* v. *Regents of the University of California*, 1990). In a few cases physicians performing for-profit scientific research have charged patient-subjects a fee to participate (Oldham, 1987). Although such entrepreneurial research is controversial, the conflicts embedded in for-profit research are not necessarily worse than those found throughout the high-pressure world of medical research (Morreim, 1991c).

Other health professionals

While physicians and dentists often are private practitioners or independent contractors, nurses, physical therapists, dietitians, and allied health professionals usually are employees of hospitals, HMOs, clinics, home health services, or public-health agencies. These professionals' conflicts of interest most often arise where their contractual duties as employees to administer the therapies ordered by a physician, or to follow established institutional rules, clash with their own beliefs about what is best for a patient. Such health professionals may suffer personal retaliation if they violate institutional mandates in order to do what seems best for the patient.

In these cases the problem begins with a conflict of obligation: One's obligations to the institution do not match one's obligations to the patient. The conflict of interest arises as one faces a personal price for favoring the patient over the institution. In other words, these professionals are caught between two obligations; the holder of one obligation, the institution, has the power to enforce its preferences by creating conflicts of interest. Thus, though conflicts of obligation are not the same thing as conflicts of interest, in these cases they are connected. For example, a nurse was fired for providing information to a patient about alternative cancer treatments (the dismissal was later vacated on procedural grounds; *Tuma v. Board of Nursing*, 1979). In another case a nurse was discharged for refusing to dialyse a patient for whom she believed the treatment was pointless and inhumane (*Warthen v. Toms River Community Mem. Hosp.*, 1985). Such clashes between administrative requirements and one's professional judgment are probably the greatest, though not the sole, source of conflicts for allied health professions.

Institutions

The interests of institutions and their administrators, like those of individual professionals, often mesh with patients' best interests. Ideally, in a competitive market where consumers seek quality and value for their dollars, a health-care institution will prosper by serving patients well. However, such a happy match does not always occur, partly because ill patients often are not equipped to appraise and challenge the quality of their care, and because generous insurance insulates many patients from caring about the costs of care. Accordingly, the financial best interests of a hospital might prompt excessive charges, inadequate staffing and equipment, bloated advertising, or the premature "dumping" of uninsured patients onto public institutions (Ansell and Schiff, 1987). Similarly, a pharmaceutical company may be financially rewarded for producing and marketing new drugs as early and as vigorously as possible, even if the drugs and their production methods are not as refined as they could be. As a result, some drugs may have more side effects, or cost more, than is necessary (Garber, 1992).

Managing conflicts of interest

The existence of a conflict of interest does not entail that a provider has mistreated or will mistreat any patient. It means only that while there is a mandate to promote the patient's (or sometimes someone else's) best interest, there are self-interested reasons to do otherwise. To be tempted is not necessarily to succumb.

Providers cannot escape conflicts of interest. If they are paid according to how many services they provide, their interest is to provide more services, with the concomitant dangers of excessive interventions, costs, and risks of iatrogenesis. If they are paid according to how many patients they care for, their financial advantage lies in taking on too many patients. Physicians who are strictly on a salary have an adverse incentive to mini-

mize their own labor, even if they cannot increase their income, by seeing fewer and less demanding patients.

Formal protections can help. Regulatory agencies such as state boards of medicine, nursing, and dentistry, and the Joint Commission on Accreditation of Health Care Organizations can establish standards of performance for individuals and institutions (Morreim, 1993a). And the legal system can redress individual cases where providers' self-interest injures patients. Antitrust law, for instance, can provide potent enforcement action against the abuses of physician investment and self-referral (Morreim, 1993b). Further, fiduciary law requires that a fiduciary in a conflict of interest must disclose that conflict fully to the beneficiary (here, the patient) and empower the latter to determine how the conflict should be resolved (*Fulton National Bank v. Tate*, 1966). Patients thus can have common-law remedies for breach of fiduciary duty, lack of informed consent, and other causes (*Moore v. Regents of the University of California*, 1990; Morreim, 1989).

Regulation and litigation are thus very important protections. They cannot supplant personal integrity, however. The prospective employee of an HMO or other institutional provider should check carefully into its incentive structure and refuse to join any organization that links financial consequences too closely to individual patient care decisions (Morreim, 1991a). The physician in private practice can refuse to accept costly gifts from drug company representatives. Those who would invest in referral facilities can first ensure that there is a genuine need for the facility and, second, empower their patients with information and freedom to make their own choices of ancillary health-care provider (Morreim, 1989, 1993b). Researchers can refrain from investing in corporations sponsoring their research, and can work with other research-sponsoring institutions to minimize conflicts. Where private industry pays university-based physicians a large per-patient fee, for example, that fee can be put into a general fund to benefit the institution after research costs are paid (Shimm and Spece, 1991). Nurses and allied health professionals can work individually or collectively for contract terms that protect their right to exercise professional integrity.

Institutions must ensure that they do not create inordinate conflicts of interest for the professionals they employ. HMOs, for instance, should refrain from instituting incentive systems that unduly influence individual patient-care decisions. They and other payers should likewise disclose to current and potential subscribers any such incentives or limits on care (Chittenden, 1991; Figa and Tag, 1990). Informed subscribers are better empowered to guard their own interests. Institutions can ameliorate their conflicts by pursuing continuous improvement, or "total quality management," as a way of promoting quality care while economizing on costs (Berwick, 1989). A focus on the success that comes from long-term quality should replace any preoccupation with short-term profitability.

Conflicts of interest affect providers pervasively, powerfully, and personally. Where once the fiduciary duty consisted mainly in refraining from vulgar exploitation, the obligation to place the patient's interests before one's own can no longer be an unlimited obligation. Providers must exercise great care to avoid conflicts where possible, and to uphold a strong fiduciary presumption to favor patients' interests over their own. However, they cannot be expected routinely to commit professional self-sacrifice in an often futile unilateral attempt to battle economic forces beyond their control. Therefore, one of the most important and difficult moral challenges of medicine's new economics is to consider not just what providers owe their patients but also the limits of those obligations (Morreim, 1991a). Under a revised health-care system of the future, perhaps patients will have greater choice and influence over the content of their health-care benefits, and thereby be more empowered to make more trade-offs between the cost and quality of care—thus alleviating at least some of the conflicts of interest that arise as providers attempt to make these trades on patients' behalf (Butler and Haislmaier, 1989; Eddy, 1990).

E. HAAVI MORREIM

Directly related to this entry is the entry DIVIDED LOYALTIES IN MENTAL-HEALTH CARE. *For a further discussion of topics mentioned in this entry, see the entries* COMMERCIALISM IN SCIENTIFIC RESEARCH; HEALTH-CARE DELIVERY; HEALTH-CARE FINANCING; LAW AND BIOETHICS; LICENSING, DISCIPLINE, AND REGULATION IN THE HEALTH PROFESSIONS; PHARMACEUTICS; PROFESSIONAL–PATIENT RELATIONSHIP; PROFESSION AND PROFESSIONAL ETHICS; RESEARCH, UNETHICAL; RESEARCH METHODOLOGY; *and* RESEARCH POLICY. *This entry will find application in the entry* ALLIED HEALTH PROFESSIONS; ANIMAL RESEARCH, *article on* LAW AND POLICY; PSYCHIATRY, ABUSES OF; *and* VETERINARY ETHICS. *For a discussion of related ideas, see the entries on* FIDELITY AND LOYALTY; HARM; RESPONSIBILITY; *and* TRUST. *See also the* APPENDIX (CODES, OATHS, AND DIRECTIVES RELATED TO BIOETHICS), SECTION II: ETHICAL DIRECTIVES FOR THE PRACTICE OF MEDICINE, *and* SECTION III: ETHICAL DIRECTIVES FOR OTHER HEALTH-CARE PROFESSIONS.

Bibliography

ANSELL, DAVID A., and SCHIFF, ROBERT L. 1987. "Patient Dumping, Implications and Policy Recommendations." *Journal of the American Medical Association* 257, no. 11:1500–1502.

Batty v. Arizona State Dental Board. 1941. 112 P.2d 870.

BERENSON, ROBERT A. 1987. "In a Doctor's Wallet." *New Republic,* May 18, pp. 11–13.

Berkey v. Anderson. 1969. 82 Cal. Rptr. 67 (Cal. App. 2 Dist.).

BERWICK, DAVID M. 1989. "Continuous Improvement as an Ideal in Health Care." *New England Journal of Medicine* 320, no. 1:53–56.

BLUM, JOHN D. 1991. "Economic Credentialing: A New Twist In Hospital Appraisal Processes." *Journal of Legal Medicine* 12:427–475.

BOCK, RANDALL S. 1988. "The Pressure to Keep Prices High at a Walk-in Clinic: A Personal Experience." *New England Journal of Medicine* 319, no. 12:785–787.

Brown v. Blue Cross & Blue Shield of Alabama. 1990. 898 F. 2d 1556 (11th Cir.).

BUTLER, STUART M., and HAISLMAIER, EDMUND F., eds. 1989. *A National Health System for America.* Critical Issues. Washington, D.C.: Heritage Foundation.

CHITTENDEN, WILLIAM A. 1991. "Malpractice Liability and Managed Health Care: History and Prognosis." *Tort and Insurance Law Journal* 26:451–496.

CHREN, MARY-MARGARET; LANDEFELD, C. SETH; and MURRAY, THOMAS H. 1989. "Doctors, Drug Companies, and Gifts." *Journal of the American Medical Association* 262, no. 24:3448–3451.

Darling v. Charleston Community Memorial Hospital. 1965. 211 N.E. 2d 253 (Ill.).

EDDY, DAVID M. 1990. "What Do We Do About Costs?" *Journal of the American Medical Association* 264, no. 9:1161,1165,1169,1170.

FIGA, S. FRED, and TAG, HOWARD M. 1990. "Redefining Full and Fair Disclosure of HMO Benefits and Limitations." *Seton Hall Legislative Journal* 14:151–157.

Fulton National Bank v. Tate. 1966. 363 F.2d 562 (4th Cir.).

GARBER, ALAN M. 1992. "No Price Too High?" *New England Journal of Medicine* 327, no. 3:1676–1678.

HILLMAN, ALAN L. 1987. "Financial Incentives for Physicians in HMOs: Is There a Conflict of Interest?" *New England Journal of Medicine* 317, no. 27:1743–1748.

HILLMAN, BRUCE J.; JOSEPH, CATHERINE A.; MABRY, MICHAEL R.; SUNSHINE, JONATHAN H.; KENNEDY, STEPHEN D.; and NOETHER, MONICA. 1990. "Frequency and Costs of Diagnostic Imaging in Office Practice—A Comparison of Self-Referring and Radiologist-Referring Physicians." *New England Journal of Medicine* 323, no. 23:1604–1608.

INSTITUTE OF MEDICINE. 1986. "Committee Report." In *For-Profit Enterprise in Health Care,* especially pp. 127–204. Edited by Bradford H. Gray. Washington, D.C.: National Academy Press.

JONSEN, ALBERT R. 1983. "Watching the Doctor." *New England Journal of Medicine* 308, no. 25:1531–1535.

KESSLER, DAVID A. 1991. "Drug Promotion and Scientific Exchange. The Role of the Clinical Investigator." *New England Journal of Medicine* 325, no. 3:201–203.

LIND, STUART E. 1990. "Finder's Fees for Research Subjects." *New England Journal of Medicine* 323, no. 24:192–195.

Lockett v. Goodill. 1967. 430 P.2d 589 (Wash.).

Moore v. Regents of the University of California. 1990. 793 P.2d 479.

MORREIM, E. HAAVI. 1989. "Conflicts of Interest: Profits and

Problems in Physician Referrals." *Journal of the American Medical Association* 262, no. 3:390–394.

———. 1991a. *Balancing Act: The New Medical Ethics of Medicine's New Economics.* Dordrecht, Netherlands: Kluwer.

———. 1991b. "Economic Disclosure and Economic Advocacy: New Duties in the Medical Standard of Care." *Journal of Legal Medicine* 12:275–329.

———. 1991c. "Patient-Funded Research: Paying the Piper or Protecting the Patient?" *IRB* 13, no. 3:1–6.

———. 1993a. "Am I My Brother's Warden? Responding to the Unethical or Incompetent Colleague." *Hastings Center Report* 23, no. 3:19–27.

———. 1993b. "Unholy Alliances: Physician Investment for Self-Referral." *Radiology* 186, no. 1:67–72.

OLDHAM, ROBERT K. 1987. "Patient-Funded Cancer Research." *New England Journal of Medicine* 316, no. 1: 46–47.

RANDALL, TERI. 1991. "Kennedy Hearings Say No More Free Lunch—or Much Else—from Drug Firms." *Journal of the American Medical Association* 265, no. 4:440–441.

RELMAN, ARNOLD S. 1983. "The Future of Medical Practice." *Health Affairs* 2, no. 2:5–19.

REYNOLDS, ROGER A.; RIZZO, JOHN A.; and GONZALEZ, MARTIN L. 1987. "The Cost of Medical Professional Liability." *Journal of the American Medical Association* 257, no. 20:2776–2781.

RODWIN, MARK A. 1993. *Medicine, Money, and Morals: Physicians' Conflicts of Interest.* New York: Oxford University Press.

SHIMM, DAVID S., and SPECE, ROY G. 1991. "Conflict of Interest and Informed Consent in Industry-Sponsored Clinical Trials." *Journal of Legal Medicine* 12:477–513.

Tuma v. Board of Nursing. 1979. 593 P.2d 711 (Id.).

Warthen v. Toms River Community Memorial Hospital. 1985. 488 A.2d 229 (N.J.Super.A.D.).

Wohlgemuth v. Meyer. 1956. 293 P.2d 316 (Cal.).

CONFUCIANISM

The following is a revision and update of the first-edition entry "Confucianism" by the same author. Portions of the first-edition entry appear in the revised version.

The effects of Confucianism on the development of health care and medical ethics in China were manifold; medical ethics was a direct outgrowth of the basic content and tendency of Confucian social theory. Decision makers of the Early Western Han dynasty (202 B.C.E.–25 C.E.) chose to recognize Confucianism (rather than any of several other social theories that were offered by philosophical schools during that time) as the most appropriate ideology to stabilize the social pattern that had emerged under their rule and to prevent social crises that might have led to social change.

Ensuing actions by Confucian policymakers consequently were strictly conservative in the sense of conserving in Chinese society the distribution pattern of resources preferred by the ruling class. Confucianists were aware that control over potentially powerful resources by specialized groups might lead to shifts in the pattern of distribution of those resources within society, with social change as the unavoidable consequence. Countless decisions were made to prevent this from happening. Deliberate measures to destroy or erode the power bases of groups that had managed to gain control over certain resources during times of administrative weakness were rather constant actions of the government. Official policy toward salt merchants, financial experts, military leaders, and other groups reveals these efforts.

Two diametrically opposed alternatives were open to Confucian politicians: either to dilute control over potentially dangerous resources among all the people, or to concentrate all control in the hands of the government, that is, the ruling bureaucracy. The resources watched most carefully included those relating to the knowledge and practice of medicine.

In the following a distinction will be made between primary and secondary medical resources. The former include medical knowledge and skills, drugs and medical technology, and medical equipment and facilities. Secondary medical resources are defined as rewards of material or nonmaterial kind, that is, money, gifts, prestige, or social power to be gained through medical practice. Access to secondary resources is generally achieved by a group only after having gained control over existing primary resources. The result is the emergence within society of an influential elite group, with consequences harmful to the continuity of social structure. Policy toward medical practice, therefore, followed the line determined by these premises.

Inherent in Confucianism is the appreciation of life and the desire to keep the body from untimely or unnecessary death. It is difficult, however, to assess all the corollaries of that basically positive attitude toward life. There is some indirect support for the assumption that children with certain congenital malformation were killed in prerepublican China, though few such cases have been recorded. Also, as sources indicate, abortion was frequently induced—a practice that evoked little, if any, concern among Confucian thinkers. Confucian ideology contains several values of bioethical relevance, for instance, *jen* (humane benevolence) and *tz'u* (compassion). These, however, were applied, at least by some dogmatists, within strict socially defined limits. Thus, some Confucians argued that a medical practitioner should not answer every call he received but should respond only to requests for help by those who were suitable for social intercourse.

Mencius (372–289 B.C.E.), an early Confucian philosopher, commented on the universality of benevolent human nature when he pointed out that anyone who happened to see a child fall into a well would certainly rush to the scene and attempt to rescue it from drowning. Furthermore, Confucianism regarded *hsiao* (filial piety) as one of the key values necessary to maintain social stability. The duty to assist one's parents and other relatives to reach advanced age without unnecessary suffering naturally entailed providing medical care for them. The Confucian tenet stressing the role of individual laypersons and their ability to assist their relatives became the focus of political efforts designed to spread control of medical resources over society as a whole in order to make the impact of medical practitioners marginal if not superfluous. Time and again statements and admonitions released by concerned Confucianists asserted that possession of sufficient medical knowledge was necessary to fulfill one's obligations of filial piety.

In spite of this attempt to distribute responsibility for primary health care, social circumstances and political expediency (the nature of which is not always entirely clear) led Confucian decision makers to promulgate a variety of public-health measures; the ensuing institutions had to be staffed with at least partially specialized personnel. Thus, ironically, the stimulus for the professionalization of a specifically trained group within Confucian society was a result of Confucian health policy. It is a moot point to what extent credit for humanitarian health-policy decisions during the imperial era can be attributed to the voluntary acts of the Confucianists and how much was forced upon them by external events. Still, the mere fact that public-health solutions to impending problems were conceived and that attempts were made to put them into practice must be regarded as an achievement of the Confucian culture. Again, today's readers of classical Chinese accounts of public-health measures must be cautioned, for such reports do not reveal much about the actual implementation of the programs decreed.

At the beginning of the Confucian era, now slightly more than two thousand years ago, medical practitioners enjoyed the status of more or less renowned craftsmen. Some of them were itinerant and offered their services to the general populace; others, whose skills had created sufficient fame for them, would approach the rulers at the many feudal courts existing during that period (Bridgman, 1955). "Medical workers" were attached to the military and to administrative posts from Han times on. Somewhat later, better-trained experts were required, and it was only natural in Confucian society that the necessary training supplement the standard education of Confucian civil servants, again as a strategy to preserve control over medical resources for the ruling class. During the early seventh century this led to the establishment of institutions for the teaching of medi-

cine outside the imperial court. By the twelfth century, medical training in certain government institutions was restructured and became even more integrated with classical nonmedical knowledge.

Possibly as a response to the opening of such an institution under Buddhist auspices in the fifth century, one finds soon thereafter the first reports of the establishment of a hospital under secular control. The competitive character of public-health policies when directed toward followers of Buddhism became even more evident in 653 C.E. when Buddhist (and also Taoist) monks and nuns were prohibited from the practice of medicine, and in 845 C.E. when all Buddhist-controlled hospitals were secularized (Needham, 1970). After a period of weakness during which even Chinese emperors had shown commitment to the Buddhist faith, this kind of loss of control over important primary and secondary medical resources could not be tolerated by a reviving Confucian society.

From the eighth through the twelfth century a mass migration of people from northern regions to southern parts of China occurred as a result of climatic changes in the north. It is estimated that previously 95 percent of the Chinese population inhabited the plains of the north, which were more favorable for husbandry and agriculture; during the period of the Southern Sung dynasty (1127–1179), approximately 45 percent of the total Chinese population lived in the south with its mountainous geography (Kracke, 1954–1955). The population shift produced unprecedented large cities, often with hundreds of thousands and, not infrequently, more than a million people crowded together. Possibly as a consequence of the living conditions in the cities, in which so many people had been uprooted from their former style of life and natural environment, a welfare program was initiated during the eleventh century that entailed the establishment of public dispensaries and state-controlled polyclinics. That system continued in operation at least until the sixteenth century, possibly even the eighteenth. The impact of these institutions cannot be regarded as decisive for public health at any time. The numbers of "offices" established were too small for this purpose. Furthermore, there were such severe scandals surrounding them that even the Confucian chroniclers could not avoid mentioning them. Not surprisingly, in a slight modification of the official title, the public dispensaries were called by the people "offices for the welfare of the bureaucrats" (Unschuld, 1979).

Public-health programs were continued even during times of alien rule over China. Reports from the time of the Mongols (Yüan dynasty, 1206–1368), for instance, show an abundance of directions to provide medical assistance to prisoners through "medical workers," the lowest category of government-employed practitioners.

The foregoing reference to examples of public-health policies in imperial China may suffice to indicate that it was possible for any medical group to achieve a higher level of professionalization and thus to become socially influential. Orthodox Confucianists, however, observed these developments closely and continuously promoted what might in effect be called an anti-medical-professionalization campaign.

By the twelfth century, three distinguishable main groups were contending for control over medical resources. The first were the free-practicing physicians outside Confucianism. This group included Taoists, Buddhists, and others who practice medicine to make a living or as a sideline when they were economically independent. Many famous physicians and medical writers belonged to the group. They should be distinguished from those favored by Confucian dogmatists, persons who used their medical abilities only to assist family members or friends in need, or during medical assignments as civil servants.

One outstanding early representative of free-practicing physicians was Sun Ssu-miao (581–682?), who possibly was the first to recognize the need of the free-practicing group for explicit medical ethics to advance in professionalization against the Confucian class. It is not surprising that many of the famous members of this group were offered official positions at the imperial court or elsewhere. This may be understood not only as an attempt by the decision makers to secure the best physicians for their own care but also as a way to alienate them from their free-practicing peers who might have gained additional status by association with outstanding personalities.

The second group is the Confucian class, whose interests have been dealt with earlier in this article. Within this group a third emerged, composed of those Confucianists who because of either an official assignment or personal interest practiced medicine outside their own families on behalf of clients of all kinds, often accepting money and other material rewards. The third group did not adhere to the famous saying of Confucius (551–479 B.C.E.): "The accomplished scholar is not a utensil!" Its strategy, carried out to gain acceptance within its own superior group and to compete successfully with the group of the free-practicing physicians, was twofold.

In their explicit medical ethics these people on the one hand had to assure the orthodox Confucianists that their medical practice was in perfect accordance with Confucian values. On the other hand they continuously stressed that "common physicians," as non-Confucian practitioners were called officially, constituted a source of permanent evil practice. In this latter effort the group was supported by the orthodox Confucianists.

A severe blow against the social acceptance of medicine as more than an ordinary craft resulted from some saying of Chu Hsi (1130–1200), the leading Confucian philosopher of his time. In commenting on the ancient classic Lun yü ("Analects"), which supposedly comprises sayings by Confucius and his disciples, compiled by the latter, Chu Hsi made some statements regarding medicine that were bound to stigmatize all who wished to practice medicine, outside the domain of their own families, as a means of earning a living.

Confucius had originally stated, "The people in the South have a saying: 'A man without persistency cannot become a sorcerer-physician.' Good!" (Legge, 1960, vol. I). There were at least two grammatically correct ways to interpret these words. Chu Hsi chose to separate the terms "sorcerer" and "physician," and commented: "Sorcerers communicate with demons and spirits; physicians are entrusted with matters of death and life. If such petty personnel [cannot do without persistency], how much more is this true for others!" (Chu Hsi, 1958, pp. 598–601). Elsewhere in the Lun yü the following remark is attributed to a disciple of Confucius: "Petty teachings certainly also contain some aspects which cannot be disregarded. But if you carry them far, you will become soiled. The noble man, therefore, does not deal with them" (Legge, 1960, vol. 1, pp. 340–341). In this case Chu Hsi wrote in his commentary: "'Petty teachings' does not mean 'strange [or heterodox] principles'; 'petty teachings' refers to 'teachings' too, but just to 'petty' ones. These are for instance: agriculture, horticulture, medicine, divination, and all other specialized occupations" (Chu Hsi, 1965, p. 23a).

These two comments exerted an almost continuous influence over most of the remaining centuries of the Confucian era. They provoked many defensive criticisms by medical writers from both the free-practicing physicians and the Confucian medical practitioners. A well-known physician named Hsü Ch'un-fu, who lived around 1556 and had served as an official at the Imperial Medical Office at court for a while, questioned Chu Hsi's interpretation of Confucius's statement and argued that "sorcerer-physicians" were to be regarded as one single category of people, namely, those who would dance, pray, and offer sacrifices to avert sickness; through this sort of practice they proved not to have any knowledge of medicine and drugs. Therefore, they should not be confused with true medical practitioners.

Later, at the end of the sixteenth century, Lai Fu-yang focused on the meaning of "petty" and argued: "If one directs his medical knowledge only on his own body, this is to be regarded as 'petty'; if one spreads the application [of his medical knowledge] all over mankind, this is not to be regarded as 'petty'!" Here Lai Fu-yang attempted to reverse completely the orthodox Confucian attitude toward medical practice.

Chang Chieh-pin (fl. 1624) is a third and last example of criticism of Chu Hsi's remarks on medicine. Chang Chieh-pin was a noted medical writer who originally was in the group of free practitioners but became a close follower of the ideas of Sung-Confucian medicine, a healing system that integrated the use of drugs into medical theories of the Confucian tradition. The use of drugs had been developed mainly in Taoist traditions. Chang Chieh-pin did not dare or did not find it effective to voice his strong criticism of Chu Hsi's comments himself. He placed his thoughts into the mouth of a "strange man," whom he allegedly met somewhere in the wilderness. This "strange man" in conversation with Chang Chieh-pin showed an outburst of anger when the latter told him that although medicine was to be regarded as a "petty teaching," he was still aware of the necessity to be careful in its application. The stranger then gave him an emphatic lecture on the importance and subtlety of medicine and admonished him to keep it in high esteem. Chang Chieh-pin as a result of this lecture felt extremely ashamed and noted it down so that it might not be forgotten.

Another dimension of the Confucian attitude toward medicine that was expressed in many ethical statements focused on what were called "heterodox" practices and beliefs. Orthodox or officially endorsed medicine consisted of theoretical foundations and actual treatments by means of acupuncture or other techniques, including drugs at a later time. All of these were related to the cosmogonic theories and philosophical concepts of nature that were also basic to the Confucian social theory.

Effective medical practice outside of those theories and philosophies might have jeopardized the validity of the Confucian paradigms as a whole and could not be tolerated. This is not surprising, for the way of life recommended by Confucian-endorsed medicine as a guarantee for physiological harmony, that is, health, is the same way of life demanded by the Confucian social theory to maintain social order and stability. It was again Sun Ssu-miao, a leading thinker critical of the Confucian way of life, who named demonic medicine as an alternative. The notion inherent in this healing system was that one is constantly subject to attacks by evil demons, which may cause diseases if one does not protect oneself carefully enough. The consequences of this theory of disease causation for individual and social behavior were quite different from those put forth by the Confucian social theory.

The resulting ideology toward heterodox knowledge and practices was part of the overall competition between Confucianists and the followers of other social theories. Shamans, Taoists, Buddhists, and often private individuals who had taken up a healing practice on their own by using charms, prayers, or other means that were not in conformity with Confucian medicine, provided the major target for accusations of heterodox practice.

The need to advance over other groups in society competing for control of secondary resources (i.e., the material or immaterial rewards to be gained from practice) is one of the major forces behind medical progress. However, several well-documented historical examples indicate that the pace of medical progress is generally retarded when the control over primary medical resources rests in the hands of a group whose access to secondary resources is not wholly dependent on the use of these primary resources and possesses other means to maintain its control over the people.

Orthodox Confucianists constituted such a group. They attempted to control primary medical resources or to spread them over society merely to prevent any specialized group from rising to influence and power in society. Their own power was by no means solely dependent on primary medical resources. Therefore, orthodox Confucianists had no interest as such in increasing or improving primary medical resources. In contrast, the free-practicing physicians and those Confucianists who practiced medicine outside their own families appear to have been genuinely interested in improving their skills and expanding the available materia medica. The resulting antagonism manifested itself, for example, in the delineation of medical jurisdiction and in repeated admonitions to practitioners not to develop new theories but to stick to the old interpretations. This restrictive policy could not prevent the invention or importation of new primary medical resources—for example, theories, drugs, techniques, and facilities. However, it is impossible to estimate to what extent it may have impeded progress and served to preserve those archaic medical paradigms that dominated Chinese medical literature up to the twentieth century.

One of the last Confucianists to resort to this kind of argument was Li Han-chang (1821–1899), elder brother of the famous statesman Li Hung-chang (1823–1901). In the preface to a medical work of a previous century, he castigated those who would originate or follow other than the classical theories, and condemned those who would try their "unintelligible prescriptions" at the cost of thousands of human lives. It is not unreasonable to assume that these criticisms were meant to discourage those practitioners who were just then experiencing the initial impact of Western surgical and pharmaceutical knowledge. A subsequently increased influx of Western primary resources of many kinds into China brought dramatic changes in the overall pattern of resource distribution. The millennia-old maxims of Confucian ideology concerning professionalization proved to be infeasible at a time when the amount and the character of primary resources available in the field of medicine and elsewhere seemed to necessitate groups of specialists to control and handle them. The Confucian social system collapsed with the revolution of 1911.

PAUL U. UNSCHULD

Directly related to this entry are the entries BUDDHISM; TAOISM; *and* MEDICAL ETHICS, HISTORY OF, *article on*

SOUTH AND EAST ASIA, *sections on* CHINA *and* SOUTH-EAST ASIAN COUNTRIES. *Other relevant material may be found under the entries* BENEFICENCE; COMPASSION; DEATH, *article on* EASTERN THOUGHT; MEDICINE AS A PROFESSION; *and* PUBLIC HEALTH. *See also the entry* ETHICS, *article on* RELIGION AND MORALITY.

Bibliography

BRIDGEMAN, ROBERT F. 1955. *La médecine dans la Chine antique.* Mélanges chinois et bouddhiques 10. Brussels: Institut belge des hautes études chinoises.

CHOU I-MOU. 1983. *Li-tai ming-i lun i-te* [Famous Physicians through the Ages on Medical Ethics]. Ch'ang-sha: Hunan Science and Technology.

CHU HSI, commentator. 1958. *Lun yü chi chu* [Commented Analects], by Confucius. 10 vols. Taipei: Chung-hua ts'ung-shu wei-yüan-hui. Translated by Pyun Yung-tai as *Analects,* by Confucius. 2 vols. Seoul: Minjungsugwan, 1960.

———. 1965. *Chu-tzu ta ch'üan* [Master Chu's Complete Works]. *Ssu-pu-pei-yao,* vols. 396–406. Taipei: Chung-hua-shu-chü.

HSÜ TA-CH'UN. 1989. *Forgotten Traditions of Ancient Chinese Medicine.* The *I-hsüeh yuan liu lun* of 1757. Translated and annotated by Paul U. Unschuld. Brookline, Mass.: Paradigm.

KRACKE, E. A., JR. 1954–1955. "Sung Society: Change within Tradition." *Far Eastern Quarterly* 14, no. 4:479–488.

LEGGE, JAMES. 1960. *The Chinese Classics.* 5 vols. Hong Kong: Hong Kong University Press.

NEEDHAM, JOSEPH R. 1970. *Clerks and Craftsmen in China and the West: Lectures and Addresses on the History of Science and Technology.* Cambridge: At the University Press.

UNSCHULD, PAUL U. 1979. *Medical Ethics in Imperial China: A Study in Historical Anthropology.* Berkeley: University of California Press. This monograph gives the original sources of all Chinese citations provided in this article.

———. 1985. *Medicine in China. A History of Ideas.* Berkeley: University of California Press.

CONSCIENCE

Matters of conscience arise with some frequency in bioethics. A health professional may cite considerations of conscience in declining to perform or participate in a certain procedure. A patient may refuse a particular treatment on grounds of conscience. And new or unanticipated circumstances may create conflicts of conscience for patients and health professionals alike. What do we mean by "conscience" in these and related contexts? Is conscience an internal moral sense sufficient for distinguishing right from wrong? Is the "voice" of conscience simply the echo of parental and social prohibitions? Or does conscience differ in important ways from

either of these? How much weight should be given in ethical reflection to claims of conscience? To what extent and for what reasons should health professionals compromise personal convenience, institutional efficiency, or medical effectiveness in order to respect individual conscience, their own or their patients'?

Three conceptions of conscience

The idea of conscience has a long and complex history (D'Arcy, 1961; Mount, 1969). The word "conscience" derives from the Latin *conscientia,* introduced by Christian Scholastics. Most generally, it refers to conscious awareness of the moral quality of some past or contemplated action and the disposition to be so aware (conscientiousness). In what follows we consider three main conceptions: (1) conscience as an inner sense that distinguishes right acts from wrong; (2) conscience as the internalization of parental and social norms; and (3) conscience as the exercise and expression of a reflective sense of integrity.

Moral sense.   Conscience is sometimes conceived as an internal moral sense sufficient for distinguishing right from wrong. The reliability of this inner sense is usually attributed to its divine origin, its reflection of our true nature, or some combination of the two. There are, however, difficulties with this conception.

Consider, first, a variation of an argument developed by Plato in his *Euthyphro.* Is what makes an act right the fact that it is endorsed by one's conscience? Or does conscience recommend a certain course of conduct because it is right? If the former, the promptings of conscience appear to be arbitrary. Whatever is urged by a person's conscience would, in this view, be right. There would be no way to assess the deliverances of conscience or to compare the consciences of, say, Hitler and Mother Teresa. If, on the other hand, conscience directs us to perform certain acts because they are right, it cannot be the principal source of moral knowledge. We must, in this event, have prior, independent criteria of rightness and wrongness that allow us to distinguish those acts that should be recommended by conscience from those that should not—in which case conscience is not sufficient to guide conduct.

A related difficulty is the prevalence of conflicts of conscience, both within persons and between them. Such conflicts are especially pronounced in bioethics, where advances in knowledge and technology confront us with unprecedented, consequential choices ranging well beyond our ethical traditions. The limitations of conscience, if it is conceived as a sufficient guide to moral decision making, may not be so noticeable in static, homogenous, insular cultures and subcultures. But where new circumstances require members of pluralistic societies to come to some agreement on bioethical questions, appeals to an internal, self-validating sense of right and wrong are apt to generate more heat than light.

Internalized social norms.   The most plausible explanation for the limitations of conscience in resolving ethical conflicts is that the "voice" of conscience is simply the echo of social and parental admonitions impressed upon the developing psyches of young children (i.e., the Freudian superego). Whatever its psychological and developmental significance, conscience so conceived has little normative import. That we have certain moral compunctions as a result of our socialization does little to establish their validity. We are bound by the voice of conscience only if we can provide independent justification of its dictates. It is the adequacy of the justification, not the persistence of the voice, that carries moral authority. Conceived as internalized social norms, then, conscience plays no direct role in ethical deliberation.

Sense of integrity.   "I couldn't live with myself if I were [or were not] to perform the abortion in these circumstances." "I can no longer participate in this treatment plan in good conscience." "How could I continue to think of myself as a Jehovah's Witness if I were to consent to the blood transfusion?" Each of these sentences expresses an appeal to conscience that is neither a deliverance of an internal moral sense nor an internalization of an external social norm. What is expressed in each case is the culmination of *conscientious* reflection about the relationship between a certain course of action and a particular conception of the self. So understood, appeals to conscience are closely connected to reflective concern with one's integrity. The focus is not so much on the objective or universal rightness or wrongness of a particular act as on the consequences for the self of one's performing it.

There is something absurd, Gilbert Ryle has observed, in saying "My conscience says that *you* ought to do this or ought not to have done that" (Ryle, 1940, p. 31). I may be troubled by your wrongdoing, but unless I have advised or assisted you, or culpably failed to prevent you from performing the act in question, my conscience will be clear. The same is not true, however, about those of *my* acts that I have determined, for one reason or another, were or would be morally wrong. Having judged a certain act to be wrong, an appeal to conscience stresses the added wrongness of my performing it. Appeals to conscience therefore presuppose a prior determination of the rightness or wrongness of an act (Childress, 1979). Moreover, one may or may not extend the standards one employs in making this assessment to others in similar situations. If, for example, the standards are universalizable principles of respect for persons, justice, or beneficence, one will maintain that anyone would do wrong in performing the act in question. But if one's standards are grounded in religious convictions, personal ideals, or a particular worldview

and way of life, one may not hold everyone else to them. What is at stake in all such appeals is one's wholeness or integrity as a person.

Integrity

"It would be better for me," Socrates says in the *Gorgias*, "that my lyre or a chorus I directed should be out of tune and loud with discord, and that multitudes of men should disagree with me rather than that I, *being one*, should be out of harmony with myself and contradict me" (Arendt, 1971, p. 439). One cannot lead a good and meaningful life, Socrates suggests, unless the self is reasonably unified or integrated—unless, that is, one's words and deeds cohere with one's basic, identity-conferring, moral, religious, and philosophical convictions. Hence the importance of critical reflection on one's life as a whole. The words, deeds, and convictions of an unexamined life are unlikely to be sufficiently integrated to constitute a singular life—let alone one worth living.

Conscience should not, therefore, be conceived as a faculty or component of the self. It is, rather, the voice of one's self as a whole, understood temporally—as having a beginning, a middle, and an end—as well as at a particular moment. Operating retrospectively, what Christian tradition calls "judicial" conscience makes judgments about past conduct. Operating prospectively, what the same tradition calls "legislative" conscience anticipates whether a prospective utterance or course of action is likely to be at odds with one's most basic ethical convictions (D'Arcy, 1961). In each case, the signal that something is wrong—that one's integrity has been, is currently, or would be compromised—is an actual or anticipatory feeling of guilt, shame, or remorse.

Consider, in this connection, the words of Aleksandr N. Chikunov, a veteran of the 1968 Soviet invasion of Czechoslovakia, as he explains sharing his experience with young soldiers called to Moscow to suppress democratic reforms during the abortive coup of August 1991: "I entered Prague in 1968 and I still have an ill conscience about it. I was a soldier then, like these guys. We were also sent like they are now, to defend the achievements of socialism. Twenty-three years have passed, and I still have an ill conscience" (*New York Times*, August 20, 1991, p. A13). Here Chikunov draws upon the lessons of his "ill" judicial conscience to inform and alert the legislative consciences of the doung soldiers. His motivation, it seems, is not only to spare them the pangs of an ill conscience but also to help heal his own (and thus to heal himself).

The authority and sanctions of conscience are, Mr. Chikunov suggests, self-imposed. No external source can create or directly relieve a troubled conscience. Nor may we easily rationalize or evade its judgments. "Other judges," as D'Arcy points out, "may be venal or partial or fallible; not so the verdict of conscience" (D'Arcy, 1961, p. 8). The oppressiveness of a guilty conscience is due in part to its identity with the self.

Conscience in bioethics

Three factors contribute to the prevalence of appeals to conscience in bioethics: (1) bioethical decision making often involves our deepest identity-conferring convictions about the nature and meaning of creating, sustaining, and ending life; (2) health-care professionals and patients and their families will occasionally have radically differing beliefs about such matters; and (3) the complexity of modern health care often requires agreement and cooperation on a single course of action.

Conflicts of conscience. Conflicts of conscience arise not only between individuals but also within them. Consider a physician whose patient, suffering greatly from the ravages of the last stages of a terminal illness, is also a longtime friend. The patient requests the physician to provide both the substance and the instruction for taking his own life. The physician finds herself torn. On the one hand, her conception of medicine and professional identity is incompatible with what appears to be physician-assisted suicide. On the other hand, the bonds of friendship and her natural sympathies strongly incline her to accede to her patient's request. The situation has, as a result, precipitated a crisis of conscience, and the physician must engage in what Charles Taylor has called "strong evaluation"—reflection about the self by the self in ways that engage and attempt to restructure one's deepest and most fundamental convictions (Taylor, 1976). Such reflection manifests an admirable concern for wholeness or integrity.

Conscientious refusal. From Socrates to Sir Thomas More to Henry David Thoreau, individuals have appealed to conscience in refusing to comply with a wide range of legal or socially mandated directives. In some cases such noncompliance may be covert and evasive—for example, a physician's providing contraceptive information to married couples in Connecticut before that state's anticontraceptive law was declared unconstitutional (Childress, 1985). In most cases, however, health professionals and patients give reasons of conscience in openly seeking personal exemption from certain standard practices.

Physicians may appeal to conscience in refusing to do procedures that are both legal and performed by their colleagues. Consider an obstetrician's refusal to perform a legal abortion or a pediatrician's refusal to prescribe human growth hormone for short, but normal, children at the behest of their anxious parents. In each case the physician's decision may be based on moral convictions or personal ideals. The obstetrician need not believe that abortion ought to be illegal or that women who request, or physicians who perform, abortions are deeply

immoral. The pediatrician may neither urge the legal prohibition of administering human growth hormone to short, but normal, children nor regard parents who request this treatment, or other pediatricians who administer it, as unethical. Both agree, however, that it would be a violation of conscience—a betrayal of their deepest personal convictions about life or the nature of medicine—if they were to perform the act in question.

Similarly, nurses appeal to conscience in seeking exemption from procedures or care plans that threaten their sense of integrity. For example, a nurse may conscientiously refuse to follow a physician's directive to remove medically administered hydration and nutrition from a patient in a persistent vegetative state. Regardless of the act's legality, the family's concurrence, and the physician's directive, given her deepest identity-conferring convictions about the nature and value of life, the nurse may be unable to carry out the action. Her reasoning, she might add, is not strong enough to condemn others who believe differently; but as for herself, she must refrain.

Patients, too, may appeal to conscience in refusing forms of medical treatment. When informed, mentally competent Jehovah's Witnesses refuse blood transfusions on religious grounds, they do not at the same time urge that blood transfusions be legally prohibited, nor do they condemn those who gratefully accept blood transfusions. What they want is not so much respect for the content of their particular convictions as much as respect for their consciences. The same is true of other patients who refuse or request certain forms of treatment on the basis of fundamental moral and religious convictions.

Respect for conscience

Respect for conscience is a corollary of the principle of respect for persons. To respect another as a person is, insofar as possible, to respect the expression and exercise, if not the content, of a person's most fundamental convictions. A society's respect for individual conscience may extend not only to religious toleration but also, for example, to exempting conscripted pacifists from direct participation in war.

In the biomedical context, respect for conscience may be inconvenient, inefficient, or detrimental to medical outcomes. Still, it must always be taken seriously and often should prevail. In some cases, respect for conscience may be balanced with biomedical goals. At a certain level of abstraction, the purpose of health care is strikingly similar to that of protecting individual conscience. Although health care is usually focused on the body, emphasis on informed consent implies that the principal function of medicine is the health or wholeness of the patient as a person. Yet a person's sense of health or wholeness may also be threatened by what the former Soviet soldier, Aleksandr Chikunov, revealingly called an "ill" conscience. The values underlying appeals to conscience within the health-care system are not, therefore, radically at odds with the values underlying medical and nursing care. In each case the aim is to preserve or restore personal wholeness. Insofar, then, as appeals to conscience and the health-care system share a fundamental commitment to preserving and restoring personal wholeness or integrity, we ought in cases of conflict to seek some sort of balance or accommodation between them.

Health professionals who refuse, withdraw, or dissociate themselves from certain practices or procedures on grounds of conscience may well be among the more thoughtful and effective members of a health-care team. Thus a health-care institution intent on retaining such nurses and physicians has prudential as well as ethical grounds for accommodating their claims of conscience even at the cost of some inconvenience or expense. Respect for conscience requires going to greater lengths for patients, however, than it does for health-care professionals. This is in part because an individual's role as a health-care professional is voluntary in a way that being a patient is not. It is one thing, for example, to respect a Jehovah's Witness patient's conscientious refusal of a blood transfusion; it is quite another to respect the conscientious refusal of a physician who is a Jehovah's Witness to administer blood transfusions. An individual whose moral or religious convictions are incompatible with a common, essential type of health care has no business seeking a position in which such care is a routine expectation.

Problems and limits

At least two important questions remain. First, how do we distinguish genuine claims of conscience from claims serving as smoke screens for laziness, cowardice, distaste for certain procedures, or dislike or prejudice toward certain patients? Second, given that a genuine act of conscience may be morally wrong, should individuals always (or always be permitted to) follow their conscience?

Genuineness. Understanding the nature and justification of conscientious refusal allows us to distinguish genuine from spurious or self-deceived appeals to conscience. In assessing the authenticity of such appeals we may, for example, inquire into (1) the underlying values and the extent to which they constitute a core component of the individual's identity; (2) the depth of the individual's reflective consideration of the issue; and (3) the likelihood that he or she will experience guilt, shame, or a loss of self-respect by performing the act in question. Such criteria have been employed with reasonable success by the U.S. Selective Service System in identifying those whose deep and long-standing moral convictions forbid direct participation in war. They can be used with similar success in identifying genuine ap-

peals to conscience in the health-care setting (Benjamin and Curtis, 1992).

Conscientious but wrong. Conscience is not an infallible guide to conduct. Even those who attend carefully to matters of integrity and who critically examine their basic convictions may, at a later date, judge some of their conscientious acts as wrong. Should one, then, always follow one's conscience? If by "conscience" we mean the exercise and expression of good-faith efforts to integrate conduct with reflective ethical conviction, the answer is "yes." Following conscience is obligatory, even if one's act turns out to be wrong, because one is doing what one reflectively believes to be right. Conversely, deliberately acting contrary to conscience is blameworthy, even if one's act turns out to be right, because one is doing what one reflectively believes to be wrong.

We must therefore distinguish the character of an agent from the rightness of a particular act. That an act is required by conscience entails neither that it is right nor that others must endorse the agent's convictions or permit the act to occur. It is difficult, for example, to question the character of Jehovah's Witness parents when they conscientiously refuse to consent to a life-saving blood transfusion for a young child. Yet if we have good reasons for believing that withholding the transfusion would be seriously wrong, we may try to persuade the parents to consent and, if necessary, seek a court order mandating treatment. Distinguishing the conscientiousness of the parents from our judgment of the act, though not eliminating the difficult question of whether, and if so, how, to intervene, enables us to attend more adequately to its complexity.

MARTIN BENJAMIN

For a further discussion of topics mentioned in this entry, see the entries AUTONOMY; ETHICS, *especially* RELIGION AND MORALITY; PERSON; PROFESSIONAL–PATIENT RELATIONSHIP; RESPONSIBILITY; VALUE AND VALUATION; *and* VIRTUE AND CHARACTER. *This entry will find application in the entries* BIOETHICS; CIVIL DISOBEDIENCE AND HEALTH CARE; CLINICAL ETHICS; MEDICINE, ART OF; *and* NURSING ETHICS.

Bibliography

ARENDT, HANNAH. 1971. "Thinking and Moral Considerations: A Lecture." *Social Research* 38:417–446. Reprinted in *Social Research* 51:7–37 (1984).

———. 1972. "Civil Disobedience." In her *Crises of the Republic: Lying in Politics, Civil Disobedience, On Violence, Thoughts on Politics and Revolution*, pp. 51–102. New York: Harcourt Brace Jovanovich.

BEAUCHAMP, TOM L., and CHILDRESS, JAMES F. 1984. *Principles of Biomedical Ethics.* 3d ed. New York: Oxford University Press.

BENJAMIN, MARTIN. 1990. *Splitting the Difference: Compromise and Integrity in Ethics and Politics.* Lawrence: University Press of Kansas.

BENJAMIN, MARTIN, and CURTIS, JOY. 1992. *Ethics in Nursing.* 3d ed. New York: Oxford University Press.

BROAD, CHARLIE DUNBAR. 1940. "Conscience and Conscientious Action." *Philosophy* 15:115–130.

BUTLER, JOSEPH. 1900. [1726]. *Fifteen Sermons.* In *The Works of Bishop Butler,* vol. 1. Edited by John Henry Bernard. New York: Macmillan.

CHILDRESS, JAMES F. 1979. "Appeals to Conscience." *Ethics* 89, no. 4:315–335.

———. 1985. "Civil Disobedience, Conscientious Objection, and Evasive Noncompliance: A Framework for the Analysis and Assessment of Illegal Actions in Health Care." *Journal of Medicine and Philosophy* 10, no. 1:63–83.

D'ARCY, ERIC. 1961. *Conscience and Its Right to Freedom.* New York: Sheed and Ward.

———. 1977. "Conscience." *Journal of Medical Ethics* 3, no. 2:98–99.

FUSS, PETER. 1964. "Conscience." *Ethics* 74, no. 2:111–120.

GARNETT, A. CAMPBELL. 1966. "Conscience and Conscientiousness." In *Insight and Vision: Essays in Philosophy in Honor of Radoslav Andrea Tsanoff,* pp. 71–83. Edited by Konstantin Kolenda. San Antonio: Trinity University Press.

GILLON, RAANAN. 1984. "Conscience, Virtue, Integrity, and Medical Ethics." *Journal of Medical Ethics* 10, no. 4: 171–172.

MAY, LARRY. 1983. "On Conscience." *American Philosophical Quarterly* 20, no.1:57–67.

McGUIRE, MARTIN. 1963. "On Conscience." *Journal of Philosophy* 60, no. 10:253–263.

MOUNT, ERIC, JR. 1969. *Conscience and Responsibility.* Richmond, Va.: John Knox Press.

RYLE, GILBERT. 1940. "Conscience and Moral Convictions." *Analysis* 7:31–39.

TAYLOR, CHARLES. 1976. "Responsibility for Self." In *The Identities of Persons,* pp. 281–299. Edited by Amelie Oksenberg Rorty. Berkeley: University of California Press.

WAND, BERNARD. 1961. "The Content and Function of Conscience." *Journal of Philosophy* 58, no. 24:765–772.

CONSENT, INFORMED

See INFORMED CONSENT.

CONSEQUENTIALISM

See ETHICS, *article on* NORMATIVE ETHICAL THEORIES; *and* UTILITY.

CONTRACEPTION

See FERTILITY CONTROL.

COST–BENEFIT ANALYSIS

See ECONOMIC CONCEPTS IN HEALTH CARE; *and* TECHNOLOGY, *article on* TECHNOLOGY ASSESSMENT.

COST-EFFECTIVENESS

See ECONOMIC CONCEPTS IN HEALTH CARE; HEALTH-CARE RESOURCES, ALLOCATION OF; *and* TECHNOLOGY, *article on* TECHNOLOGY ASSESSMENT.

CREATIONISM

See EVOLUTION; *and* PHILOSOPHY, BIOLOGY OF.

CRYONICS

The term "cryonics" refers to the practice of freezing dead human bodies or even separated heads in the hope of achieving a temporary but lengthy suspension of life functions. The freezing of persons who are not already legally dead is considered to be homicide.

Cryonics was popularized as a theory by Robert C. W. Ettinger in 1964. His assumption was that frozen human beings could eventually be revived through the use of advanced scientific techniques. Although practiced on a limited scale, cryonics has received extensive popular attention (e.g., Vogel, 1988) and has some scientific supporters (e.g., Wowk and Darwin, 1989). Because its methodology does not involve the testing of results, thus differing significantly from tissue- and organ-freezing studies, cryonics is not accepted as a true science by most low-temperature scientists and their official organization, the Society for Cryobiology.

Freezing objects for various purposes has been a useful practice for many centuries, but it was not until 1940 that Basile Luyet and P. N. Gehenio compiled the first comprehensive survey on the survival of organisms at low temperatures. In 1964, an increasing volume of research on low-temperature biology precipitated the founding of *Cryobiology,* a journal that continues to serve as an important source of research reports. The journal will not accept articles on cryonics.

Human beings, like other mammals but unlike most animal species, normally maintain their body temperature within very narrow limits. In all species a decline in body temperature is accompanied by a corresponding reduction in vital activities. Actual freezing essentially suspends all life processes.

Scientists have frozen and successfully recovered many segregated mammalian cells and tissues. The freezing of most mammalian cells, however, without previous exposure to cryoprotective agents, like glycerol or dimethyl sulfoxide, results in their death due to irreversible structural and biological changes.

No one has ever succeeded in the more ambitious cryonic goal of maintaining the whole body or the separated head of a human in the frozen state and eventually resuscitating it. Indeed, there are no scientific data that promise success, and even if a whole body somehow survived, the likelihood of significant debilitating injury would be great. Nevertheless, there are those who believe resuscitation will be possible at some distant time when science is further advanced and when both the pathology that caused the death and any injury resulting from the freezing process can be reversed. Those who are interested in using cryonic interment have founded d'cryonics," or "life extension," societies and have forecast its eventual widespread application.

In cases of long-term human cryonic preservation, as soon as the subject is pronounced legally dead, various stabilizing medications, including anticoagulants, are administered in order to minimize damage from reduced circulation. A heart/lung machine is employed to maintain oxygenated circulation while the body is being cooled externally. Selected blood vessels are permeated with a cryoprotective agent until the replacement of blood is complete. The subject is then cooled further and immersed in a container of liquid nitrogen at −196°C (Wowk and Darwin, 1989), or in the vapor phase of liquid nitrogen at −150°C. More economical though somewhat less cold mechanical freezers may also be used.

In any case, the expense of maintaining a body in this state for a long time is high, and some form of endowment or insurance policy must be available for support.

Possible low-temperature states

There are three low-temperature states that might theoretically be considered for the long-term maintenance of a human body in a reduced or halted metabolic condition: hypothermia, hibernation, and freezing. Each has severe limitations.

Hypothermia.   Hypothermia involves the cooling of the body to a temperature below normal but above freezing. This can take place when the body temperature–regulating mechanisms fail, or the heat production of an individual does not compensate for the heat loss resulting from exposure to cold. Although some persons have survived after accidentally becoming deeply hypothermic for brief periods, whole-body hypothermia, even under controlled conditions, cannot be maintained successfully for much over twenty-four hours. However, experiments on dogs cooled to an unusually deep hypothermia, a few degrees above freezing, for several hours following the substitution of a well-balanced artificial

solution for the animal's blood, have resulted in successful revival (Bailes et al., 1991). These are very promising experiments.

The failure of tissues to receive an adequate supply of oxygenated blood is the primary cause of damage or death. In medical usage, regional or differential hypothermia is generally preferred over whole-body cooling. Hypothermia has been found useful to preserve isolated organs, such as the kidney and heart, prior to transplantation, and to minimize trauma during some surgical procedures.

Hibernation.   Hibernation, a state of greatly reduced body temperature, occurs naturally in some mammals and birds (French, 1988). The hibernating animal retains the capability of spontaneously rewarming to its normal level of around 37°C (98°F) by a mechanism of internal heat production without absorbing heat from its environment. Hibernating animals are able to recover fully from weeks-long periods of profound torpor—a state in which the temperature of the entire body falls to within a few degrees of freezing, heart rate is slowed to a few beats per minute, and metabolism is depressed as much as 99 percent. Under certain medical circumstances it would be useful to be able to produce a state of hibernation in a patient, but the mechanism of hibernation is unknown. Science is far from solving this mystery and, in any case, hibernation would not completely succeed in halting the aging process, a goal of cryonicists.

Freezing.   If healthy recovery could be accomplished, total-body freezing presumably would be the best method for long-term preservation of human bodies in a totally inactive state. If only the head is frozen, as has been done in several cases, reconnection following defrosting would itself present a formidable challenge. Such practices at the present time are simply hopes lacking a sufficient scientific foundation.

On the other hand, cryopreservation of individual human cells, such as ova and spermatozoa, some tissues, and embryos (but not fetuses), has met with considerable success (Lieber, 1989; Malinin et al., 1991). This is primarily due to their small size, which facilitates total treatment; their resistance to damage; and their capacity for recovery. The use of controlled rates of cooling and cryoprotective solutions generally are necessary. If injury occurs it is usually in the early stages of freezing; the duration of freezing below −100°C seems to be of little significance. Numerous attempts to freeze complete human organs for possible transplantation have not yet succeeded despite controlled rates of cooling, the use of a wide variety of cryoprotective agents, and repeated testing of freezing organs while they are still in the donor body or after they have been removed. Research continues with isolated organs, including efforts to avoid some of the damaging effects of freezing by preventing fracturing and crystallization (Fahy et al., 1990).

Probably because of its complexity, the freezing of whole mammals has received relatively little serious attention from scientists. Extensive studies were conducted on a hibernator, the golden hamster, by Audrey U. Smith (1970), but full recovery of a completely frozen mature mammal has not been demonstrated. It should be noted, however, that many nonmammalian species survive freezing, a fact that has often led to public confusion about the viability of frozen mammals.

In summary, attempts to preserve humans by freezing must be regarded as based on unfounded hopes. There is essentially no material "prospect of immortality" for bodies frozen by the cryonic methods now employed.

Ethical issues in human freezing

Moral concerns about cryoscience and its application in cryogenic projects focus on its value in enabling the achievement of a more human future; the question of human nature and destiny; concern about personal freedom and fulfillment; and the commitment to justice and the common good.

The values of cryoscience.   Cryobiology as a biomedical enterprise shares the two basic values of human science—the amelioration of human disease and suffering, and the longer-range achievement of a better life for humankind. Derivative from this salutary impulse, but more ethically problematic, the technological imperative says that things that can be done, should be done. Some immediate and near-range goals of cryoscience are morally valid. Human experimentation of all sorts often serves elusive and futuristic goals, such as the ability to survive long periods of time in space with minimal bodily atrophy and aging. Some argue that the survival of the human race will be made possible by cryopreservation chambers acting as a Noah's Ark and saving the germ cells of the plant and animal kingdoms in the face of a nuclear holocaust. We may question whether the human purposes of science include ensuring that all to come after us will be just like us or, worse yet, that our own clone or cryborg will live forever. Freezing and maintaining in perpetuity someone once dear to us may both violate our sense of the particular and precious in a life's story and impose a burden of anxiety and false expectation that saps joy from our life as we experience its possibility and limitation. If awareness of mortality and the values derived from one's finitude are part of traditional humanistic wisdom, then the quest for physical immortality is ethically disorienting.

Human nature and destiny.   The question of scientific purpose is ultimately grounded in the question of human identity and purpose. Is the raison d'être of human existence the conquest of disease and death, and the implied achievement of immortality, or is it the achievement of more modest and humane goals?

While the philosophy favoring cryonic stabilization and interment seems to be contrary to religious understandings of the purpose of life and the meaning of death, Ettinger (1964) understands cryonic interment to be an "urgent spiritual goal," and proposes a "religious" vision of "supermen" greatly enriched by biological techniques.

If perfected, preservation for periods of years or decades might be defined in circumstances such as long space flights, expectation of new medical developments, or even historical continuity of mankind. Each situation would have to be evaluated individually. Widely applied long-term human preservation, however, would confront us with a very different and highly ambiguous set of moral concerns.

According to Vaux (1974), humans, as social beings, must learn to die for the sake of the future. He maintains that we must learn that death energy is creative. We face population and ecological disaster if we disrupt the evolutionary death now in process without simultaneously disrupting birth. The success of the freezing procedure would not of itself mean that the actual, active, human biological life would be significantly extended, although the chronological life span would be increased. It could mean that age proportions in our population would be disrupted. Perhaps our concentration on health care would be even more emphasized, to the diminution of other values (Caplan, 1992). Unless there is some limit to birthrate and unless the death rate is at least maintained in step with this limit, the quality of life on this planet may be radically altered.

Personal freedom and fulfillment.   Modern bioethics is strongly influenced by commitments to autonomy and the rights of persons to act upon and dispose of their own bodies as they wish. Cryonics could enhance or erase human freedom. The right to die could be violated, the consent of the individual be abrogated. In the frozen state, where there can be no dialogue with the individual, rights could easily be neglected. A variety of questions pertaining to property and family relationships would also be raised. Cryopreservation of germ cells and embryos has already raised these questions of rights. Does anyone own the person?

A person's behavior is dependent on constant interactions with surrounding objects and actions that impinge upon him or her. One might hope to be unchanged after a long period of preservation, but ambience, historical context, and associations would be radically disrupted. What would be the effect on personal development? What would be the effect of a long cessation of biological rhythms, so essential for a balanced human existence? What subtle behavioral variations might result in an individual or a population? Long-term preservation would probably produce individuals out of step with human historical development. And, of course, it is more than likely that the preservation procedures would be at least slightly imperfect and would yield many mentally or physically unhealthy individuals. Would society accept a moral responsibility to see that such defective persons are cared for until they die naturally? Such biomedical activity forces the question of whether personal freedom and fulfillment are found in self-preservation or self-sacrifice.

Justice and the common good. The ultimate ethical question raised by the cryonics project is the social justice of such exotic procedures for some while the more basic needs of many go unattended. In a freedom-infused, entrepreneurial world, persons can do with their bodies as they please and corporations can market their wares—even the package of biological resurrection. But if, as is increasingly the case, we find ourselves in a resource-limited and interdependent world, considerations of justice will ask whether limited resources ought to be diverted in this direction. The immediate benefits of preserving cells, tissues, and organs by low-temperature methodologies are obvious and compelling. Moral questions become much more complex and problematic when the goal of such procedures becomes hubristic challenge to the life–death rhythm of human existence.

J. A. PANUSKA AND KENNETH L. VAUX

For a further discussion of topics mentioned in this entry, see the entries AUTONOMY; DEATH, *articles on* WESTERN PHILOSOPHICAL THOUGHT, *and* WESTERN RELIGIOUS THOUGHT; FUTURE GENERATIONS, OBLIGATIONS TO; HEALTH-CARE RESOURCES, ALLOCATION OF, *article on* MICROALLOCATION; *and* TECHNOLOGY, *article on* TECHNOLOGY ASSESSMENT. *This entry will find application in the entry* ORGAN AND TISSUE TRANSPLANTS, *article on* MEDICAL OVERVIEW; *and* REPRODUCTIVE TECHNOLOGIES, *article on* CRYOPRESERVATION OF SPERM, OVA, AND EMBRYOS. *For a discussion of related ideas, see the entries* DEATH, ATTITUDES TOWARD; HUMAN NATURE; JUSTICE; *and* VALUE AND VALUATION.

Bibliography

BAILES, JULIAN E.; LEAVITT, MARC L.; TEEPLE, EDWARD, JR.; MAROON, JOSEPH C.; SHIH, SHOU-REN; MARQUARDT, MERLIN; EL RIFAI, AMR; and MANACK, LEO. 1991. "Ultraprofound Hypothermia with Complete Blood Substitution in a Canine Model." *Journal of Neurosurgery* 74, no. 5:781–788.

CAPLAN, ARTHUR. 1992. "Is Aging a Disease?" In *If I Were a Rich Man Could I Buy a Pancreas?: And Other Essays on the Ethics of Health Care.* Bloomington: Indiana University Press.

Cryobiology, International Journal of Low Temperature Biology and Medicine. San Diego, Calif.: Academic Press.

ETTINGER, ROBERT C. W. 1964. *The Prospect of Immortality.* Garden City, N.Y.: Doubleday.

FAHY, GREGORY M.; SAUR, JOSEPH; and WILLIAMS, ROBERT J. 1990. "Physical Problems with the Vitrification of Large Biological Systems." *Cryobiology* 27:492–509.

FRENCH, ALAN R. 1988. "The Patterns of Mammalian Hibernation." *American Scientist* 76:568–575.

LIEBER, JAMES. 1989. "A Piece of Yourself in the World." *Atlantic Monthly,* June, pp. 76–80.

LUYET, BASILE, and GEHENIO, MARIE PIERRE. 1940. *Life and Death at Low Temperatures.* Normandy, Mo.: Biodynamica.

MALININ, THEODORE I.; THOMSON, CATHERINE B.; and BROWN, MARK D. 1981. "Freeze-dried Tissue Allografts in Surgery." In *Organ Preservation for Transplantation,* pp. 677–689. 2d ed. Edited by Armand M. Karow and David E. Pegg. New York: Marcel Dekker.

RAMSEY, PAUL. 1970. "The Ethics of Genetic Control: Shall We Clone a Man?" In *Who Shall Live?: Medicine, Technology, Ethics,* pp. 77–113. Edited by Kenneth Vaux. Philadelphia: Fortress.

SMITH, AUDREY U. 1970. "Frostbite, Hypothermia, and Resuscitation After Freezing." In *Current Trends in Cryobiology,* pp. 181–208. Edited by Audrey U. Smith. New York: Plenum.

VAUX, KENNETH. 1974. *Biomedical Ethics: Morality for the New Medicine.* New York: Harper & Row.

VOGEL, SHAWNA. 1988. "Cold Storage." *Discover* 9:52–54.

WOWK, BRIAN, and DARWIN, MICHAEL. 1989. *Alcor: Threshold to Tomorrow.* 2d ed. Riverside, Calif.: Alcor Life Extension Foundation.

CRYOPRESERVATION OF SPERM, OVA, AND EMBRYOS

See REPRODUCTIVE TECHNOLOGIES, *article on* CRYOPRESERVATION OF SPERM, OVA, AND EMBRYOS, *and also the articles on* ETHICAL ISSUES, *and* LEGAL AND REGULATORY ISSUES.

CUBA

See MEDICAL ETHICS, HISTORY OF, *section on* THE AMERICAS, *article on* LATIN AMERICA.

CYPRUS

See MEDICAL ETHICS, HISTORY OF, *section on* EUROPE, *subsection on* CONTEMPORARY PERIOD, *articles on* SOUTHERN EUROPE, *and* CENTRAL AND EASTERN EUROPE.

CZECHOSLOVAKIA

See MEDICAL ETHICS, HISTORY OF, *section on* EUROPE, *subsection on* CONTEMPORARY PERIOD, *article on* CENTRAL AND EASTERN EUROPE.

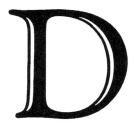

DEATH

I. ANTHROPOLOGICAL PERSPECTIVES

For all peoples, death embodies problems of existential meaning. Death is known and anticipated in all human societies as the extinction of life and takes on meanings associated with the defeat or frustration of valued life activities. Whether the activities involve religious, familial, communal, political, military, or economic importance, death constitutes a final loss of an individual's capacity to achieve them. Death is associated with sickness and pain, homicide and war, pestilence and famine, agony and grief. Accordingly, all societies exercise institutional controls to preserve and protect the lives of their members, controls supported by dread of death as well as by attachments to persons who are members of the community (Durkheim, 1951).

In all cultures, efforts to understand why evils exist and afflict human communities focus in large measure on death and its finality (Weber, 1963). Yet not only is death feared as an evil, but it may also be seen as an end or culmination or life and as a release from burdens and sufferings. Death may assume highly positive significance as a liberation in situations where the struggles and pains of life have become so exacerbated as to be intolerable. Societies that embrace elaborate cultural sentiments regarding the sufferings of life often also emphasize the attractions of death, weaving positive meanings of death dialectically through their institutional protections of life. In Hindu culture, for example, persons who have been dutiful to the customs of their "castes" are believed to gain reincarnation as members of higher "castes" or even to escape the burdens of rebirth to worldly suffering (Zimmer, 1956).

As Max Weber and later Karl Jaspers argued, the greatest divide in human experience originated with the emergence of "world religions" based on sustained, transgenerational, rational reflection on problems of religious ethics (Weber, 1946, 1963; Jaspers, 1949). Ever since the "axial age" from approximately 800 B.C.E. to 300 B.C.E., when several civilizations independently created religiophilosophical conceptions of a transcendental order and began to revitalize their ethical and normative orders in terms of these compelling ideals, human experience has been broadly divided between social orders legitimated through one or more of the world religions, and social orders legitimated through folk cultures (Bellah, 1970; Nelson, 1981). On the one side, social values and institutions have been rooted in philosophical reflection about the transcendental significance of life and death, good and evil, the sacred and the profane. On the other side, worldly and often magical conceptions make the sacred a more immediate and transfigurable force in daily life (Weber, 1963). The sacred may be encountered at nearly any time and in any of a great many guises, and it may present tangible threats to life unless special measures are adopted to ward it away (Durkheim, 1965). The continuities of life in the course of everyday routines are experienced as resting upon religiomagical rituals and protections and otherwise being vulnerable to the sorcery or witchcraft of others (Mauss, 1975; Evans-Pritchard, 1937).

While other articles in this entry are devoted to cultural and social orientations toward death in the great civilizations of antiquity, the East, and the West, this article focuses on death as a phenomenon among the thousands of tribal, folk, and archaic communities of the present and the past that have lacked cultural grounding in transcendental belief systems. Attention will also be given to the folk communities of peasants and the urban poor who in contemporary developing nations live partly in the culture of twentieth-century rationalism and partly in the magical or "enchanted" (Weber, 1963) outlooks of archaic cultures.

Death and sacred culture

Since Emile Durkheim, anthropologists have widely held that the core of every culture is made up of beliefs concerning the sacred and the profane (Levi-Strauss, 1963). The sacred entails special powers and commands extraordinary respect and awe. In treating the sacred with respect, members of society elevate it above the profane, or mundane, sphere of life and make it a higher source of meaning for their own lives. Sacred myths, beliefs, symbols, objects, and practices may have no apparently ethical nature, yet in maintaining various standards of respectful conduct toward the sacred, communities establish the moral authority and normative quality of traditional social orders, or at least central domains of them (Durkheim, 1965). It is thus important that in all societies human individuals and various groupings of individuals (lineages, clans, age grades, warrior fraternities, cult groups, and so forth) are viewed as participating under certain circumstances in the sacred. Although the routines of everyday life are profane, the individual is understood to have a soul or spirit that figures in the sacred domain and its awesome dignity. The sacred quality of the soul imparts social respect to the life of each individual. The soul is an essence of the individual that kin, friends, rivals, and enemies are all bound to respect; if not, they must fear the conse-

quences of having alienated a sacred power (Durkheim, 1965; Mauss, 1975; Turner, 1969).

Societies may differ substantially not only in ritual practices concerning death, but also in the underlying cultural outlooks they adopt toward its sacred implications. Anthropologists have characterized the cultural tempers of some New Guinea tribes as almost obsessive and even paranoid because of the worry their members invest in protecting themselves against the black magic or sorcery of others and against possible harms from the souls of the dead (Bateson, 1958; Berndt, 1962). Not only is there fear of the dead, but individuals feel intense anxiety over their own immediate vulnerability to disease, accidents, and death. Deaths are thus followed by elaborate rituals intended to protect from various dangers a number of classes of persons—a deceased person's spouses and affines, siblings and kin, and, hardly less, their rivals or enemies. As compared with this intense worry, the people of Java relinquish their dead with calm and cultivated dispassion (Geertz, 1960). Consistent with the generalized fatalism of Javanese values, individuals view the possibility of their own death without overt anxiety or fear. Warriors among the tribes of the North American plains were socialized to face pain and death fearlessly and with pride in their inner fortitude, although not with the passivity or resignation of the Javanese. The deaths of kin, therefore, were customarily mourned with strong emotion and open feelings of loss (Wallace, 1965).

Australian anthropologists have long reported on the many ways in which members of aboriginal societies experience personal access to the sacred domain (Warner, 1958; Elkin, 1954; Stanner, 1963). The sacred founding of society is believed to have occurred in a mythical time through the action of awesome figures. These figures are understood to be ancestral, hence dead, but on ritual occasions their sacred activities are enacted by living individuals and groups. Major life-cycle rituals, in particular, involve enthusiastic participation in the sacred realm. Intense emotion is released by the excitement of actually taking part in the key events of the mythical time (Stanner, 1963). In a significant sense, the bonds of society are reforged when individuals—in the roles of the mythical beings and as members of kinship, age-grade, and ritual groups—act out the stories of the founding of their societies (Warner, 1958). The awesome quality of the sacred then legitimates not only the conventional practices of initiation, marriage, and mourning, but equally the underlying relationships between kinship and ritual groups. Individual participants gain a revitalized reverence for, but also kinship and familiarity with, the sacred figures. Elders in particular are respected for their close relations with the sacred figures and for their ability to speak for the latter's sacredly endowed ways of life. When rituals are performed successfully, with each of the requisite groups fulfilling an appointed role, the participants experience a renewed respect for one another's souls or spirits, for the sacred qualities that dwell within members of the community. Lives, traditional ways of life, and communal sharing of the lifeways created by the figures in the sacred myths are affirmed and the solidarity of the community is strengthened (Durkheim, 1965; Warner, 1958).

The experience of proximity to the sacred can also be a source of existential insecurity. Life in Australian societies is vulnerable to black magic, the self-interested invoking of sacred powers to bring harm to others. Elders and adepts whose familiarity with the sacred enables them to use black magic are likely to be feared (Cowan, 1989). When conflicts emerge among groups that depend upon one another for trade, cooperative work, ritual exchanges, and intermarriage, sorcery is expected, and the resulting fears may leave many people anxious over possible sickness and death (Warner, 1958). When illness or death occurs, the causes are thus sought in the realm of black magic. The actions and motives of rival groups and individuals are scrutinized for signs of sorcery. Efforts to heal persistent illness focus on identifying a cause in the black magic of rivals. If death occurs, near kin may be expected to retaliate through sorcery or even direct personal aggression, and such retaliation may carry the legitimacy of legal sanction (Elkin, 1954).

Larger-scale archaic societies—with the authority of chiefs or kings to centralize political power; privileged status groups encompassing the leadership of many local communities; institutions for producing, collecting, and redistributing economic surpluses; and specially educated priesthoods—developed very different conceptions of the sacred and its relations to mundane society (Moret and Davy, 1970; Hubert and Mauss, 1964; Parsons, 1966). Sacred orders may be conceived in terms of an immense cosmos, vast periods, and multiple cycles of intricate myths—cycles often interpreted by the priesthoods as revealing various aspects of a mysterious reality accessible only to initiates (Schele and Miller, 1986; Frankfort, 1948). In most archaic traditions, gods were conceptualized as figures with extraordinary powers and the will to favor or harm humans, individually and collectively, in ways that could lead to prosperity or poverty, great power or enslavement, health or suffering, long life or immediate death.

As Henri Hubert and Marcel Mauss (1964) emphasized, religious concerns in archaic societies focused on propitiating gods to secure earthly well-being. Sacrifice—the offering of gifts to the gods in order to compel their favor by reciprocation—was thus the primary form of archaic religiosity. Often sacrifice was carried out on a large scale to demonstrate quantitatively the extreme honor being shown to the gods and to impress on a population the power and wealth of the noble figures on whose behalf a sacrifice was performed. Monumentality is thus a theme of archaic religiosity, visible in the temples and pyramids of Egypt, the ancient palaces of the Mesopotamian states, the burial sites of the early Chinese kings, or the temples and palaces of Central American civilizations.

Sacrifices might be acts of individuals designed to obtain personal or familial advantages, but they were often elaborate institutional performances guided by priestly guilds to secure cosmic beneficence for the entire community. Kings and royal lineages typically assumed central roles in mediating the relationships between the cosmic and social orders. In his classic study of Mesopotamian kingship and Egyptian pharaonic institutions, Henri Frankfort (1948) contrasted two modes of such mediation. In Mesopotamia, kings were chief propitiators of the gods and even portrayed ritually as consorts of great goddesses, highly privileged in their ability to secure divine beneficence. Good weather and bountiful crops, freedom from epidemics, the success of trading expeditions, and victory in battle were all attributed in part to the favor of gods secured ritually by the king, with the assistance of his priests. Famine, pestilence, losses in battle, and so forth brought out vigorous and, if persistent, eventually desperate efforts to propitiate the gods. The death of a king placed the entire society in a situation of peril until a suitable succession, involving at a crucial phase the ritual marriage of king with goddess, had been accomplished.

In Egypt, the pharaohs were regarded as divine beings, playing direct and essential roles in the cosmic order itself. Deaths of pharaohs thus appeared to be disruptions of the divine order, hence occasions fraught with dangers of cosmic as well as political evils. The funerary rites of the pharaohs were typically prepared over many years and involved substantial portions of the society's wealth, as the construction of the great pyramids or the collection of the burial treasures of Tutankhamen indicate. The rituals of pharaonic succession were closely tied to myths of transformation central to the Egyptian understanding of the cosmos. As Frankfort explicates the Memphite Theology, the most sophisticated variant of the myths, the pharaoh is Horus, son of Osiris and empowered by Osiris, a commanding figure in the cosmos; but after death the pharaoh becomes Osiris and ritually empowers his son as his successor and Horus. Horus rules with the sacred powers conveyed by his procreator, Osiris, and thus brings the divine beneficence of the entire cosmos to Egypt and its people, ordered by his rule (Frankfort, 1948).

Nearly all the major archaic civilizations appear to have practiced the sacrifice of living human individuals as part of key rituals. Human sacrifice has been amply documented for many ancient societies of the Middle

East, India, China, and the Mediterranean (Tierney, 1989). Ritual sacrifices of captives after battle and of personal retainers as part of the funerary rites of kings have been frequently noted. Recent studies have documented the large role of human sacrifice in the religiopolitical institutions of pre-Columbian Andean civilization; they also suggested that in some remote areas children and young women are even today occasionally sacrificed by shamans as part of propitiatory cults descended from Incan civilization (Tierney, 1989).

Aztec, Mayan, and related civilizations elaborated the sacrificial cult to a far greater degree. The Mayan cosmology stressed the fearsome importance of powerful gods who demanded blood sacrifices in return for favoring the city-state in its relationship with the cosmos or entire human environment. Kings, their wives, and their extended families were responsible for providing the blood to propitiate the major gods in elaborate rituals. Their own bloodletting rites were central to this propitiation. However, kings also needed to offer up the blood of great captives in their rituals. Both accession to the throne and various rites of the renewal of royal powers required the blood of captives (Schele and Miller, 1986). Battles were fought not only for domination of new territories and peoples, but also to acquire captives—preferably powerful chiefs or kings themselves—for the sacrificial cult. Warriors captured in battle were taken back to the palaces and ritual centers for ceremonies of personal humiliation and bloodletting. It appears that many captives were subjected to the rites of bloodletting and often extremely painful torture a number of times over periods of several years or more. Eventually, however, the captives were sacrificed, with their chests cut open, their hearts ripped out, and the flowing blood burned as offering to the gods (Schele and Miller, 1986).

Among the Aztecs, the cult of human sacrifice evolved in a different direction. Although the Aztec sacrifice was also a sequel to battle, it was not so strongly focused on ritualizing a particular relation between the conquering king and his captive. Accordingly, humiliation and torture were not emphasized, and death by sacrifice was even regarded as an honorable end for a brave member of the warrior class (Soustelle, 1970). Warriors were socialized to view their fates as glorious and take part in the sacrifice with resigned dignity, although they typically did so after drink or drugs and lengthy ceremonies had produced an ecstatic possession to ease their inevitable surrender to the knives of the priests (Clendinnen, 1991). However, the Aztec sacrifice escalated geometrically as the size, power, and social complexity of the empire grew. Aztec armies employed special tactics to maximize the number of captives gained in battle and they ranged over a large territory in search of communities to conquer. The loose hegemony under which the Aztecs managed the dependent peoples of their empire created many opportunities for battle and the taking of captives. In later times, Aztec merchant groups also seem to have sought social honor by trading for slaves whom they could contribute to the public sacrifice. The high god Uitzilopotchli was believed to need the placation of thousands of warrior sacrifices at a number of times during the year, but the ritual calendar also required sacrifices of appropriately prepared slaves and even children of the community to honor a number of other gods as well (Soustelle, 1970; Coe, 1962; Clendinnen, 1991).

The social regulation of life and death

Emile Durkheim introduced the insight that under everyday conditions societies impose firm obligations on individuals to respect and protect their own lives and the lives of others (Durkheim, 1965). In Durkheim's view, there is no such thing as a "natural" life cycle because lives are always the result of socially enjoined efforts to extend them. Even before birth, individuals depend on the efforts of parents and others to nurture and protect them, efforts supported by strongly institutionalized expectations. Care in avoiding danger and in helping others to avoid danger is enjoined as part of the socialization process in all communities. By adulthood, men and women have typically assumed responsibilities to protect themselves and others from a variety of practical threats to life—threats of accidents, disease, lack of food or shelter, forces of nature, and so forth. Moreover, in all societies, the lives of members are protected by the regulations of law and custom, supported by powerful moral sentiments that ordinarily prohibit purposeful aggression and conspiracy on the part of others. Yet societies exhibit great variation in the details of the normative protections they extend to life and in defining the circumstances under which such protections may be suspended. The normative orders of all societies recognize conditions that justify and may even valorize aggression against the lives of others or the offering of one's own life (Durkheim, 1951).

The normative protections that communities extend to the lives of their individual members vary with such factors as social status, gender, and stage of the life cycle. In the legal systems of ancient Mesopotamian societies, for example, the legal codes provided that criminal sanctions for assaults and bodily injuries depended upon the social classes of both the assailant and the person attacked (Saggs, 1962). Thus, the penalty for breaking another person's leg depended on whether the person was a member of a noble lineage, a commoner, or a servant. A commoner who assaulted a person of like status would receive a lesser penalty than a servant, but a greater penalty than a nobleman. Among most peoples, as for the Mundurucu of Brazil, the social roles of women have carried less prestige than those of men, and accordingly a variety of normative arrangements have extended firmer protections to men (Murphy and Murphy, 1985). Some of these arrangements are mundane, though of considerable practical importance, such as priority in the distribution of food. Other arrangements concern such matters of the sacred as privileges of ritual protection against sorcery. In most societies, the strongest protections are extended to men and women in middle adulthood who bear the major institutional responsibilities in their households and communities. By contrast, the relatively inactive or "retired" elderly are often viewed as nearing the completion of life and of less social importance. However, some societies extend deference and protective respect to the elderly, even to the infirm, as has been true in China since early antiquity (Granet, 1958).

Birth is not only a time of high natural risk for a child, but one in which social protections for life are often limited. Many societies expose to the elements children with birth defects or without parents to take responsibility for their care. Moreover, particularly in areas with high infant mortality rates, children are often not extended full protection as members of society until they have shown their viability by living for some months or even years. Their kin may meliorate the pains of losing young children by regarding them as only provisional members of society, not yet qualified to be strongly cathected (Warner, 1958). Only after a rite of passage into societal membership, signified, for example, by formal naming, are more complete and unconditional affective attachments made to the children. In a variant of such practices, the Mundurucu offer protection only to those newborns who are free of the physical anomalies of major birth defects and twinship as well as the social anomaly of illegitimacy (Murphy and Murphy, 1985). Babies whose mothers have not been married are anomalous in the sense that they lack the social identity of clanship and hence their relationships with others, including future marriageability, are undefined. They are killed after birth because they have no determinate place in the society (Murphy and Murphy, 1985).

The suicides of lonely and depressed individuals, perhaps the most common type of suicide in contemporary Western societies, appear to have been rare in folk and archaic societies until recent times, possibly because the forms of social integration in the older communities provided more immediate and tangible support. Altruistic suicides by individuals responding to social obligations to terminate their lives were more frequent (Durkheim, 1951). Historically, the retainers who gave up their lives to be buried with great chiefs or kings may have fit the altruistic type, as did women who accompanied royal husbands in funeral pyres or burials.

Among the Inuit, the elderly who exposed themselves on the ice rather than continuing to consume resources, feeling themselves no longer able to contribute effectively to the household, were altruistic suicides (Poncins, 1941). Defeated or occasionally traitorous generals who deliberately sought death in battle or by their own swords rather than returning alive to their commanders or fellow citizens were familiar suicides in antiquity, perhaps especially among the Greeks (Ehrenberg, 1960).

In many contemporary folk communities located at the social margins of large-scale modern societies, alcoholism that appears "suicidal" has become not uncommon. For much of the twentieth century, alcoholism has been an immense public-health problem among indigenous peoples of North America, regions of Central and South America, South Africa, and Australia. People have turned to alcohol seeking consolation or escape from the emotional pain that accompanies intense anomie, the loss of coherence in traditional communities and the eroding of traditional lifeways. Caught between commitment to social orders that are no longer viable and an absence of opportunities in the larger societies, many such people have found their lives purposeless and frustrating. In situations like these, the alternatives to aimless drink may appear to lack in moral authority. The resulting loss of life, whether due to direct effects of alcohol, to malnutrition, or to infectious disease after weakening of the body, has been immense in many parts of the world. In many communities, revitalization movements have emerged in response to the widespread alcoholism and the underlying anomic social conditions, though with highly variable degrees of success (Wallace, 1956; Lanternari, 1963).

Anthropologists have generally maintained that homicide within the community is prohibited by established norms backed by public sanction in every known society (Hoebel, 1954). Yet all or nearly all societies permit homicide under specific circumstances—for example, self-defense, defense of spouse or kin, defense of sacred objects or places, and, in archaic societies, defense of privileged persons. Infractions of law, ranging from profanation of sacred objects to adultery to abandonment of fellow warriors in circumstances of peril, may justify homicide as sanction in support of tradition and law. In many societies, the right to self-defense entails a right of action against persons believed to have exercised sorcery against oneself, one's kin, or sacred emblems with which one is identified. Ambiguity about when sorcery has been employed may in some societies permit the rather free justification of homicide against rivals. However, beliefs in the efficacy of black magic can also enable a person to sanction another effectively without resorting to a direct confrontation with its risks of physical injury (Fallers, 1969). Where cultures do not distinguish between "natural" causes of diseases, accidents, and deaths, and willful harm imposed by others through black magic, such events as epidemics, storms, crop failures, and accidental injuries may result in exchanges of sorcerous acts, eventually escalating to personal attacks and homicide. As Edward Evan Evans-Pritchard demonstrated in his classic study of the East African Azande, complicated subcultures of witchcraft and divination with trained specialists may be needed to guide the ordinary member of the community in determining what has befallen him or her, who has been behind it and with what intent, what alternatives for responding are appropriate, and what outcomes may be expected (Evans-Pritchard, 1937).

In the legal systems of most folk societies, a death attributed to the acts of another person obligates the kin of the deceased to exercise revenge. In taking revenge, however, the kin may create new obligations of retribution against themselves. In parts of New Guinea, the duties of revenge have been nearly absolute despite the dangers of reciprocal retribution. The reciprocal taking of revenge traditionally defined relationships between proximate villages over long periods of time and stood as an established, virtually unchangeable feature of everyday life (Berndt, 1962). In other societies, revenge has been less automatic. A group of kin might acknowledge the justice of an action against one of its members and forbear to strike back. In some cases, gifts of valued objects or the performance of rituals of respect for the deceased might allay the need for revenge. Informal mediation by elders of other groups might also encourage a settlement without retaliation. In societies with court systems, as in many parts of Africa, one party might bring the entire conflict to a court for resolution and gain a decision forestalling the threatened or expected revenge (Fallers, 1969). In other societies, the court powers of a chief or king might be drawn in partisan fashion into conflicts between rival groups. In archaic kingdoms fragmented into semiautonomous, competing fiefdoms by various economic and political forces, such outcomes were especially common (Bloch, 1961). The Merovingian royal kindred of sixth- to eighth-century France, for example, was torn by treacherous and deadly conspiracies among its rival branches, each with its own territorial base, in their power struggles with one another over several generations.

Warfare has historically played a prominent role in most folk and archaic societies. In many small-scale societies, the role of warrior was normative for most adult men; and socialization to warrior lifeways, with their ethic of ascetic perseverance in the face of injury and pain as well as resignation to the possibility of eventual death in battle, typically began early in life for boys. For many New Guinea villagers, a number of North American tribes, and peoples in some parts of Africa, conflict or potential conflict with surrounding groups was a nearly constant feature of life. Villagers needed to be alert for possible raids from hostile groups on a routine basis, while their men planned and sought favorable opportunities for raids on other villages or tribes. Capture of food, domesticated animals, craft goods, and often children who could be raised as contributing members of the community, were a major source of wealth. Participation in and especially leadership of raids on rival groups became important sources of social prestige for men. Often enhanced status followed from killing enemies and particularly from such outward signs of magical domination over the souls of enemy warriors as possessing scalps or "shrunken heads." In some societies, the magical dominance that accompanied the taking of scalps constituted a primary basis of a shaman's or chief's powers. Studies in New Guinea have shown how the interweaving of duties to revenge killed or wounded kin, rivalries among villages, and advantages in terms of magic and power gained by men successful in battle could sustain cycles of attack and counterattack across generations (Berndt, 1962).

Archaic societies commonly developed semiprivileged or privileged classes whose men were devoted in large degree to warrior roles. The citizens of the early Hellenic city-states are a prime example of a privileged class devoted to advancing the well-being of the community politically and militarily. Organized in terms of lineage and geographic ties as well as in terms of social rank and often heritable rights to leadership, the body of male citizens took collective responsibility for protecting the city (Ehrenberg, 1960; Gernet, 1981). Given the rivalries among as well as within city-states, politics and diplomacy were major instrumentalities for fulfilling the duties of citizens. Some states favored developing alliances to stabilize complicated diplomatic situations and to maintain peace. Yet male citizens were educated methodically as warriors in the expectation that going to war would likely be necessary in every generation. The solidarity of the phalanx, or tightly ranked battle group, was a primary consideration in all relationships among male citizens, with the core of personal honor based on a reputation for courage in protecting one's fellow warriors during the perils of closely engaged battle. The Greek warrior was trained to step forward instantly into the thrust of a spear or a sword to protect the life of the next person in the phalanx. In Sparta, ascetic training of citizens to develop a capacity for self-sacrifice in the service of military discipline began early in childhood and continued through active manhood.

In a number of historical epochs, warfare among archaic societies has caused extensive devastation and misery while also comprising a major force of social change. The dominant powers of the ancient Middle East—the Babylonian, Assyrian, and Persian empires, for example—were created in environments of many competing states, partly by threat and forceful diplomacy but largely by brutal conquest (Moscati, 1962). Chronicles that reported tens of thousands of inhabitants put to the sword after their cities were pillaged and burned may have exaggerated at times. Frequently, captives were not killed but were taken off for sale as slaves, enriching the conquering commanders. Yet the scale of brutality and loss of life often must have been immense. Similar customs of warfare and conquest were involved in the expansion of the Roman Empire and later its fragmentation over several centuries through the "barbarian" invasions. A common feature of the invasions was the organization of highly mobile, disciplined, and cunning warrior groups anxious to gain the benefits of settlement on empire territories and capable of concentrating their forces to exploit the weaknesses of peripheral defenses (Lot, 1961).

Rituals of death and survival

The soul is rarely conceived as coming to rest immediately after death. In most societies, the soul is believed to remain active and to require scrupulous attention and management by the living. In the symbolic dimension, mortuary rites are typically thought to care for the deceased, but also to protect the living from possible harm by the soul of the deceased. The kin of the deceased are in practically all societies required to fulfill the most elaborate duties, with fulfillment of these duties believed necessary for the soul to achieve its final rest, such as rebirth in an afterlife or, in some societies, rebirth in a next generation of its kindred (Metcalf and Huntington, 1991). An offended soul, prevented from achieving appropriate repose through the dereliction of its kin, may be greatly feared as a trickster or sorcerer wielding sacred forces and capable of imposing sickness, sterility, famine, or failure in battle. Thus, a major emphasis of ritual is often to ensure that the spirit of the deceased has made a transition from the world of the living to a world of the dead where it can no longer interfere in everyday affairs, at least not without special invocation or cause. Mourners are often motivated not only by a concern for the well-being of the soul of the deceased, but also by an interest in separating themselves from a sacred, powerful, and potentially harmful spirit. Not only kin are at risk from the soul, however. Rivals or enemies may also fear the soul's revenge and be obliged to undertake elaborate rites of protection, such as the rituals used by warriors to demonstrate their respect for, and thereby placate the souls of, persons they have killed in battle.

Death may also be thought to threaten orderly relations between the entire sacred and profane spheres. In some small-scale societies, when a number of people die through related events, whether diseases, storms, accidents, or enemy raids, the disfavor of gods or other sacred forces may be perceived as the actual cause. Propitiating the sacred forces through special rites may then assume priority for the entire community. Nearly all routine activities may be halted until such rites have been successfully performed. In the archaic societies of antiquity, as already noted, deaths of chiefs or kings were often viewed as precipitating crises in the relations between the society and the cosmic order. Ritual renewals involving the succession of a new leader and the securing of favorable relations with the sacred for his rule then became urgent measures for the well-being of the entire society. Moreover, favorable outcomes of the rituals were often closely linked to matters of practical politics. The failure of a dependent group to give proper tribute, for example, might spoil a ritual and at the same time signal the start of a rebellion designed to exploit a period of political weakness. A population experiencing a lack of ritually validated political order during an interregnum might suffer an existential precariousness in which none of the traditional truths seemed secure (Wilson, 1951).

As Arnold Van Gennep (1960) and Victor Turner (1969) emphasized, the recently deceased person is in a liminal state between life and death, the profane and the sacred. Although no longer living, the person has not yet been assimilated to the sacred status or company of the dead. Mortuary rituals are an institutional means of addressing this liminal condition and transforming the person's status into that of the dead (Metcalf and Huntington, 1991). This may be conceived as a process of liberating the soul or spirit from the body, as fulfilling or gaining release from certain meaningful relations to the living, as entering an afterlife or realm of the dead, or as a combination of these possibilities. In some societies, mortuary rites may be initiated before death, when an individual seems mortally ill or wounded. The rites may then express the moral support of the community in order to ease the process of dying.

Anthropologists have also observed the induction of death among previously healthy individuals through rituals of black magic. In such cases, the rituals dramatize a community's withdrawal of support for the continued life of an individual and may precipitate an overwhelming anxiety leading to death; it has also been suggested, however, that some victims of black magic may die of dehydration after losing the right to drink fluids (Warner, 1958; Metcalf and Huntington, 1991). Whether rituals are easing, imposing, or acknowledging a death, the liminality of the dead or dying person imparts an intense moral and sentimental power to the proceedings.

Mortuary and funerary rituals are typically complex, involving a series of separate rites that make different contributions to the overall transformation of the deceased person and thus are carried out on separate occasions. The component rites nearly always follow a principle of structure common to status-transforming rituals, including initiations (Durkheim, 1965; Hertz, 1960; Turner, 1969). From their profane status at the start, the mourners and other participants are gradually sacralized through a sequence of prescribed enactments. When thus prepared to engage the sacred, they perform the central actions of the ritual—the ones that contribute directly to a particular phase of the transformation of the liminal person from the living to the dead. After completing the central and most sacred acts involved in the ritual, the participants perform a series of desacralizing acts that return them to the profane world and ensure that they will not disrupt mundane activities and relationships.

A cycle of mortuary rites may be completed in some societies within days or weeks, while in other societies the whole sequence of ceremonies may extend over several years (Hertz, 1960). Customs of "secondary burial" of an individual's bones, months or years after primary burial and the resulting decay of the flesh, are found in many parts of the world. Such practices often carry the dual significance of placing the remains of the deceased finally to rest, assuring his or her soul that it, too, can be at peace in its afterlife, while also showing that the surviving groups, particularly kinship groups, have completed their transition in membership and survived the loss of the deceased. Both meanings may depend upon affirmation that revenge has been taken against enemies of the deceased.

Mourning is itself, in Van Gennep's sense, a liminal status, and individuals and groups who have been closely identified with a deceased person are generally treated with caution (Turner, 1969). Mourners may be regarded as having altered, even unbalanced, relations with the sacred. The special duties associated with mourning may change their day-to-day lives for extended periods. Other members of the community may expect them to be preoccupied with the emotions of mourning and thus neither fully in charge of their faculties nor fully responsible for their conduct. Moreover, mourners are often in a process of assuming a new social status, such as widow, head of family, or heir to a position of leadership. They may be in the midst of reorganizing households, redistributing property, and reallocating rights of authority, and may be preoccupied with these tasks for weeks, months, or even years. In most cases, release from these interrelated elements of liminal status can be gained only by completing the process of mourning and discharging ritual obligations to the deceased.

In most societies, mourning rituals are intensely emotional occasions, combining the grief of loss with pride in identification with the deceased and particularly the social persona of the deceased; Durkheim (1965) called them "sad celebrations." Mourning is almost everywhere viewed both as a burden and as an occasion for the expression of sympathy to the mourners. People in mourning are seen as going through a difficult trial and in need of the social support of others with whom they enjoy close relationships. Yet the affective temper of mourning varies markedly from culture to culture. In some societies, grief is expressed by loud wailing; in others, by quiet displays of sadness. Ecstatic possession may be expected in some societies, while utter self-control is required in others. Conformity with these expectations is generally important to mourners, as the propriety of their conduct is usually scrutinized by the community at large. As with other rituals, violations of the rules of proper conduct in mortuary rites are typically viewed as sacrileges occasioning serious sanctions (Metcalf and Huntington, 1991). Violations may result in the enmity of other participants, the scorn or disrespect of the community, and even an expectation that harm will be brought about by sacred forces, whether spirits of the dead, gods, or an impersonal fate (Malinowski, 1948).

Death, contemporary anthropology, and bioethics

Anthropologists have generally maintained that the ethics of any community can properly be assessed only in the context of a detailed understanding of that community's broader social and cultural patterns. Accordingly, the anthropological impetus in bioethics has been in the first instance ethnographic, emphasizing that empirical study of the views of life and death in a community constitutes an essential foundation for any effort to resolve its problems or issues. In this perspective, each human community has its own beliefs about the conditions under which termination of life may be legitimate, and bioethical investigation must carefully relate its prescriptive efforts to the beliefs and practical life circumstances of the particular community it is addressing. Only by understanding what it means in the terms of the local culture to be sick, infirm, or disabled; to be judged criminal, mad, or sacrilegious; to be friend or enemy; to be wealthy and privileged or poor and dispossessed; and to be young or elderly, can the bioethicist grasp what will be at issue when members of a community make life-and-death decisions about particular individuals. Social scientists have thus tried to clarify ways in which bioethical dilemmas can be addressed from within the frameworks of meaning, belief, and sentiment of a community, but have been skeptical about generalized claims of validity for specific principles or standards (Fox and Swazey, 1992).

Yet from the earliest times of their discipline, anthropologists have also been advocates for the peoples and communities they study. Acutely aware of the deprivations suffered by tribal and folk communities when they must compete with larger, wealthier, and more powerful societies for resources, anthropologists have used their international influence to extend at least some protection. Anthropology has thus developed its own "bioethics" that emphasizes helping dispossessed and culturally isolated peoples who cannot protect themselves in modern political arenas. Moreover, study of the cultural, social, and personal havoc often wrought in many tribal and folk communities by their weak positions in large nations and global economic systems has in recent decades become a major field in anthropology (Eder, 1987).

As documented since 1977 in *Cultural Survival Quarterly*, tribal societies and folk communities living on the brink of ecological extinction are found in nearly every region of the world. Many suffer from extremes of political oppression and economic destitution, but the fragmentation of traditional normative orders, institutions of social control, and religiomoral cultures is hardly less destructive. Life under these conditions tends to be short, with hunger, infection, alcoholism, and homicide all taking heavy tolls. The cost to humankind appears inevitably to include a vast diminution in the variety of cultures that will be sustained as frameworks for human life past the early decades of the twenty-first century.

A pathbreaking bioethical–anthropological work on the dispossessed of the Third World is Nancy Scheper-Hughes's study of the high mortality among children in the slums of a Brazilian city (1992). Scheper-Hughes focuses on mothers who raise children in the slums and on the ways in which their relationships with their young children are affected as the children starve to death or, weakened by lack of nutrition, succumb to infections. In the background is a system of medical care that prevents doctors and nurses from providing effective treatment for slum-dwelling patients. The lack of sanitation and other public-health measures leaves the slum-dwellers susceptible to infections. Health clinics are physically and often socially inaccessible, and the middle-class practitioners, not comprehending the living conditions of their patients, are often ineffective in prescribing treatments. Frequently, children are so severely malnourished that, saved from one infection, they die from the next, without their lack of nourishment being addressed. Mothers who cannot afford the costs of medical care or food for a child may, at the cost of personal humiliation, approach employers or political patrons for financial help. But the personal relationships of patronage generally place limits on the scope and frequency of a supplicant's requests for help as well as on a patron's concern to be helpful.

Conclusion

In all societies, the meanings of death are the subject of established cultural beliefs. These beliefs constitute generalized orientations toward death and also relate death to a number of other matters essential to human society.

All cultures thus provide guidance concerning a wide range of human problems associated with death and, in doing so, draw strength from shared beliefs about the sacred as a source of values, about the enduring purposes of life activities, about the normative obligations to protect life, and about the significance of losses of life. Ideas found in many societies about afterlife as a final realization of complicated hopes of the living exemplify the ways in which meanings of death may be shaped through the confluence of many cultural elements. In providing guidance toward issues of life and death, individual cultures express their orientations in deeply characteristic ways, and these orientations may differ vastly from one another, as noted above in discussions of Aztecs, Mayans, ancient Egyptians and Mesopotamians, the Balinese, and peoples of New Guinea.

In every society, deaths are commonly viewed as losses that communities must endure. The universal psychological mechanisms of attachment among persons involve processes of justification, exaggeration, repression, displacement, and projection. Losses of valued persons to death thus raise complicated issues of the dynamics of affect and sentiment. Individuals who have been personally close to the deceased may suffer profound emotions of loss, but so also may individuals whose relations to the deceased were largely symbolic, as when peasants participate in mourning for a distant noble or king. The feelings of loss that are involved in mourning are also especially susceptible to symbolic transformation, and hence may involve reversals of love into fear or hate (or vice versa), become masked by denial, and/or fuel intense projections of malevalence onto others, typically social rivals or enemies. Because of the lability of both individual affect and collective sentiment, times of loss and mourning can be socially explosive. The social institutions of mourning thus generally emphasize social support for groups suffering loss, fulfillment of duties to the deceased, reforging of community solidarity, and eventual return to everyday social roles. Thus, institutions of mourning respond to social stress with intense social control.

The anthropology of tribal and folk societies teaches that death figures essentially in the human condition. Death occurs to all living beings and is expected for all human individuals. People typically expect death for themselves and it is always expected for them by others. Yet, death often occurs without immediate anticipation, whether due to sudden disease, accident, or the acts of others. Interpreting the significance or meaning of a death poses difficulties, and all cultures contain elaborate beliefs about its causes, consequences, and social sequellae. All communities exercise social control in response to death as a necessarily troubling and potentially disruptive occasion through institutions permeated by local culture. The complexity of the social and cultural means for addressing death requires that ethical judgment be involved in their use. In this sense, bioethics of a sort are involved in the magical or enchanted cultures with which Australian and New Guinea tribespeople defend themselves against sorcery, the Aztecs of past centuries operated their institutions of sacrifice, and ancient Mesopotamians ensured the continuities of life through symbolic marriages of kings with goddesses.

If we view such cultures as bioethical, however, we must also note differences from modern bioethics. In the tribal and archaic societies of the past, the institutions of modern medicine and biomedical technology did not exist, nor did their cultural resources for understanding death in "natural" terms. In particular, it was not possible to conceive of death as due to "natural" or even impersonal causes or as a natural completion of a full life span. Death was necessarily understood as caused by magical forces and/or the motivated conduct of one or more other persons. Discussion over the rights or wrongs of protecting or ending a life quickly escalated to political issues and could threaten the solidarity of the community. The typical response to a death was actual or symbolic retribution against persons deemed responsible, including magical action against them. There was no frame of reference for the impersonal, technical, case-focused bioethical decision making of the modern kind.

Scheper-Hughes's study of death among children in Brazilian slums suggests that the presence of an autonomous frame of reference for bioethical thought cannot be taken for granted, despite the presence of modern medical technology, where folk communities lack strong connection to rationalistic and activistic culture of the Western type. Anthropological studies may in the coming decades clarify a variety of such cultural, medical-technical, and social class parameters of the functioning of bioethics in the modern sense. Understanding of these parameters will be of special importance to the use of bioethical thought in developing nations in Latin America, Africa, and Asia, where cultural traditions and social structure often differ radically from the North American and European settings in which bioethics originated. However, comparative research may be equally important for creating more detailed knowledge of the respects in which Western bioethics has been dynamically related to cultural premises of rationalism, individualism, and naturalism as well as to the more readily apparent technical proficiency of modern medicine.

VICTOR LIDZ

Directly related to this article are the other articles in this entry: EASTERN THOUGHT, WESTERN PHILOSOPHICAL THOUGHT, WESTERN RELIGIOUS THOUGHT, *and* DEATH IN THE WESTERN WORLD (*with its* POSTSCRIPT). *Also directly related to this article are the entries* HEALTH AND DISEASE, *article on* ANTHROPOLOGICAL PERSPECTIVES; BODY, *article on* CULTURAL AND RELIGIOUS PERSPECTIVES; DEATH, ATTITUDES TOWARD; DEATH: ART OF DYING; *and* DEATH, DEFINITION AND DETERMINATION OF, *especially the articles on* LEGAL ISSUES IN PRONOUNCING DEATH *and* PHILOSOPHICAL AND THEOLOGICAL PERSPECTIVES. *For a further discussion of topics mentioned in this article, see the entries* AGING AND THE AGED, *article on* SOCIETAL AGING; FAMILY; HEALING; HOMICIDE; INFANTS, *especially the article on* HISTORY OF INFANTICIDE; LIFE; MARRIAGE AND OTHER DOMESTIC PARTNERSHIPS; NATIVE AMERICAN RELIGIONS; PAIN AND SUFFERING; SEXISM; SUBSTANCE ABUSE, *especially the article on* ALCOHOLISM; SUICIDE; *and* WARFARE. *Other relevant material may be found under the entries* BODY, *article on* SOCIAL THEORIES; DEATH AND DYING: EUTHANASIA AND SUSTAINING LIFE, *article on* HISTORICAL ASPECTS; DEATH EDUCATION; ETHICS, *article on* RELIGION AND MORALITY; HUMAN NATURE; MEDICINE, ANTHROPOLOGY OF; PUBLIC HEALTH; *and* WOMEN, *article on* HISTORICAL AND CROSS-CULTURAL PERSPECTIVES.

Bibliography

BATESON, GREGORY. 1958. *Naven.* 2d ed. Stanford, Calif.: Stanford University Press.

BELLAH, ROBERT N. 1970. "Religious Evolution." In *Beyond Belief: Essays on Religion in a Post-Traditional World,* pp. 20–50. New York: Harper & Row.

BERNDT, RONALD M. 1962. *Excess and Restraint: Social Control Among a New Guinea Mountain People.* Chicago: University of Chicago Press.

BLOCH, MARC. 1961. *Feudal Society.* Translated by L. A. Manyon. Chicago: University of Chicago Press.

CLENDINNEN, INGA. 1991. *Aztecs: An Interpretation.* Cambridge: At the University Press.

COE, MICHAEL. 1962. *Mexico.* Mexico City: Ediciones Lara.

COWAN, JAMES. 1989. *Mysteries of the Dream-Time: The Spiritual Life of Australian Aborigines.* New York: Avery.

DURKHEIM, EMILE. 1951. *Suicide: A Study in Sociology.* Translated by John A. Spaulding and George Simpson. Glencoe, Ill.: Free Press. First published in French.

———. 1965. *The Elementary Forms of the Religious Life.* Translated by Joseph Ward Swain. New York: Free Press.

EDER, JAMES F. 1987. *On the Road to Tribal Extinction: Depopulation, Deculturation, and Adaptive Well-Being Among the Batak of the Philippines.* Berkeley: University of California Press.

EHRENBERG, VICTOR. 1960. *The Greek State.* Oxford: Basil Blackwell.

ELKIN, ADOLPHUS PETER. 1954. *The Australian Aborigines: How to Understand Them.* 3d ed. London: Angus and Robertson.

EVANS-PRITCHARD, EDWARD EVAN. 1937. *Witchcraft, Oracles, and Magic Among the Azande.* Oxford: At the Clarendon Press.

FALLERS, LLOYD A. 1969. *Law Without Precedent: Legal Ideas in*

Action in the Courts of Colonial Busaga. Chicago: University of Chicago Press.

Fox, Renée C., and Swazey, Judith P. 1992. *Spare Parts: Organ Replacement in American Society.* New York: Oxford University Press.

Frankfort, Henri. 1948. *Kingship and the Gods: A Study of Ancient Near Eastern Religion as the Integration of Society and Nature.* Chicago: University of Chicago Press.

Geertz, Clifford. 1960. *The Religion of Java.* Glencoe, Ill.: Free Press.

———. 1980. *Negara: The Theater State in Nineteenth-Century Bali.* Princeton, N.J.: Princeton University Press.

Gernet, Louis. 1981. *The Anthropology of Ancient Greece.* Translated by John Hamilton and Blaise Nagy. Baltimore: Johns Hopkins University Press.

Granet, Marcel. 1958. *Chinese Civilization.* New York: Meridian.

Hertz, Robert. 1960. [1907]. *Death and the Right Hand.* Translated by Rodney Needham and Claudia Needham. Glencoe, Ill.: Free Press.

Hoebel, E. Adamson. 1954. *The Law of Primitive Man: A Study in Comparative Legal Dynamics.* Cambridge, Mass.: Harvard University Press.

Hubert, Henri, and Mauss, Marcel. 1964. *Sacrifice: Its Nature and Function.* Translated by W. D. Halls. Chicago: University of Chicago Press.

Jaspers, Karl. 1949. *Von Ursprung und Ziel der Geschichte.* Munich: R. Piper.

Lanternari, Vittorio. 1963. *The Religions of the Oppressed: A Study of Modern Messianic Cults.* New York: Knopf.

Levi-Strauss, Claude. 1963. *Totemism.* Translated by Rodney Needham. Boston: Beacon Press.

Lot, Ferdinand. 1961. *The End of the Ancient World and the Beginnings of the Middle Ages.* New York: Harper & Row.

Malinowski, Bronislaw. 1948. *Magic, Science, and Religion and Other Essays.* Garden City, N.Y.: Doubleday.

Mauss, Marcel. 1975. *A General Theory of Magic.* Translated by Robert Brain. New York: Norton.

Metcalf, Peter, and Huntington, Richard. 1991. *Celebrations of Death: The Anthropology of Ritual.* 2d ed. New York: Cambridge University Press.

Moret, Alexander, and Davy, George. 1970. *From Tribe to Empire: Social Organization Among Primitives and in the Ancient East.* Translated by V. Gordon Childe. New York: Cooper Square.

Moscati, Sabati. 1962. *The Face of the Ancient Orient: A Panorama of Near Eastern Civilizations in Pre-Classical Times.* Garden City, N.Y.: Anchor.

Murphy, Yolanda, and Murphy, Robert F. 1985. *Women of the Forest.* 2d ed. New York: Columbia University Press.

Nelson, Benjamin. 1981. *On the Roads to Modernity: Conscience, Science, and Civilizations: Selected Writings.* Edited by Toby Huff. Totowa, N.J.: Rowman and Littlefield.

Parsons, Talcott. 1966. *Societies: Evolutionary and Comparative Perspectives.* Englewood Cliffs, N.J.: Prentice-Hall.

Poncins, Gontran de Montaigne. 1941. *Kabloona.* New York: Reynal and Hitchcock.

Saggs, H. W. F. 1962. *The Greatness that Was Babylon: A Sketch of the Ancient Civilization of the Tigris-Euphrates Valley.* New York: Hawthorn.

Schele, Linda, and Miller, Mary Ellen. 1986. *The Blood of Kings: Dynasty and Ritual in Maya Art.* London: Thames and Hudson.

Scheper-Hughes, Nancy. 1992. *Death Without Weeping: The Violence of Everyday Life in Brazil.* Berkeley: University of California Press.

Soustelle, Jacques. 1970. *Daily Life of the Aztecs: On the Eve of the Spanish Conquest.* Translated by Patrick O'Brian. Stanford, Calif.: Stanford University Press.

Stanner, W. E. H. 1963. *On Aboriginal Religion.* Sydney: University of Sydney.

Tierney, Patrick. 1989. *The Highest Altar: Unveiling the Mystery of Human Sacrifice.* New York: Penguin.

Turner, Victor. 1967. *The Forest of Symbols: Aspects of Ndembu Ritual.* Ithaca, N.Y.: Cornell University Press.

———. 1969. *The Ritual Process: Structure and Anti-Structure.* Chicago: Aldine.

Van Gennep, Arnold. 1960. *The Rites of Passage.* Translated by Monica B. Vizedom and Gabrielle L. Caffee. Chicago: University of Chicago Press.

Wallace, Anthony F. C. 1956. "Revitalization Movements." *American Anthropologist* 58, no. 2:264–281.

———. 1965. *Religion: An Anthropological View.* New York: Random House.

Warner, W. Lloyd. 1958. *A Black Civilization: A Social Study of an Australian Tribe.* Rev. ed. New York: Harper.

Weber, Max. 1946. "Religious Rejections of the World and Their Directions." In *From Max Weber: Essays in Sociology,* pp. 323–359. Edited by H. H. Gerth and C. Wright Mills. New York: Oxford University Press.

———. 1963. *The Sociology of Religion.* Translated by Ephraim Fischoff. Boston: Beacon Press. First published in German.

Wilson, John. 1951. *The Burden of Egypt: An Interpretation of Ancient Egyptian Culture.* Chicago: University of Chicago Press.

Zimmer, Heinrich. 1956. *Philosophies of India.* New York: Meridian.

II. EASTERN THOUGHT

Unlike other species, humans can reflect on death. One response to the mystery and fear humans associate with death is to create systems of religious meaning that give purpose to life in the face of death. A corollary of the fact that people can reflect on death is their realization that it is possible for them intentionally to end life. Religion constrains this possibility in the interest of human survival; only a few exceptions to the taboo against killing humans are allowed. Animals, by contrast, cannot decide to kill themselves and seldom kill members of their own species.

Concepts of death in Asian religions include two basic types: natural—for example, death by disease and old age; and unnatural—for example, death by an accident, by the intention of another person (homicide), or by one's own intention. The latter, here called self-willed death, may be subdivided into three types: (1)

suicide (self-willed death out of depression or passion, an irrational and private act); (2) heroic (self-willed death by warriors, and sometimes their wives, to avoid being killed or captured by an enemy, and therefore shamed; or to follow a leader in death because of loyalty); and (3) religious (self-willed death as a rational and public act sanctioned by a religion; for example, in cases of terminal illness or debilitating old age, or as a means to achieve heaven or enlightenment).

Hinduism

The concept of natural death. In no small measure, Vedic (Brahmanical) religion (1500–600 B.C.E.), its sequel now called Hinduism, and other Indian religions (Jainism and Buddhism) inherited views of death from the Indo-Europeans who came to India, probably from eastern Anatolia. Because life expectancy in the prehistoric world was about thirty years, on account of disease, natural calamities, and warfare, people turned to religion for help, performing rituals for health, physical security, longevity, or immortality.

A proto–Indo-European myth about death involved a primordial sacrifice in which Manu (literally Man), the first priest, sacrificed Yemo, his twin and the first king, to create the cosmos, including the realm of the dead. Located to the south, symbolizing warmth, the realm of the dead was described as a paradise where cold, suffering, labor, injustice, evil, darkness, aging, sickness, and death were unknown (Lincoln, 1991). According to one Indian version found in the *Rgveda* (10.13.4)—the earliest and most authoritative Hindu scripture—Manu sacrificed King Yama, who showed the path to where the forebears of old had gone: The *Rgveda* considered this place either the southern world or the highest region—a paradise with light, beauty, and joy. (In later texts, Yama was demoted to preside over a hell; the fetters that once bound him as the sacrificial victim for creation were now used by him to fetter sinners.) In another early Indian version, the Purusasūkta (*Rgveda*, 10.90), Man, the sacrificial victim, was bound, killed, and dismembered. His mind became the moon; his eye, the sun; his mouth, the fire; his breath, the wind; his feet, the earth. Henceforth, each sacrifice repeated the cosmogonic one, with animals representing the human victims of earlier Indo-European myths or rituals, to ensure the continued existence of the cosmos. A symbolic reenactment of the cosmogonic sacrifice occurred in the funeral ritual; according to *Rgveda* 10.16, different parts of a dead person went to various parts of the universe.

The Vedas prescribed a life of one hundred years, indicating a desire for longevity and natural death. For those who died a natural death, the funeral ritual (*śrāddha*) would be performed; this would provide them the status of ancestor, ensuring rebirth as a human or existence as a god (hence creating a double buffer against death as annihilation).

Drawing on their pastoral practice of seasonal migration, the Indo-Europeans referred to the dead as traveling along a pathway. In India, the Vedas also referred to the paths of the dead. The straight and easy one ascended to a luminous paradise where the gods lived; the tortuous and difficult one descended to a dark netherworld. By performing sacrifices and funerals, people gained access to the former (*Rgveda*, 10.2.3). The most common Indo-European image of the dead following a path involved crossing a river or ocean by means of a ferry guided by a ferryman, the personification of old age, to paradise (Lincoln, 1991). During their migrations into India, the Indo-Europeans conquered settlements at fords (*tīrtha*) to cross rivers. A popular Vedic myth alludes to this: The warrior god Indra killed the native serpent demon Vrtra, thus creating a passage from drought to water, barrenness to prosperity, death to survival, danger to security, darkness to light, and chaos to order (Young, 1980). Hence the Vedic notion of figuratively crossing over dangers to arrive happily on the other shore, to make a way through experience or suffering, and to penetrate the real or the true.

Some of these ideas prefigured a new worldview that led to a dramatic transformation of Vedic religion and the birth of two new religions (Jainism and Buddhism) around the sixth century B.C.E. This period witnessed a great increase in life expectancy. Seeing the miseries of frailty and old age, however, led many people to increasing anxiety over the end of life (Tilak, 1987). This gave rise to reflections on old age, the meaning and purpose of life, and ways to move beyond death. The path no longer led to another realm *within* the cosmos; it now *crossed* the cosmos (symbolized as the ocean of *samsāra*, characterized by the cycles of time, rebirth, finitude, suffering, and ignorance) to liberation.

One of the Vedic texts that elaborated on the ritual, the *Śatapatha Brāhmaṇa*, said the Vedic sacrifice was a boat; the priests, oars; and the patron, a passenger who would reach heaven if no error were made in performing the ritual (4.5.10). Sacrifice also became a way of overcoming death by moving beyond *samsāra*, the cycles of death and rebirth (2.3.3.7). A personification of death demanded what would happen to him. He was told by the other gods that he had dominion over the body but not over immortality, which would occur without him. In other words, the god of death controlled the process and time of dying, but he could not influence those who attained enlightenment because they were beyond the cycles of death and rebirth (10.4.3.1–9).

In the *Upaniṣads* (philosophical speculations said to reveal the supreme truth of the Vedas but, from a historical perspective, beginning the transformation of Vedic religion to Hinduism), this extracosmic liberation (*mokṣa*) was characterized by the realization of eternal consciousness, called Brahman. This could be achieved during life; at death the body would disappear forever. Or it could be achieved by a postmortem passage to a supreme heaven where there would be eternal life with a supreme God. Some Upaniṣadic texts spoke of sacrifice leading to the path of the forefathers (*pitṛyāna*) and thus to rebirth (indicating a demotion of the status of Vedic rituals), whereas others spoke of self-knowledge leading to the path of the gods (*devayāna*). Still others spoke of a passage to liberation made possible by religious discipline (*sādhana*) and the guidance of a teacher (guru) leading to supreme knowledge. This notion was expressed as a boat guided by a pilot, ferrying the individual across to the other shore. In *Kauṣītaki Upaniṣad* 1.4, for example, the deceased proceeded to the river Vijarā (literally, "apart from old age"), shaking off their good and bad deeds. Their good deeds were transferred to relatives for a better rebirth; their bad ones, to other people. Beyond deeds and dualities, the deceased approached the god Brahmā. Although the human body represented bondage, it also provided the only opportunity for liberation (an argument that was probably necessary to inspire humans to pursue a path to liberation in this life, because they might be reborn as plants or animals).

Closely associated with this development was the law of karma, according to which actions (karma) determined destiny. People were reborn higher or lower in the scale of beings (from high-caste people down to plants), depending on the quantity of good (*puṇya*) or bad (*pāpa*) karma they had accumulated. With an excess of good karma, they had a temporary vacation in a paradise; with an excess of bad karma, they descended to a hellish realm. But with an extraordinary religious effort (based on knowledge or devotion), they could negate the law of karma by removing the bondage of action and the perpetual cycles of rebirth. Despite the highly individualistic nature of this karma doctrine (people reap what they sow), some versions allowed the transfer of merit from an extraordinary person, or divine grace from a deity, in order to redirect destiny and ultimately achieve liberation.

After the sixth century B.C.E, the idea of crossing over, signified in the term *tīrtha*, became associated with various bodies of water; these were sacred places where people could cross over to a better rebirth, a vacation in a cosmic paradise (*svarga*), or liberation beyond the cosmos (*mokṣa*). To facilitate crossing over, they followed a religious path characterized by action (*karmayoga*), knowledge (*jñānayoga*), and devotion (*bhaktiyoga*); different schools order the three in different ways.

Even today, most Hindus want to die on the banks of the Ganges—believed to be the river of heaven, the nectar of immortality, a goddess, a mother, or even a physician, since this allows them to cross over to liberation. From all parts of India, the dying come to Banaras to live on its banks. They spend their final days in a hospice where spiritual help but no medicine is provided. Hearing the names of the gods chanted continually, they eat sacred *tulsī* leaves and drink Ganges water, focusing their thoughts exclusively on God. Śiva, Lord of Death, whispers the ferryboat mantra into their ears. After they die, their corpses are taken to the cremation ground, given a final bath in the Ganges, decked with garlands of flowers, and honored as a guest or deity. Then the last sacrifice (*antyeṣṭi*) is performed. The eldest son circumambulates the corpse counterclockwise (reversal symbolizing death) and lights the pyre. Relatives are silent, for wailing is inauspicious or even painful for the dead. Finally, the eldest son turns his back to the pyre, throws water over his shoulders to douse the embers, and leaves the pyre without looking back. For the next eleven days, during the performance of the *śrāddha* rituals, ideally at Banaras or another holy place, rice balls are offered to the dead; on the twelfth day, the departed soul reaches its destination (Eck, 1982). It is said that when people die in Banaras, their souls attain liberation—though the idea that transitional souls (*preta*) are transformed into ancestors (*pitṛ*) is also maintained, as are a host of other ideas about destiny.

If dying by the Ganges is impossible, dying at some other *tīrtha* in India may be a substitute, for the Ganges is said to be there, too, just as all rivers are said to be in the Ganges. And if even that is impossible, simply thinking about the Ganges at the moment of death may influence destiny. Casting the bones that remain after cremation into a *tīrtha* is also effective. Ascetics are buried, however, because they have given up their *śrauta* fires (the locus of the Vedic rituals) and their sacrificial implements (Kane, 1973). Hindus perform the annual *śrāddha* ceremonies for the dead (offering rice balls to three generations of male ancestors, *pitṛs*) at the Ganges or any other *tīrtha*, since this will either sustain the ancestors until rebirth as humans or allow them a long vacation as gods (*viśvadeva*) in heaven. In short, the Hindu tradition offers a number of safeguards against annihilation at death: rebirth, a visit to another realm, liberation. Individuals can influence destiny or others can help them by the transfer of merit. Gods, through their grace, also may influence an individual's destiny. There is always hope. The sting is taken out of death, for it is said that even mosquitoes are liberated in Banaras (Eck, 1982).

The concept of self-willed death in Hinduism. According to the traditional law books, funeral rituals were not to be performed for those who died in unnatural ways. This may have been used as a deterrent against suicide; the Hindu tradition disapproved of suicide, which was defined as killing oneself because of depression, passion, or uncontrollable circumstance. But unnatural death was not always viewed negatively; death by violence (war, murder, or accident) was viewed as powerful, leading to heaven or deification. The type of unnatural death that has relevance for bioethics is the self-willed death, which is given religious sanction. During the late classical and medieval periods, Hinduism came to accept a rational decision either (1) to kill oneself as a way to destroy bad karma, create good karma, and thus attain heaven or liberation; or (2) if liberated in life, to remove the body. Such self-willed death (istamṛtyu), took many forms. People could walk without food or drink until they dropped dead (mahāprasthāna); bury themselves alive and meditate (samādhimāraṇa); abstain from food and wait in a seated posture for the approach of death (prāyopaveśana); or jump into fire, over a cliff, into sacred water, or under the wheels of a temple cart. The terminally ill and the extremely old who were no longer able to perform their religious duties and rituals sometimes killed themselves by one of these methods. Such self-willed death was religiously permitted. Sati (a woman's self-immolation on the funeral pyre of her husband) was a variant of self-willed death that produced a surplus of merit that ensured heaven for both spouses. Despite efforts to prevent abuse, it appears that there was some, for by the tenth century, with the Kalivarjya Prohibitions, all forms of killing oneself—except sati—were prohibited (in theory though not in practice).

Some families continued to endorse sati because the alternative was lifelong support for widows or, as in Bengal, a share in the inheritance. After additional criticism by both Muslims and Christians in the following centuries, this practice virtually ended. The Indian Penal Code in 1860 made suicide and abetting suicide crimes; judges interpreted suicide as any form of self-willed death and used that interpretation to stop sati as well as other practices of self-willed death (Young, 1989). There have been isolated incidents since then, including the widely publicized case of Roop Kanwar in 1987. Almost 160 years after sati was declared culpable homicide, Roop Kanwar, an eighteen-year-old Rajasthani woman, performed sati. The government alleged that she was forced onto the pyre and pinned down with heavy firewood. This caused the Indian parliament to pass another law in December 1987 to check the practice. According to the new law, the death penalty is imposed for those who help carry out the ritual of sati; the woman who tries to perform sati may be sentenced to six months in jail; those who glorify sati may be given prison sentences up to seven years; and the government is em-

powered to dismantle memorials and temples related to sati. Accordingly, her brother-in-law, who lit the pyre, was charged with murder and twenty-two others received lesser charges.

Implications of Hindu views of death for bioethics. According to the Caraka Samhitā (a classical text on medicine with religious legitimation written about the first century B.C.E.), physicians were not to treat incurable diseases (a policy to establish the benefits of the fledgling science of medicine and to protect the physician's reputation as a healer). This refusal could provide traditional religious legitimation for modern withdrawal of treatment by physicians in cases of terminal disease.

Physicians also were not to reveal the possibility of impending death, unless there was a specific request, so that negative thoughts would not be imposed on the patient that might create bad karma and hasten death. Rather, the process of death should be peaceful and auspicious, because it was the prelude to rebirth or final liberation. The implication of this view for modern medicine is that pain relief provided by a physician might make the dying process peaceful and therefore auspicious in Hindu terms; however, the refusal to inform the patient about terminal illness unless directly asked would be against the modern concept of mandatory truth-telling by the physician and the patient's right to know the prognosis. But another view also existed in traditional Indian religions: a person's last thought influences destiny. In this case, the individual should know of impending death and should not allow anything to cloud the mind. The implication of this view for modern medicine is that pain relief should be given only to the extent that the person remains alert.

Finally, the long tradition of self-willed death, especially fasting to death, in cases of terminal illness or debilitating old age, can be used to give religious legitimation for refusal or withdrawal of treatment in modern India, for it accords with the voluntary and public nature of living wills requesting refusal or withdrawal of treatment and nutrition. Whether it will be used to invoke precedent for active euthanasia depends on the assessment of assistance and whether there had been a slippery slope in the practice of self-willed death. As for the first issue, the Hindu tradition was quite careful to insist on the voluntary nature of self-willed death, though once there was a public declaration and the person could not be discouraged from his or her decision, assistance was allowed, at least in the case of sati. For instance, priests were allowed to hold a woman down during her self-immolation if they had been convinced that the decision for sati had been her own. As for the second issue, the types of self-willed death and possibly their numbers increased over the centuries; since there was criticism of the practice internal to the religion by the tenth century, there was probably the perception of a slippery slope.

Jainism

The concept of natural death. Jainism is an Indian religion that developed about the sixth century B.C.E. The Jains speak of the twenty-four *tīrthaṅkaras*, such as their founder Mahāvīra, who are the makers of the path or causeway to liberation, enabling people to cross over *saṁsāra*. The Jain view of death is related to its view of liberation: Because karmas (actions) cause bondage in the cycles of existence (reincarnation), they should be eliminated by fasting and meditation leading to the realization of liberation, the radical autonomy of pure consciousness (*kaivalya*).

The Jain concept of self-willed death. According to tradition, Mahāvīra fasted to death. Henceforth, the ideal form of death for Jain monastics was a "final fast" to death known by different names—*bhakta-pratyākhyāna, inginī, prāyopagamana, samādhi, pañcapada, sallekhanā, ārādhanā*—depending on variants in the practice such as whether there is the assistance of others, whether one dies meditating or chanting, whether the body is to be eliminated by emasculation after initiation, or whether death occurs after the attainment of wisdom (Settar, 1990). Jainism was the first Indian religion to legitimate self-willed death. Initially, the fast to death was to be done only by monastics late in life but before debilitating old age or terminal illness, so that they would be in full control of the meditative and fasting process. Some centuries later, however, the practice was extended to the Jain laity as a legitimate form of death in times of public crisis (natural calamities and military defeat) or personal crisis (debilitating old age and terminal illness).

Implications of Jain views of death for bioethics. Although self-willed death is illegal in India today, Jains are arguing for the decriminalization of suicide so that they can restore the traditional practice of fasting to death. They argue that this practice legitimates refusal or withdrawal of nutrition and life-support systems in modern medical contexts for the terminally ill. They also argue that prolongation of the dying process is immoral, because it increases suffering or depletes the resources of the family or community; thus the fast to death is a way to "permit oneself the honour of dying without undue prolongation of the process" (Bilimoria, 1992). But since the fast to death was also practiced traditionally in nonmedical contexts, it was not always a way to avoid the prolongation of dying; on the contrary, it was a way of hastening death by the cultural act of fasting when the body was not about to die of natural causes. Although the fast to death was generally under-

stood to be voluntary and planned (and in a category distinct from both homicide and suicide), there were several exceptions. According to some, severely handicapped newborns were allowed to die (*bālamaraṇa*) when permission was given by parents or a preceptor. In the *Bhāva Pāhuḍa Ṭīku, bālamaraṇa* is classified as: "The death of the ignoramus, or a foolish process of meeting death . . . *Bāla* means childish, undeveloped, or yet-to-be-developed, premature and silly" (Settar, 1990, p. 15). It includes the death of infants and those who have an infantile knowledge—who are ignorant, who do not understand the moral codes, or who have a wrong notion of the faith and kill themselves by fire, smoke, poison, water, rope, suffocation, or jumping. While the original classification indicated simply a subdivision of natural death that would lead to rebirth, it seems that at some point in the tradition or perhaps in the modern period, the classification *bāla-maraṇa* has been reinterpreted. Accordingly, Bilimoria (reporting on statements made by Jain informants) observes that "in principle there appeared to be no reason why a child afflicted with or suffering from the kinds of conditions described earlier should not be given the terminal fast (*sallekhanā*). Parental permission would be required where there is contact, failing which a preceptor (for instance in an ashram) may be in a position to make a pronouncement. Consent of the recipient is not necessary (hence, a case of *nonvoluntary* terminal fast). One who has fallen in a state of unconsciousness, again, can be given the fast . . . even if the person had made no requests while she was conscious, though parents or kin would be consulted. It seemed evident that 'consent,' either of the individual or a proxy, or of the parent, does not seem to be a necessary condition for commending [a] final fast. This would seem to constitute a case of *involuntary sallekhanā*. . . . When . . . asked whether it would be acceptable to inject lethal poison to bring on the impending death, the response was that under extreme conditions where the pain and suffering is unendurable and not abating. . . ." (Bilimoria 1992, p. 347).

It is currently argued by Jains that the history of fasting to death demonstrates that self-willed death need not lead to other forms of self-willed or other-willed death. While it is true that in the past there were a number of safeguards (permission of the head of the monastery, a formal public vow, established ascetic discipline, evidence of courage and will rather than cowardice) and the history of fasting to death was without any extreme abuse in India, there was still a change in the number of groups involved (from monastics to lay people) indicating extension or popularization of the practice. Moreover, the fact that Jainism was the first Indian religion to legitimate a form of self-willed death means that it set an example, which may have inspired legitimation of self-willed death without such careful safeguards by other Indian religions (Young, 1989). In other words, its indirect contribution to a slippery slope in Indian religions cannot be ruled out despite Jain disclaimers. When the Indian penal code made suicide illegal, fasting to death was included. Despite the fact that any form of self-willed death is still illegal in India, there are between six and ten reported Jain fasts to death annually (Bilimoria, 1992).

Buddhism

The concept of natural death.
The imagery of crossing the ocean or river of *saṁsāra* to the other shore of enlightenment is used by Buddhists as well as Hindus. Theravāda (one of the main branches of Buddhism, which purportedly continues the early tradition and is still found in Sri Lanka, Burma, Thailand, Cambodia, and Vietnam) metaphorically considers the Buddha's teaching (*dhamma*) a boat and the individual its pilot. For instance, in Burma, a coin called "ferry fare" is placed in the mouth of a dead person (Spiro, 1970).

The Buddha thought often about the nature of death. According to Aśvaghoṣa's version of his life, the *Buddhacarita*, the future Buddha was surrounded by royal luxury as a youth, sealed off from the real world in a palace. When he finally ventured into the world, he was overwhelmed by his first sight of a sick person, an old person, and a dead person. These shocking revelations about dimensions of human existence beyond anything he had known so troubled him that he left his life of ease to become an ascetic and search for meaning. Later, on the verge of enlightenment, he recalled his own previous lives, meditated on the cycles of rebirth common to all creatures, and came to understand that all beings are propelled into repeated lives by ignorance and desire. The Buddha spent his life teaching others how to blow out (*nibbāna*) the flame of ignorance and desire by realizing that all beings are composite and impermanent (subject to suffering, decay, and death). In the final analysis, there was no "person" who died; there was only the process of dying. As narrated in the *Mahāparinibbāna Sutta*, written down about the first century B.C.E., the Buddha attained final release from his body (*parinibbāna*) at the age of eighty. After falling ill, he chose the time and place of his departure: Telling those present that all composite things must pass away and advising them to strive diligently for liberation, he meditated with complete equanimity and took his last breath.

Despite the Buddha's emphasis on liberation, subsequent generations of monks and nuns took precautions in case they were to be reborn. The *Mulāsarvāstivāda-vinaya* (a text composed at the end of the seventh century) describes the monastic funeral: A gong was sounded; the body was taken to the cremation ground and honored; verses on impermanence were recited;

merit from this act was transferred to the deceased, suggesting extra insurance in case the monastic was to be reborn; ownership of property was transferred; and cremation was performed. Finally, Buddhist sacred monuments (*stūpa* or *caitya*) were worshiped by the living, who then took a sacred bath (Schopen, 1992). Laypeople tried to attain a better rebirth by practicing morality, accumulating merit, reflecting on the nature of suffering, and disengaging from activities during old age. They were helped by merit transferred to them through the religious activities of families and friends, especially during the dying process, the funeral, and subsequent ancestral rituals.

As in Hinduism, the moment of death was important, because the final thought influenced rebirth. Even today, according to the popular religion of Burma, relatives chant Buddhist texts or have monks chant the *paritta*, canonical verses for protection against danger, to calm those who are dying; good thoughts thus arise and lead them either to a better rebirth or to a heavenly reward (Spiro, 1970). In popular forms of Theravāda Buddhism, ideas of the soul often replace the doctrine of no soul (*anatta*). The soul, or ghost, lurks around the house for some days after death and must be ritually fed, placated, and induced to leave the world of the living. Death rituals, ideally involving food and gifts for the monks, not only eliminate the danger posed by a ghost but also allow for the transfer of merit to the dead person, as do rituals performed by relatives on the anniversaries of the death.

Mahāyāna (the other main branch of Buddhism, which originated in India but eventually became popular in Tibet, China, Korea, and Japan) also conceives of the teaching as a boat, but views the pilot as a *bodhisattva*, a salvific figure who refuses enlightenment until all sentient creatures are saved, graciously steering the boat across to the other shore. Nevertheless, Mahāyāna maintains that ultimately there is no boat, no pilot, and no shore, since all is nothingness (*śunyatā*).

In Tibet, monastics meditated on death and simulated the process of dying to attain enlightenment; they also protected themselves against a bad rebirth by certain funerary rituals. Laypeople focused mainly on rebirth and sought help to ensure a good destiny. A spiritual teacher performed the ritual *gzhan po wa*, by which a disciple went to a paradise. Or the *Tibetan Book of the Dead*, which describes the journey from the moment of death through an intermediate state to rebirth, was read to the deceased over a number of days. Each of the three stages, or *bardos*, offered an experience of past karma along with a vision of both peaceful and wrathful divine figures. These provided more opportunities to attain enlightenment (Buddhahood) or a better rebirth, even though each succeeding one was more difficult than the last. Only by recognizing that the deities were ultimately illusory, for all was emptiness (śūnyatā), would one attain liberation. These beliefs and practices are still found in Tibetan communities.

In China, Mahāyāna views of death were reinterpreted in several ways: (1) The notion of heaven was modeled on both Taoist ideas of paradise and its images of Confucian kingdoms complete with palaces, courts, and bureaucracy; the notion of hell was based on Taoist hells and Confucian prisons. (2) Some Chinese argued that the existence of a soul was implied in the theory of reincarnation, in the storehouse of consciousness, or in the Buddhahood of all living creatures. (3) Transferring merit from monastics or relatives became extremely popular. Buddhist monks instituted the annual All Souls festival based on the story of Maudgalyāyana (Mu-lien), who rescued his mother from the lowest hell, as told in the *Ullambana Sūtra* of Central Asian origin (Smith, 1974). Food, clothing, and other gifts were offered to rescue seven generations of ancestors from their sufferings in various hells, and the story was reenacted at Chinese funerals (Berling, 1992). (4) Pure Land Buddhism, which became particularly popular in China, promoted, in some versions, an otherworldly paradise attained through faith in Amida (a savior whose grace allows people to be reborn in a paradise called the Land of Bliss until they reach *nirvāna*) and calling out his name at the moment of death. According to Pure Land philosophers, this paradise was not real, however, but a product of the mind. (6) Ch'an claimed that the Buddha nature was in all sentient beings, truth was near at hand, and Earth was the Lotus Land; enlightenment was the realization that nothing existed beyond the realm of *samsāra*. Consequently, death meant reabsorption into nature.

Just as Chinese Buddhism had absorbed Taoist ideas of death and native Confucian ancestor worship, so Japanese Buddhism assimilated, in turn, native Shintō views of death and ancestor worship. According to ancient Shintō, death was a curse; the corpse, polluting; and the spirit of the deceased, frightening. Buddhism contributed rituals to purify the spirits of the dead and transform them into gods: Spirits were deified thirty-three years after death and henceforth worshipped with the Shintō *kami* (entities with a spiritual function that inspire awe). In the seventh century, Empress Saimei ordered that the *Ullambana Sūtra* be taught in all the temples of the capital and that offerings be made on behalf of the spirits of the dead. The Japanese version of the All Souls festival, called Bon, dates from this time. The association of Buddhism with ancestor worship was reinforced in the anti-Christian edicts of the seventeenth century, which insisted on the formal affiliation of every Japanese household with a Buddhist temple and its death rituals (Smith, 1974).

Modern Japanese Buddhism has been primarily associated with death: In addition to funerals, there are seventh-day, monthly, hundredth-day, seventh-month, and annual rituals (Smith, 1974). Besides these, the collectivity of the spirits of the household dead is given daily offerings and honored at festival times. The Japanese hold conflicting opinions about where the spirits live: (1) Spirits may live peacefully in ancestor tablets on the altar in the home. (2) As depicted in Nō plays, those who suffered tragedy during life or died violently haunt their graves or former homes. (3) Spirits may have a continued existence as buddhas. Curiously, the dead are referred to as buddhas (*hotoke*). The Japanese misunderstood the term *nibbāna*, "to blow out" (in Japanese, *nehan*). Whereas in Indian Buddhism it expressed the metaphorical idea of blowing out the flames of desire in life and thereby achieving enlightenment, in Japanese Buddhism it was understood literally: People attained continued existence as buddhas when life was "blown out," a euphemism for death (Smith, 1974); this may have inspired self-willed death. (4) By chanting Amida's mantra (according to Hōnen) or having faith in him (according to Shinran), spirits enter paradise. (5) Spirits go to mountains such as Osore or Morinoyama with its Sōtō Zen and Jōdo-shin shrines. Today many of these beliefs and rituals are dying out. The breakdown of the extended family due to mobility and urbanization has contributed to the lessening of interest in ancestor worship. Now, memory and prayers are for the immediate ancestors; tablets and altars, therefore, are becoming smaller (Smith, 1974).

Buddhist views of self-willed death.   Despite his discussion of the body as the locus of suffering, the Buddha did not endorse self-willed death for everyone. He himself lived out his natural life span. An incident is recorded in the *Pārājika* (a text of the Pāli Canon, the scripture of Theravāda Buddhism) about how, when some monks became depressed in their meditation on the impurity of their bodies, a sham monk encouraged them—up to sixty in one day—to take their lives or be killed by him so that they could cross *samsāra* immediately. When he heard about this, the Buddha changed the form of meditation to a breathing exercise and declared that intentionally encouraging or assisting another person to die would lead to expulsion from the monastery. The Buddha also condemned, on the basis of nonviolence (*ahimsā*), any monk who told people to do away with their wretched lives. It is possible that the Buddha, known as the "good physician," allowed one exception to this general principle: From the accounts of the cases of Vakkali, Godhika, Channa, Assaji, Anāthapindika, and Dīghāvu, it seems that if people were experiencing unbearable pain in dying, they could kill themselves. There is some controversy over such an interpretation, however, for good palliative care had been offered and there were serious attempts to dissuade people from taking their lives. Moreover, neither the Buddha nor the monks gave explicit permission for these monastics and laypeople to take their lives, although the account implies that the act was condoned, perhaps because there were no options aside from physical force to restrain them.

According to an observation of I-Ching, a Chinese pilgrim who traveled to India (671–695), the practice of self-willed death was not popular among the Buddhists in India. Several centuries later, however, its popularity may have grown. In China, some Buddhist monks chose the time, place, and manner of death to bring its uncertainty under their control. It is possible that a story in the *Saddharmapuṇḍarīka* about how the *bodhisattva* Bhaiṣajyarāja, who was so dissatisfied with his worship that he set himself on fire, may have inspired the Chinese practice. But the fact that Chinese monks fasted to death in a yogic posture in underground pits (as in the Indian *samādhimāraṇa*), and after death their bodies were smoked, wrapped, lacquered, and installed in temples as objects of great veneration (Welch, 1967), suggests a different Indian Buddhist influence. This may have been combined with Taoist techniques to achieve immortality. Finally, it has been argued that self-willed death was popularized in China by a misunderstanding of Pure Land Buddhism, which suggested that people should kill themselves to reach the Pure Land more quickly. Shan-Tao's disciple, for example, jumped out of a tree to reach the Pure Land (Kato, 1990).

Some sects of Japanese Pure Land continued this idea. Kūya (903–972) and Ippen (1239–1289), both charismatic leaders among the masses, killed themselves by drowning in order to reach the Pure Land. Before his death Ippen instigated Nyudo to drown while meditating on Amida (a story illustrated on many scrolls). Ippen's death prompted six disciples to drown in sympathy. These examples were further popularized by a tradition of drowning to reach the Pure Land; ordinary people who lost their nerve would be hauled ashore by a rope attached around their waist (Becker, 1990). Devotees were told to "Delight in dying" and "Hasten your death" (Kato, 1990).

These Pure Land practices inspired more secular forms of self-willed death. There are over forty-five terms in Japanese to describe the various forms of self-willed death; for example, the tradition of parents killing first their children and then themselves to avoid further suffering; the tradition of abandoning old women in distant mountains; and the tradition of *joshi* or love-killing, also known as *oshinjuo* or *aitai-shi* (a death pact between two people, such as lovers who want to attain a happier realm) (Kato, 1990). Such practices (which also included death by fasting or fire), collectively called *sha-shinojo*, came under scrutiny by subsequent Pure Land

leaders who argued that such acts of self-willed death were a denial of Amida's grace.

Some views held by Zen leaders may have been misinterpreted, inspiring self-willed death; Dogen, for example, says to throw away your "body-mind." Zen inspired the samurai warriors and helped them cultivate a stoicism to face death. In medieval Japan, *harakiri* or *seppuku* was practiced by warriors to expiate crimes, apologize for errors, escape disgrace, redeem friends, or express devotion to their master by following him in death. These forms of warrior self-willed death are similar to the forms of heroic death by warriors in India. Sometimes *seppuku* was assisted by a relative or friend. By the Tokugawa period (1603–1867), it involved an elaborate ceremony and, for the famous, burial in a Buddhist tomb.

The popularity of self-willed death in Japan may have been derived in part from ancient Shintō views of death. The lack of a definitive boundary between life and death led to a feeling of intimacy with death and a desire to take refuge in holistic being, understood as *kami* (nature). This Shintō idea was combined with the concept of the Tao (the transcendent and immanent reality of the universe, represented by vacuity or emptiness because of its being formless and imperceptible) or the concept of the Buddha as nothingness (*śūnyatā*), pure consciousness, or nature. It was also combined with the Buddhist idea of life as suffering and transience, which could be escaped by attaining the Pure Land (Kato, 1990).

The Buddhist practice of self-willed death has acquired political significance in the modern period. Known as "falling down like cherry blossoms" or "dying with a smile" (Kato, 1990), this way of dying belonging to *bushido*, the way of the warriors, contributed to the psychology of the Japanese kamikaze pilots of World War II. In Vietnam, the monk Thich Quang Duc's self-immolation in Saigon (1963) focused world attention on the plight of the Vietnamese under Ngo Dinh Diem's oppressive regime.

Implications of Buddhist views of death for bioethics. Assessments of the importance of Buddhist views of death for bioethics vary considerably, depending on whether Theravāda or Mahāyāna is the focus and what the commentator thinks about issues such as withdrawal of treatment and euthanasia. Pinit Ratanakul (1988) observes, for instance, that in Thailand the Buddhist principle of the sanctity of life is maintained and self-willed death is not condoned as a rule, even in cases of pain and suffering. Two reasons are given: (1) suffering is a way for bad karma to come to fruition rather than be transferred to the next life; and (2) a person who assists suicide or performs euthanasia will be affected by such an act, since it involves repugnance toward suffering and his or her own desire to eliminate that which arouses a disagreeable sensation. But one exception is allowed: self-willed death when incurably ill, in order to attain enlightenment. These comments suggest that Thailand has maintained a reluctance to endorse self-willed death, in line with its Theravāda tradition, but continues to acknowledge the precedent established by the cases of the terminally ill Vakkali, Godhika, Channa, and others reported in the Pali Canon.

Current Japanese views show a greater acceptance of euthanasia, which is to be predicted, given the history of self-willed death in Japanese Buddhism. It is striking that the modern word for euthanasia is *anraku-shi* (literally, "ease—pleasure—death"), also a name for the Pure Land, though now some Japanese prefer the term *songen-shi* (death with dignity). Carl B. Becker, a Western scholar who has discussed this topic with Japanese people, argues that the Buddha accepted or condoned "many" cases of suicide but gives only three examples. He also argues that Buddhists view death as a transition, not an end; therefore, it is the state of mind at the moment of death that is important, not whether the body lives or dies. Those who are not fruitful members of society should be able to die, according to his assessment of Japanese views. Once consciousness (which he takes as brain activity) has permanently dissociated itself from the body, there is no reason to maintain the body, "for the body deprived of its *skandhas* [the constituents of human existence] is not a person" (Becker, 1990, p. 554). In short, all that matters is clarity of mind at the moment of death. (We must be careful in using Becker's analysis of the data. In point of fact, the Buddha was very reluctant to condone self-willed death if indeed he did so; it was only a few people who possibly killed themselves with the Buddha's blessing, because they were suffering from terminal illness and because they desired enlightenment. The other examples were simply threats. Becker also ignores the fact that the Buddha called the mere encouragement for others to perform self-willed death—or to provide the means—a deplorable act that would lead to expulsion from the monastery. One traditional commentator on the Parājita includes poison in the list of means. Because Buddhist monks were often physicians in ancient India, it is noteworthy that they were told not to perform abortions nor provide the means or even information to facilitate it; moreover, they must not help a family to kill a physically dependent member. This amounts to a strong position against physician-assisted suicide.

Shigeru Kato is much more cautious in his assessment of the Japanese practice of self-willed death and current Japanese interest in self-willed death, but for different reasons. After noting that some prominent Japanese jurists are advocating the legalization of euthanasia,

he reflects on Japan's reputation of being "a kingdom of suicides" and relates the fact that it has the largest number of suicides among all Buddhist countries to its tendency to beautify suicide or absolve it of a sense of wrong. Kato argues that "Human beings have no right to manipulate arbitrarily and selfishly their 'own' lives, which are transiently borrowed and must be returned soon to the holistic Being" (Kato, 1990, p. 71). He opines that "We can never dismiss this religious holism as an outdated superstition; we must keep it as a brake against the drive toward euthanasia" (Kato, 1990, pp. 78–79). He also looks to the formation of a better hospice organization in Japan in the 1980s as a way of resolving the "euthanasia problem" through the practice of withdrawal of treatment combined with dialogue and religious and aesthetic care. In the final analysis, however, he is willing to entertain active euthanasia as the right to die "with dignity" and to consider the merits of each case.

Confucianism and Taoism

Concepts of natural death. Confucian concepts of death are closely associated with ancestor worship, which was practiced as early as the first historical dynasty, the Shang (ca. 1500–1045/1046 B.C.E.). Judging from the written record provided by inscriptions of oracles written on bones, the dead were consulted by means of divination, as if they were living. Everything needed for the next life was put in the tombs of the kings and nobles. Originally servants, entertainers, and others were buried with them. Later, pottery figures were substituted. (In modern times, paper effigies of servants are used.) The cult of the ancestors must also have been practiced by commoners, because it was considered an ancient and widespread practice by Confucius in the sixth century B.C.E.

The ancestor cult was based on rituals, or *li*. It assumed the continuity of life after death, communication between the living and the dead, the legitimacy of a social hierarchy, and a virtual deification of the ancestors. In his *Analects*, Confucius upheld the ancient practices, refusing to shorten the period of mourning (XVII.21). Nevertheless, he taught that the spirits should be kept at a distance, so as not to preoccupy the living (VII.20; XI.11). He also thought that mourning rituals should be moderate; they should express grief rather than fear (III.3). Four centuries later, details of the mourning rituals were described in the ritual text *Yi Li*. Now elaborate, they were to last for three years. During the first year, the eldest son (as chief mourner) had to wear sackcloth, live in a hut outside the home, wail periodically, and eat very little food. Over the next two years, the restrictions were gradually lifted. Even after life returned to normal, though, he reported family business to the ancestors. In Confucianism, as in other patrilineal traditions, the performance of funerary and ancestral rites by the eldest son has contributed to a preference for sons. As a result, female infanticide has sometimes been practiced unofficially.

The Chinese developed two other perspectives on death: a return to nature and physical immortality. The Taoist philosopher Chuang Tzu (365–290 B.C.E.) wrote that life and death were two aspects of the same reality, mere differences of form. Death was a natural and welcomed release from life, and was to be neither feared nor desired. Because individuals were reabsorbed into nature, both birth and death were as natural as the progression of the four seasons. Other Taoists were interested in alchemy, macrobiotic diets, exercises, fasting, and meditation. Besides desiring health, youth, and longevity, they wanted immortality. They had several views of the latter: the physical body would rise to heaven; the "real body," not the physical one in the tomb, would rise; the physical body would go to the Isles of the Blessed, said to be off the northeast coast of China; or the self would emerge from the body at death, like the butterfly from its cocoon, to wander freely about the universe or go to the realm of the immortals.

In Taiwan, the Chinese still practice ancestor worship. They believe that people are related to common ancestors and to each other by an elaborate kinship system in which status is symbolized by the length of time spent mourning and authority is passed through the eldest son. They also believe in two souls: the *hun*, living in a tablet at the shrine, and the *p'o*, living in the grave. Both souls may influence the living. Kin meet periodically in the ancestral temple for sacrifices to the *hun*; the latter are offered wine, food, rice, and first fruits in exchange for health, longevity, prosperity, offspring, virtue, and a peaceful death. They are also remembered by preserving extensive genealogical records and documents written by the deceased. Families visit graves to communicate with or pay respect to the *p'o* and thus ensure the *p'o*'s goodwill toward the living.

The Taiwanese euphemistically call death "longevity"; after fifty, a person begins to prepare for death by making "longevity clothes" in the Han style of the second century B.C.E., a coffin, and if possible, a tomb. At the time of death, the eldest son of the deceased person eats "longevity noodles" and puts on the "longevity clothes" inside out. Then he puts these garments on the corpse, whose personal name henceforth may not be spoken. Other family members don sackcloth, leave their hair uncombed, and wail periodically (Thompson, 1975). The *hun* is first given a temporary resting place in a paper sword, placed in front of the corpse to receive prayers. After processions to and from the grave, this sword is transferred to a home shrine where the son and

relatives offer it food. Finally it is burned, and the spirit is thus transferred to a permanent tablet in the shrine. To keep the *p'o*, the body's orifices are plugged. The body is then rubbed with an elixir, placed in a coffin, and buried. Sometimes it is placed in a strong, watertight tomb to prevent decay. Coffins and graves are positioned according to exact rules for magical protection. If mistreated, the *p'o* causes trouble and threatens to become a ghost (*kuei*). Ritual specialists are then asked to inspect the grave, coffin, or bones to see why the *p'o* is unhappy (Berling, 1992). Taoist and Buddhist priests participate in the rituals of families who can afford them. For instance, priests hold services for seven weeks, during which they chant and pray for the soul to pass quickly through purgatory. Clearly, the Taiwanese try to ensure every advantage for the soul by incorporating practices from many religions.

In Taiwan, death remains associated with the ancestor cult. In the People's Republic of China, by contrast, there have been attempts to reform and even destroy ancestor worship. Communists have argued that traditional funeral rites and customs are remnants of the feudal economy and social structure; those lower in the clan hierarchy are exploited, and women, who cannot attend banquets in the ancestral temple, are excluded. Mourning clothes, moreover, waste cotton; wooden coffins waste timber; graves and tombs waste land; lavish funerals put families into debt; and beliefs in the afterlife instill superstition. Consequently, Communists have recommended the following: simple memorial services for the cadre, factory, village, or cooperative; the replacement of mourning clothes by arm bands; and the introduction of cremation (MacInnis, 1972).

Chinese concepts of self-willed death. Some of these concepts have already been discussed in the section on Buddhism. But it is important to point out that there were practices of self-willed death in the warrior circles of China as well. In fact, it was the obligation, not only the privilege of warriors to practice self-willed death under certain circumstances. This tradition, which had once been found among the elite, became common among the lower classes when warriors began to be recruited from them in the late Chou Dynasty. Later, members of the Mohist school of philosophy, which had links with the lower-class warriors, maintained a tradition of absolute loyalty to their leader. In one incident, eighty-three disciples followed their leader in death (Fung Yu-lan, 1953, p. 83).

Implications of Chinese views of self-willed death for bioethics. According to a report by Shi Da Pu (1991), euthanasia in China, once a taboo topic, has been discussed since the 1980s in the magazine *Medicine and Philosophy*. After the controversial case of the active euthanasia of a patient named Xia in 1986, which led to a court case being filed by her two daughters against their brother, who had authorized it, the topic was hotly debated in the media. It was also debated by the Chinese Dialectical Institute and Beijing Medical Ethics Academy, which concluded that active euthanasia was permissible for patients with no hope of cure. When the widow of former premier Zhou En-lai wrote that euthanasia was a "proper point of dialectical materialism" in need of discussion, there followed even more public debate. Some argued that it represented the height of civilization because it was a pure act of freedom; others, that it was "the result of the infection in the area of medicine from sick Western customs and morality . . . sharply against our socialist ethical values" (Shi Da Pu, 1991, p. 133). In 1988, a survey of 400 people (health professionals and nonprofessionals) showed that 80 percent were in favor of euthanasia. Both withdrawal of treatment and active euthanasia are being quietly practiced; though they are illegal, no one has been charged. Shi Da Pu concludes that most experts in China think that euthanasia should be regarded as part of the agenda of modernization, that the country should develop appropriate legislation to legalize it, and that the press should be enlisted to spread the dialectical materialist teaching about it (Shi Da Pu, 1991).

Conclusion

Four major views of natural death emerge when Asian religions are compared: (1) the cosmic, (2) the existential, (3) the familial, and (4) the natural. Hinduism has focused on the cosmic dimension of death, though it has also included the familial in connection with ancestor worship and the existential because of its long interaction with Buddhism. Buddhist views of death are existential in philosophical texts and some monastic circles; cosmic in the popular religion of both Theravāda and Mahāyāna countries; and familial (in countries with traditions of ancestor worship). Chinese religions emphasize the familial aspect of death, though cosmic dimensions are derived from Buddhism and popular Taoism, along with natural ones from philosophical Taoism.

Some of the Asian religions legitimated self-willed death (and sometimes assistance) in certain circumstances—such as a way to attain heaven or enlightenment, or a way to cope with a crisis such as terminal disease or extreme old age—as an exception to natural death. Although there were attempts to distinguish such self-willed death and assistance from suicide and homicide, respectively, some of the religions decided that the practice had created problems over time.

Each religion has a tendency to assimilate many, often contradictory, views, as if these provide extra antidotes against death. When views are too this-worldly—for example, the desire to eliminate suffering or mundane problems—or too otherworldly—for example, promises of easy heaven or liberation by self-willed death—premature death may occur. People, it seems, need to balance respect for the body and transcendence of it in order to live with health and purpose, thereby doing justice to their full humanity.

KATHERINE K. YOUNG

Directly related to this article are the other articles in this entry: ANTHROPOLOGICAL PERSPECTIVES, WESTERN PHILOSOPHICAL THOUGHT, WESTERN RELIGIOUS THOUGHT, *and* DEATH IN THE WESTERN WORLD (*with its* POSTSCRIPT). *Also directly related are the entries* DEATH, ATTITUDES TOWARD; DEATH AND DYING: EUTHANASIA AND SUSTAINING LIFE, *article on* ETHICAL ISSUES; HINDUISM; JAINISM; BUDDHISM; TAOISM; CONFUCIANISM; *and* SIKHISM. *For a discussion of related ideas, see the entries* DEATH, DEFINITION AND DETERMINATION OF; DEATH: ART OF DYING; HARM; HEALTH AND DISEASE, *article on* HISTORY OF THE CONCEPTS; HOSPICE AND END-OF-LIFE CARE; INFANTS; *article on* HISTORY OF INFANTICIDE; PERSON; *and* SUICIDE. *Other relevant material may be found under the entry* MEDICAL ETHICS, HISTORY OF, *section on* SOUTH AND EAST ASIA.

Bibliography

BECKER, CARL B. 1990. "Bioethics and Brain Death: The Recent Discussion in Japan." *Philosophy: East and West* 40, no. 4:543–556.

BERLING, JUDITH A. 1992. "Death and Afterlife in Chinese Religion." In *Death and Afterlife: Perspectives of World Religions*, pp. 181–192. Edited by Hiroshi Obayashi. New York: Greenwood Press.

BILIMORIA, PURUSHOTTAMA. 1992. "A Report from India: The Jaina Ethic of Voluntary Death." *Bioethics* 6, no. 4:331–355.

BLACKBURN, STUART H. 1985. "Death and Deification: Folk Cults in Hinduism." *History of Religions* 24, no. 3:255–274. Chicago: University of Chicago Press.

CAILLAT, COLETTE. 1977. "Fasting unto Death According to Āyaraṅga-Sutta and to Some Paninṇayas." In *Mahāvīra and His Teachings*, pp. 113–117. Edited by Adinath N. Upadhye et al. Bombay: Bhagavan Mahāvīra 2500th Nirvana Mahotsava Samiti.

ECK, DIANA L. 1982. *Banaras: City of Light*. Princeton, N.J.: Princeton University Press.

FUNG YU-LAN. 1953. *History of Chinese Philosophy*. 2 vols. Princeton, N.J.: Princeton University Press.

FUSÉ, TOYOMASA. 1980. "Suicide and Culture in Japan: A Study of Seppuku as an Institutionalized Form of Suicide." *Social Psychiatry* 15:57–63.

GUNARATNA, V. F. 1966. *Buddhist Reflections on Death*. Kandy, Ceylon: Buddhist Publication Society.

HOLCK, FREDERICK H., ed. 1974. *Death and Eastern Thought: Understanding Death in Eastern Religions and Philosophies.* Nashville, Tenn.: Abingdon Press.

JAINI, PADMANABH S. 1979. *The Jaina Path of Purification.* Berkeley: University of California Press.

KALTENMARK, MAX. 1969. *Lao Tzu and Taoism.* Translated by Roger Greaves. Stanford, Calif.: Stanford University Press.

KANE, PANDURANG VAMAN. 1968. *History of Dharmaśāstra: Ancient and Mediaeval Religious and Civil Law.* 2d ed. Poona, India: Bhandkarkar Oriental Research Institute.

KATO, SHIGERU. 1990. "Japanese Perspectives on Euthanasia." In *To Die or Not To Die? Cross-Disciplinary, Cultural, and Legal Perspectives on the Right to Choose Death,* pp. 85–102. Edited by Arthur S. Berger and Joyce Berger. New York: Praeger.

KEITH, ARTHUR BERRIEDALE. 1961. "Suicide (Hindu)." In vol. 12 of *Encyclopaedia of Religion and Ethics,* pp. 33–35. Edited by James Hastings, john A. Selbie, and Louis H. Gray. New York: Charles Scribner's Sons.

LATI, RINBOCHAY, and HOPKINS, JEFFERY. 1985. *Death, Intermediate State and Rebirth.* Ithaca, N.Y.: Snow Lion.

LAY, ARTHUR HYDE. 1974. "A Buddhist Funeral in Traditional Japan." In *Religion in the Japanese Experience: Sources and Interpretations,* pp. 62–64. Edited by H. Byron Earhart. Encino, Calif.: Dickenson.

LINCOLN, BRUCE. 1991. *Death, War, and Sacrifice: Studies in Ideology and Practice.* Chicago: University of Chicago Press.

LODRU, LAMA. 1987. *Bardo Teachings: The Way of Death and Rebirth.* Ithaca, N.Y.: Snow Lion.

MacINNIS, DONALD E., comp. 1972. *Religious Policy and Practice in Communist China: A Documentary Reader.* New York: Macmillan.

MULLIN, GLENN H. 1985. *Death and Dying: The Tibetan Tradition.* London: Arkana.

OBAYASHI, HIROSHI, ed. 1992. *Death and Afterlife: Perspectives of World Religions.* New York: Greenwood Press.

POUSSIN, LOUIS DE LA VALLÉE. 1961. "Suicide (Buddhist)." In vol. 12 of *Encyclopaedia of Religion and Ethics,* pp. 24–26. Edited by James Hastings, John A. Selbie, and Louis H. Gray. New York: Charles Scribner's Sons.

PU, SHI DA. 1991. "Euthanasia in China: A Report." *Journal of Medicine and Philosophy* 16, no. 2:131–138.

RATANAKUL, PINIT. 1988. "Bioethics in Thailand: The Struggle for Buddhist Solutions." *Journal of Medicine and Philosophy* 13, no. 3:301–312.

REYNOLDS, FRANK E., and WAUGH, EARLE H., eds. 1977. *Religious Encounters with Death: Insights from the History and Anthropology of Religions.* University Park: Pennsylvania State University Press.

SCHOPEN, GREGORY. 1992. "On Avoiding Ghosts and Social Censure: Monastic Funerals in the *Mūlasarvāstivada-Vinaya.*" *Journal of Indian Philosophy* 20, no. 1:1–39.

SETTAR, SHADAKSHARI. 1989. *Inviting Death: Indian Attitude Towards the Ritual Death.* Leiden: E. J. Brill.

———. 1990. *Pursuing Death: Philosophy and Practice of Voluntary Termination of Life.* Dharward, India: Institute of Indian Art History, Karnatak University.

SHARMA, ARVIND; RAY, AJIT; HEJIB, ALAKA; and YOUNG, KATHERINE K. 1988. *Sati: Historical and Phenomenological Essays.* Delhi: Motilal Banarsidass.

SMITH, ROBERT J. 1974. *Ancestor Worship in Contemporary Japan.* Stanford, Calif.: Stanford University Press.

SPIRO, MELFORD E. 1970. *Buddhism and Society: A Great Tradition and Its Burmese Vicissitudes.* New York: Harper & Row.

THAKUR, UPENDRA. 1963. *The History of Suicide in India, an Introduction.* Delhi: Munshi-ram Manohar-lal.

THAPAR, ROMILA. 1981. "Death and the Hero." In *Mortality and Immortality: The Anthropology and Archaeology of Death,* pp. 293–315. Edited by Sarah C. Humphreys and Helen King. London: Academic Press.

THOMPSON, LAURENCE G. 1975. *Chinese Religion: An Introduction.* 2d ed. Encino, Calif.: Dickenson.

TILAK, SHRINIVAS. 1987. *Religion and Aging in the Indian Tradition.* Albany: State University of New York Press.

TUKOL, T. K. 1976. *Sallekhanā Is Not Suicide.* Ahmedabad: L. D. Institute of Indology.

WELCH, HOLMES. 1967. *The Practice of Chinese Buddhism: 1900–1950.* Cambridge, Mass.: Harvard University Press.

WILTSHIRE, MARTIN G. 1983. "The 'Suicide' Problem in the Pāli Canon." In *Journal of the International Association of Buddhist Studies* 6, no. 2:124–140.

WOOS, FLEUR. 1993. "Pokkuri-Temples and Aging: Rituals for Approaching Death." In *Religion and Society in Modern Japan: Selected Readings.* Edited by Mark R. Mullins, Shimazono Susumu, and Paul L. Swanson. Berkeley, Calif.: Asian Humanities Press.

YOUNG, KATHERINE K. 1980. "*Tīrtha* and the Metaphor of Crossing Over." *Studies in Religion* 9, no. 1:61–68.

———. 1989. "Euthanasia: Traditional Hindu Views and the Contemporary Debate." In *Hindu Ethics: Purity, Abortion, and Euthanasia,* pp. 71–130. Edited by Harold G. Coward, Julius J. Lipner, and Katherine K. Young. Albany: State University of New York Press.

———. 1993. "Hindu Bioethics." In *Religious Methods and Resources in Bioethics,* pp. 3–30. Edited by Paul F. Camenisch. Dordrecht, Netherlands: Kluwer.

———. 1994. "A Cross-Cultural Historical Case Against Planned Self-Willed Death and Assisted Suicide." *McGill Law Journal* 39, no. 3(Sept.).

III. WESTERN PHILOSOPHICAL THOUGHT

For both humankind generally and each living person individually, the recognition of the universality and inevitability of death is but the beginning of the problem of death. Indeed, recognizing death as the individual and collective fate of human beings, and of all living creatures, creates the problem of death: Why does it happen? What does it mean? Is death final? Is death a good thing or a bad thing? At least as often these questions emerge for us in their mirror image, still provoked by death: What is the meaning of life, its purpose? Can life be meaningful if it ends in death? What purposes could outlast the inevitability of my death?

Philosophers have struggled with a human fear of death. Recognizing the inevitability of death is very different from supposing death is final. At a very general level, philosophical reflections on death divide those who deny the finality of death and suppose there is ongoing, usually individual, self-consciousness after death, and those who regard bodily death as final, as the destruction of consciousness, but who offer consolation meant to assuage fear of the inevitability of personal extinction. A very few philosophers have found death to be inevitable, final, and horrible. What binds all together in a recognizably "Western" tradition are the analytically and argumentatively philosophical approaches each group takes and the exclusively human-centered character of their views.

Probably the single most persistent theme in Western philosophical reflection on death is the view that death is not the annihilation of the self but its transformation into another form of existence. The conviction that individual human beings survive death, perhaps eternally, has been very differently grounded and elaborated in the history of philosophy, but in some form has persisted and frequently dominated through antiquity, the long era of Christian theologizing, modernity, and into contemporary "postmodern" thinking. Considerably less attended to is the attempt to reconcile human beings to death's finality, to death as the end of individual human experiencing beyond which there exists no consciousness.

The pre-Socratic philosophers

The tension in Western philosophy between regarding death as transformation and thinking of death as final appears at the very outset of what is conventionally regarded as the beginning of Western philosophy, in the fragmentary remains of writing that have survived from thinkers in the early Greek colonies of Asia Minor, especially the Ionians. Anaximander (ca. 610–547 B.C.E.) and Heraclitus (ca. 533–475 B.C.E.) in particular were singularly impressed with the transitoriness of all things, as captured in the best-known corruption of a Heraclitean fragment, "One cannot step into the same river twice" (cf. Kirk and Raven, 1960, fr. 217). The attempt to reconcile opposites—such as life and death— and to perceive the underlying unity, even harmony, in all of reality was preeminent for the pre-Socratics.

The very earliest surviving pre-Socratic fragment, from a book attributed to Anaximander, contains a passage that allows one to see both of the subsequent views about death—death as final and death as transitory— that have dominated Western thinking:

> And the source of coming-to-be for existing things is that into which destruction, too, happens, "according

to necessity; for they pay penalty and retribution to each other for their injustice according to the assessment of Time." (Kirk and Raven, 1960, fr. 112)

Jacques Choron, to whom all subsequent accounts of death in Western philosophy are indebted, reads this passage as evidence of how impressed Anaximander was with the terrible fact that things perish, but also as expressing the hope "that somewhere and somehow death shall have no dominion" (1963, p. 35). Further, there is the suggestion that despite appearances, death is not annihilation: In the everlasting boundlessness (aperion), individual death is not meaningless, perhaps not even final.

In what is now southern Italy, Pythagoras (ca. 572– 497 B.C.E.) struggled with these same realities, teaching that the soul suffered from embodiment, longed for release and reunion with the divine, possibly at death experienced transmigration into possibly other life forms, and could be purified in part through the process of rebirth. For the purification needed to overcome death and to be evermore united with the divine, it was most important to live a philosophical life, especially one that paid considerable attention to the contemplation of mathematical truth. This very abstract, highly intellectual element in Pythagoreanism distinguished it from the Orphic cults and Dionysian predecessors that so influenced it, and gave Pythagoreanism considerable appeal for Plato.

Continuity and change, constancy through flux, permanence and impermanence, death, extinction, and recurrence are the enduring concerns of pre-Socratic philosopher/scientists. If, as Alfred North Whitehead has suggested, the whole of Western philosophy is but a series of footnotes to Plato, it might equally be said that the history of Western philosophy on death is but a series of footnotes to Plato's predecessors.

Socrates, Plato, and Aristotle

What we know of Socrates' (ca. 470–399 B.C.E.) view of death is largely detached from a theoretical context replete with ontological and metaphysical doctrines. His views seem to be rooted in the immediacy of his experience and circumstances, at a time when he is first anticipating, then under, a death sentence. It is the example Socrates sets, more than the words that Plato (or Xenophon) reports him to have said, that have influenced generations of students.

Early in Apology (29Aff.), Socrates is tentative in his assertions about death, saying only that "To be afraid of death is only another form of thinking that one is wise when one is not; it is to think that one knows what one does not know." Later, having been sentenced to death, Socrates ventures that death is either dreamless sleep from which, it seems, we do not awaken (annihilation) or transport to a place where we might ever after commune with those who precede us in death. The first is not fearsome; the second is to be joyfully celebrated (41B–42A). Socrates' deepest and most influential conviction, however, may have been that "Nothing can harm a good man, either in life or after death" (Plato, 1961).

Socrates' courage and equanimity in the face of a manifestly unjust death sentence is universally admired. But exactly why he was so compliant with injustice at the end of his life is a continuing mystery (cf. Momeyer, 1982).

Less mysterious is how Socrates could go from the cautious and skeptical views on death expressed in *Apology* to the far more metaphysically burdened opinions of *Phaedo*. The accepted explanation here is that in *Phaedo*, written later than *Apology* and *Crito*, Socrates has been transformed into a spokesperson for Plato (ca. 428–348 B.C.E.). As such, *Phaedo* is best read as the most complete case that Plato makes for his views on the immortality of the soul, with only the final death scene bearing any likely resemblance to Socrates's actual words.

Plato's view of death is inseparable from his doctrine of the soul, his identification of the soul with personhood, and ultimately the theory of Forms. Curiously, Plato's arguments are directed more to establishing the immortality of the soul than to the logically prior task of showing that the soul is the person. Whether the soul is identical to the person is a matter of continuing controversy today in bioethical debates over the definition of death and criteria for personhood.

In *Phaedo*, Plato reminds readers that knowledge is recollection and shows that the soul must have existed before birth and embodiment in order for us to know most of what we do know during life. While this does not show that the soul survives death, it is suggestive in that it implies the soul's independence from the body. Other arguments attempt to show that the soul is "simple," that is, not composed of parts and hence not subject to dissolution; that the soul resembles immortal gods in ruling the body; and that since the essence of the soul is life, it cannot admit of its negation or opposite any more than fire can be cold. Similarly, Plato holds that since the soul is capable of apprehending the eternal and immutable Forms or Ideas, it must be of a similar nature, eternal and divine.

It is not clear how seriously Plato intends most of these arguments to be taken, nor how seriously he himself takes them. But at least two central Platonic views are relevant and seriously maintained. The first is the reality of ideas, a domain of pure, unchanging essences the apprehension of which, however imperfect, is as close to real knowledge as living human beings can get.

Second, Plato's suspicion of the body—construed by much later followers to be outright disdain—and his longing to be free of its burdens are consistent throughout his work. In Plato's judgment, intellectual pursuits are the most noble, but these are consistently and constantly hindered by bodily appetites and bodily limitations of sensory experience. Hence the true philosopher aspires to death, we are assured in *Phaedo*, and lives to die, in the expectation that only the soul's liberation from embodiment will make possible the fullest attainment of knowledge.

Plato's premier student began his own philosophizing in *Eudemos*, espousing Platonic views on the immortality of the soul and how individual selves survive death. Soon, however, Aristotle (384–322 B.C.E.) departed substantially from his mentor, and in *De anima* sees the soul as almost entirely physical, the entelechy of the body. More than being physically inseparable from the body, Aristotle argues, the soul is logically inseparable, as vision is logically inseparable from the seeing eye. The closest Aristotle will allow us to come to immortality is in the same fashion other creatures experience it, in successive generations of progeny. (Aristotle, 1941).

Aristotle does allow for the possibility that part of the soul survives death, the part that distinguishes us from other animals: reason, our divine element. But Aristotle's writings on these matters are fraught with ambiguity, and it is not clear that he thinks there is any survival of individual personalities.

In any case, the strongest imperative for Aristotle is to live a life of reason, an important part of which requires one to overcome a natural fear of death through courage and virtue. It seems to be Aristotle's considered judgment that individual selves do not survive death, and no benign deity watches over us; yet life is still meaningful so long as we are awed by the beauty and order of nature, and meet life's misfortunes with courage and perseverance.

Aristotle's death in 322 B.C.E. brought an appropriate close to the Hellenic period of philosophizing and provided some of the central themes in reflections on death for the Hellenistic schools that followed. Chief among these were Epicureanism and Stoicism.

Hellenistic schools: Epicureanism and Stoicism

Where death had been a distinctly secondary concern for Socratic thinking, it soon became a primary one for Hellenistic philosophers. For Epicurus, Lucretius, and Zeno, then Seneca, Epictetus, and Marcus Aurelius, discovering how to live life and confront death were the central tasks of philosophy.

Although Epicureans and Stoics differed on what

they most valued in life, they equally valued attaining equanimity in the face of imminent death. Epicureans in particular saw no reason to fear death, believing that at death the soul, composed of the finest atoms, simply dissipated, so that there was nothing left to have experiences. Epicurus argued that one need not fear an unpleasant afterlife, for there was no afterlife; nor need one fear death as annihilation, for as soon as it occurred, one no longer existed to suffer anything. Epicurus's view is well captured in his memorable letter to Menoecus, in which he asserts:

> Death . . . is nothing to us, since so long as we exist, death is not with us; but when death comes, then we do not exist. It does not then concern either the living or the dead, since for the former it is not, and the latter are no more. (Epicurus, 1926, p. 85)

Epicurus may well be on strong ground in urging us to regard death as final and afterlife as nonexistent, for this claim at least is supportable by overwhelming empirical evidence: People die, and they do not return. His second assurance, however—that the living need not fear death because once it occurs, they no longer exist to experience it—is far more problematic.

Epicurus's argument seems to be the following: Only that which is experienced can be evil and fearful. But death is a condition in which nothing is experienced, for the subject of experience no longer exists. Hence, it is unreasonable to fear death.

The problematic assumption here is that only that which is experienced is harmful. Deception, betrayal, and ridicule behind one's back are all capable of doing great harm, though one may never be aware of them, know of the damage they do, or be able to mind the harm. Consequently, it is legitimate to argue, contrary to Epicurus, that death is a harm (even though not experienced) precisely because it is the irrevocable loss of opportunity, of the continued good of life. Death is the deprivation of life, and were one not dead, possibilities for satisfying experiences could be realized (cf. Nagel, 1979).

The Stoics pursued a rather different strategy than the Epicureans in attempting to accommodate people to their mortality. Though we have only the most minimal fragments from the early Stoics—Zeno of Citium (ca. 336–264 B.C.E.), Cleanthes of Assos (ca. 331–232 B.C.E.), and Chrysippus of Soli (ca. 280–206 B.C.E.)—it is clear that they were much influenced by Heraclitus and emphasized discoveries in logic and cosmology. In ethics, they were early natural-law theorists, urging the unity of physical and moral universes and the duty to live a life as orderly as the cosmos, always striving for *autarkeia* (autonomy) of the virtuous person. Socrates, especially during his trial and execution, was a model and inspiration for Stoics of all eras.

Most closely identified with Stoicism today are the later Stoics of the first two centuries of the Christian era in imperial Rome. The most prominent of these were Seneca (ca. 4 B.C.E.–65 C.E.), Epictetus (ca. 50–130), and Marcus Aurelius (121–180). What bound these philosophers together was their commitment to virtue, understood as willing behavior in accord with reason (or nature) and unresisting resignation before what was uncontrollable.

The art of mastering the fear of death is not easily learned. Stoics recommend emulating great men [sic], virtuously living the life of a philosopher, and always remembering that living well is by far the most important thing. Reminders of the futility of fearing or resisting death are also prevalent in their writings. For all of its inevitability, death need not be our imposed fate before which impassibility is required. No philosopher more than Seneca recommended so enthusiastically and vigorously, nor practiced so decisively, taking control of death by choosing it in the form of suicide. In one remarkable letter (no. 70), he says the following:

> For mere living is not a good, but living well. Accordingly, the wise man will live as long as he ought, not as long as he can. . . . As soon as there are many events in his life that give him trouble and disturb his peace of mind, he sets himself free. . . . It is not a question of dying earlier or later, but of dying well or ill. And dying well means escape from the danger of living ill. . . . Just as I shall select my ship as I am about to go on a voyage . . . so shall I choose my death when I am about to depart from life. . . . Every man ought to make his life acceptable to others besides himself, but his death to himself alone. The best form of death is one we like. (Seneca, 1970)

Seneca was not, in practice, so casual about self-killing as some of the above implies. Still, when Nero accused him of conspiring against the state, and ordered him to take his own life, Seneca is reported to have paused only long enough to remind his followers of the philosophical precepts they had striven to live by before slashing his wrists and bleeding to death.

The long transition to a modern view of death

In tracing our theme through Western philosophy—whether death is final or whether some notion of afterlife is envisioned—there is very little more to say about this between the time of Stoicism's greatest influence and the onset of a secular, scientific modern renaissance. For over 1,200 years Christian religious views held sway, and philosophy, dominated by theology, had little of substance and still less that was novel to say about death. Enormously important philosophical work was done during this long era, but little of it had much new to contribute to Western philosophical thought on death.

Western philosophical thought on death did not take a turn back to the secular until Francis Bacon (1561–1626) promoted an increasingly scientific methodology and worldview, and René Descartes (1596–1650) reordered the philosophical agenda. Both reflect on death with the aim of excising the fear of death (which in the late Middle Ages, overwhelmed by both plague and superstition, reached new heights). Bacon, however, does so by emphasizing the continuity of dying with living, such that once we learn to live fearlessly, we will be assured of dying fearlessly. Descartes chooses to assuage fears of death by the now more traditional route of arguing for the immortality of the soul. And as is well known, Descartes's argument to this end relies upon a radical division of persons into different substances, body and soul, mysteriously and problematically united, which sets the stage for much subsequent philosophizing.

Most of modern philosophy pursues Cartesian themes, and the variety of responses is considerable. Rationalist philosophers have generally sought to salvage hopes of surviving death. (Benedict Spinoza [1632–1677] is a notable exception.) But the philosophes of the eighteenth century, and the empiricists they often looked to, came to regard doctrines of the immortality of the soul as "priestly lies." Voltaire (1694–1778), through Candide's misadventures in "the best of all possible worlds," savagely ridicules Gottfried Wilhelm Leibniz's (1646–1716) faith in universal harmony, and other philosophes look back to the Epicureans and Stoics for inspiration on how to face the prospects of death as annihilation (Voltaire, 1966).

But it was David Hume (1711–1776) who most systematically and rigorously called into question doctrines of the soul's immortality. His attack is two-pronged: First he argues against the notion of substance, specifically the self as a substance, and second, he directs a series of arguments against the notion that some part of a person survives death.

In "On Immortality" (1777), Hume characterizes "substance" as a "wholly confused and imperfect notion," an "aggregate of particular qualities inhering in an unknown something." As for the self as a substance, he states in *A Treatise of Human Nature* (1739):

> There is no impression constant and invariable. Pain and pleasure, grief and joy, passions and sensations, succeed each other, and never all exist at the same time. It cannot therefore be from any of these impressions, or from any other, that the idea of self is derived; and consequently there is no such idea. (Hume, 1978, bk. I, pt. 4, sec. 6)

Hume claims to be "insensible of *myself*," for the self is "nothing but a bundle or collection of different perceptions which succeed each other with an inconceivable rapidity, and are in a perpetual flux and movement." All that binds perceptions together is memory and constancy, but it is futile to ask what it is that "has" memory or experiences constancy of conjoined perceptions (Hume, 1978, bk. I, pt. 4, sec. 6).

Hume's more vigorous critique of immortality is reserved for benighted attempts to settle questions of fact by a priori metaphysical speculation, which is what is done by all doctrines of "immaterial substance" and all attempts to identify personhood with an immaterial "soul" substance that is individuated and survives the demise of the body. Placing his faith in the conviction that all natural processes have some point (if not purpose), Hume notes the universal fear of death and remarks that "Nature does nothing in vain, she would never give us a horror against an *impossible* event."

The only admissible arguments on such a question of fact as whether human beings survive death are those from experience, and these, Hume asserts, are "strong for the mortality of the soul." What possible argument could prove a "state of existence which no one ever saw and which in no way resembles any that ever was seen?" Body and mind grow together, age together, ail together, and, from all experience conveys to us, perish together.

Moral arguments that turn on a just Deity's desire to punish the wicked and reward the good fare no better than metaphysical ones when attempting to prove immortality. It would be a "barbarous deceit," "an injustice in nature," Hume asserts, to restrict "all our knowledge to the present life if there be another scene still waiting us of infinitely greater consequence." Still worse, it would be monstrous for a loving God to base a judgment of how each of us will spend eternity upon the all too finite experience of one human lifetime.

Notwithstanding that in Immanuel Kant's own words, reading Hume "awakened me from my dogmatic slumbers," Kant (1724–1804) advanced his own version of a moral argument for the immortality of the human soul. Kant agrees with Hume that no argument from nature (i.e., experience) can demonstrate the immortality of a human soul, and he even concedes that "pure reason" is not up to the task. Nonetheless, Kant is firmly convinced that a compelling metaphysical/moral argument will do the job.

Kant apparently never doubted his belief in human immortality, and his argument to show the soul's immortality is both elegant in its simplicity and rich in the number of fundamental Kantian tenets that it incorporates or presupposes. Kant asserts in the *Critique of Practical Reason* (1788) that the most basic requirement of the moral law is the attainment of perfection. Such an achievement is not possible in a finite life, however. But the moral law can command only what it is possible for moral agents to do. Hence the necessity of an immortal soul so that moral agents will have the opportunity to do what they ought to do (Kant, 1949).

One of the more interesting features of Kant's "proof" is that it breaks with the long tradition that sees afterlife as occurring in paradise. In Kant's moral universe, there must still be pain and suffering in the hereafter, for these are inseparable features of the moral life. Further, doubt, uncertainty, and struggle for constant improvement must accompany our disembodied journey through eternity. The moral law would appear to be nearly as powerful as God.

The soundness of Kant's argument turns on the truth of at least the following Kantian doctrines: Objective reality must conform to the essential structure of the human mind; moral certainty is as sure a route to knowledge as the logical demonstrations of reason; moral perfection is required of all who would live a moral life; human beings exist, simultaneously, in two worlds, one phenomenal, the other noumenal. If any of these dogmas fail—and all have been extensively criticized—Kant's argument for the immortality of the human soul fails as well. Any number of philosophers after Kant, less enamored of metaphysical arguments, have turned his argument around and observed that if perfection is not possible in a human life span, the moral law cannot require perfection of human beings. Far from showing human immortality, Kant's insight into morality shows the limits of what a reasonable morality can demand of mortal creatures.

Toward postmodernism. Variations on religious, usually Christian, views of death and immortality continued in the writings of eighteenth- and nineteenth-century philosophers, including most notably the idealism of Georg W. F. Hegel (1770–1831) and the atheistic pessimism of Arthur Schopenhauer (1788–1860). Not until a real break with modern thought occurred did genuinely novel views about the significance of death and the possibility of immortality arise. In the thought of Friedrich Nietzsche (1844–1900) many now find both the culmination of ancient and modern approaches to death and the transition to a postmodern worldview. And it is certainly true that in Nietzsche's various writings, one can find many different historically grounded and historically transcendent approaches to the problem of death.

While still a student, Nietzsche read Schopenhauer's *The World as Will and Idea*. Profoundly moved and deeply disturbed, he sought escape from Schopenhauer's pessimism and atheism, and saw the task of philosophy as overcoming the former while taking responsibility for the latter (*Ecce Homo*). Physical pain and mental suffering were lifelong companions; staring into the abyss of despair and coping with the guilt of killing God, Nietzsche tried a number of different strategies for finding life worth continuing.

Through classical studies and art, Nietzsche supposed, one might escape the profound misery of existence (*The Birth of Tragedy*). The consolations of "beautiful dreams" soon faded, however, and Nietzsche turned to a detached, critical search for knowledge, and the "*interesting* illusion of science replaces the *beautiful* illusion of art" (Choron, 1963, p. 201).

Objective knowledge, or its semblance, proved unsatisfying as well, and Nietzsche then began to develop the idea of the "superman" as the disciplined Dionysian man capable of living a pain-filled life with full creativity. Truth is painful and, to all but the superman, unbearable. Above all, one must love fate (*amor fati*), which becomes possible with the Eternal Recurrence of the Same:

> Everything goes, everything returns; eternally rolls the wheel of existence. Everything dies, everything blossoms forth again; eternally runs the year of existence. . . . All things return eternally and we ourselves have already been numberless times, and all things with us. (*Also Sprach Zarathustra*, quoted by Choron, 1963, p. 202)

At least Heraclitus's voice seems to recur here.

How such a view of the one life we have and the one death we experience, albeit endlessly repeated, solves the problem of death is not clear. Sometimes Nietzsche suggests that recognizing the Eternal Recurrence of the Same should lead us to passionately embrace and affirm life, to live with as much conviction and determination as we can muster, for life might otherwise be all the more miserable for its endless repetition. But Nietzsche, who attempted suicide three times, must have been terrified at the prospect of such recurrence. It is the ultimate test of the superman to love fate while recognizing precisely what fate has in store.

Contemporary philosophy. The problem of death has not often been seen by contemporary philosophers as a choice between devising consolations for our finitude and demonstrations of our eternalness. For many, perhaps most, philosophers late in the twentieth century, the death of God is a century past, the grieving finished nearly half a century ago. The problem of death, understood as the struggle to make life meaningful in an increasingly secular age plagued by the temptations of nihilism, continues. The little that philosophers in the present time have had to say about death—outside of chiefly moral concerns centering on choosing death—has tended to suppose death is final, not, in any form, to be survived.

It has been the French existentialists—chiefly Jean-Paul Sartre (1905–1980), Simone de Beauvoir (1908–1986), and Albert Camus (1913–1960)—who have had some of the most distinctive things to say about the problem of death in the twentieth century. Building on Nietzsche's alienation from convention, despair at the death of God, and attraction to nihilism, and struggling with revelations of the distinctly human capacity for genocide revealed during the Holocaust and the era of nuclear weaponry, existentialists have sought ways to affirm against all odds the meaningfulness of individual human existence. A good deal of the spirit of this distinctive approach to death is captured in de Beauvoir's unsettling judgment on the very difficult dying of her mother:

> There is no such thing as a natural death: nothing that happens to a man is ever natural, since his presence calls the world into question. All men must die: but for every man his death is an accident and, even if he knows it and consents to it, an unjustifiable violation. (Beauvoir, 1965, p. 123)

Far from providing assurances of immortality or consolations designed to meet death with equanimity, existentialists recommend a rebellious, often angry response to the "cosmic injustice" that human beings die. Rebellion against or resistance toward death, however, is not recommended as a strategy for overcoming death; no illusions are allowed as to the inevitability and finality of death. Rather, for Albert Camus especially, such resistance is recommended as an affirmation of one's decency, caring about life, and personal integrity. Nowhere is this better illustrated than in Camus's novel *The Plague*, an extended allegory about any number of evils, not the least of which is death itself. Dr. Bernard Rieux and his closest friend, Jean Tarrou, struggle mightily against the ravages of the plague in the seaside town of Oran in Algeria. In time, however, Tarrou succumbs to the plague, and Rieux reflects on what it means:

> Tarrou had lost the match, as he put it. But what had he, Rieux, won? No more than the experience of having known plague and remembering it, of having known friendship and remembering it, of knowing affection and being destined one day to remember it. So all a man could win in the conflict between plague and life was knowledge and memories. But Tarrou, perhaps, would have called that winning the match. (Camus, 1948, p. 262)

Afterword

Most Western philosophical views on death have been singularly human-centered, driven by the assumption of human uniqueness. Even atheistic existentialists, for whom God is displaced altogether from the universe, seem lost with no center, and substitute human beings and a kind of humanism as their moral center.

We have only just begun to explore the post-Darwinian implications of regarding human beings as a natural kind—as creatures like other creatures known to us, evolved from simpler life forms without conscious direction. The moral implications of such a change in worldview are getting considerable attention from philosophers at present—in reflections on ecology and the moral status of nonhuman animals, in more sympathetic treatments of rational suicide and euthanasia, in greater openness about the difficulties of dying—but the larger ontological and metaphysical consequences are infrequently addressed. If there is to be any substantial breakthrough in our philosophical thinking about death, it might well come only with the displacement of human self-centeredness, with seeing human beings as one among many natural kinds on a solitary planet in an ordinary solar system that is on the fringes of one of many billions of galaxies in an apparently infinite universe. Such a potentially revitalized naturalism need not imply that life is meaningless for solitary, mortal human beings, nor does it guarantee significant life, but it might suggest that our plight is not unique, not unshared by others, and not, finally, to be resolved (or dissolved) by exclusive self-centered speciesist concerns.

But maybe not. Even such a revitalized naturalism might prove to be but one more variation on one side of the recurrent debate between those who seek a satisfactory means to reconcile each of us to the finality of death, and those who, on the other hand, seek to sustain the hope that life does not end with death and that individual consciousness continues beyond the grave.

RICHARD W. MOMEYER

Directly related to this article are the other articles in this entry: ANTHROPOLOGICAL PERSPECTIVES, EASTERN THOUGHT, WESTERN RELIGIOUS THOUGHT, *and* DEATH IN THE WESTERN WORLD (*with its* POSTSCRIPT). *Also directly related to this article are the entries* DEATH, ATTITUDES TOWARD; DEATH, DEFINITION AND DETERMINATION OF, *article on* PHILOSOPHICAL AND THEOLOGICAL PERSPECTIVES; DEATH: ART OF DYING; *and* LIFE. *For a discussion of related ideas, see the entries* BODY, *article on* EMBODIMENT: THE PHENOMENOLOGICAL TRADITION; HUMAN NATURE; INTERPRETATION; PERSON; *and* TRAGEDY. *Other relevant material may be found under the entries* DEATH AND DYING: EUTHANASIA AND SUSTAINING LIFE, *article on* HISTORICAL ASPECTS; HOSPICE AND END-OF-LIFE CARE; JUDAISM; ROMAN CATHOLICISM; *and* SUICIDE.

Bibliography

ARISTOTLE. 1941. *The Basic Works of Aristotle.* Edited by Richard McKeon. New York: Random House.

BEAUVOIR, SIMONE DE. 1965. *A Very Easy Death.* Translated by Patrick O'Brien. New York: Penguin.

CAMUS, ALBERT. 1948. *The Plague.* Translated by Stuart Gilbert. New York: Modern Library.

CHORON, JACQUES. 1963. *Death and Western Thought.* New York: Collier Books.

EPICURUS. 1926. *Epicurus, the Extant Remains.* Translated by Cyril Bailey. Oxford: At the Clarendon Press.

GUTTMANN, JAMES. 1978. "Death: Western Philosophical Thought." In *The Encyclopedia of Bioethics,* pp. 235–243. Edited by Warren T. Reich. New York: Macmillan.

HUME, DAVID. 1978. *A Treatise of Human Nature.* 2d ed. Edited by L. A. Selby-Bigge. Oxford: At the Clarendon Press.

———. 1985. *Essays: Moral, Political and Literary.* Edited by Eugene F. Miller. Indianapolis, Ind.: Liberty Classics.

KANT, IMMANUEL. 1949. *Critique of Practical Reason and Other Writings in Moral Philosophy.* Translated and edited by Lewis White Beck. Chicago: University of Chicago Press.

KIRK, GEOFFREY S., and RAVEN, JOHN E., trans. and eds. 1960. *The Presocratic Philosophers.* Cambridge: At the University Press.

MOMEYER, RICHARD W. 1982. "Socrates on Obedience and Disobedience to Law." *Philosophy Research Archives* 8:21–54.

———. 1988. *Confronting Death.* Bloomington: Indiana University Press.

NAGEL, THOMAS. 1979. "Death." In his *Mortal Questions.* Cambridge: At the University Press.

NIETZSCHE, FRIEDRICH WILHELM. 1977. *A Nietzsche Reader.* Translated and edited by R. J. Hollingdale. New York: Penguin.

OATES, WHITNEY JENNINGS, ed. 1940. *The Stoic and Epicurean Philosophers: The Complete Extant Writings of Epicurus, Epictetus, Lucretius, Marcus Aurelius.* New York: Random House.

PLATO. 1961. *The Collected Dialogues of Plato.* Edited by Edith Hamilton and Huntington Cairns. Princeton, N.J.: Princeton University Press.

SENECA, LUCIUS ANNAEUS. 1970. "On the Proper Time to Slip the Cable." In vol. 2 of *Ad Lucillum Epistulae Morales.* Translated by Richard M. Gummere. Cambridge, Mass.: Harvard University Press.

VOLTAIRE. 1966. *Candide.* Translated and edited by Robert M. Adams. New York: Norton.

IV. WESTERN RELIGIOUS THOUGHT

Death in biblical thought

There is no "biblical view of death" as such. This lack of a single scriptural understanding of death is hardly surprising, given the fact that the Bible is sacred scripture for three world religions and that its contents were written and compiled over a period of a thousand years or more. But the history of literary and religious development embedded within the Bible itself does allow for a kind of "archaeology" of death in biblical thought. Though admittedly vastly over-simplified, the following narrative of the Bible's evolving views on death can be traced backward through their random branchings and read forward toward their studied convergences.

Put in its simplest terms, an ancient desert god named Yahweh came to be regarded not only as the national god of a holy nation, but ultimately as the one and only God of the universe. These momentous shifts in the biblical understanding of God were paralleled by remarkable changes in biblical views of death, beginning with the denial and concluding with the affirmation of individual postmortem existence.

The Hebrew Bible. Hebrew religion emerged out of the tribal polytheisms of ancient Mesopotamia. The protagonists of Yahwism only gradually succeeded in establishing their deity as the national god of the various Semitic tribes that were finally welded together, during the latter half of the second millennium B.C.E., into the people known as the Israelites. A key weapon in their struggle to establish Yahweh's supremacy was the suppression of prevailing beliefs and practices dealing with death. In two very different responses to death, Mesopotamian culture had preserved primitive notions of life after death as a continuation of the life before death. On the one hand, mortuary cults affirmed a significant afterlife for the powerful and privileged who commanded the worship and fealty of the living. On the other hand, postmortem existence was limited to an awful underworld where the departed dead were shrouded in darkness and subsisted on clay. In either case, the realm of the dead was under the control of the gods of the underworld. For that reason, the champions of Yahwism denounced the polytheistic beliefs and practices of both the mortuary cults and the "house of dust."

Against the mortuary cults, the Yahwists presented a view of human nature and destiny that undercut all ancestor worship and necromancy. In the Yahwist creation myth, the protohuman couple was created from the soil and destined to return to the soil (Gen. 3:19). Human beings are material bodies animated by a life force (*nephesh* or *ruach*) residing in the breath or the blood. Death comes when the life force leaves the body and returns to Yahweh. Thus, a common fate awaits all persons upon death—master and slave, rich and poor, good and bad—all descend beneath the earth to the place of the dead called She'ol, where they continue a shadowy existence, but only for a brief period of time. This land of the dead was variously described as an awful pit shrouded in darkness or a walled city covered with dust. Although reminiscent of the Mesopotamian underworld, the Yahwist notion of She'ol excluded any divine

ruler of the infernal regions. Neither a god of the underworld nor Yahweh himself was involved with the
denizens of She'ol. Yahweh reigned supreme over the
community of the living, meting out collective rewards
and punishments only in the present life. In other
words, mortality was accepted as a fact of life. Premature
and violent deaths were feared as great evils and regarded as punishments for sin. As such, the untimely or
agonizing death remained under the control of Yahweh
(Isa. 45:7). But death at the end of a long and happy
life was accepted, if not welcomed (Gen. 25:8; Job
5:26). What mattered were those things which survived
the mortal individual: a good reputation (Prov. 10:7),
male offspring (Isa. 56:3–5), the promised land (Gen.
48:21), and the God of Israel (Ps. 90).

Precisely this emphasis on present existence contributed to the eventual transformation of Yahwism. The
naive assumption that Yahweh rewards the pious with
prosperity and a long life while punishing the wicked
with misfortune and a brief life was obviously contradicted by communal and individual experience. Especially the disasters that befell Israel between the eighth
and the sixth centuries B.C.E. raised radical doubts about
Yahweh's justice and omnipotence, because the entire
social and religious order of Israel was disrupted and
eventually destroyed.

This massive destruction evinced two distinctive
responses. On the one hand, most of the great prophets
of Israel responded to these dire circumstances by reaffirming collective retribution and promising collective
restoration (Isa. 11:10–16; Ezek. 36:16–36). Some
prophets moved beyond communal responsibility and
punishment (Jer. 21:3), but their new emphasis on the
individual only heightened the tension between divine
power and justice in the face of innocent suffering (Job
10:2–9). On the other hand, an apocalyptic school of
thought slowly emerged that anticipated a miraculous
deliverance of the faithful living and dead at the end of
time. Envisioned in this apocalyptic outlook was the final defeat of death itself, which had increasingly been
personified as a destructive evil force. Thus, by the end
of the second century B.C.E., two sharply contrasting
views of death dominated the Hebraic worldview. The
older notion that death marked the end of life remained
the traditional view among those who came to be known
as the Sadducees. The newer view that affirmed postmortem divine judgment and human resurrection flourished among such sectarian movements as the Pharisees
and the Essenes. For these sectarians, the powers of
death would eventually be overcome by the power of
God.

The intertestamental literature. This sectarian transformation of the Hebraic view of death during
the so-called intertestamental period was immense (ca.
200 B.C.E. to 50 C.E.). A number of disparate ideas were
combined into a dramatically new eschatology. The
Book of Daniel marked a watershed in Hebrew religious
thought by promising Yahweh's final intervention in history to rescue his people from their enemies and to res-
urrect past generations from the dead to participate in
this ultimate restoration. To be sure, this final restoration was limited to the nation of Israel. But, under the
impact of speculative thought and foreign influences
concerning life after death, the prospect of a final resurrection and judgment for all humankind appeared in
the later apocalyptic literature, much of which is contained in the Apocrypha. In this apocalyptic literature,
human consciousness and the life force were fused into
an entity (*psyche* or *pneuma*) which, unlike the earlier
conceptions of *nephesh* or *ruach*, survived the cessation
of bodily functions in some spiritual fashion. She'ol was
reconceived as a holding place for the dead until their
ultimate fate was decided at a final judgment. More significantly, She'ol was divided into compartments reflecting the moral character of the dead, wherein
rewards and punishments were already meted out in anticipation of the catastrophic end of the existing world
order (Enoch 22:9–14). Thus, death held no terror for
the righteous. In fact, death through martyrdom was
seen as a seal of divine favor (2 Macc. 6:30–31) and
even premature death from serious illness freed the righteous from further suffering (Wisd. of Sol. 4:11). Death
was only a threat and curse to the wicked. Reminiscent
of the older Yahwist traditions, the apocalyptic emphasis
remained largely on the collective aspects of human destiny, for it is the nations that are arraigned for the final
judgment (2 Ezd. 7:32–38). The postmortem survival of
the individual became an affirmation of faith within certain Jewish circles only following the shattering of the
Jewish state in 70 C.E.

The New Testament. Primitive Christianity
emerged out of Jewish apocalyptic expectations of the
catastrophic end of the existing world order and the final
judgment of the living and the dead. These apocalyptic
expectations had been joined in the popular imagination
with the older prophetic Messianic traditions in which
a divinely appointed and endowed figure would crush
the enemies and restore the glories of Israel. So far as
the New Testament Gospels allow for historical reconstruction, the message of Jesus centered in the nearness
of the Day of the Lord, when the chosen people of Yahweh would be vindicated before the nations of the
world. Jesus called his compatriots to prepare themselves
for the Coming Judgment through repentance and obedience to the written and oral Law of God. But, unlike
the earlier nationalistic preoccupations of Jewish apocalypticism, this newer eschatology emphasized the eternal destiny of individuals in accordance with their moral
achievements (Matt. 25:40–46). After his death and
resurrection, the followers of Jesus identified him as the

promised Messiah who would restore the righteous and judge the wicked. This same "Christianized" apocalyptic tradition informs the Revelation to John, which so profoundly influenced later Christian views of human death and destiny. Here the "end of the world" was described in elaborate detail as a cataclysmic establishment of the millennial reign of Christ and the saints on earth, after which the righteous are rewarded with eternal life and the wicked are punished with eternal death. Thus, the earliest Christian view of life after death was heavily influenced by, but not identical with, Jewish apocalypticism. Jesus was heralded by his early followers as their resurrected Lord who would shortly return in supernatural power and glory to preside over the Final Judgment of the living and the dead.

A somewhat different interpretation of the message and mission of Jesus was offered by Paul in his outreach to a Gentile audience. Paul regarded the death of Christ as a divinely planned event to rescue humankind from enslavement to the demonic powers of evil and death that ruled the world. Although influenced by apocalyptic thought, Paul's interpretation of a divine Savior's death and resurrection involved an eschatology very different from the apocalyptic scheme of things. No longer was obedience to the Twofold Law the basis on which the living and the dead would be judged; instead, faith in the crucified and risen Lord became the crucial factor. The ritual of baptism, which reenacted the death, burial, and resurrection of Christ, initiated believers into immortal life while still living in their material bodies. The baptized Christian, having become a new creation *in Christo*, had already passed from death to life. Thus, the imminent return of Christ and the end of the world held no fear for baptized believers, for their final judgment and destiny had already been settled.

With the Roman overthrow of the Jewish state in 70 c.e., the Mother Church of Jerusalem disappeared and eventually Pauline Christianity became the normative interpretation of Christ. Elements of the earlier apocalyptic eschatology were carried over into this form of faith. Christianity became a salvation religion centered in a Savior God who would shortly return to bring the existing world to a catastrophic end and to judge those who had oppressed the faithful. But the continuing delay of the second coming of Christ forced the Church to rethink its notions of eschatological fulfillment. The Church could no longer think of itself as an eschatological community awaiting the imminent return of their Lord. Rather, the Church developed a hierarchical structure and a sacramental system to shepherd believers through the perils and pitfalls of life from birth to death. Accordingly, Christ was reconceived as the heavenly mediator between God and humankind. Despite these doctrinal and ecclesiological developments, the apocalyptic vision of the catastrophic end of the

world was retained, raising anew all sorts of problems about the status of the dead before the final day of resurrection and judgment. Over time, these problems were resolved in ever more vivid and complicated schemes of postmortem paradisal bliss for the saints and purgatorial torment for the sinners until the day of Final Judgment (Luke 16:19–26).

Ethical implications.   As noted above, the Bible is a diverse literature containing a variety of religious perspectives on death. Religious affirmation of the triumph of life over death is a common theme running through the whole of scripture, but how, where, and when this victory is won differs dramatically among biblical perspectives. For that reason, the Bible offers no consensus of direct guidelines on death and dying. Nevertheless some application of the biblical tradition to modern "end of life" ethical issues can be ventured.

1. Biblical views of death are greatly influenced by the wider cultural milieu. As human conditions and needs changed, so did prevailing religious beliefs and practices concerning death. Thus, the Bible itself seems to allow for changing definitions and responses to death in the light of new social conditions, scientific knowledge, and religious insights.

2. The biblical tradition's intimate connection between body and spirit is not only a mandate for medical care as treatment of the whole person but also grounds for regarding human life as more than biological functioning. While the Bible does not authoritatively establish when death occurs, it defines death as the separation of the spirit from the body. Thereby, the Bible provides indirect warrants for withholding or withdrawing extraordinary means of life support when the vital bond between body and spirit has been dissolved or destroyed.

3. The biblical tradition never accords absolute power or independent status to death. Death, whether viewed as a natural event or an evil force, is always subordinated to the power and purposes of God. While the Bible speaks of sin as both a cause and a consequence of death, even the death of the sinner remains under divine control and serves the divine will. God's sovereignty over death serves as a caution against simplistic religious warrants for directly or indirectly terminating the lives of the suffering.

4. Biblical support can be found both for death as a natural part of life and death as an evil power opposed to life. Those who regard death as an "enemy" that must be battled at all costs will find more support for their view in the New Testament. Those who see death as a "friend" that can be welcomed at the end of life will feel more kinship with the Hebrew Bible. But both Jewish and Christian scriptures regard untimely and violent deaths as evils to be avoided and enemies to be combatted by all legitimate means that do not compromise re-

ligious or moral duties. Of course, death by coercive martyrdom can be affirmed as a seal of great faith, and even premature death from debilitating illness can be welcomed by the believer as a deliverance from great suffering.

5. Taken as a whole, the Bible does not unambiguously affirm individual life after death. But where postmortem existence is affirmed in the Bible, the grounds are theological rather than anthropological. The individual's survival beyond death is a divine possibility rather than a human certainty. Immortal life is a "supernatural" endowment rather than a "natural" attribute. In other words, a belief in life after death is neither a given of human nature nor a constant of human culture. Thus, the idea of life after death cannot become an explicit warrant for public policies or ethical decisions regarding "end of life" issues in a pluralistic society.

Death in systematic religious thought

The classical doctrines and rituals of Judaism and Christianity are no less complicated and diverse than their biblical backgrounds. Neither the Judaic nor the Christian tradition is monolithic. Both faiths have been developed over extended periods of time in response to changing historical circumstances and cultural influences. But these theological complexities can be simplified for purposes of comparing and contrasting their respective views of death. Just as there are elements of continuity and mutuality within the Hebrew Bible and the New Testament, so are there broad similarities between Judaism and Christianity in their traditional beliefs and practices regarding death.

Postbiblical Jewish beliefs and practices.   A long and slow transformation took place from the completion of the Hebrew Bible (ca. 200 B.C.E.) to the completion of the Talmud (ca. 500 C.E.), during which time biblical Hebraism emerged as rabbinic Judaism. The Talmud brought together eight hundred years of rabbinic commentary on scripture which was broadly categorized as *halakhah* (law) and *haggadah* (story), the former describing the obligations, the latter explaining the meaning of God's covenant with Israel. This massive compendium of rabbinic thought explicated the scripture's "moralization" of life and death in vast and vivid detail. For example, heaven (*Gan Eden*) and hell (*Gehinnom*) were each divided into five separate chambers, reflecting different levels of eternal rewards for the righteous and punishments for the wicked. Similarly, the rabbis described 903 forms of death. The hardest way of dying is by asthma and the easiest, which is reserved for the righteous, is "like drawing a hair from milk." Death following five days of illness was considered ordinary. Death after four days or less indicated increasing degrees of divine reprimand. Those who died before fifty were

"cut off," sixty years was "ripe age," and above seventy was "old age." Despite all this moralizing about death, comparatively few rabbis held that death as such was the wages of sin. Against those who taught that Adam's sin brought death into the world, the majority of rabbis taught that Adam's mortality was given with his creation. Death was an integral part of the good world that God created in the beginning. Thus, sin hastens death but does not cause it in the first place.

In other words, only the timing and manner of death are affected by moral conditions. Acts of benevolence and confessions of sins can delay the hour of death as surely as sins of impurity and injustice can speed it. But there is no avoiding death once the angel of death receives the order from God. Given God's permission to destroy, the angel of death makes no distinction between good and bad, but wields the sword against royalty and commoner, old and young, pious and pagan, animal and human alike. While both the wicked and the righteous must die, their deaths are as different as their lives. The wicked perish to pay for their sins while the righteous die to be freed from their sins. Death is a punishment for the sins of the wicked but an atonement for the sins of the righteous. Put another way, the righteous are still alive even though dead, while the wicked are already dead though still alive.

When death occurs, the soul leaves the body with a silent cry that echoes from one end of the world to the other. The soul's departure from the body is marked by the absence of breathing, heartbeat, and pulse. The slightest sign of movement is an indication that death has not yet occurred. Where the soul goes was a matter of considerable dispute among the rabbis. Some taught that the soul sleeps until the resurrection of the dead and the final judgment. Others believed that the soul passes into an interim state of consciousness and activity. But they all agreed that the body that remains must be treated with dignity and given a proper burial. Desecration of the body, such as mutilation or burial with missing body parts, is forbidden, and burial must be before nightfall if possible. Interment must be in the ground to fulfill the biblical mandate ("Dust you are and to dust you shall return") and to complete the atoning process ("May my death be an atonement for all my sins"). A speedy and simple burial also accorded with widespread popular beliefs that the soul is free to complete its journey to the other world only when the body has decomposed.

These beliefs about death were reflected in a number of customs and rituals surrounding the dying and mourning process. A dying person (*goses*) was given special consideration by loved ones who gave support and comfort during the last hours. The dying person was never to be left alone. Last wishes and spiritual advice were to be faithfully observed. When nearing the end, the dying were encouraged to make a confession such as the following: "I acknowledge unto Thee, O Lord my God, and God of my fathers, that both my cure and my death are in Thy hands. May it be Thy will to send me a perfect healing. Yet if my death be fully determined by Thee, I will in love accept it at Thy hand. O, may my death be an atonement for all my sins, iniquities, and transgressions of which I have been guilty against Thee." This confession was followed with the traditional Jewish affirmation of faith: "Hear, O Israel: The Lord is our God, the Lord is One" (Deut. 6:4).

When death had occurred, the eyes and mouth were closed by the eldest son or nearest relative. The arms were extended alongside the body, which was placed on the floor with the feet toward the door and covered by a sheet. A lighted candle was placed close to the head. Mirrors were turned to the wall or covered. Water in the death room was poured out, reflecting the ancient legend that the angel of death washes its bloody sword in nearby water. The windows of the death chamber were opened to allow the spirits to enter and depart. The dead body was never left alone, whether on weekdays or the Sabbath, until the funeral. Thus, the entire deathbed drama was structured to allow the dying to face the future realistically, yet within a reassuring framework of family and faith.

The theological and literary diversity of the talmudic period yielded two very different developments of the Jewish tradition during the Middle Ages (ca. 1100–1600). A mystical school emerged whose teachings concerning death and the afterlife went far beyond rabbinical Judaism. An emphasis on divine immanence and human transcendence lay at the heart of the *Kabbalah*, the most commonly used term for the esoteric teachings of medieval Judaism. Human life is the journey of the soul from God and back to God. During the interim period of life on earth and in the body, the soul must attain the "knowledge of the mysteries of the faith," which will purify and prepare it for its return to God. Since this esoteric knowledge is seldom learned in a single life, the soul transmigrates from one embodiment to another until all sins are purged and all duties fulfilled. In this mystical scheme of things, death is simply a threshold marking the passage from one life to another in the soul's ascent to God.

By contrast, a scholastic approach emerged, which codified talmudic beliefs and practices concerning death and dying. The greatest halakist of medieval Judaism was Rabbi Joseph Caro. His sixteenth-century work, *Shulhan Arukh*, became the authoritative code of Jewish law by synthesizing and reconciling the three giants of medieval *halakhah*—Isaac Alfasia, Moses Maimonides, and Asher B. Jehiel. Unlike Maimonides, who reinterpreted traditional Jewish teachings in Aristotelian terms, Caro did not subject Jewish law to speculative criticism. Rather,

he brought order out of chaos by investigating each stage of development of every single law, finally arriving at a decisive interpretation and application of that law. His work has remained the indispensable guide to the development and interpretation of Jewish laws and customs for two millennia. Included in *Shulhan Arukh* are the detailed halakic rites and duties surrounding death, burial, and mourning observed throughout Orthodox Jewry to this day.

In the modern period, a variety of reform movements have modified many traditional Jewish beliefs and practices concerning death. Orthodox Jews have for the most part remained loyal to rabbinic eschatology, with its emphasis on the final resurrection, but they diverge on whether the resurrection awaits all humankind, the righteous of every age, or only the Jewish people. These otherworldly notions of Messianic redemption and divine judgment have largely faded into the background for Conservative Jewish thinkers. They interpret the Messianic Hope historically in terms of the restoration of the nation of Israel, and spiritually in terms of the immortality of the soul. References to the resurrection of the dead in Jewish rituals of death, burial, and mourning are retained, but the language of resurrection is assimilated to teachings about the immortality of the soul.

Reform Judaism has gone even further in rejecting doctrines of bodily resurrection and the Messianic Age. The "Pittsburgh Platform" of Reformed Judaism (1885) excluded all bodily notions of heaven and hell as abodes for everlasting punishment and reward. Indeed, some liberal Jewish thinkers have rejected the idea of individual immortality entirely, though they affirm the lasting value of each human life within the everlasting life of God. These reformulations of Jewish belief have also produced liberalizations in the areas of Jewish death, burial, and mourning rites. Curiously enough, this turn away from the otherworld and afterlife has fueled a profound concern for the salvation of humankind in the full reality of their historical existence. Thus, many Reformed Jews have returned full cycle to the essentially "humanistic" outlook of the great prophets of ancient Israel.

Postbiblical Christian beliefs and practices. The traditional Christian understanding of death developed largely in response to two challenges facing the Church at the close of the first century. Internally, the delay of the second coming of Christ forced Christian thinkers to deal with the state of the soul between death and resurrection. For the most part, primitive Christians believed that the dead slept until the Last Day, at which time they would be resurrected from the grave to receive their everlasting rewards or punishments. But, as this period of time lengthened, questions about the interim between individual death and universal judgment became ever more pressing. Externally, the pervasive view of death in Hellenistic religion and philosophy called for some theological response. The Greeks believed that the immortal soul is released from its bodily entrapment by death. This understanding of death was so widespread that some Christian assimilation of the soul's immortality and the body's inferiority was inevitable. Taken together over time, the delay of the return of Christ and the appropriation of Greek ideas of immortality fostered an elaborate system of Christian beliefs and practices concerning the active life of the soul during the period between one's death and the general resurrection at the end of the age. In time, this new eschatology displaced the apocalyptic vision of the Last Days, which vision survived for the most part in millenarian or chiliastic sects, who looked forward to the return of Christ and the establishment of the Kingdom of God on earth.

The church fathers adopted many of the categories of Greek philosophy but retained most of the substance of Pauline Christianity. They affirmed the immortality of the soul but rejected the ultimate separability of soul and body, along with all Hellenistic notions of reincarnation and immediate judgment. The soul is the vivifying principle and as such is incomplete without a body. Indeed, had Adam and Eve not sinned, humankind never would have experienced death. But all must suffer the separation of soul and body in death as punishment for their sins. Their souls, however, cannot perish because they are immortal. Therefore, these souls must eventually be reunited with "the dust of bodies long dead" (Augustine) in order to receive their final inheritance of everlasting salvation or eternal damnation. Surprisingly, there was little speculation among the church fathers about this interim between individual death and general resurrection. Since the soul is immaterial during this period, the dead could experience no sense of place or time, no awareness of comfort or pain, until the resurrection.

Given its finality, death thus became a decisive moment in the soul's destiny. The hour of death sealed the fate of the saved and damned alike. Those who died with their sins forgiven were destined for heaven's bliss. Those who died "while yet in their sins" were condemned to hell's agony. This emphasis on penance in relation to God's mercy and judgment fueled the more elaborate view of heaven, hell, and purgatory that characterized medieval Christianity. The materials for that view were already available in the earlier periods, but an adequate conceptual framework was lacking. The notion of a fire that cleanses the righteous and consumes the wicked at the final resurrection belonged to the earliest biblical traditions. Pushing this purgation of sins back from the final judgment into the interim period after death was encouraged by pietistic and penitential practices. Prayers to the saints and masses for the dead whose sins require expiation implied an active existence for

souls following death and suggested a postmortem purgation of sins. But these implications were not fully worked out until the High Middle Ages (1200–1500).

Drawing on Aristotelian philosophy, Thomas Aquinas worked out an eschatology that combined an active spiritual afterlife with the traditional biblical notions of a general resurrection and last judgment. While the soul actualizes the body as its matter, it contains within itself to a degree all the perfections of physical and spiritual existence. Thus, the infliction of punishment or the bestowal of reward on the soul begins immediately after its separation from the body. But neither ultimate happiness nor ultimate misery is possible for a disembodied soul and, therefore, both must await the reunion of soul and body at the resurrection. Moreover, the soul that is ultimately rewarded must be entirely purified, either during or after this life. In other words, the existence of purgatory was a logical correlate of the immortal soul and the sacrament of penance, which requires contrition and satisfaction for all sins committed after baptism.

This thirteenth-century theological synthesis ineluctably shifted the emphasis to the individual's judgment at death rather than the universal judgment of humankind at the final resurrection of the dead. The Church's official view retained the two judgments, but in popular belief and practice they were in effect merged into one. People simply went to heaven, hell, or purgatory at the moment of death. Accordingly, the hour of death became overloaded with urgency. Dying in a state of grace meant eternal salvation, in a state of sin, eternal damnation, while dying with unconfessed sin required purgatorial cleansing. Thus, dying became more important than living. This focus on death was most obvious in the medieval *Ars moriendi* art of dying manuals that gave step-by-step advice to the dying and to the persons attending the dying to ensure a "good death." Of greater significance was the increasing importance of the sacrament of extreme unction, which was administered to the dying for all sins of sight, hearing, smell, speech, touch, and action. For those believers who died ill-prepared, there were masses for the dead and indulgences for the remission of sin for those in purgatory. In other words, a whole arsenal of beliefs and practices were mobilized against the terror of dying outside the state of grace.

What was developed in the thirteenth century as gifts of divine grace became in the fourteenth and fifteenth century marks of human folly. Or so the Protestant reformers claimed. Abuses surrounding the sacraments and indulgences for the dying were rife in the late medieval Church. These abuses were a precipitating cause of the sixteenth-century reform movements that swept both church and society. In point of fact, neither Luther nor Calvin broke with the fundamental worldview of medieval Christianity. Both challenged current beliefs and practices from within the medieval tradition. Thus, with regard to eschatology, the reformers retained the concept of the soul's immortality and eternal destiny. But they both undercut the entire penitential system with a different understanding of divine mercy and justice. The blood of Christ is the sole satisfaction for the sins of believers. Thus, medieval notions of a purgatorial state and a treasury of merits fell to the ground because these practices compromised the sole ground of salvation in Christ through faith. What remained for the reformers was an affirmation of the imperishable soul, which immediately enters its eternal reward or punishment upon separation from the body in death. The older idea of a general resurrection and judgment at the End of the Age was retained, but this last state of the soul only ratifies and perfects the fate of the saved and the damned at death.

In the modern world, mainline Catholic theologians have for the most part remained faithful to the position of Thomas Aquinas. The lurid images and frantic piety surrounding death and the afterlife in the Middle Ages have long since been rejected by educated Catholics. But the devout Catholic can still face the enemy of death armed with the traditional sacramental graces and doctrinal truths of life everlasting. To be sure, some contemporary Catholic theologians interpret these traditional beliefs and practices in symbolic rather than literal terms. For them, the experience of death is viewed as pilgrimage in faith rather than punishment for sin. Death is seen as "the law of human growth," whereby each stage of growth requires a tearing away from previous environments, which have become like so many prisons. In death, one's own body, like the mother's body at birth, is abandoned so that personal growth may continue. Alternatively, death allows the soul to enter into a new all-embracing unity. At death the soul is freed from the limitation of being related to one particular human body and becomes related to the whole universe. The pouring out of the self at death leads to a pan-cosmic level of personal and communal existence. But for the most part, contemporary Roman Catholics simply "look forward to the resurrection of the dead and the life of the world to come," in the words of the Nicene Creed.

Modern Protestant theologians have been even more innovative than their Catholic counterparts. To be sure, mainline Protestants have followed the guidelines laid down by the Reformers. They have combined an emphasis on postmortem rewards and punishments for the soul at death with some notion or another of a Final Consummation of the Age. But a growing freedom from ecclesiastical authority and biblical literalism allowed for a wide range of Protestant theological innovations. These new theologies were usually developed in response to the challenges of modern science and in partnership with one or another modern philosophy. Beginning in the eighteenth century, the Christian faith was interpreted within such diverse philosophical frameworks as rationalism, romanticism, empiricism, existentialism, and process thought. Not surprisingly, each philosophical theology has dealt with the problem of death and the afterlife in its own distinctive way. These liberal theological experiments share certain convictions about life after death. They reject apocalyptic schemes of history and literalistic views of the afterlife. They empty the afterlife of all ideas of eternal torment, preferring instead to speak of either the total annihilation or eventual salvation of the wicked. But their concrete notions of eternal life run the gamut from the soul's immaterial existence in heaven to the self's authentic existence while on earth. Despite these wide-ranging theological reflections on death, most present-day Protestants hold to the idea of death as the soul's passage to its immortal destiny, either in eternal communion with or eternal separation from God and the people of God.

Ethical implications. The long histories of Judaism and Christianity reveal disagreements within as well as differences between these religious traditions. And yet there are striking parallels between the ways they deal with death over the centuries. Of course, both traditions come out of the same Hebraic background and confront the same broad cultural challenges. But of greater importance is the fact that both traditions are preoccupied with the issue of theodicy. There must be some ultimate justification of the brute fact that the righteous suffer and die along with the wicked. The stubbornly moral character of the Judaic and Christian traditions militates against either indiscriminate immortality or universal annihilation. Thus, for all their differences, Judaism and Christianity are bound together by their efforts to reconcile ethics and eschatology. Not surprisingly, Judaism and Christianity respond in similar ways to a number of "end of life" ethical issues.

1. For the most part, Judaism and Christianity traditionally define death as the moment the spirit leaves the body. The accepted signs of the spirit's departure are the absence of breathing, heartbeat, and pulse. But there is nothing in these theological traditions that directly rules out more precise empirical signs of death, such as a flat brain wave. Most Christian theologians, and many Jewish thinkers, have accepted a brain-oriented definition of death, but some, especially within Orthodox Judaism, oppose such a definition, focusing instead on breathing as the definitive indicator of life. Some contemporary theologians are openly embracing higher-brain oriented definitions of death as modern equivalents of the departure of the spirit from the body.

2. Regardless of the etiology of death, the Jewish and Christian traditions regard death as an evil to be endured rather than a good to be embraced. Though

death is inevitable, it is an event to be held at bay by every possible and honorable means that is not excessively burdensome or morally ambiguous. Therefore, most traditional Jews and Christians are categorically opposed to suicide and active euthanasia, or "mercy killing." Since martyrdom is not considered suicide, choosing death over life in service to one's faith or for the sake of others is allowable if it cannot be avoided in an honorable way.

3. Although all must die, not all deaths are the same in the Jewish and Christian traditions. Clearly, there are better and worse ways of dying. The best of deaths is the death of a person at peace with God who is "full of years," relatively free of pain, and surrounded by loved ones. The worst of deaths is to die "before your time," in rebellion against God, and alienated from family and friends. Recognition of these different ways of dying lends at least indirect religious sanctions to modern-day concerns about the "good death." There are no clear-cut religious obligations to prolong the dying process by extraordinarily burdensome means of life support. Indeed, the moral permissibility of withholding or withdrawing heroic means of life support from the terminally ill enjoys wide support among contemporary Jews and Christians alike, even though some Jewish scholars, particularly among the Orthodox, prefer to provide support, whenever possible, until the patient is moribund.

4. For both Jews and Christians, death is a reality that cannot be ignored or wished away. Whether death comes slowly or suddenly, the worst time to deal with death is after it happens. Believers should be prepared to deal with the heartache and havoc it brings before illness or tragedy strikes. We are ready to live only when we are prepared to die. While such preparation need not require the cultivated preoccupation with death of the medieval *Ars moriendi*, it should include a recognition of human mortality and an acceptance of human limits. In principle, such preparation might include the execution of advanced directives regarding terminal care.

5. Although the soul is infinitely more valuable than the body, the bodies of the dead deserve to be treated with care and love. For traditional Jews, such respect for the human body ordinarily excludes mutilation of the body, although sanctions against autopsies and dissection may yield to the superior value of protecting life or punishing crime. Some contemporary Jewish thinkers extend this overriding obligation to preserve life to the justification of organ harvesting for transplantation. Despite centuries of theological opposition, traditional Christians have reconciled themselves to the legitimacy of anatomical dissection and organ harvesting in the interests of science and medicine, perhaps reflecting the Christian view that the resurrected body is a new creation of God. But more liberal Jews and Christians are untroubled by any of these postmortem procedures,

provided they do not disgrace the corpse or disturb the family.

6. Both the Jewish and Christian emphasis on death is, in reality, the obverse of an even greater emphasis on life. At best, death serves as a motive for a creative and responsible life. At worst, death looms as a menace to a courageous and generous life. Either way, death lends an urgency to life that would be utterly lacking without it. Death enhances rather than cheapens the value of life.

7. For both Jews and Christians, there is hope that death does not have the final word in human experience. For many, death is a corridor that leads to a life free of sorrow, suffering, and separation. For others, death is powerless to cut off the faithful from the life of the community and the life of God. On either reckoning, death is incorporated as a meaningful stage in the life cycle. Both the Jewish and Christian traditions, strengthened by centuries of suffering and surviving, provide a variety of ways of affirming life in the face of death.

LONNIE D. KLIEVER

Directly related to this article are the other articles in this entry: ANTHROPOLOGICAL PERSPECTIVES, EASTERN THOUGHT, WESTERN PHILOSOPHICAL THOUGHT, *and* DEATH IN THE WESTERN WORLD (*with its* POSTSCRIPT). *Also directly related are the entries* DEATH: ART OF DYING; DEATH AND DYING: EUTHANASIA AND SUSTAINING LIFE; DEATH, ATTITUDES TOWARD; DEATH, DEFINITION AND DETERMINATION OF; JUDAISM; ROMAN CATHOLICISM; PROTESTANTISM; *and* EASTERN ORTHODOX CHRISTIANITY. *For a discussion of related ideas, see the entries* HARM; HEALTH AND DISEASE, *article on* HISTORY OF THE CONCEPTS; PERSON; SUICIDE; *and* TRAGEDY. *Other relevant material may be found under the entries* HOSPITAL, *article on* MEDIEVAL AND RENAISSANCE HISTORY; *and* MEDICAL ETHICS, HISTORY OF, *section on* EUROPE, *subsections on* ANCIENT AND MEDIEVAL, *and* RENAISSANCE AND ENLIGHTENMENT.

Bibliography

Biblical thought

BAILEY, LLOYD R., SR. 1979. *Biblical Perspectives on Death.* Philadelphia: Fortress Press.

BRANDON, SAMUEL GEORGE FREDERICK. 1967. *The Judgment of the Dead: An Historical and Comparative Study of the Idea of a Post-Mortem Judgment in the Major Religions.* London: Weidenfeld and Nicolson.

BRUEGGEMAN, WALTER. 1976. "Death, Theology of." In *The Interpreter's Dictionary of the Bible: An Illustrated Encyclopedia, Supplementary Volume,* pp. 219–222. Edited by Keith Crim, Lloyd R. Bailey, Sr., Victor P. Furnish, and Emory S. Bucke. Nashville, Tenn.: Abingdon.

CHARLES ROBERT HENRY. 1963. *Eschatology: A Doctrine of a Future Life in Israel, Judaism, and Christianity: A Critical History.* New York: Schocken.

JACOB, EDMOND. 1962a. "Death." In vol. 1 of *The Interpreter's Dictionary of the Bible: An Illustrated Encyclopedia,* pp. 802–804. Edited by George Arthur Buttrick, Thomas S. Kepler, John Knox, Herbert G. May, Samuel Terrien, and Emory S. Bucke. Nashville, Tenn.: Abingdon.

———. 1962b. "Immortality." In vol. 2 of *The Interpreter's Dictionary of the Bible: An Illustrated Encyclopedia,* pp. 688–690. Edited by George Arthur Buttrick, Thomas S. Kepler, John Knox, Herbert G. May, Samuel Terrien, and Emory S. Bucke. Nashville, Tenn.: Abingdon.

KAISER, OTTO, and LOHSE, EDUARD. 1981. *Death and Life.* Translated by John E. Seely. Nashville, Tenn.: Abingdon.

KECK, LEANDER E. 1969. "New Testament Views of Death." *Perspectives on Death,* pp. 33–98. Edited by Liston O. Mills. Nashville, Tenn.: Abingdon.

SILBERMAN, LOU H. 1969. "Death in the Hebrew Bible and Apocalyptic Literature." *Perspectives on Death,* pp. 13–32. Edited by Liston O. Mills. Nashville, Tenn.: Abingdon.

Postbiblical Judaism

GORDON, AUDREY. 1975. "The Jewish View of Death: Guidelines for Mourning." In *Death: The Final Stage of Growth,* pp. 44–51. Edited by Elisabeth Kübler-Ross. Englewood Cliffs, N.J.: Prentice-Hall.

HELLER, ZACHARY I. 1975. "The Jewish View of Death: Guidelines for Dying." In *Death: The Final Stage of Growth,* pp. 38–43. Edited by Elisabeth Kübler-Ross. Englewood Cliffs, N.J.: Prentice-Hall.

JAKOBOVITS, IMMANUEL. 1959. *Jewish Medical Ethics: A Comparative and Historical Study of the Jewish Religious Attitude to Medicine and Its Practice.* New York: Bloch.

KAYSER, RUDOLF. 1972. "Death." In vol. 5 of *Encyclopaedia Judaica,* pp. 1419–1427. New York: Macmillan.

KOHLER, KAUFMANN. 1964. "Death, Angel of." In vol. 4 of *The Jewish Encyclopedia,* pp. 480–482. Edited by Cyrus Adler and Isidore Singer. New York: Ktav.

KOHLER, KAUFMANN, AND EINSTEIN, J. D. 1964. "Death, Views and Customs Concerning." In vol. 4 of *The Jewish Encyclopedia,* pp. 482–486. Edited by Cyrus Adler and Isidore Singer. New York: Ktav.

LAMM, MAURICE. 1969. *The Jewish Way in Death and Mourning.* New York: J. David.

RIEMER, JACK, ed. 1974. *Jewish Reflections on Death.* New York: Schocken.

SCHOLEM, GERSHOM. 1972. "Kabbalah." In vol. 10 of *Encyclopaedia Judaica,* pp. 490–654. New York: Macmillan.

WEISS, ABNER. 1991. *Death and Bereavement: A Halakhic Guide.* Hoboken, N.J.: Ktav.

Postbiblical Christian thought

BADHAM, PAUL. 1987. "The Christian Hope Today." *Death and Immortality in the Religions of the World,* pp. 37–50. Edited by Paul Badham and Linda Badham. New York: Paragon House.

GATCH, MILTON McCORMICK. 1969. *Death: Meaning and Mortality in Christian Thought and Contemporary Culture.* New York: Seabury.

HICK, JOHN. 1976. *Death and Eternal Life.* New York: Harper & Row.

McGOWN, THOMAS. 1987. "Eschatology in Recent Catholic Thought." *Death and Immortality in the Religions of the World,* pp. 51–70. Edited by Paul Badham and Linda Badham. New York: Paragon House.

MILLER-McLEMORE, BONNIE J. 1988. *Death, Sin and the Moral Life: Contemporary Cultural Interpretations of Death.* Atlanta, Ga.: Scholars Press.

Comparative studies

ARIES, PHILIPPE. 1974. *Western Attitudes Toward Death: From the Middle Ages to the Present.* Translated by Patricia M. Ranum. Baltimore: Johns Hopkins University Press.

CHORON, JACQUES. 1963. *Death and Western Thought.* New York: Macmillan.

ECKARDT, A. ROY. 1972. "Death in the Judaic and Christian Traditions." *Social Research* 39, no. 3:489–514.

HOCKEY, JENNIFER LORNA. 1990. *Experiences of Death: An Anthropological Account.* Edinburgh: University Press.

STANNARD, DAVID E., ed. 1975. *Death in America.* Philadelphia: University of Pennsylvania Press.

STEPHENSON, JOHN S. 1985. *Death, Grief, and Mourning: Individual and Social Realities.* New York: Free Press.

V. DEATH IN THE WESTERN WORLD

This article, by the late Talcott Parsons, is reprinted from the first edition. It is followed immediately by a Postscript, prepared by Victor Lidz for purposes of updating the original article.

That the death of every known human individual has been one of the central facts of life so long as there has been any human awareness of the human condition does not mean that, being so well known, it is not problematical. On the contrary, like history, it has needed to be redefined and newly analyzed, virtually with every generation. However, as has also been the case with history, with the advancement of knowledge later reinterpretations may have some advantages over earlier ones.

Some conceptualization, beyond common sense, of a human individual or "person" is necessary in order to understand the set of problems presented by death. Therefore, a few comments on this topic are in order before proceeding to a reflection on some of the more salient features of death as it has been understood in the Western world.

The person and the problematic of death

The human individual has often been viewed in the Western world as a synthesized combination of a living organism and a "personality system" (an older terminology made the person a combination of "body" and "mind" or "soul"). It is in fact no more mystical to conceive of a personality analytically distinct from an organism than it is to conceive of a "culture" distinct from the human populations of organisms who are its bearers. The primary criterion of personality, as distinct from organism, is an organization in terms of symbols and their meaningful relations to each other and to persons.

Human individuals, in their organic aspect, come into being through a process of bisexual reproduction. They then go through a more or less well-defined "life course" and eventually die. That human individuals die as organisms is indisputable. If any biological proposition can be regarded as firmly established, it is that the mortality of individual organisms of a sexually reproducing species is completely normal. The death of individuals has a positive survival value for the species.

As Sigmund Freud said, organic death, while a many-faceted thing, is in one principal aspect the "return to the inorganic state." At this level the human organism is "made up" of inorganic materials but is organized in quite special ways. When that organization breaks down—and there is evidence that this is inevitable by reason of the aging process—the constituent elements are no longer part of the living organism but come to be assimilated to the inorganic environment. Still, even within such a perspective on the human individual as an organism, life goes on. The human individual does not stand alone but is part of an intergenerational chain of indefinite durability, the species. The individual organism dies, but if he or she reproduces, the line continues into future generations.

But the problematic of human death arises from the fact that the human individual is not only an organism but also a user of symbols who learns symbolic meanings, communicates with others and with himself or herself through them as media, and regulates his or her behavior, thought, and feelings in symbolic terms. The individual is an "actor" or a "personality." The human actor clearly is not born in the same sense in which an organism is. The personality or actor comes into being through a gradual and complicated process sometimes termed "socialization."

Furthermore, there is a parallel—in my judgment, something more than a mere analogy—between the continuity of the actor and that of the organism. Just as there is an intergenerational continuity on the organic side, so is there an intergenerational continuity on the personality or action side of the human individual. An individual personality is generated in symbiosis with a growing individual organism and, for all we know, dies with that organism. But the individual personality is embedded in transindividual action systems, both social and cultural. Thus the sociocultural matrix in which the individual personality is embedded is in an important

sense the counterpart of the population-species matrix in which the individual organism is embedded. The individual personality dies, but the society and cultural system, of which in life he or she was a part, goes on.

But what happens when the personality dies? Is the death of a personality to be simply assimilated to the organic paradigm? It would seem that the answer is yes, for just as no personality in the human sense can be conceived as such to develop independently of a living organism, so no human personality can be conceived as such to survive the death of the same organism. Nevertheless, the personality or actor certainly influences what happens in the organism—as suicide and all sorts of psychic factors in illnesses and deaths bear witness. Thus, although most positivists and materialists would affirm that the death of the personality must be viewed strictly according to the organic paradigm, this answer to the problem of human death has not been accepted by the majority in most human societies and cultures. From such primitive peoples as the Australian aborigines to the most sophisticated of the world religions, beliefs in the existence of an individual "soul" have persisted, conceivably with a capacity both to antedate and to survive the individual organism or body. The persistence of that belief and the factors giving rise to it provide the framework for the problematic of death in the Western world.

Christian orientations toward death

Because the dominant religious influence in this history of the Western world has been that of Christianity, it is appropriate to outline the main Christian patterns of orientation toward death.

There is no doubt of the predominance of a duality of levels in the Christian paradigm of the human condition, the levels of the spiritual and the material, the eternal and the temporal. On the one hand, there is the material-temporal world, of which one religious symbol is the "dust" to which humankind is said to return at death. On the other hand, there is the spiritual world of "eternal life," which is the location of things divine, not human. The human person stands at the meeting of the two worlds, for he or she is, like the animals, made of "dust," but is also, unlike the animals, made in the image of God. This biblical notion of humanity, when linked to Greek philosophical thought, gave rise to the idea in Catholic Christianity that the divine image was centered in the human soul, which was conceived as in some sense an emanation from the spiritual world of eternal life. Thus arose the notion of the "immortal soul," which could survive the death of the organism, to be rejoined to a resurrected body. The hope of the resurrection, rooted in the Easter faith of the Christian community, was from the beginning a part of the Christian faith and provided another dimension behind the teaching on the immortality of the soul.

The Christian understanding of death as an event in which "life is changed, not taken away," in the words of the traditional requiem hymn, *Dies irae*, can be interpreted in terms of Marcel Mauss's paradigm of the gift and its reciprocation (Parsons et al., 1972). Seen in this way, the life of the individual is a gift from God, and like other gifts it creates expectations of reciprocation. Living "in the faith" is part of the reciprocation, but, more important to us, dying in the faith completes the cycle. The language of giving also permeates the transcendental level of symbolism in the Christian context. Thus, Mary, like any other woman, *gave* birth to Jesus, God also *gave* his only begotten Son for the redemption of humankind. Finally, Jesus, in the Crucifixion and thus the Eucharist, *gave* his blood for the same purpose. By the doctrine of reciprocation humankind assumes, it may be said, three principal obligations: to accept the human condition as ordained by the Divine Will, to live in the faith, and to die in the faith (with the hope of resurrection). If these conditions are fulfilled, "salvation," life eternal with God, will come about.

This basically was the paradigm of death in Catholic Christianity. Although the Reformation did collapse some elements in the Catholic paradigm of dualism between the eternal and the temporal, it did not fundamentally alter the meaning of death in societies shaped by the Christian faith. Still, the collapse of the Catholic paradigm did put great pressures on the received doctrine of salvation. The promise of a personal afterlife in heaven, especially if this were conceived to be eternal—which must be taken to mean altogether outside the framework of time—became increasingly difficult to accept. The doctrine of eternal punishment in some kind of hell has proved even more difficult to uphold.

The primary consequence of this collapsing was not, as it has often been interpreted, so much the secularization of the religious component of society as it was the sacralization of secular society, making it the forum for the religious life—notably, though by no means exclusively, through work in a "calling" (as Max Weber held).

Though John Calvin, in his doctrine of predestination, attempted to remove salvation from human control, his doctrine could not survive the cooling of the effervescence of the Reformation. Thus, all later versions of Protestantism accepted some version of the bearing of the individual's moral or attitudinal (faith) merit on salvation. Such control as there was, however, was no longer vested in an ecclesiastical organization but was left to the individual, thus immensely increasing religious and moral responsibility.

The concept of a higher level of reality, a supernatural world in which human persons survived after death,

did not give way but became more and more difficult to visualize by simple extrapolation from this-worldly experience; the same problem occurred with the meaning of death as an event in which one gave life back to its Giver and in return was initiated into a new and eternal life. In addition to the changes in conceptualization set in motion by the Reformation, the rise of modern science, which by the eighteenth century had produced a philosophy of scientific materialism, posed an additional challenge to the Christian paradigm of death, manifesting itself primarily in a monism of the physical world. There was at that time little scientific analysis of the world of action, and there was accordingly a tendency to regard the physical universe as unchanging and hence eternal. Death, then, was simply the return to the inorganic state, which implied a complete negation of the conception of eternal life, since the physical, inorganic world was by definition the antithesis of life in any sense.

Contemporary scientific orientations

The subsequent development of science has modified, or at least brought into question, the monistic and materialistic paradigm generated by the early enthusiasm for a purely positivistic approach. For one thing, beginning in the nineteenth century and continuing into the twentieth, the sciences of organic life have matured, thanks largely to placing the conception of evolutionary change at the very center of biological thought. This resulted in the view, which we have already noted, that death is biologically normal for individual members of evolving species.

A second and more recent development has been the maturing of the sciences of action. Although these have historical roots in the humanistic tradition, they have only recently been differentiated from the humanistic trunk to become generalizing sciences, integrating within themselves the same conception of evolutionary change that has become the hallmark of the sciences of life.

The development of the action sciences has given rise, as already noted, to a viable conception of the human person as analytically distinct from the organism. At the same time these sciences, by inserting the person into an evolutionary sociocultural matrix analogous to the physico-organic species matrix within which the individual organism is embedded, have been able to create an intellectual framework within which the death of the personality can be understood to be as normal as the death of the organism.

Finally, the concept of evolutionary change has been extended from the life sciences (concerned with the organism) and the action sciences (concerned with the person-actor) to include the whole of empirical reality. And at the same time we have been made aware—principally by the ways in which Einstein's theory of relativity modified the previous assumptions of the absolute empirical "givenness" of physical nature in the Newtonian tradition—of the relative character of our human understanding of the human condition.

Thus there is now a serious questioning of absolutes, both in our search for absolutely universal laws of physical nature and in our quest for metaphysical absolutes in the philosophical wake of Christian theology.

The Kantian impact and the limits of understanding

The developments in a contemporary scientific understanding of the human condition are both congruent with, and in part anticipated and influenced by, Immanuel Kant, whose work during the late eighteenth century was the decisive turning point away from both physical and metaphysical absolutism. Kant basically accepted the reality of the physical universe, as it is humanly known, but at the same time he relativized our knowledge of it to the categories of the understanding, which were not grounded in our direct experience of physical reality but in something transcending this. At the same time Kant equally relativized our conceptions of transcendental reality, whose existence he by no means denied, to something closer to the human condition. Indeed, it may be suggested that Kant substituted procedural conceptions of the absolute, whether physical or metaphysical, for substantive propositions.

While relativizing our knowledge both of the physical world, including the individual human organism, and of the metaphysical world, with its certitude about the immortality of the soul, Kant nonetheless insisted on a transcendental component in human understanding and explicitly included belief in personal immortality in the sense of eternal life.

With respect to the bearing of Kant's thought and its influence through subsequent culture on the problem of the meaning of death, I have already noted that he prepared the way, procedurally, for the development of the action sciences and their ability to account intellectually for the personality or actor experienced as one aspect of the human individual without the need to infer, of necessity, the existence of a spiritual soul existentially and not merely analytically distinct from the living organism. The action sciences, in a very real sense, attempt to provide a coherent account of human subjectivity, much as Kant attempted to do in his *Critique of Judgment,* without collapsing the difference of levels between the physical and what may be called the telic realm.

The framework provided by Kant's thought is indeed congenial to the scientific perspective on the normality of the death of a person, conceived as an actor whose coming into existence is in symbiosis with a growing individual organism and whose individual personality, while continuing into a new generation in the same sociocultural system, can be understood to die in symbiosis with the same organism. Nonetheless, if Kant was right in refusing to collapse the boundaries of the human condition into the one vis-à-vis the physical world, the meaning of human individual death can no more be exhausted by that of the involvement of the human individual in a sociocultural system of more comprehensive temporal duration than can the meaning of our sensory experience of empirical reality be exhausted by the impressions emanating from that external world, or even the theoretical ordering of those impressions.

If Kant's fundamental position is accepted, then his skepticism about absolutes must apply to both sides of the fundamental dichotomy. Modern biology certainly must be classed as knowledge of the empirical world in his sense, and the same is true of our scientific knowledge of human action. In his famous terminology, there is no demonstrable knowledge of the thing in itself in any scientific field.

In empirical terms organic death is completely normal. We have, and according to Kant we presumably can have, no knowledge of the survival of any organic entity after death, except through the processes of organic reproduction that enable the genetic heritage to survive. Kant, however, would equally deny that such survival can be excluded on empirical grounds. This has an obvious bearing on the Christian doctrine of the resurrection of the body. If that is meant in a literal biological sense (though this is by no means universally the way in which Christians understand it), then the inference is clearly that it can never be proved, but it can still be speculated about and can be a matter of faith, even though it cannot be the object of either philosophical or scientific demonstration.

The same seems to hold for the personality-action component of the human individual. Empirically, the action sciences can account for its coming-to-be and its demise without postulating its survival. But they cannot exclude the possibility of such survival. Thus the eternal life of the individual soul, although metaphysically unknowable, can, like resurrected bodies, be speculated about and believed in as a matter of faith.

Thus, included in the victims of Kant's skepticism or relativization is belief in the cognitive necessity of belief in the survival of human individuality after death as well as belief in the cognitive necessity of belief in the nonsurvival of human individuality after death. Kant's relativization of our knowledge, both empirical and metaphysical, both closed and opened doors. It did, of course, undermine the traditional specificities of received beliefs; but at the same time, and for the very same reason, it opened the door, by contrast to scientific materialism, not merely to one alternative to received Christian belief but to a multiplicity of them.

This leaves us with the position that the problem of the meaning of death in the Western tradition has, from a position of relative closure defined by the Christian syndrome, been "opened up" in its recent phase. There is above all a new freedom for individuals and sociocultural movements to try their hands at innovative definitions and conceptions. At the same time, the viability of their innovations is subject to the constraints of the human condition, both empirical and transcendental, noted by Kant.

The grounding of this door-opening process lies in Kant's conception of freedom as the central feature of what he called "practical reason." In essence, the human will, as he called it, can no more be bound by a set of metaphysical dogmas than a person's active intellect can be bound by alleged inherent necessities of the empirical, relevant *Ding an sich*. This doctrine of freedom, among other things, opens the door to Western receptivity to other, notably Oriental, religious traditions. Thus, Buddhist tradition, on the whole by contrast with Christian, stresses not individuality except for this terrestrial life but, rather, the desirability of absorption, after death, into an impersonal, eternal matrix (as opposed to a personal eternal life). The recent vogue of Oriental religion in Western circles suggests that this possibility has become meaningful in the West.

The problem of the meaning of death in the West is now in what must appear to many to be a strangely unsatisfactory state. It seems to come down to the proposition that the meaning of death is that, in the human condition, it cannot have any "apodictically certain" meaning without abridgment of the essential human freedom of thought, experience, and imagination. Within limits, its meaning, as it is thought about, experienced for the case of others, and anticipated for oneself, must be autonomously interpreted. But this is not pure negativism or nihilism, because such openness is not the same as declaring death, and of course with it individual life, to be meaningless.

Conclusion

So far as Western society is concerned, I think the tolerability of this relatively open definition of the situation is associated with the activistic strain in our values, the attitude that human life is a challenging undertaking that in some respects may be treated as an adventure— by contrast with a view that treats human life as a matter of passively enduring an externally imposed fate. Even though Western religion has sometimes stressed humanity's extreme dependency on God, and indeed the sinfulness of asserting independence, on the whole the activistic strain has been dominant. If this is the case, it seems that humans can face their deaths and those of others in the spirit that whatever this unknown future may portend, they can enter upon it with good courage.

Insofar as it is accessible to cognitive understanding at all, the problem of the meaning of death for individual human beings must be approached in the framework of the human condition as a whole. It must include both the relevant scientific understanding and understanding at philosophical levels, and must attempt to synthesize them. Finally it must, as clearly as possible, recognize and take account of the limits of both our scientific and our philosophical understanding.

We have contended that the development of modern science has so changed the picture as to require revision of many of the received features of Christian tradition, both Catholic and Protestant. This emergence of science took place in three great stages marked by the synthesis of physical science in the seventeenth century, that of biological science in the nineteenth, and that of the action sciences in the nineteenth to twentieth.

The most important generalizations seem to be the following. First, the human individual constitutes a unique symbiotic synthesis of two main components, a living organism and a living personality. Second, both components seem to be inherently limited in duration of life, and we have no knowledge that indicates their symbiosis can be in any radical sense dissociated. Third, the individualized entity is embedded in, and derives in some sense from, a transgenerational matrix that, seen in relation to individual mortality, has indefinite but not infinite durability.

From this point of view, death, or the limited temporal duration of the individual life course, must be regarded as one of the facts of life that is as inexorable as the need to eat and breathe in order to live. In this sense, death is completely normal, to the point that its denial must be regarded as pathological. Moreover, this normality includes the consideration that, from an evolutionary point of view, which we have contended is basic to all modern science, death must be regarded as having high survival value, organically at least to the species, actionwise to the future of the sociocultural system. These scientific considerations are not trivial, or conventional, or culture-bound but are fundamental.

There is a parallel set of considerations on the philosophical side. For purposes of elucidating this aspect of the problem complex, I have used Kant's framework as presented in his three critiques. On the one hand, this orientation is critical in that it challenges the contention that absolute knowledge is demonstrable in any of the three aspects of human condition. Thus, any conception like that of the ontological essence of nature, the idea of God, or the notion of the eternal life of the human soul is categorized as *Ding an sich*, which in principle is not demonstrable by rational cognitive procedures.

At the same time, Kant insisted, and I follow him here, on the cognitive necessity of assuming a transcendental component, a set of categories in each of the three realms, that is not reducible to the status of humanly available inputs from either the empirical or the absolute telic references of the human condition. We have interpreted this to mean that human orientation must be relativized to the human condition, not treated as dogmatically fixed in the nature of things.

The consequence of this relativization that we have particularly emphasized is that it creates a new openness for orientations, which humans are free to exploit by speculation and to commit themselves in faith, but with reference to which they cannot claim what Kant called apodictic certainty.

If the account provided in the preceding sections is a correct appraisal of the situation in the Western world today, it is not surprising that there is a great deal of bafflement, anxiety, and downright confusion in contemporary attitudes and opinions in this area. Any consensus about the meaning of death in the Western world today seems far off, although the attitude reflected in this article would seem to be the one most firmly established at philosophical levels and the level of rather abstract scientific theory.

A very brief discussion of three empirical points may help to mitigate the impression of extreme abstractness. First, though scientific evidence has established the fact of the inevitability of death with increasing clarity, this does not mean that the experience of death by human populations may not change with changing circumstances. Thus, we may distinguish between inevitable death and "adventitious" death, that is, deaths that are premature relative to the full life span, and in principle preventable by human action (Parsons and Lidz, 1967). Since about 1840, this latter category of deaths has decreased enormously. The proportion of persons in modern populations over sixty-five has thus increased greatly, as has the expectancy of life at birth. This clearly means that a greatly increased proportion of modern humans approximate to living out a full life course, rather than dying prematurely. Individuals living to "a ripe old age" will have experienced an inevitably larger number of deaths of persons who were important to them. These will be in decreasing number the deaths of persons younger than themselves, notably their own children, and increasingly deaths of their parents and whole ranges of persons of an older generation, such as teachers, senior occupational associates, and many public figures. Quite clearly these demographic changes will have a strong effect on the balance of experience and expectations, of the deaths of significant others, and of anticipation of one's own death.

Second, one of the centrally important aspects of a

process of change in orientation of the sort described should be the appearance of signs of the differentiation of attitudes and conceptions with regard to the meaning of the life cycle. There has already been such a process of differentiation, apparently not yet completed, with respect to both ends of the life cycle (Parsons et al., 1972). With respect to the beginning, of course, this centers on the controversy over the legitimacy of abortion and the beginning of life. And concomitant with this controversy has been an attempt at redefinition of death. So far the most important movement has been to draw a line within the organic sector between what has been called brain death, where irreversible changes have taken place, destroying the functioning of the central nervous system, and what has been called metabolic death, where, above all, the functions of heartbeat and respiration have ceased. The problem has been highlighted by the capacity of artificial measures to keep a person alive for long periods after the irreversible cessation of brain function. The main point of interest here is the connection of brain function with the personality level of individuality. An organism that continues to live at only the metabolic level may be said to be dead as an actor or person.

Third, and finally, a few remarks about the significance for our problem of Freud's most mature theoretical statement need to be made. It was printed in the monograph published in English under the title *The Problem of Anxiety*. In this, his last major theoretical work, Freud rather drastically revised his previous views about the nature of anxiety. He focused on the expectation of the loss of an "object." For Freud the relevant meaning of the term "object" was a human individual standing in an emotionally significant relation to the person of reference. To the growing child, of course, the parents became "lost objects" in the nature of the process of growing up, in that their significance for the growing child was inevitably "lost" at later ages. The ultimate loss of a concrete human person as object—of cathexis, Freud said—is the death of that person. To have "grown away" from one's parents is one thing, but to experience their actual deaths is another. Freud's account of the impact on him of the death of his father is a particularly relevant case in point.

Equally clearly, an individual's own death, in anticipation, can be subsumed under the category of object loss, particularly in view of Freud's theory of narcissism, by which he meant the individual's cathexis of his or her own self as a love object. Anxiety, however, is not the actual experience of object loss, nor is it, according to Freud, the fear of it. It is an anticipatory orientation in which the actor's own emotional security is particularly involved. It is a field of rather free play of fantasy as to what might be the consequences of an anticipated or merely possible event.

Given the hypothesis that, in our scientifically oriented civilization, there is widespread acceptance of death—meant as the antithesis of its denial—there is no reason why this should lead to a cessation or even substantial diminution of anxiety about death, both that of others and one's own. Indeed, in certain circumstances the levels of anxiety may be expected to increase rather than the reverse. The frequent assertions that our society is characterized by pervasive denial of death may often be interpreted as calling attention to pervasive anxieties about death, which is not the same thing. There can be no doubt that in most cases death is, in experience and in anticipation, a traumatic event. Fantasies, in such circumstances, are often characterized by strains of unrealism, but the prevalence of such phenomena does not constitute a distortion of the basic cultural framework within which we moderns orient ourselves to the meaning of death.

Indeed, the preceding illustrations serve to enhance the importance of clarification, at the theoretical and philosophical levels, to which the bulk of this article has been devoted. This is essential if an intelligible approach is to be made to the understanding of such problems as shifts in attitudes toward various age groups in modern society, particularly the older groups, and the relatively sudden eruption of dissatisfaction with the traditional modes of conceptualizing the beginning and the termination of a human life, and with allegations about the pervasive denial of death, which is often interpreted as a kind of failure of "intestinal fortitude." However important the recent movements for increasing expression of emotional interests and the like, ours remains a culture to which its cognitive framework is of paramount significance.

TALCOTT PARSONS

DEATH IN THE WESTERN WORLD: A POSTSCRIPT

Talcott Parsons's article "Death in the Western World" addresses the changing and conflicting orientations toward death in contemporary culture. Parsons sought to connect these orientations to broad cultural frameworks that have shaped Western civilization over hundreds of years. His effort was an extension of his previous writings on American orientations toward death and on more general patterns of Western civilization (Parsons and Lidz, 1967; Parsons, 1971).

In the 1960s and 1970s, a number of authors argued that Americans defensively "deny" death (Mitford, 1963; Becker, 1973). They cited certain funeral customs and mourning practices as evidence, especially the preparing of remains to appear lifelike and peaceful for ritual viewing and the expectation that formal mourning need divert the family of a deceased person from other social obligations for only a brief period. Parsons, how-

ever, perceived that a generalized denial of death would conflict with a pragmatic realism deeply rooted in American culture since Puritan times.

Max Weber characterized the Puritan religious ethic as an "inner-worldly asceticism" that engaged the harsher realities of life to transform them into elements of the "kingdom of God on earth" (Weber, 1950). Parsons preferred the term "instrumental activism" to underscore that American civilization had secularized the Puritan emphasis on mastery over the given conditions of life. Following Weber, he noted that secular variants of the mastery ethic legitimized science and technology, formally rational law and bureaucracy, the market system and entrepreneurship, and motives of self-discipline and improvement (Parsons, 1971). Emphasizing consistency within these cultural themes, Parsons found not "denial" of death but mastery over its disrupting effects on social life.

While death is inevitable, its social impact is meliorable. Parsons explored two respects in which this is true (Parsons and Lidz, 1967; Parsons et al., 1972). First, medical and public-health technologies have reduced premature death and now typically enable members of society to use "God-given" talents to advance their vocations in good health over long careers. The demographic changes of the late nineteenth and twentieth centuries, and related efficiencies in the use of human talents, thus flow from an effort to master death. Second, when individuals die, the resulting social losses can be minimized. Measures ranging from life insurance to psychotherapy to retirement planning in business to estate planning in personal affairs reduce the harm ensuing from deaths (Zelizer, 1983). Similarly, American mourning customs emphasize austerely supporting the bereaved in overcoming grief and guilt, so they can return to their routine social duties without long delay.

Parsons recognized that, despite sharing the values of "instrumental activism," Americans disagree over many matters related to death. Abortion, capital punishment, licensing of firearms, euthanasia, medical care for the terminally ill, and organ transplantation, for example, have long been controversial. "Death in the Western World" attempts to explain why this particular domain of contemporary culture has been chronically ridden with controversy. Parsons sought an answer in the rationalism of the Enlightenment, focusing on its synthesis in Immanuel Kant's philosophy.

Kant epitomized the Enlightenment's elevation of Reason as a force of human betterment and a method of transforming culture (Cassirer, 1955). Parsons used Kant's writings to explicate the foundation established in the Enlightenment for new intellectual disciplines and ideologies. Kant's critique of Newtonian physics became a model for assessing the intellectual legitimacy of new disciplines. The domain of methodically developed and evaluated knowledge was opened to new forms, and, from Kant's time to ours, there has been continuous growth in specialized disciplines. Kant's critiques of the human faculties of judgment and practical reason proved no less important. They legitimated the voice of moral Reason while also, as Parsons emphasized, undercutting all claims to ultimate certainty. Ever since, Western civilization has been engulfed in ever-renewed moral and ideological controversies on almost every topic of social import. Orientations toward death, given their irreducible significance to humanity, have been caught up in many of the controversies.

Although Parsons expected death-related matters to remain controversial, he could not foresee the recent evolution of cultural conflicts. The intense social criticism of funeral and mourning customs has subsided, though practices have changed little. How "life" and the "living being" should be defined before birth and at the approach of death remains an effervescent issue. Public debates over abortion not only have persisted but have grown in bitterness and political prominence. The health-food, antismoking, physical exercise, environmental, and indeed animal-rights movements have altered activities of everyday life as parts of what Parsons would have characterized as an ongoing effort to increase mastery over death. The public attends with ever greater interest to advances in medicine, with new findings and procedures featured routinely on television and in newspapers. Coverage of heroic lifesaving procedures resonates deeply in American moral culture, dramatizing shared beliefs that emphasize the unique value of each life.

Despite impressive institutions to master death, contemporary civilization remains acutely insecure over life (Fox and Swazey, 1992). Mass media have grown increasingly attentive to medicine, and in concentrating on life-threatening conditions have left the public less secure about health and more readily mobilized into panic over environmental threats and even endemic conditions such as breast cancer. Matters of personal habit and lifestyle, including diet, exercise, work schedules, and even sexual practices, are viewed as regimens to be adjusted whenever new knowledge emerges about their possible effects on longevity. In attending patients with elaborately cultivated medical insecurities, physicians have a limited fund of trust to draw upon and are constrained to practice "defensive medicine." They may thus use new and expensive technologies for diagnosis or treatment even when older and cheaper procedures would likely serve as well. When the lives of patients are genuinely at risk, pressures build to use "heroic measures" in order to show that everything possible is being attempted, regardless of the chances of success or the quality of the lives that may be extended. These tendencies persist while the public also worries greatly over the rising costs of medical care.

In the mid-1990s, national policy has engaged the issue of democratizing access to medical care. Political leadership has focused public awareness on the large sectors of the population who have lacked medical insurance and, thus, reliable access to expensive health care. The desirability of providing better care to citizens of modest means and the poor is generally accepted, but proposals about how to manage its costs are controversial. Proposals that are perceived as potentially restricting the freedom of relationships between patients and practitioners, whether the rights of patients to select personal practitioners or the rights of practitioners to treat patients as they believe correct, generate widespread opposition. Moreover, new plans for cost containment have not directly confronted public sentiment favoring use of "heroic measures" and experimental procedures, regardless of cost—sentiment that becomes especially forceful when physicians and family members face a patient's impending death. Although eventual national policy is uncertain, the United States is clearly embarking on a major extension of "instrumental activism" in the medical field, with the goal of devising institutions to offer more secure protection from illness, suffering, and death for many millions of the nation's less affluent citizens.

Parsons believed, along with many scientists, that modern medicine verged on conquering all infectious epidemics, at least for societies with effective systems of sanitation and public-health services. The appearance in the 1980s of the human immunodeficiency virus (HIV) and the acquired immunodeficiency syndrome (AIDS) has shaken such optimism more and more rudely as it has become clear that humankind faces a major pandemic that, despite modern science and technology, will take tens of millions of lives on all continents. Neither a vaccine nor an effective cure has been found, despite vast research efforts and early hopes for success. Clinicians have devised inventive treatments for many of the secondary infections in the AIDS syndrome. Good clinical care now reduces the pains and discomforts of the disease and extends the lives of many AIDS patients substantially longer than could be achieved early in the epidemic. Yet scarcities of resources and lack of political will to reallocate resources still leave many of the afflicted to die with minimal care. While prevention programs have at their best been guided by a liberal and tolerant understanding, they have frequently failed to communicate effectively with the people most seriously at risk, leaving them poorly protected from the epidemic. In some African and Asian nations, HIV has spread rapidly and with little control, and the epidemic may change the demographic structures and even common life-cycle patterns of a number of societies during the next few decades.

In Parsons's terms, a major feature of HIV as an epidemic is that it has afflicted many young adults and people in early middle age. The individuals who become diseased and die would otherwise typically expect to live several decades longer. Their deaths represent unfulfilled lives, with future achievements, relationships, and experiences all lost. In Western societies, where homosexual men and injection drug users have had the highest rates of infection, the transmission of HIV has in most instances involved unconventional and widely disapproved personal behavior. Although homosexuals and drug users previously bore burdens of public disfavor, HIV has added to their stigmas the ugly image of a wasting, disfiguring, and dementing disease. In many cases, people with HIV disease have experienced intense feelings of guilt and self-blame as an added dimension of their suffering. In social circles where HIV has become common, many individuals still in early adulthood have lost large numbers of friends and associates, otherwise a rare experience in modern societies. They may feel numbed and disoriented, burdened by the "survivors' guilt" typical among people who live through disasters that have claimed the lives of many others (Erikson, 1976). They often find that any attempt at a spirited resumption of everyday activities is complicated by feelings that their futures are hopeless or meaningless without the individuals who have been lost. Even people not infected may feel that they will inevitably become diseased—indeed, that they are already "dead," although still walking around. Efforts to change personal conduct in order to avoid exposure to HIV may be complicated by a belief that it is impossible to stay well or even feelings that it would be better to accompany one's friends in heroic suffering and death (Weitz, 1991). In some Western communities and in Third World nations, lassitude engendered by the HIV epidemic, through social loss, fear of death, and guilt, may cause immense social dislocation in the future.

Parsons's article highlighted the distinctive pattern of Western institutions relating to death. In comparative perspective, Parsons argued, the modern West has uniquely endeavored to "master" death. Such mastery has involved a range of institutions, including scientific medicine and public-health services designed to protect life; insurance, retirement, and estate planning designed to manage the practical consequences of deaths; and funeral and mourning customs that emphasize recovery of survivors' abilities to perform ordinary social roles soon after the death of family members, friends, and associates. Some elements of these institutions are closely tied to the "instrumental activism" of Western cultural values; while other elements, such as the techniques of scientific medicine or the actuarial tables and formulas of the insurance industry, have a universal or transcultural validity now that they have been developed. A matter for future investigation concerns the ways in which

these universal elements will be institutionalized in sociocultural settings where they may be disconnected from Western value orientations. Scientific medicine, for example, is now practiced almost the world over—but in many non-Western societies it is generally reserved for patients from elite status groups and provided to common citizens only in emergency conditions, combined with traditional healing in ways that create different doctor–patient roles, or even are contingently linked with personal relationships of political patronage (Kleinman, 1980; Scheper-Hughes, 1992). In these settings, the bioethical cultures that emerge may be very different from the frameworks that have emerged in the West over the past several decades, not least because they rest upon different value orientations toward life and death. Comparative study of these bioethical cultures may now constitute the most powerful way of building upon, correcting, or refining the analysis developed by Parsons in his writings on American and Western orientations toward death.

VICTOR LIDZ

Directly related to this article are the other articles in this entry: ANTHROPOLOGICAL PERSPECTIVES, EASTERN THOUGHT, WESTERN PHILOSOPHICAL THOUGHT, *and* WESTERN RELIGIOUS THOUGHT. *Also directly related to this article are the entries* BODY, *article on* CULTURAL AND RELIGIOUS PERSPECTIVES; DEATH, ATTITUDES TOWARD; DEATH: ART OF DYING, *article on* ARS MORIENDI; LIFE; *and* PERSON. *For a further discussion of topics mentioned in this article, see the entries* AGING AND THE AGED, *article on* LIFE EXPECTANCY AND LIFE SPAN; AIDS; *and* DEATH AND DYING: EUTHANASIA AND SUSTAINING LIFE, *article on* HISTORICAL ASPECTS. *For a discussion of related ideas, see the entries* BODY, *article on* EMBODIMENT: THE PHENOMENOLOGICAL TRADITION; HEALTH AND DISEASE; HUMAN NATURE; *and* MEDICINE, SOCIOLOGY OF. *Other relevant material may be found under the entries* PROTESTANTISM; ROMAN CATHOLICISM; *and* TRAGEDY.

Bibliography

BELLAH, ROBERT N. 1964. "Religious Evolution." *American Sociological Review* 29, no. 3:358–374.

BURKE, KENNETH. 1961. *The Rhetoric of Religion: Studies in Logology.* Boston: Beacon Press.

CHOMSKY, NOAM. 1957. *Syntactic Structures.* Janua Linguarum no. 4. The Hague: Mouton.

DURKHEIM, ÉMILE. 1933. *The Division of Labor in Society.* Edited and translated by George Simpson. Glencoe, Ill.: Free Press Paperbacks.

———. 1976. *The Elementary Forms of the Religious Life.* Translated by Joseph Ward Swain. 2d ed. London: Allen and Unwin.

———. 1974. *Sociology and Philosophy.* Enl. ed. Translated by D. F. Pocock. New York: Free Press.

FREUD, SIGMUND. 1955–1974. [1920]. *Beyond the Pleasure Principle.* In vol. 18 of *The Standard Edition of the Complete Psychological Works of Sigmund Freud,* pp. 7–64. Edited by James Strachey, Anna Freud, Alix Strachey, and Alan Tyson. London: Hogarth.

———. 1955–1974. [1923]. *The Ego and the Id.* In vol. 19 of *The Standard Edition of the Complete Psychological Works of Sigmund Freud,* pp. 12–66. Edited by James Strachey, Anna Freud, Alix Strachey, and Alan Tyson. London: Hogarth.

———. 1955–1974. [1926]. *Inhibitions, Symptoms and Anxiety.* In vol. 20 of *The Standard Edition of the Complete Psychological Works of Sigmund Freud,* pp. 77–156. Edited by James Strachey, Anna Freud, Alix Strachey, and Alan Tyson. London: Hogarth.

———. 1955–1974. [1927]. *The Future of an Illusion.* In vol. 21 of *The Standard Edition of the Complete Psychological Works of Sigmund Freud,* pp. 5–56. Edited by James Strachey, Anna Freud, Alix Strachey, and Alan Tyson. London: Hogarth.

———. 1954. *The Origins of Psycho-analysis: Letters to Wilhelm Fliess, Drafts and Notes, 1887–1902.* Edited by Marie N. Bonaparte, Anna Freud, and Ernst Kris. Translated by Eric Mosbacher and James Strachey. New York: Basic Books.

———. 1955–1974. *The Standard Edition of the Complete Psychological Works of Sigmund Freud.* 24 vols. Edited by James Strachey, Anna Freud, Alix Strachey, and Alan Tyson. London: Hogarth Press.

HENDERSON, LAWRENCE JOSEPH. 1913. *The Fitness of the Environment: An Inquiry into the Biological Significance of the Properties of Matter.* New York: Macmillan.

———. 1917. *The Order of Nature: An Essay.* Cambridge, Mass.: Harvard University Press.

———. 1935. *Pareto's General Sociology: A Physiologist's Interpretation.* Cambridge, Mass.: Harvard University Press.

KANT, IMMANUEL. 1929. *Critique of Pure Reason.* Translated by Norman Kemp Smith. London: Macmillan.

———. 1949. *Critique of Practical Reason and Other Writings in Moral Philosophy.* Translated and edited by Lewis White Beck. Chicago: University of Chicago Press.

———. 1952. *Critique of Judgment.* Translated by James Creed Meredith. Oxford: At the Clarendon Press.

LEACH, EDMUND R. 1969. *Genesis as Myth and Other Essays.* Cape Editions no. 39. London: Jonathan Cape.

LÉVI-STRAUSS, CLAUDE. 1963. *Structural Anthropology.* Translated by Claire Jacobson and Brooke Grundfest Schoepf. New York: Basic Books.

LOVEJOY, ARTHUR ONCKEN. 1936. *The Great Chain of Being: A Study of the History of an Idea.* Cambridge, Mass.: Harvard University Press.

MAUSS, MARCEL. 1954 [1925]. *The Gift: Forms and Functions of Exchange in Archaic Societies.* Translated by Ian Cunnison. Glencoe, Ill.: Free Press.

NOCK, ARTHUR D. 1933. *Conversion: The Old and the New in Religion from Alexander the Great to Augustine of Hippo.* London: Oxford University Press.

PARSONS, TALCOTT. 1977. *Social Systems and the Evolution of Action Theory.* New York: Free Press.

PARSONS, TALCOTT; FOX, RENÉE C.; and LIDZ, VICTOR M. 1972. "The 'Gift of Life' and Its Reciprocation." *Social Research Experience* 39:367–415. Repr. in *Death in American Experience,* pp. 1–49. Edited by Arien Mack. New York: Schocken.

PARSONS, TALCOTT, and LIDZ, VICTOR. 1967. "Death in American Society." In *Essays in Self-Destruction,* pp. 133–170. Edited by Edwin S. Shneidman. New York: Science House.

WARNER, WILLIAM LLOYD. 1959. *The Living and the Dead: A Study of the Symbolic Life of Americans.* Yankee City Series vol. 5. New Haven, Conn.: Yale University Press.

WEBER, MAX. 1930. *The Protestant Ethic and the Spirit of Capitalism.* Translated by Talcott Parsons. London: George Allen and Unwin.

———. 1963. *The Sociology of Religion.* Translated by Ephraim Fischoff. Boston: Beacon Press.

Bibliography (*Postscript*)

BECKER, ERNEST. 1973. *The Denial of Death.* New York: Free Press.

CASSIRER, ERNST. 1955. *The Philosophy of the Enlightenment.* Boston: Beacon Press.

ERIKSON, KAI T. 1976. *Everything in Its Path: Destruction of Community in the Buffalo Creek Flood.* New York: Simon and Schuster.

FOX, RENÉE C. 1979. "The Medicalization and Demedicalization of American Society." In her *Essays in Medical Sociology: Journeys into the Field,* pp. 465–483. New York: Wiley.

FOX, RENÉE C., and SWAZEY, JUDITH P. 1992. *Spare Parts: Organ Replacement in American Society.* New York: Oxford University Press.

KLEINMAN, ARTHUR. 1980. *Patients and Healers in the Context of Culture: An Exploration of the Borderland Between Anthropology, Medicine, and Psychiatry.* Berkeley: University of California Press.

MITFORD, JESSICA. 1963. *The American Way of Death.* New York: Simon and Schuster.

PARSONS, TALCOTT. 1971. *The System of Modern Societies.* Englewood Cliffs, N.J.: Prentice-Hall.

PARSONS, TALCOTT; FOX, RENÉE C.; and LIDZ, VICTOR M. 1972. "The Gift of Life and Its Reciprocation." *Social Research* 39, no. 3:367–415.

PARSONS, TALCOTT, and LIDZ, VICTOR M. 1967. "Death in American Society." In *Essays in Self-Destruction,* pp. 133–170. Edited by Edwin S. Shneidman. New York: Science House.

SCHEPER-HUGHES, NANCY. 1992. *Death Without Weeping: The Violence of Everyday Life in Brazil.* Berkeley: University of California Press.

WEBER, MAX. 1950. *The Protestant Ethic and the Spirit of Capitalism.* Translated by Talcott Parsons. New York: Scribners.

WEITZ, ROSE. 1991. *Life with AIDS.* New Brunswick, N.J.: Rutgers University Press.

ZELIZER, VIVIANA. 1983. *Morals and Markets: The Development of Life Insurance in the United States.* New Brunswick, N.J.: Transaction Books.

DEATH, ATTITUDES TOWARD

Although death is a fact, something that happens to all, dying and grieving are activities in which one engages according to the attitudes one holds about them. An attitude about death, dying, and bereavement, a more or less enduring readiness to behave in a characteristic way, does not differ from other attitudes. One is socialized into it by a culture.

A death attitude system

The set of attitudes by which one experiences dying and grieving has been called a "death system" (Kastenbaum and Aisenberg, 1972). A death attitude system is cognitive, affective, and behavioral, that is, it teaches what to think about death, how to feel about it, and what to do regarding it. It comprises one's orientation to the persons, places, ideas, traditions, acts, omissions, and emotions associated with death and the statements made about death. In other words, it is the total picture of questions related to death, dying, bereavement, suicide, and euthanasia in a given culture at a given time.

Attitudes toward death are multilayered rather than single responses. They contain feelings about dependency, pain, indignity, isolation, separation, possible rejection, leaving loved ones, afterlife, finality of death, facing the unknown, and the fate of the body (Leming, 1979–1980). The difficulty of categorizing such diverse attitudes with any exactness is compounded by the fact that one may be very open about death and bereavement on a verbal level but quite anxious below the level of consciousness or at the fantasy level (Feifel, 1990).

Whatever the contemporary attitudes toward death, there are other ways of looking at death, dying, and bereavement than the ones prominent in the West. Though these are found in the West today to a modest degree, they are not dominant (but they have been dominant at other times and are still dominant in other settings). Death attitudes in most cultures have changed since the beginning of the twentieth century. They changed after World War II, and again after the 1960s as a result of hospices and what has been called the death awareness movement. This article will discuss the historical development of Western attitudes toward death, examine the effects of the death attitude system by showing the interaction between the North American death system and those most affected by it (the dying, the bereaved, and health-care professionals), and propose suggestions for an appropriate death attitude system.

Western attitudes in history

The French historian Philippe Ariès (1981) postulated that attitudes toward death over the centuries are indications of the person's awareness of himself or herself, and of his or her degree of individuality. In other words, attitudes about death and bereavement differ because of differing conceptions of what it is to be a person and the relationship of the person to his or her community, to the world, and to God. Ariès groups these attitudes historically around four basic orientations that he calls "tamed death," "the death of the self," "the death of the other," and "death denied" (Ariès, 1981, p. 602).

Ariès characterizes as "the unchronicled death throughout the long ages of the most ancient history" the orientation he calls tamed death, which dominated until the late Middle Ages (Ariès, 1981, p. 5). Since life was, as Thomas Hobbes wrote, "solitary, poor, nasty, brutish and short" (Hobbes, 1968, p. 95), one was constantly exposed to, and therefore familiar with, death as "a knife at our throat or a scourge at our child's bedside" (Ariès, 1981, p. 206). The effects of this "uncontrolled mortality" were that since child and maternal deaths were common, one did not spend much time in preparation for adulthood: Courtships were short, relationships were understood to be limited, education was minimal. Such familiarity with death seemingly effected a more conscious dying than many persons experience today. Death was not viewed as some remote possibility but as a dominant fact of life. Having seen relatives and friends die, the dying person knew the role and prepared for it, saying good-byes, commending himself or herself to God, even lying in bed with arms crossed. Such role enactment continued at least until the Civil War in the United States, when soldiers prepared themselves in a like manner (Callahan, 1993). Death was public; family members were present, as were the neighbors who came to accompany the dying person in this last stage of life's journey. Care for the dying and funeral arrangements were the tasks of the family, not of professionals outside the family. Family members had as their role models the relatives and neighbors they had seen confront loss by death. Death was a familiar, if not always welcome, neighbor.

In the second historical period, which Ariès dates from approximately the twelfth to the fifteenth century, the individual became aware of himself or herself as distinct from the community. Whereas the earlier period emphasized familiarity with death, the second orientation, called "my death," emphasized the termination of one's own life, one's personal death. Death was the last act of a personal drama. This is the period of the *Ars moriendi* genre, manuals on dying that were meant to guide the reader's behavior as he or she faced the end of life. Elaborate tombs memorializing the life became common, as did placing these tombs in churches of various sizes.

One of the consequences of the awareness of personal death was concern about the judgment of the soul. Each moment of life would be weighed before all the powers of heaven and hell: The just would be rewarded, and the wicked would be condemned. The Latin hymn from the liturgy for the dead, *Dies irae,* which solicits mercy for the dead, dates from this period. Both the individual and his or her family prayed for conversions, even at the point of death. Wills, especially those that arranged for prayers by the living for the deceased as he or she met God, were common.

In the nineteenth century, the ideas of "death as a neighbor" and "death as the personal end" declined in favor of a third orientation, "death of the other." Life was viewed as having meaning, primarily through relationships. Thus death was perceived as the loss of that relationship. It was no longer as public because privacy had become necessary for a relationship to develop. Dying was not mourned as the loss of community, as the end of life, or as judgment, but as physical separation from the beloved. The image of the beyond in the earlier periods, which had ranged from eternal sleep to a glorious heaven or damned hell, became in the nineteenth century the scene of the reunion of those whom death had separated. Wills became less common, for one had put his or her physical and spiritual affairs in the trust of the beloved without the necessity of a written document.

Contemporary Western death attitudes

At least the remnants of the above three orientations to death are sufficiently familiar in the twentieth century that death is sometimes viewed as a familiar guest, as the last act of a personal drama, or as the ending of an important relationship. However, the present Western death culture differs significantly from those that preceded it. Ariès names the twentieth century the period of "death denied." To understand this designation, one must look at the parameters of contemporary death attitudes. They differ among cultures because of four major factors: exposure to death, life expectancy, perceived control over the forces of nature, and the understanding of what it is to be a human being (Ariès, 1981).

Exposure to death. Exposure to death and bereavement constitutes the first element in an understanding of death. If one has little experience of the loss of significant others, death attitudes will be limited by

that inexperience. Earthquakes in Mexico, volcanic eruptions in the Philippines and Central America, and chemical and nuclear disasters in India and Russia indicate that even the twentieth century is subject to uncontrolled mortality. However, these events create headlines precisely because they are unusual. In most Western settings, children grow up protected from death. In other parts of the world, the young are exposed to death quite early through war and starvation. Even in the West, exposure varies. Persons living in inner cities, especially those of African descent, may have an awareness of death vastly different from that of most suburbanites (Barrett, 1993). The child whose parents die early, or the child of a funeral director or an emergency room physician, grows up with a greater exposure to death than does the average North American.

Since formal education about death and bereavement is not a common part of the school curriculum, and since the churches no longer have the educational influence they once did, the entertainment media have been the main teachers of death attitudes. According to recent studies, television has taught three messages about death and bereavement. The first is that death is entertainment: Cartoon characters systematically annihilate one another, only to reappear unscathed in the next episode. The second lesson is that life is brutal and lethal: Young males kill or are killed through the malevolence of others with little grief entailed. The third is that death, when it actually occurs, occurs elsewhere and mostly to foreigners, to people alien in appearance, language, and national ideology (Fulton and Owen, 1994). North Americans have become uncomfortable with bodily processes that forebears viewed as natural and manageable. There is an ideology of personal happiness which holds that life consists of a series of snares to be avoided and problems to be solved (Brody, 1992).

Today at least 75 percent of persons die in hospitals; thus actual death is seen by few persons. Fewer persons die at home, much less in public, as they might have during the Black Plague. The very appearance of death has changed. At one time one could "put his finger" on death by feeling for a pulse. Death has an increasingly technology-defined dimension, making it more isolating and ambiguous than in the past. One is now aware of "cardiac death" and "brain death," and only doctors can certify that the various types of death have occurred. In earlier days the physician's primary role was to be with the sick, to encourage the body's recuperative powers, and as Paul Ramsey (1970) stated, "to (only) care for the dying." Today, doctors deal as much with drugs and machines as with people. In prolonging life, medical technology has separated the chronically ill and the dying from their families. This medicalization of death has affected the entire Western culture's view of death.

A 1991 Gallup poll indicated that most Americans

do not think about death. "Miracle" drugs and organ transplantation have become sufficiently common that the expectation is that an illness is always curable. Thus personal experience and the notion that a cure is readily available (Beck, 1991) teach that accidents, disease, and death happen to others. When one finally has personal exposure to death, often as late as the third decade of life, it appears as unusual and thus cruel. This innocence of death is compounded by what has been called an oxymoronic view: The four leading causes of death across all age groups in the West are heart disease, cancer, stroke, and accidents, causes that are partly of human origin (Beck, 1991). Vast resources are spent to save lives at the same time that even greater resources are spent on weapons of mass destruction or on polluting the planet.

Life expectancy.   Exposure to death is related to life expectancy. Most babies born in North America can be expected to live to their late seventies. The latter part of the twentieth century is a period of increased longevity and predictable age-specific death rates due to fewer neonatal and maternal deaths, better sanitation and food supplies, and improved medical care. The discovery that contagious diseases could be prevented through inoculation neutralized diseases that sometimes killed whole populations in earlier times. Consequently, in developed countries, it is today reasonable to assume that most mothers will not die from infections contracted as a result of childbirth and that most children will live to maturity.

Around the turn of the twentieth century, the death rate was approximately seventeen per thousand live population in the United States, whereas in the 1990s the figure is less than eight per thousand live population. The very old constitute the fastest-growing segment of the population; 10 percent of those over sixty-five years of age have a child who also is over sixty-five (Kowalski, 1986). As the population ages, the rate of death will increase, especially because the birth rate is too low to replace these additional deaths. Women outlive men, as they have always. The age-adjusted mortality rate in the United States, which fell 26 percent for elderly males between 1940 and 1980, dropped 48 percentage points for elderly females in the same period (Kowalski, 1986).

More and more the elderly are living in "homes" or retirement communities, where they will be seen only by other elderly persons or by professional caregivers. As the mobility of society increases, the aged are not seen or visited on a regular basis by their families; they live physically and psychologically removed from their children and grandchildren. The medical technology that makes possible the prolongation of life has also resulted in extended separations of chronically ill or elderly persons from their families. This disengagement of the aged

from their families prior to their death means that their death may have little effect on the day-to-day life of the family, thereby depriving the elderly of traditional family assistance and depriving children of the opportunity to see the aging process. Dying appears to be not a gradual process but a telephone call in the night. Role models are scarce for the dying process and for the grief experienced and shown at the time of death.

Although death rates have declined in the population as a whole, the benefits are not shared equally. Nonwhite race, poverty, and poor education are predictors of early death. Poor and poorly educated persons have higher death rates than wealthier and better-educated persons, and these differences increased from 1960 to 1986 (Pappas et al., 1993). The mortality rate from heart disease in 1986 was 2.3 times higher for unskilled workers and 1.3 times higher for blacks than for whites (Navarro, 1991). From 1983 to 1988 the percentage of individuals with an annual income over $60,000 who had limited activity due to a chronic condition declined, and for those with incomes less than $10,000 it increased.

Perceived control over nature.   Attitudes toward death are particularly shaped by one's view of the world and one's place in and perceived control of it. One who believes that persons are entirely subject to the "laws" of nature will have a death attitude different from one whose view is that he or she has significant control over the forces of nature. In the West the dominant attitude is that nature exists to be used and controlled. Other cultures do not share that view. Those who live on the floodplain of Bangladesh or in the shadow of Mount Pinatubo in the Philippines have a different perception of their relationship to nature than do those who move about in climate-controlled cars and reside in air-conditioned and insulated offices and homes. Persons who believe they can be "protected" from nature have less respect for the power of nature over life.

Perception of the person.   The most important element in the development of attitudes toward death is the perception of what it is to be a person. Most people in the West today believe that the person is unique, what Ernest Becker refers to as "the ache of cosmic specialness" (Becker, 1973, p. 4). In a culture that emphasizes the individual and individual rights, persons will have a different orientation toward death than will members of a culture that perceives each individual as having meaning primarily as a part of the whole, whether religious or political, or perhaps as not having any meaning at all. Those who believe that each life is unique will perceive the end of that life as a different order of loss than those who perceive that a life has meaning only within a whole.

William James wrote that the word "good" fundamentally means "destined to survive" (James, 1959, p.

13). When an individual says that something is good, he or she implicitly affirms that the thing ought to exist. The effect of this self-awareness is the following enigma: "I am. I am good. Yet I shall die." This awareness is, in the words of William James, "the worm at the core of our pretensions to happiness" (Becker, 1973, p. 15). Death ultimately is the proof that no matter what powers humans have or develop, they still are not God (Parsons et al., 1972). If James is right that good means "destined to survive," then death is nature's way of saying that humans are not absolutely good.

Denial.   Ariès referred to contemporary death attitudes as "death denied." This denial of death is not cognitive. Living in the shadow of the Holocaust and possible nuclear destruction, people in the twentieth century have seen more real and threatened deaths than any people in the previous history of the human race (Ariès, 1981). No one doubts the validity of the syllogism "All persons are mortal, I am a person, therefore I am mortal." Indeed, the evidence is that college students think about death more often than did their grandparents (Lester and Becker, 1992–1993). Rather, death is denied in the psychological sense. Contemporary Western culture does not seem to take seriously the fact that death is the end of possibilities, the collapse of personal space and time, the end of all relationships. As death is removed from daily consciousness, it appears to be less appropriate and thus contributes to more cases of complicated mourning (Rando, 1992–1993).

The community seemingly no longer thinks it necessary to defend itself against a nature that has been domesticated by the advance of technology. Even community in the traditional sense of the word—persons with common interests coming together to live their lives in common—has been replaced by atomized individuals. Death is a slap in the face of the great North American dream that time and money can remove all obstacles to human enjoyment. As Herman Feifel put it:

> We witnessed a shift from spiritual mastery over self to physical conquest of nature. A major consequence was that we became impoverished in possessing religious or philosophic conceptual creeds, except nominally, with which to transcend death. Death became a "wall" rather than a "doorway." A taboo of considerable measure was placed on death and bereaved persons. Death and its concomitants were sundered off, isolated, and permitted into society only after being properly decontaminated. In this context, further circumstances making the area uncomfortable to deal with were (a) an expanding industrial, impersonal technology that steadily increased fragmentation of the family and dismantled root neighborhoods and kinship groups with more or less homogeneous values . . . thus depriving us of emotional and social supports with which to cushion the impact of death when it intruded into our lives; (b) a spreading

deritualization of grief, related to criticism of funerary practices as being overly expansive, baroque, and exploitive of the mourner's emotions; (c) a gradual expulsion of death from everyday common experience; death has developed into a mystery for many people, increasingly representing a fear of the unknown, and has become the province of the "professional," whose mastery, unfortunately, is more technical than human these days; and (d) in a modern society that has emphasized achievement, productivity, and the future, the prospect of no future at all, and loss of identity, has become an abomination. Hence, death and mourning have invited our hostility and repudiation. (Feifel, 1990, p. 537)

One indication of the death denial of contemporary North Americans can be found in the media coverage of the Gulf War (Operation Desert Storm). The public has a stake in denying that death occurs in a war. The words "death," "die," and "kill" rarely appeared in media reports; euphemisms for death were used instead (Umbertson and Henderson, 1992). The contemporary view of death in the West is that every death is contingent, a matter of chance, and that in principle there is no reason why any particular cause or disease cannot be overcome (Callahan, 1993).

There is substantial evidence that the violence that grows daily, addiction, and poverty are results of the refusal to take seriously the human reality of death (Leviton, 1991). Not taking death seriously allows one to risk the lives of unknown others, loved ones, and oneself. Violence exists in spite of the fact that for millennia the great religions have taught responsibility for others and that the Creator can be seen in the least of one's neighbors. Apart from religion, philosophical systems have agreed with Immanuel Kant that one ought never to use another person as a means. Violence, according to Becker, is "a symbolic solution of a biological limitation" (Becker, 1973, p. 99). It is easy to believe that one is master of his or her own life when one holds someone else's fate in one's hands.

Effects of the death attitude system

When one considers the persons, places, objects, and roles related to death, one becomes aware of the breadth of influence that death attitudes have on everyone in the culture. It is virtually impossible to read a newspaper or watch a television set without being aware of death, euthanasia, suicide, funerals, or questions of ultimate value. While everyone is affected by, and in turn affects, the death system, it is instructive to focus on the effects that death attitudes have on those most immediately involved: the dying, the bereaved, and health-care workers.

Effects on the dying.   Although the culture as a whole denies the importance or reality of death, the dying and the bereaved cannot do so. The effect of this situation is to alienate the dying and the bereaved from the support they have a right to expect. Most dying patients do not expect "miracles" to reverse their biological condition. What is essential is care and concern. The hospice movement has shown that when the physical and emotional needs of dying patients are attended to, there is less depression, blaming, and guilt for the patient and for the family, and death is the death of a person rather than an illness (Lamers, 1990). Most persons arrive at some sense of acceptance: a realization that time is limited, that one's work is complete, and that one's life has been good.

The most important element of the Western view of life and death is that life and death are profoundly different and completely unrelated states; that once one is born, one maintains a constant state of life until the moment of death, and that once one is dead, one maintains a constant state of being dead; and that the event of death is an instantaneous leap from one state to the other—there is no transitional state, no gray or ambiguous area (Ramsdem, 1991). Those who tend to infuse death with a sense of purpose or meaning, who see it as an event that leads to some form of continued existence, find more meaning (Holcomb et al., 1993). The major question to be faced by the dying is whether death is to be understood as within or outside of human life (Callahan, 1993). There is a major difference between seeing death as a wall and seeing death as a door. For those who see death as a wall, death entails self-annihilation, loss of self-fulfillment, and loss of identity (Florian and Mikulincer, 1992–1993). For those who see death as a door, death is a transformation of life's meanings (Ross and Pollio, 1991).

Effects on the bereaved. Although bereavement is one of life's greatest stressors, most of the bereaved have found that within one year, the death of a loved one has been an opportunity for growth. The main goal of the bereaved is to seek a meaning in the death (Gallagher et al., 1989). The discovery of the meaning of the death, as well as the sense of purpose in their own lives, is the major factor that brings a satisfactory adjustment.

Effects on health-care professionals. Medicine and religion have much in common. Both address the fears of humanity and the meaning of events surrounding life and death. Religion has responded to these needs by constructing theologies; medicine, by providing a scientific theory of health and sickness (Brody, 1992). Labeling a biological state as a disease is akin to declaring that there is an evil that ought to be eliminated. The rescue fantasy, that one can "snatch the patient away from the jaws of death" (Brody, 1992, p. 139), is an important part of medical culture and the popular folklore about physicians. As Becker (1973) has pointed out, all power is ultimately viewed as power over

death; thus the conceptions of the physician's powers flow from the view that medicine is a priesthood with power over evil. Cardiopulmonary resuscitation is an example of the rescue fantasy's becoming a reality. Cardiopulmonary resuscitation was developed for a select group of patients with temporary cardiac arrhythmias who would die without resuscitation. The procedure became standard practice, and now the presumption is that no one should be allowed to die in a hospital without an attempt at resuscitation even though less than 20 percent survive (Brody, 1992).

Medical and nursing cultures attach value to lifesaving activity. To the physician, the inability to prevent or slow a patient's death represents the loss of power and control. This is especially true when the death is of a "significant patient" (Benoliel, 1982), one in whom the practitioner has invested a great deal of time or clinical effort. In addition, caregivers not only have to deal with critically ill and dying people but also have to face several people dying at one time (Vachon, 1987). As a protection from loss of professional control, nurses and doctors may become "impermeable." This reaction of building a wall between oneself and the patient is caused by the heavy workload, the emotional demands of frequent contact with dying patients, dealing with the adjustment problems of the patients and their families, and their own anxieties and uncertainties. The role that has been historically assigned to medical doctors is that of suprahuman mediator between life and death (Family, 1992–1993).

If the purpose of life is to live well, then the patient has a right to a medical relationship that ensures that he or she will be treated with respect and that medical knowledge will be used to further his or her life plans and values (Brody, 1992). The ongoing personal relationship with each patient is the corresponding tool of the trade for the primary-care physician.

Toward an appropriate death attitude system

Death becomes acceptable, according to Daniel Callahan (1993), when it comes at the point in a life when (1) further efforts to deter dying are likely to deform the process of dying, or (2) there is a good fit between the biological inevitability of death in general and the particular timing and circumstances of that death in the life of an individual. The achievement of such a peaceful death should be a goal of life, and therefore of medicine. The process of dying is deformed when it is extended unduly by medical interventions or when there is an extended period of loss of consciousness well before one is actually dead.

An integrated death system would enable individuals to achieve such an acceptable death by thinking, feeling, and behaving with respect to death in ways that they might consider effective and appropriate. Avery Weisman (1978) outlined what he considered the parameters of an appropriate death. They include (1) relative freedom from pain, (2) control of social and emotional impoverishment, (3) resolution of residual conflicts, (4) satisfaction of those ego ideals consistent with the dying person's present condition, (5) the yielding of control to others, and (6) maintaining or severing key relationships. In judging the helpfulness of attitudes to death, one should ask if this death attitude system promotes the type of death that Weisman describes.

Because there can be no guarantee that an acceptable or peaceful death will be available, some store of courage must be available (Callahan, 1993).

JOHN D. MORGAN

Directly related to this entry are the entries DEATH; DEATH, DEFINITION AND DETERMINATION OF; DEATH: ART OF DYING; DEATH AND DYING: EUTHANASIA AND SUSTAINING LIFE; DEATH EDUCATION; *and* LIFE. *For a further discussion of topics mentioned in this article, see the entries* AGING AND THE AGED, *articles on* LIFE EXPECTANCY AND LIFE SPAN, *and* SOCIETAL AGING; CARE; COMPASSION; ETHICS, *article on* RELIGION AND MORALITY; FAMILY; HOMICIDE; HOSPICE AND END-OF-LIFE CARE; MEDICAL ETHICS, HISTORY OF, *section on* EUROPE; MEDICINE, SOCIOLOGY OF; PAIN AND SUFFERING; PERSON; RISK; SUICIDE; *and* TECHNOLOGY. *For a further discussion of related ideas, see the entries* CHILDREN, *article on* HISTORY OF CHILDHOOD; DEATH PENALTY; ENVIRONMENTAL ETHICS; ENVIRONMENTAL HEALTH; HEALTH AND DISEASE; INFORMATION DISCLOSURE; INJURY AND INJURY CONTROL; JUDAISM; LIFE, QUALITY OF; LONG-TERM CARE, *especially the article on* NURSING HOMES; MEDICINE, ANTHROPOLOGY OF; RACE AND RACISM; *and* WARFARE. *Other relevant material may be found under the entries* ABORTION; AIDS; CRYONICS; ENVIRONMENT AND RELIGION; FETUS; INFANTS, *article on* HISTORY OF INFANTICIDE; *and* NARRATIVE.

Bibliography

ARIÈS, PHILIPPE. 1981. *The Hour of Our Death.* Translated by Helen Weaver. New York: Knopf.

BARRETT, RONALD K. 1993. "Psychocultural Influences on African-American Attitudes Toward Death, Dying and Funeral Rites." In *Personal Care in an Impersonal World: A Multidimensional Look at Bereavement,* pp. 213–230. Edited by John D. Morgan. Amityville, N.Y.: Baywood.

BECK, KENNETH H. 1991. "Human Response to Threat." In *Horrendous Death, Health, and Well-Being,* pp. 31–47. Edited by Daniel Leviton. New York: Hemisphere.

BECKER, ERNEST. 1973. *The Denial of Death.* New York: Free Press.

BENOLIEL, JEANNE QUINT, ed. 1982. *Death Education of the Health Professional.* Washington, D.C.: Hemisphere.

BRODY, HOWARD. 1992. *The Healer's Power.* New Haven, Conn.: Yale University Press.

CALLAHAN, DANIEL. 1993. *The Troubled Dream of Life: Living with Mortality.* New York: Simon and Schuster.

FAMILY, GILLA. 1992–1993. "Projected Image and Observed Behaviors of Physicians in Terminal Cancer Care." *Omega* 26, no. 2:129–136.

FEIFEL, HERMAN. 1990. "Psychology and Death: Meaningful Rediscovery." *American Psychologist* 45, no. 4:437–543.

FLORIAN, VICTOR, and MIKULINCER, MARIO. 1992–1993. "The Impact of Death-Risk Experiences and Religiosity on the Fear of Personal Death: The Case of Israeli Soldiers in Lebanon." *Omega* 26, no. 21:101–110.

FULTON, ROBERT L., and OWEN, GREG. 1994. "Death in Contemporary American Society." In *Death and Identity.* 3d ed., pp. 12–27. Edited by Robert Fulton and Robert Bendiksen. Philadelphia: Charles.

GALLAGHER, DOLORES; LOVETT, STEVEN; HANLEY-DUNN, PATRICIA; and THOMPSON, LARRY W. 1989. "Use of Select Coping Strategies During Late-Life Spousal Bereavement." In *Older Bereaved Spouses: Research with Practical Applications,* pp. 111–121. Edited by Dale A. Lund. New York: Hemisphere.

HOBBES, THOMAS. 1968. [1651]. "The Leviathan." In *Philosophical Classics,* pp. 82–107. Edited by Walter Kauffman. Engelwood Cliffs, N.J.: Prentice Hall.

HOLCOMB, LAURA E.; NEIMEYER, ROBERT A.; and MOORE, MARLIN K. 1993. "Personal Meanings of Death: A Content Analysis of Free-Response Narratives." *Death Studies* 17, no. 4:299–318.

JAMES, WILLIAM. 1948. [1879]. "The Sentiment of Rationality." In *Essays in Pragmatism by William James,* pp. 3–36. Edited by Alburey Castell. New York: Hafner.

KASTENBAUM, ROBERT, and AISENBERG, RUTH. 1972. *The Psychology of Death.* New York: Springer.

KOWALSKI, N. CLAIRE. 1986. "Anticipating the Death of an Elderly Parent." In *Loss and Anticipatory Grief.* Edited by Therese A. Rando. Lexington, Mass.: Lexington.

LAMERS, WILLIAM M. 1990. "Hospice: Enhancing the Quality of Life." *Oncology* (May).

LEMING, MICHAEL R. 1979–1980. "Religion and Death: A Test of Homans' Thesis." *Omega* 10, no. 4:347–364.

LESTER, DAVID, AND BECKER, DEANNE M. 1992–1993. "College Students' Attitudes Toward Death Today as Compared to the 1930s." *Omega* 26, no. 3:219–222.

LEVITON, DANIEL, ed. 1991. *Horrendous Death, Health and Well-being.* New York: Hemisphere.

NAVARRO, VINCENTE. 1991. "The Class Gap." *Nation,* April 8, pp. 436–448.

PAPPAS, GREGORY; QUEEN, SUSAN; HADDEN, WILBUR; and FISHER, GAIL. 1993. "The Increasing Disparity in Mortality Between Socioeconomic Groups in the United States, 1960 and 1986." *New England Journal of Medicine* 329, no. 2:103–109.

PARSONS, TALCOTT; FOX, RENÉE C.; AND LIDZ, VICTOR M. 1972. "The Gift of Life." *Social Research* 39, no. 3:367–415.

RAMSDEM, PETER G. 1991. "Alice in the Afterlife: A Glimpse in the Mirror." In *Coping with the Final Tragedy: Cultural Variation in Dying and Grieving*, pp. 27–41. Edited by David R. Counts and Dorothy A. Counts. Amityville, N.Y.: Baywood.

RAMSEY, PAUL. 1970. *The Patient as Person: Explorations in Medical Ethics*. New Haven, Conn.: Yale University Press.

RANDO, THERESE A. 1992–1993. "The Increasing Prevalence of Complicated Mourning: The Onslaught Is Just Beginning." *Omega* 26, no. 1:43–60.

ROSS, LAWRENCE M., AND POLLIO, HOWARD R. 1991. "Metaphors of Death: A Thematic Analysis of Personal Meanings." *Omega* 23, no. 4:291–307.

UMBERTSON, DEBRA, and HENDERSON, KRISTIN. 1992. "The Social Construction of Death in the Gulf War." *Omega* 25, no. 1:1–150.

VACHON, MARY L. S. 1987. *Occupational Stress in the Care of the Critically Ill, the Dying, and the Bereaved*. New York: Hemisphere.

WEISMAN, AVERY. 1978. "An Appropriate Death." In *Death and Dying: Challenge and Change*, pp. 193–194. Edited by Robert L. Fulton, Eric Markusen, Greg Owen, and Jane L. Scheiber. Reading, Mass.: Addison-Wesley.

DEATH, DEFINITION AND DETERMINATION OF

I. Criteria for Death
   Ronald E. Cranford
II. Legal Issues in Pronouncing Death
   Alexander Morgan Capron
III. Philosophical and Theological Perspectives
   Karen Grandstrand Gervais

I. CRITERIA FOR DEATH

Prior to the middle of the twentieth century, there was no major dispute over the criteria for death. In the nineteenth century several isolated cases of premature burial from around the world did raise some alarm, and safeguards (e.g., coffins equipped with alarms) were established to minimize the possibility of this unfortunate practice. But concern about the accuracy of diagnosing death had largely abated by the turn of the twentieth century.

However, beginning with the advent of more effective artificial respirators in the 1940s, major technological breakthroughs in modern medicine raised serious questions about the traditional ways of diagnosing death. Prior to the widespread use of respirators, defibrillators, intensive-care units, and cardiopulmonary resuscitation, failure of cardiac, respiratory, and neurologic functions were closely linked. When one system

failed, the other two inevitably failed as well. But respirators and other advanced life-support systems can now sustain cardiac, respiratory, and other autonomic functions for prolonged periods of time even after neurologic functions have ceased.

Terminology

With the advent of these new technologies, neurological specialists became aware of some new neurologic syndromes, to which an array of confusing and inconsistent terms were applied.

Several landmark medical events stand out in the early days of these new neurologic syndromes. In 1959, the French first described the syndrome of brain death (*coma dépassé*) (Mollaret and Coulon); in 1968, a special committee of the Harvard Medical School formulated specific neurologic criteria to diagnose brain death ("The Definition of Irreversible Coma," 1968); and in 1972, Bryan Jennett of Scotland and Fred Plum of the United States first described and originated the term "persistent vegetative state," or PVS (Jennett and Plum). A variety of terms have been used to describe the medical syndrome of brain death: cerebral death, *coma dépassé*, and irreversible coma. Terms used as imprecise equivalents for the persistent vegetative state have included: apallic state, neocortical death, irreversible coma, and permanent unconsciousness. It also became necessary to distinguish these new neurologic syndromes from already common and well-accepted neurologic conditions, such as coma and dementia. Many newer terms—for example, persistent vegetative state—were used solely to describe the clinical condition. Others, like the apallic state or neocortical death, attempted to correlate the loss of neurologic functions with the underlying pathologic changes in the brain.

As of 1994, there are two different legal/philosophical positions about what it means to be dead in terms of brain functions. One, the whole-brain-oriented position, considers a person dead if there is an irreversible loss of all functions of the entire brain (brain death). The other, which is not currently law in any jurisdiction, would pronounce a person dead when there is an irreversible loss of higher brain functions (permanent unconsciousness).

Recent dilemmas surrounding these new syndromes, such as when it is appropriate to stop treatment and when death has occurred, have also raised fundamental questions about the meaning of such medical concepts as consciousness, awareness, self-awareness, voluntary interactions with the environment, purposeful movement, pain, and psychological and physical suffering.

Neurological specialists are achieving a much greater understanding of these syndromes and their similarities and differences, and are reaching some consensus on terminology. However, they have not reached universal agreement on several major issues primarily related to the persistent vegetative state. A historical example illustrates how difficult it can be to reach consensus on terminology. The Harvard Committee equated irreversible coma with brain death, as did many neurological specialists in the 1970s. Others, equally knowledgeable and experienced, equated irreversible coma with the persistent vegetative state. Still others used the term in a much broader fashion to denote any form of permanent unconsciousness. Since this term has gathered so many different and contradictory meanings, the only reasonable alternative among neurological specialists was to drop it entirely.

Traditional criteria

With all the controversy surrounding neurologic criteria for death, the traditional criteria related to heartbeat and breathing have remained largely unchanged and undisputed, except for the University of Pittsburgh Medical Center's program to take organs from certain patients as soon as possible after expected cardiopulmonary death (Lynn, 1993). No major legal or ethical concerns have been raised about the traditional criteria for death. Medical organizations around the world have not felt it necessary to establish specific clinical criteria for the diagnosis of death based on the irreversible loss of cardiac and respiratory functions. The medical consultants to the President's Commission for the Study of Ethical Problems in Medicine and Biomedical and Behavioral Research (President's Commission) recommended that the clinical examination disclose at least the absence of consciousness, heartbeat, and respiratory effort, and that irreversibility be established by persistent loss of these functions for an appropriate period of observation and trial of therapy ("Guidelines for the Determination of Death," 1981). But these consultants recommended no length of time for this period of observation.

Brain death

The neurologic syndrome of brain death has now been accepted by the medical profession as a distinct clinical entity that experienced clinicians can diagnose with an extremely high degree of certainty, and can usually easily distinguish from other neurologic syndromes. Brain death is defined as the irreversible cessation of all functions of the entire brain, including the brain stem. If the brain can be viewed simplistically as comprising two parts—the cerebral hemispheres (higher centers) and the brain stem (lower centers)—then brain death is the destruction of the entire brain, both the cerebral hemispheres and the brain stem. In contrast, in the permanent vegetative state, the cerebral hemispheres are

extensively and permanently damaged, but the brain stem is relatively intact (Cranford, 1988).

An understanding of the pathologic sequence of events that leads to brain death is essential to appreciate fully why brain death is such a unique syndrome and why it can be readily differentiated from other neurologic syndromes with such a high degree of certainty. Although a variety of insults can cause the brain to die, head trauma, cardiorespiratory failure, and intracerebral hemorrhage are the most common causes. Whatever the underlying cause, the pathologic sequence is essentially the same in almost all cases. The acute massive insult to the brain causes brain swelling (cerebral edema). Since the brain is contained within an enclosed cavity, this brain swelling gives rise to a massive increase in intracranial pressure. In brain death, this increased intracranial pressure becomes so great that it exceeds the systolic blood pressure, thus causing a loss of blood flow to both the cerebral hemispheres and the brain stem. Whatever the primary cause of brain death, this end result of loss of blood flow results in massive destruction of the entire brain. This sequence of events usually occurs within a matter of hours after the primary event, so that brain death can be diagnosed within a short period of time with an extraordinarily high degree of certainty.

The loss of both cerebral hemisphere and brain stem functions is usually quite evident to the experienced clinician from the clinical bedside exam. The patient is in a coma—the deepest possible coma, a sleeplike state associated with a loss of all brain stem functions such as pupillary reaction to light; gag, swallowing, and cough reflexes; eye movements in response to passive head turning (oculocephalic response) and in response to cold caloric stimulation (oculovestibular response); and spontaneous respiratory efforts. However, while respirations are completely dependent upon the functioning of the brain stem, cardiac function can continue independent of brain destruction, since the heart has an independent mechanism for spontaneously firing (semiautonomous functioning). With modern life-support systems, continued cardiac and blood pressure functions can persist for hours, days, or even longer. Extremely rare cases of continued cardiovascular functions for over a year in the presence of a loss of all brain functions have been reported.

In the 1970s and 1980s, numerous medical organizations in the United States and around the world developed specific medical criteria for the diagnosis of brain death (Bernat, 1991). In the United States, major criteria were published by Harvard University, the University of Minnesota, the National Institutes of Health, Cornell University, and the President's Commission. Major international criteria emerged from Sweden, Japan, the United Kingdom, and Canada. All these standards essentially agreed on three clinical findings: coma, apnea (loss of spontaneous respirations), and absence of brain stem reflexes.

The critical issue distinguishing these international criteria was not the clinical findings, but how best to establish irreversibility. The United Kingdom, deemphasizing the use of laboratory studies such as electroencephalography, focused on the basic diagnosis as clinical and asserted that the best way to establish irreversibility was to preclude any reversible processes prior to a final determination of brain death (Conference of Royal Colleges, 1976). Reversible processes that could mimic brain death include a variety of sedative medications and hypothermia (low body temperature—below 32.2° C). The British also recommended a period of observation of at least twelve hours. In contrast, the Swedish criteria focused less on the period of observation and more on the need for definitive laboratory studies to document a loss of blood flow to the brain, as with intracranial angiography. In the United States, the earlier standards emphasized the use of electroencephalography to establish electrocerebral silence (a loss of all electrical activity of the brain); more recent standards focused on establishing a loss of intracranial circulation by means of radioisotope angiography. The 1981 report of the medical consultants to the President's Commission, which became the definitive medical standard in the United States, recommended a period of observation of at least six hours when combined with a confirmatory study, such as tests measuring intracranial circulation ("Guidelines for the Determination of Death," 1981). If no confirmatory laboratory studies were performed, then an observation period of at least twelve hours was suggested—assuming that all reversible causes of loss of brain functions had been excluded. In cases of damage to the brain caused by the lack of blood or oxygen (hypoxic-ischemic encephalopathy), the consultants recommended an observation period of at least twenty-four hours if confirmatory studies were not performed.

The diagnosis of brain death in newborns, infants, and children is often more difficult than in adults. A major reason for this difficulty is that the usual pathologic sequence of events in adults, leading to increased intracranial pressure and loss of all blood flow to the brain, does not apply to the newborn and infant because the cranial cavity has not yet closed completely. Thus, the mechanism for brain death in newborns and infants may be different than it is in older children and adults.

To address this question, a task force for the determination of brain death in children representing several neurological and pediatric specialty organizations in the United States developed specific diagnostic criteria in the younger age groups (Task Force for the Determination of Brain Death in Children, 1987). This task force stated that it would be extremely difficult to establish brain death in newborns less than seven days old. The

task force recommended that in infants seven days to two months of age, there should be two separate clinical examinations and two electroencephalograms separated by at least forty-eight hours; for infants two months to one year of age, two clinical examinations and two electroencephalograms separated by at least twenty-four hours; and for children over one year in age, criteria similar to those established in adults.

Permanent unconsciousness

The syndromes of permanent unconsciousness include two major types. The first is a permanent coma: an eyes-closed, sleeplike, unarousable unconsciousness. The second is the permanent vegetative state: an eyes-open, wakeful unconsciousness (U.S. President's Commission, 1993). This article takes no position on the ethical and legal issues involved in choosing between the whole-brain and higher-brain formulations of death, but describes the neurologic syndromes of permanent unconsciousness that would be considered the medical basis for the higher-brain formulation of death.

A permanent coma is an uncommon neurologic syndrome because most patients with damage sufficient to cause brain stem impairment resulting in permanent coma die soon—either naturally or because decisions are made to discontinue treatment due to the poor prognosis. Cases of prolonged (more than a few weeks) permanent coma do occur but are extremely uncommon.

The vegetative state has three major classes, depending on the temporal profile of the onset and progression of the brain damage. The first is the acute vegetative state. This occurs when the onset of brain damage is sudden and severe, such as with head trauma (traumatic vegetative state) or loss of blood flow to the brain caused by sudden cardiorespiratory insufficiencies (hypoxic-ischemic vegetative state). The second is the degenerative, or metabolic, vegetative state, where the brain damage begins gradually and progresses slowly over a period of months to years. In adults, the most common form of the degenerative vegetative state is the final stage of Alzheimer's disease, whereas in children it is the final stage of a variety of degenerative and metabolic diseases of childhood. The third form is the congenital vegetative state, secondary to a variety of severe congenital malformations of the brain present at birth, such as anencephaly.

The vegetative state is considered persistent when it is present longer than one month in the acute form, and permanent when the condition becomes irreversible. The exact prevalence is unknown, but it is estimated that in the United States there are approximately 10,000–25,000 adults and 4,000–10,000 children in a vegetative state (Multisociety Task Force on PVS, 1994). This syndrome—when it becomes permanent—

is the major neurologic condition that is the prototype for the higher-brain formulation of death.

Vegetative state

The vegetative state is characterized by the loss of all higher brain functions, with relative sparing of brain stem functions. Because brain stem functions are still present, the arousal mechanisms contained in the brain stem are relatively intact, and therefore the patient is not in a coma. The patient has sleep/wake cycles but at no time manifests any signs of consciousness, awareness, voluntary interaction with the environment, or purposeful movements. Thus, the patient can be awake but is always unaware—a mindless wakefulness.

Unlike brain death, where the pathology and sequence of changes are relatively uniform regardless of the primary cause of the brain damage, the pathologic changes in the vegetative state vary substantially with the cause of the unconsciousness. While there is a variety of causes, the two most common causes of the acute form are head trauma and hypoxic-ischemic encephalopathy. In head trauma, the major damage is due to tearing injuries to the subcortical white matter (the fiber tracts connecting the cell bodies of the cerebral cortex with the rest of the brain) of the cerebral hemispheres. With hypoxic-ischemic encephalopathy, the primary damage is to the neurons themselves in the cerebral cortex. These different patterns of brain damage are important for several reasons, among them that the chances for recovery of neurologic functions and the time necessary to establish irreversibility vary according to the underlying cause.

For patients—adults and children—in an hypoxic-ischemic vegetative state longer than three months, the prognosis for recovery is uniformly dismal. The vast majority who recover and do well after an hypoxic-ischemic insult to the brain are those who have regained consciousness in the first three months. For adults in a traumatic vegetative state, the majority who do well will usually have regained consciousness within six months of the injury. The prognosis for recovery of children in a traumatic vegetative state is slightly more favorable than for adults (Council on Scientific Affairs and Council on Ethical and Judicial Affairs, 1990). However, in both children and adults, a period of observation of at least twelve months may be appropriate before establishing permanency (The Multi-Society Task Force on PVS, 1994).

While specific medical criteria have been established for brain death by numerous organizations around the world, no comparable criteria have been established for the diagnosis of the vegetative state. It is unlikely that any criteria as specific as those for brain death will be formulated in the near future, because the diagnosis of the vegetative state is not nearly as precise and definitive. The determination of irreversibility in brain death usually takes hours and does not vary according to etiology, whereas it may take months to establish irreversibility in the permanent vegetative state, and the time necessary to establish this irreversibility varies substantially with cause and age (Institute of Medical Ethics Working Party, 1991).

Because all vegetative state patients are unconscious, they are unable to experience suffering of any kind—psychological or physical. These patients normally manifest periods of eyes opening and closing with accompanying sleep/wake cycles. They also may demonstrate a variety of facial expressions and eye movements that originate from the lower centers of the brain and do not indicate consciousness. They may appear at times to smile and grimace, but observation over prolonged periods of time reveals no evidence either of voluntary interaction with the environment or of self-awareness (Executive Board, American Academy of Neurology, 1989). Neuroimaging studies, such as computerized axial tomography (CAT) and magnetic resonance imaging (MRI), may be helpful in establishing the severity and irreversibility of the brain damage. After several months in a vegetative state, the brain begins to show progressive shrinkage (atrophy), primarily of the cerebral hemispheres. The loss of consciousness and the inability to experience suffering, established on the basis of clinical observations, have been supported by measuring metabolism of glucose and oxygen at the level of the cerebral cortex by positron emission tomography (PET) scanning. These studies have shown a 50–60 percent decrease in cerebral cortical metabolism, a level consistent with unconsciousness and deep anesthesia (Levy et al., 1987).

Long-term survival of vegetative state patients at all ages is drastically reduced compared to the normal population. Life expectancy in adult patients is generally about two to five years; the vast majority will not live longer than ten years. In elderly patients, the prognosis for survival is even worse; many do not survive for more than a few months. Infants and children may survive longer than adults, but probably not significantly so. Some studies have shown the average life expectancy to be four years for infants up to two months of age, and about seven years for children seven to eighteen years old (Ashwal et al., 1992). Cases of prolonged survival—longer than twenty years—have been reported but are rare. The longest reported survivor is in her forty-second year in the vegetative state; another patient lived for 37 years and 111 days without regaining consciousness. Considering the total estimated number of patients in a persistent vegetative state, and the small number of well-documented cases of survival beyond fifteen years, the probability of an individual patient having such a prolonged survival is extremely low, probably less than 1/15,000 to 1/75,000 (The Multi-society Task Force on PVS, 1994).

The diagnosis of the vegetative state in newborns and infants is more difficult to make. Generally the diagnosis cannot be made below the age of three months, except for the condition of anencephaly. Anencephaly is the congenital malformation form of the permanent vegetative state (Stumpf et al., 1990). This extensive and severe congenital malformation of the brain can be diagnosed with an extraordinarily high degree of certainty. At birth, it is readily apparent by visual observation alone that the child has only rudimentary cerebral hemispheres and no skull except in the rear of the head. These children have variable degrees of brain stem functions but usually not enough functions to sustain life for any period of time. The vast majority are dead within two months, most within a few weeks.

Conclusion

The criteria for diagnosing cardiorespiratory death and brain death have now been well established and accepted by the medical profession. Even though there are differences in how physicians may apply these criteria in individual cases, and the standards around the world may vary somewhat, there are no major disputes about the medical diagnosis itself.

The syndromes of permanent unconsciousness, on the other hand, are much more variable than those of brain death. The three major forms of the vegetative state—acute, degenerative, and congenital—are substantially different in terms of causes, type of brain damage, and length of time necessary to establish irreversibility. Thus, the criteria for a higher-brain formulation of death are far more complex and uncertain than those for the whole-brain formulation of death.

RONALD E. CRANFORD

Directly related to this article are the other articles in this entry: LEGAL ISSUES IN PRONOUNCING DEATH, *and* PHILOSOPHICAL AND THEOLOGICAL PERSPECTIVES. *For a further discussion of topics mentioned in this article, see the entry* DEATH. *This article will find application in the entries* INFANTS, *article on* MEDICAL ASPECTS AND ISSUES IN THE CARE OF INFANTS; *and* ORGAN AND TISSUE PROCUREMENT, *especially the article on* ETHICAL AND LEGAL ISSUES REGARDING CADAVERS. *For a discussion of related topics, see the entries* LIFE; PAIN AND SUFFERING; PERSON; *and* UTILITY.

Bibliography

ASHWAL, STEPHEN; BALE, JAMES F., JR.; COULTER, DAVID L.; EIBEN, ROBERT; GARG, BHUWAN P.; HILL, ALAN; MYER, EDWIN C.; NORDGREN, RICHARD E.; SHEWMON, D. ALAN; SUNDER, THEODORE R.; and WALKER, RUSSELL W. 1992. "The Persistent Vegetative State in Children: Report of the Child Neurology Society Ethics Committee." *Annals of Neurology* 32, no. 4:570–576.

BERNAT, JAMES L. 1991. "Ethical Issues in Neurology." In *Clinical Neurology,* pp. 1–105. Edited by Robert J. Joynt. Philadelphia: J.B. Lippincott.

CONFERENCE OF ROYAL COLLEGES AND FACULTIES OF THE UNITED KINGDOM. 1976. "Diagnosis of Brain Death." *Lancet* 2:1069–1070.

COUNCIL ON SCIENTIFIC AFFAIRS AND COUNCIL ON ETHICAL AND JUDICIAL AFFAIRS, AMERICAN MEDICAL ASSOCIATION. 1990. "Persistent Vegetative State and the Decision to Withdraw or Withhold Life-Support." *Journal of the American Medical Association* 263, no. 3:426–430.

CRANFORD, RONALD E. 1988. "The Persistent Vegetative State: Getting the Facts Straight (The Medical Reality)." *Hastings Center Report* 18:27–32.

"The Definition of Irreversible Coma: Report of the Ad Hoc Committee of the Harvard Medical School to Examine the Definition of Brain Death." 1968. *Journal of the American Medical Association* 205, no. 6:337–340.

EXECUTIVE BOARD, AMERICAN ACADEMY OF NEUROLOGY. 1989. "Position of the American Academy of Neurology on Certain Aspects of the Care and Management of the Persistent Vegetative State Patient." *Neurology* 39, no. 1:125–126.

"Guidelines for the Determination of Death: Report of the Medical Consultants on the Diagnosis of Death to the U.S. President's Commission for the Study of Ethical Problems in Medicine and Biomedical and Behavioral Research." 1981. *Journal of the American Medical Association* 246, no. 19:2184–2186.

INSTITUTE OF MEDICAL ETHICS WORKING PARTY ON THE ETHICS OF PROLONGING LIFE AND ASSISTING DEATH. 1991. "Withdrawal of Life-Support from Patients in a Persistent Vegetative State." *Lancet* 337, no. 8733:96–98.

JENNETT, BRYAN, and PLUM, FRED. 1972. "Persistent Vegetative State After Brain Damage: A Syndrome in Search of a Name." *Lancet* 1, no. 7753:734–737.

LEVY, DAVID E.; SIDTIS, JOHN J.; ROTTENBERG, DAVID A.; JARDEN, JENS O.; STROTHER, STEPHEN C.; DHAWAN, VIJAY; GINOS, JAMES Z.; TRAMO, MARK J.; EVANS, ALAN C.; and PLUM, FRED. 1987. "Differences in Cerebral Blood Flow and Glucose Utilization in Vegetative Versus Locked-in Patients." *Annals of Neurology* 22, no. 6:673–682.

LYNN, JOANNE. 1993. "Are the Patients Who Become Organ Donors Under the Pittsburgh Protocol for 'Non-Heart Beating Donors' Really Dead?" *Kennedy Institute of Ethics Journal* 3, no. 2:167–178.

MOLLARET, PIERRE, and COULON, M. 1959. "Le Coma dépassé." *Revue Neurologique* 101:5–15.

The Multi-Society Task Force on PVS (American Academy of Neurology, Child Neurology Society, American Neurological Association, American Association of Neurological Surgeons, American Academy of Pediatrics). 1994. "Medical Aspects of the Persistent Vegetative State. *New England Journal of Medicine* 330, no. 2:1499–1508, 1572–1579.

Stumpf, David A.; Cranford, Ronald E.; Elias, Sherman; Fost, Norman C.; McQuillen, Michael P.; Meyer, Edwin C.; Poland, Ronald; and Queenan, John T. 1990. "The Infant with Anencephaly." *New England Journal of Medicine* 322, no. 10:669–674.

Task Force for the Determination of Brain Death in Children (American Academy of Neurology, American Academy of Pediatrics, American Neurological Association, Child Neurology Society). 1987. "Guidelines for the Determination of Brain Death in Children." *Neurology* 37, no. 6:1077–1078.

U.S. President's Commission for the Study of Ethical Problems in Medicine and Biomedical and Behavioral Research. 1983. *Deciding to Forego Life-Sustaining Treatment: Ethical, Medical, and Legal Issues in Treatment Decisions.* Washington, D.C.: U.S. Government Printing Office.

II. LEGAL ISSUES IN PRONOUNCING DEATH

The following is a revision and update of the first-edition article "Death, Definition and Determination of, II. Legal Aspects of Pronouncing Death" by the same author.

The capability of biomedicine to sustain vital human functions artificially has created problems for the public and its legal institutions as well as for medical practitioners. In some cases, determining that people have died is no longer the relatively simple matter of ascertaining that their heart and lungs have stopped functioning. Mechanical respirators, electronic pacemakers, and drugs that stimulate functioning and affect blood pressure can create the appearance of circulation and respiration in what is otherwise a corpse. The general public probably first realized that public policy concerning when and how death could be declared needed to be changed when Christiaan Barnard performed the first human-to-human heart transplant in Cape Town, South Africa, on December 3, 1967. Beyond amazement at the technical feat, many people were astonished that a heart taken from a woman who had been declared dead conferred life on a man whose own heart had been removed.

Cardiac transplantation provides the most dramatic illustration of the need for clear standards to classify the outcomes of intensive medical support (e.g., respirators). But only a handful of the moribund, unconscious patients maintained through intensive support long after they formerly would have ceased living become organ donors (U.S. President's Commission, 1981). Sometimes such medical intervention is ended because it has succeeded in enabling the patient to recover; sometimes it is terminated because the patient's bodily systems have collapsed so totally that circulation and respiration cannot be maintained. But for a significant number of patients, artificial support could be continued indefinitely with no prospect that consciousness would ever return. For some of this latter group of patients—especially those who can eventually be weaned from the respirator and require only nutrition and hydration by tube—the question arises whether to withdraw treatment and allow death to occur. But for others who have suffered great brain damage, the need arises to recognize that death has occurred and that further attempts to keep the patient alive are therefore no longer appropriate even before the point (usually within several weeks) at which it becomes impossible to maintain physiological processes in the body.

Beginning in the 1960s, the response of the medical profession was to develop new criteria, such as those articulated in 1968 by an ad hoc committee at Harvard Medical School. Experts in the United States tend to rely on certain clinical signs of the absence of any activity in the entire brain (Ad Hoc Committee, 1968); British neurologists focus on the loss of functioning in the brain stem, while doctors in certain European countries search for conditions for brain function, such as intracranial blood circulation (Van Till, 1975). Despite differences in technique, the medical profession arrived at a consensus that the total and irreversible absence of brain function is equivalent to the traditional cardio-respiratory indicators of death (Medical Consultants, 1981).

The story of the law's response to these new medical criteria can be divided into three parts. The first, largely played out in the late 1960s and the 1970s, concerned an issue of process—how ought society respond to the divergence between new medical precepts and practices, on the one hand, and the common understanding of the lay public of rules embodied in custom and law, on the other? (Anglo-American common law, for example, had traditionally defined death as the total cessation of all vital functions.) The second phase, from the 1970s through the 1980s, centered on the specific changes that should be made in the law. In the third period, which is still continuing, commentators (principally philosophers and a few physicians) have raised questions about the appropriateness of the legal standards that have been adopted and call for various changes in those standards.

Phase one: Framing definitions

A medical matter? A number of routes were advanced for arriving at what was often termed a new definition of death that would encompass the neurological understanding of the phenomenon of death that emerged in the 1960s and has since been further refined. (The commonly employed phrase "definition of death" is useful shorthand, but should not be taken to mean the explanation of a fact but rather a choice about the significance of certain facts in the task of determining whether, and when, a person has died.) Early commentators proposed that the task should be left to physicians, because the subject is technical and because the law might set the definition prematurely, leading to conflicts with developments that will inevitably occur in medical techniques (Kennedy, 1971). Yet the belief that defining death is wholly a medical matter misapprehends the undertaking. At issue is not a biological understanding of the inherent nature of cells or organ systems but a social formulation of humanhood. It is largely through its declaration of the points at which life begins and ends that a society determines who is a full human being, with the resulting rights and responsibilities.

Since physicians have no special competence on the philosophical issue of the nature of human beings and no special authority to arrogate the choice among definitions to themselves, their role is properly one of elucidating the significance of various vital signs. By the 1970s, it became apparent that a new definition should be forthcoming, not simply to accommodate biomedical practitioners' wishes but as a result of perceived social need and of evidence that tests for brain function were as reliable as the traditional heart-lung tests.

Judicial decisions?   If not physicians, then who should frame the definition? One answer was, "Let the courts decide." In the United States and other common-law countries, law is to be found not only on the statute books but in the rules enunciated by judges as they resolve disputes in individual civil and criminal cases. Facing a factual situation that does not fit comfortably within the existing legal rules, a court may choose to formulate a new rule in order to more accurately reflect current scientific understanding and social viewpoints.

Nonetheless, problems of principle and practicality emerged in placing primary reliance on the courts for a redefinition of death. Like the medical profession, the judiciary may be too narrowly based for the task. While the judiciary is an organ of the state with recognized authority in public matters, it still has no means for actively involving the public in its decision-making processes. Judge-made law has been most successful in factual settings embedded in well-defined social and economic practices, with the guidance of past decisions and commentary. Courts operate within a limited compass—the facts and contentions of a particular case—and with limited expertise; they have neither the staff nor the authority to investigate or to conduct hearings in order to explore such issues as public opinion or the scientific merits of competing "definitions." Consequently, a judge's decision may be merely a rubber-stamping of the

opinions expressed by the medical experts who appeared in court. Moreover, testimony in an adversary proceeding is usually restricted to the "two sides" of a particular issue and may not fairly represent the spectrum of opinion held by authorities in the field.

Furthermore, in the U.S. cases in which parties first argued for a redefinition, the courts were unwilling to disturb the existing legal definition. Such deference to precedent is understandable, because people need to be able to rely on predictable legal rules in managing their affairs. As late as 1968, a California appellate tribunal, in a case involving an inheritorship issue, declined to redefine death in terms of brain functioning despite the admittedly anachronistic nature of an exclusively heart-lung definition (Cate and Capron, 1992).

The unfortunate consequences for physicians and patients of the unsettled state of the common-law definition of death in the 1970s is illustrated by several cases. In the first, *Tucker v. Lower,* which came to trial in Virginia in 1972, the brother of a man whose heart was taken in an early transplant operation sued the physicians, alleging that the operation was begun before the donor had died. The evidence showed that the donor's pulse, blood pressure, respiration, and other vital signs were normal but that he had been declared dead when the physicians decided these signs resulted solely from medical efforts and not from his own functioning, since his brain functions had ceased. The trial judge initially indicated that he would adhere to the traditional definition of death; but he later permitted the jurors to find that death had occurred when the brain ceased functioning irreversibly, and a verdict was returned for the defendants. However, since the court did not explain its action, the law was not clarified.

The other two cases arose in California in 1974, when two transplant operations were performed using hearts removed from the victims of alleged crimes. The defendant in each case, charged with homicide, attempted to interpose the action of the surgeons in removing the victim's still-beating heart as a complete defense to the charge. One trial judge accepted this argument as being compelled by the existing definition of death, but his ruling was reversed on appeal, and both defendants were eventually convicted. This graphic illustration of legal confusion and uncertainty led California to join several other jurisdictions in the United States, Canada, and Australia that, beginning in 1970, followed a third route to redefining death, the adoption of a statutory definition.

Statutory standards?   The legislative process allows a wider range of information to enter into the framing of standards for determining death, as well as offering an avenue for participation of the public. That is important because basic and perhaps controversial choices among alternative definitions must be made. Because they provide prospective guidance, statutory standards have the additional advantage of dispelling public and professional doubt, thereby reducing both the fear and the likelihood of cases against physicians for malpractice or homicide.

Not all countries have adopted legislation. In Great Britain, for example, rather than a statute, the standards for determining death reside in medically promulgated codes of practice, which have been indirectly accepted in several judicial decisions (Kennedy and Grubb, 1989). Yet in the United States and among most commentators internationally, the first period in policymaking on a new definition of death produced wide agreement that an official response was necessary in light of the changes wrought by medical science, and that this response ought to be statutory. By 1979 four model statutes had been proposed in the United States; in addition to those from the American Bar Association (ABA), the American Medical Association (AMA), and the National Conference of Commissioners of Uniform State Laws (NCCUSL), the most widely adopted was the Capron–Kass proposal, which grew out of the work of a research group at the Hastings Center (U.S. President's Commission, 1981). Ironically, the major barrier to legislation became the very multiplicity of proposals; though they were consistent in their aims, their sponsors tended to lobby for their own bills, which in turn produced apprehension among legislators over the possible importance of the bills' verbal differences. Accordingly, the President's Commission worked with the three major sponsors—the ABA, the AMA, and the NCCUSL—to draft a single model bill that could be proposed for adoption in all jurisdictions. The resulting statute—the Uniform Determination of Death Act—was proposed in 1981 and is now law in more than half of U.S. jurisdictions, while virtually all the rest have some other, essentially similar statute. In four states the law consists of a decision by the highest court recognizing cessation of all functions of the brain as one means of determining death (Cate and Capron, 1992).

Phase two: The contours of a statute

The Uniform Determination of Death Act (UDDA) provides that an individual who has sustained either (1) irreversible cessation of circulatory and respiratory functions, or (2) irreversible cessation of all functions of the entire brain, including the brain stem, is dead. A determination of death must be made in accordance with accepted medical standards. This statute is guided by several principles. First, the phenomenon of interest to physicians, legislators, and the public alike is a human being's death, not the "death" of his or her cells, tissues, or organs. Indeed, one problem with the term "brain death" is that it wrongly suggests that an organ can die;

organisms die, but organs cease functioning. Second, a statute on death will resolve the problem of whether to continue artificial support in only some of the cases of comatose patients. Additional guidance has been developed by courts and legislatures as well as by professional bodies concerning the cessation of treatment in patients who are alive by brain or heart-lung criteria, but for whom further treatment is considered (by the patients or by others) to be pointless or degrading. This question of "when to allow to die" is distinct from "when to declare dead."

Third, the merits of a legislative definition are judged by whether its purposes are properly defined and how well the legislation meets those purposes. In addition to its cultural and religious importance, a definition of death is needed to resolve a number of legal issues (besides deciding whether to terminate medical care or transplant organs) such as homicide, damages for the wrongful death of a person, property and wealth transmission, insurance, taxes, and marital status. While some commentators have argued that a single definition is inappropriate because different policy objectives might exist in different contexts, it has been generally agreed that a single definition of death is capable of being applied in a wide variety of contexts, as indeed was the traditional heart-lung definition. Having a single definition to be used for many purposes does not preclude relying on other events besides death as a trigger for some decisions. Most jurisdictions make provision, for example, for the distribution of property and the termination of marriage after a person has been absent without explanation for a period of years, even though a person "presumed dead" under such a law could not be treated as a corpse were he or she actually still alive (Capron, 1973).

Fourth, although dying is a process (since not all parts of the body cease functioning equally and synchronously), a line can and must be drawn between those who are alive and those who are dead (Kass, 1971). The ability of modern biomedicine to extend the functioning of various organ systems may have made knowing which side of the line a patient is on more problematic, but it has not erased the line. The line drawn by the UDDA is an arbitrary one in the sense that it results from human choice among a number of possibilities, but not in the sense of having no acceptable, articulated rationale.

Fifth, legislated standards must be uniform for all persons. It is, to say the least, unseemly for a person's wealth or potential social utility as an organ donor to affect the way in which the moment of his or her death is determined. One jurisdiction, in an attempt to accommodate religious and cultural diversity, has departed from the general objective of uniformity in the standards for determining death. In 1991, New Jersey adopted a statute that allows people whose religious beliefs would be violated by the use of whole-brain criteria to have their deaths declared solely on the traditional cardio-respiratory basis (New Jersey Commission, 1991).

Sixth, the UDDA was framed on the premise that it is often beneficial for the law to move incrementally, particularly when matters of basic cultural and ethical values are implicated. Thus, the statute provides a modern restatement of the traditional understanding of death that ties together the accepted cardiopulmonary standard with a new brain-based standard that measures the same phenomenon.

Finally, in making law in a highly technological area, care is needed that the definition be at once sufficiently precise to determine behavior in the manner desired by the public and yet not so specific that it is tied to the details of contemporary technology. The UDDA achieves this flexible precision by confining itself to the general standards by which death is to be determined. It leaves to the developing judgment of biomedical practitioners the establishment and application of appropriate criteria and specific tests for determining that the standards have been met. To provide a contemporary statement of "accepted medical standards," the U.S. President's Commission assembled a group of leading neurologists, neurosurgeons, pediatricians, anesthesiologists, and other authorities on determination of death (Medical Consultants, 1981). Their guidelines, which provide the basis for the clinical methodology used in most American institutions, have since been supplemented by special guidance regarding children (Task Force, 1987).

Phase three: The continuing points of debate

As a practical matter, the law nearly everywhere (the major exception being Japan) now recognizes that death may be diagnosed based upon the determination that the brain as a whole has ceased functioning. In the United States, this consensus is embodied in the UDDA, which has therefore become the focus of criticism from certain people—principally some philosophers, but also physicians and lawyers—who are not comfortable with this consensus. Their objections can be summarized in three challenges to the UDDA.

Whole-brain versus higher-brain death. The strongest position against the UDDA is mounted by those who would substitute for its "whole brain" standard a "higher brain" standard. Many philosophers have argued that certain features of consciousness (or at least the potential for consciousness) are essential to being a person as distinct from merely a human being (Veatch, 1976; Zaner, 1988). The absence of consciousness and cognition—as occurs, for example, in patients in the permanent vegetative state (PVS)—thus results in the

loss of personhood. A related argument rests on the ontological proposition that the meaning of being a person—that is, a particular individual—is to have a personal identity, which depends on continuity of personal history as well as on self-awareness. The permanent loss of consciousness destroys such identity and hence means the death of that person, even if the body persists.

Consideration of the implications of these theories for determination of death takes several forms. On a conceptual level, the specific characteristics deemed by philosophers to be essential for personhood have varied widely from John Locke's focus on self-awareness to Immanuel Kant's requirement of a capacity for rational moral agency (Lizza, 1993). Thus, while certain definitions would exclude only those who lack any capacity for self-knowledge, such as PVS (persistent vegetative state) patients, other conceptions would encompass senile or severely retarded patients who cannot synthesize experience or act on moral principles.

On a practical level, trying to base a definition of death on cessation of higher-brain functions creates at least two problems. The first is the absence of agreed-upon clinical tests for cessation of these functions. Although certain clinical conditions such as PVS that involve the loss of neocortical functioning when brainstem functions persist can be determined sufficiently reliably for prognostic purposes (such as when deciding that further treatment is no longer in the best interests of a dying patient), the greater complexity and uncertainty that remain prevent testing with the same degree of accuracy as with the whole-brain standards. The practical problems increase enormously if the higher-brain definition is grounded on loss of personhood or personal identity, because loss of such a characteristic is not associated with particular neurologic structures.

More fundamentally, patients who are found to have lost (or never to have had) personhood because they lack higher-brain functions, or because they no longer have the same personal identity, will still be breathing spontaneously if they do not also meet whole-brain standards such as those of the UDDA. While such entities may no longer be "persons," they are still living bodies as "living" is generally understood and commonly used. "Death can be applied directly only to biological organisms and not to persons" (Culver and Gert, 1982, p. 183). To regard a human being who lacks only cerebral functions as dead would lead either to burying spontaneously respiring bodies or to having first to take affirmative steps, such as those used in active euthanasia, to end breathing, circulation, and the like. Neither of these would comport with the practices or beliefs of most people despite widespread agreement that such bodies, especially those that have permanently lost consciousness, lack distinctive human characteristics and need not be sustained through further medical interventions. Perhaps for this reason, in proposing a statute that would base death on cessation of cerebral functions, Robert Veatch condones allowing persons, while still competent, or their next of kin to opt out of having their death determined on the higher-brain standard (Veatch, 1976). No state has adopted a "conscience clause" of this type, and the New Jersey statute mentioned above does not endorse the higher-brain standard (Olick, 1991).

The major legal evaluation of the higher-brain standard has arisen in the context of infant organ transplantation because of several highly publicized attempts in the 1980s to transplant organs from anencephalic infants (babies born without a neocortex and with the tops of their skulls open, exposing the underlying tissue). In 1987–1988, Loma Linda Medical Center in California mounted a protocol (a formal plan for conducting research) to obtain more organs, particularly hearts, from this source. The protocol took two forms. At first, the anencephalic infants were placed on respirators shortly after birth; but such infants did not lose functions and die within the two-week period the physicians had set, based on historical experience that virtually all anencephalics expire within two weeks of birth. In the second phase of the protocol, the physicians delayed the use of life support until the infants had begun experiencing apnea (cessation of breathing). Yet by the time death could be diagnosed neurologically in these infants, the damage to other organs besides the brain was so great as to render the organs useless. No organs were transplanted under the Loma Linda protocol.

Proposals to modify either the determination of death or the organ-transplant statutes to permit the use of organs from anencephalic infants before they meet the general criteria for death have not been approved by any legislature, nor was the Florida Supreme Court persuaded to change the law in the only appellate case regarding anencephalic organ donation. In that case, the parents of a child prenatally diagnosed with anencephaly requested that she be regarded as dead from the moment of birth so that her organs could be donated without waiting for breathing and heartbeat to cease. The Florida statute limits brain-based determinations of death to patients on artificial support. Turning to the common law, the court held that it established the cardiopulmonary standard, and the court then declined to create a judicial standard of death for anencephalics in the absence of a "public necessity" for doing so or any medical consensus that such a step would be good public policy (T.A.C.P., 1992).

Although the Loma Linda protocol for using anencephalic infants as organ sources attempted to comply with the general consensus on death determination, it also proved that the "slippery slope" is not merely a hypothetical possibility. While the program was ongoing and receiving a great deal of media attention, the neonatologist who ran the pediatric intensive-care unit where potential donors were cared for reported receiving offers from well-meaning physicians of infants with hydrocephalus, intraventricular hemorrhage, and severe congenital anomalies. These physicians found it difficult to accept Loma Linda's rejection of such infants, whom the referring physicians saw as comparable on relevant grounds to the anencephalic infants who had been accepted. Beyond the risk of error in diagnosing anencephaly, it is hard to draw a line at this one condition, since the salient criteria—absence of higher-brain function and limited life expectancy—apply to other persons as well. The criterion that really moves many people—namely, the gross physical deformity of anencephalic infants' skulls—is without moral significance. Thus, a decision to accept anencephaly as a basis for declaring death would imply acceptance of some perhaps undefined higher-brain standard for diagnosing any and all patients.

Changing clinical criteria. Some medical commentators have suggested that the society should rethink brain death because studies of bodies determined to be dead on neurological grounds have shown results that fail to accord with the standard of "irreversible loss of all functions of the entire brain" (Truog and Fackler, 1992). Specifically, some of these patients still have hypothalamic-endocrine function, cerebral electrical activity, or responsiveness to the environment.

Although the technical aspects of these various findings differ, similar reasoning can be applied to assessing their meaning for the concept of brain death. For each, one must ask first, are such findings observed among patients diagnosed through cardiopulmonary as well as neurological means of diagnosing death? Second, are such findings inconsistent with the irreversible loss of integrative functioning of the organism? Finally, do such findings relate to functions that when lost do not return and are not replaceable?

If some patients diagnosed dead on heart-lung grounds also have hypothalamic-endocrine function, cerebral electrical activity, or environmental responses, then the presence of these findings in neurologically diagnosed patients would not be cause for concern that the clinical criteria for the latter groups are inaccurate, and no redefinition would be needed.

Plainly, in many dead bodies some activity (as opposed to full functions) remains temporarily within parts of the brain. The question then becomes, for example, whether the secretion of a particular hormone (such as arginine vasopressin, which stimulates the contraction of capillaries and arterioles) is so physiologically integrative that it must be irreversibly absent for death to be declared. Depending upon the answer, it might be appropriate to add to the tests performed in diagnosing death measurements of arginine vasopressin or other tests and procedures that have meaning and significance consistent with existing criteria.

Such a modest updating of the clinical criteria is all that is required by Truog and Fackler's data and is preferable to the alternative they favor, modifying the conceptual standards to permanent loss of the capacity for consciousness while leaving the existing criteria for the time being. Not only does this change fail to respond to their data that testing can evoke electrical activity in the brain stem, despite the absence of such activity in the neocortex (called electrocerebral silence); it also has all the problems of lack of general acceptability that attach to any standard that would result in declaring patients with spontaneous breathing and heartbeat dead because they are comatose (i.e., deeply unconscious).

The meaning of irreversibility. The final challenge to the UDDA is less an attempt to refute its theory than it is a contradiction of the standards established by the statute and accompanying medical guidelines. Under a protocol developed at the University of Pittsburgh in 1992, a patient who is dependent on life-support technology for continued vital functions and who desires to be an organ donor would be wheeled into the operating room and the life support disconnected, leading to cardiac arrest. After two minutes of asystole (lack of heartbeat), death would be declared based upon the "irreversible cessation of circulatory and respiratory functions," at which point blood flow could be artificially restored to the organs which are to be removed for transplantation (Youngner et al., 1993). Yet the failure to attempt to restore circulatory and respiratory functions in these patients shows that death had not occurred according to the existing criteria. The requirement of "irreversible cessation" must mean more than simply the physician "chose not to reverse." If no attempt is made to restore circulation and respiration before organs are removed it is not appropriate to make a diagnosis of death—merely a prognosis that death will occur if available means of resuscitation continue not to be used.

The reason for alternative standards for determining death is not because there are two kinds of death. On the contrary, there is one phenomenon that can be viewed through two windows, and the requirement of irreversibility ensures that what is seen is virtually the same thing through both. To replace "irreversible cessation of circulatory and respiratory functions" with "choose not to reverse" contradicts the underlying premise, because in the absence of the irreversibility there is no reason to suppose that brain functions have also permanently ceased.

Conclusion

The movement toward a modern legal formulation of the bases for pronouncing death has not been completed. In some societies that task may be left to the medical profession, since the problems faced in medical practice have provided the impetus for change. Tradition as well as sound policy suggests, however, that the ground rules for decisions about individual patients should be established by public authorities. Whether the new legal definition of death emerges from the resolution of court cases or from the legislative process, it will be greatly influenced by opinion from the medical community. Recognition that the standards for determining death are matters of social and not merely professional concern only serves to underline the education of the public on this subject as an important ethical obligation of the profession.

ALEXANDER MORGAN CAPRON

Directly related to this article are the other articles in this entry: CRITERIA FOR DEATH, *and* PHILOSOPHICAL AND THEOLOGICAL PERSPECTIVES. *Also directly related are the entries* DEATH; ORGAN AND TISSUE PROCUREMENT, *articles on* MEDICAL AND ORGANIZATIONAL ASPECTS, *and* ETHICAL AND LEGAL ISSUES REGARDING CADAVERS; *and* LIFE. *For a further discussion of topics mentioned in this article, see the entries* HOMICIDE; PERSON; *and* VALUE AND VALUATION. *For a discussion of related ideas, see the entries* ARTIFICIAL ORGANS AND LIFE-SUPPORT SYSTEMS; DEATH AND DYING: EUTHANASIA AND SUSTAINING LIFE, *article on* ETHICAL ISSUES; *and* LAW AND BIOETHICS.

Bibliography

AD HOC COMMITTEE OF THE HARVARD MEDICAL SCHOOL TO EXAMINE THE DEFINITION OF BRAIN DEATH. 1968. "A Definition of Irreversible Coma." *Journal of the American Medical Association* 205, no. 6:337–340. The original guidance on the means for determining an irreversible loss of total brain functioning, unfortunately mislabeled "irreversible coma."

CAPRON, ALEXANDER MORGAN. 1973. "The Purpose of Death: A Reply to Professor Dworkin." *Indiana Law Journal* 48(4):640–646. Argues for developing a definition that comports with social reality and that can be employed in as many legal settings as it suits.

CAPRON, ALEXANDER MORGAN, and KASS, LEON R. 1972. "A Statutory Definition of the Standards for Determining Human Death: An Appraisal and a Proposal." *University of Pennsylvania Law Review* 121:87–118. Discusses the procedures and objectives for lawmaking and provides a model that was widely adopted.

CATE, FRED H., and CAPRON, ALEXANDER MORGAN. 1992. "Death and Organ Transplantation." In *Treatise on Health Care Law*, pp. 45–60. Edited by Michael G. Macdonald, Robert M. Kaufman, Alexander M. Capron, and Irwin M. Birnbaum. New York: Matthew Bender.

CULVER, CHARLES M., and GERT, BERNARD. 1982. *Philosophy in Medicine: Conceptual and Ethical Issues in Medicine and Psychiatry.* New York: Oxford University Press.

Kass, Leon R. 1971. "Death as an Event: A Commentary on Robert Morison." *Science* 173, no. 998:698–702. Refutes Morison's thesis that death does not occur at an identifiable time and explores the social rules that follow from this view.

Kennedy, Ian McColl. 1971. "The Kansas Statute on Death: An Appraisal." *New England Journal of Medicine* 285, no. 17:946–949. Criticizes the first American statute and urges that defining death be left in medical hands.

Kennedy, Ian McColl, and Grubb, Andrew. 1989. *Medical Law: Text and Materials.* London: Butterworths.

Lizza, John P. 1993. "Persons and Death: What's Metaphysically Wrong with our Current Statutory Definition of Death?" *Journal of Medicine and Philosophy* 18, no. 4:351–374.

Medical Consultants on the Diagnosis of Death to the President's Commission for the Study of Ethical Problems in Medicine and Biomedical and Behavioral Research. 1981. "Guidelines for the Determination of Death." *Journal of the American Medical Association* 246, no. 19:2184–2187. This statement, signed by nearly all the leading American authorities on the subject, became the prevailing standard for pronouncing death.

New Jersey Commission on Legal and Ethical Problems in the Delivery of Health Care. 1991. *The New Jersey Advance Directives for Health Care and Declaration of Death Acts: Statutes, Commentaries and Analysis.* Trenton, N.J.: Author. Proposes and defends state's unique statute on determination of death.

Olick, Robert S. 1991. "Brain Death, Religious Freedom, and Public Policy: New Jersey's Landmark Legislative Initiative." *Kennedy Institute of Ethics Journal* 1, no. 4:275–288. Discusses New Jersey's religious exemption and offers a defense of the conscience clause in law and policy.

T.A.C.P., In re. 1992. 609 So.2d 588-95 (Fla. Sup. Ct.).

Task Force for the Determination of Brain Death in Children. 1987. "Guidelines for the Determination of Brain Death in Children." *Annals of Neurology* 21, no. 6:616–621. Provides special standards for pediatric death determination.

Truog, Robert D., and Fackler, James C. 1992. "Rethinking Brain Death." *Critical Care Medicine* 20, no. 12:1705–1713.

U.S. President's Commission for the Study of Ethical Problems in Medicine and Biomedical and Behavioral Research. 1981. *Defining Death: Medical, Legal, and Ethical Issues in the Determination of Death.* Washington, D.C.: U.S. Government Printing Office. Explanation of concepts and rationale for Uniform Determination of Death Act by federal bioethics commission, which operated from 1980 to 1983.

Van Till-d'Aulnis de Bourouill, Adrienne. 1975. "How Dead Can You Be?" *Medicine, Science and the Law* 15, no. 2:133–147. Compares American diagnostic criteria with those used in France, Austria, and Germany; also differentiates ceasing artificial maintenance from murder or active euthanasia.

Veatch, Robert M. 1976. *Death, Dying, and the Biological Revolution: Our Last Quest for Responsibility.* New Haven, Conn.: Yale University Press. Argues for regarding death as the loss of cerebral functions and provides a statute to achieve this end.

Youngner, Stuart, and Arnold, Robert M., for the Working Group on Ethical, Psychosocial, and Public Policy Implications of Procuring Organs from Non-Heart-Beating Cadaver Donors. 1993. "Ethical, Psychosocial, and Public Policy Implications of Procuring Organs from Non-Heart-Beating Cadaver Donors." *Journal of the American Medical Association* 269, no. 21:2769–2774. Reviews issues that are raised by using as organ donors patients whose hearts stop beating when life-sustaining treatment is discontinued.

Zaner, Richard M., ed. 1988. *Death: Beyond Whole-Brain Criteria.* Dordrecht, Netherlands: Kluwer Academic Publishers. A symposium on the debate between whole- and higher-brain standards, with essays favoring the latter by such leading figures as Edward T. Bartlett and Stuart J. Youngner, H. Tristram Engelhardt, Robert M. Veatch, and Richard M. Zaner.

III. PHILOSOPHICAL AND THEOLOGICAL PERSPECTIVES

The bioethics debate concerning the definition and criteria of human death emerged during the rise of organ transplantation in the 1960s, prompted by the advent of functional mechanical replacements for the heart, lungs, and brain stem, and by the ability to diagnose the pervasive brain destruction that is now termed "brain death." Previously, there had been no need to explore the conceptual or definitional basis of the established practice of declaring death when the heart and lungs ceased to function, or to consider additional criteria for determining death, since the irreversible cessation of either heart or lung function was quickly followed by the permanent loss of any other functioning deemed important to human life.

Now, however, such functional mechanical replacements as the respirator, as well as advances in resuscitation, have permitted the dissociated functioning of some of these bodily systems. In particular, we have experienced the phenomenon of a mechanically sustained patient whose whole brain is dead, and we have been led to ask, Is whole-brain death, death? Should we adopt a brain-death criterion for determining death?

Further, there is an increasing number of patients whose bodies have been resuscitated to the status of spontaneously functioning organisms but whose higher brains have permanently lost the capacity for conscious awareness. In these cases we are led to ask, Is higher-brain death, death? Should we adopt a higher-brain-death criterion for determining death?

In short, we must decide upon the relevance of the permanent loss or absence of various aspects of brain functioning as direct evidence that death has occurred.

Such a decision cannot be made without a clear understanding or concept of human death. It is difficult to understate the importance of clarifying our underlying cultural definition of death. Any criteria used to determine that a human being has died lack justification without an explicit foundation in a clear concept or definition of human death. Moreover, practices dependent on a determination that a person has died, such as negotiations with families of prospective organ donors concerning donation consequent to brain death, will be confused and confusing.

Defining death is a philosophical/theological activity, while determining and applying the criteria for declaring that someone has died are medical activities. Since a definition of death is informed by basic beliefs and values, people may hold different understandings of death. In a culture premised on the toleration of conscientiously held beliefs, a policy concerning the determination of death must in some way honor, or at a minimum acknowledge, the plurality of concepts of death among its citizens while still articulating an adequate societal standard.

Brain basics

The definition-of-death debate requires a rudimentary understanding of the brain and its connection to the other vital systems of the body. First, when a healthy human organism functions as an integrated whole, there is an ongoing interaction between the lower brain or brain stem, the lungs, and the heart. As long as the lungs receive appropriate direction from the brain stem, they continue to supply oxygenated blood to the heart, and the heart continues its circulatory activity, supplying oxygenated blood to the organism as a whole. This cycle of biological activity constitutes the integrated functioning of the organism as a whole and supports the possibility of consciousness.

Second, the higher brain centers are the locus of human consciousness. If these centers are destroyed through trauma or oxygen deprivation, the individual will never again be conscious or aware of self, others, or environment. Since these higher centers are functionally distinct from the brain stem, it is easy to see how a patient could be permanently unconscious yet exhibit spontaneous integrated functioning of the organism as a whole. Since such integrated functioning requires no more than a well-functioning brain stem, however, difficult debates about the life/death status have arisen about infants born without a higher brain (anencephaly) and individuals with higher-brain destruction that has left them permanently unconscious.

The central understandings about the brain, then, are these: The human being can survive as an integrated organism in the absence of consciousness. Survival as

an integrated organism can occur either naturally or through mechanical means. If there is no damage to the brain stem, heart, or lungs, the integration is natural. But if there is damage to any one of these, such that a mechanical replacement must be used (e.g., the respirator for the brain stem) the organism still functions as an integrated whole, but by artificial means. It is in such cases as these that the question originally arose, What loss of function is so essentially significant to human life that its permanent loss constitutes human death?

In 1968, the Ad Hoc Committee of the Harvard Medical School to Examine the Definition of Brain Death suggested that the death of the whole brain is such a significant functional loss that it should be considered direct and sufficient evidence of the death of a patient. Thus arose the suggestion that in addition to the traditional heart and lung criteria for determining death, a whole-brain death criterion ought to be used to determine death for a special category of cases: brain-dead patients who were respirator-dependent. The apparent integrated functioning of the organism as a whole, mediated through the respirator rather than the brain stem, was thereby defined to be an artifact, not a genuine instance of the integrated functioning of the organism as a whole. Hence, the Harvard Committee recommended that it be considered death.

Thus began the bioethics discussion referred to as "the definition-of-death debate." Several questions went unspoken and unaddressed by the Harvard Committee. What is death, such that either the traditional criteria or the brain-death criterion is sufficient indication of its occurrence? Do the traditional criteria and the brain-death criterion presuppose the same answer to this question, that is, the same definition of death? The Harvard Committee report was a clinical recommendation, not a philosophical discussion. It gave rise to a philosophical/theological discussion that is ongoing and remains centered on the question, What is so essentially significant to the nature of a human being that its irreversible loss should be considered human death?

The literature has been replete with answers to this question. For example, the irreversible loss of the flow of vital fluids, the irreversible departure of the soul from the body, the irreversible loss of the capacity for bodily integration, the irreversible loss of function of the organism as a whole, and the irreversible loss of the capacity for consciousness or social interaction. Without such an account of what is essentially significant, the criterion used as a basis for determining death lacks an explicit foundation.

Yet this normative question concerning what is essentially significant to the nature of the human being requires a prior account of the nature of the human being. In philosophical and theological terms, such an account of the nature of a being is referred to as an ontological account. One's view of the nature of the human being is informed by philosophical and/or theological perspectives on the nature of human existence, its essentially significant characteristics, and the nature of its boundary events. The goal of this essay is to explain the essential role of philosophical and theological reflection in the selection of adequate criteria for determining death, and of appropriate public policy on the determination of death in a pluralistic society.

Three levels of the debate

As the definition-of-death debate matured throughout the 1970s and 1980s, it became clear that it has three logically connected levels: (1) the conceptual or definitional level, (2) the criteriological level, and (3) the medical diagnostic level. There are important disagreements among those qualified to speak at each of these three levels, and there remains substantial uncertainty among professional practitioners concerning the appropriateness of using various criteria and the rationales for doing so.

The debate as a whole has proved intractable because there is no agreement at the definitional or conceptual level, where philosophical/theological beliefs exert their impact. In short, since the initial suggestion in 1968 that a brain-death criterion be used for the unique case of a respirator-dependent, brain-dead patient, practitioners still lack a unified sense of the concept of death that supports this practice; and some of them disagree with the understanding of death this practice seems to them to entail. Such confusion and lack of clarity is intolerable when families are being asked to comprehend a situation sufficiently to decide whether to donate organs of their loved ones.

By recognizing the three levels of the definition-of-death debate, one is able to identify the root confusion as lying at the definitional or conceptual level. The debate is a philosophical/theological conundrum rendered even more difficult to resolve in a pluralistic society. Let us first identify its levels.

The conceptual level. At this level the concept or definition of human death itself is philosophically and/or theologically informed. This concept answers the question, What is human death? This question can be answered in a general, provisional way by saying that human death is the irreversible loss of that which is essentially significant to the nature of the human being. But this merely sets the stage for the essential philosophical/theological task: to determine what the distinctive nature of the human being is, and what its essentially significant characteristic(s) is (are).

People differ radically in their answers to this most fundamental question of the definition-of-death debate.

Why do they do so? As a result of fundamental philosophical and theological perspectives on human nature will show, the human being can be thought of as a wholly material or physical entity, as a physical/mental amalgam, or as an essentially spiritual (though temporarily embodied) being. Depending on the frame chosen at this ontological level, the normative choice concerning that which is so essentially significant to human life that its permanent absence constitutes death will be affected. The definition of human death chosen will be the framework for evaluating criteria for determining death.

The criteriological level. Based on the resolution of the ontological and normative questions (the conceptual or philosophical/theological level), a criterion for determining that an individual has died, reflecting the functional characteristics deemed essentially significant, is specified. That is, the essentially significant human characteristic(s) delineated at the conceptual level is (are) located in (a) functional system(s) of the human organism. The traditional criteria center on heart and lung function, suggesting that the essentially significant characteristics are respiration and circulation. The brain-death criterion is said to focus on the functioning of the organism as a whole, and hence on the brain's role in the integrated functioning of the organism and consciousness.

The diagnostic level. At this level are the medical diagnostic tests to determine that the functional failure identified as the criterion of death has in fact occurred. These tests are used by medical professionals to determine whether the criterion is met, and thus that death should be declared. As technological development proceeds, diagnostic sophistication increases. The ability to diagnose brain death led to the suggestion that the brain-death criterion for determining death be used in addition to the traditional criteria in special cases of respirator dependency. As skill in reading the condition and capacities of the body improves, new questions are bound to arise: Is life still present? Has death already occurred?

These three levels—conceptual, criteriological, and diagnostic—provide a crucial intellectual grid for following the complex definition-of-death debate since 1968. The debate encompasses all three levels. In any reading and reflection associated with this complex debate, it is essential to remember what level of the debate one is on, and what sort of expertise is required on the part of those party to the debate at that level. For example, philosophers and theologians are best suited to work at the conceptual level. But work at the criteriological level without corresponding philosophical/theological reflection is intellectually ungrounded. As David Hume said centuries ago, "Concepts without percepts are blind." In our time, a criterion for determining death without a philosophical/theological analysis of what constitutes death is equally blind.

Moreover, any analysis and critical assessment of suggested criteria for determining death require that one attend to the important interconnections among tests, criteria, and concepts. Criteria without tests are useless; criteria without concepts lack justification. It is the philosophical/theological task of constructing an adequate concept or definition of human death that becomes central to the development of adequate criteria for the determination of death.

To put this in more specific terms: If a particular criterion (for example, the brain-death criterion) is used to determine death, there should be some agreed-upon answer to the question, Why should the condition identified by that criterion (of being brain dead) be considered human death?

To answer this question, thinking of a philosophical/theological sort is required. First, there must be the consideration of the kind of entity the human being is, and second, of the normative problem of the essentially significant characteristics of the human being. In the next section of this essay, the range of possible philosophical/theological perspectives that might be brought to bear on these ontological and normative problems will be summarized. In the final section, the bioethics debate about the criteria for determining death will be described and assessed relative to the philosophical/theological background, and considerations pertinent to public-policy formation will be raised.

Philosophical and theological perspectives: Preliminaries

Human groups engage in different behaviors upon the death of one of their members. They do so because they have different understandings of the nature of the individual self and, consequently, of the death of the self. Yet every human society needs a way of determining when one of its members has died, when the quantum change in the self that both requires and justifies "death behaviors" has occurred, when the preparation of the bodily remainder of the individual for removal from the sphere of communal interaction both may and must begin.

This need for a line of demarcation between life and death suggests that for societal purposes, the death of an individual must be a determinable event. There has been debate, however, about whether death is an event or a process. Those engaged in this debate have appealed to the biological phenomena associated with the shutting down of a living organism. Some of them have argued that death is a discrete biological event; others,

that it is a biological process. In fact, neither biological claim settles the philosophical question of whether death is an event or a process. We decide whether to view the biological phenomena associated with death as an event or a process. For societal/cultural reasons, it is essential that some terminus be recognized.

Death is a biological process that poses a decisional dilemma because, arguably, the biological shutdown of the organism is not "complete" until putrefaction has occurred. Human communities have a need to decide when, in the course of the process of biological shutdown, the individual should be declared dead; they must decide which functions are so essentially significant to human life that their permanent cessation is death. For a variety of reasons, we have come to associate death with the permanent cessation of functions we consider vital to the organism rather than with the end of all biological functioning in the organism. These vital functions play a pervasive and obvious role in the functioning of the organism as a whole, and so their use as lines of demarcation is reasonable. With their cessation, the features of human life we value the most cease forever, and it is reasonable to regard that as the event of a person's death. Advances in medical technology, permitting the mechanical maintenance of cardiac and respiratory functions in the absence of consciousness, force us to evaluate the functions we have always associated with life, and to choose which of them are essentially significant to human life or so valuable to us that their permanent loss constitutes death. The ancient and (until recently) reasonable assumption has been that death is an irreversible condition, so it should not be declared until the essentially significant functions have irreversibly ceased.

In pretechnological cultures, humans undoubtedly drew on the functional commonalities between other animal species and themselves to decide that the flow of blood and breathing were essentially significant functions. When either of these functions stopped, no other "important" functions continued, and predictable changes to the body ensued. Since it was beyond human power to alter this course of events, the permanent cessation of heart and lung functioning became the criterion used to determine that someone had died.

This choice has clearly stood the test of time. Often referred to as the traditional heart and lung criteria, there is certainly no reason to impugn this choice for a society lacking the technological life-support interventions characteristic of modern medicine. But it is important to see that even in a pretechnological culture, the choice of the traditional cardiopulmonary criteria was a choice, an imposition of values on biological data. It was a choice based on a decision concerning significant function, that is, a decision concerning what is so essentially significant to the nature of the human being that its irreversible cessation constitutes human death. Such a decision is informed by fundamental beliefs and values that are philosophical or theological in nature.

If a technologically advanced culture is to update its criteria for declaring death, it must reach to the level that informs such a decision. Deciding the normative issue concerning the essentially significant characteristic of a human being is impossible without an ontological account of the nature of the human being. The assumptions and beliefs we hold on these matters form the combined philosophical/theological basis upon which we dissect the biological data and eventually bisect them into "life" and "death."

Such assumptions and beliefs constitute our most fundamental understandings and function as the often unseen frame through which we view, assess, and manipulate reality. As a rule, this frame is inculcated through the broad range of processes that a social group uses to shape its members. The frame itself consists of philosophical/theological assumptions and beliefs that we use to organize and interpret experience. They are deeply yet pragmatically held beliefs that may be adjusted, adapted, discarded, or transformed when they cause individual or social confusion, cease to be useful, or no longer make sense. Arguably, changes in our capacity to resuscitate and support the human body in the absence of consciousness have brought our culture to such a point of non-sense. To respond fully to this crisis, we have to consider the various philosophical and theological perspectives in our culture that inform thinking about human nature and death.

Representative philosophical and theological perspectives

"Death" is the word we use to signify the end of life as we know it. As stated above, individuals and groups hold different understandings of the existence and the death of the self. These understandings are the background for the "nuts and bolts" medical decision that a person has died, when death should be declared, and what ought/ought not be done to and with the physical remains of the person who has died.

As individuals and as cultural groups, humans differ in their most basic assumptions and beliefs about human death. For some, the death of the body marks the absolute end of the self; for others, it is a transition to another form of existence for the continuously existing self. This transition may be to continued life in either a material or an immaterial form. Despite these differences, every human community needs a way of determining when one of its members has died, a necessary and sufficient condition for considering the body as the

remainder of the individual that can now be treated in ways that would have been inappropriate or immoral before, and for preparing the body for removal from the communal setting. Different philosophical and theological perspectives on the nature of death, the individual self, and the death of the self will yield different choices of criteria for the determination of death, just as these differing perspectives yield very different death practices or death behaviors. To see why this is the case, let us look at various philosophical and theological views of death and the self.

In the Hebrew tradition of the Old Testament, death is considered a punishment for the sin of disobedience. It is an absolute punishment. This tradition does not hold a concept of an afterlife following the punishment of death. But it would be misleading to say that this tradition has no conception of immortality, since the communal setting of the individual's experience and life remains the arena of that person's identity and impact, even after the death of the body. Although the conscious life of the person ceases, the person lives on in the collective life, unless he or she lived badly. Thus, immortality is the community's conscious and unconscious memory of the person.

Another view, originating in Platonic philosophy and found in Christian and Orthodox Judaic thought, and in Islam and Hinduism, holds that death is not the cessation of conscious life. The conscious self, often referred to as the soul, survives in a new form, possibly in a new realm. The experience of the self after the death of the body depends on the moral quality of the person's life. The body is the soul's temporary housing, and the soul's journey is toward the good, or God, or existence as pure rational spirit without bodily distractions. Thus, death is the disconnection of the spiritual element of the self (mind, soul, spirit) from the physical or bodily aspect of the self.

Traditions believing in eternal life differ in their view of the soul and its relationship to the body. This has implications for the criteria that might be used to determine death, as well as for the appropriate treatment of the body after death. The soul is viewed by some as separate and capable of migrating or moving into different bodies as it journeys toward eternal life. The Christian tradition, by contrast, posits the self as an eternally existing entity created by God. The death of the body is just that—the person continues, with body transformed, either punished in hell for living badly or rewarded in heaven for having faith and living righteously. These diverse views have a common belief: everyone survives death in some way. This may influence the understanding of what constitutes the death of the body as well as of what ought/ought not to be done to the body of the person who has died. For some traditions, certain bodily functions are indicative of life, whether or not those functions are mechanically supported, and damage to the body is damage to the self.

In contrast to these theological conceptions of death and the self, three philosophical perspectives, secular in that they hold materialist views of the self, figure in Western thought: the Epicurean, the Stoic, and the existential. A materialist view of the self considers the human to be an entirely physical or material entity, with no soul or immaterial aspect. The Epicurean view of the self holds that humans are fully material beings without souls. The goal of life is to live it well as it is and not to fear death since death is the end of experience, not something one experiences. Therefore, there is no eternal life for souls; the body dies and disintegrates back into the material nature from which it sprang. The death of the body marks the end of consciousness, and thus the death of the self. A materialist holding a view such as this could conclude that the cessation of consciousness itself should be considered death, whether or not the body continues to function in an integrated manner.

The Stoic view acknowledges death as the absolute end of the conscious self but directs persons to have courage about its inevitability and to resign to it creatively. This creative resignation is achieved by focusing on the inevitability of death in such a way that one treats every moment of life as a creative opportunity. The necessity of death becomes the active inspiration for the way one lives. Like the Epicurean view, the Stoic conception ties the self to the body; the end of the self to the death of the body. But it is the consciousness supported by the body that is the creative self.

In contrast, existential thought believes that the absoluteness of death renders human life absurd and meaningless. The other materialist views of the self saw death as the occasion for meaning in life, not the denial that life has meaning. Rather than infusing meaning into life and inspiring a commitment to striving, existentialism holds that death demonstrates the absurdity of human striving. While individuals may pursue subjective goals and try to realize subjective values during their lives, there are no objective values in relation to which to orient one's striving, and so all striving is ultimately absurd. Since death is the end of the self, there is nothing to prepare for beyond the terms of physical existence and the consciousness it supports.

Without critiquing these theological and philosophical perspectives on death and the self, we can ask why their diversity is relevant to a discussion of the debate in bioethics about the criteria for determining that a human being has died. The earlier demonstration that the criteria rest on a decision of functional significance, and that a decision of functional significance is philosophically/theologically informed, coupled with this demonstration of philosophical/theological diversity on the fundamental concepts of self and the death of the self, together show that criteria are acceptable only if they are seen to be consistent with an accepted philosophical/theological frame, and that what is acceptable in one frame may be unacceptable in another.

Further, while it might be the case that virtually every tradition has agreed on the appropriateness of the traditional heart and lung criteria for declaring death, they may do so for vastly different reasons deriving from their specific understanding of death and the self. There may be ways of reconciling virtually every ontological view to the use of the traditional criteria but not to the use of consciousness-centered criteria like the higher-brain-death criterion, or even the brain-death criterion (which appears, to a tradition like Orthodox Judaism, to deny that the still-functioning body is indicative of life, even when the entire brain is dead).

Philosophical and theological commitments relate centrally to our death practices, including our conclusions concerning the acceptability of traditional, whole-brain, and higher-brain formulations of death. How philosophically and theologically sophisticated has the bioethics debate on the definition of death been, over the years?

The definition-of-death debate

Whole-brain-death formulations. In 1968, the Ad Hoc Committee of the Harvard Medical School to Examine the Definition of Brain Death recommended that a whole-brain-death criterion be used to determine death in respirator-dependent patients, thus creating an exception to the use of the traditional heart and lung criteria for a specific category of patients. The brain-death criterion was said to measure the death of the entire brain, including the brain stem.

In its historic report, the Harvard Committee provided a diagnostic protocol for establishing brain death. It further recommended that brain death be adopted as a criterion for determining death in respirator-dependent patients. But the questions the Harvard Committee never asked or answered were philosophical/theological: Why is the brain-dead patient dead? Why is brain death, death? What concepts of human death and self underlie the use of the brain-death criterion? In short, the Harvard Committee delineated the diagnostic tests for an alternative criterion for determining death but did not justify the use of that criterion by explaining the concepts of self and human death it presupposed.

It is now common knowledge that the Harvard tests for determining brain death do not in fact reflect the permanent cessation of functioning throughout the entire brain. Rather, the clinical tests are said to reflect the permanent cessation of all brain functioning essential to the integrated functioning of the organism as a whole. While there may be residual cellular and subcellular activity occurring when the criterion now referred to as the brain-death criterion is fulfilled, those advocating a whole-brain formulation of death have deemed it to be irrelevant to the determination of the life/death status of the patient. In their view, the brain-death criterion reflects an adequate concept of human death: the irreversible cessation of the integrated functioning of the organism as a whole.

Defenders of the brain-death criterion, or any whole-brain formulation of death (the British use a brain-stem death criterion that is a variant of the whole-brain formulation), reason that because the integration between the brain stem, lungs, and heart is no longer "real," but rather an artifact of the respirator's functioning, brain death is death. It is a bit like saying, "In the situation of brain death, if the respirator were not taking over the role of the brain stem, the lungs would not be working, and therefore the heart would not be beating. Hence, brain death is the irreversible loss of the integrated functioning of the organism as a whole, just as the permanent cessation of integrated brain stem, lung, and heart functioning is."

When the Harvard Committee initially proposed the brain-death criterion, which it misleadingly labeled "a definition of irreversible coma," controversy arose over whether the adoption of this criterion constituted a departure from the concept of death implicit in the use of the traditional heart and lung criteria for the determination of death. Some saw this new basis for determining death as a blatant and unfounded maneuver to increase the availability of transplantable organs. They opposed it because it was inconsistent with their philosophical/theological view of the human self and disrespectful to dying patients. While others agreed that the neurological focus represented an alternative understanding of the self, they saw the move to be eminently logical: What argument could one reasonably have with the notion that someone whose whole brain is dead, is dead?

Some of the staunchest defenders of the brain-death criterion have argued that it represents no change in our understanding of death as the permanent cessation of integrated organismic functioning. What their assertion overlooks, however, is the profound difference between conceiving of human life as a heart-centered reality and as a brain-centered reality. The shift to a neurological focus on the human that is made with the adoption of the brain-death criterion is at the same time a discounting of the relevance of the spontaneous beating of the heart and the mechanically sustained functioning of the lungs. There remain cultures and faith traditions that

cannot make this leap, suggesting that there is a radically different way of thinking of the human self at issue.

Thus, not everyone has agreed that the traditional criteria and the brain-death criterion share the same underlying concept of human death. Some resist the adoption of the brain-death criterion for this reason, considering the shift to a new understanding of human death to be philosophically/theologically unjustifiable. However, others have welcomed the change: Reflecting on the contingency of the definition of death under circumstances of technological change, some have argued in favor of redefining death even further. In their view, the philosophical concept of death said to underlie the brain-death criterion inadequately reflects the essentially significant characteristic of human existence: existence as an embodied consciousness. A more adequate concept of human death, they contend, would center on the permanent cessation of consciousness (requiring a higher-brain-death criterion), not on the permanent cessation of the integrated functioning of the organism. Their view is that the whole-brain criterion unjustifiably defers to the characteristics biological organisms have in common and ignores the relevance of distinctively human characteristics like consciousness to our concepts of life and death.

In 1981, the President's Commission for the Study of Ethical Problems in Medicine and Biomedical and Behavioral Research published its report, *Defining Death: A Report on the Medical, Legal, and Ethical Issues in the Determination of Death*, giving the states guidelines for enacting brain-death legislation. That model law, called the Uniform Determination of Death Act, is widely accepted by relevant professional groups (health-care, law, ethics). It recognizes the traditional criteria and the brain-death criterion, and it concludes that the adoption of the brain-death criterion does not entail a change in our concept of death as the irreversible loss of the integrated functioning of the organism.

There are at least three significant questions to pursue in relation to the adoption of the brain-death criterion and its alleged conceptual base. First, given that the brain-death criterion does not measure the death of the entire brain, as it was originally said to do, on what basis is the distinction between residual and nonresidual brain functioning drawn? On what basis is "residual" brain functioning determined to be irrelevant so far as a determination of brain death is concerned? In point of fact, advocates of whole-brain formulations have failed to provide a nonquestion-begging, principled basis for this important discrimination.

Second, as long as the respirator is functioning, it seems something of a word game to say that the organism is not functioning as an integrated whole. True, the brain stem is no longer playing its linking role in the triangle of function along with lungs and heart. But the respirator is standing in for the brain stem, just as it might if there were only partial brain destruction in the area of the brain stem. If the patient were conscious, but just as dependent on the respirator in order to continue functioning as an organism, one doubts there would be any inclination to pronounce the patient dead. Hence, it would seem that even the brain-dead patient is exhibiting integrated organismic functioning until the respirator is turned off, the lungs stop, and the heart eventually stops beating.

Third, as the last point makes clear, the real reason so many people are inclined to agree that the brain-dead patient is dead has much more to do with the fact that the brain-dead patient is permanently unconscious than with the facts of brain stem destruction and respirator dependency. It is this loss of the self, the loss of consciousness and thus of embodiment as a self, that is for the vast majority of us a good reason to consider the brain-dead patient dead. This suggests that the concept of human death underlying people's willingness to adopt the brain-death criterion has more to do with the loss of the capacity for embodied consciousness than with the loss of the capacity for integrated organismic functioning.

Higher-brain formulations. Some contributors to the definition-of-death debate have found the emphasis on the death of the whole brain to be philosophically/theologically indefensible. They propose instead a higher-brain-death criterion for the determination of death. Philosophically/theologically, they contend that this criterion presupposes a different and preferable view of what is essentially significant to the nature of the self. They hold that consciousness, sometimes characterized as a capacity for social interaction, is the sine qua non of human existence, and that the criterion used to determine death should reflect this. In their view, requiring that the brain-death criterion be used when the patient is permanently unconscious is biologically reductionistic. That is, the brain-death criterion, requiring the death of the lower brain, reduces the human being to the status of a mere organism, in effect saying that what is essentially significant to life as a human being is the basic functioning of the organism and not the conscious capacity that functioning supports. Unless our concept of human death reflects what is essentially significant to the nature of the human being—conscious awareness—it fails to provide a community with an effective moral divide between the living and the dead.

Critics of the higher-brain formulations object that the emphasis on consciousness and person-centered functions of the human being places us on a "slippery slope" that will eventually lead to a broadening of the definition of death to include those who are severely demented or only marginally or intermittently conscious. They argue further that the adoption of a higher-brain

basis for determining death would require us to bury spontaneously respiring (and heart beating) "cadavers."

These arguments have little to recommend them. First, there is a bright and empirically demonstrable line between those who are in a permanent vegetative state (recall the cases of Karen Quinlan, Paul Brophy, Nancy Cruzan, and others) and those who retain the capacity for higher-brain functioning. The "slippery slope" worry that we would begin to declare conscious patients dead is unfounded. By contrast, the "slippery slope" objection *is* telling in relation to the brain-death criterion, which does not in fact measure the death of the brain in its entirety. Whole-brain death adherents have failed to show that there is a bright line between residual and nonresidual brain functions, so the opportunity for the unprincipled enlargement of the "residual functioning" category is ever present.

Finally, for aesthetic reasons as well as reasons of respect, we do not permit certain forms of treatment of the dead. There is no reason to think that a new definition of death would require us to set aside such considerations since they constitute the dignified and appropriate treatment of the body of the deceased person. We would not bury a spontaneously breathing body any more than we would bury a brain-dead body still attached to a respirator. And stopping residual heart and lung function would be as morally appropriate in the case of a permanently unconscious patient as is the discontinuation of the respirator in the case of a brain-dead patient.

Non-heart-beating cadaver donors. In the early 1990s, yet another determination-of-death strategy was introduced for the purpose of increasing the quantity and quality of transplantable organs. The University of Pittsburgh Medical Center proposed a protocol for organ procurement from persons who have been "dead" according to the traditional heart and lung criteria for two minutes. In contrast with brain-dead organ donors, these organ donors are called non-heart-beating cadaver donors. They are patients who have elected not to receive life-sustaining treatment, or whose families have done so on their behalf. Similar proposals have been made for unsuccessfully resuscitated trauma victims.

While this organ-procurement strategy does not affect the criteria presently in place for the determination of death, it represents change at the diagnostic level and raises questions of a philosophical/theological nature. After two minutes, resuscitation efforts could be attempted and might be successful. Should we discard one of our age-old assumptions about death, its irreversibility? Or do we maintain that such deaths are de facto irreversible because a decision has been made not to resuscitate?

Further, this new strategy for determining death raises interesting issues about the overall consistency of criteria for determining death. It has always been the case that a patient declared brain dead could not be declared dead using the traditional criteria, since the respirator was maintaining lung and heart functions. Yet after only two minutes of cardiopulmonary cessation, the patient is arguably not brain dead, raising a question: Which way of being determined dead is more morally appropriate when surgery to procure organs is to be undertaken?

The persistence of the debate

Why do arguments concerning the definition and criteria of death persist? The debate has been intractable since 1968. One important reason is that the concepts of self and death that inform the various positions in the debate are based on fundamental beliefs and values that are seldom held up to rational scrutiny and are often irreconcilably different. While it is true that persons holding different philosophical/theological premises may assent to the use of the same criteria for determining death, they may well do so for very different reasons. Because of this, it is reasonable to seek and adopt a broadly acceptable societal standard for the determination of death.

For example, the several materialist views of the self that were examined earlier suggest a consciousness-centered concept of self and death that further recommends a higher-brain formulation of death. But equally, the prevailing Judeo-Christian understandings of the self and death—that of death as the dissociation of consciousness from the body, the end of embodied consciousness—are also compatible with a higher-brain formulation of death.

Some traditions, like Orthodox Judaism, and certain Japanese and Native American perspectives, resist the use of the brain-death criterion because they understand death to be a complete stoppage of the vital functions of the body. The self is not departed until such stoppage has occurred. Such groups will be uncomfortable with the use of the brain-death criterion because it permits the determination of death while vital functions continue. This kind of philosophical/theological difference in perspective on the human self, intimately linked to a person's religious and cultural identity, raises serious questions about how a pluralistic culture should deal with deeply held differences in designing a policy for the determination of death.

Given that there are a finite number of possible perspectives on the human person and on human death, and given the rootedness of these perspectives in conscientiously held philosophical and religious views and cultural identities, public policy on the determination of death in a complex and diverse culture could well manage to service conscience through the addition of a conscience clause in a determination-of-death statute. Similar to and perhaps in conjunction with a living will, a person could execute a conscience-clause exclusion to the statute's implicit concept of death. For instance, an Orthodox Jew could direct that death be determined using the traditional criteria alone, and also indicate personal preferences concerning the use of life-sustaining treatment such as ventilator support in the situation of brain death.

The fact that a conscience clause would permit some to reject the use of the brain-death criterion need not hinder the law from specifying punishable harms against others on the basis of considerations additional to whether death was caused. The exotic life-sustaining technologies now available have already generated arguments concerning whether the person who causes someone to be brain dead or the person who turns off the ventilator on that brain-dead patient causes the patient's death.

Life-sustaining technologies as well as the alternative concepts of death among us underscore the need for more precise legal classifications of punishable harms to persons. Such a classification should recognize permanent loss of consciousness as a harm punishable to the same extent as permanent stoppage of the heart and lungs.

The self can be thought of in a variety of ways: as an entirely material entity, as an essentially mental entity, and as a combined physical/mental duality. In contemporary language, the human being may be thought of as a physical organism, as an embodied consciousness (which we often call "person"), or as an amalgam of the two. As one examines the definition-of-death debate, one sees that fundamentally different ontological perspectives on the human have been taken.

Once such an ontological perspective on the human being has been chosen, a further decision as to what is essentially significant to the nature of the human being can be made. When a conclusion is reached as to which function is essentially significant to the human being, the potential exists for settling on the criterion (or criteria) for determining death. To the extent that these two steps of philosophical analysis support attention to the brain as the locus of the relevant human functions, views may divide on whether a whole-brain or a higher-brain formulation of death is adopted.

A complex entity that manifests its aliveness in a variety of ways has the potential to engender dispute about the ontological perspective that should be taken toward it, as well as about what is essentially significant to it. Hence, there may be no agreement on the definition of death that should be applied. Instead, our greatest achievement may be to articulate a policy on the determination of death that honors a plurality of philosophical/theological perspectives.

KAREN GRANDSTRAND GERVAIS

Directly related to this article are the other articles in this entry: CRITERIA FOR DEATH, *and* LEGAL ISSUES IN PRONOUNCING DEATH. *Also directly related are the entries* DEATH; DEATH, ATTITUDES TOWARD; DEATH AND DYING: EUTHANASIA AND SUSTAINING LIFE; *and* LIFE. *For a further discussion of topics mentioned in this article, see the entries* ARTIFICIAL ORGANS AND LIFE-SUPPORT SYSTEMS; HINDUISM; HUMAN NATURE; ISLAM; JUDAISM; NATIVE AMERICAN RELIGIONS; ORGAN AND TISSUE PROCUREMENT, *especially the articles on* MEDICAL AND ORGANIZATIONAL ASPECTS, *and* ETHICAL AND LEGAL ISSUES REGARDING CADAVERS; PAIN AND SUFFERING; PROTESTANTISM; *and* ROMAN CATHOLICISM. *For a further discussion of related ideas, see the entries* AGING AND THE AGED, *article on* HEALTH-CARE AND RESEARCH ISSUES; ARTIFICIAL HEARTS AND CARDIAC-ASSIST DEVICES; CONFLICT OF INTEREST; CRYONICS; DEATH: ART OF DYING; DEATH EDUCATION; DEATH PENALTY; HARM; HOMICIDE; *and* ORGAN AND TISSUE TRANSPLANTS. *Other relevant material may be found under the entries* ABORTION; ANIMAL WELFARE AND RIGHTS, *articles on* HUNTING, *and* VEGETARIANISM; DOUBLE EFFECT; *and* VALUE AND VALUATION.

Bibliography

AD HOC COMMITTEE OF THE HARVARD MEDICAL SCHOOL TO EXAMINE THE DEFINITION OF BRAIN DEATH. 1968. "A Definition of Irreversible Coma: A Report of the Ad Hoc Committee." *Journal of the American Medical Association* 205, no. 6:337–340.

BECKER, LAWRENCE C. 1975. "Human Being: The Boundaries of the Concept." *Philosophy and Public Affairs* 4, no. 4:335–359.

"Declaration of Death." 1994. *New Jersey Statutes Annotated.* Title 26, ch. 6A. St. Paul, Minn.: West.

DE VITA, MICHAEL A., and SNYDER, JAMES V. 1993. "Development of the University of Pittsburgh Medical Center Policy for the Care of Terminally Ill Patients Who May Become Organ Donors After Death Following the Removal of Life Support." *Kennedy Institute of Ethics Journal* 3, no. 2:131–143.

GERVAIS, KAREN G. 1986. *Redefining Death.* New Haven, Conn.: Yale University Press.

———. 1989. "Advancing the Definition of Death: A Philosophical Essay." *Medical Humanities Review* 3, no. 2:7–19.

GREEN, MICHAEL, and WIKLER, DANIEL. 1980. "Brain Death and Personal Identity." *Philosophy and Public Affairs* 9, no. 2:105–133.

HOFFMAN, JOHN C. 1979. "Clarifying the Debate on Death." *Soundings* 62, no. 4:430–447.

LAMB, DAVID. 1985. *Death, Brain Death and Ethics.* Albany: State University of New York Press.

TRUOG, ROBERT D., and FACKLER, JAMES C. 1992. "Rethinking Brain Death." *Critical Care Medicine* 20, no. 12:1705–1713.

U.S. PRESIDENT'S COMMISSION FOR THE STUDY OF ETHICAL PROBLEMS IN MEDICINE AND BIOMEDICAL AND BEHAVIORAL RESEARCH. 1981. *Defining Death: A Report on the Medical, Legal, and Ethical Issues in the Determination of Death.* Washington, D.C.: Author.

VEATCH, ROBERT M. 1989. *Death, Dying, and the Biological Revolution: Our Last Quest for Responsibility.* Rev. ed. New Haven, Conn.: Yale University Press.

———. 1992. "Brain Death and Slippery Slopes." *Journal of Clinical Ethics* 3, no. 3:181–187.

YOUNGNER, STUART J. 1992. "Defining Death: A Superficial and Fragile Consensus." *Archives of Neurology* 49, no. 5:570–572.

ZANER, RICHARD M., ed. 1988. *Death: Beyond Whole-Brain Criteria.* Dordrecht, Netherlands: Kluwer.

DEATH: ART OF DYING

I. *Ars Moriendi*
    Brian Copenhaver
II. Contemporary Art of Dying
    James F. Bresnahan

I. ARS MORIENDI

The *Ars moriendi* (The Art of Dying) is an important subgenre of late medieval conduct literature. Like similar treatises on courtesy, courtship, education, recreation, and warfare, these little manuals on dying were meant to guide the reader's behavior on an occasion of considerable importance. Today, about 300 manuscripts of the *Ars moriendi* survive along with 100 or so incunabula (books printed before 1500), including both block books (books printed from engraved wood blocks) and editions printed with movable type. The best evidence indicates that the first woodcut edition appeared by 1465, and the fact that some 20 percent of all surviving block books are *Artes moriendi* is enough to show the extraordinary importance of this subgenre for the history of late medieval and early modern thought. Both Latin and vernacular texts (in seven modern languages, eventually) had appeared in both woodcut and printed form by 1475. Their striking illustrations of the deathbed surrounded by agents of heaven and hell extended the impact of these popular little works beyond the ranks of the literate.

The *Ars moriendi* occurs in longer and shorter versions. The long versions are divided into six sections: (1) a miscellany of quotations on death from Christian authorities; (2) advice to the dying person (*Moriens*) on overcoming temptations to faithlessness, despair, impatience, pride, and worldliness; (3) catechetical questions whose correct answers lead to salvation; (4) prayers and rules for imitating the dying Christ; (5) advice to persons attending the dying person; and (6) prayers to be said by the attendants.

The shorter *Ars moriendi* treatises seem to be abridged derivatives of the longer, which are about triple their size. The smaller works occur in almost all the woodcut editions. A brief introduction and conclusion summarize the material contained in the first, third, fourth, and fifth sections of the longer versions. The body of the shorter versions corresponds to the second section of the longer, but this material is transformed and dramatized as a *psychomachia*, a struggle between angels and demons for the dying person's soul. *Moriens* (the dying person) must choose either the five vices mentioned in the longer text or their contrary virtues: faith, hope, love, humility, and detachment. In one extant shorter *Ars moriendi*, eleven graphic woodcuts in the fifteenth-century Flemish style illustrate the fight against temptation: five cuts for the virtues, five for the vices, and one for the eventual delivery of *Moriens*'s soul to the good angel.

The origins of the *Ars moriendi* as a subgenre are in the various compendia of piety and doctrine that appeared when later medieval church councils mandated a greater effort to educate the laity in the fundamentals of Christianity. Jean Gerson's *Opus tripartitum* (before 1408) grew out of such concerns, and the third part of this work, titled *De arte moriendi*, is the source of much of the *Ars moriendi*. Other important sources are to be found in the Bible, the church fathers, medieval liturgies, papal and conciliar statements, medieval patristic collections, and later medieval devotional and doctrinal literature. The authorship of the earliest longer version of the *Ars moriendi* remains in doubt, but there is good reason to locate its composition in southern Germany, at the time of the Council of Constance (1414–1418), with the Dominican Order. The earliest shorter version appeared in the mid-fifteenth century.

From a religious point of view, the gravest concern of the dying person was the prospect of the soul's judgment and the body's resurrection. Resurrection awaited the end of time, a postponement that contributed to the ascetic Christian view of the earthly body, in sickness or in health. But judgment came in two phases: personal judgment of the individual sinner immediately after death, and general judgment of all humans at the Second Coming. Late medieval emphasis on personal piety naturally concentrated on the first judgment, whose proper stage was domestic, the familiar bedroom scene rather than the grander cosmic setting where all the "sheep" would eventually take leave of all the "goats."

The main actors in the small drama of *Moriens* were supernatural: the Devil and evil demons tempting him to worldly avarice, despair, and damnation; Christ, the Virgin, and good angels urging him to otherworldly detachment, hope, and salvation. In the context of im-

mediate judgment and eventual resurrection, traditional Christian virtue ethics as expressed in the *Ars moriendi* counseled the dying person to be hopeful and not to despair, advice based on a virtue/vice opposition that foreshadowed the ultimate choice of heaven or hell. Since heaven and hell were to last forever, following the painful interlude of purgatory, the dying person was advised to shun the vice of avarice because the very impulse to hang on to family, friends, and property was a sinful miscalculation of the stakes in the game of eternity.

Both the fifth section of the longer *Ars moriendi* and Gerson's *De arte moriendi* advise those who attend the dying man against reinforcing one special kind of hope, the false hope of regaining the health of the body. This is a commentary not only on the state of medicine in the late Middle Ages and on contemporary attitudes toward it, but also on the Christian view of the death of the body. Since physical death was a beginning, not an end, there was no reason to take heroic measures to forestall it. Pope Innocent III, the effects of whose legislation found their way into the *Ars moriendi*, warned that none were to administer bodily medicine to *Moriens* until the ills of the soul had been cared for. In the thirteenth century, Innocent wrote a treatise, *On the Misery of the Human Condition*, that loathed the body in terms too lurid for the refined Platonist immaterialism of Giovanni Pico della Mirandola, whose *Oration on the Dignity of Man* expresses fifteenth-century attitudes less austere than those presented by the *Ars moriendi*. And yet Pico, a lay humanist, chose to die in the robes of a monk. That such spiritual therapy was more important than medicine for the body was an idea as old as Plato (*Charmides* 156–157) and the Gospels (Matt. 8:5–13; John 5:1–14).

A woodcut that depicts *Moriens*'s faith being tempted also sets deathbed medicine in a problematic light. Three learned persons, apparently physicians, stand in consultation at *Moriens*'s right while a demon points at them and whispers the words "infernus factus est" (hell has been prepared) into the dying patient's ear. In light of what the *Ars moriendi* says elsewhere about corporeal medicine, it is likely that the demon is enticing *Moriens* into the error of caring for his bodily health just at the moment when spiritual health ought to be his chief concern. The demon raises the prospect of damnation in order to frighten *Moriens* into clinging to his worldly goods and thus losing his chance of a good Christian death.

The "good death" became an ideal more visible in the literature of personal piety after time had softened the harsh message and stark images of the *Ars moriendi*. Although the *Ars moriendi* certainly aimed to make the Christian's death a good one in its outcome, nevertheless it left the impression that death was a "last ordeal," an exit that would sober rather than edify its audience.

Fifteenth-century humanist moral thought encouraged a different and more genteel treatment of death, as when Coluccio Salutati compared Petrarch's end to the noble departure of the dying Hermes as reported in the medieval *Liber Alcidi*. Johan Huizinga (1949) and other modern authorities on the late Middle Ages have mentioned the *Ars moriendi* in the same breath with the *danse macabre*, plague books, grisly funerary art, and other manifestations of an obsession with death in the late Middle Ages, an obsession consequent, perhaps, upon the great plague, which arrived in Europe in 1348 and recurred for several centuries. While the great popularity of the *Ars moriendi* may support such a view, its contents generally do not. True, crowds of demons populate its woodcuts, *Moriens* looks like a dying person, and its graphic style resembles that of the darker Dance of Death literature. But on the whole there is little terror in the advice given by the *Ars moriendi*, which was meant to point the way toward an afterlife of bliss. It ended in the expectation of heaven, not with the horrors of hell. For a society whose members viewed death as a passage to an afterlife, a manual on the art of dying had an eminently practical function. Seeing the *Ars moriendi* as the nightmare of a necrophile culture may tell us more about modern anxieties than about medieval mentalities.

The theological roots of the *Ars moriendi* extend back through the entire history of Christianity's emphasis on the inestimably greater value of the life of the soul than the life of the body, and hence the paramount importance of a spiritually salutary death. An emphasis on a good death has remained a central characteristic of theological and pastoral concerns. Instructions for Christians' preparing for death continued to be written after the end of the Middle Ages, either as sections of larger theological and pastoral manuals or, more rarely, as separate treatises. Nevertheless, as a distinct subgenre, the *Ars moriendi*, a significant example of the religious homogeneity of the late Middle Ages, essentially ended with the breakdown of that homogeneity in the sixteenth century.

BRIAN COPENHAVER

Directly related to this article is the companion article in this entry: CONTEMPORARY ART OF DYING. *Also directly related is the entry* DEATH EDUCATION. *For a further discussion of topics mentioned in this article, see the entry* DEATH, *article on* WESTERN RELIGIOUS THOUGHT. *For a discussion of related ideas, see the entries* DEATH AND DYING: EUTHANASIA AND SUSTAINING LIFE, *article on* HISTORICAL ASPECTS; MEDICAL ETHICS, *section on* EUROPE, *subsection on* ANCIENT AND MEDIEVAL, *article on* MEDIEVAL CHRISTIAN EUROPE; *and* ROMAN CATHOLICISM. *See also the entries* LITERATURE; NARRATIVE; *and* VIRTUE AND CHARACTER.

Bibliography

ARIES, PHILIPPE. 1981. *The Hour of Our Death*. Translated by Helen Weaver. New York: Knopf.

BEATY, NANCY LEE. 1970. *The Craft of Dying: A Study in the Literary Tradition of the* Ars moriendi *in England*. New Haven, Conn.: Yale University Press.

BOASE, THOMAS SHERRER ROSS. 1972. *Death in the Middle Ages: Mortality Judgment and Remembrance*. London: Thames and Hudson.

HUIZINGA, JOHAN. 1949. *The Waning of the Middle Ages: A Study of the Forms of Life, Thought and Art in France and the Netherlands in the XIVth and XVth Centuries*. Translated by F. Hopman. New York: Longmans Green.

MCNEILL, JOHN T. 1951. *A History of the Cure of Souls*. New York: Harper & Row.

O'CONNOR, MARY CATHARINE. 1942. *The Art of Dying Well: The Development of the Ars Moriendi*. New York: Columbia University Press.

TENENTI, ALBERTO. 1952. *La Vie et la mort à travers l'art du XVe siècle*. Paris: Armand Colin.

———. 1957. *Il senso della morte e l'amore della vita nel Rinascimento*. Turin: G. Einaudi.

II. CONTEMPORARY ART OF DYING

The *Ars moriendi*, as a literature dealing with attitudes and actions preparing for one's dying, was a development of the last stages of a distinctly Christian, religiously homogeneous society. By contrast, within contemporary North American culture, a search to find and to express a deep meaning in one's dying has emerged, manifested in a great variety of ways. Some of these ways are religious, but they reflect an enormous pluralism of religious belonging; others are not overtly religious and reflect a thoroughly secularized worldview. Each of these ways reciprocally influences the others to varying degrees.

A spirituality of dying

A contemporary art of dying can be described generically as a spirituality of dying. In this culture, such a spirituality expresses an effort by reflection and action to achieve a subjectively but deeply held ideal or aspiration with the aim of fulfilling what Paul Tillich has spoken of as one's "ultimate concern"—in the inclusive sense cited approvingly by the U.S. Supreme Court in recognizing a secular basis in law for conscientious objection to war (United States v. Seeger, 380 U.S. 163 (1964) at 187). A spirituality of dying, therefore, presupposes that one understands one's dying to involve a final free effort to achieve personal expression of one's deepest value commitment.

As held by the individual, this ideal of fulfillment, though personally appropriated, may be strongly influenced by a community of belief or ideology. A spirituality of dying involves more than the effort to observe moral obligations, though it is intimately related to that effort. A spirituality of dying seeks to achieve, not only as a moral obligation but also as an aspiration toward personal excellence in one's dying, an ultimate fulfillment of the personal self. A spirituality of dying includes a quest both for reflective understanding and for ways of behaving that express in action one's deep commitment.

Often in American culture, however, this personal search to discover and affirm an ultimate meaning in one's dying is avoided or evaded as long as death is not imminent, not only by patients but also by family and friends and by medical caregivers. Because a majority of those dying of a diagnosed illness die within a medical institution rather than (as in former times) at home, the individual's reluctance to deal seriously with the future event of death is often influenced by how medical caregivers view the meaning of their professional activity. Since the antibiotic revolution of midcentury, a tendency has existed within high-technology medical caregiving to emphasize quantitative prolongation of life achieved by treatments aimed at cure. This has produced a proclivity in many caregivers toward "medical vitalism" (seeking to prolong biological survival at any cost in suffering), and so contributes to what Ernest Becker (1973) has described as "denial of death." The qualitative improvement of life of the incurable, which palliative medicine aims to achieve for the dying, has taken second place.

Reconstructing the art of dying

Several developments serve to counteract these influences and so to encourage a revival of explicit expressions of a spirituality of dying. First, Elisabeth Kübler-Ross (1969, 1983) has studied and described the different forms that the struggle to deal with dying actually takes in both adults and children. She found that the dying were very often shunned by caregivers and even family. Kübler-Ross observed that persons dying under medical care very often were not allowed to admit their awareness of approaching death or to voice openly their struggle to find and express meaning in their dying. When allowed to do so, however, the dying were found to be commonly struggling through what Kübler-Ross described insightfully as five typical stages: denial and isolation, anger, bargaining, depression, and finally acceptance. (Kübler-Ross does *not* make a normative claim with respect to the sequence of these stages or the moral value of the struggle of the dying person in each.) Thus, Kübler-Ross has promoted renewed recognition of an empirically observable, basic human need to transcend denial of death and to seek human sharing of one's dying quest for meaning with friends and caregivers.

Second, Kübler-Ross's psychological analysis seems to offer support to the experience of the hospice move-

ment in caring for the dying. Cicely Saunders founded hospice as a compassionate, medically sophisticated way of responding to the needs of the terminally ill. Hospice caregivers have observed that the terminally ill commonly want to interact in very personal, intimate ways with family, friends, and caregivers. Through these intimate relational interactions, the dying person often seeks what will make more or deeper sense of the life that has gone before and of its imminent ending (e.g., sometimes verbally through what is called "life review," often through a final caring by the dying person for family and caregivers). This hospice approach to care of the dying, therefore, includes sophisticated use of all available palliative medical measures as well as personal psychological and spiritual support of the dying person's autonomy in these personal interactions ending life.

Third, Eric J. Cassell (1991) has urged that all medical caregivers, in acute-care settings as well as formal hospice programs, should recognize that relief of suffering, which is more than relief of pain, constitutes a goal of medicine equally primary with prolongation of life. This comfort care should take priority as the more important goal shaping care of the dying. Cassell thus argues that giving priority to relief of suffering should be considered entirely respectable clinical medical practice in care of the dying. Explicit attention to protecting patient autonomy in the search for meaning in one's dying is thus supported across the spectrum of high-technology health caregiving.

Finally, the federal Patient Self-determination Act of 1990 has mandated that medical institutions receiving federal funds communicate to patients information about legal options available to them in their particular local jurisdiction to prepare an "advance directive" (typically, the "living will" or durable agency for health-care decision making). A number of jurisdictions also legally authorize "surrogate decision-making" procedures to be employed in the absence of written advance directives, and these encourage attention to unwritten expressions of how one would want to die while receiving health care. These legal measures, too, contribute to the growing realization of many people, outside as well as within the medical community, that, given the capacity of modern medicine to prolong dying, one needs to take responsibility in freedom for one's dying lest it be more burdened than benefited by medical care. All of these developments stimulate persons in our culture to reflect on their personal spirituality of dying.

Until recently, a person's struggle to develop and express a spirituality of dying under medical care became explicit as an effort to strike some balance between expressing courage in cooperating with caregivers in a "fight" to achieve cure, on the one hand, and expressing a trust and peaceful acceptance of, even submissive surrender to, death, on the other. Some medical caregivers (especially among physicians) communicate their expectation that the good patient will unconditionally endure suffering under treatments aimed at prolonging life—nurses generally are more often concerned to recognize and affirm the need of the patient for relief from suffering. Patients respond to both of these cues. Dying patients respond to Western religious traditions or to secular philosophies influenced by these traditions as well. The exercise of one's freedom in dealing with the approach of death has generally been interpreted to be virtuous not only when one resists death and endures suffering as part of treatment, but also when one accepts one's mortality by submitting to a divine providence or to an inevitable but impersonal human fate. A spirituality of dying also has often included recognizing acceptance of dying as the gracious receiving of the "gift" of a final relief from suffering—whether from providence or fate. Arthur Frank speaks of "a struggle, not a fight," in which the seriously ill or dying person has the "opportunity" through "acceptance" to "achieve something," to "organize the experience of grave illness," "to make our lives meaningful" (Frank, 1991, pp. 89–90).

Control over the hour of death: Is it artful?

In the last two decades of the twentieth century, however, the personal struggle to deal with human dying has begun to involve a third alternative. Increasingly the claim is made by such groups as the Hemlock Society and by some medical caregivers that competent patients who so choose have a moral right, and should have a legal right, to physician intervention that deliberately shortens the suffering involved in dying by initiating a new lethal process. Such claims of a right to precipitate one's own death seem to derive from two rather disparate but related developments in how one understands living and dying under medical care.

First, within medical ethics, a very strong emphasis has developed on the primacy of patient autonomy as the dominant value, over against values of caregiver nonmaleficence and beneficence formerly given priority. To the extent that patient autonomy is conceived of primarily or exclusively as the exercise of freedom in the form of *control,* and given moral pluralism as to the normative content of this control, patient autonomy can be claimed to include the choice of killing oneself as just another treatment to which subjects who are suffering in their dying can give their informed consent. If rational self-killing is claimed, at least implicitly, as a final step in achieving a deeply held ideal, an ultimate concern, it becomes a component of a new, third kind of spirituality of dying.

Second, these claims of the right to medical assistance in precipitating one's death seem also to derive from unfortunate experiences of prolonged dying under high-technology medical care. Many medical professionals and laypersons believe that a significant number of medical caregivers do not know how to stop aggressively cure-oriented medical treatments at an appropriate point and are simply unable to give priority to the goal of comfort of the dying and hospice-type care. Thus, they fear dying under high-technology medical care that they cannot prevent from being torturously prolonged. Disproportionate increase of suicide among the aging in our culture is seen to derive from this fear. The lengthening survival of aged persons in a severely compromised or progressively demented state also confirms this fear, as does the prolonged survival of the permanently unconscious through use of medically engineered nutrition and hydration and antibiotics. The right to suicide can appear, therefore, to be needed as a measure of preemptive self-defense that qualifies the older spiritualities' enjoining virtuous submission to death.

The troubling question of the conflicting spiritualities of dying described by a modern art of dying is now posed in a new way: Is an appropriate way to fulfill one's spiritual ideal of living and dying expressed when some persons exercise their autonomy by seeking to control decisively their moment of dying through a final decision seeking medically assisted self-killing? Or, if this does not express a high spiritual ideal, is self-killing at least sometimes morally justified as a desperate measure no longer to be judged wholly inconsistent with traditional ideals of submission to death—given our increasingly impersonal, technologically driven, cure-obsessed medical-care culture? These questions are about competing commitments to conflicting conceptions of ultimate concern, and thus also about the deepest meaning of freedom and about the ideals and limits of exercising freedom in shaping one's self according to one's ultimate concern.

This new option in the struggle to achieve meaning and fulfillment in dying according to one's ultimate concern has begun to affect the older ethic of medical care that excluded inflicted death as treatment. Conflict among these spiritualities of dying may even produce separate systems of health care and other kinds of social and political institutional diversity. If so, the *ars moriendi* of the future will be a story not only about the diverse ways in which individuals pursue their personal quest for a deeply meaningful way to be and to act in their dying, but also about a conflict of human institutions tailored to support these diverse final expressions of ultimate concern.

JAMES F. BRESNAHAN

Directly related to this article is the companion article in this entry: ARS MORIENDI. *Also directly related is the entry*

DEATH EDUCATION. *For a further discussion of topics mentioned in this article, see the entries* AUTONOMY; BENEFICENCE; DEATH AND DYING: EUTHANASIA AND SUSTAINING LIFE, *articles on* HISTORICAL ASPECTS, ETHICAL ISSUES, *and* ADVANCE DIRECTIVES; HOSPICE AND END-OF-LIFE CARE; *and* SUICIDE. *For a discussion of related ideas, see the entries* AGING AND THE AGED, *articles on* SOCIETAL AGING, HEALTH-CARE AND RESEARCH ISSUES, *and* OLD AGE; DEATH, *article on* DEATH IN THE WESTERN WORLD (*with its* POSTSCRIPT); *and* DEATH, ATTITUDES TOWARD.

Bibliography

BECKER, ERNEST. 1973. *The Denial of Death*. New York: Free Press.

BRESNAHAN, JAMES F. 1991. "Catholic Spirituality and Medical Interventions in Dying." *America* 164 (June 22–29):670–675.

CASSELL, ERIC J. 1991. *The Nature of Suffering and the Goals of Medicine*. New York: Oxford University Press.

FRANK, ARTHUR W. 1991. *At the Will of the Body: Reflections on Illness*. New York: Houghton Mifflin.

HAMEL, RONALD P., ed. 1991. *Choosing Death: Active Euthanasia, Religion, and the Public Debate*. Philadelphia: Trinity Press International.

KÜBLER-ROSS, ELISABETH. 1969. *On Death and Dying*. New York: Macmillan.

———. 1983. *On Children and Death*. New York: Macmillan.

QUILL, TIMOTHY E. 1993. "Doctor, I Want to Die. Will You Help Me?" *Journal of the American Medical Association* 270, no. 7:870–873.

STODDARD, SANDOL. 1992. *The Hospice Movement: A Better Way of Caring*. Rev. ed. New York: Vintage.

WANZER, SIDNEY H.; FEDERMAN, DANIEL D.; ADELSTEIN, S. JAMES; CASSEL, CHRISTINE K.; CASSEM, EDWIN H.; CRANFORD, RONALD E.; HOOK, EDWARD W.; LO, BERNARD; MOERTEL, CHARLES G.; SAFAR, PETER; STONE, ALAN; and van EYS, JAN. 1989. "The Physician's Responsibility Toward Hopelessly Ill Patients: A Second Look." *New England Journal of Medicine* 320:844–849.

DEATH AND DYING: EUTHANASIA AND SUSTAINING LIFE

I. Historical Aspects
   Harold Y. Vanderpool
II. Ethical Issues
   Dan W. Brock
III. Advance Directives
   Joanne Lynn
   Joan M. Teno
IV. Professional and Public Policies
   Alexander Morgan Capron

I. HISTORICAL ASPECTS

Drawn from the Greek language (*eu* for good or noble, and *thanatos* for death), the English word "euthanasia" was coined by Francis Bacon (1561–1626) in the seventeenth century and referred to an easy, painless, happy death. Although the term euthanasia is no longer used as Bacon defined it, the concept of "good death" appears in many historical settings and encompasses a variety of beliefs and practices.

Four long-standing meanings of *euthanatos* are historically traced in this essay: (1) inducing death for sufferers; (2) ending the lives of the unwanted; (3) caring for the dying; and (4) letting persons die. In keeping with contemporary definitions and common usage, this article restricts the use of the term "euthanasia" to the first two meanings. To preserve historical usage, the word "euthanatos" is coined to refer to all four meanings, including the third, care-for-the-dying tradition called "euthanasia" by Bacon and many others well into the twentieth century, and the fourth, letting-die tradition that has been variously called "indirect," "negative," or "passive" euthanasia since 1960. Ideas and practices regarding the prolongation of human life are also discussed in their relevant historical settings.

This exploration of four thousand years of human history centers on the meanings of euthanatos within the West's major religious and secular traditions. The historic and living traditions discussed here include Hebraic-Jewish, Graeco-Roman, Christian, and Enlightenment-secular heritages through the nineteenth century, as well as certain medical, national, and philosophical traditions in the nineteenth and twentieth centuries.

Hebraic and Jewish perspectives

Preserving stories and teachings as ancient as the second millennium B.C.E., the Hebrew Scriptures proclaim an understanding of human life that has been immensely influential in Christian, Islamic, and Western history. Humans are created by God (Gen. 2:2–27); life and consciousness are precious gifts of God; and as Lord of life, God alone should determine when and how humans die (Job 1:21). As God's property, no individual has the right to destroy his or her life as if it were self-owned. Nor is it lawful wantonly to take the life of another person (Ex. 20:13, Gen. 9:5–6). The Hebraic heritage does not, however, elevate the sanctity or intrinsic value of human life over all other values (cf. Brody, 1989; Jakobovits, 1959). Death penalties are decreed for those guilty of transgressing divine laws (Ex. 21:12–17); Israel's opponents can be destroyed (Deut. 2 and 3), and

King Saul was not criticized after he killed himself to avoid mockery and death at the hands of the enemy (1 Sam. 31:3–4, 2 Sam. 2:17–23).

Yet for the Hebrews, life is inherently precious. Received as a divine gift, life should never be destroyed without divine warrant. Although life is brief and frail for all (Ps. 103:15–16), longevity is prized as a reward for righteousness (Gen. 25:7–8; Ps. 34:15–22), while early death is often attributed to disobedience and sin (Job 22:16; Ps. 37:35–37).

Predicated on this legacy, Jewish tradition values human life by requiring that when life is threatened by illness or injury, it must be sustained if possible. Jews were and are positively obligated to prolong their lives by seeking medical treatment when needed, and they are not to settle in communities where no physician is available. Obligations to save and extend life are drawn from Scripture: "You shall not stand idly by the blood of your neighbor" (Lev. 19:16). Advanced medical interventions are urged for critically ill persons as long as there is good reason to believe that such treatment will save or prolong life (Bleich, 1979). Rabbinic debate continues over those situations in which life can be prolonged for a while, but only at the expense of great pain with no hope for real cure. Past and present Jewish authorities have held that active pain relief can be undertaken at the risk of the patient's dying sooner (Jakobovits, 1959; Brody, 1989).

Death must never be hastened by intention. Physicians who kill patients in order to spare them from pain are considered murderers (Ex. 20:13, and Carmi, 1984). To end the lives of those who might be viewed as socially unwanted is absolutely prohibited. This includes killing or neglecting severely deformed newborns (Bleich, 1979).

While forbidding euthanasia, Judaism nevertheless accepts two meanings of euthanatos: caring for dying persons and letting terminally ill persons die. The meaning of "honorable death" (Mita Yafa) in the Talmud centers on merciful dying, not mercy killing (Carmi, 1984). Each dying person (goses) should be comforted by the prayers and presence of relatives, friends, and physicians. Prayers for life to end are permissible. Once the patient is goses, treatments that interrupt or prolong dying and hinder the soul's departure should be discontinued (Bleich, 1979).

Graeco-Roman antiquity

By the fifth century B.C.E., Greek physicians and the aristocracy were heralding health as a human value par excellence. Accompanying this ideal, Greeks ascribed superior status to the healthy and regarded sick persons as weak and inferior (Edelstein, 1967). To promote health and preserve life, rules regarding food, drink, exercise, hygiene, sleep, and the emotions were assiduously cultivated. This regimen lay at the heart of the physician's art, the ultimate goals of which were "to bring health in all cases of sickness [and] preservation of health to those who are well" ("Regimen in Acute Diseases," 4th c. B.C.E., p. 71). As reflected in the influential writings of Galen (131–201 C.E.), these Grecian ideals and approaches were adapted to Roman life and its institutions.

As cultivators of health through comparatively mild, dietetic measures, Greek physicians were urged to recognize the limitations of their art. Modestly conceived, their goals were "to do away with the sufferings of the sick, to lessen the violence of their diseases, and to refuse to treat those who are overmastered by their diseases" ("The Art," 5th c. B.C.E., p. 193). Persons with dire prognoses could, and apparently often did, seek cures through religious means—in particular, by sojourning in the temples of Asclepius, god of healing. But medical practitioners believed they would abuse their art and ruin their reputations if they sought to prolong the lives of the severely ill and injured.

Graeco-Roman views of euthanasia harmonized with these understandings of health, healing, and human excellence. Ordinary Greek practitioners, Socrates (ca. 470–399 B.C.E.), Plato (ca. 427–348 B.C.E.), and Stoic philosophers from Zeno (ca. 336–264 B.C.E., Greece) to Seneca (4 B.C.E.–65 C.E., Rome) justified induced death for severely sick and suffering humans. Predicating human worth on social usefulness and accenting the welfare of the city, the polis, Socrates and Plato believed that chronically sick persons were expendable. Unable to carry out active, socially useful lives, these persons consumed the vital resources of family and community. With or without their requests and consent, their lives could be ended justifiably (Carrick, 1985). Seneca and earlier Stoics praised the capacity of humans to choose how to end their lives. Humans ought to quit life nobly, rather than passively await the cruel endings "either of disease or of man" (Seneca in Carrick, 1985, p. 145). Preferring voluntary death to extended agony, sufferers of dreadful injuries and diseases were readily given life-extinguishing poisons—in particular, hemlock—by willing physicians (Edelstein, 1967). Elite citizens, virgins, married women, slaves, common persons, and soldiers ended their lives when faced with humiliation, fearful futures, illness, and old age (van Hooff, 1990).

These strands of opinion and practice display how Graeco-Roman thought and practice endorsed the permissibility of euthanasia both in the form of voluntary death for sufferers and in the form of extinguishing the lives of unwanted humans involuntarily. This view included putting to death deformed and sickly infants. Such infants were usually killed by exposure, either before they were first fed—at which time they were not considered fully human—or after being fed, if they were chronically and pitifully sick (Carrick, 1985). Plato justified euthanasia for sick and defective infants, whom he regarded as too great a burden for the polis. By law in Sparta, newborns were examined by nonparents for anatomical flawlessness and vigor to determine which should be exposed (Amundsen, 1987).

Certain individuals and schools of thought, however, opposed induced death for sufferers. Holding that death is "the most terrible of all things," Aristotle (384–322 B.C.E.) withstood the willful ending of life in the face of dire infirmity, even though he, too, justified infanticide for defective newborns (Amundsen, 1987; Carrick, 1985). Aristotle's objections to induced death reflected his notions of human virtue—the nobility of facing death bravely rather than cowardly quitting life when faced with pain.

The Hippocratic Oath, vastly influential in Western history, has physicians swear "neither to give a deadly drug to anybody if asked for it, nor . . . [to] make a suggestion to this effect" (Edelstein, 1967, p. 6). Wrongly attributed to Hippocrates (469–399 B.C.E.) until the 1960s, the oath reflects Pythagorean or partly Pythagorean origins (Edelstein, 1967; Carrick, 1985). In contrast to the dominant Greek traditions sketched above, Pythagoreans opposed physician-assisted euthanasia in an almost Hebraic sense. With the gods "our keepers" and we "one of their possessions," we sin against our masters if we seek to escape from our posts in life. Like Judaism before and Christianity thereafter, this view rests on the premise that God or gods exist, that humans must obey divine commands, and that one of these commands bars humans from taking early leave from earthly existence (Carrick, 1985).

Christian views

Christianity emerged from Judaism and matured within the Graeco-Roman world. Christians viewed Hebrew scripture as the Word of God, but they reinterpreted its meaning in light of the actions, teachings, death, and resurrection of Jesus the Christ. Within three centuries, the orthodox Church developed a thoroughgoing critique of many features of Greco-Roman culture.

Early Christianity. Like their Jewish predecessors, Christians regarded God as the sovereign creator and sustainer of human life, whose commandments must be obeyed. From its beginnings, Christianity opposed self-induced death out of suffering or despair. Contrary to the myth that many people committed suicide to escape from life and be with God, Christ, and departed loved ones, early Christians ardently opposed self-induced death (cf. Amundsen, 1989; Beauchamp, 1989).

Christianity added new themes to Jewish criticisms of suicide and euthanasia. With the suffering and death of Jesus as their model, Christians accented the redemptive dimensions of suffering (2 Cor. 12:7–10, Heb. 12:5–11). In the face of pain and death, they, too, should exclaim, "Not my will, but thine, be done" (Luke 22:42). Beginning with the early church (Jas. 5:10) and extending through writings of Christian theologians from the second century to the time of Augustine (354–430 C.E.), Christians praised the example of Job, who endured grave suffering steadfastly (Amundsen, 1989). Patience and steadfastness were valued all the more in the face of frequent persecutions from Christianity's opponents (1 Pet. 4:12–5:1). Faith and hope sustained throughout adversity would help secure the reward of eternal blessing at the great judgment day at the end of time (Matt. 25:31–46, Rom. 8:16–36).

Bodily existence was not to be despised (1 Cor. 6:19–20). Christian accents on the intrinsic worth of life were rooted in Jesus' teaching that all humans are the daughters and sons of a loving Father (Luke 15) as reflected in his ministry to the sick, infirm, and dying (e.g., Luke 4:16–21, 8:26–56). The power to heal was conveyed to the leaders of the early church (Luke 10; Acts 3ff.), who cultivated the virtues of mercy, compassion, and love for the sick and poor (Matt. 5:7; Luke 6:36, 10:29–37).

These themes informed early Christian critiques of Graeco-Roman society (1 John 2:15–4:21). By the second and third centuries, Christianity's defenders were condemning gladiatorial spectacles, abortions, infanticide, a host of sexual sins, and self-induced death (Amundsen, 1989). No human group was considered unwanted or unworthy of life and nurturing. Like the Neoplatonists, Christians reasoned that no person should separate one's divinely co-joined body and soul by self-killing (van Hooff, 1990).

Augustine. In the fourth century, Augustine's elaborate criticisms of suicide, including ending one's life because of raging pain, appealed to the Bible as authoritative and addressed justifications of self-induced death by Stoics and others (Amundsen, 1989; van Hooff, 1990). Like Aristotle, Augustine regarded self-inflicted death as cowardly. He viewed it as contrary to the sixth commandment, "Thou shall not kill." He also regarded self-killing as an egregious sin because it excluded the possibility of repentance (Amundsen, 1989). With the establishment of Christianity as the officially sanctioned religion of the Roman Empire after 325, self-killing became equated with homicide. Within central and northern Europe, the property of suicides was confiscated, their corpses were desecrated, and they were excluded from Christian burial grounds.

Aquinas and modern Roman Catholicism. Thomas Aquinas (1225–1274) and later Catholic theologians followed this reasoning. Aquinas also expanded upon past arguments against suicide in ways that deeply inform Roman Catholic perspectives to the present time. Suicide, and, by extension, euthanasia for sufferers, were and are viewed as contrary to Christian tradition, to natural law, to the well-being of civil society, to Christian compassion, and, most important, to the dominion of God over human life (Beauchamp, 1989; Sullivan, 1975; Sacred Congregation, 1980).

While forbidding the intentional killing (euthanasia) of all innocent human beings, contemporary Roman Catholicism permits letting grievously and terminally ill persons die by forgoing life-sustaining measures. While ordinary means of prolonging life are required, technical measures that impose strain or suffering disproportionate to foreseen benefits may be discontinued. This prescription includes refusing "forms of treatment that would only secure a precarious and burdensome prolongation of life" in the face of inevitable death (Sacred Congregation, 1980, p. 156).

Protestantism. On matters of life and death, the major Protestant Reformers of the sixteenth century differed little from their Catholic predecessors. By the seventeenth century, however, differences appeared in Protestant thought. Although they still regarded suicide as contrary to the sixth commandment and against natural law, Lutheran and Puritan divines argued that some self-inflicted deaths stemmed from mental imbalance. Against Catholic notions of suicide as an unforgivable sin, they held that the soul's eternal destiny was for God alone to decide (Ferngren, 1989). Deviating further from Christianity's orthodox legacy, the English poet and Anglican prelate John Donne (1572–1631) sought to prove that certain instances of suicide did not violate natural law, human reason, Scripture, or the dominion of God over human life. Although other Protestants, John Locke (1632–1704) included, continued to condemn self-killing as contrary to nature, opposed to the commandments of God, and cowardly, this standard Protestant view emerged: Mitigating circumstances must be permitted, and those who take their own lives should be entrusted to the mercy of God (Ferngren, 1989).

Modern Protestants remain divided on the morality of self-ended life for the terminally ill. While Paul Ramsey and Arthur J. Dyck oppose voluntary euthanasia, other Protestant ethicists as diverse as Joseph Fletcher and Paul D. Simmons defend the morality of euthanasia for persons suffering from painful and fatal disease. Fletcher and Simmons maintain that biblical and humanistic notions of mercy, love, and the worth and dignity of each individual justify ending life when personal existence is degraded and demoralized by terminal disease (Fletcher, 1954; Simmons, 1983).

Regarding the morality of letting persons die, Protestants generally agree that in instances when life is being prolonged by advanced technology without the possibility of restoring meaningful health, treatment can be discontinued. In his influential early work on medical ethics, Paul Ramsey discussed "only caring for the dying." For Ramsey, this phrase denoted: (1) stopping useless treatments predicated on the notion that "death is always a disaster"; (2) never ending life directly; and (3) "positively to care, to comfort, to be humanly present" with dying persons (Ramsey, 1970, pp. 118, 160).

Ramsey's admonitions introduce the third meaning of euthanatos in the Catholic and Protestant West—ease and comfort for dying persons, short of hastened death. Good Christian dying became the focus of popular medieval Catholic manuals respecting Ars moriendi, The Art of Dying. This religious tradition of good dying centered on the weighty concerns of the time: caring for one's eternal soul, rather than falling into the error of dwelling on bodily health with the scant aid of medieval medicine (Copenhaver, 1995). Catholics and Protestants alike fostered notions of good dying through ensuing centuries of theological change and transformations in medical practice. Countless publications explained how to care for dying persons, as well as how to provide solace and inspiration to families and the faithful (Vanderpool, 1986).

Secular and Enlightenment legacies through the nineteenth century

As minority points of view within the dominant framework of Judeo-Christian culture, various secular thinkers from the sixteenth through the nineteenth centuries spoke of the permissibility of inducing death for seriously sick and injured persons.

Montaigne. Sickened by the heretic hunting, torturing, and massacres that marked the age in which he lived, Michel de Montaigne (1533–1592) professed to be a Catholic but voiced tolerance, neutrality, and scepticism. He summarized Catholic orthodoxy as a view widely supported:

> For many maintain, that we cannot quit this garrison of the world without the express command of him who has placed us here . . . it is for God, who sent us into this world, . . . to give us our discharge when it pleases him, and not for us to take it. (Montaigne, 1580, p. 339)

But, enamored with Greco-Roman thought and custom, Montaigne also espoused unorthodox views: "The most voluntary death is the finest"; and "God gives us permission enough [to take our lives] when he reduces us to such a condition that living is worse than dying" (Montaigne, 1580, p. 338). After elaborating on the numerous reasons for and ways of exchanging painful life for death, he remarked at the end of one of his essays, "Intolerable pain and the fear of a worse death appear to me to be the most excusable inducements" (Montaigne, 1580, p. 351).

The reigning religious orthodoxy of his time greatly limited Montaigne's immediate influence. But his skepticism, secular interests, and accent on personal pleasure were increasingly well received in England and France during the seventeenth and eighteenth centuries. In addition to John Donne, discussed above, English playwrights such as John Dryden (1631–1700) and Deists such as Charles Blount (1654–1693) defended certain suicides motivated by honor, suffering, lost love, or self-willed destiny (Ferngren, 1989). These themes informed the thought of one of the Enlightenment's greatest representatives, David Hume (1711–1776).

Hume.   In contrast to Montaigne, Hume began his essay "On Suicide" (1783) with a frontal attack on "superstition and false religion," which compels a person to prolong "a miserable existence . . . lest he offend his Maker" (Hume, 1783, pp. 252–253). Hume proposed to examine "all the common arguments against suicide" and show that it can be free "from every imputation of guilt or blame." Critiquing Thomas Aquinas's main arguments against suicide and voluntary active euthanasia, Hume held that sickness, overwhelming suffering, and accompanying wishes to die should be regarded as calling persons from life "in the clearest and most express terms" (Hume, 1783, pp. 253, 259).

Expressing views similar to those of Socrates and Plato, Hume predicated the morality of self-killing on one's duties to society. He reasoned that persons plagued with suffering to the point of negating their social usefulness were under no moral obligation to prolong their lives. Freed from social obligation, each person's "native liberty" consists of carrying out an autonomous course of action in keeping with one's "chance for happiness" (Hume, 1783, p. 261).

Throughout the eighteenth and nineteenth centuries, Hume's arguments were often opposed as the pernicious opinions of a Scottish infidel. Hume's critics included Immanuel Kant (1724–1824), who viewed self-killing as immoral because it cannot be willed as a universal course of action without undermining the very possibility of morality, namely the existence of rational beings. Kant also viewed voluntary euthanasia as a violation of one's duty to God, the sovereign of all life (Beauchamp, 1989).

Nineteenth century

Not until the end of the nineteenth century did arguments similar to Hume's enter the realm of public debate and advocacy respecting voluntary euthanasia. This debate emerged as the intellectual and social power of religion waned at the hands of biblical critics and evolutionists (Vanderpool, 1973). Like Hume, Arthur Schopenhauer (1788–1860), Friedrich Nietzsche (1844–1900), and others who advocated induced death appealed to the right of autonomous persons to end their lives when terminal disease extinguishes pleasure and social usefulness (Battin, 1995). Debates over the permissibility of physician-induced death for incurable sufferers first ensued in Great Britain and the United States in the last decades of the nineteenth century. Although the waning influence of religion in the face of secular onslaughts made the debate possible, discussion centered on doctors because they could diagnose incurability with far greater accuracy, and armed with chloroform and hypodermic morphine, first isolated in 1816, they could end pain—and life—with ease (Fye, 1978).

Moreover, physicians had become associated with death and the care of the dying. Rather than shunning cases of incurable illness as they had in antiquity and the Middle Ages, doctors by mid-century agreed, as in the Code of Ethics of the American Medical Association of 1847, that they

> ought not to abandon a patient because the case is deemed incurable; for [their] attendance may continue to be highly useful . . . even to the last period of a fatal malady, by alleviating pain and other symptoms, and by soothing mental anguish.

In effect, physicians in Germany, Great Britain, and the United States reformulated, then assumed control over, the centuries-old *Ars moriendi* tradition of the West's religious heritages. Employing the term "euthanasia" as it was first coined by Francis Bacon, physicians such as Carl F. H. Marx (1796–1877) practiced "that science . . . which checks oppressing features of illness, relieves pain, and renders the supreme and inescapable hour a most peaceful one" (Marx, 1826, p. 495). A number of the physicians who cultivated the "science" of diagnosing terminal illness, maintaining hope, and alleviating pain criticized religious traditions of good dying (Vanderpool, 1981). In keeping with the tenets of Judaism and Christianity, however, the great majority of physicians ardently opposed induced death, a legacy that extends to the present (Reiser, 1975).

Physician supervision at the time of death apparently met with little opposition. Hand in hand with their expanding diagnostic and therapeutic capabilities, physicians championed an all-pervasive social ideal, the prolongation of human life. While physicians in the Greco-Roman eras delimited medical interventions to restoring health within the constraints of nature, physicians in the seventeenth century and thereafter sought to gain greater command over nature. Personifying this trend, Francis Bacon called for a new branch of medicine: prolonging life by finding remedies for conditions considered incurable (Amundsen, 1978; Gruman, 1966). Life prolongation converged with the notion of progress that became an article of secular faith after the seventeenth century (Gruman, 1966; Webster, 1975).

In the eighteenth century, humane societies were established throughout the Western hemisphere for the purpose of saving persons who appeared to be dead from drowning, suffocation, and other causes. Many means were discovered by which to prolong life: manually induced breathing, smelling salts, ammonia, blood-letting, doses of strychnine, and tongue stretching. The duty to sustain life legitimated the supervisory roles of physicians at the bedsides of those thought to be dying. Confident that their diagnostic skills and messages of hope "happily prolonged" many lives, notable physicians consciously assumed these roles (Hooker, 1849, p. 353; Vanderpool, 1981).

Twentieth-century developments

In the twentieth century the word "euthanasia" became equated with hastened or induced death. Replacing its historic usage with phrases like "care for the dying," physicians in the early decades of the century continued to publish books and journal articles on their diagnostic, therapeutic, and emotional responsibilities with dying patients and family members (Worcester, 1935).

Technical pursuit of sustaining life. By the middle decades, however, physician control was directed toward sustaining life by technical means. Noting how medical practice had "deteriorated" with respect to "the art of caring for the dying," Alfred Worcester chastised his peers for their overuse of "modern methods of resuscitation." In "defiance of Nature" and against the "merciful release" of death, "too many of our profession," Worcester warned, feel "duty bound to do their utmost. They ought to know better" (Worcester, 1935, p. 47).

Such warnings often went unheeded as attempts to prolong life grew increasingly heroic and technologically complex. In the early 1900s, artificial circulation by cardiac massage and injections of epinephrine to the heart were introduced. Various types of mechanical respirators were employed in the 1930s, and in response to the polio epidemic of the early 1950s, the use of iron lung respirators became common. From the 1950s through the 1980s, enormous energy was expended on perfecting endotracheal and masked ventilators. With the discovery of anticoagulants (1916), blood oxygenators were developed and employed in surgery by the mid-1950s. Modern closed-chest cardiopulmonary shock devices were in place by the 1960s (Hermreck, 1988).

In the United States, the physician's duty to sustain life achieved increasing preeminence from the 1940s through the 1960s. Lest they betray the ideals and dynamics of their training and the common expectations of family members, many doctors felt that they should do everything possible to sustain life, rather than "just let the patient die" (Glaser and Strauss, 1965, p. 196; Ramsey, 1970). Even in the face of dire prognoses, heroic treatments were frequently continued until the patient's organ systems deteriorated, extensive pain was experienced, the patient's family members reached "an advanced stage of grieving," or one's colleagues intervened (Glaser and Strauss, 1965, p. 199).

Questioning the reign of technology. A broadly shared revulsion against undignifying, expensive, and often futile attempts to prolong human life began at the end of the 1960s. Revulsion was fueled by a resurgence of interest in death and dying, a broad-based advocacy of patients' rights, and the establishment of free-standing hospices and hospital-based palliative care units (Vanderpool, 1981). Aimed at recovering the tradition of humanely caring for and comforting dying persons, these post-1960 developments sought to free terminal patients from having to endure life-sustaining measures as standard treatment.

As noted, the permissibility of letting terminally ill persons die by forgoing life-sustaining measures accorded with Jewish, Catholic, and Protestant traditions. It also harmonized with the dominant principle of post-1970 secular medical ethics: respect for the autonomous choices of patients (Vanderpool, 1981). And it agreed with the principles of individual freedom and privacy inherent in Anglo-American law. From removing the respirator of Karen Ann Quinlan (1975) to removing hydration and nutrition from Claire Conroy (1983), patients and families have secured the right to forgo medical treatment in the face of catastrophic illness (Winslade and Ross, 1986).

Reappearance of inducing death. Not accented since Greco-Roman times, the second meaning of euthanatos—ending the lives of unwanted human beings—reappeared in the twentieth century. Convinced that human evolution depended upon the survival of the fittest (Darwinism), that a population's hereditary endowment could be improved by selective breeding (eugenics), and that heredity accounted for such conditions as "feeblemindedness," alcoholism, and criminality, numerous spokespersons and organizations successfully lobbied for forcible sterilization laws in the United States, England, and western Europe by the early 1930s (Garver and Garver, 1991).

Germany. An influential voice in Germany by the turn of the century, Ernst Haeckel (1834–1919) used eugenics and social Darwinism to argue that Germany's physical and mental incurables ought to be "delivered from evil" by being put to death painlessly. Haeckel praised the Spartans for killing their deformed and weak children—in contrast to "antiselection" stemming from exaggerated Christian compassion for the infirm and sickly (Van Der Sluis, 1979; Lifton, 1986).

Others regarded Germany as a new polis, the health and destiny of which rendered individual existence insignificant. Physicians should view this national polis as a patient. Each doctor should become a "physician to the *Volk*" for the "promotion and perfection of the health of the German people . . . to ensure . . . the full potential of their racial and genetic endowment" (Lifton, 1986, p. 30). After suffering the loss of so many young men during World War I and from scarcity and famine thereafter, the body politic should be healed and invigorated through programs of racial hygiene and physical fitness. Positive racial hygiene included marriage inducements for the fit, while negative hygiene moved from sterilization to induced death for those deemed inferior. By 1920 the eminent professor–lawyer Karl Binding and the professor-psychiatrist Alfred Hoche jointly sanctioned the destruction of "lives not worth living." They primarily had in mind the "completely worthless" and economically burdensome lives of severely retarded and deformed children. In the place of continued suffering and struggling deaths, their lives should be ended painlessly (Van Der Sluis, 1979).

These beliefs were widely accepted by physicians, academicians, and scientists within Germany before their adoption by Adolf Hitler (1889–1945) as a feature of National Socialist (Nazi) policy. Shortly before Germany's invasion of Poland in September 1939, Hitler directed that children with severe mongolism, hydrocephaly, paralysis, and deformities must be registered. In about thirty newly established pediatric departments all over Germany, physicians supervised the registering, sorting out, and euthanizing of some 5,000 children, most of whom were killed by drinking overdoses of the sedative sodium phenobarbital (Lauter and Meyer, 1982). Within months, Hitler issued a brief decree that mentally ill adolescents and adults should be killed—in his words, that those "considered incurable according to the best available human judgment . . . be granted a mercy death." This decree created an agency that orchestrated physician-directed killing of 80,000 to 100,000 persons in gas chambers disguised as showers (Lifton, 1986, p. 63).

A minority of Catholic and Protestant clergy publicly and passionately opposed this program of involuntary euthanasia. Once they were stereotyped as destructive to the health of the body politic, Jews, Gypsies, and others were consigned to a massive, bureaucratic, doctor-run extermination program modeled on its medical predecessors. Although all these programs lasted only six years, they remained forever etched in the minds of those who debated the morality of euthanasia thereafter.

Anglo-American developments. After World War II, the World Medical Association, along with several national medical associations, condemned the Nazi extermination programs, including the killing of defective and incurably sick children and adults. After 1960, however, the development and use of dramatic, new life-saving techniques for premature and severely defec-

tive newborns again raised poignant questions as to the permissibility of involuntary euthanasia for infants. In the United States, debate ensued over the morality of allowing a child with Down syndrome and an intestinal blockage to starve to death. After the 1971 filming and popularizing of this "Johns Hopkins Case," Raymond S. Duff and A. G. M. Campbell published a survey of the treatments and moral dilemmas in the special-care nursery of the Yale-New Haven Hospital. They indicated that between 1970 and 1972, 14 percent of the severely impaired infants in that nursery were allowed to die from withdrawal of treatment (Duff and Campbell, 1973). In light of the Nazi past, discussion centered on the morality of passively allowing infants with multiple anomalies to die, rather than actively ending their lives. The debate also sought to reject the values on which Nazi policy had been based—eugenics, race, and national costs. Those who defend the morality of allowing certain infants to die focus on limiting the extent to which the new technology should be used for those who manifest no potential for human relationships (McCormick, 1974) or for those whose existence is continually painful to self and severely burdensome to the family (Engelhardt, 1975).

The turmoil that began at the end of the nineteenth century over induced death for willing, terminally ill adults continued in the twentieth century. In England, bills favoring the legalization of physician-administered voluntary euthanasia were introduced in the House of Lords in 1936, 1950, and 1969. In the United States, similar measures were introduced in the state legislatures of Ohio (1906), Iowa (1906), Nebraska (1937), New York (1947), Idaho (1969), Oregon (1973), Washington (1991), and California (1992). Though promulgated by clergy, physicians, writers, and members of England's Voluntary Euthanasia Legalization Society (founded in 1935), the Euthanasia Society of America (1938), and the Hemlock Society (1980), none of these bills passed.

The issues behind all these initiatives have remained surprisingly consistent over time. Proponents have appealed to respect for personal autonomy, ideals of peaceful death, the hope of freeing patients from painful and undignifying disease, the need to protect compassionate physicians from homicide charges, and the virtue of mercy. Opponents have held that the legalization of active euthanasia undermines physicians' historic healing roles and the trust inherent in the doctor–patient relationship; falsely assumes that terminally sick patients can make clear moral judgments; heightens already-present feelings of guilt and burdensomeness on the part of patients; may give rise to involuntary euthanasia for vulnerable humans who are severely physically and emotionally compromised but not terminally ill; and opposes Jewish and Christian traditions ("Voluntary Euthanasia," 1936; Breo, 1991).

During the last three decades of this century, public

opinion in the United States has been shifting in favor of legalized euthanasia. Asked whether doctors should be allowed legally to end the lives of incurably sick persons when they or their families request it, 63 percent of Americans responded "yes" in several national opinion surveys conducted between 1983 and 1991—in contrast to 36 percent in 1950 (Blendon, 1992). This shift in attitudes resulted primarily from patients' fears of being burdensome to the family, their fears of being forced to live in pain and dependency on life-prolonging machines, and the degree to which euthanasia has been discussed and advocated in scholarly circles (Fletcher, 1954; Engelhardt, 1986), the press, and best-seller publications (Humphry, 1991). Popular rhetoric now refers to physician-performed voluntary euthanasia not as aid-in-death, but as "aid-in-dying," a phrase that euphemistically associates mercy killing with the tradition of "caring for the dying" advanced by physicians after the seventeenth century.

The Netherlands.   That the Netherlands had legalized active euthanasia by the early 1990s was widely rumored and reported, but false. In fact, the Netherlands' penal code during that time stated that anyone who takes another's life, even upon that person's serious and explicit request, can be imprisoned for up to twelve years. Without reforming that code, the Dutch nevertheless made it possible for physicians to end the lives of incurably sick and suffering patients. A nationwide study indicated that 54 percent of Dutch physicians had practiced euthanasia and that the lives of 1.8 percent of Dutch citizens were ended by lethal drugs upon request (Van Der Mass et al., 1991). Physicians can escape state prosecution if they act in accord with criteria developed in case law and established as precise guidelines in Holland's medical institutions. These guidelines hold that patients must be incurably sick, must be experiencing unbearable suffering, and must clearly and persistingly request that their lives be ended. The Netherlands' quasi-legal allowance of active euthanasia rests on a four-centuries-old tradition of tolerance and on the secular assumption that humans are responsible for their own lives—and deaths. Leading opponents of attempts to decriminalize mercy killing in the Netherlands appeal to the horrors of Nazism and to Judeo-Christian teaching: Active euthanasia is a slippery slope toward "mercy killing" on a massive scale, and humans are creatures of God who have no right to end their own lives (Pence, 1988).

Perspectives

Against this historical backdrop, it is clear that contemporary debates over physician-induced voluntary euthanasia in the United States and continental Europe still pit Jewish and Christian traditionalists against those espousing secular and Enlightenment versions of Greco-Roman thought. All those persons debating the issue must also take into account the Nazi atrocities as well as organized medicine's longstanding commitments and practices.

The different concepts and practices of euthanatos surveyed here emerged from particular understandings of the world, each of which embeds meanings of life and death in some overarching vision of human worth and destiny. Reformulated in the face of cultural and historical change, most of the historical visions described still survive in the modern West. They are perpetuated by historically shaped, like-minded social groups through which persons secure self-identity—Catholic, or Protestant, or in the camp of Kant or Hume, or loyal to the Hippocratic Oath. Coexisting within national boundaries, these groups make up Western pluralism.

This pluralism accounts for the nature of present-day public discourse whereby persons of differing persuasions register their opinions freely and seek to persuade others to adopt their views. Widespread discussion enabled persons of various persuasions to discover that they could agree on ways to care for the dying as well as on the morality of withdrawing life-sustaining medical interventions at the end of life. Common fears over being forced to become machine-dependent or tube-fed at the end of life have motivated disparate groups to lobby for the right to die more naturally and peacefully.

But no common ground has been found with respect to physician-supervised voluntary euthanasia. While the permissibility of forgoing life-sustaining treatment accorded with the basic premises and aims of the West's major cultural heritages, euthanasia kindles conflict rather than compromise.

Western pluralism sanctions endless arguing over euthanasia, but the arguments of respective groups readily pass over the others' heads. Until the discussion deepens to an exchange that deals with the frameworks of meaning that undergird the opposing views, disagreement over induced death is unlikely to end.

HAROLD Y. VANDERPOOL

Directly related to this article are the other articles in this entry: ETHICAL ISSUES, ADVANCE DIRECTIVES, *and* PROFESSIONAL AND PUBLIC POLICIES. *Also directly related are the entries* DEATH: ART OF DYING; DEATH, *article on* WESTERN RELIGIOUS THOUGHT; SUICIDE; HOMICIDE; *and* HOSPICE AND END-OF-LIFE CARE. *For a further discussion of topics mentioned in this article, see the entries* AUTONOMY; JUDAISM; NATURAL LAW; PAIN AND SUFFERING; PATERNALISM; PROTESTANTISM; ROMAN CATHOLICISM; *and* VALUE AND VALUATION. *For a discussion of related ideas, see the entries* AGING AND THE AGED, *articles on* HEALTH-CARE AND RESEARCH ISSUES, *and* OLD AGE; EUGENICS; LIFE; LIFE, QUALITY OF; MEDICAL CODES AND OATHS, *article on* HISTORY; MEDICAL ETHICS, HISTORY

OF, *section on* EUROPE, *especially the article on* THE BEN-
ELUX COUNTRIES, *and section on* THE AMERICAS; *and*
NATIONAL SOCIALISM. *See also the* APPENDIX (CODES,
OATHS, AND DIRECTIVES RELATED TO BIOETHICS),
SECTION II: ETHICAL DIRECTIVES FOR THE PRACTICE OF
MEDICINE, OATH OF HIPPOCRATES, *and* CODE OF ETHICS
[1847] OF THE AMERICAN MEDICAL ASSOCIATION.

Bibliography

AMUNDSEN, DARREL W. 1978. "The Physician's Obligation to
Prolong Life: A Medical Duty without Classical Roots."
Hastings Center Report 8, no. 4:23–30.
———. 1987. "Medicine and the Birth of Defective Children:
Approaches of the Ancient World." In *Euthanasia and the
Newborn: Conflicts Regarding Saving Lives*, pp. 3–22. Ed-
ited by Richard C. McMillan; H. Tristram Engelhardt,
Jr.; and Stuart F. Spicker. Dordrecht, Netherlands: D.
Reidel.
———. 1989. "Suicide and Early Christian Values." In *Suicide
and Euthanasia: Historical and Contemporary Themes*, pp.
77–153. Edited by Baruch A. Brody. Dordrecht, Nether-
lands: Kluwer.
"The Art." 1923. *Hippocrates*, II, pp. 186–217. Translated by
W. H. S. Jones. Cambridge, Mass.: Harvard University
Press.
BATTIN, MARGARET PABST. 1995. "Suicide." In *Encyclopedia
of Bioethics*, 2d ed. Edited by Warren Reich. New York:
Macmillan.
BEAUCHAMP, TOM L. 1989. "Suicide in the Age of Reason."
In *Suicide and Euthanasia: Historical and Contemporary
Themes*, pp. 183–219. Edited by Baruch A. Brody. Dor-
drecht, Netherlands: Kluwer.
BLEICH, J. DAVID. 1979. "The Obligation to Heal in the Ju-
daic Tradition: A Comparative Analysis" In *Jewish Bioeth-
ics*, pp. 1–44. Edited by Fred Rosner and J. David Bleich.
New York: Sanhedrin Press.
BLENDON, ROBERT J. et al. 1992. "Should Physicians Aid
Their Patients in Dying? The Public Perspective." *Journal
of the American Medical Association* 267, no. 19:2658–
2662.
BREO, DENNIS L. 1991. "MD-Aided Suicide Voted Down:
Both Sides Say Debate to Continue." *Journal of the Amer-
ican Medical Association* 266, no. 20:2895–2896, 2899–
2900.
BRODY, BARUCH A. 1989. "An Historical Introduction to Jew-
ish Casuistry on Suicide and Euthanasia." In *Suicide and
Euthanasia: Historical and Contemporary Themes*, pp. 39–
75. Edited by Baruch A. Brody. Dordrecht, Netherlands:
Kluwer.
CARMI, A. 1984. "Live Like a King: Die Like a King." In *Eu-
thanasia*, pp. 3–28. Edited by A. Carmi. New York:
Springer-Verlag.
CARRICK, PAUL. 1985. *Medical Ethics in Antiquity: Philosophical
Perspectives on Abortion and Euthanasia*. Dordrecht, Neth-
erlands: D. Reidel.
COPENHAVER, BRIAN P. 1995. "Death: Art of Dying: I. Ars
Moriendi." In *Encyclopedia of Bioethics*, 2d ed. Edited by
Warren Reich. New York: Macmillan.

DUFF, RAYMOND S., and CAMPBELL, A. G. M. 1973. "Moral
and Ethical Dilemmas in the Special-Care Nursery." *New
England Journal of Medicine* 289, no. 17:890–894.
EDELSTEIN, LUDWIG. 1967. In *Ancient Medicine: Selected Papers
of Ludwig Edelstein*. Edited by Owsei Temkin and C. Lilian
Temkin. Baltimore: Johns Hopkins Press.
ENGELHARDT, H. TRISTRAM, JR. 1975. "Ethical Issues in Aid-
ing the Death of Young Children." In *Beneficent Eutha-
nasia*, pp. 180–192. Edited by Marvin Kohl. Buffalo,
N.Y.: Prometheus Books.
———. 1986. *The Foundations of Bioethics*. New York: Oxford
University Press.
FERNGREN, GARY B. 1989. "The Ethics of Suicide in the Re-
naissance and Reformation." In *Suicide and Euthanasia:
Historical and Contemporary Themes*, pp. 155–181. Edited
by Baruch A. Brody. Dordrecht, Netherlands: Kluwer.
FLETCHER, JOSEPH. 1960 [1954]. *Morals and Medicine*. Boston:
Beacon Press.
FYE, W. BRUCE. 1978. "Active Euthanasia: An Historical Sur-
vey of Its Conceptual Origins and Introduction into Med-
ical Thought." *Bulletin of the History of Medicine* 52, no.
4:492–502.
GARVER, KENNETH L., and GARVER, BETTYLEE. 1991. "Eugen-
ics: Past, Present, and the Future." *American Journal of
Human Genetics* 49, no. 5:1109–1118.
GLASER, BARNEY G., and STRAUSS, ANSELM L. 1965. *Aware-
ness of Dying*. Chicago: Aldine.
GRUMAN, GERALD J. 1966. "A History of Ideas About the Pro-
longation of Life." *Transactions of the American Philosoph-
ical Society*, new series 56, part 9:3–102.
HERMRECK, ARLO S. 1988. "The History of Cardiopulmonary
Resuscitation." *The American Journal of Surgery* 156, no.
6:430–436.
HOOKER, WORTHINGTON. 1972 [1849]. *Physician and Patient:
Or a Practical View of the Mutual Duties, Relations, and In-
terests of the Medical Profession and the Community*. New
York: Arno Press.
HUME, DAVID. 1963 [1783]. In *Hume on Religion*. Edited by
Richard Wollheim. New York: World Publishing.
HUMPHRY, DEREK. 1991. *Final Exit: The Practicalities of Self-
Deliverance and Assisted Suicide for the Dying*. Eugene,
Ore.: Hemlock Society.
JAKOBOVITS, IMMANUEL. 1959. *Jewish Medical Ethics*. New
York: Bloch Publishing.
LAUTER, H., and MEYER, J. E. 1982. "Mercy Killing Without
Consent: Historical Comments on a Controversial Issue."
Acta Psychiatria Scandinavica 65, no. 2:134–141.
LIFTON, ROBERT JAY. 1986. *The Nazi Doctors: Medical Killing
and the Psychology of Genocide*. New York: Basic Books.
MARX, CARL F. H. 1977 [1826]. "Medical Euthanasia." In
*Ethics in Medicine: Historical Perspectives and Contemporary
Concerns*, pp. 495–497. Edited by Stanley Joel Reiser, Ar-
thur J. Dyck, and William J. Curran. Cambridge, Mass.:
MIT Press.
McCORMICK, RICHARD A. 1974. "To Save or Let Die: The
Dilemma of Modern Medicine." *Journal of the American
Medical Association* 229, no. 2:172–176.
MONTAIGNE, MICHEL. 1946 [1580]. "A Custom of the Island
of Cea." In *The Essays of Montaigne*. Translated by Emit
Julius Trechmann. New York: Oxford University Press.

PENCE, GREGORY E. 1988. "Do Not Go Slowly into That Dark Night: Mercy Killing in Holland." *American Journal of Medicine* 84:139–141.

RAMSEY, PAUL. 1970. *The Patient as Person: Explorations in Medical Ethics.* New Haven, Conn.: Yale University Press.

"REGIMEN IN ACUTE DISEASES." 1923. In *Hippocrates,* II, pp. 62–125. Translated by W. H. S. Jones. Cambridge, Mass.: Harvard University Press.

REISER, STANLEY JOEL. 1975. "The Dilemma of Euthanasia in Modern Medical History: The English and American Experience." In *The Dilemmas of Euthanasia,* pp. 27–49. Edited by John A. Behnke and Sissela Bok. New York: Anchor Press.

SACRED CONGREGATION FOR THE DOCTRINE OF THE FAITH. 1980. "Vatican Declaration on Euthanasia." *Origins* 10, no. 10:154–157.

SIMMONS, PAUL D. 1983. *Birth and Death: Bioethical Decision-Making.* Philadelphia: Westminster.

SULLIVAN, JOSEPH V. 1975. "The Immorality of Euthanasia." In *Beneficent Euthanasia,* pp. 12–33. Edited by Marvin Kohl. Buffalo, N.Y.: Prometheus.

VAN DER MAAS, PAUL J.; VAN DELDEN, JOHANNES J. M.; PIJNENBORG, LOES; and LOOMAN, CASPAR W. N. 1991. "Euthanasia and Other Medical Decisions Concerning the End of Life." *Lancet* 338, no. 8768:669–674.

VANDERPOOL, HAROLD Y. 1973. *Darwin and Darwinism.* Lexington, Mass.: D.C. Heath.

———. 1981. "The Responsibilities of Physicians Toward Dying Patients." In *Medical Complications in Cancer Patients,* pp. 117–133. Edited by Jean Klastersky and Maurice J. Staquet. New York: Raven Press.

———. 1986. "The Wesleyan-Methodist Tradition." In *Caring and Curing: Health and Medicine in the Western Religious Traditions,* pp. 317–353. Edited by Ronald L. Numbers and Darrel W. Amundsen. New York: Macmillan.

VAN DER SLUIS, I. 1979. "The Movement for Euthanasia, 1875–1975." *Janus* 66, no. 1–3:131–172.

VAN HOOFF, ALTON J. L. 1990. *From Autothanasia to Suicide.* London: Routledge.

"VOLUNTARY EUTHANASIA: DEBATE IN THE HOUSE OF LORDS." 1936. *British Medical Journal* 2:1232–1234.

WEBSTER, CHARLES. 1975. *The Great Instauration.* London: Gerald Duckworth.

WINSLADE, WILLIAM J., and ROSS, JUDITH WILSON. 1986. *Choosing Life or Death.* New York: Free Press.

WORCESTER, ALFRED. 1935. *The Care of the Aged, the Dying and the Dead.* Springfield, Ill.: Charles C. Thomas.

II. ETHICAL ISSUES

Ethical and legal norms exist in virtually all societies to help protect human life and regulate when taking or not prolonging life is ethically permissible. In most Western societies, the Judeo-Christian religious tradition has given great importance to the sanctity of life. Modern medicine has also gained extraordinary new powers to prolong life. Within the last few decades, medical treatments such as kidney dialysis, cardiopulmonary resuscitation, organ transplantation, respirator support, and even provision of food and water by artificial means have become common in hospitals.

While these new treatments often benefit patients, restoring them to well-functioning lives, they often can be employed in circumstances where they may be neither a benefit to nor wanted by patients. Where once pneumonia was the "old man's friend," the way in which "nature" ended a life that had become seriously debilitated, now the time and manner of death has been brought increasingly under human control. In coming to grips with sustaining, taking, or not prolonging life, medicine has drawn on both its own ethical traditions and society's broader ethical and religious traditions.

This article will first develop an ethical framework for life-sustaining-treatment decisions around which a considerable, though hardly universal, consensus has developed, and contrast it with the distinction between ordinary and extraordinary care. It will then consider broad alternative positions on the morality of taking life and some of their implications for care of the dying. Focusing on more specific controversies, it will then address the intentional taking of life versus pain relief that hastens death, killing and allowing to die, not starting versus stopping treatment, and two prominent examples of life-sustaining treatment—resuscitation and artificially administered food and water. Finally we will conclude with discussions of life-sustaining treatment and suicide and of physician-assisted suicide and voluntary euthanasia.

An ethical framework for life-sustaining-treatment decisions

Competent patients. In the United States in the twentieth century, health-care-treatment decision making has come increasingly under the dominion of the ethical and legal doctrine of informed consent. This doctrine requires that treatment not be administered without the informed and voluntary consent of a competent patient. From a paternalistic and authoritarian tradition, in which the physician made almost all treatment decisions and the patient's role was to follow the doctor's orders, a new ideal has emerged that involves shared treatment decision making between physicians and patients. Physicians use their knowledge, experience, and training to determine the patient's diagnosis and prognosis with different possible alternative treatments, and the risks and benefits of each, including the alternative of no treatment. Patients, on the other hand, use their own aims and values to discern and decide which option is best for them. Shared decision making is based on the recognition that sound, individualized treatment decision making requires both contributions.

The principal ethical values that underlie shared decision making are promoting the patient's well-being while respecting his or her self-determination or autonomy. The term "well-being" is meant to signal that what is best for a particular patient depends not only on the "medical facts," but also on the patient's own aims and values. It is also meant to signal the extremely important point that preserving or sustaining life is not always a benefit to patients; whether it is depends on the nature of life sustained and whether the patient values that life. Self-determination is the interest ordinary persons have in making important decisions about their lives for themselves and according to their own values or conception of a good life. The capacity for self-determination allows people to take control over and responsibility for their lives and the kind of persons they become. The fundamental importance of self-determination has consistently been the central appeal in the United States both in the long line of informed-consent legal cases going back at least as far as Schloendorf, and in the more recent life-sustaining-treatment cases (*Schloendorf* v. *Society of New York Hospital*, 1914).

On the basis of these two values, as well as the ideal of shared decision making and the requirement of informed consent they support, competent patients have the right to weigh the benefits and burdens of alternative treatments, including the option of no treatment, and to make their own selection. While this ethical framework applies to any treatment, it provides especially strong support for patients deciding about life-sustaining treatment. When forgoing life-sustaining treatment is seriously in question, the patient is often critically or terminally ill and near death and also often in a seriously debilitated state. Whether continued life is, on balance, a benefit and wanted, or a burden and unwanted, will depend on how the particular patient evaluates that life. Likewise, self-determination on so important a decision as when and in what ways one's life comes to an end or is sustained by medical treatment is of especial importance.

Incompetent patients. When forgoing life-sustaining treatment is seriously in question, patients are often—probably usually—incompetent to make the decision for themselves, and so another person must decide for them. Bioethics and the law have given much attention to who should decide about life support for incompetent patients and what standards should be used. A number of ethical grounds support the common practice, employed by physicians and sanctioned by the courts, of turning to a close family member of the patient, when one is available. Most patients would want such a person to make these decisions for them when they are unable to do so; in most cases, then, turning to a close family member respects the patient's self-determination. Moreover, a close family member will usually know the patient best, and will therefore be in the best

position to determine what the patient would have wanted. This person is also likely to care most about doing what is best for the patient. Turning to him or her thus promotes both the patient's self-determination and the patient's well-being. Finally, in most societies the family is the social unit in which important social bonds and responsibilities to care for dependent members are developed; one exercise of this responsibility is to serve as surrogate for an incompetent family member. These ethical grounds usually, but do not always, apply and so can be thought of as establishing an ethical presumption that a close family member is the appropriate surrogate to make life-sustaining-treatment decisions for an incompetent patient. When these reasons do not apply—for example, when there is evidence that the patient would have wanted someone else to serve as surrogate or there is a serious conflict of interest between the family member and surrogate—then the presumption in favor of the family member as surrogate can be rebutted and another should be selected to serve instead.

How should a surrogate make life-sustaining-treatment decisions for an incompetent patient? A significant consensus has developed, both in ethics and in law, that there are three standards for a surrogate's decisions. First, if the patient has made an advance directive (e.g., a "living will" or a "durable power of attorney for health care") that includes instructions about his or her wishes as to the decision in question, then the patient's choice expressed in the advance directive should be followed, with only limited qualifications. Second, since most patients do not have advance directives, the "substituted judgment" standard should be used, which directs a surrogate to attempt to make the decision that the patient would have made, in the circumstances that then obtain, if the patient were competent. More informally, the surrogate should use his or her knowledge of the patient and the patient's values and wishes to attempt to decide what the patient would have wanted. Third, when there is no knowledge available of the patient and the patient's values that bear on the decision at hand, the "best-interest" standard should be used. Here, the surrogate should determine what is in the patient's overall best interests by a more objective and communal conception of best interest. This often amounts to asking what most reasonable persons would want; in the absence of available evidence about how, in relevant respects, the patient is different from most people, this is justified. These three standards constitute a way to promote patient well-being and self-determination to the extent possible when the patient lacks capacity to make decisions.

These standards have not gone unchallenged (Meisel, 1992; Veatch, 1993). For example, especially in the case of young children, parents are given significant discretion in deciding what would be best for their child and are permitted to give some weight to the effects of different options on important interests of other family members. The authority of both advance directives and substituted judgment have also been challenged when following them would conflict with important interests of the now-incompetent patient and when the patient has undergone such profound mental changes that he or she appears to be a "new person" with new interests. Despite the substantial consensus on the ethical framework sketched above, it is not uncontroversial.

This ethical framework for life-sustaining-treatment decisions by competent and incompetent patients does give weight to a narrowly focused quality-of-life judgment: Is the best life possible for the patient with treatment sufficiently poor, according to the patient's evaluation of that quality, that it is worse than no further life at all? No weight is given, on the other hand, to the fact that the patient's quality of life may have diminished from what it once was or from most people's lives, or to any evaluation of the social worth or social value of the patient. The fundamental feature of this ethical framework is that it entitles the patient or surrogate to weigh the benefits and burdens of possible treatments, including the option of no treatment, according to the patient's aims and values, and to select from among available treatments or to refuse any treatment. This decision-making framework has largely supplanted the distinction between ordinary and extraordinary treatment.

Ordinary versus extraordinary care

The distinction between ordinary and extraordinary care has its origins in Roman Catholic moral theology, where it is employed to distinguish between obligatory care—ordinary—and care that may be permissibly forgone—extraordinary. The two central issues about this distinction are: What is the difference between ordinary and extraordinary care? and Why should that difference determine whether care is morally obligatory or optional?

The distinction itself has been criticized as unclear because it results in confusion and controversy about how it should be applied (U.S. President's Commission, 1983). For example, it has been used to mark the difference between statistically usual or unusual care (perhaps the most commonly held understanding of the terms), between treatments that are noninvasive or highly invasive, or between treatments that employ low- or high-technology interventions, and so forth. Because the distinction has many different, natural understandings, confusion often arises about what it means. None of the possible meanings of the distinction explains why the difference itself should determine whether the treatment is morally obligatory or optional. For example, treatment that is statistically common or involves the use of low technology might be beneficial to a particular patient in particular circumstances, but not beneficial or,

perhaps, even burdensome to another patient in different circumstances.

The correct understanding of the traditional distinction is the difference between treatment that is beneficial or treatment that is unduly burdensome (or without benefit) to a patient. Of course, treatment is only unduly burdensome when the benefits it provides are insufficient to warrant its burdens. Unlike the other interpretations noted above, this interpretation of the ordinary—extraordinary distinction does mark a morally significant difference. Understood in this way, however, no general list of kinds of treatments that would be consistently ordinary or consistently extraordinary is possible; any treatment may be beneficial in some circumstances but not in others. More important, when the distinction is understood in this way it ceases to be an alternative to the benefit–burden framework. The judgment that a treatment is "extraordinary" places a label on treatment already and independently determined to be without benefit or unduly burdensome to the patient. The benefit–burden assessment does the substantive work in assessing treatments. For this reason, many commentators have given up the ordinary–extraordinary analysis in favor of the clearer and more direct appeal to the assessment of the benefits and burdens of treatment to a particular patient.

Of course, no ethical framework of the sort sketched here can be applied mechanically to make decisions to forgo life-sustaining treatment easy and unambiguous; even with the best efforts and the clearest reasoning, many decisions remain ethically problematic and emotionally wrenching. While this is also true of many decisions about treatment that is not life-sustaining, decisions concerning whether to sustain or shorten life raise several special ethical issues. In the 1960s and 1970s, it was common to distinguish between "active" and "passive" euthanasia. Passive euthanasia was understood to include forgoing life-sustaining treatment, either by stopping it or by not starting it. Active euthanasia was understood to be a deliberate intervention to end a patient's life, for example, by administering a lethal injection. Since euthanasia is often understood to be only active euthanasia, it has become common to refer to forgoing life-sustaining treatment, avoiding the term passive euthanasia. Most of these additional ethical issues raised about life-sustaining treatment represent special constraints or limits to be considered regarding the ethical framework just discussed for decisions where life itself is at stake.

The morality of taking life

Any view about the morality of forgoing life-sustaining treatment or of euthanasia will depend in large measure on the basic moral principle presupposed concerning the taking of human life. This principle will differ depending on the general moral theory or conception of which it is a part or from which it is derived. Moral conceptions regarding taking life and killing may be divided into those that are goal-based, duty-based, and rights-based. A goal-based position, of which utilitarianism is the best-known variant, prohibits taking life when doing so fails to maximize the goals or consequences the position holds to be valuable, for example, human happiness or the satisfaction of people's desires. In this view it is a factual matter whether any particular killing produces better consequences than any other available alternative. Because this position not only permits but requires taking an innocent person's life when doing so will produce the greatest balance of benefits over harms, it is in sharp conflict with the patient-centered, ethical framework, which does not permit sacrifice of the patient for the benefit of others.

In a duty-based view, taking life is wrong because it violates a fundamental moral duty not to take innocent human life intentionally. This view looks not to the consequences produced by a particular killing but to the action itself, which is prohibited by the duty not to kill. It is often found within religions that view life as a gift from God, and therefore subject only to God's decision about when to take it. Perhaps the most serious difficulty for this view is its failure to give moral weight to the consent of the person whose life may or may not be taken. In this view, a competent patient's free request that another take his or her life need not morally justify doing so; instead, it is a request or temptation to do evil and should be resisted by a moral person.

In a rights-based view, taking human life is morally wrong because it violates a basic moral right not to be killed. In this view, killing is morally wrong because it denies the person a future, together with all that the person wanted to pursue or achieve in that future. In contrast with the duty-based view, however, when a competent individual freely requests that another person take his or her life because that life has become a burden and no longer a good for the individual, acceding to that request would be understood to be waiving his or her right not to be killed.

The most important, substantive moral difference between duty-based and rights-based views is whether an individual's free and informed consent can justify taking his or her life. The distinction between duty-based and rights-based views is a natural way in which this moral difference is often expressed. However, the duty not to kill could be understood to apply only to individuals who wish to live, and the right not to be killed could be understood to be unwaivable, as many in the right-to-life movement understand it. The distinction between rights-based and duty-based accounts of the morality of killing is used in this article only to distinguish whether an individual's consent to be killed does or does not make killing him or her morally permissible.

Which of these alternative positions is correct is controversial and raises general questions of moral theory that cannot be addressed here. An ethical position that gives fundamental ethical importance to individual self-determination—as the ethical framework for life-sustaining-treatment decisions sketched above does—is most naturally formulated as a rights-based position. Whichever basic view is adopted, however, two important questions are: What actions are included under the moral prohibition of taking life, broadly construed? and Is this prohibition absolute or does it have exceptions? The duty-based view is sometimes understood to make absolute the prohibition of intentionally taking human life; but it also typically distinguishes acts that intentionally take life from acts in which death is a foreseen but unintended consequence. Both duty-based and rights-based views about the morality of taking life tend to share the position that allowing to die is a less serious wrong than taking a life by killing.

Intended versus foreseen but unintended taking of life

When caring for dying patients, health professionals frequently take actions that may and sometimes do shorten the patient's life. They may, for example, provide larger and larger doses of morphine when necessary to relieve a patient's pain, and in doing so, risk bringing on respiratory depression and earlier death. When this is done with the patient's or surrogate's knowledge of the risk and with his or her consent, it is morally justified. For the rights-based moral view about taking life, consent to the risk is crucial. In many duty-based positions, however, the consent of the victim does not justify taking human life, and a distinction is drawn between whether the resulting death was intended, or whether it was only foreseen but unintended.

This intended/foreseen distinction has a long history. Invoked by Thomas Aquinas in the thirteenth century to justify killing in self-defense, the distinction is central to the Roman Catholic doctrine of double effect. In some form, it is also common in much secular thinking about the morality of taking life.

Two central questions must be answered in order to evaluate whether this distinction really can or should be used to distinguish some morally permissible from impermissible taking of life. First, what precisely is the nature of the difference between "intended" and "foreseen"? Second, why is this difference morally important? In treating a dying cancer patient's pain, it may seem clear that the physician's primary or direct intention is to treat the pain; the death from respiratory depression caused by the morphine the physician prescribes to treat the pain is, at most, a secondary or indirect intention, or more accurately, a foreseen but unintended consequence. Many physicians would not give this same patient a lethal injection if all other means of pain relief had failed, because then the death would be intended. Yet the physician's primary intention in the case of killing by lethal injection might also be to relieve the patient's pain, though then the means of doing so is to kill the patient. This distinction between what is intended as a means and what is a foreseen but unintended consequence, however, is not always clear. Killings that seem plainly wrong because they are an impressible means to a good end can be redescribed as only a foreseen but unintended consequence of achieving the good end, and therefore, morally permissible. An extreme example will illustrate the point. Suppose a renowned transplant surgeon removes the heart and liver from a healthy person without his or her consent in order to transplant them in two patients who otherwise will die from heart and liver failure. Such killing is wrong even though it as a means of saving a greater number of persons. But suppose the surgeon denies the killing is the means of saving other patients: The means of saving the other patients, he claims, was by removing the healthy person's organs and transplanting them, whereas the death of the healthy person was merely foreseen but not intended. Proponents of this distinction have not clarified it in a way that prevents such unwelcome misuse of it.

In many cases, such as giving morphine as opposed to a lethal injection, there is agreement about how to apply the intended-versus-foreseen-but-unintended distinction. The question then arises, what is its moral significance? Critics of the distinction note that in each case the physician's end is to relieve suffering, and that to gain such relief, both physician and patient are prepared to accept the patient's earlier death. Whether by morphine or a lethal injection, relieving the patient's suffering will bring about an earlier death. These similarities cast doubt on the moral importance of this difference. In the case of morphine, there may be only a risk of death, whereas in the case of a lethal injection the death is certain. However, sometimes the amount of morphine necessary makes the likelihood of earlier death extremely high, and then this small difference in probabilities is too slim a foundation for the very great moral difference between permissible and impermissible killings. In any event, this is a difference in the certainty or risk of the outcome of death, not in whether it is intended or unintended.

Critics of the distinction between intended and foreseen deaths argue that physicians are morally responsible for all foreseen or foreseeable consequences of their actions, whether intended or foreseen but unintended, because foreseeability brings these consequences under the control of physicians and so makes physicians responsible for them. This disagreement in medical contexts about the moral importance of whether death is intended is often a particular instance of a broader dis-

agreement between goal-based or utilitarian theorists who are concerned only with good results and duty- or rights-based theorists who place moral restrictions on how good results may be brought about.

Killing and allowing to die

Many moral theorists distinguish between duties not to kill, called negative duties, and duties to save or not to allow to die, called positive duties. They argue that, unless this distinction is used to set reasonable moral limits, moral responsibilities will extend far beyond what they are usually thought to be and will deeply limit people's pursuit of their various life plans. Persons can usually satisfy the duty not to kill simply by pursuing their particular aims and purposes, although these goals may be altered if necessary to avoid killing. But if there is an equally stringent duty not to allow to die, it might seem that people must likewise set aside nearly all their usual aims and activities and devote their lives to saving those whose lives are in peril, such as victims of famines or extreme poverty. The implications of whether killing is morally worse than allowing to die are far-reaching both within and outside of medicine.

There are again two distinct issues. First, what makes one particular "doing," understood to include both acts and omissions, a killing, and another, an allowing to die? Once the difference is clear, the second issue is whether and why this difference between killing and allowing to die is morally important. Killing is usually distinguished from allowing to die by establishing whether something was done, or not done, that resulted in death. A person who kills performs an action that causes a person to die in a way and at a time that the person would not otherwise have died. For example, two people are in a boat; Person 1 cannot swim. Knowing this, Person 2 pushes Person 1 out of the boat; Person 1 drowns.

A person who allows another to die knows that there is an action he or she could perform that would prevent another's death, but does not take this action, and the person dies. For example, Person 1 accidentally falls out of the boat. Person 2 does not throw out an available life preserver, and Person 1 drowns. Some philosophers have argued that if the difference between killing and allowing to die is predicated on acting or not acting, killing is not morally worse than allowing to die.

The meaning of this claim has often been misunderstood. The claim is that the mere fact that one doing is a killing, while the other is an allowing to die, does not make one morally better or worse than the other, or make one morally justified or permissible when the other is not. This is compatible with saying that a particular killing, all things considered, is morally worse than, or not as bad as, a particular allowing to die because of other differences between the two, such as the motives of the agents or the presence or absence of the consent of the victim. This is also compatible with holding that most killing, all things considered, is morally worse than most allowing to die, but once again, that must be because of other morally important differences between them.

The usual argument for the position that killing is not in itself morally worse than allowing to die has consisted of comparing two cases that differ in no other morally relevant respect except that one is a killing, the other an allowing to die. Such a comparison helps focus on whether this difference by itself is morally important. Here is a well-known example:

> In the first [instance], Smith stands to gain a large inheritance if anything should happen to his six-year-old cousin. One evening, while the child is taking his bath, Smith sneaks into the bathroom and drowns the child, and then arranges things so that it will look like an accident.
>
> In the second, Jones also stands to gain if anything should happen to his six-year-old cousin. Like Smith, Jones sneaks in planning to drown the child in his bath. However, just as he enters the bathroom Jones sees the child slip and hit his head, and fall face down in the water, Jones is delighted; he stands by, ready to push the child's head back under if it is necessary, but it is not necessary. With only a little thrashing about, the child drowns all by himself, "accidentally," as Jones watches and does nothing (Rachels, 1975, p. 79).

While Smith killed, Jones allowed to die. James Rachels argues that there seems to be no basis for saying that what Smith did was any worse than what Jones did; there must be other factors in real cases that account for any moral differences. The conclusion that killing is not, in itself, morally worse than allowing to die remains controversial. Those who hold that there is a significant moral difference between the two argue that it is important to establish which, if any, forgoing of life support comes under the stronger moral prohibition against killing. Since forgoing life support includes both not starting treatment and stopping treatment, we can pursue whether either is equivalent to killing by asking whether or not starting life support and stopping life support are morally different.

Not starting treatment and stopping treatment

When a decision is made not to initiate some form of life-sustaining treatment, such as kidney dialysis or respirator support, and the patient dies as a result, this is commonly understood to be an omission and so and allowing to die. Even if active killing is wrong, its prohibition does not apply to not initiating life support. But what of stopping life support—for example, stopping respirator support at the persistent, voluntary request of a clearly competent and respirator-dependent patient who is terminally ill and undergoing suffering that cannot be adequately relieved? If such action is taken by the physician with the intent of respecting the patient's right to decide about his or her treatment, most people would consider it a morally justified instance of allowing the patient to die. If only killing, but not allowing to die, is prohibited, then stopping life support and not starting it are both allowing to die and morally permitted.

But some philosophers have argued that stopping this patient's respirator is killing, not allowing to die (Brock, 1993). Suppose, for example, the patient has a greedy son who mistakenly believes that his mother will never decide to stop treatment and that even if she did, her physicians would not comply with her wishes. Afraid that his inheritance will be exhausted by a long hospitalization, he enters his mother's room while she is deeply sedated, removes her from the respirator, and she dies. If upon being found out, the son protested, "I didn't kill her; I merely allowed her to die; it was her disease that caused her death," this claim would be rejected. The son went into his mother's room and deliberately killed her.

Does the physician who did just the same thing, performed the same physical action, kill the patient as well? Even if the physician in such a case does kill, other moral differences make the physician's killing morally justified, while the son's is morally wrong. The physician acts with a good motive, to respect the patient's wishes, with the patient's consent, and in a professional role in which he or she is socially and legally authorized to so act; the son acts with a bad motive, without consent, and with no social or legal authorization to do so. But these do not appear to be differences in whether either kills or allows to die: One can kill or allow to die with a good or bad motive, with or without consent, and in or not in a role that authorizes the action.

Those who reject this analysis and hold that stopping life support is allowing to die usually have a different account of the kill/allow-to-die difference than the act/omission account offered in the last section. They hold that when a patient has a lethal illness like lung disease, whose usual fatal outcome is being held off by a life-sustaining treatment such as a respirator, removing this artificial intervention amounts to allowing the patient to die by letting the disease process proceed unimpeded to death. But this account is problematic, not least because it requires us to accept that the greedy son also allows to die, but does not kill.

Whether stopping life support is killing or allowing to die, some physicians and others believe it is an ethically graver matter to stop a life-sustaining treatment than not to start it, or that it is permissible not to start it in circumstances in which it would not be justified to stop it. But consideration of cases like the following has led many persons to reject the argument that stopping life support is different from or more serious morally from not starting it:

> A gravely ill patient, Mr. S, arrives at the hospital in respiratory distress and is sent to the intensive care unit (ICU) to be intubated and placed on a respirator. Before he is intubated, his family and physician arrive at the ICU and inform the staff that while clearly competent Mr. S, after extensive consideration and because of his debilitated and terminal condition, had firmly rejected being put on a respirator under any circumstances. The ICU staff respect his wishes, keep him comfortable, and he dies of respiratory failure. Now suppose instead that heavy traffic had delayed the family and the physician and they arrive at the ICU just after Mr. S is put on the respirator. His treatment now must be stopped instead of not started as before. (Brock, 1993)

It is hard to see why the same factors that morally justified not starting his treatment do not equally, morally justify stopping it.

Those who hold that stopping life support is not different ethically from not starting it usually stress two bad effects of an unwillingness to stop life support. First, it will result in continuing treatment beyond the point at which it is a benefit to or still wanted by the patient. Second, and less obvious but at least as important, knowing that it will be harder to stop life support once it is begun can make physicians, patients, and family members all reluctant to try treatment when its benefits are uncertain or unlikely, for fear that if it proves not to be beneficial it will not be able to be stopped and the patient will end "stuck on machines." The result is to deny patients possibly beneficial life-sustaining treatment.

In fact, there is often better reason to stop a life-sustaining treatment than not to start it. Often, before a life-sustaining treatment is started, it is uncertain whether it will bring the hoped-for benefits to the patient. Once it has been tried, and it is clear that it does not produce the benefits sought, a reason exists for stopping it that did not exist for not starting it. This supports the use of time-limited trials of life-sustaining treatment, with the understanding that if the treatment does not prove to be beneficial it will be stopped.

Sustaining food and water

Two forms of life-sustaining treatment that have received special attention are resuscitation and artificial nutrition and hydration. Life-sustaining-treatment debates in the United States during the 1970s and 1980s often focused on the use of cardiopulmonary resuscitation (CPR) for persons who suffer cardiac or pulmonary arrest. Since CPR, to be effective, must be administered immediately after a patient suffers an arrest, hospitals have developed policies generally requiring that CPR be administered to any such patient, unless there is a "do not resuscitate" (DNR) order already in effect for the patient. The presumption of these policies—that anyone in medical need of resuscitation would receive CPR unless there was a prior order not to use it—made CPR different from many other life-sustaining treatments, which required a physician's explicit order to start them.

CPR is the most prominent example of a class of emergency procedures for which consent is presumed unless the patient or the patient's surrogate has explicitly refused it beforehand. Since CPR in the hospital is usually not successful, is associated with significant morbidity for the patient even when it is successful, and often would, at best, extend the lives of dying patients only briefly, there is widespread consensus that forgoing it is often ethically justified so long as patients or their surrogates agree and explicitly withdraw the presumption of consent for it. As a result, resuscitation, or "code status," is probably the most frequently raised life-sustaining treatment decision.

Those who seek to limit the life-sustaining treatments for which it is ethically permissible for patients or their surrogates to decide to forgo have usually focused on the provision of nutrition and hydration by artificial means, such as intravenous nasogastric, and other forms of tube feeding. Some people have argued that food and water are not medical treatment but are instead the most basic form of caring for dependent persons; all people, not just medical patients, need food and water. Others argue that when the patient's medical condition necessitates the artificial provision of food and water, and when this is done by medical personnel using medical means, there is not much difference between this situation and the provision of oxygen by respirators to patients with lung disease.

Other opponents of forgoing food and water focus not on the issue of whether it is medical treatment, but on the strong symbolic meaning and importance of feeding those in need. However, the usual symbolism of food and water may be misleading in the circumstances in which the question arises in medicine. There the cultural and social symbolism and meaning associated with eating and feeding are largely absent, as is the suffering typically associated with starvation. Applying the benefits-and-burdens analysis, food and water should only be forgone if doing so would not cause significant suffering to the patient. The benefits-and-burdens analysis will support forgoing nutrition and hydration either when continued life itself is burdensome or not a benefit to the patient, or when providing nutrition and hydration increases, rather than decreases, the patient's suffering. For example, many patients in a persistent vegetative state (PVS)—that is, those who have permanently and completely lost the capacity for any conscious experience—would not want nor consider it a benefit to have their lives continued. Consequently, treatment that sustains life is not beneficial, and its withdrawal cannot impose any burden on a PVS patient. In other cases, providing normal levels of nutrition and hydration may increase the awareness and suffering of some dying patients; for these patients, feelings of thirst can be assuaged, for example, with ice chips, without providing a level of hydration that would make their dying less peaceful and comfortable (Lynn, 1986). In still other cases, the benefits of continued life for seriously demented patients must be weighed against the burdens of physician restraints necessary to keep them from removing feeding tubes.

Life-sustaining treatment and suicide

Suicide is difficult to define precisely, but is usually understood as the intentional taking of one's own life. In some religious traditions, suicide has long been and continues to be prohibited and considered a sin, and some important moral philosophers such as Immanuel Kant have held that suicide is morally wrong (Battin, 1982). Historically, the law often reflected these views, although in the United States no states criminalize suicide or attempted suicide, and a majority but not all prohibit assisting in suicide.

The different, basic moral positions discussed earlier on the morality of taking human life have different implications for the morality of suicide. Despite these differences, most people agree that a public policy of seeking to prevent most suicide attempts is morally justified. Even strong defenders of individual self-determination generally agree that most suicide attempts are dramatic pleas for help and that they occur when a person's decision-making capacity is seriously disordered by such conditions as depression. These features justify intervention to prevent the suicide, so as to determine if the patient is competent and not subject to impaired decision making, in which case, some believe, others should cease coercive interference.

Since a patient's decision to forgo treatment correctly believed to be life-sustaining will result in the patient's death, the question arises whether this is suicide. In some cases, the patient may not intend his or her own death, or seek death, but only be unwilling to undergo the burdens of a particular life-sustaining treatment. In other cases, however, the patient's decision may also be made in the interest of seeking an end to an excessively burdensome existence, and so with the intent to cause one's own death, making it hard to differentiate from suicide. Many legal decisions about life-sustaining treatment, and most Western religious traditions, have sought to distinguish forgoing life support from suicide,

often by characterizing the former as an exercise of self-determination about one's medical treatment, not intentional self-destruction. (The courts may have sought to distinguish forgoing life support from suicide to protect participating physicians and others from potential prosecution under legal statutes prohibiting assisting in suicide.) Yet the normative judgment a competent person makes justifying each act is often essentially the same: The best future life possible for me (with life-sustaining treatment, in the case of a decision to forgo treatment) is so bad that it is worse than no further life at all. The principal difference between some cases of forgoing life-sustaining treatment and suicide appears to be only a difference in the means a person uses to bring about his or her death. However, even if some or all forgoing of life support is essentially suicide, it need not, for that reason, be morally wrong, but instead a justified exercise of self-determination.

Physician-assisted suicide

In nearly all countries, neither professional practice nor the law permits physicians to grant patients' requests for physician-assisted suicide or voluntary euthanasia. An example of physician-assisted suicide is when a patient ingests a lethal substance provided by a physician for that purpose; voluntary euthanasia, by contrast, would be the physician administering the lethal substance. In both cases, the choice rests fully with the patient, and the patient can change his or her mind up until the moment the lethal process become irreversible. The only difference need be who performs the last physical action of administering the lethal dose, for example, placing potassium chloride in the patient's intravenous line. This small difference in the part played by the physician in the causal process leading to death seems not to support a substantial moral difference between physician-assisted suicide and voluntary euthanasia.

Those who nevertheless believe that it is morally worse for physicians to perform voluntary euthanasia than physician-assisted suicide can argue that in the former, the physician kills the patient, while in the latter, the patient kills himself or herself. But it may be more accurate to say that in physician-assisted suicide, the physician and the patient together kill the patient—a case of joint action for which both together bear responsibility. This suggests that physician-assisted suicide and voluntary euthanasia may not be substantially different morally.

Voluntary, active euthanasia

Considerable public and professional attention, spurred by publicity about the practice in the Netherlands (Van Der Maas et al., 1991) and several notorious cases in the United States, such as those of Dr. Jack Kevorkian, has focused on voluntary, active euthanasia. In significant part, the public concern with euthanasia reflects fear of loss of control and of undergoing substantial pain and suffering while dying. It also reflects a recognition that the same values of patient self-determination and well-being that have been accepted as guiding treatment decision making in general, and decisions about life-sustaining treatment in particular, can in some cases support voluntary, active euthanasia as well. If this positive support for voluntary euthanasia is granted, opponents have in general offered two kinds of arguments against it.

The first argument is that any individual instance of euthanasia is morally wrong because it violates the duty not to kill human beings. As noted earlier, in some duty-based accounts of the wrongness of killing, the consent of the one killed does not make the killing permissible. However, given the centrality of the patient's consent in ethical accounts of the permissibility of forgoing life-sustaining treatment, some special argument is needed for why consent has no relevance for euthanasia. Moreover, if the argument in the section above on killing and allowing to die is correct—that some stopping of life support is justified killing—then euthanasia cannot be morally condemned simply because it is killing. Many duty-based moral accounts of the wrongness of killing either implicitly or explicitly depend on theological premises that give God sole dominion over life and death. However, in pluralistic societies that respect religious freedom, public policy should not be based on religious beliefs that are not shared by many members of that society. The rights-based account of the wrongness of killing, however, gives decisive weight to the consent and self-determination of the patient who seeks it.

The other general kind of argument against euthanasia is that although it may be morally permissible in some individual cases, nonetheless it would be bad public policy to permit voluntary, active euthanasia. This argument depends on an assessment of the likely good and bad consequences of permitting euthanasia, only a few of which can be noted here. Among the potential good consequences that proponents cite are: respecting the self-determination of those who request euthanasia but have not been able to get it; assuring the much larger number of people who believe it should be permitted that should they request it, it would be available; ending the pain and suffering of dying patients that cannot be relieved by any other means; and providing a more humane and peaceful death than some patients would otherwise have.

Among the potential bad consequences opponents cite are: its apparent incompatibility with the aim of medicine of protecting life in all its frailty; erosion of the trust of patients in their physicians as caregivers; in

an era of cost containment, erosion of the social commitment to provide appropriate care to the dying if euthanasia is seen as an acceptable and cheaper alternative; and fear that permitting voluntary euthanasia would, over time, lead to permitting nonvoluntary euthanasia of incompetent patients, which would be wrong and subject to serious abuse. Evaluating the likelihood and relative seriousness of these and other possible good and bad consequences of permitting voluntary euthanasia is difficult and controversial. Whether it should be permitted remains one of the most deeply controversial issues in medical ethics.

Conclusion

Since the 1960s, the capacity of medicine to prolong patients' lives has steadily increased, making the time and circumstances of people's death increasingly a matter of human choice and control. The debates considered and the ethical framework for life-sustaining-treatment decisions sketched in this article have been responses to this new control over how and when we die. Perhaps the central feature and accomplishment of the great public and professional attention to death and dying in recent decades has been securing the rights of patients or their surrogates to decide about care near the end of life.

Three likely features of attention to death and dying in coming years can already be anticipated. The first will be increased attention to physician-assisted suicide and euthanasia, the natural culmination of the movement to secure patients' and surrogates' control over the end of life. The second will be attempts to define the limits of patients' and, especially, families' rights to force physicians to provide life-sustaining treatment that the physicians judge to be futile; this issue may help in gaining a deeper and more subtle understanding of what shared decision making between physicians and patients or their surrogates should be. The third will be the need to clarify and decide about relative priorities in care of the dying as countries around the world limit care in order to control the growth of health-care costs. The deeply personal, emotionally complex, and ethically controversial nature of these decisions means they will continue to be a prominent part of bioethics.

DAN W. BROCK

Directly related to this article are the other articles in this entry: HISTORICAL ASPECTS, ADVANCE DIRECTIVES, *and* PROFESSIONAL AND PUBLIC POLICIES. *For a further discussion of topics mentioned in this article, see the entries* COMPETENCE; DOUBLE EFFECT; HOMICIDE; INFORMED CONSENT; *and* SUICIDE. *For a discussion of related ideas, see the entries* AGING AND THE AGED, *article on* HEALTH-CARE AND RESEARCH ISSUES; ETHICS, *article on* NORMA-

TIVE ETHICAL THEORIES; LIFE; LIFE, QUALITY OF; PROFESSIONAL–PATIENT RELATIONSHIP; *and* VALUE AND VALUATION.

Bibliography

BATTIN, MARGARET PABST. 1982. *Ethical Issues in Suicide.* Englewood Cliffs, N.J.: Prentice-Hall.

BOLE, THOMAS J., ed. 1991. "Double Effect: Theoretical Function and Bioethical Implication." *Journal of Medicine and Philosophy* 16, no. 5:467–585.

BROCK, DAN W. 1993. *Life and Death: Philosophical Essays in Biomedical Ethics.* Cambridge: At the University Press.

BRODY, BARUCH A., ed. 1989. *Suicide and Euthanasia: Historical and Contemporary Themes.* Dordrecht, Netherlands: Kluwer.

BUCHANAN, ALLEN E., and BROCK, DAN W. 1989. *Deciding for Others: The Ethics of Surrogate Decision Making.* New York: Cambridge University Press.

GLOVER, JONATHAN. 1977. *Causing Death and Saving Lives.* New York: Penguin.

HARRIS, JOHN. 1985. *The Value of Life.* London: Routledge & Kegan Paul.

HASTINGS CENTER. 1987. *Guidelines on the Termination of Life-Sustaining Treatment and the Care of the Dying.* Bloomington: Indiana University Press.

KAMM, F. M. 1993. *Morality, Mortality. Volume I: Death and Whom to Save from It.* Oxford: Oxford University Press.

KANT, IMMANUEL. 1967. *The Moral Law: Kant's Groundwork of the Metaphysic of Morals.* Translated and edited by Herbert James Paton. New York: Barnes and Noble.

KUHSE, HELGA. 1987. *The Sanctity-of-Life Doctrine in Medicine: A Critique.* Oxford: Oxford University Press.

KUHSE, HELGA, and SINGER, PETER. 1985. *Should the Baby Live? The Problem of Handicapped Infants.* Oxford: Oxford University Press.

LYNN, JOANNE, ed. 1986. *By No Extraordinary Means: The Choice to Forgo Life-Sustaining Food and Water.* Bloomington: Indiana University Press.

MEISEL, ALAN. 1992. "The Legal Consensus About Foregoing Life-Sustaining Treatment: Its Status and Its Prospects." *Kennedy Institute of Ethics Journal* 2, no. 4:309–345.

RACHELS, JAMES. 1975. "Active and Passive Euthanasia." *New England Journal of Medicine* 292, no. 2:78–80.

———. 1986. *The End of Life: Euthanasia and Morality.* Oxford: Oxford University Press.

Schloendorf v. Society of New York Hospital. 1914. 211 N.Y. 125, 105 N.E. 92, 95.

STEINBOCK, BONNIE, ed. 1980. *Killing and Letting Die.* Englewood Cliffs, N.J.: Prentice-Hall.

U.S. PRESIDENT'S COMMISSION FOR THE STUDY OF ETHICAL PROBLEMS IN MEDICINE AND BIOMEDICAL AND BEHAVIORAL RESEARCH. 1983. *Deciding to Forego Life-Sustaining Treatment: A Report on the Ethical, Medical, and Legal Issues in Treatment Decisions.* Washington, D.C.: Author.

VEATCH, ROBERT M. 1993. "Forgoing Life-Sustaining Treatment: Limits to the Consensus." *Kennedy Institute of Ethics Journal* 3, no. 1:1–19.

VAN DER MAAS, PAUL J.; VAN DELDEN, JOHANNES J. M.; and PIJNENBORG, LOES. 1991. "Euthanasia and Other Medical Decisions Concerning the End of Life." *Lancet* 338, no. 8768:669–674.

WEIR, ROBERT F. 1989. *Abating Treatment with Critically Ill Patients: Ethical and Legal Limits to the Medical Prolongation of Life.* New York: Oxford University Press.

III. ADVANCE DIRECTIVES

In 1914, Justice Benjamin Cardozo declared, "Every human being of adult years and sound mind has a right to determine what shall be done with his own body." In 1990, the U.S. Supreme Court endorsed this claim in the *Cruzan* case, ruling that nutritional support sustaining a young adult with severe neurological injury could be discontinued if it were clear that she would have chosen to do so. This principle underlies contemporary authoritative guidelines and official statements on decision making and forgoing life-sustaining treatment (U.S. President's Commission, 1983; Hastings Center, 1987; National Center for State Courts, 1991).

How to enable a patient to exercise this control when the patient is adult but not "of sound mind" has been a common but intractable problem. Most deaths now occur after a decision has been made to forgo life-sustaining therapy such as cardiopulmonary resuscitation (Bedell et al., 1986). Often those decisions are made by someone else, since the patient is no longer able to do so. Three million to six million people in the United States are incapacitated for decision making because of substantial dementia, and the number is expected to grow as the population ages (Buchanan and Brock, 1989). Probably at least as many people will experience a period of being incapable of bearing responsibility for their own decisions, either transiently during illness or when near death.

Decision making in such situations must rely upon one of the three available strategies: (1) decisions directed by the patient's own preferences, stated in advance of decisional incapacity; (2) decisions made by a surrogate (who may be a family member, a friend, or a court-appointed guardian); or (3) decisions directed by community and professional guidelines and practices. The opportunity that patient directives stated in advance offer for individualizing choice, combined with the uncertainties and insensitivities of the other two approaches, have encouraged substantial enthusiasm for what have come to be called advance directives. The increase of chronic disease in the population also grants patients the opportunity to become knowledgeable about the expected course of illness and the merits of alternative plans of care for anticipated future situations, thus enabling their giving informed directions about future choices.

Advance directives originated in public outcry regarding overly burdensome medical technology that seemed to serve only to prolong the dying process. In 1969, Luis Kutner proposed the "living will," a document directing that medical treatment should cease if the patient were vegetative and unable to regain his or her mental and physical capacity (Kutner, 1969). The plight of the Quinlan family in trying to remove a ventilator from their daughter Karen Ann, who was in a persistent vegetative state, inspired the first U.S. state law granting legal status to living wills (U.S. President's Commission, 1983). Since then, nearly every state in the United States has passed legislation authorizing living wills. Since these aim to allow patients to die "naturally," they are often called natural-death acts. Living wills are usually composed in such broad terms that they require substantial interpretation. In response to the ambiguities that arise in interpreting living wills, the U.S. President's Commission for the Study of Ethical Problems in Medicine and Biomedical and Behavioral Research in 1983 advocated the use of existing durable power-of-attorney statutes. This approach allows the patient to name a surrogate decision maker, whose enhanced authority is often recognized by being called a proxy. Having a person named to substitute for the patient in making judgments can allow sensitive interpretation and responsiveness over a full range of decision making, rather than being limited to stopping life-supporting treatments for dying or permanently unconscious patients (U.S. President's Commission, 1983).

Types of advance directives

Advance directives provide instructions regarding a person's preferences, goals, and values while competent, in anticipation of a future period of decisional incapacity. Thereby, the preferences and values of once-competent persons can continue to direct their medical care, even when the patients cannot do so directly. An advance directive can designate another person to make decisions (a proxy directive), or can provide instructions about the patient's values and goals or treatment preferences (an instruction directive), or can do both (a combined directive). These are specifically authorized in the laws of most states and are probably enforceable in all states. Some newer formats, such as the "medical directive" (Emanuel and Emanuel, 1989), have encouraged the patient to consider a variety of concrete future possibilities and to give directions about each. Others have encouraged a more detailed but less decision-oriented "values history" (Gibson, 1990) that would serve as advice to a surrogate. Each approach will probably prove to have a role for some patients.

Directives are also classified as formal (e.g., a signed and legally authorized written document, such as a living will or durable power of attorney for health care) or informal (e.g., oral communication with family or health-care provider). Allan Buchanan and Dan Brock (1989) have identified several advantages of formal advance directives over informal communications. First, the implementation of formal directives may be more likely to entail careful deliberations about preferences and values. Second, these directives provide more reliable evidence of the patients' preferences. Third, formal directives invoke a legal practice that commits all future decision makers to a course of action and offers legal enforcement for patients' preferences. On the other hand, formal documents may command undue respect when adequate counseling has not occurred or the language is imprecise, and therefore the documents fail to convey the preferences of informed patients.

Considerations in using advance directives

Advance directives cannot reproduce the contemporaneous decision making of a competent individual, and thus cannot have quite the degree of authority granted to a patient's own decisions. The moral importance of an advance directive should increase to the degree to which it replicates a thoughtful, informed, contemporaneous decision by the patient. This is most likely when the patient clearly understood the clinical situation that was likely to occur, the directive itself is readily understood, the treatment possibilities have not changed substantially since the patient's directive was written (e.g., by an advance in medical therapy possibilities), the discretion allowed to contemporaneous decision makers is clear, and the choices articulated are congruent with what is otherwise known about the patient. Advance directives will always be somewhat more open to interpretation or being set aside than are contemporaneous decisions of competent adults (Schneiderman and Arras, 1985).

The classic living will includes phrasing similar to "If I am permanently unconscious or there is no reasonable expectation for my recovery from a seriously incapacitating or lethal illness or condition, I do not wish to be kept alive by artificial means" (U.S. President's Commission, 1983). This language may be effective as the initiation of a conversation about the patient's preferences, but virtually every word requires interpretation, a fact that limits its utility. Without further explication, the surrogate who is doing the interpretation effectively determines the content. The durable power of attorney evades problems of interpretation, but it provides no real direction for decisions beyond the naming of a proxy. Ordinarily, some combination of the naming of a proxy and the giving of instructions to that proxy should serve patients best. How much instruction is given will depend upon the trustworthiness of the proxy and his or her knowledge of the patient's preferences, as well as the clarity and durability of those preferences. If a patient has no one to name as proxy, then instruction directives should be more carefully considered and more detailed. In general, instruction directives should focus upon goals and values more than on specific medical interventions, for each medical intervention can ordinarily be desirable in some circumstances and repugnant in others (Brett, 1991).

Utilization and impact of advance directives

Until recently, advocacy of advance directives rested upon conceptual claims that they should improve self-determination. Recent research suggests that significant barriers exist to having advance directives achieve morally important goals.

Health-care providers, patients, and the general public in the United States report positive attitudes toward and are generally aware of written advance directives (Harvey et al., 1989; U.S. President's Commission, 1983; Teno et al., 1994). Yet the widespread endorsement and positive attitudes have not translated into frequent utilization of advance directives. With the exception of patients with HIV-related disease (Steinbrook et al., 1986; Teno et al., 1990), in typical populations less than one-fifth have a formal advance directive (Emanuel et al., 1991; Davidson et al., 1989; Harvey et al., 1989; Teno et al., 1994; High, 1993). Written advance directives have not been shown to play a major role in shaping treatment decisions to withhold or withdraw life-sustaining treatment (Smedira et al., 1990; Lo et al., 1985; Teno et al., 1994; Schneiderman et al., 1992). This lack of effect may arise because patients stayed competent through virtually all of their course of treatment, because decisions made by others would not have differed much, or because patients preferred that treatment choices be made by others, even though they were willing to state their own choices in advance (Sehgal et al., 1992). Of course, a lack of effect may also arise because written advance directives are not known to the care providers (Teno et al., 1994).

Increasing the prevalence of formal advance directives may be quite difficult. Jan Hare and Carrie Nelson (1991), utilizing printed materials and physician-initiated counseling, stimulated only eight of fifty-two patients to complete a living will, a rate similar to that reported by Greg Sachs and colleagues (1991). One small but highly successful intervention was reported by Lawrence Markson and Knight Steel (1990), who found that forty-eight of seventy-four of their homebound patients completed a durable power of attorney when counseled and encouraged by their physician. One study found that patients did not see the need for written directives because they expected and trusted that family members would make decisions for them (High, 1987). The understanding of why patients do or do not complete written directives is still quite incomplete.

Only a few studies have examined the impact of advance directives on medical decision making. Open-ended interviews with fifty-seven physicians in California and Vermont found advance directives to have minor impacts on medical decision making (Zimberg, 1988). Nevertheless, questionnaires mailed to physicians in Arkansas revealed that physicians felt advance directives aided decision making; most who had experience with them stated that their experience was positive (Davidson et al., 1989). In a study of advance directives articulated by 126 competent nursing-home residents and the surrogates of 49 incompetent nursing-home residents, researchers found that care consistent with these treatment preferences was provided 75 percent of the time when an outcome event (hospitalization or death in the nursing home) occurred (Danis et al., 1991). Most of the inconsistencies were in withholding CPR or hospitalization from an incompetent patient whose advance directive had not advised this course. The authors noted that some of these inconsistencies may have been appropriate if the clinical situation had substantially changed so that the likelihood of successful treatment was no longer substantial. Joan Teno et al. have reported that seriously ill patients with written advance directives generally or living wills specifically are not much more likely than those without them to have "do not resuscitate" orders or, indeed, to prefer to forgo resuscitation (1994). Whether advance directives are or can be important in shaping care plans is not yet clear.

Recent research has illuminated three additional areas of concern with advance directives. First, patient preferences regarding life-sustaining treatment have only a moderate degree of stability over time (Everhart and Pearlman, 1990). Second, patients and surrogates disagree so often in their responses to formal interviews asking about treatment choices that the ability of surrogates to make substituted judgments is called into question (Seckler et al., 1991). Third, advance directives with similar content may well be meant to carry quite disparate degrees of discretion in regard to whether they are binding upon surrogates (Sehgal et al., 1992). Since many patients expect their surrogates to overrule their written instructions some of the time, this consideration probably will have to come to be included in the advance directive itself.

These concerns, demonstrated through empirical research, combine with certain conceptual problems to restrain enthusiasm for advance directives as a solution for decision making for incompetent adults. Allan Buchanan and Dan Brock (1989) and Rebecca Dresser (1989) have addressed the troubling concern that the preferences, values, and best interests of people may change substantially over time, sometimes quite radically. Should a healthy person be able to dictate his or her own treatment during a future illness, when his or her own concerns and priorities may be quite different? For example, a demented patient who is happy and cheerful might have dictated the nontreatment of a painful condition through an advance directive written when he or she was well. Following such a dictate is and should be troubling, but deciding whether to override it is also troubling. No adequate guidance has yet been developed.

In addition, advance directives commonly speak as if all of the decisions articulated are centrally important to the author. This is probably not the case: Some preferences arise from deep commitments and contravening them is a serious affront, while others are trivial or transient choices, and the author would not feel wronged to find that they had not been honored.

Finally, the traditional scope of advance directives may not include some issues that are of great importance in patient choice. Some patients may prefer decisions to be made so as to spare the family certain emotional or financial costs, or so as to grant family the opportunity to pursue a reasonable self-interest (Buchanan and Brock, 1989; Lynn, 1991). Some might be more concerned with spiritual issues or location of care. These and similar concerns are not barred from advance directives; they just are not ordinarily included.

Policy and practice

What role should advance directives play in decision making for incompetent adults? Some patients are certainly best served by having formal advance directives: those with unusual preferences for proxy or for treatment goals, those with unusually clearly considered preferences, and those with no natural proxy. Virtually all patients are well served by continually formulating appropriate oral advance directives, which should generally be documented by caregivers in the medical record. Yet advance directives are unlikely to resolve all decisions for those who have directives, and most patients are likely not to have any advance directive applicable to their current situation. Advance directives can even be hazardous if written without understanding, or if inappropriately specific or excessively vague. Good practice and public policy for decision making for incompetent adults will require establishing how to combine the use of all three of the available elements: (1) advance directives when possible and appropriate; (2) family and other surrogate decision makers to interpret advance directives and to make decisions in their absence; and (3) reasonable community and professional standards, at least for those situations where the patient has no history, no advance directives, and no natural proxy.

The merit of statutes and regulations is unclear. Natural-death acts formulated in response to the plight of Karen Quinlan would not have helped decision making for her case. These acts often established significant barriers to patient autonomy. For example, California's Natural Death Act of 1976 did not allow the document to become effective until fourteen days after the patient's condition was determined to be terminal and required that the person be competent at that time (Buchanan and Brock, 1989). Many individuals die or become incompetent during this waiting period, and having to attend to this sort of requirement makes implementing an advance directive seem incomprehensible to patients and care providers alike. In fact, although much effort has been expended upon obtaining statutory authority for advance directives, their utility does not seem to be linked to their having such a statutory basis.

The quest for unambiguous and readily enforceable directives may be detrimental. For example, a standard of "clear and convincing evidence" of the patient's own preferences has sometimes been advocated for decision making for incompetents (Cruzan v. Director, 1990). This could be interpreted to require written or quite formal statements of patient preferences in advance. While it may seem a reasonable standard to err on the side of life, ordinarily the trade-off for affected patients is between an earlier death and a small delay in dying, bought with great suffering by the patient and family. In these circumstances, the burden of proof for a proposed course of care should be more neutral. To require explicit advance directives before allowing a life-sustaining treatment to be forgone would often mean imposing a seriously harmful treatment.

The U.S. Patient Self-Determination Act, implemented December 1, 1991, requires notice to all adult patients, on admission to a health-care facility, of their rights to make decisions and to write advance directives. The merits of this approach are under examination.

Conclusions

Decision making for incompetent adults remains a perplexing problem. Written and oral advance directives provide a way to exercise control over decision making, allowing people to shape their medical treatment even when they become incapable of contemporaneous decision making. Health-care providers and patients need to learn how to accomplish appropriate advance planning for care, often using oral or written directives concerning proxies, goals, or treatments. Advance directives are limited by being no better than the counseling that preceded them; thus, appropriate counseling is an important obligation of caregivers. Some patients may not want or benefit from articulating preferences in an instruction directive. Most patients are well advised to seek to identify their preferred surrogate decision maker. Continued policy innovation and empirical research are needed for further guidance on practice.

Given the low rate of completion of advance directives, they cannot be expected to obviate the need for surrogate decision making that is not guided by direct patient instruction. Advance directives also cannot replicate the authority that is granted to contemporaneous decision making by competent adults. However, the standards and procedures for overriding an advance directive and substituting surrogate decision making have not yet been well articulated.

Advance directives offer an opportunity to direct or shape decisions so that the patient's preferences continue to be honored even when the patient cannot directly make the decisions. The United States has embarked upon an implicit social experiment to assess the potential for advance directives. Evaluation of that experiment over the coming years ought to shape the practices used in advance care planning and the balance in clinical practice among decision-making possibilities for incompetent adults: directives made in advance, decision making by family or surrogates, and decision making by guidelines and professional practices.

JOANNE LYNN
JOAN M. TENO

Directly related to this article are the other articles in this entry: HISTORICAL ASPECTS, ETHICAL ISSUES, *and* PROFESSIONAL AND PUBLIC POLICIES. *Also directly related to this article are the entries* DEATH: ART OF DYING, *article on* CONTEMPORARY ART OF DYING; HOSPICE AND END-OF-LIFE CARE; INFORMED CONSENT, *articles on* MEANING AND ELEMENTS OF INFORMED CONSENT, *and* CLINICAL ASPECTS OF CONSENT IN HEALTH CARE; *and* RIGHTS, *article on* RIGHTS IN BIOETHICS. *For a discussion of related ideas, see the entries* BIOETHICS; CONFLICT OF INTEREST; DEATH; DEATH, ATTITUDES TOWARD; FREEDOM AND COERCION; *and* LAW AND BIOETHICS. *Other relevant material may be found under the entries* FAMILY; HOSPITAL, *article on* CONTEMPORARY ETHICAL PROBLEMS; *and* PATIENTS' RIGHTS, *article on* ORIGIN AND NATURE OF PATIENTS' RIGHTS.

Bibliography

BEDELL, SUSANNA E; PELLE, DENISE; MAHER, PATRICIA L.; and CLEARY, PAUL D. 1986. "Do-Not-Resuscitate Orders for Critically Ill Patients in the Hospital: How Are They Used and What Is Their Impact?" *Journal of the American Medical Association* 256, no. 2:233–237.

BRETT, ALAN S. 1991. "Limitations of Listing Specific Medical Interventions in Advance Directives." *Journal of the American Medical Association* 266, no. 6:825–828.

BUCHANAN, ALLEN E., and BROCK, DAN W. 1989. *Deciding for Others: The Ethics of Surrogate Decisionmaking.* Cambridge: At the University Press.

CARDOZO, BENJAMIN. 1914. Dissenting opinion in *Schloendorff v. Society of New York Hospital.* 211 N.Y. 125, 105 N.E. 92.

Cruzan v. Director, Missouri Department of Health. 1990. 110 S. Ct. 2841.

DANIS, MARION; SOUTHERLAND, LESLIE I.; GARRETT, JOANNE M.; SMITH, JANET L.; HIELEMA, FRANK; PICKARD, C. GLENN; EGNER, DAVID M.; and PATRICK, DONALD L. 1991. "A Prospective Study of Advance Directives for Life-Sustaining Care." *New England Journal of Medicine* 324, no. 13:882–888.

DAVIDSON, KENT W.; HACKLER, CHRIS; CARADINE, DEBRA R.; and McCORD, RONALD S. 1989. "Physicians' Attitudes on Advance Directives." *Journal of the American Medical Association* 262, no. 17:2415–2419.

DRESSER, REBECCA S. 1989. "Advance Directives, Self-Determination, and Personal Identity." In *Advance Directives in Medicine,* pp. 155–170. Edited by Chris Hackler, Ray Moseley, and Dorothy E. Vawter. New York: Praeger.

EMANUEL, LINDA L.; BARRY, MICHAEL J.; STOECKLE, JOHN D.; ETTELSON, LUCY M.; and EMANUEL, EZEKIEL J. 1991. "Advance Directives for Medical Care—A Case for Greater Use." *New England Journal of Medicine* 324, no. 13:889–895.

EMANUEL, LINDA L., and EMANUEL, EZEKIEL J. 1989. "The Medical Directive: A New Comprehensive Advance Care Document." *Journal of the American Medical Association* 261, no. 22:3288–3293.

EVERHART, MARIA A., and PEARLMAN, ROBERT A. 1990. "Stability of Patient Preferences Regarding Life-Sustaining Treatments." *Chest* 97, no. 1:159–164.

GIBSON, JOAN. 1990. "National Values History Project." *Generations* 14 (Suppl.):51–63

HARE, JAN, and NELSON, CARRIE. 1991. "Will Outpatients Complete Living Wills? A Comparison of Two Interventions." *Journal of General Internal Medicine* 6, no. 1:41–46.

HARVEY, LYNN K.; SHUBAT, STEPHANIE C.; and FRESHNOCK, LARRY J. 1989. *Physician and Public Attitudes on Health Care Issues.* Chicago: American Medical Association.

HASTINGS CENTER. 1987. *Guidelines on the Termination of Life-Sustaining Treatment and the Care of the Dying.* Bloomington: Indiana University Press.

HIGH, DALLAS M. 1987. "Planning for Decisional Incapacity: A Neglected Area in Ethics and Aging." *Journal of the American Geriatrics Society* 35, no. 8:814–820.

———. 1993. "Advance Directives and the Elderly: A Study of Intervention Strategies to Increase Use." *Gerontologist* 33, no. 3:342–349.

KUTNER, LUIS. 1969. "Due Process of Euthanasia: The Living Will, a Proposal." *Indiana Law Journal* 44, no. 4:539–554.

LO, BERNARD; SAIKA, GLENN; STRULL, WILLIAM; THOMAS, ELIZABETH; and SHOWSTACK, JONATHAN. 1985. "'Do Not Resuscitate' Decisions: A Prospective Study at Three Teaching Hospitals." *Archives of Internal Medicine* 145, no. 6:1115–1117.

LYNN, JOANNE. 1991. "Why I Don't Have a Living Will." *Law, Medicine and Health Care* 19, nos. 1–2:101–104.

MARKSON, LAWRENCE, and STEEL, KNIGHT. 1990. "Using Advance Directives in the Home-Care Setting: A Pilot Project." *Generations* 14 (Suppl.):25–29.

NATIONAL CENTER FOR STATE COURTS, COORDINATING COUNCIL OF LIFE-SUSTAINING MEDICAL TREATMENT DECISION MAKING BY THE COURTS. 1991. *Guidelines for State Court Decision Making in Authorizing or Withholding Life-Sustaining Medical Treatment.* Williamsburg, Va.: Author.

SACHS, GREG A.; MILES, STEVEN H.; and LEVIN, REBEKAH A. 1991. "Limiting Resuscitation: Emerging Policy in the Emergency Medical System." *Annals of Internal Medicine* 114, no. 2:151–154.

SACHS, GREG A.; STOCKING, CAROL B.; and MILES, STEVEN H. 1992. "Empowerment of the Older Patient? A Randomized, Controlled Trial to Increase Discussion and Use of Advance Directives." *Journal of the American Geriatrics Society* 40, no. 3:269–273.

SCHNEIDERMAN, LAWRENCE J., and ARRAS, JOHN D. 1985. "Counseling Patients to Counsel Physicians on Future Care in the Event of Patient Incompetence." *Annals of Internal Medicine* 102, no. 5:693–698.

SCHNEIDERMAN, LAWRENCE J.; KRONICK, RICHARD; KAPLAN, ROBERT M.; ANDERSON, JOHN P.; and LANGER, ROBERT D. 1992. "Effects of Offering Advance Directives on Medical Treatments and Costs." *Annals of Internal Medicine* 117, no. 7:599–606.

SECKLER, ALLISON B.; MEIER, DIANE E.; MULVIHILL, MICHAEL; and PARIS, BARBARA E. 1991. "Substituted Judgement: How Accurate Are Proxy Predictions?" *Annals of Internal Medicine* 115, no. 2:92–98.

SEHGAL, ASHWINI; GALBRAITH, ALLISON; CHESNEY, MARGARET; SCHOENFELD, PATRICIA; CHARLES, GERALD; and LO, BERNARD. 1992. "How Strictly Do Dialysis Patients Want Their Advance Directives Followed?" *Journal of the American Medical Association* 267, no. 1:59–63.

SMEDIRA, NICHOLAS G.; EVANS, BRADLEY H.; GRAIS, LINDA S.; COHEN, NEAL H.; LO, BERNARD; COOKE, MOLLY; SCHECTER, WILLIAM P.; FINK, CAROL; EPSTEIN-JAFFE, EVE; MAY, CHRISTINE; and LUCE, JOHN M. 1990. "Withholding and Withdrawal of Life Support from the Critically Ill." *New England Journal of Medicine* 322, no. 5:309–315.

STEINBROOK, ROBERT; LO, BERNARD; MOULTON, JEFFREY; SAIKA, GLEN; HOLLANDER, HARRY; and VOLBERDING, PAUL A. 1986. "Preferences of Homosexual Men with AIDS for Life-Sustaining Treatment." *New England Journal of Medicine* 314, no. 7:457–460.

TENO, JOAN; FLEISHMAN, JOHN; BROCK, DAN W.; and MOR, VINCENT. 1990. "The Use of Formal Prior Directives Among Patients with HIV-Related Diseases." *Journal of General Internal Medicine* 5, no. 6:490–494.

TENO, JOAN; LYNN, JOANNE; PHILLIPS, RUSSELL S.; MURPHY, DONALD; YOUNGHER, STUART J.; BELLAMY, PAUL; CONNERS, ALFRED F., JR.; DESBIENS, NORMAN A.; FULKERSON, WILLIAM; and KNAUS, WILLIAM A. 1994. "Do Formal Advance Directives Affect Resuscitation Decisions and the Use of Resources for Seriously Ill Patients?" *Journal of Clinical Ethics* 5, no. 1:23–61.

U.S. PRESIDENT'S COMMISSION FOR THE STUDY OF ETHICAL PROBLEMS IN MEDICINE AND BIOMEDICAL AND BEHAVIORAL RESEARCH. 1983. *Deciding to Forego Life-Sustaining Treatment: A Report on the Ethical, Medical, and Legal Issues in Treatment Decisions.* Washington, D.C.: U.S. Government Printing Office.

ZIMBERG, JOEL M. 1988. "Decisions For the Dying: An Empirical Study of Physicians' Responses to Advance Directive." *Vermont Law Review* 13:455–491.

IV. PROFESSIONAL AND PUBLIC POLICIES

The rise of explicit policies

The development of professional and public policies on forgoing life-sustaining treatment and on euthanasia has paralleled the transformation of death and dying since the middle of the twentieth century. The process of dying and the moment of death were once visible and familiar events in people's lives, even from an early age. Deaths outside of a hospital were the norm, not only sudden or accidental deaths but those that followed long illnesses or the gentle decline into old age. When pneumonia, "the old man's friend," came to call, it usually found him at home, with his family holding vigil, bolstered by the presence of a priest or a physician. Until recently, physicians could usually do little more than family members could do. They could give comfort measures and wait and see, for example, if the fever broke and the patient survived. If the patient did not survive, there was nothing more for the physician to do than declare death and let the process of grieving begin.

Potent means have emerged to overcome many acute causes of death such as kidney failure, cardiopulmonary arrest, and bacterial infections, and to sustain patients for long periods afterwards, with artificial replacement of organ functions and enteral and parenteral nutrition. The locus of dying has shifted to health-care facilities, where the course of illness can be managed and, with good luck, even reversed. "Perhaps 80% of the deaths in the United States now occur in hospitals and long-term care institutions, such as nursing homes" (U.S. President's Commission, 1983, pp. 17–18).

In the process, however, dying has become a less familiar part of life for most people; even when visiting a dying patient in the hospital, laypeople now find many barriers—from medical technology to medical personnel—between themselves and the patient. Furthermore, with people living longer, a growing number of patients are old and frail and, most important, virtually alone. "Dying in one's own bed" increasingly means dying in a long-term or other health-care facility rather than at home surrounded by family and friends.

In the earlier era there was little need for formal policies. Control of the dying process—to the extent that any human control or choice was exercised—rested with patients, who were usually awake and competent until the final hours, and their next of kin. Physicians followed the Hippocratic dictate to do what was best for their patients, meaning to forestall death if possible and to provide comfort measures in any event. These efforts were usually appreciated; indeed, physicians' comfort and compassion for dying patients, including long hours at their bedsides, accounted for much of the respect physicians enjoyed in their communities. Moreover, since they were expected, most deaths were not seen by others, nor were they usually experienced by physicians as failures, nor did they need outside review.

The move to institutions may have made dying less visible to laypeople, but it opened each death to the eyes of many more professionals. Indeed, more people—other physicians, nurses, and paramedical and administrative personnel—became directly involved in caring for each patient. Policies and procedures were thus needed to make sure all personnel understood what was to be done in each case: What medications are to be given on what schedule? Is resuscitation to be attempted if the patient's breathing stops?

The very existence of myriad means of medical intervention transformed what had been matters of fate into matters of choice and hence, also matters about which the people involved (e.g., patients, families, physicians, and nurses) could disagree, which they did with increased frequency. Anxiety among physicians and other health-care providers over the rising number of tort suits and actual or potential disagreement about what treatments to use or to forgo, led either to decision-making paralysis, to review by an institutional ethics committee or consultant, or to the courthouse to await a judge's ruling, especially before discontinuing life support. As a result, beginning in the 1970s, the existing practice of deferring to private decision making by patients and their families, guided by medical conventions and ethical standards, was replaced with more detailed policies that combine patients' right to self-determination, the state's interest in protecting human life, and health-care professionals' collective and personal norms.

In the 1950s professional and public policies were meager and largely implicit; today they are voluminous, detailed, and explicit, still evolving and sometimes contradictory. Public policy was once largely deferential to professional policies and actions; in many jurisdictions it now contains detailed prescriptions for what physicians and other professionals may or must do, as well as restrictions on and empowerment of patients and those who act as surrogate decision makers on patients' behalf.

Public policies on euthanasia and sustaining life intersect with professional policies in complex ways. While the two categories of policies are usually congruent, at times they balance the fundamental objectives of well-being and self-determination in dissimilar ways. Moreover, they rest on different grounds and are articulated through diverse means.

Professional policies

Each profession reflects certain important policies in its basic ethical code. In the case of medicine, the Hippocratic Oath contains both the general pledge to "follow that system of regimen which, according to my ability and judgment, I consider for the benefit of my patients, and abstain from whatever is deleterious and mischievous" and the specific injunction against giving a deadly drug if asked and against suggesting its use. As much as any technical skill, commitments of this sort define a profession by stating the objectives for, and limitations on, using the knowledge and techniques that members of the profession hold in common. Over time, through the writings of influential commentators on the profession and its practices and through explicit decisions of professional associations, the policies of the profession are further elaborated. Again, those policies that are central to the professional role become part of the self-definition of that profession and hence part of the standard of conduct and mode of analysis commonly found among members of the profession. The provisions of a professional code and the policies they generate not only provide the basis for group cohesion but also reveal the profession's ethical assumptions and standards to outsiders.

Self-determination. The codes of the health professions are more strongly committed to promoting patients' well-being than enhancing their autonomy, although nurses' codes contain explicit commitment to honoring the latter. In the United States, the official statements of the medical profession mention involving patients in decision making about their care, but the medical profession's age-old ambivalence about the possibility, or even desirability, of patient self-determination is well documented (Katz, 1984). Moreover, the commitment in the American Medical Association's (AMA) *Principles of Medical Ethics* that physicians will "deal honestly with patients," "respect the rights of patients," and "make relevant information available to patients" (AMA, 1988) does not provide a level of specificity that matches the law's or that provides much guidance either to physicians or to those who wish to evaluate their compliance with the profession's ethical dictates.

Sustaining life and relieving suffering. The devotion of health-care professionals to their patients' welfare is not usually questioned, even by those who object to certain interventions as unauthorized or ill-suited to fulfill their own sense of patient welfare under the circumstances. But when cure of a lethal condition is unlikely or worse, the meaning of "above all, do no harm" becomes cloudy. Does this injunction mean that medical and nursing interventions should be limited to comfort measures, or are steps to extend life also permitted or even required?

The extent to which the health professions' ethical codes commit members to the use of life-prolonging treatment is debated. The equation of harm prevention with life extension lacks classical roots and enjoys only minority support. As early as 1981, well before physicians had generally begun questioning their enthusiasm for aggressive death-delaying tactics in all cases, Robert Veatch concluded that "Only one important twentieth-century code commits the physician to the preservation of life, the World Medical Association's International Code of Medical Ethics, and that seems highly qualified with exceptions . . ." (Veatch, 1981, pp. 22–23). In the succeeding years, professional associations have made explicit that the commitment to the patient's well-being is not violated by ceasing life-prolonging care. For example, the Council on Ethical and Judicial Affairs, the arm of the AMA that interprets its *Principles of Medical Ethics,* has concluded that "For humane reasons, with informed consent, a physician may do what is medically necessary to alleviate severe pain, or cease or omit treatment to permit a terminally ill patient whose death is imminent to die" (AMA, 1988, p. 3).

Physicians clearly distinguish between, on the one hand, measures such as morphia that are intended to relieve pain but that also risk causing death because they suppress respiratory effort and the gag reflex, and on the other hand, measures such as lethal injections or administration of carbon monoxide that provide relief only by causing death. The former are permitted, but the latter are not according to the formal declarations of most health-care professional associations around the world. The AMA's Council on Ethical and Judicial Affairs, for example, reaffirmed in 1992 its strong opposition to "mercy killing." It concluded that "Physicians must not perform euthanasia or participate in assisted suicide" because the "societal risk of involving physicians in medical interventions to cause patients' deaths is too great in this culture" (1992, p. 2230). "The British Medical Association, the National Council of the French Medical Association, the Medical Council in the Federal Republic of Germany, and the Swedish Commission on Terminal Care, and the views of physicians in Denmark, Australia, and New Zealand presented in a 1988 British Medical Association Report also oppose physicians' performance of direct, active euthanasia" (Shapiro et al., 1994, p. 583). Among exceptions to this stance are the Royal Dutch Medical Association, which in 1984 endorsed guidelines under which it is deemed legitimate for physicians to perform active euthanasia (de Wachter,

1989), and the Michigan Nurses Association, which in 1994 differed with the state's medical society and supported a recommendation that physician-assisted suicide be legalized.

Respect for the law.   Finally, health-care professionals are committed to respecting the laws of the jurisdiction in which they practice; indeed, such respect is expected by society in exchange for allowing professionals a great deal of autonomy in organizing and overseeing their own work. It might therefore seem that as professional and public policies intersect, the professional are subordinated to the public. In fact, to a large degree, public policies on life-sustaining treatment and euthanasia have long deferred to professionally formulated ethical policies and standards of behavior. For example, in 1992 a commission of the Japan Medical Association concluded that a patient's expression of a wish to die with dignity should be respected but that active euthanasia should not be approved. Two years later, the Science Council, the principal governmental body for all matters affecting medical research and the life sciences, approved a report of its Special Committee on Death and Medical Treatment advocating removal of life support for patients in a deep, irreversible coma if they had previously stated their opposition to life-prolonging measures.

Public policies: Sources

The term "public policy" encompasses both explicit legal rules and the practices and procedures of individuals and groups that are recognized and sanctioned by society. To take a simple example, it has long been the practice of physicians and others in health care to obtain consent for procedures from the next-of-kin of adult patients who are unable to communicate their own wishes because of their illness or because of the effects of treatment itself. In the United States, until the mid-1980s, however, this practice seems simply to have been accepted, without any express judicial holding, much less any specific statutory basis. Even so, it would have been accurate to say that the policy was to allow medical interventions to proceed on adult patients who lack decision-making capacity when consent was obtained from their relatives (or, in certain circumstances, their closest friend).

Nonetheless, when speaking of public policy, what is usually intended are the more formal and explicit manifestations of the society's will. An examination of public policy on euthanasia and life support should therefore begin by looking at the ways in which such policies take formal shape in constitutions, court decisions, legislation, and regulations before turning to the objectives and values that guide these policies. The examination should result in the specific manifestation of these policies, which are closely intertwined with the professional policies previously described.

Constitutions.   Most legal systems in the world now operate according to a basic charter that guarantees certain positive and negative rights, particularly through limiting the government's powers. The U.S. Constitution is the world's oldest such document. Although limitations on governmental power may not directly control the relationship of private parties such as physicians and patients, constitutional rights may restrict the actions of health-care providers by limiting their ability to enforce their will on patients through legal proceedings or, conversely, may reassure health-care providers that they will not be at legal risk for following instructions of patients or their surrogates to forgo life support. The extent to which people's right to make choices about their lives is found to be outweighed by the state's authority to protect other interests may nonetheless limit professional authority, since health-care professionals have no greater right to be free of state interference in treating patients than the latter have over their own lives.

Judicial decisions.   In countries whose legal systems derive from that of Great Britain (including the United States), judicial decisions are an important source of law on life support and euthanasia. Judges in these countries not only interpret statutes (as they do in the code-based legal systems found on the European continent, in the former European colonies of South America and Africa, and in Japan), they also make law interstitially and incrementally as they resolve new issues that arise in individual cases. Such cases are particularly likely to arise when substantial changes occur in underlying practices, such as in how dying patients are treated. New practices, which by definition are not a settled part of how a field operates and hence cannot be assumed to be an implicit part of public policy, are more likely to clash with the expectations and wishes of people both in and outside of the profession and therefore to generate issues in need of resolution.

If the resulting uncertainty is great enough, those involved in providing health services may refuse to act without advance judicial review of the legality of the proposed steps. It is proper to seek judgment when a genuine question exists as to the identity of the appropriate decision maker for a patient who lacks decisional capacity or when such a decision maker insists on a course of action that appears, to the health-care providers, to be manifestly contrary to a patient's interests or express wishes. Courts ought not entertain cases involving merely providers' disagreement with competent patients or cases with no genuine dispute between an incapacitated patient's authorized surrogate decision maker and the health-care professionals. "Some providers have sought judicial review, for example, not because they disagreed with the patient's or surrogate's decision or judgment, but because they wanted a guarantee that no criminal or civil liability would flow from the implementation of the treatment decision. Judicial involvement is generally inappropriate in such cases, because no genuine issue exists" (Coordinating Council, 1993, pp. 33–34). Cumulatively, judicial resolution of individual cases amounts to a set of common-law precedents, which in turn guide the decisions of subsequent cases and the development of doctrines that have an effect on professional practices comparable with the effect of statutory requirements.

Statutes.   Unlike most areas of health care, the statutes that affect decision making about life-sustaining treatment and euthanasia are predominantly criminal, specifically those on homicide and suicide (analyzed in the next section). Statutory rules and standards for judicial protection of the rights and welfare of incompetent persons are sometimes important in contributing to policies in this field as well.

In addition, many technical, economic, and organizational aspects of health care are covered by statutory provisions, as is the operation of agencies that license and supervise the practice of medicine and other professions. The latter statutes are generally procedural in nature and leave a good deal of discretion to the agencies in establishing relevant standards and processes through regulations. In dealing with complex fields, legislatures typically frame the basic legal structure and delegate the task of filling in the details to those with greater time and expertise at the administrative level.

Regulations.   As a general matter, health professionals are licensed by the state upon fulfilling specified educational and training requirements and passing examinations. The state also licenses health-care facilities, which themselves establish requirements to be met by the people whom they employ or allow to practice in the facility. Both the state agencies and health-care facilities rely in turn on private organizations to accredit and credential practitioners and institutions. The standards employed by accrediting and credentialing organizations are usually entirely within their own control, although they may be adjusted to meet the perceived or expressed needs or demands of society. While privately formulated, such standards become part of public policy as expressions of society's expectations for the competencies and behavior of institutions that have been approved. Unlike a license, accreditation or credentials are not needed as a matter of law, but their possession may become so closely linked to other decisions (such as obtaining privileges to practice in a particular facility or to be reimbursed by an insurance company) that they take on something akin to legal force.

In addition to ensuring that professionals possess the knowledge and technical abilities appropriate to their areas of practice, these various official and private standard-setting and enforcing bodies also typically establish basic ethical expectations for practitioners and facilities. Most of the increasingly detailed and voluminous rules and regulations deal primarily with the economics and organization of health care (such as prohibitions on self-dealing, kickbacks, and financial conflicts of interest) and only a small portion relates directly to end-of-life decision making. The core standard, common to most regulatory schemes, subjects physicians to discipline and loss of license for "unprofessional conduct." In itself this does little to determine whether it is unacceptable for a physician to discontinue life-sustaining treatment or to administer a lethal injection in order to provide a patient with a swift and painless death. In reaching a determination on this point, licensing bodies look not only to the rules established by statute or other direct expressions of societal expectations but also to the opinions of professional bodies, such as the AMA's Council on Ethical and Judicial Affairs.

Public policies: Values and objectives

Although the core values in this arena of public policy—personal autonomy, protection of human life and well-being, and respect for professional integrity—coincide with those that undergird professional policies, they receive a slightly different emphasis here. Health-care professionals' belief that they "serve patients best by maintaining a presumption in favor of sustaining life" is constrained by the basic principles that "[t]he voluntary choice of a competent and informed patient should determine whether or not life-sustaining therapy will be undertaken" and that those involved in health care "should try to enhance patients' abilities to make decisions . . . and to promote understanding of available treatment options" (U.S. President's Commission, 1983, p. 3).

Self-determination and bodily integrity. The primacy of personal autonomy in public policy on all aspects of health care has two legal roots, in addition to the substantial support provided by bioethicists. The first of these is the common law's firm and long-standing protection of bodily integrity against unconsented interference, even interference with benevolent motives. Perhaps recognizing the great powers that medicine was beginning to possess, courts from the beginning of this century enunciated protection against abuse of these powers in terms that resonate with the shield the law erects against official harms. As the Illinois Court of Appeals declared in a landmark decision, "the free citizen's first and greatest right, which underlies all others—the right to the inviolability of his person, in other words, his right to himself—is the subject of universal acquiescence, and this right necessarily forbids a physician

or surgeon, however skillful or eminent . . . to violate without permission the bodily integrity of his patient . . ." (*Pratt v. Davis*, 1905, p. 166).

Beginning with a 1957 California appellate decision (*Salgo v. Leland Stanford Jr. University Board of Trustees*, 1957), American courts required physicians and others, when obtaining consent, to disclose the risks and benefits of the proposed medical intervention and other principal options. In the succeeding years, most commentary on "informed consent" has focused on the disclosure requirement and on the ways in which it was translated into law and became—or failed to become—an actual part of health-care practices (Faden et al., 1986).

In the context of euthanasia and life support, the obligation of disclosure, while not unimportant, should not obscure the limited context within which the "consent" half of the doctrine was first developed, namely, not as an absolute right of self-determination but as a barrier to being subjected to a medical intervention to which one has not agreed. Taken as a whole and stripped of rhetoric, then, public policy proceeds from the position that each adult should be given an opportunity to learn about and freely choose among available medical options.

The second root of self-determination is specific to systems that have constitutions, such as the United States, that protect a range of activities from interference by the government. As with the protection that informed consent provides against unwanted private interventions, the exact contours of this constitutional protection have evolved substantially in the past quarter century, and their impact on health care remains uncertain. It is apparent, however, that the relevant interest in personal liberty—which in the United States was denominated the "right to privacy" in the context of contraception and abortion—is not absolute, though it does guard certain basic choices about one's life and body from state interference without sufficient justification. Plainly, then, the major issue in applying this objective in framing public policy lies in determining which state interests are sufficient to justify restricting individuals in the choices they make about their lives.

Protection of human life (and well-being). The cardinal interest that is weighed against self-determination in the context of life-sustaining treatment and euthanasia is the protection of life. The state supports this interest by marshaling resources to advance biomedical science and to apply existing knowledge in preventing and curing illness. But of even greater symbolic importance in affirming the sanctity of human life is the protection provided by the criminal law of homicide and suicide, through which the state attempts to prevent both the intentional and negligent infliction of potentially lethal harm.

Homicides can be divided in several ways according to their severity. Such divisions are very important for the law but of little relevance to public policy on forgoing treatment and euthanasia. In brief, the distinguishing feature of murder "is an intent to kill or a disregard of so plain a risk of death to another that it is treated as the equivalent of an intent to kill," whereas voluntary and involuntary manslaughter both depend on a death "lacking the very high degree of culpability which characterizes the capital offense of murder but not so lacking in culpability as to be noncriminal altogether" (Weinreb, 1983, pp. 858 and 862). Four features of homicide law are nevertheless of potential salience to public policy in this area.

First, unlike in civil litigation, the consent of the victim is not a defense or a legal justification to a charge of murder or manslaughter (Capron, 1983). Second, while some Continental legal systems, such as the Dutch, have recognized euthanasia—"the active killing of a patient at his or her request by a physician" (de Wachter, 1989, p. 3316)—as a lesser category of homicide, euthanasia is not a separate criminal category under the common law. Thus, neither the status of the defendant as a physician nor of the victim as a patient requesting death would be enough to bar a charge of criminal homicide.

Third, the imminence of a patient's death from an underlying disease or injury is of no importance to the law, which protects all human lives equally. "Courts have repeatedly held that any active shortening of life constitutes homicide, no matter how brief a time the victim would have lived if the defendant had not acted" (Capron, 1983, p. 711). The fourth and final feature of homicide law—namely, that the state must prove beyond a reasonable doubt that the defendant's act caused the victim's death—has entered into several acquittals in "mercy killing" cases in which the jurors were apparently persuaded of the possibility that the patient had died of his or her underlying condition almost instantaneously with the defendant administering a lethal injection (Sanders, 1969).

Typically, homicide is a larger concern to society than suicide, as well as being a topic of greater legal interest, scholarly as well as practical. But in some ways, suicide plays a disproportionate role in thinking about dying patients, perhaps because personal choice, which is so central in suicide, is a major tenet of bioethics. Debate about suicide in the context of health care is increasing as a result of physicians' growing willingness to express interest in, or even admit experience with, assisting patients in committing suicide (Quill, 1993).

Although suicide has been part of human experience since ancient times and was even approved by some groups, such as the Greek Stoics, it has typically been met with fear and condemnation. For many years in Western nations, suicide was viewed both as a sin and an offense against the civic order, comparable with other forms of homicide. In England, the bodies of suicides could not be buried on consecrated ground (the custom was burial in the public highway with a stake driven through the body) and their estates were seized by the Crown. Although it is not possible to punish a dead person directly, it was thought that the prospect of leaving one's family poor and in disgrace would deter people who were thinking of committing the crime.

By the 1960s, however, criminal law reformers had concluded that the people most affected by the prohibition were those who attempted suicide but failed. Reformers felt suicide-attempters, rather than being turned over to public prosecutors, should be evaluated and treated for mental illness. Today, suicide is no longer a felony in any jurisdiction in the United States. Nevertheless, in forty-four states, assisting a suicide is a crime under statutory or common law. Why is it criminal to aid in the commission of a noncrime?

The answer lies in the very reason why suicide was removed from the statute books: not because society approved of suicide or even regarded it neutrally, but because society recognized that such an act, in the face of the instinct for self-preservation, typically resulted from distressing circumstances, depression, or other forces or conditions that can overwhelm a person's judgment and will to live. Many people are caught up by such collection of forces at some time in their lives. At that moment, they are vulnerable to suggestion and domination. Someone desiring to kill a person could thus manipulate the situation so that the potential victim carries out the act. By criminalizing aid or encouragement to suicide, society attempts to prevent people from pushing others into an act of self-destruction. The prohibition is also intended to discourage people with good motives from bringing about suicides, since a person pondering suicide may not really be determined to take his or her own life unless someone else provides sanction for him or her to do so. Indeed, having received the aid (such as poison or a large quantity of medicine) that he or she solicited, the person thinking of suicide may even feel obligated to carry through with the act.

Respect for professional integrity. The third major value that enters into public policy on euthanasia and life support is the integrity of the medical profession. The state has two objectives here. The first is to encourage responsible behavior by health-care professionals by recognizing and reinforcing their own ethical standards which, as described above, are integral to the existence and cohesion of the professions themselves. By establishing ethical commandments, a profession in effect places limits on the use of the expert skill and knowledge that defines the profession from a technical viewpoint. Thus, these limits are essential to a full definition of the profession and they must be respected both by members of the profession in good standing and by the state if the profession is going to exist as a distinctive group, able to select (and demit) those who are qualified to operate within its unique field of action.

Second, in addition to collective ethical standards, individual practitioners may place personal limits on conduct in which they are willing to engage. Unless professionals are to be treated as people with lesser rights to control their own lives than others have, the state should also respect their ethical objections to carrying out steps that they may technically be qualified to execute. The primary qualification typically enunciated here is that in refusing to provide medically appropriate treatment, professionals may not abandon their patients (recognizing that the effect of such "abandonment" may actually seem more like imprisonment for the patient). For example, a physician who is unwilling to prescribe doses of morphine adequate to palliate a hospitalized patient's cancer pain, or who is unwilling to withdraw a respirator at the request of a competent patient, would have to arrange the patient's transfer to another physician rather than simply leaving the patient trapped without the medical assistance he or she has a right to receive.

Public policies on allowing to die

Over the past fifty years, the transformation of the process of dying has also produced an intricate, if not totally consistent, corpus of policies about allowing patients to die and actively ending their lives. These policies have arisen from various antecedents, both explicit (constitutions, judicial decisions, statutes, and regulations) and implicit (including professional policies), which have brought together the major ethical values or objectives of protecting individual self-determination, defending human life, and respecting the law and the integrity of health-care professionals. The subject of forgoing life support—that is, either withholding a new medical intervention or withdrawing an existing one—has been more fully developed in policy terms, while the subject of euthanasia is much more in flux.

Patients with decisional capacity. By the early 1990s, the policy accepted in virtually all jurisdictions held that competent adults are entitled to refuse treatment even when doing so results in their death; furthermore, not only are health-care professionals who comply with the patient's instructions not liable civilly or criminally, but failing to comply is itself a wrong. These policies were first articulated in the United States beginning with the landmark *Quinlan* decision by the New Jersey Supreme Court in 1976, but the policies have now gained widespread acceptance on two grounds. First, these policies are the logical corollary of the doctrine of informed consent: the right to consent has meaning only if the patient possesses the right not to consent. Second, in jurisdictions with a written constitution to protect personal liberty, the right recognized in *Quinlan* is one manifestation of what some courts labeled a "right of privacy," although the United States Supreme Court now describes it as a "protected liberty interest" in avoiding unwanted medical interventions, including "artificially delivered food and water essential to life" (*Cruzan*, 1990, p. 279). Regarding competent patients' own treatment, the right to make choices about health care is not limited by the patient's prognosis (e.g., the patient need not have a "terminal condition") or the type of treatment being passed up (e.g., "heroic measures") (*Bouvia* v. *Superior Court*, 1986).

The primary forum for the development of these policies was the courthouse, as judges balanced individuals' interests in self-determination and bodily integrity against the state's interest in the preservation of life and prevention of suicide, the protection of the well-being of third parties (such as the minor child at risk of losing a parent), and the ethical integrity of health-care professionals. Prior to *Quinlan*, these interests were found to outweigh personal choice in some cases that typically involved an otherwise healthy person's religiously motivated refusal of a blood transfusion needed to prevent death from a curable, acute condition. Since then courts and commentators substantially agree that the interests of the state in opposition to competent persons' right to refuse treatment "are virtually nonexistent" (Meisel, 1994, p. 27).

Although the state has a strong interest in preserving the life of the individual and in upholding the sanctity of all human life, even that fails "because the life that the state is seeking to protect in such a situation is the life of the same person who has competently decided to forgo the medical intervention" (*Conroy*, 1985, p. 1223). Furthermore, the courts concluded that in rejecting life-prolonging treatment patients were not committing suicide and thus health-care providers were not aiding suicide when they agreed to the patients' wishes. Protection of third parties is the state interest responsible for more judicial overrulings of treatment refusal than any other, but most have been "in cases in which the patient's condition is such that he can probably be returned to status quo ante if treatment is administered" (Meisel, 1989, p. 103). Finally, explicit changes in the policies of the medical profession, which now accepts the refusal of even life-sustaining treatment by patients, remove any interest the state has in this regard, although the courts continue to recognize that health-care professionals or institutions that object to the course chosen by a patient should not usually be forced to participate.

Patients without decisional capacity. Adults (and certain minors who live independently or take on adult responsibilities) are presumed to be competent unless it is shown that they have lost the ability to understand and reason about the particular choices in question. While competence is a legal determination, in medical settings it is recognized that certain medical conditions—most definitively, a permanent loss of consciousness—can deprive patients of their decisional capacity. Policies have now been developed through judicial decisions, statutes, and regulations, on the effect of decisional incapacity on patients' right to have treatment suspended.

The interest of incompetent patients who are dying or permanently unconscious in avoiding a long and undignified dying process is such that the persons who act as their surrogate decision makers may order life-sustaining treatment suspended when the patient expressed such a wish while still competent. Moreover, in most jurisdictions, even when such desires are not spelled out, the surrogate can direct that treatment be stopped either when doing so best approximates what the patient would have decided based on what is known of the patient's values and preferences (under the "substituted judgment" standard), or when the burdens of continued treatment outweigh the benefits (under the "best interests" standard).

Although many courts have asserted that an "incompetent's right to refuse treatment should be equal to a competent's right to do so" (*Grant*, 1987, p. 449), the U.S. Supreme Court in *Cruzan* made clear that the state may limit the actions of those who make choices for incompetent patients in the service of several interests. Foremost among these is protection of human life. This entitles the state to insist (although few have chosen to do so) that the wishes of the patient be proven by "clear and convincing evidence" (rather than a mere "preponderance of the evidence"). Moreover, the state is actually protecting autonomy when it insists on proof of the patient's wishes, for the right to choose is a personal one, and forgoing treatment when an incompetent patient actually would have chosen to have it continued does not respect autonomy. Nonetheless, most states recognize that patients who persist in an unconscious state for a long period might be said to have lost all interests, other than the interest in avoiding a mistake in prognosis (U.S. President's Commission, 1983). For these patients, it is the next of kin whose interests are primarily affected by prolonged treatment, and they are usually regarded as the appropriate surrogates in the absence of manifest unfitness or a clear conflict of interest.

In furtherance of the interest in protecting patients' well-being and the integrity of the health-care professions, facilities have established institutional ethics committees charged not only with helping to prepare local policies on end-of-life decision making and to educate personnel about such policies and the issues involved, but also to play a role in situations in which disputes have arisen about such decisions, particularly when the patient lacks the capacity to participate in decisions about forgoing treatment. Such committees have been required by accrediting bodies (Joint Commission on Accreditation of Healthcare Organizations, 1994), as well as by courts in some jurisdictions since *Quinlan*, to review the prognosis and the reasoning that goes into decisions to forgo life support. Also, federal regulations promulgated in response to instances of alleged "medical negligence" of newborn babies with life-threatening anomalies in effect treat ethics committee review as evidence of good faith and an absence of wrongdoing.

Although rather confused in the way they express this point, the courts and legislatures, in developing law on treatment cessation for incompetent patients, have distinguished treatments that are lifesaving (in the sense of restoring the patient to a relatively healthy condition, with indefinite survival) from those that are merely life-prolonging (especially when the patient is expected to remain unconscious). Such distinctions are problematic not merely because of difficulties in accurate prognosis but because they ignore considerations other than length of life that are of great importance to many people. Nonetheless, many judges and legislators seem to regard the state's interest in preservation of life as stronger when the treatment in question could preserve a relatively normal life for an indefinite period, and hence they are more willing to override decisions to forgo treatment, at least those made by surrogates for incompetent patients. Of course, the same result would probably be reached if the surrogates were operating under either the substituted judgment or best interests standard because it is hard to believe that most people would want to forgo a curative or highly restorative treatment or that the burdens of such treatment would outweigh the benefits.

Since 1976, when California (in light of the problems made apparent by the *Quinlan* case) adopted the first statute giving legal effect to advance directives, statutes have been adopted in all American jurisdictions to make decision making about incompetent patients both easier and more reflective of patients' wishes. Under these statutes persons while still competent may appoint a health-care agent whose authority persists beyond, or takes effect upon, the person's becoming incompetent (in legal terms, the agency is "durable"), or they may provide instructions about the care they want at the end of life (particularly when efforts to prolong life are to be limited—such documents are known as "living wills"), or they may combine the two. Although it is sometimes loosely said that such statutes make advance directives "binding," their enforcement provisions are weak. There is little indication that legal actions are frequently employed either to enforce such documents (except where a dispute has arisen about who is authorized to act under the document or what its provisions mean) or to recover damages from physicians or others after the fact for failing to honor the document. Instead, the effect of the statutes seems to be to provide reassurance to physicians and others that they are at no legal risk for following the instructions contained in the directive, as well as to console all involved that however difficult the decision to cease treatment may be, it was the patient's wish.

Public policy strongly favors the use of advance directives, even though relatively little is known about the efficacy of directives among different population groups and despite the fact that most people do not execute advance directives. To encourage their use, the U.S. Congress in 1990 adopted the Patient Self-Determination Act, which requires that persons being admitted to hospitals, home-health agencies, hospices, and nursing homes, and those joining health maintenance organizations, be informed of their rights under state law to make an advance directive and that the institution inquire whether they have such a document (McCloskey, 1991). Furthermore, in her concurring opinion in the *Cruzan* case, Justice Sandra Day O'Connor suggested that decisions made by a surrogate pursuant to an advance directive might be constitutionally protected against state interference.

Categorical distinctions.   In the process of reaching the present policy, the courts took note of the four principal points that have arisen in bioethical examinations of the subject.

Acts versus omissions.   Although bioethicists have sometimes distinguished acts that cause death, which are taken to be forbidden, from omissions that are acceptable because they merely "allow the patient to die," the law realizes that all results have multiple causes and the distinction between acting and omitting can be very artificial. Instead, the relevant question is which among many causes are morally or legally culpable, recognizing that an intentional omission to act could be as culpable as a negligent action that caused a comparable harm. Thus, in the only case in which American physicians have been prosecuted for homicide for discontinuing life support, the appellate court dismissed the indictment, but not on the ground that the defendants had merely let the patient die rather than killing him. Instead, the court held that the patient's death would have been wrongful only if the physicians' failure had breached a duty to continue treatment and no such duty remained once appropriate surrogates for the patient requested that the ventilator and later the hydration and nutrition tubes be removed (*Barber v. Superior Court,* 1983).

Not starting versus stopping.   A similar duty-based analysis has led courts to reject the putative "not starting versus stopping" distinction that would make withholding treatment less a source of civil or criminal liability than withdrawing the same treatment that has already started. The distinction had been adopted by administrative officials, such as the U.S. Department of the Army, which decreed that life support once begun could not be stopped without a court order (*Tune v. Walter Reed Army Medical Hospital,* 1985). But while acknowledging its psychological underpinnings, courts have rejected it (*Satz v. Perlmutter,* 1978), pointing out that "from a policy standpoint, it might well be unwise to forbid persons from discontinuing a treatment under circumstances in which the treatment could permissibly be withheld. Such a rule could discourage families and doctors from even attempting certain types of care and could thereby force them into hasty and premature decisions to allow a patient to die" (*Conroy,* 1985, p. 1234).

Public policies on active euthanasia and physician aid in suicide

The legality of physicians' performing active euthanasia or aiding their patients to commit suicide (for example, by prescribing medication sufficient for a lethal overdose) is one of the most controversial areas in bioethics. Although public policy on forgoing treatment is sometimes said to affirm a "right to die," in fact, it only establishes a "right to choose" among available medical options. Thus, the questions become whether active euthanasia and assisted suicide fall within the practice of medicine, and if at least some physicians think so, whether laws that preclude them from acting on their beliefs ought to be changed or swept aside. On the first point, the euthanasia debate demonstrates that professional policies may have a large, perhaps decisive impact on public policy. At the moment, the official position of the health-care professions against euthanasia and aid-in-suicide is shared by leading commentators (Gaylin et al., 1988). If care is administered properly at the end of life patients should not be so distressed that they desire suicide, but in rare cases this will occur, and some commentators argue that it is not necessarily wrong for physicians to assist (Wanzer et al., 1989). Indeed, some have argued that a wider range of options should be legalized for physician assistance to dying patients (Quill, 1993).

Even most opponents of legalizing euthanasia recognize that in circumstances of great and unrelievable suffering, the case for mercifully easing a patient across the threshold of death can seem compelling enough not only to lead physicians to participate but to make prosecutors unwilling to charge the physicians and jurors unwilling to convict them. Provided that such cases remain rare, they do not alter the underlying policy, and the presumption remains that physicians (like other people) are not authorized to take the life of another person directly.

In one legal system, however, first the courts and then the legislature have altered the presumption. Active voluntary euthanasia has been openly practiced in the Netherlands since 1973, when a Dutch physician who had been found guilty of participating in a mercy killing was given a suspended sentence, based on the court concluding that the physician had met four conditions that made euthanasia acceptable: (1) the patient's condition is incurable; (2) the patient's suffering is unbearable; (3) the patient requests euthanasia in writing; and (4) a physician performs the euthanasia (de Wachter, 1989). In that same year the Royal Dutch Medical Association issued a statement asserting that euthanasia is justifiable in some circumstances, but that it should remain illegal. A government-commissioned study of the practice of euthanasia in 1991 found that 3 percent of all Dutch deaths annually are caused by active euthanasia or assisted suicide. The totals—2,300 cases of voluntary euthanasia, 400 of physician-assisted suicide, and 1,000 of involuntary euthanasia—were far lower than predicted. However, doubts about controlling the practice arose because the requirement that physicians report each case of euthanasia to the local prosecutor for investigation had not been met in most cases. Furthermore, euthanasia had been performed 1,000 times without the persistent request of the patient, apparently in cases where the physician believed that it would be too burdensome to the patient to discuss euthanasia, where the patient became unconscious before the discussion could be made, or where the patient was a child incapable of making a competent choice (Gomez, 1991).

In February 1993 the Dutch Parliament approved legislation codifying and strengthening the existing euthanasia guidelines, and immunizing from prosecution physicians who follow them. The law requires that the patient voluntarily request euthanasia repeatedly over a period of time, be mentally competent, and have a terminal disease accompanied by unbearable physical or mental suffering. The physician must consult a colleague experienced in euthanasia and submit a documented report stating the patient's medical history and the circumstances of the euthanasia. Once the patient has died, the doctor must submit a report to the coroner's office. As long as the report shows that the guidelines were followed and that there is no evidence of malpractice, the doctor will remain immune from prosecution.

Euthanasia or direct assistance in committing suicide had not become official policy in any other country by 1994, although proposed legislation for physician-performed euthanasia had been submitted through referenda to voters in Washington State in 1991 and California in 1992, and the proponents planned to place a proposal on the ballot in Oregon to legalize physician assistance in suicide.

U.S. courts have also had occasion to review the issue. Between June 1990 and November 1993, Jack Kevorkian, a retired pathologist, helped twenty people commit suicide in Michigan using various devices to provide a lethal injection or carbon monoxide gas. When the state found that he could not be prosecuted under its murder statute (because the final act of administering the deadly substance was always taken by the victim rather than by Kevorkian), it adopted a statute specifically banning assistance in suicide. In May 1994 Kevorkian was acquitted of violating that statute, but the jury's decision seems to have turned on the technical defenses he raised. Thus, his highly conspicuous activities have not provided a clear test of his claim that he should be free of prosecution for effectuating his patient's "right to die."

In 1994 a group of patients, physicians, and an organization that supports "terminally ill adults considering suicide" brought suit in the U.S. District Court for the Western District of Washington. It challenged the Washington state statute that makes it a felony knowingly to aid another person in committing suicide "insofar as it bans physician-assisted suicide by mentally competent, terminally ill adults who knowingly and voluntarily choose to hasten their death" (*Compassion in Dying* v. *Washington*, 1994). In early May, Chief Judge Barbara J. Rothstein declared the law unconstitutional because it violated two Fourteenth Amendment rights of this group of patients. First, reasoning that the intimate personal decision to commit suicide "falls within the realm of the liberties constitutionally protected under the Fourteenth Amendment," Judge Rothstein concluded that the Washington statute places an "undue burden" on the exercise of a protected liberty. Yet the holding of the Supreme Court in *Cruzan* made clear that the state need only have a good (not a compelling) reason for restricting conduct that directly threatens its interest in protecting the sanctity of life. Indeed, shortly after deciding *Roe* v. *Wade*, the Court rejected the argument that conduct involving "consenting adults" is beyond state regulation, and cited as "unchallenged" a number of laws outlawing conduct in which adults engage in private, including suicide (Capron, 1994).

Second, Judge Rothstein held that the statute violated the right to equal protection by treating terminally ill patients—who want physicians to help them take their lives—differently from patients who are permitted to die by refusing life-sustaining treatments. Yet the cases cited by the court all involve situations in which one group of people is treated differently than another group that is in all relevant respects identical. In the present context, crucial differences do exist between the relative handful of people who would die quickly were it not for medical interventions and the potentially limitless number of people whose suffering seems to them a rational ground for suicide. More to the point, the two groups are seeking different, not similar, treatment by the state. Although Judge Rothstein claimed to limit her decision to helping terminally ill patients commit suicide, certainly those persons who need active euthanasia (because, for example, a physical impediment precludes their taking the final step toward death) could rely on the judge's reasoning to show that a legal system that allows active steps to aid suicide but not active euthanasia does not treat them equally.

Unlike their role in making common law in a factually grounded and incremental fashion, judges, in ruling on the constitutionality of statutes, regulate broadly. Thus, problems will arise when the propriety and success of a practice depend upon the details: under what circumstances, with what review, following what procedures and safeguards, and so forth, would physicians be able to help what group of patients? It is the difficulty of ensuring that any system of legalized euthanasia applies only to voluntary, rational patients with truly untreatable pain and no prospect of long-term survival or recovery that helps explain why courts as well as legislatures in most jurisdictions have been unwilling to make exceptions to the laws on murder and aiding suicide. Suicide is rare among the terminally ill, and most people who want to commit suicide do not suffer from a terminal condition but from a treatable mental illness, albeit one that their family and even physician may not recognize as such (New York State Task Force on Life and the Law, 1994). No one is more vulnerable than a sick person, and it is a very short distance from the triumphant right to control the time and manner of self-death to feeling an obligation to succumb to the apparent preferences of one's caregivers in order to end the misery.

Public policy not only supports the preservation of life, it also strongly promotes patients' well-being, including the relief of suffering. Those who argue for actively ending life on this ground "overlook the potential of contemporary medicine to provide palliation and pain relief to those who are dying. . . . Health care professionals have a moral duty to provide adequate palliative care and pain relief, even if such care shortens the patient's life" (Hastings Center, 1987). Legalizing physician aid-in-dying would probably undermine, rather than reinforce, the development of public and professional policies that attempt to balance respect for patient's autonomy with preservation of the sometimes fragile web that protects the vulnerable in society.

ALEXANDER MORGAN CAPRON

Directly related to this article are the other articles in this entry, especially the articles on ETHICAL ISSUES, *and* ADVANCE DIRECTIVES. *Also directly related are the entries* LICENSING, DISCIPLINE, AND REGULATION IN THE HEALTH PROFESSIONS; DEATH, ATTITUDES TOWARD; HOSPICE AND END-OF-LIFE CARE; *and* AGING AND THE AGED, *articles on* SOCIETAL AGING, HEALTH-CARE AND RESEARCH ISSUES, *and* OLD AGE. *For a further discussion of topics mentioned in this article, see the entries* ACTION; AUTONOMY; COMPETENCE; HEALTH OFFICIALS AND THEIR RESPONSIBILITIES; HOMICIDE; INFORMED CONSENT, *especially articles on* HISTORY OF INFORMED CONSENT, LEGAL AND ETHICAL ISSUES OF CONSENT IN HEALTH CARE (*with its* POSTSCRIPT), *and* ISSUES OF CONSENT IN MENTAL-HEALTH CARE; MEDICAL CODES AND OATHS; PROFESSIONAL–PATIENT RELATIONSHIP; *and* SUICIDE. *For a discussion of related issues, see the entries* LAW AND BIOETHICS; LAW AND MORALITY; MEDICAL ETHICS, HISTORY OF, *section on* EUROPE, *subsection on* CONTEMPORARY PERIOD, *article on* THE BENELUX COUNTRIES; PRIVACY IN HEALTH CARE; *and* PUBLIC POLICY AND BIOETHICS. *See also the* APPENDIX (CODES, OATHS, AND DIRECTIVES RELATED TO BIOETHICS), SECTION II: ETHICAL DIRECTIVES FOR THE PRACTICE OF MEDICINE, *especially the* OATH OF HIPPOCRATES, *and* INTERNATIONAL CODE OF MEDICAL ETHICS *of the* WORLD MEDICAL ASSOCIATION.

Bibliography

AMERICAN MEDICAL ASSOCIATION, COUNCIL ON ETHICAL AND JUDICIAL AFFAIRS. 1988. "Report 12: Euthanasia." In *Code of Medical Ethics: Reports of the Council on Ethical and Judicial Affairs*. Chicago: American Medical Association (loose leaf). An interpretation of the association's ethical principles as applied to life-prolonging treatment and active euthanasia; relies on two Opinions that the Council issued in 1986, Section 2.18 and 2.19 in its compilation, *Current Opinions of the Council on Ethical and Judicial Affairs.*
———. 1992. "Decisions Near the End of Life." *Journal of the American Medical Association.* 267, no. 16:2229–2233.
———. 1994. *Code of Medical Ethics: Current Opinions with Annotations.* 1994 ed. Chicago: Author.
Barber v. Superior Court. 1983. 147 Cal. App. 3d 1006–1022; 195 Cal. Rptr. 484–494.
Bouvia v. Superior Court (Glenchur). 1986. 179 Cal. App. 3d 1127–1148; 225 Cal. Rptr. 297–308.
CAPRON, ALEXANDER MORGAN. 1983. "Euthanasia." In *Encyclopedia of Crime and Justice*, pp. 709–715. Edited by Sanford H. Kadish. New York: Free Press.
———. 1994. "Easing the Passing." *Hastings Center Report* 24, no. 4:25–26.
Compassion in Dying v. State of Washington. 1994. No. C94-119R, (W.D.Wash., 3 May).
Conroy, In re. 1985. 98 N.J. 321–399; 486 A.2d 1209–1250.
COORDINATING COUNCIL ON LIFE-SUSTAINING MEDICAL TREATMENT DECISION MAKING BY THE COURTS. 1993.

Guidelines for State Court Decision Making in Life-Sustaining Medical Treatment Cases. 2d ed. St. Paul, Minn.: West Publishing. Suggestions for trial judges about how to handle a set of relatively rare but important and urgent cases, from assuming jurisdiction of the case through the hearing and rendering of judgment; contains special advice on cases involving minors, analysis of underlying ethical principles and distinctions, and explanations of the practices and policies of health-care institutions.

Cruzan v. *Director, Missouri Department of Health.* 1990. 110 S.Ct. 2841–2892.

FADEN, RUTH R., and BEAUCHAMP, TOM L. 1986. *A History and Theory of Informed Consent.* New York: Oxford University Press. A magisterial analysis of the precedents—historical, philosophical, and legal—for the requirements of disclosure and consent in health care, and a thorough exploration of the conceptual issues raised.

GAYLIN, WILLARD; KASS, LEON R.; PELLEGRINO, EDMUND D.; and SIEGLER, MARK. 1988. "'Doctors Must Not Kill'." *Journal of the American Medical Association* 259, no. 14:2139–2140.

GOMEZ, CARLOS F. 1991. *Regulating Death: Euthanasia and the Case of the Netherlands.* New York: Free Press.

Grant, In re Guardianship. 1987. 109 Wash. 2d 545–580; 747 P.2d 445–464; modified, 757 P.2d 534 (1988).

HASTINGS CENTER. 1989. *Guidelines on the Termination of Life-Sustaining Treatment and the Care of the Dying.* Briarcliff Manor, N.Y.: Author.

JOINT COMMISSION ON ACCREDITATION OF HEALTHCARE ORGANIZATIONS. 1994. *Accreditation Manual for Hospitals.* 2 vols. Oakbrook Terrace, Ill.: Author.

KATZ, JAY. 1984. *The Silent World of Doctor and Patient.* New York: Free Press. A thoughtful examination of the physician-patient relationship and especially of the barriers to candid and complete disclosure and informed, voluntary consent.

McCLOSKEY, ELIZABETH LIEBOLD. 1991. "The Patient Self-Determination Act." *Kennedy Institute of Ethics Journal* 1, no. 2:163–169.

MEISEL, ALAN. 1989, 1994. *The Right to Die: 1994 Cumulative Supplement.* New York: John Wiley & Sons. A complete compilation and analysis of statutes and judicial decisions on forgoing life support and euthanasia; regularly updated.

NEW YORK STATE TASK FORCE ON LIFE AND THE LAW. 1994. *When Death Is Sought: Assisted Suicide and Euthanasia in the Medical Context.* New York: Author.

Pratt v. *Davis.* 1905. 118 Ill. App. 161–184, affirmed, 224 Ill. 300–310, 79 N.E. 562–565 (1906).

QUILL, TIMOTHY E. 1993. *Death and Dignity: Making Choices and Taking Charge.* New York: W. W. Norton.

Quinlan, In re. 1976. 70 N.J. 10–55, 355 A.2d 647–672, certiorari denied, 429 U.S. 922.

Salgo v. *Leland Stanford Jr. University Board of Trustees.* 1957. 154 Cal. App. 2d 560; 317 P. 2d 170–182 (Cal. App.).

SANDERS, JOSEPH. 1969. "Euthanasia: None Dare Call It Murder." *Journal of Criminal Law, Criminology, and Police Science* 60:351–359. Demonstrates the diversity of treatment received by defendants in "mercy killing" cases.

Satz v. *Perlmutter.* 1978. 362 So.2d 160–164 (Fla. Dist. Ct. App.), affirmed, 379 So.2d 359–361 (Fla. 1980).

SHAPIRO, ROBYN S.; DERSE, ARTHUR R.; GOTTLIEB, MARK; SCHIEDERMAYER, DAVID; and OLSON, MARY. 1994. "Willingness to Perform Euthanasia: A Survey of Physician Attitudes." *Archives of Internal Medicine* 154, no. 5:575–584.

Tune v. *Walter Reed Army Medical Hospital.* 1985. 602 F.Supp. 1452–1456 (D.D.C.).

U.S. PRESIDENT'S COMMISSION FOR THE STUDY OF ETHICAL PROBLEMS IN MEDICINE AND BIOMEDICAL AND BEHAVIORAL RESEARCH. 1983. *Deciding to Forego Life-Sustaining Treatment: A Report on the Ethical, Medical, and Legal Issues in Treatment Decisions.* Washington, D.C.: Author.

VEATCH, ROBERT M. 1981. *A Theory of Medical Ethics.* New York: Basic Books. A pioneering and comprehensive analysis of health-care ethics that draws on an eclectic mix of philosophical and religious theories to argue for assigning patients greater responsibilities and rights.

WACHTER, MAURICE A. M. DE. 1989. "Active Euthanasia in the Netherlands." *Journal of the American Medical Association* 262, no. 3:3316–3319.

WANZER, SIDNEY H.; FEDERMAN, DANIEL D.; ADELSTEIN, S. JAMES; CASSEL, CHRISTINE K.; CASSEM, EDWIN H.; CRANFORD, RONALD E.; HOOK, EDWARD W.; LO, BERNARD; MOERTEL, CHARLES G.; SAFAR, PETER; STONE, ALAN; and VAN EYS, JAN. 1989. "The Physician's Responsibility Toward Hopelessly Ill Patients." *New England Journal of Medicine* 320, no. 13:844–849.

WEINREB, LLOYD L. 1983. "Homicide: 2. Legal Aspects." In *Encyclopedia of Crime and Justice,* pp. 855–866. Edited by Sanford H. Kadish. New York: Free Press.

WILLIAMS, GLANVILLE L. 1957. *The Sanctity of Life and the Criminal Law.* New York: Alfred A. Knopf.

DEATH EDUCATION

Education, the process by which one develops one's potential for one's own sake as well as for that of society, has included education about death and grief since prehistoric times. Different cultures have introduced their young to the realities of ultimate loss as a part of tribal or religious custom and, more recently, through formal teaching.

The term "death education" has many meanings, but three seem basic. In analogy to many specific forms of education, such as medical education, death education has the sense of "preparation for death." The *I Ching, The Tibetan Book of the Dead,* the *Ars moriendi* literature, and the Hebrew-Christian Bible have, to a greater or lesser degree, the purpose of preparing the person for death and for death-related issues such as immortality, funeral rites, and bereavement behaviors. Since each of the great religions—Hinduism, Buddhism, Islam, Judaism, and Christianity—teaches that the person in this life is in a transition to another life, one can argue that one of the purposes of all religion has been the preparation for death.

The second meaning of death education is education for those decisions affected by actual or possible death. The practice of medicine and nursing, law, religious ministry, counseling, the military, law enforcement, fire-fighting, and funeral direction are all affected by the possibility of preventing or causing death, and by the consequences of a death. The training of practitioners in these careers would be incomplete if it did not include serious discussion of the definitions of death and of the personal, moral, legal, and economic issues involved in the death-related decisions made by these professionals.

The third meaning of death education, and the one that is the primary focus of this article, refers to a course or part of a course focusing on the meaning of death, attitudes toward death, and ways of coping with death. Such courses often have as their purpose the realization that (a) death is a part of the natural life cycle, (b) dying persons are still fully alive and have unique needs in the terminal stage of their illnesses, (c) the bereaved have normal reactions and needs, (d) the needs of the dying and bereaved can be satisfied by a supportive community, and (e) children have the right to know about the fullness of the life cycle, including death and bereavement. Death education differs as it is taught in elementary, high school, and university programs, but the above five elements are common enough to be considered a general orientation.

The need for formal death education

In earlier centuries, one did not have to live too many years before being exposed to the death of a sibling, a parent, a grandparent, or a neighbor. Today, due to longer life as well as the professionalization of death-related activities such as medical care and funeral direction, death is less frequently experienced in an immediate manner. It is common in the developed world to grow into one's twenties or even thirties without having experienced the death of a significant other. In a questionnaire John Morgan distributed between 1975 and 1993 to over 2,000 Canadian students whose ages ranged from seventeen to forty-four, the answer to the question "What was your first experience of death?" was rarely a family member or friend. Vanderlyn Pine notes that "for American [university] students, death courses, formal instruction, seminars, projects, minicourses, and so forth, provide an opportunity for the acquisition of experiential knowledge regarding dying and death. Given the other institutional structures existing today, such educational socialization seems essential" (Pine,

1977, p. 77). Since it is less known than other aspects of a human life, death is less accepted as an integral part of it.

Contemporary formal education about death and bereavement is primarily a North American phenomenon. A 1993 survey found that education about death and bereavement occurs in Europe, Africa, and Australia as part of religious education, professional ethics, and, to a lesser extent, the training of the health-care professional. However, education about death and bereavement for the average elementary, high school, or college student has developed only in Australia and North America. One possible reason for this is that with the exception of Quebec, the hospice movement began as an English-speaking movement and remained so until fairly recently. The hospice movement—the establishment of programs to provide only supportive care for persons with advanced progressive disease—started in England with the work of Cicely Saunders and was brought to Canada and the United States in the 1970s. Only since 1985 have there been hospices in Europe, South America, and Asia.

Death education as we know it today began in universities and colleges, and later filtered into elementary and high schools. While Vanderlyn Pine, Donald Irish, and others have sponsored seminars dealing with death, Robert Fulton seems to have offered the first formal course at the graduate level at the University of Minnesota in the early 1960s. The first undergraduate course was offered in 1968 at Loyola College in Montreal by John Morgan. For the most part, death education at the university level seems to be limited to one or two courses in departments of sociology, psychology, religion, or philosophy. Even in medicine, nursing, or social work, few formal courses exist, and what training there is in the psychosocial aspects of death and bereavement occurs at the discretion of the instructor. Only Brooklyn College, New York University, and the College of New Rochelle, all three in the New York City area, offer formal degree programs with a focus on thanatology—death studies—at the graduate level. A thanatological orientation may be found in the sociology program at the University of Minnesota, the Educational Psychology Department of the University of Florida, and the Psychology Department at York University in Toronto. The University of Western Ontario began a certificate program in palliative care and thanatology in 1994.

The death-awareness movement has been highly influenced by women, starting with Cecily Saunders who was responsible for the establishment of St. Christopher's Hospice in London, and Elisabeth Kübler-Ross, whose many books and lectures have reintroduced death into popular consciousness as witnessed in films and on television. The movement, both in theory and in practice, has a commitment to caring for the individual person, which Jeanne Quint Benoliel believes is a direct result of the feminine influence (Benoliel, 1993). Seventy-five percent of the membership of the Association for Death Education and Counseling, a professional organization that, among other functions, certifies persons as professional death educators and/or professional counselors, is female. About 60 percent of the literature in the field has been written by women. Perhaps women are over-represented in death-related areas because of their roles as mothers, as well as their careers in nursing, medicine, social work, and teaching (Benoliel, 1993).

Few formal courses devoted to death education exist in elementary and high schools. What are found are modules, or units within courses, that deal with loss and grief. There are three basic orientations to education about death and bereavement below the university level. The first and most common form of death education, at least at the level of secondary schooling, is suicide prevention. Staffs in schools are deemed by the courts to be responsible if they do not act in "a reasonably prudent manner" in reporting possibly suicidal behavior (Leenaars and Wenckstern, 1991, p. xiii), so school boards across North America have emphasized the importance of education as a form of suicide prevention. The second most common form of death education is an immediate response to a tragic event, such as the death of a child, a teacher, or a parent. Literature dealing with the support of the bereaved child in the classroom is now well developed. Since a curriculum is a statement of priorities, the third form of death education, proactive learning prior to a loss, would be the most important. It is, however, the least developed form of death education.

The aims of death education

Judith Stillion has pointed out that "rarely has a course been called upon to meet such variety of expectations: to teach people to live peacefully with each other, to appreciate life, and to give service to others as they seek meaning in living and dying. All this plus teaching a body of knowledge and research are the tasks of the death educators" (Stillion, 1979, p. 158). Since death education involves coming to understand one's place in the world, and the reality of ultimately limited resources, such knowledge should contribute to general education as a basis for personal development.

Many goals have been established for death education. The list below represents what has occurred in the literature since 1977; however, one must not assume that every course, much less every module, effects these goals. The goals cited are: (1) to remove the taboo aspect of death language; (2) to promote comfortable and intelligent interactions with the dying; (3) to educate children about death so they develop a minimum of death-related anxieties; (4) to understand the dynamics of grief; (5) to understand and be able to interact with a suicidal person; (6) to understand the social structure of dying (the "death system"); and (7) to recognize the variations involved in aspects of death both within and among cultures (Leviton, 1977). In reality, most courses effect no more than an understanding of the definitions of death, the meaning and necessity of palliative care, funerals, the dynamics of grief, and children's awarenesses of death (Morgan, 1990).

The curriculum

The death-education curriculum has a cognitive aspect that includes the development of a body of knowledge and an affective aspect that includes changes in attitudes and values. The International Work Group on Death, Dying and Bereavement has recommended the following criteria for education about death and bereavement: (1) that it be based on the current state of knowledge from a variety of disciplines; (2) that it integrate theory and practice; (3) that it promote sensitivity, awareness, and skills development through role modeling and supervised practice; and (4) that it provide emotional support and foster confidence (Corr et al., 1994).

One of the first topics in death education is the understanding of the death system, that is, the manner in which the traditions of a culture create and reinforce attitudes and behaviors regarding death and bereavement. Second, death education provides structured experiences of death. Since young persons have seldom had direct confrontation with death, some confrontation in the classroom is necessary to establish a starting point. Third, such education attempts to teach the dynamics of working with the dying and the bereaved in a sensitive yet helpful way. Fourth, death education addresses moral decisions about both life and death.

The educators

There are several types of death educators. Pioneers such as Herman Feifel, Robert Fulton, Vanderlyn Pine, Hannelore Wass, and Charles Corr started in the 1950s and 1960s and were still involved as of the early 1990s. Those who have taken courses in death and bereavement at colleges and universities as part of a program in another discipline form the bulk of death educators today. Since 1984 the Association for Death Education and Counseling has offered certification in both death education and death counseling. Many others, however, having read one or two books about death and bereavement, believe they are qualified to teach the subject. This is usually not a problem if death education is restricted to a unit in a family studies or religion course, or a "teachable moment"—that is, taking the opportunity to discuss death and bereavement when it arises through the death of a pet, in the news, or in the literature discussed by the class.

Teacher, nursing, and physician preparation programs offer virtually no education about death and bereavement, despite the fact that teachers, doctors, and nurses will be expected not only to teach and council about death and bereavement, but also to cope personally when someone dies.

Death education and ethics

One must distinguish ethics *in* death education from the ethics *of* death education. First, religious traditions have based many of their commandments on the view that death is not the end for persons and that the consequences of moral decisions transcend the grave. Second, a body of ethical literature has developed in law, medicine, and philosophy because of the possibility of causing death through human decision making. Formal death and bereavement education reflects these concerns, especially in dealing with informed consent, suicide, and euthanasia.

In addition to ethical issues found in death education, there are ethical principles in education about death and bereavement. Since all education is a form of normative ethics, the view that a balanced education ought to include issues of loss and grief is itself normative. In addition to this primary value, there is the issue of using students as subjects in research dealing with bereavement and grief reactions. This is an especially thorny issue because while most students claim to take death-education courses for professional reasons, the professional reasons have often proven to be only the excuse to address personal issues. In a group of 2000 students between 1975 and 1993, 2 percent were themselves terminally ill, and over 30 percent were coping with the recent or anticipated death of a loved one.

The need for evaluation

Death education has not been universally accepted. From a practical standpoint, it is one more thing to be added to the already overcrowded general or professional curriculum. While there is some resistance to formal death-education programs, death education within the discussion of literature, family life, or health has found more acceptance. There have been abuses in death-education courses—for example, the practice of taking students to funeral homes and encouraging them to lie in coffins without adequate preparation. Only since 1989 has the Association for Death Education and Counseling had a code of ethics.

The code of ethics of the Association for Death Education and Counseling demands that members maintain competence in the field and act responsibly toward their clients, their employers, and society as a whole, since death-related anxieties and guilt have a ripple effect that affects many. In addition, death educators are enjoined to make sure that assistance is available to students when exercises used in the course may evoke memories or other reactions that are threatening. Educators are reminded to be honest in the claims that their courses make about their content, to be responsible for the accuracy of that content, and to be attentive to the development of appropriate skills for those students who may be preparing to do sensitive work with the young, the dying, or the bereaved. Finally, death educators are expected to be aware of their own limitations and to refer students to appropriate professionals when necessary (Association for Death Education, 1993–94).

The future of death education

If education about death and bereavement is to fulfill its possibilities, those engaged in it must examine more clearly the goals they wish to accomplish. It is impossible for a single course or unit of study to accomplish all that is expected from death education, from transmitting a body of research to improving the lot of the dying and the bereaved, to reducing violence in the world. More attention must be paid in teacher education programs to the importance of education about death and bereavement, so that the discussion of such matters is not left to the discretion of teachers who are inexperienced in death-related issues. There must be greater concern for the effectiveness of death education. The few studies that have been done are inconclusive. Persons who take death-education courses are more comfortable with the reality of death in life, but it is not known if this acceptance of death is an effect or a cause of taking such courses. Finally, there must be more stress on the discussion of ethical issues in all death-related courses or units—not just those that are formally described as such—with the hope that more focused ethical discussion will bring greater depth to the public debate on such important topics as grief, suicide, and euthanasia.

JOHN D. MORGAN

Directly related to this entry is the entry DEATH: ART OF DYING. *For a further discussion of topics mentioned in this article, see the entries* CARE; COMPASSION; DEATH AND DYING: EUTHANASIA AND SUSTAINING LIFE; EMOTIONS; HOSPICE AND END-OF-LIFE CARE; LITERATURE; *and* SUICIDE. *For a discussion of related ideas, see the entries* DEATH, DEFINITION AND DETERMINATION OF; LIFE; *and* WOMEN, *section on* WOMEN AS HEALTH PROFESSIONALS.

Bibliography

ARIES, PHILIPPE. 1981. *The Hour of Our Death.* New York: Alfred A. Knopf.

ASSOCIATION FOR DEATH EDUCATION AND COUNSELING. 1993–1994. "Code of Ethics." In *Directory of Members.* Hartford, Conn.: Author.

BENOLIEL, JEANNE QUINT. 1993. "Personal Care in an Impersonal World." In *Personal Care in an Impersonal World: A Multidimensional Look at Bereavement.* Edited by John D. Morgan. Amityville, N.Y.: Baywood.

CORR, CHARLES A.; MORGAN, JOHN D.; and WASS, HANNELORE. 1994. *International Work Group on Death, Dying, and Bereavement: Statements on Death, Dying, and Bereavement.* London, Ontario: King's College.

FULTON, ROBERT, and BENDIKSEN, ROBERT. 1994. *Death and Identity.* 3d ed. Philadelphia: Charles.

IRISH, DONALD P., and LUNDQUIST, KATHLEEN F., eds. 1993. *Ethnic Variations in Death, Dying and Grief: Diversity in Universality.* Washington: Taylor & Francis.

LEENAARS, ANTOON A., and WENCKSTERN, SUZANNE, eds. 1991. *Suicide Prevention in Schools.* Washington, D.C.: Hemisphere.

LEVITON, DANIEL. 1977. "The Scope of Death Education." *Death Studies* I, no. 1:41–56.

MORGAN, JOHN D. 1990. *Death Education in Canada: Survey, Curricula, Protocols, Bibliography.* London, Ontario: King's College.

PINE, VANDERLYN. 1977. "A Socio-Historical Portrait of Death Education." *Death Studies* I, no. 1:57–84.

STILLION, JUDITH M. 1979. "Discovering the Taxonomies: A Structural Framework for Death Education Courses." *Death Education* 3, no. 2:157–164.

WASS, HANNELORE; CORR, CHARLES A.; PACHOLSKI, RICHARD A.; and FORFAR, CAMERON S., eds. 1985. *Death Education II: An Annotated Resource Guide.* Washington, D.C.: Hemisphere.

DEATH PENALTY

Fewer and fewer crimes are punishable by death even in countries where execution is legal, and crimes that are widely considered to be extremely serious, such as murder, often lead to prison sentences rather than capital punishment. In 1991, offenses under the laws of over ninety countries carried a penalty of death. In eighty-five, execution was illegal or had ceased to be imposed. These included virtually all of the nations of western Europe, as well as Canada, Australia, Hungary, and Czechoslovakia. In the United States, in addition to military and federal jurisdictions, thirty-six states impose the death penalty. Not all of these states do so regularly, however; and in those where capital punishment has become routine, it is sometimes a relatively new development. From 1967 to 1977 there were no executions in the United States; between 1977 and 1992, there were 190, and over 2,500 people in 34 states were on death row. In a few countries in which the death penalty was still used in the 1980s—Brazil, Argentina, and Nepal—it had been reintroduced (in Brazil and Argentina by military governments) after a long period of abolition.

The reintroduction of capital punishment after centuries of decline has once again raised the question of the morality of execution. No code of law now prescribes death for the theft of fruit or salad, as Draco's code did in ancient Athens; and boiling to death is no longer a recognized punishment for murder by poisoning, as it was in England under the Tudors and Stuarts. Can a principle that explains why these developments are good also explain why it is good that some codes of law no longer prescribe death as punishment for murder? Or can a principle that condemns the death penalty for some crimes also support its imposition for others? These are live questions, for one of the arguments commonly presented against the death penalty turns on the suggestion that retaining it or reintroducing it is a case of being morally behind the times. According to this argument, standards of humane punishment have now risen to a point where killing a human being—even one who is guilty of a terrible crime—can only be understood as cruel, and therefore immoral. Such an argument is sometimes used to counter another that is perhaps even more familiar: that the death penalty is justified because of its power to deter people from violent crime. The argument from deterrence will be examined later.

The argument from cruelty

The language of this argument is sometimes taken from the Eighth Amendment of the U.S. Constitution ("Excessive bail shall not be required, nor excessive fines imposed, nor cruel and unusual punishments inflicted"); or from human-rights declarations that outlaw "cruel, inhuman or degrading" treatment or punishment. Thus, a brochure titled *When the State Kills,* issued by the British Section of Amnesty International (1990), contains the following passage under the heading "Cruel, Inhuman and Degrading": "International law states that torture or cruel, inhuman or degrading punishments can never be justified. The cruelty of the death penalty is self-evident."

Certain methods of execution are quite plausibly said to be so painful that any application of them must be cruel. Amnesty International cites the case of a Nigerian military governor who in July 1986 ordered successive volleys of bullets to be fired at convicted armed robbers. The shots would first be aimed at the ankles, to produce painful wounds, and only gradually would the firing squad shoot to kill. Other methods, believed by some authorities to be painless, can undoubtedly cause suffering when clumsily applied. According to eyewitness reports, the first death sentence carried out by use of the electric chair in the United States; in August 1890, was very painful. But these ill effects may not be typical. Certainly the electric chair was not introduced because it was thought to be painful; on the contrary, along with other methods of execution, such as the guillotine, it was thought to spare the convicted person suffering.

Execution by lethal injection is the latest in a series of supposedly humane methods of execution to be introduced. It is now being used in a number of states in the United States. Is this technique cruel? Perhaps not, if severe pain is the test of cruelty. Deliberate poisoning is normally cruel, and Amnesty International classifies the use of lethal injection as deliberate poisoning. But is it clear that poisoning in the form of lethal injection is always cruel? What if the injection is self-administered in a suicide or given at the request of someone who is dying in intense pain? If poisoning is always cruel, then it must be so in these cases. On the other hand, if it is not cruel in these cases, then it is not necessarily cruel in the case of execution. It is true that execution is usually not in line with the wishes of the convicted person, as it is when poison is administered to someone at his or her request. But that by itself cannot make execution cruel, unless virtually all punishment is cruel: Virtually all punishment is inflicted on people against their wishes. If it is not pain and not the unwillingness of the criminal to undergo it that makes lethal injection cruel, then what does? If nothing does—if lethal injection is sometimes painless and not cruel in other respects—then there may be principles that consistently explain why it is good for murderers, for example, to be punished with death (severe crimes deserve severe punishments); why it was bad for murderers to be put to death in the past by boiling (torture is wrong); and why it is not necessarily bad for murderers to be put to death today by lethal injection.

Arguments from finality and arbitrariness

Arguments against the death penalty sometimes emphasize its finality. There are several versions of the argument from finality, some religious, some secular. One religious version has to do with the way the death penalty removes all possibility of repentance or a saving change of heart on the part of the offender (Carpenter, 1969). Capital punishment writes off the offender in a way that, for example, imprisonment combined with education or religious instruction does not. It arguably refuses the offender the sort of love that Christianity enjoins, and it presumes to judge once and for all—a prerogative that may belong to God alone.

Secular arguments from finality are almost always combined with considerations about the fallibility of judicial institutions and doubt whether people who are accused of crimes are fully responsible agents. In some views, society contributes to the wrongdoing of criminals (Carpenter, 1969), so that they are not fully responsible and should not be punished. This argument shows sympathy for those who are accused of wrongdoing, but because it does not take wrongdoers as full-fledged agents it may not show them as much respect as apparently harsher arguments do. As for fallible judicial institutions, certain factors—such as prejudice against some accused people, and poor legal representation—can produce wrong or arbitrary verdicts and sentences; even conscientious judges and juries can be mistaken. When errors occur and the punishment is not death, something can be done to compensate the victims of miscarriages of justice. The compensation may never make up entirely for what is lost, but at least a partial restitution is possible; but where what is lost is the accused person's life, on the other hand, the possibility of compensation is ruled out. This argument is particularly forceful where evidence exists that certain groups (black males in the United States, Tibetans in China) are disproportionately represented among those receiving harsh sentences, including the death sentence (Amnesty International, 1991; Wolfgang and Reidel, 1987). In these cases, the possibility of an error with disastrous consequences starts to grow into something like a probability. What is more, the evidence of certain groups being disproportionately represented suggests that the law is not being applied justly. This adds to the argument that the death penalty should not be applied, for it suggests that people are fallible, the background conditions for the existence of justice are not being met, and consequently that some miscarriages of justice result from factors other than honest error.

Arguments from side effects

Effects on professionals.   Executions are carried out by officials who are not always hardened to their task, and at times they rely on the services of medical people, who have sworn to preserve life. The burdens of those who officiate and serve in these ways; the suffering of those who are close to the convicted person; and the ill effects on society at large of public hangings, gassings, or electrocutions are sometimes thought to constitute an argument against capital punishment over and above the argument from cruelty to the offender.

The side effects on medical personnel have recently been brought into prominence in the United States by the use of lethal injection. The method involves intravenous injection of a lethal dose of barbiturate as well as a second drug, such as tubocurarine or succinylcholine, that produces paralysis and prevents breathing, leading to death by asphyxiation. Doctors have sometimes had to check that the veins of the convicted person were suitable for the needle used and, where death took longer than expected, to attend and give direction during the process of execution. In Oklahoma, which was the first state to adopt lethal injection as a method of execution, the medical director of the Department of Corrections is required to order the drugs to be injected; the physician in attendance during the execution itself has to inspect the intravenous line to the prisoner's arm and also pronounce him dead.

Of course, doctors have been in attendance at executions carried out by other methods, and some of the moral objections to their involvement are applicable no matter which method is used. What is different about intravenous injection, in the opinion of some writers (e.g., Curran and Cassells, 1980), is that it involves the direct application of biomedical knowledge for the taking of life. This practice is often said to be in violation of the Hippocratic Oath (Committee on Bioethical Issues of the Medical Society of the State of New York, 1991); and many national and international medical associations oppose the involvement of doctors in the death penalty. The fear that nurses might assist at executions led the American Nurses Association in 1983 to declare it a "breach of the nursing code of ethical conduct to participate either directly or indirectly in legally authorized execution."

The conflict between providing medical services to further an execution and abiding by the Hippocratic Oath makes the moral problem facing doctors particularly sharp, but other professionals may face difficulties as well. Judges and lawyers may be caught up unwillingly or reluctantly in prosecutions that will lead to the imposition of the death sentence. They, too, have a reason for withdrawing their services if they are sincerely opposed to capital punishment; but if all the professionals with qualms acted upon them, the legal process, and the protections it extends to those accused of capital crimes, might be compromised as well (Bonnie, 1990). This argument probably understates the differences between legal and medical professionals: the latter recognize a duty of healing and of relieving pain; the former are committed to upholding the law and seeing that justice is done, which does not necessarily conflict with participation in a regime of execution.

Effects on persons close to the condemned and on society. In addition to the effects of the death penalty on involved professionals, the effects on persons close to condemned prisoners are sometimes cited in utilitarian arguments against the death penalty (Glover, 1977). These effects are undoubtedly unpleasant, but it is unclear whether they are to be traced to the existence of capital punishment or to the commission of the crimes classified as capital. As for the effects on society at large, they are harder to assess. Samuel Romilly, who campaigned successfully for a reduction in the very large number of capital offenses recognized in English law at the beginning of the 1800s, maintained that "cruel punishments have an inevitable tendency to produce cruelty in people." In fact, Romilly's success in law reform owed something to the benevolence of juries, who had consistently, and often against evidence, found accused people innocent of capital offenses as minor as shoplifting. Whoever was made cruel by the existence of cruel punishments, it was not ordinary English jurors. Judges avoided imposing the death penalty for minor crimes by transporting criminals to the colonies.

Deterrence

The death penalty has often been introduced to act as a strong deterrent against serious crime, and the deterrence argument is commonly used to justify reintroduction. In a British parliamentary debate on the reintroduction of capital punishment in May 1982, one legislator said, "The death penalty will act as a deterrent. A would-be murderer will think twice before taking a life if he knows that he may well forfeit his own in so doing" (Sorell, 1987, pp. 32–33). He went on to argue that the absence of the death penalty had been associated with a rise in the number of ordinary murders, and an increase in the rate of murder of police officers. But the evidence for its having the power to discourage, or for its having a greater such power than imprisonment, is inconclusive (Hood, 1989). Indeed, deterrence generally seems to depend on potential offenders expecting to be caught rather than on their judging the punishment for an offense to be severe (Walker, 1991). In the case of murder, the deterrent effect is particularly doubtful: Murder is often committed in a moment of high passion or by those who are mentally disturbed (Sorell, 1987). Either way, the serious consequences of the act are unlikely to register so as to make the agent hesitate. An American review of statistical studies concludes that the deterrent effect of capital punishment is definitely not a settled matter, and that the statistical methods necessary for reaching firm conclusions have yet to be devised (Klein et al., 1978).

Incapacitation

A purpose of punishment that is more convincingly served by the death penalty is the incapacitation of offenders. The death penalty undoubtedly does incapacitate, but this is just another aspect of its finality, which has already been seen to be morally objectionable from some points of view. Again, for incapacitation to be a compelling general ground for the imposition of the death penalty—that is, a ground that justifies the imposition of the penalty in more than the occasional case—there has to be strong evidence that people who have the opportunity to repeat capital crimes frequently do so. Although killers sometimes kill again, it is not clear that they are *likely* to reoffend. Finally, life imprisonment without parole may be sufficiently incapacitating to make the death penalty unnecessary.

Retribution

Another argument in favor of the death penalty is based on the value of retribution. Here the idea is that the evil of a crime can be counterbalanced or canceled out by an appropriate punishment, and that in the case of the most serious crime, death can be the appropriate punishment because it is deserved. Appropriateness should be understood against the background of the thought that penal justice requires what Immanuel Kant called an "equality of crime and punishment." His examples show that he meant an act of punishment not identical to the crime but proportionate to its severity; Kant held that death was uniquely appropriate to the crime of murder (Kant, 1965). John Stuart Mill, in a famous speech in favor of capital punishment delivered in the British House of Commons in 1868, argued that only those guilty of aggravated murder—defined as brutal murder in the absence of all excusing conditions—deserved to be executed. Mill called the punishment "appropriate" to the crime and argued that it had a deterrent effect. He meant "appropriate" in view of the severity of the crime.

Retribution should not be confused with revenge. It is generally considered revenge, not retribution, when there is love or sympathy for the one who has suffered an injury; retribution requires a response even to injuries of people no one cares about. Its impersonality makes the injuries of the friendless have as much weight as the injuries of the popular. Again, revenge is still revenge when the retaliation is utterly out of proportion to the original injury, but the retributivist *lex talionis*—an eye for an eye—limits what can be done in return.

One question raised by the retributivist defense of capital punishment is how a punishment can counterbalance or cancel out an evil act. Retributivists sometimes refer in this connection to the ideal case in which the offender willingly undergoes a punishment as a sign of remorse and of wishing to be restored to a community from which he or she has been excluded due to a criminal act (Duff, 1986). In that case the punishment is supposed to counterbalance the crime. But it is unnecessary for retributivism to be committed to the idea that a punishment cancels out an offense. One can appeal instead, as Kant did, to a punishment's fitting an offense—being proportional in quality to the quality of the offense—and one can justify the imposition of punishment by reference to the following three considerations: (1) laws have to promise punishment if people who are not wholly rational and who are subject to strong impulses and temptations are to obey the laws, and promises must be kept; (2) offenders who are convicted of breaking laws in a just society can be understood to have been party to a social contract designed to protect people's freedom; and (3) threats of punishment in a just society are intended to prevent encroachments on freedom.

This is not a justification of capital punishment, until one specifies a crime that capital punishment uncontroversially fits. Murder is not always the right choice, since such factors as provocation, the numbers of people who die, and the quality of the intention can make some murders much more serious than others; while crimes other than murder—crimes in which, despite the criminal's best efforts, the victim survives—can be as bad as or worse than those in which death occurs. Aggravated murder is, as Mill maintained, a more plausible candidate for capital crime than is plain murder. But execution even for aggravated murder has something to be said against it: the danger of executing the innocent in error, and the suspicion—which goes to the heart of retributivism—that it is bad for pain or unpleasantness to be visited even on wrongdoers.

TOM SORELL

Directly related to this entry is the entry PRISONERS, *article on* TORTURE AND THE HEALTH PROFESSIONAL. *For a further discussion of topics mentioned in this article, see the entries* MEDICINE AS A PROFESSION; NURSING AS A PROFESSION; NURSING ETHICS; *and* PROFESSION AND PROFESSIONAL ETHICS. *For a discussion of related ideas, see the entries* ETHICS, *article on* NORMATIVE ETHICAL THEORIES; HARM; JUSTICE; LAW AND BIOETHICS; LAW AND MORALITY; PAIN AND SUFFERING; *and* WARFARE, *article on* MEDICINE AND WAR. *See also the* APPENDIX (CODES, OATHS, AND DIRECTIVES RELATED TO BIOETHICS), SECTION II: ETHICAL DIRECTIVES FOR THE PRACTICE OF MEDICINE, OATH OF HIPPOCRATES, *and* SECTION III: ETHICAL DIRECTIVES FOR OTHER HEALTH-CARE PROFESSIONS, CODE FOR NURSES *of the* INTERNATIONAL COUNCIL OF NURSES, *and* CODE FOR NURSES *of the* AMERICAN NURSES' ASSOCIATION.

Bibliography

AMNESTY INTERNATIONAL. 1989. *When the State Kills: The Death Penalty v. Human Rights.* London: Author.

———. 1991. *Death Penalty: Facts and Figures.* London: Author.

BEDAU, HUGO A. 1987. *Death Is Different: Studies in the Morality, Law, and Politics of Capital Punishment.* Boston: Northeastern University Press.

————, ed. 1982. *The Death Penalty in America*. 3d ed. New York: Oxford University Press.

BONNIE, RICHARD I. 1990. "Medical Ethics and the Death Penalty." *Hastings Center Report* 20, no. 3:12–18.

CARPENTER, CANON E. F. 1969. "The Christian Context." In *The Hanging Question: Essays on the Death Penalty*, pp. 29–38. Edited by Louis J. Blom-Cooper. London: Duckworth.

COMMITTEE ON BIOETHICAL ISSUES OF THE MEDICAL SOCIETY OF THE STATE OF NEW YORK. 1991. "Physician Involvement in Capital Punishment." *New York State Journal of Medicine* 91, no. 1:15–18.

CURRAN, WILLIAM J., and CASSELLS, WARD. 1980. "The Ethics of Medical Participation in Capital Punishment by Intravenous Drug Injection." *New England Journal of Medicine* 302, no. 4:226–230.

DUFF, R. ANTONY. 1986. *Trials and Punishments*. Cambridge: At the University Press.

GLOVER, JONATHAN. 1977. *Causing Death and Saving Lives: A World-Wide Perspective*. Harmondsworth, U.K.: Penguin.

HOOD, ROGER G. 1989. *The Death Penalty*. Oxford: At the Clarendon Press.

KANT, IMMANUEL. 1965. *The Metaphysical Elements of Justice: Part 1 of The Metaphysics of Morals*. Translated by John Ladd. Indianapolis, Ind.: Bobbs-Merrill.

KLEIN, LAWRENCE; FORST, BRIAN; and FILATOV, VICTOR. 1978. "The Deterrent Effect of Capital Punishment: An Assessment of the Estimates." In *Deterrence and Incapacitation: Estimating the Effects of Criminal Sanctions on Crime Rates*, pp. 336–361. Edited by Alfred Blumestein, Jacqueline Cohen, and Daniel Nagin. Washington, D.C.: National Academy of Sciences.

MILL, JOHN STUART. 1868. In *Hansard's Parliamentary Debates*. 3d series. London: Hansard.

NATHANSON, STEPHEN. 1987. *An Eye for an Eye? The Morality of Punishing by Death*. Totowa, N.J.: Rowman & Littlefield.

SORELL, TOM. 1987. *Moral Theory and Capital Punishment*. Oxford: Basil Blackwell.

VAN DEN HAAG, ERNEST. 1991. *Punishing Criminals: Concerning a Very Old and Painful Question*. New York: University Press of America.

WALKER, NIGEL. 1991. *Why Punish?* Oxford: Oxford University Press.

WOLFGANG, MARVIN E., and REIDEL, M. 1982. "Racial Discrimination, Rape and the Death Penalty." In *The Death Penalty in America*. 3d ed. Edited by Hugo Bedau. New York: Oxford University Press.

WOLPIN, KENNETH I. 1978. "An Economic Analysis of Crime and Punishment in England and Wales, 1894–1967." *Journal of Political Economy* 86, no. 5:815–840.